Johnson's Psychiatric–Mental Health Nursing

◆ NURSING CARE PLANS

6–1	Sample	105	24–2	The Client With Bipolar Disorder in the Manic Phase	507
17–1	The Sexual Trauma Survivor	340	25–1	The Client With a Thought Disorder	544
18–1	The Client With Post-Traumatic Stress Disorder	360	26–1	The Aggressive, Potentially Violent Client	567
19–1	The Client With Somatoform Disorder	387	27–1	The Client With Alcoholism	598
20–1	The Client With Erectile Dysfunction	415	28–1	The Client With Delirium	615
21–1	The Client With Dissociative Identity Disorder	430	28–2	The Client With Early-Stage Alzheimer's Disease	631
22–1	The Client With Schizoid Personality Disorder	448	29–1	The Child With ADHD	661
23–1	The Client With Anorexia Nervosa	470			
24–1	The Client With Depression	506			

◆ THERAPEUTIC COMMUNICATION

4–1	Exploring the Need for Treatment	67	22–1	The Client With Antisocial Personality Disorder	450
4–2	Encouraging Formulation of a Plan	69	23–1	Moving With Resistance	465
10–1	Involving Families in the Client's Treatment	176	24–1	The Suicidal Client	510
10–2	Family Consultation	182	25–1	Language Problems in Schizophrenia	548
18–1	The Client With Generalized Anxiety Disorder	367	27–1	A Cocaine Abuser in Denial	601
19–1	Addressing Somatization Disorder	389	28–1	A Client With Dementia	635
20–1	Respecting a Client's Wishes Regarding Sexual Issues	413	29–1	Discussing Peer Pressure and Substance Use With Adolescents	672
21–1	The Client With a Dissociative Disorder	432			

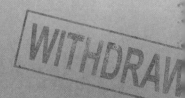

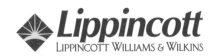
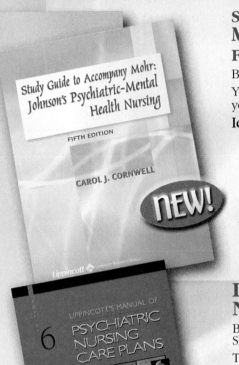
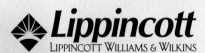

Johnson's
Psychiatric-Mental Health Nursing

FIFTH EDITION

Wanda K. Mohr, PhD, RN, FAAN

Rutgers University
College of Nursing
Newark, New Jersey

 LIPPINCOTT WILLIAMS & WILKINS
A **Wolters Kluwer** Company

Philadelphia • Baltimore • New York • London
Buenos Aires • Hong Kong • Sydney • Tokyo

Acquisitions Editor: Margaret Zuccarini
Developmental Editor: Renee Gagliardi
Senior Editorial Coordinator: Helen Kogut
Production Editor: Debra Schiff
Senior Production Manager: Helen Ewan
Design Coordinator: Brett MacNaughton
Manufacturing Manager: William Alberti
Indexer: Ellen Brennan
Compositor: Peirce Graphic Services
Printer: Quebecor-Versailles

5th Edition

9 8 7 6 5 4 3 2 1

Library of Congress Cataloging-in-Publication Data

Johnson's psychiatric-mental health nursing / [edited by] Wanda K. Mohr.—5th ed.
   p. ; cm.
   Rev. ed. of: Psychiatric-mental health nursing / [edited by] Barbara Schoen Johnson.
   Includes bibliographical references and index.
   ISBN 0-7817-1984-4 (alk. paper)
   1. Psychiatric nursing.   I. Title: Psychiatric-mental health nursing.   II. Mohr, Wanda K.
III. Johnson, Barbara Schoen.
   [DNLM: 1. Mental Disorders—nursing. 2. Psychiatric Nursing—methods. WY 160 J71 2003]
RC440 .P737 2003
610.73'68—dc21
                                                                              2002069434

Care has been taken to confirm the accuracy of the information presented and to describe generally accepted practices. However, the authors, editors, and publisher are not responsible for errors or omissions or for any consequences from application of the information in this book and make no warranty, express or implied, with respect to the content of the publication.

The authors, editors, and publisher have exerted every effort to ensure that drug selection and dosage set forth in this text are in accordance with the current recommendations and practice at the time of publication. However, in view of ongoing research, changes in government regulations, and the constant flow of information relating to drug therapy and drug reactions, the reader is urged to check the package insert for each drug for any change in indications and dosage and for added warnings and precautions. This is particularly important when the recommended agent is a new or infrequently employed drug.

Some drugs and medical devices presented in this publication have Food and Drug Administration (FDA) clearance for limited use in restricted research settings. It is the responsibility of the health care provider to ascertain the FDA status of each drug or device planned for used in his or her clinical practice.

LWW.com

Contributors

Jeffrey A. Anderson, PhD
Assistant Professor and Area Coordinator for Special Education
School of Education at Indiana University Purdue University Indianapolis
Indianapolis, Indiana

Jeanneane L. Cline, MS, RN, CS, APN, CHTP, LCDC LMFT
Clinical Instructor, Lead Teacher
Psychiatric-Mental Health Nursing
University of Texas at Arlington
Arlington, Texas

Victoria Conn, MN, MA
Psychiatric Rehabilitation and Family Consultant
NAMI Pennsylvania Training Institute
Harrisburg, Pennsylvania

Phyllis M. Connelly, PhD, RN, CS
Professor and Graduate Coordinator
School of Nursing
San Jose State University
San Jose, California

Carol J. Cornwell, PhD, MS, CS
Director of Center for Nursing Scholarship
Assistant Professor of Nursing
Georgia Southern University School of Nursing
Statesboro, Georgia

Barbara Tunley Crenshaw, BSN, MS
Professor Emerti
Front Range Community College
Westminster, Colorado

Sherill Nones Cronin, PhD, RN, C
Professor of Nursing
Bellarmine University
And
Nurse Researcher
Jewish Hospital
Louisville, Kentucky

Janet Dalsheimer, MS, RN
Graduate Student
Texas Woman's University
Denton, Texas

Susan Dee Decker, RN, MSN, PhD
Associate Professor of Nursing
University of Portland
Portland, Oregon

Catherine Deering, PhD, RN, CS
Professor of Psychology and Nursing
Clayton College and State University
Morrow, Georgia

Kathleen R. Delaney, RN, DNSc
Associate Professor of Nursing
Rush College of Nursing
Chicago, Illinois

Cheryl S. Detwiler, RN, BSN, MSN
Associate Professor
Department of Nursing
Jackson State Community College
Jackson, Tennessee

Robin S. Diamond, MSN, JD, RN, CPHQ, CNAA
Risk Manager and Health Care Consultant
Proassurance, Inc.
Coppell, Texas

Delia Esparza, PhD, APRN, BC, LMFT
Nurse Clinical Specialist in Psychiatric Mental Health
Department of Veterans Affairs
Austin Veteran Center
Austin, Texas

Jane Frederick, PhD, RN
Former Assistant Professor of Nursing
Clayton College and State University
Morrow, Georgia

Judith A. Greene, PhD, RN-CS, APRN
Psychiatric Nurse Practitioner
Volunteer Behavioral Health
Cleveland, Tennessee

Diane Hinderliter, RN, BS, MS, DNSc
Director of Professional Services and Women's and Children Services
OSF Saint Anthony Medical Center
Rockford, Illinois

Mildred O. Hogstel, PhD, RN, C
Professor Emeritus of Nursing
Harris School of Nursing
Texas Christian University
Fort Worth, Texas

Anita G. Hufft, PhD, RN
Associate Dean of Academic Programs
Louisiana State University Health Sciences Center School of Nursing
New Orleans, Louisiana

Mary Huggins, RN, BA, MA, CPRP
Program Manager
Children, Family and Adult Services Department, Hennepin
    County
Maples, Minnesota

Barbara Schoen Johnson, PhD, RN, CS, PMHNP
Child Psychiatric Nurse Practitioner
Behavioral Health Services
Cook Children's Health System
Fort Worth, Texas

Nina A. Klebanoff, PhD, APRN, BC, LPCC
Director, Behavioral Health Services
St. Vincent Hospital
Sante Fe, New Mexico

Karen V. Lamb, ND, RN, CS
Associate Professor
Rush College of Nursing
Chicago, Illinois

Gwen Larsen, PhD, RN, CS
Assistant Professor
University of Nebraska Medical Center, College of Nursing
Omaha, Nebraska

Susan Ellen Margolis, PhD, RN, CNS-P/MH
Director of Geriatric Services
Psychiatric Center of North Texas
DeSoto, Texas

Sue Ellen Odom, RN, DSN
Associate Professor
School of Health Sciences, Nursing Department
Clayton College and State University
Morrow, Georgia

Geraldine S. Pearson, PhD, RN, MSN, CS
Nurse Clinical Specialist
Riverview Hospital for Children and Youth
Middletown, Connecticut
And
Clinical Faculty
University of Connecticut School of Nursing
Storrs, Connecticut

Suzanne Perraud, RN, PhD
Associate Chair and Assistant Professor
Community and Mental Health Nursing
Rush University, College of Nursing
Chicago, Illinois

Cindy A. Peternelj-Taylor, BScN, MSc, RN
Professor
College of Nursing
University of Saskatchewan
Saskatoon, Saskatchewan, Canada

Kay Peterson, MS, RN, CS
Psychiatric Nurse Practitioner
Cascadia Behavioral Healthcare
Portland, Oregon

**Bonnie Rickelman, EdD, MEd, BSN, APRN, BC, CNS,
    LMFT, CGP**
Associate Professor, Division of Holistic Adult Health and
    Mental Health Nursing
The University of Texas at Austin School of Nursing
Austin, Texas

Janet M. Stagg, MS, RN, CNS
Director of Education, Kindred Hospital
Psychiatric-Mental Health Nurse Consultant
Guest Lecturer
Texas Woman's University
Dallas, Texas

Reviewers

Janet A. Ambrogne, PhD, ARNP
Assistant Professor
Seattle University
Postdoctoral Fellow
University of Washington
Seattle, Washington

David J. Anna, MSN
Assistant Professor
School of Nursing
Medical College of Georgia
Augusta, Georgia

Nancy L. Cowan, RN, MSN, EdD
Director/Coordinator Nursing Program
Chabot College
Hayward, California

Denise H. Elliott, RN, MSN
Director, Department of Nursing Education
Wallace State Community College
Hanceville, Alabama

Karen K. Fritz, RN, DNSc
Assistant Professor of Nursing
Augustana College
Sioux Falls, South Dakota

Amy L. Govoni, RN, MSN, CS
Assistant Professor
Cleveland State University, Department of Nursing
Cleveland, Ohio

Joann Lavin, RN, EdD, CS
Professor
Kingsborough Community College
Brooklyn, New York

Gwen Larsen, PhD, RN, CS
Assistant Professor
College of Nursing
University of Nebraska Medical Center
Lincoln, Nebraska

Preface

GUIDING THE TEXT

While the history of mental health research is at least 200 years old, the heavy work commenced during the 21st century. The biochemical, physiological, pharmacological, and structural features of the brain have been described and in many instances defined. So too have the basic perceptual, emotional, attentional, and cognitive functions. In the past 20 years, these fundamentals have accelerated exponentially, providing the field of mental health research and service provision a wealth of new knowledge.

In addition to this explosion of knowledge, the economics of healthcare have changed dramatically during the past few decades. The interaction of new science and new economic pressures brings with it an urgency for psychiatric-mental health nursing to begin articulating a new paradigm redefining how psychiatric nursing is conceptualized, taught, and practiced. Susan McCabe (2000) argued that psychiatric nursing might be in danger of extinction as a specialty unless the specialty can let go of what may be historically interesting, but no longer clinically relevant. In addition to letting go of the old, she points out that the time has also come to incorporate the new.

My vision for this book was to begin to let go of the old and articulate the new. While paying homage to historical figures and concepts, the text minimizes such information, making clear what practices are current, and, more importantly, which are based in empirical research. Since it is clear that the major conceptual approach of the 21st century to psychiatry is grounded in molecular biology, we have devoted a chapter to explaining concepts such as neuroplasticity and genetic expression. Because evidence is increasing that "mental states" have their representation in brain neuronal anatomy and functioning, the text focuses on those psychotherapeutics that have a solid grounding in research.

In addition to focusing on the latest research in neurobiology, physiology, and psychopharmacotherapeutics, the book articulates service provision changes that have taken place, emphasizing the shift toward care of clients in their community settings and with their families. Special consideration is given to portraying persons suffering from mental illnesses and their families as human beings who are reacting normally to very stressful and overwhelming experiences.

Attention is also paid to the role of nurses as key members of the psychiatric team and the different contributions they can make to client care at varying levels of practice. Knowing from experience how frightening the word "theory" can be, I hope that students will be empowered by the down-to-earth discussion of theory and theoretical frameworks. Ever mindful of the strong role of the therapeutic alliance, the text conceptualizes psychotherapy as a process of learning new thinking and new behaviors rather than as a "talking cure," thereby taking the mystery out of it and placing it in understandable terms for students who can in turn demystify it to clients.

Our team at Lippincott decided early that we wanted to produce a textbook that was concise, current, and readable. We carefully edited for redundant material as well as for material that constituted a "nice to know" as versus a "need to know." Some of the chapters may seem truncated or condensed to readers from what they have seen in previous editions of this text. All the requisite elements and subject matter, however, are present. For example, suicide is discussed in the context of mood disorders, homelessness and forensics are discussed in the chapter on working with special populations, and child maltreatment and violence against women are discussed in the context of community violence.

For every silver lining there seems to be a dark side. The exciting new knowledge presented in this book represents a revolution in the arena of the behavioral sciences, one that is analogous to the revolution that came about in orthopedics with the development of radiology. We live in an era in which scientific advances frequently make even the most recent scientific books and journals dated soon after their publication. Our team recognizes that what was written may have been timely when we wrote it, but may be out of date in a decade given the explosion of knowledge in the field. This underscores the importance and indispensability of reading and keeping abreast of new publications and new editions of texts as they are published.

Researching and writing this textbook was both tedious and exhilarating. During my research I was struck by the complexity of the emergent knowledge but at the same time excited by its possibilities. My reading highlighted the intricacies of the human condition and made me very aware of how specialized psychiatric mental health nursing can be. This awareness gave rise the urgency for providing these vulnerable clients with competent caregivers. It also underscored the importance for this nursing specialty to survive and thrive.

EXAMINING THE CONTENTS

The textbook is organized into five units:

- Unit I, *Foundations of Psychiatric-Mental Health Nursing,* contains material basic to the study of psychiatric-mental health nursing. Topics include the introduction to the field, neurobiology, conceptual frameworks, therapeutic communication and relationships, culture, nursing process, and legal and ethical issues.
- Unit II, *Conceptual Bases of Treatment,* discusses methodologies of care and treatment. Chapters focus on working with individuals, groups, and families; adapting care in special environments; psychopharmacology; spiritual care; and complementary and alternative treatments.
- Unit III, *Continuum of Care,* emphasizes the importance of the community as the setting for care delivery. Chapters focus on community mental health, support, and rehabilitation; behavioral health home care; and violence within the community.
- Unit IV, *Nursing Care for Clients with Psychiatric Disorders,* explores the spectrum of psychiatric disorders according to the following classifications: anxiety, somatoform, sexual and gender, dissociative, personality, eating, mood, thought, anger and aggression, substance abuse, and cognitive.
- Unit V, *Nursing Care for Special Populations,* presents mental health issues pertinent to children and adolescents and older adults.

FOCUSING ON FEATURES

- **Key Terms.** Each chapter opens with an alphabetical list of essential terminology and accompanying definitions for quick study and reference. In text, key terms are distinguished in raspberry-colored ink. All key terms and definitions are also found in the end-of-book glossary.
- **Learning Objectives.** This bulleted list highlights the main ideas for students to know or accomplish after reading the chapter.
- **Clinical Examples.** These displays are found throughout chapters and focus on the history, symptoms, and progress of a client's condition. Many have accompanying "Points for Reflection and Critical Thinking" that challenge students to form opinions or make judgments based on their understanding of the information provided and cumulative learning in the text. In Units IV and V, a Clinical Example appears at the beginning of each chapter and is connected with that chapter's Nursing Care Plan and Reflection and Critical Thinking Exercises. This connection helps students to follow a client's progression and better understand how specific disorders are handled.
- **Nursing Care Plans.** Found throughout Units IV and V and connected with Clinical Examples, Nursing Care Plans outline appropriate diagnoses, goals, interventions, rationales, and evaluation based on the particulars of a client's assessment data, signs and symptoms, and psychiatric disorder.
- **Disorder Information Maps.** Found in Units IV and V, these maps present important information related to the group of disorders under discussion: prevalence, criteria based on *DSM-IV-TR,* prevention strategies, and resources for more information.
- **Therapeutic Communication.** This feature provides sample dialogues to assist nurses in understanding effective versus ineffective communication. Reflection and Critical Thinking at the end help students make choices and interpret why certain communication styles succeed or fail for clients with psychiatric problems.
- **Historical Capsules.** This feature contains historical discussions related to conditions and issues in the chapter.
- **Client and Family Education.** These boxes contain client- and family-focused teaching points and related resources (eg, Web sites, organizations, books) for the condition under discussion.
- **Implications for Nursing Practice.** These boxes of bulleted points describe important considerations to help nurses provide focused client care.
- **Research Studies.** These displays present research studies and findings relevant to the chapter content.
- **Reflection and Critical Thinking Questions.** These questions challenge students to expand their thinking about issues discussed within each chapter.
- **Chapter Summary.** At the end of each chapter, this bulleted list of summary points connects with the chapter's learning objectives to ensure full understanding and continuity.
- **Review Questions.** Each chapter contains several NCLEX-style, multiple-choice questions to test students' knowledge of the chapter's content. Additionally, answers with rationales for both right and wrong answers appear in Appendix A.
- **Full four-color art and design program.** Color is used throughout to highlight important concepts and enhance the visual appeal for students.

TEACHING-LEARNING PACKAGE

- For the first time, a Study Guide is available to accompany this text. Based on the text and designed to build from simple to complex, the Study Guide provides several activities designed to meet a wide range of learning approaches and help students make the transition from textbook theory to clinical application. Examples of features include learning objectives, key terms and definitions, chapter outlines, and care plan development exercises tied into case-study scenarios. The guide incorporates various learning tools including discussion questions, critical thinking and self-evaluation exercises, matching, short-answer, multiple choice, NCLEX-style questions, and diagram labeling.

- The Instructor's Resource CD-ROM contains an Instructor's Manual and Testbank. The Instructor's Manual provides chapter-by-chapter teaching strategies, suggestions for movies that help illustrate a variety of disorders, and additional references. The Testbank provides a Word file of over 400 NCLEX-style test items that can be cut and pasted into an existing testbank. The test items are analysis and application focused questions requiring higher cognitive skills to answer.

- The Connection Web site (connection.lww.com/ go) provides many faculty and student resources, Web URL hotlinks to newly approved drugs, and systematically updated content to assist in keeping your textbook current.

Wanda K. Mohr

McCabe, S. (2000). Bringing psychiatric nursing into the 21st century. *Archives of Psychiatric Nursing, 14*(3), 109–116.

Dedication and Acknowledgments

I would like to acknowledge and dedicate this book to two important men in my life. The first is my husband and sometimes co-author, Brian, whose confidence in me and ceaseless cheerleading gave me the energy and self-assurance to reach even higher than the last time. The second is my research colleague and friend, Professor John W. Fantuzzo of the University of Pennsylvania. John taught me much during our long association—the most important lesson being how to think critically.

I would also like to acknowledge my friends from the National Alliance for the Mentally Ill (NAMI) who work tirelessly against stigma and on behalf of research and education. As mental health consumers and family members they have taught me valuable lessons about the devastation of mental illness and the courage of those who suffer from it.

An effort such as this book is made possible by the hard work of dozens of people, the chapter authors, as well as the developmental editors. I wish to specifically acknowledge the following folks at Lippincott Williams and Wilkins who provided timely advice, emotional support, and help and hundreds of hours of reading and re-reading: the Editorial team consisting of Renee Gagliardi, Tracey Hopkins, Helen Kogut, Sarah Kyle, and Margaret Zuccarini and the production team consisting of Helen Ewan, Debra Schiff, and Carolyn O'Brien.

Wanda K. Mohr

LWW ACKNOWLEDGMENT

Lippincott Williams & Wilkins would like to acknowledge and thank Barbara Schoen Johnson for conceiving the project, striving to perfect its development, and nurturing *Psychiatric-Mental Health Nursing* through four editions. Her hard work and dedication has provided a firm foundation for the fifth edition. LWW greatly appreciates her contribution towards the education of psychiatric-mental health nursing students over the past 16 years.

We would also like to express our appreciation and thanks to Cheryl Anderson, PhD, RN; Celeste Johnson, MSN, RN; and Evelyn Labun, DNSc, RN, for the time and expertise that they graciously gave to the text.

Contents

▼ UNIT I
Foundations of Psychiatric-Mental Health Nursing   1

CHAPTER 1
Introduction to Psychiatric-Mental Health Nursing   3
Barbara Schoen Johnson; Wanda K. Mohr

MENTAL HEALTH AND MENTAL ILLNESS   3
  The Mental Health-Illness Continuum   4
  Mental Health: A Report of the Surgeon General   4
  Elements of Mental Health   5
  Influences on Mental Health   5
  Incidence and Prevalence of Mental Illness   5
  Etiology of Mental Illness   6
  Diagnosis of Mental Illness   6
  Prevention and Treatment of Mental Illness   8
    Problems in Treating Mental Illness   8
      Cost-Related Issues   8
      Stigma   9
      Revolving Door Treatment   9
      Lack of Parity   9
      Limited Access to Services   9
    Goals of Care and Methods of Achievement   9
      Beyond Response to Recovery   10
      Reintegration into Society   10
      Mental Health Parity   10
      Culturally Competent Care   10
      Medication Adherence   10
    Self-Help Movements and Advocacy   11
      National Alliance for the Mentally Ill   11
      Family Advocacy Movement   11
      Psychiatric Advanced Directives   11
PSYCHIATRIC-MENTAL HEALTH NURSING   12
  Nursing Process and Standards of Care   12
  Levels of Practice   12
  Guiding Principles   13
  The Role of the Psychiatric Nurse as a Team Member   13
    Learning to Provide Appropriate Care   16
    Understanding the Client's View of Mental Healthcare   17
    Managing Stress and Burnout   17

CHAPTER 2
Neuroscience: Biology and Behavior   21
Wanda K. Mohr

NEUROANATOMY AND NEUROPHYSIOLOGY   22
  Neurons   22
    Neurotransmission   22
    Plasticity   24
  Central Nervous System   24
    Spinal Cord   25
    The Brain   25
      Organization and Structure   25
      Brain Development   28
      Neuroplasticity   29
  The Role of Genetics   30
    Genetics and Psychiatric Disorders   31
    Interactions Between Genes and Environment   32
OTHER TOPICS IN NEUROSCIENCE   32
  Memory, Repetition, and Learning   32
  Circadian Rhythm   32
  Psychoneuroimmunology   33
  Neuroimaging Techniques   33

CHAPTER 3
Conceptual Frameworks and Theories   37
Wanda K. Mohr

THEORIES: WHO CARES AND SO WHAT?   38
THEORIES OF HUMAN BEHAVIOR   39
  Psychoanalytic Perspective   39
    General Principles   40
    Critiques of Psychoanalytic Theory   40
  Behavior Theory   41
    General Principles   42
      Conditioning   43
      Reinforcement   43
      Punishment   43
      Generalization and Discrimination   43
      Modeling and Shaping   44
    Applied Behavior Analysis   44
  Cognitive-Behavior Theory   44
  The Humanistic Perspective   45
  The Interpersonal Perspective   46
  The Biophysiological Perspective   46
  The Sociocultural Viewpoint   47

TOWARD A COMPREHENSIVE, MULTIDISIPLINARY
UNDERSTANDING OF PSYCHOPATHOLOGY 47
  The Emergence of Mental Illness 49
  Multidimensionality of Assessment (Assessing
    Multiple Systems) 49
    Family Characteristics (Microsystem) 49
    Community Characteristics (Exosystem) 49

CHAPTER 4

Therapeutic Relationships and Communication

Catherine Deering; Jane Frederick

THERAPEUTIC RELATIONSHIPS 54
  Essential Elements 55
    Trust 55
    Professionalism 55
    Mutual Respect 55
    Caring 56
    Partnership 57
  Obstacles to Establishing a Therapeutic
    Relationship 57
    Judgmental Analysis 57
    Excessive Probing 58
    Lack of Self-Awareness 59
  Phases of the Therapeutic Relationship 60
    Introductory Phase 60
    Middle or Working Phase 62
    Termination Phase 63
THERAPEUTIC COMMUNICATION 63
  Theoretical Framework and Communication
  Model 64
  Listening 64
  Assertiveness 70
  Confrontation and Limit Setting 70
  Self-Disclosure 71
  Therapeutic Communication in Special Situations 72
    Clients With Anxiety 72
    Clients With Psychoses 72
    Families 72

CHAPTER 5

Culture 77

Mary Huggins

CULTURE 79
  Changing Demographics and Cultural Awareness 79
    Assimilation 80
    Implications for Healthcare 80
  Culturally Competent Healthcare 81
    Cultural Congruence 82
    Culture Care Theory 84
DISPARITIES IN MENTAL HEALTH AND BARRIERS
TO EFFECTIVE TREATMENT 84
  Variability and Vulnerability 84
  Accessibility 85

    Racial Bias 85
    Religious and Spiritual Influences 86
SOCIOCULTURAL VARIATIONS IN RESPONSE TO
MENTAL HEALTHCARE 87
  African-American Clients 87
  Native-American Clients 87
  Hispanic and Latino Clients 88
  Asian and Pacific Islander Clients 88
CULTURALLY COMPETENT AND CONGRUENT
NURSING CARE 88
  Essential Skills 88
  Phases of Transcultural Nursing Knowledge 90
  Transcultural Assessment 90
  Building Cultural Awareness 90
  Cultural Self-Awareness 91

CHAPTER 6

*The Nursing Process in Psychiatric-Mental
Healthcare* 95

Suzanne Perraud

STEPS OF THE NURSING PROCESS 96
  Assessment 97
    Components of the Psychosocial Assessment 97
      Interview 97
      Health History 97
      Mental Status Examination 99
  Nursing Diagnosis 102
    The NANDA Taxonomy 102
    Choosing and Formulating the Nursing
      Diagnosis 102
    Nursing Diagnosis and Psychiatric Diagnosis 103
  Planning 104
    Identifying Outcomes 104
    Selecting Interventions 107
      Standardized Care Plans 108
      Clinical or Critical Pathways 108
  Implementation 108
    Intervention Strategies for Beginning
      Practitioners 109
    Supervision 109
  Evaluation 109

CHAPTER 7

*Legal and Ethical Aspects of Psychiatric-Mental
Health Nursing* 113

Robin S. Diamond; Gwen Larsen

LEGAL ISSUES IN PSYCHIATRIC-MENTAL HEALTH
NURSING CARE 114
  Nurse Practice Acts and the Expanding Role of
    Nursing 116
  Malpractice 116
  Obtaining Legal Counsel 117

Basic Rights of Clients Receiving Psychiatric Care 117
Informed Consent 118
Special Considerations in Psychiatric Settings 120
Substituted Consent 120
Confidentiality 121
Responsible Record Keeping 121
Privileged Communication 121
Evolving Legal Rights 122
Right to Treatment 122
Right to Treatment in the Least Restrictive Environment 122
Right to Refuse Treatment 122
Right to Aftercare 122
Client Status and Specific Legal Issues 122
Voluntary Admissions 122
Emergency Admissions 123
Involuntary Admissions 123
Legal Issues and Special Client Populations 124
Forensic Clients 124
Competency to Stand Trial 124
Pleas of Insanity or Mental Illness 124
Minors 124
ETHICAL ISSUES IN PSYCHIATRIC-MENTAL HEALTH NURSING CARE 125
Bioethical Principles in Psychiatric Nursing Practice 126
Autonomy 126
Beneficence and Paternalism 126
Veracity and Fidelity 126
Justice 127
Nursing Ethics in Community Mental Health 127
Boundaries in Ethical Nursing Care 127

UNIT II
Conceptual Bases of Treatment 133

CHAPTER 8
Working With Individuals 135
Jeanneane L. Cline

COLLABORATIVE GOALS OF INDIVIDUAL THERAPY 136
TYPES OF INDIVIDUAL PSYCHOTHERAPY 136
Classic Psychoanalysis 138
Cognitive Therapy 138
Issues Identified by Cognitive Therapy 139
Cognitive Therapy Treatment Approach 139
Behavioral Therapy 139
Behavioral Theory 141
The Process of Behavioral Therapy 142
Cognitive-Behavioral Therapy 143
Rational Emotive Behavior Therapy 143
Choice Therapy 144
Brief, Solution-Focused Therapy 144
THE NURSE'S ROLE 145
Levels of Clinical Nursing Practice 145
Therapeutic Interventions in Nursing 146

CHAPTER 9
Working With Groups 151
Barbara G. Tunley Crenshaw

GROUP PROCESS 152
What Is a Group? 152
Characteristics of Groups 152
Types of Groups 152
Group Norms 152
Group Leadership 152
Styles of Group Leadership 153
Decision Making 153
Structuring the Group 153
Group Roles 154
Group Task Roles 154
Group Building and Maintenance Roles 154
Individual Roles 154
Group Communication 154
Latent and Manifest Communication 154
Content and Process Communication 154
Transference and Countertransference 156
Communication Themes 157
Stages of Group Development 157
Initial Stage 157
Working Stage 157
Mature Stage 157
Termination Stage 157
GROUP THERAPY 158
Purposes 158
Advantages and Disadvantages 158
Therapeutic Factors of Group Therapy 160
Instillation of Hope 161
Universality 161
Imparting of Information 161
Group Cohesiveness 161
Catharsis 161
Existential Factors 161
Types of Therapy Groups 161
Psychotherapeutic Groups 161
Growth Groups 162
NURSES AND GROUP PROCESS AND THERAPY 162
Group Process and Therapy in Nursing Education 162
Group Process and Therapy in Nursing Practice 164
Historical Perspective 164
Contemporary Nursing Groups 164

CHAPTER 10
Working With Families 169
Victoria Conn

FAMILY CAREGIVING FROM 1850 TO 2000 170
FAMILY BURDEN 170

Objective Burden   171
Subjective Burden   173
Iatrogenic Burden   175
Confidentiality Issues   175
Involuntary Treatment Statutes   175
Discrimination   175
Burden Attributable to Professionals   175
FAMILY RESILIENCE   178
NEEDS OF FAMILIES FOR SECONDARY
PREVENTION   178
Families as a Population at Risk   178
Family Consultation   179
Family Consultation Versus Family Therapy   180
Components of Family Consultation   180
The Nurse as Family Consultant   180
Family Empowerment   183
Family Education   183
Family Education Versus Family
Psychoeducation   183
Components of Family Education   183
The Nurse as Family Educator   184
Peer-Taught Family Education   184
Psychotherapy and Medication   185

CHAPTER 11

Working With Special Environments:
Forensic Clients, Crisis Intervention, and
the Homeless   191

Cindy A. Peternelj-Taylor, Anita G. Hufft, Phyllis M.
Connolly, and Kay Peterson

FORENSIC NURSING   191
Forensic Settings   192
Factors Contributing to Incarceration   192
Characteristics of the Forensic Population   193
Effects of Incarceration on Mental Health   196
Characteristics of Forensic Psychiatric Nurses   196
Application of the Nursing Process to the Forensic Client   197
Assessment   198
Nursing Diagnosis   198
Planning   198
Implementation   199
Evaluation   201
NURSING CARE FOR THE CLIENT IN CRISIS   201
Crisis Theory   202
Crisis Prevention   204
Crisis Intervention and Stabilization   204
Application of the Nursing Process to the Client in Crisis   206
Assessment   206
Nursing Diagnosis   207
Planning   208
Implementation   209
Evaluation   210
NURSING CARE OF HOMELESS CLIENTS   210
Demographics   210

Homeless Mentally Ill People   210
Application of the Nursing Process to the Homeless Client   215
Assessment   215
Nursing Diagnosis   215
Planning   216
Implementation   217
Evaluation   217

CHAPTER 12

Psychopharmacology   223

Geraldine Pearson

IMPORTANT PRINCIPLES OF
PSYCHOPHARMACOTHERAPEUTICS   224
Agonists   224
Antagonists   224
Affinity   224
Efficacy   225
Potency   225
Target Symptoms   225
Refractoriness   225
Polypharmacy   225
IMPORTANT PSYCHOTHERAPEUTIC DRUGS   226
Medications for Mood Disorders   227
Antidepressants   227
Tricyclic Antidepressants   227
Atypical Antidepressants   232
Monoamine Oxidase Inhibitors   232
Selective Serotonin Reuptake Inhibitors, Selective
Reuptake Inhibitors, and Selective
Norepineprine Reuptake Inhibitors   233
Mood Stabilizers   234
Lithium Carbonate   234
Anticonvulsants   234
Medications for Refractory Mania   236
Anxiolytics   237
Buspirone   237
Benzodiazepines   237
Antipsychotic (Neuroleptic) Agents   239
Typical or Traditional Antipsychotics   240
Low-Potency Typical Antipsychotics   240
High-Potency Typical Antipsychotics   244
Atypical Antipsychotics   244
Clozapine   244
Risperidone   245
Olanzapine   245
Quetiapine   245
Stimulants   245
Application of the Nursing Process to Clients Receiving
Psychopharmacologic Agents   246
Assessment   247
Nursing Diagnosis   248
Planning   248
Prescribed and Maximum Dose   248
Method of Administration   248
Expected Drug Action   249

Side Effects   249
Adverse Effects   249
Implementation   252
Promoting Adherence to the Medication Regimen   253
Factors Contributing to Nonadherence   253
Implications for Practice   253
Working With the Family   254
Performing Self-Clarification   254
Evaluation   255
IMPORTANT ISSUES RELATED TO
PSYCHOPHARMACOLOGY AND NURSING
MANAGEMENT   255
Lifespan Considerations   255
Pregnant and Lactating Women   255
Children and Adolescents   256
Older Adults   256
Use of Alternative Agents to Treat Psychiatric
Illness   257
Nursing Research   257

CHAPTER 13

Spirituality in Psychiatric Care   263

Wanda K. Mohr

SPIRITUALITY AND RELIGION   264
SPIRITUALITY, RELIGION, AND MENTAL HEALTH AND
ILLNESS   264
Illness Prevention   264
Spirituality, Religion, and Mental Illness   265
RELIGIOUS AND SPIRITUAL INTERVENTIONS IN
MENTAL HEALTH CARE   266
Changing Attitudes and Philosophies   266
Clarifying Values   266
The Role of Clergy in Mental Healthcare   266
The Role of the Nurse in Mental Healthcare   267
Spiritual Assessment   267
Spiritual Coping Practices and Interventions   268
Prayer   268
Bibliotherapy With Sacred Writings   268
Contemplation and Meditation   268
Repentance and Forgiveness   268
Worship and Rituals   269
Fellowship and Altruistic Service   269
Journal Writing   269
ETHICAL CONCERNS   269

CHAPTER 14

Complementary and Alternative Medicine   275

Jeanneane Cline

OVERVIEW OF COMPLEMENTARY AND ALTERNATIVE
MEDICINE   275
National Center for Complementary and Alternative
Medicine and CAM Expansion   276
Prevalence of Complementary and Alternative
Medicine   276
Research Studies   276
Ethical and Legal Considerations   276
CLASSIFICATION OF COMPLEMENTARY AND
ALTERNATIVE MEDICINE   277
Alternative Systems of Medical Practice   277
Traditional Chinese Medicine   277
Acupuncture   277
Ayurvedic Medicine   278
Naturopathy   278
Homeopathy   278
Mind-Body Interventions   279
Meditation   279
Imagery   279
Music Therapy   279
Spiritual Healing and Prayer   279
Biological-Based Therapies   280
Herbal Therapies   280
Aromatherapy   280
Manipulative and Body-Based Methods   283
T'ai Chi   283
Yoga   284
Massage   284
Energy Therapies   284
Biofield Therapies   284
Healing Touch and Therapeutic Touch   284
Reiki   284
Bioelectromagnetic-Based Therapies   285
THE NURSE'S ROLE   285

UNIT III
Continuum of Care   291

CHAPTER 15

Community Mental Health, Support, and Rehabilitation   293

Mary Huggins, Jeffrey A. Anderson, and Sue Ellen Odom

COMMUNITY MENTAL HEALTH   294
Historical Perspective   294
Levels of Prevention   295
Primary Prevention   295
Secondary Prevention   297
Tertiary Prevention   297
COMMUNITY SUPPORT SYSTEMS   297
Components of a Community Support
System   297
Guiding Principles   298
Program Models   298
Psychosocial Rehabilitation Model   299
Fairweather Lodge Model   299
Training in Community Living Model   299
Consumer-Run Alternative Models   299
Community Worker Models   299

Community Support Programs   300
Child and Adolescent Service System
    Program   300
Public Policy and Trends   301
    Chronicity of Severe Mental Illness   301
    Stalled Resources   302
    Poverty   302
    Reinstitutionalization   302
    Education   302
    Stigma   302
    Reforms   303
        Safety Net Services   303
        Legislation   303
        Public Policy   303
Application of the Nursing Process to Community Settings   304
    Assessment   304
    Nursing Diagnosis   305
    Planning   305
    Implementation   306
    Evaluation   306

CHAPTER 16

Behavioral Health Home Care   311

Nina A. Klebanoff

FOUNDATIONS OF BEHAVIORAL HEALTH HOME
CARE   312
    History of Behavioral Health Home Care   312
    Principles of Behavioral Health Home Care   312
    Home Care Services   312
    Home Care Providers   313
    Goals of Behavioral Health Home Care   313
BEHAVIORAL HEALTH HOME CARE NURSING   313
    Behavioral Health Clinical Nurse Specialists   314
    Attitudes and Feelings   315
    The Nursing Process and Behavioral Health Home
        Care   315
        Assessment   315
            Indicators and Standards of Care   315
            Data to Collect   315
            Data Gathering Methods   315
        Nursing Diagnosis   315
        Planning   315
        Implementation   319
        Evaluation   319
    Trends in Behavioral Health Home Care Nursing   320

CHAPTER 17

Violence and Abuse Within the Community   323

Kathleen R. Delaney, Delia Esparza, Diane Hinderliter,
Karen Van Dyke Lamb, and Wanda K. Mohr

THE ECOLOGICAL MODEL OF VIOLENCE   324
    Macrosystem   324
    Microsystem   324
    Exosystem   325
    Ontogenic Development   325
PUBLIC HEALTH APPROACH TO VIOLENCE
PREVENTION   325
YOUTH VIOLENCE   325
    Risk and Protective Factors for Youth Violence   326
        Individual Risk Factors   326
        Family Risk Factors   326
        Peer Risk Factors   326
        Neighborhood Risk Factors   327
        Protective Factors   327
    Public Health Approach to Youth Violence   327
    Nurses' Role in Youth Violence Prevention
        Efforts   328
FAMILY VIOLENCE   328
    Intimate Partner Violence   328
        Defining the Scope of Intimate Partner
            Violence   328
        Cost to Children   328
        Addressing Intimate Partner Violence   329
            Problems With Detection and
                Screening   329
            Importance of Screening   330
        Nurses' Role in Identification and Treatment of
            Intimate Partner Violence   330
    Child Maltreatment   331
        Effects of Maltreatment on Child Function   331
            Social Functioning   331
            Behavioral Functioning   331
            Emotional and Intellectual Functioning   332
            Health and Physical Functioning   332
            Family Functioning and Parenting
                Practices   333
        Nurses' Role in the Identification of
            Maltreatment   333
    Elder Abuse   333
        Types of Elder Abuse   333
        Causes of Elder Abuse   334
        Nurses' Role in the Identification and Treatment of
            Elder Abuse   334
RAPE AND SEXUAL ASSAULT   335
    Types of Rape   335
        Rape by a Stranger   335
        Date Rape and Acquaintance Rape   335
        Marital Rape   335
    Rape Trauma Syndrome   336
    Additional Ramifications of Rape   336
    Treatment for Survivors of Rape or Sexual
        Assault   337
        Psychopharmacologic Interventions   337
        Psychological Interventions   337
    Rape Prevention   337
    Nurses' Role in the Assessment and Treatment of
        Survivors of Rape Trauma   338
        Assessment   338
        Treatment   339

▼ UNIT IV
Nursing Care for Clients with Psychiatric Disorders   347

CHAPTER 18

The Client With an Anxiety Disorder   349

Judith A. Greene

ANXIETY   350
  The Continuum of Anxiety   350
    Effects on Sensation   350
    Effects on Cognition   350
    Effects on Verbal Ability   351
  Normal Versus Abnormal Anxiety   351
ANXIETY DISORDERS   351
  Etiology   352
    Neurological Theories   352
    Psychological Theories   352
  Signs and Symptoms/Diagnostic Criteria   353
    Generalized Anxiety Disorder   353
    Phobic Disorders   357
      Agoraphobia   357
      Social Phobia   357
      Specific Phobia   358
    Panic Attacks   358
    Panic Disorder   358
    Obsessive-Compulsive Disorder   358
    Post-Traumatic Stress Disorder   359
    Acute Stress Disorder   361
  Comorbidities and Dual Diagnoses   361
  Implications and Prognoses   361
  Interdisciplinary Goals and Treatment   362
    Psychodynamic Therapies   362
      Basic Cognitive Therapy Techniques for
        Anxiety   362
      Systematic Desensitization and Exposure
        Treatment   363
      Relaxation Techniques and Breathing
        Retraining   363
    Pharmacologic Treatment   364
      Selective Serotonin Reuptake
        Inhibitors   364
      Benzodiazepines   365
      Buspirone   365
      Beta Blockers   365
      Tricyclic Antidepressants   365
Application of the Nursing Process to the Client With an Anxiety
Disorder   366
  Assessment   366
  Nursing Diagnosis   366
  Planning   366
  Implementation   366
    Alleviating Anxiety   367

    Initiating a Therapeutic Dialogue   367
    Countering Faulty Thinking   368
    Managing Hyperventilation   368
    Suggesting Lifestyle Changes   368
  Teaching Adaptive Coping Strategies   368
    Teaching Relaxation   368
    Teaching Problem-Solving Skills   369
  Evaluation   369

CHAPTER 19

The Client With a Somatoform Disorder   373

Carol J. Cornwell

SOMATOFORM DISORDERS   374
  Epidemiology   375
  Cultural Considerations   375
  Etiology   375
  Signs and Symptoms/Diagnostic Criteria   377
    Primary and Secondary Gain   377
    Somatization Disorder   377
    Undifferentiated Somatoform Disorder   380
    Conversion Disorder   380
    Pain Disorder   381
    Hypochondriasis   381
    Body Dysmorphic Disorder   381
    Somatoform Disorder Not Otherwise
      Specified   381
  Comorbidities and Dual Diagnoses   381
  Implications and Prognosis   381
  Interdisciplinary Goals and Treatment   382
    Individual and Group Psychotherapies   383
    Somatic Therapies   383
Application of the Nursing Process to the Client With a
Somatoform Disorder   383
  Assessment   383
    Psychological Assessment   383
      Behavior   384
      Mood and Affect   385
      Thought Process and Content   385
      Intellectual and Cognitive Processing   385
      Insight and Judgment   385
      Suicidal Ideation   385
    Physical Examination   385
      Vegetative Signs   385
      Energy and Psychomotor Functioning   385
    Social Assessment   385
  Nursing Diagnoses   386
  Planning   386
  Implementation   386
    Establishing a Trusting Relationship   386
    Managing Ineffective Coping   388
    Addressing Powerlessness and Dependency
      Issues   391
    Enhancing Self-Esteem   391
    Reducing Anxiety   391

Reestablishing Social Activities 391
Reestablishing Functional Family Processes 391
Evaluation 392

CHAPTER 20
The Client With a Sexual or Gender Disorder 397

Delia Esparza

NORMAL HUMAN SEXUALITY 398
Sexual Expression 398
Effects of Sexual Orientation on Sexual
Expression 399
Sexual Preference 399
Gender Role 400
Sexual Identity 400
Effects of Culture on Sexual Expression 400
Effects of Ill Health on Sexual Expression 400
Sexual Response 401
Human Sexual Response Phases 401
Desire 402
Excitement 402
Orgasm 402
Normal Age-Related Sexual Changes 402
SEXUAL AND GENDER DISORDERS 402
SEXUAL DYSFUNCTION DISORDERS 403
Etiology 403
Signs and Symptoms/Diagnostic Criteria 403
Desire Disorders 403
Arousal Disorders 403
Orgasmic Disorders 405
Pain Disorders 405
Interdisciplinary Goals and Treatments 405
Pharmacologic Therapy 409
Sex Therapy 409
Application of the Nursing Process to the Client With Sexual Dysfunction 409
Assessment 409
Nursing Diagnosis 412
Planning 413
Implementation 414
Counseling the Client With a Sexual Dysfunction
Disorder 414
Enhancing Self-Esteem 414
Evaluation 416
PARAPHILIAS 416
Signs and Symptoms/Diagnostic Criteria 416
Interdisciplinary Goals and Treatment 416
GENDER IDENTITY DISORDERS 417
Signs and Symptoms/Diagnostic Criteria 417
Interdisciplinary Goals and Treatment 417
Sex Reassignment Surgery 417
Hormone Treatment 417
Psychotherapy 417

CHAPTER 21
The Client With a Dissociative Disorder 421

Jan Dalsheimer; Janet Stagg

DISSOCIATIVE DISORDERS 422
Epidemiology 422
Cultural Considerations 423
Etiology 423
Biologic Factors 423
Psychological and Social Factors 423
Role of Family Dynamics 424
Signs and Symptoms/Diagnostic Criteria 424
Comorbidities and Dual Diagnoses 424
Interdisciplinary Goals and Treatment 424
Treatment Approach 426
Individual Therapy 427
Group Therapy 427
Pharmacotherapy 427
Art Therapy 427
Milieu Management 428
Family Education 428
Application of the Nursing Process to the Client With a Dissociative Disorder 428
Assessment in Adults 428
Assessment in Children 429
Nursing Diagnosis 429
Planning 429
Implementation 429
Evaluation 431

CHAPTER 22
The Client With a Personality Disorder 437

Judith Greene

PERSONALITY DISORDERS 437
Etiology 438
Signs and Symptoms/Diagnostic Criteria 438
Cluster A Personality Disorders 438
Paranoid Personality Disorder 442
Schizoid Personality Disorder 442
Schizotypal Personality Disorder 442
Cluster B Personality Disorders 442
Antisocial Personality Disorder 442
Borderline Personality Disorder 442
Histrionic Personality Disorder 442
Narcissistic Personality Disorder 443
Cluster C Personality Disorders 443
Avoidant Personality Disorder 443
Dependent Personality Disorder 443
Obsessive-Compulsive Personality Disorder 443
Comorbidities and Dual Diagnoses 444
Implications and Prognosis 444
Interdisciplinary Goals and Treatment 444
Individual Psychotherapy 444

Group Therapy 445
Family Education and Therapy 445
Application of the Nursing Process to a Client With a Personality Disorder 446
Assessment 446
Nursing Diagnoses 447
Planning 447
Implementation 447
Promoting Participation in Treatment 447
Enlisting the Family in the Treatment Plan 447
Improving Coping Skills 447
Reducing Inappropriate Behaviors 447
Confronting the Client 448
Setting Limits 449
Providing for Physical Safety 449
Evaluation 451
Nurse's Self Care 451

CHAPTER 23
The Client With an Eating Disorder 455
Susan D. Decker
EATING DISORDERS 456
Etiology 456
Biologic Theories 456
Behavioral Theories 458
Sociocultural Theories 458
Family-Based Theories 458
Signs and Symptoms/Diagnostic Criteria 459
Anorexia Nervosa 459
Bulimia Nervosa 459
Comorbidities and Dual Diagnoses 459
Implications and Prognosis 462
Interdisciplinary Goals and Treatment 462
Behavioral Therapy 462
Cognitive Therapy 462
Cognitive-Behavioral Therapy 462
Interpersonal Therapy 462
Solution-Focused Brief Therapy 463
Family Therapy 463
Group Therapy 463
Pharmacologic Interventions 463
Application of the Nursing Process to Clients With Eating Disorders 464
Assessment 464
History and Physical Examination 464
Psychosocial Assessment 464
Nursing Diagnosis 467
Planning 468
Implementation 468
Restoring Nutritional Balance 469
Encouraging Realistic Thinking Processes 469
Improving Body Image 472
Building Self-Esteem 472
Exploring Feelings of Powerlessness 473

Encouraging Effective Coping 473
Restoring Family Processes 473
Enmeshments and Overprotectiveness 473
Conflict Avoidance and Rigidity 473
Evaluation 473

CHAPTER 24
The Client With a Mood Disorder 479
Carol J. Cornwell
MOOD DISORDERS 480
Epidemiology 480
Etiology 481
Genetic Factors 481
Physiologic Factors 482
Biogenic Amines 482
Psychoneuroendocrine and Immune Relationships 483
Psychological Factors 484
Psychodynamic Factors 485
Learned Helplessness 485
Cognitive Factors 485
Feminist Factors 486
Signs and Symptoms/Diagnostic Criteria 486
Major Depressive Disorder 486
Dysthymic Disorder 487
Bipolar Disorders 490
Bipolar I Disorder 490
Bipolar II Disorder 491
Cyclothymic Disorder 492
Implications and Prognosis 492
Interdisciplinary Goals and Treatment 492
Psychotherapy 492
Cognitive-Behavioral Therapy 492
Pharmacologic Therapy 494
Antidepressants 494
Mood Stabilizers 497
Medications for Refractory Mania 499
Somatic Nonpharmacologic Interventions 500
Electroconvulsive Therapy 500
Phototherapy 500
Sleep Deprivation 501
Transcranial Magnetic Stimulation 501
Vagus Nerve Stimulation 501
Application of the Nursing Process to the Client With a Mood Disorder 501
Assessment 501
Safety Assessment 501
Suicide Risk Assessment 501
Violence Assessment 502
Mental Status Examination 502
Appearance and General Behavior 503
Mood and Affect 503
Thought Process and Content 503
Perceptual Disturbances 503

Judgment and Insight 503
Physiological Stability Assessment 503
Family Issues Assessment 504
Nursing Diagnoses 504
Planning 504
Implementation 504
Protecting the Client from Suicide 504
Managing the Potential for Violence 509
Maintaining Physical Health and Personal Hygiene 509
Enhancing Thought Processes 512
Self-Esteem Issues 512
Anxiety and Agitation 512
Encouraging Treatment and Medication Adherence 513
Evaluation 513

CHAPTER 25

The Client With a Thought Disorder 521

Barbara Schoen Johnson; Geraldine S. Pearson

SCHIZOPHRENIA AND OTHER THOUGHT
DISORDERS 522
The Stigma of Schizophrenia 523
Etiology 523
Biologic Theories 526
Genetic Influences 526
Neurochemical and Neuroanatomic Changes 528
Psychosocial Theories 529
Signs and Symptoms/Diagnostic Criteria 530
The Disorganization Dimension 530
Disorganized Speech 530
Disorganized Behavior 532
Incongruous Affect 532
The Psychotic Dimension 533
Delusions 533
Hallucinations 533
The Negative Dimension 533
Other Symptoms 534
Subtypes of Schizophrenia 534
Water Intoxication in Schizophrenia 534
Comorbidities and Dual Diagnoses 535
Implications and Prognosis 535
Interdisciplinary Goals and Treatment 535
Pharmacological Interventions 537
Traditional (Conventional) Antipsychotics 537
Atypical (Novel) Antipsychotics 539
Psychosocial Interventions 540
Milieu Management 540
Individual and Group Therapy 540
Cognitive-behavioral Therapy 540
Vocational Rehabilitation 540
Continuum of Care 541
Discharge Planning 541
Care in the Community 541
Application of the Nursing Process to the Client With a Thought Disorder 542

Assessment 542
Assessing Mood and Cognitive State 542
Assessing Potential for Violence 542
Assessing Social Support 543
Assessing Knowledge 543
Nursing Diagnosis 543
Planning 543
Implementation 543
Intervening in Disturbed Thought Processes and Sensory Perceptions 546
Reinforcing Reality 546
Understanding Language Content 546
Intervening in Hallucinations 546
Managing Violent Behavior 547
Lessening Social Isolation 547
Developing Trust 547
Initiating Interaction 547
Modeling Affect 547
Promoting Adherence to Medication Regimens 547
Promoting Improved Individual Coping Skills 549
Strengthening Family Processes 549
Providing Client and Family Education 550
Teaching Symptom Management 550
Evaluation 550

CHAPTER 26

The Client Who Displays Angry, Aggressive, or Violent Behavior 555

Bonnie Louise Rickelman

AGGRESSIVE BEHAVIOR, HOSTILITY-RELATED
VARIABLES, AND VIOLENCE 556
Profiles of Aggressive and Violent Behaviors in Persons
With Psychiatric Diagnoses 556
Sociodemographic Factors 556
Inpatient Factors 557
Outpatient Factors 557
Family Factors 557
Determinants of Aggression 557
Neurobiologic Factors 558
Psychological Factors 558
Temperament Theory 558
Cognitive Theory 558
Social-Environmental Factors 559
Legal Issues 559
Interdisciplinary Goals and Treatment 560
Verbal Interventions 560
Limit Setting 560
Cognitive Interventions 560
Guided Discovery 560
Anger Management 560
Behavior Therapy: Token Economy 560
Group and Family Therapy 561
Pharmacological Intervention 561
Seclusion and Restraint 561

Outpatient Management   564
*Application of the Nursing Process to the Client Displaying
Angry, Aggressive, or Violent Behavior*   565
   Assessment   565
   Nursing Diagnosis   565
   Planning   565
   Implementation   565
      Maintaining the Safety of Clients and Staff   566
      Defusing Anger and Aggression through Verbal
      Interventions   566
      Setting Limits to Prevent Violent Behavior   568
      Teaching Anger Management and Coping Skills   568
   Evaluation   569

CHAPTER 27
The Client Who Abuses Drugs and Alcohol   575
Carol J. Cornwell
SUBSTANCE ABUSE AND DEPENDENCY   576
   Historical Context   576
   Epidemiology   576
   Prenatal Alcohol and Drug Abuse   578
   Cultural Considerations   581
   Etiology   581
      Psychosocial and Behavioral Factors   581
      Biological Factors   581
      Theoretical Concepts   582
   Comorbidities and Dual Diagnoses   582
   Implications and Prognosis   582
   Signs and Symptoms/Diagnostic Criteria   583
      Alcohol Abuse and Dependency   583
         Chemical Properties of Alcohol   583
         Alcohol Concentration in the Body   584
         Tolerance   585
         Blackout   585
         Alcohol-Induced Disorders   585
         Medical Consequences of Alcohol Abuse and
         Dependency   586
      Controlled Substances   586
   Interdisciplinary Treatment   589
      Medical Detoxification from Alcohol   589
      The Rehabilitation Process   591
      Medications Used to Treat Drug
      Dependency   591
      Self-Help Groups   591
*Application of the Nursing Process to the Client With a
Substance-Related Disorder*   593
   Assessment   593
      Physical Examination   595
      Psychosocial Assessment   595
   Nursing Diagnoses   595
   Planning   595
   Implementation   595
      Maintaining Safety   595
      Breaking Through Denial   599

Managing Anxiety   600
      Teaching Effective Coping Strategies   600
      Improving Family Processes   600
      Enhancing Self-Esteem   600
      Promoting Healthy Activities   603
   Evaluation   603

CHAPTER 28
The Client With a Cognitive Disorder   607
Cheryl Detwiler
COGNITIVE DISORDERS   608
DELIRIUM   609
   Etiology   609
   Signs and Symptoms/Diagnostic Criteria   610
   Implications and Prognosis   611
   Interdisciplinary Goals and Treatment   611
      Medical Interventions   611
      Environmental Interventions   611
      Cognitive Interventions   611
      Psychological Interventions   613
*Application of the Nursing Process to the Client With
Delirium*   613
   Assessment   613
   Nursing Diagnosis   614
   Planning   614
   Implementation   614
      Managing Confusion   614
      Providing a Safe Environment   617
      Helping the Client With Personal Care   617
      Providing Client and Family Education   617
   Evaluation   617
DEMENTIA   618
   Signs and Symptoms/Diagnostic Criteria   618
      Learning and Retaining New Information   618
      Handling Complex Tasks   618
      Reasoning Ability   618
      Spatial Ability and Orientation   618
      Language   618
      Behavior   618
   Types of Dementia   621
      Alzheimer's Disease   621
      Vascular Dementia   624
      Parkinson's Disease   624
      Huntington's Chorea   624
      Human Immunodeficiency Virus   624
      Pick's Disease   624
      Creutzfeldt-Jakob Disease   625
   Implications and Prognosis   625
   Interdisciplinary Goals and Treatment   625
      Medical and Supportive Interventions   625
      Psychosocial Interventions   626
*Application of the Nursing Process to the Client With
Dementia*   626
   Assessment   626

Behavior   626
Mental Status   626
Perceptual Problems   626
Orientation   626
Memory   626
Family   626
Education   629
Nursing Diagnoses   630
Planning   630
Implementation   630
Managing the Client's Health   630
Enhancing Sensory Capabilities   633
Meeting the Client's Physical Needs   633
Encouraging Appropriate Behaviors   634
Modifying the Environment   634
Performing Pharmacologic Interventions   634
Preventing Injury   636
Preserving the Family Unit   636
Evaluation   636
AMNESTIC DISORDERS   636

▼ UNIT V
Nursing Care for Special Populations   641

CHAPTER 29
Working With Pediatric Clients   643
Barbara Schoen Johnson, Wanda K. Mohr,
and Sherill Nones Cronin

OVERVIEW OF MENTAL HEALTH AND
PSYCHIATRIC DISORDERS IN CHILDREN
AND ADOLESCENTS   644
Theories of Child Development   644
Psychoanalytic Perspectives   645
Sigmund Freud's Psychosexual Theory   645
Erik Erikson's Psychosocial Theory   645
Piaget's Cognitive-Developmental Theory   645
Contemporary Approaches to Child
Development   646
Risk Factors for Child and Adolescent Mental
Disorders   647
Biological Influences   647
Psychosocial Influences   647
Stressors   647
Divorce   648
Child Abuse   648
Protective and Resilient Influences for Mental Health in
Children and Adolescents   648
General Interventions for Child and Adolescent Mental
Disorders   649
The Interdisciplinary Team and Coordination of
Care   649

Treatment Settings and Continuum of
Care   649
Wrap-Around Services and Systems-of-Care
Approaches   649
Prevention and Early Identification   649
Types of Therapies   650
Special Education   651
Community-Based Services   651
Pharmacologic Therapy   651
Nursing Care   651
Assessment   651
Interventions   652
COMMON PSYCHIATRIC DISORDERS OF CHILDREN
AND ADOLESCENTS   653
DISRUPTIVE BEHAVIOR DISORDERS   658
ATTENTION-DEFICIT HYPERACTIVITY DISORDER
AND ATTENTION-DEFICIT DISORDER   658
Etiology   658
Signs and Symptoms/Diagnostic Criteria   658
Comorbidities   658
Interdisciplinary Goals and Treatment   659
Pharmacologic Therapy   659
Psychosocial Interventions   659
Application of the Nursing Process to a Client With
ADHD   659
Assessment   659
Nursing Diagnosis   660
Planning   660
Implementation   660
Educating the Family About Treatment and Behavioral
Strategies   660
Helping Families Cope   662
Managing Developmental and Academic Issues   662
Teaching Social Skills   663
Improving Self-Esteem   663
Evaluation   663
OPPOSITIONAL DEFIANT DISORDER   663
CONDUCT DISORDER   664
ADJUSTMENT DISORDERS   664
ANXIETY DISORDERS   664
OBSESSIVE-COMPULSIVE DISORDER   664
PHOBIAS   665
SOCIAL ANXIETY DISORDER (SOCIAL PHOBIA)   665
GENERALIZED ANXIETY DISORDER   665
SEPARATION ANXIETY DISORDER   665
POST-TRAUMATIC STRESS DISORDER   666
MOOD DISORDERS   666
DEPRESSION   666
Etiology   667
Signs and Symptoms   667
Comorbidities   668
Prevention   668
Interdisciplinary Goals and Treatment   668
Cognitive-Behavioral and Family
Consultation   668
Pharmacologic Therapy   668
BIPOLAR DISORDER   668

Etiology 668
Signs and Symptoms 669
Interdisciplinary Goals and Treatment 669
Importance of Early Identification and
Treatment 669
Pharmacologic Therapy 669
AUTISM SPECTRUM DISORDERS 670
AUTISM 670
ASPERGER SYNDROME 670
Interdisciplinary Goals and Treatment 670
EATING DISORDERS 671
SUBSTANCE ABUSE 671
Etiology 671
Prevention of Drug and Alcohol Abuse 671
Interdisciplinary Goals and Treatment 672
TIC DISORDERS 672
TRICHOTILLOMANIA 673
SUICIDE 673
Signs 673
Prevention 673
Interdisciplinary Goals and Treatment 674
CHILDREN WITH MEDICAL ILLNESS OR
DISABILITY 674
*Application of the Nursing Process to the Child or Adolescent
With Medical Illness or a Disability* 674
Assessment 674
Characteristics of the Disease 674
Family Assessment 675
Nursing Diagnosis 676
Planning 676
Implementation 676
Evaluation 678
NURSES' SELF-CARE 679

CHAPTER *30*
Working With Older Adults 685
Mildred O. Hogstel; Susan E. Margolis
DEMOGRAPHICS OF AGING AND FUTURE
TRENDS 686
PSYCHOSOCIAL ISSUES AND INFLUENCES 686
Retirement 686
Relocation 686
Bereavement 687
Spirituality 687
Issues Related to Ethnicity and Language Barriers 687

COMMUNICATING EFFECTIVELY WITH OLDER
ADULTS 687
Techniques 688
Terminology 688
ISSUES RELATED TO OLDER CLIENTS WITH
PSYCHIATRIC DISORDERS 688
Ageism, Myths, and Prejudices 690
Settings for Care 690
Specific Mental Health Disorders 690
Treatment 690
Assessment 693
Psychotropic Medications 693
Methods of Administration 693
Polypharmacy 694
Pharmacokinetics and Pharmacodynamics 694
Adverse and Side Effects 695
Role of the Nurse 695
PROMOTING MENTAL HEALTH AND WELLNESS IN
OLDER ADULTS 696
Nutrition and Fluids 696
Mental and Physical Activities 696
Support Systems 696

*Appendix A Review Question Answers with
Rationales* 701
*Appendix B DSM-IV-TR Classification:
Axes I and II Categories and Codes* 735
*Appendix C NANDA-Approved Nursing
Diagnoses* 743
*Appendix D Canadian Standards of Psychiatric
and Mental Health Nursing Practice* 745
Appendix E Additional Resources 749
*Appendix F Nursing Interventions and Outcomes
Related to Psychiatric Disorders* 755
*Appendix G Commonly Used Assessment
Tools* 759
Glossary 763
Index 773

UNIT **I**

Foundations of Psychiatric–Mental Health Nursing

Introduction to Psychiatric-Mental Health Nursing

BARBARA SCHOEN JOHNSON; WANDA K. MOHR

▼ KEY TERMS

Altruism—The desire to contribute something valuable to society.

Culturally competent care—Care provided in a manner acceptable to a client's cultural background, regardless of whether the healthcare professional who delivers the care is from the same ethnic or minority group as the client.

Dual diagnosis—Diagnosis of both a mental disorder and a co-occurring substance abuse problem.

Horizontal violence—Anger or negativity a nurse directs toward another nurse.

Medication adherence—The actual taking of medications as prescribed; also called *medication compliance*.

Mental disorders—Health conditions marked by alterations in thinking, mood, or behavior that cause distress, impair ability to function, or both.

Mental health—The successful performance of mental function, resulting in productive activities, fulfilling relationships, and the ability to adapt to change and cope with adversity.

Mental health nursing—The care of well and at-risk populations to prevent mental illness or provide immediate treatment for those with early signs of a psychiatric disorder.

Mental illness—A clinically significant behavioral or psychological syndrome experienced by a person and marked by distress, disability, or the risk of suffering, disability, or loss of freedom.

Psychiatric-mental health nursing—The diagnosis and treatment of human responses to actual or potential mental health problems.

Psychiatric nursing—The care and rehabilitation of people with identifiable mental illnesses or disorders.

Tautology—A logical error in reasoning.

▼ LEARNING OBJECTIVES

On completion of this chapter, you should be able to accomplish the following:

- Define mental health and mental illness.
- Discuss the significance of *Mental Health: A Report of the Surgeon General*.
- Explain the purposes of the multiaxial diagnostic system used in the *Diagnostic and Statistical Manual of Mental Disorders,* 4th edition, text revision (DSM-IV-TR).
- Discuss trends, problems, and goals related to the delivery of mental healthcare and treatment of mental illness.
- Discuss the contributions of self-help organizations and advocacy movements to understanding client and family adaptation to mental illness.
- Describe the functions and levels of practice of psychiatric-mental health nurses.
- Apply the principles guiding psychiatric nursing to clinical examples.
- Identify stressors that affect the practice of psychiatric-mental health nurses and ways to prevent or decrease the effects of such stressors.

This chapter introduces the concepts of mental health and mental illness. It explains how mental illnesses are prevented, diagnosed, and treated and the many problems such conditions pose for clients who have them and their families. It also introduces the world of psychiatric-mental health nursing and how nurses will work with clients facing psychiatric problems. The topics discussed in this chapter will be relevant throughout this entire textbook.

MENTAL HEALTH AND MENTAL ILLNESS

The World Health Organization (WHO) defines *health* as a state of complete physical, mental, and social wellbeing. Health is not only the absence of disease or infirmity, but also a sense of satisfaction with and enjoyment of self and the environment.

Mental health is defined as the successful performance of mental function, resulting in productive activities, fulfilling relationships, and the ability to adapt to change and cope with adversity. Mental health provides people with the capacity for rational thinking, communication skills, learning, emotional growth, resilience, and self-esteem (U.S. Department of Health and Human Services, 1999). People experiencing emotional well-being or mental health function comfortably in society and are satisfied with their achievements.

For the purposes of this chapter, **mental disorders** are generally defined as health conditions marked by alterations in thinking, mood, or behavior that cause distress, impair ability to function, or both (U.S. Department of Health and Human Services, 1999). **Mental illness** is considered a clinically significant behavioral or psychological syndrome experienced by a person and marked by distress, disability, or the risk of suffering, disability, or loss of freedom (American Psychiatric Association [APA]). The syndrome is not merely a cultural expectation. In other words, the behavioral or psychological problem must result from brain functioning or dysfunctioning, and it must cause the person distress, impairment, or both. It cannot be a cultural practice to which the majority culture in a society objects or that might cause nonmembers of the cultural group distress. For example, some cultures believe that women should be subservient to men and expect the behavior of both sexes to reflect this idea. People of Western cultures might view such women as dependent or codependent, yet the behavior of these women is perfectly normal within the parameters of their own culture.

Precise definitions of mental disorders and mental illness are elusive and impractical. The conditions and consequences that people with mental disorders experience are much more complicated than a list of symptoms. Healthcare professionals must understand that while a person may have a diagnosis of schizophrenia or depression, the person is *not* a "schizophrenic" or "depressive." He or she is a person with schizophrenia or depression. That is, the person is separate and different from his or her diagnosis.

The Mental Health-Illness Continuum

Because mental illnesses are brain illnesses, one might think of mental health as complete structural and functional brain integrity. But mental health encompasses much more than brain functioning. Experts in the field of mental health and mental illness agree that the two are *not* polar opposites. Having said this, they also most often think of mental health and mental illness as end points on a continuum. Considering health and illness as points along a continuum is useful in communicating that neither state exists in isolation from the other. Mental illness is associated with distress and impaired functioning. These alterations in thinking, mood, and behavior contribute to a host of other problems in the person's life. Some such problems might include loss of personal freedom or heightened risk of death. Somewhere between optimal functioning (mental health) and functional impairment (mental illness), people can experience distressful states that are of insufficient intensity to qualify as mental illness. Nevertheless, using a "continuum" model also presumes that there is a pure state called "mental health" that can serve as a basis for comparison. Yet mental health is not easy to define, and built into any definition of mental health are overt and covert values. Furthermore, a concept has meaning only with reference to a certain culture.

However one chooses to view the complex issues of mental health and mental illness, nurses must remember that these issues are not completely one or the other. Much in the same way that health and illness in their broadest sense are not opposite poles, neither is a person completely well or completely ill. Seemingly healthy persons still have conditions such as acne and problems such as conflicts with siblings and friends. Likewise persons with a diagnosed illness who might be thought of as functionally impaired (eg, a person with controlled chronic schizophrenia) may function in a most optimal way in terms of his or her well-being.

Mental Health: A Report of the Surgeon General

In *Mental Health: A Report of the Surgeon General* issued in December 1999, Dr. David Satcher made mental health a national priority. The report addressed the need to eradicate the stigma attached to mental illness and emphasized the hope that treatment can offer. In fact, the strong message of the report is "There are effective treatments for mental illness" (U.S. Department of Health and Human Services, 1999). This historic document, which was the first report ever to address mental health and mental illness, focused national attention on the following messages:

- Mental health is fundamental to and necessary for a healthy life.
- Mental disorders are real health conditions with enormous consequences for individuals, families, communities, and the nation.
- Effective treatments for mental disorders are available. Most effective treatments combine psychosocial treatments (eg, behavioral therapy, counseling) with psychopharmacotherapy.
- A range of treatment options is available for most mental disorders.
- Those who have mental disorders or symptoms should seek treatment, because it can help. (U.S. Department of Health and Human Services, 1999).

Elements of Mental Health

Mental health implies mastery in the areas of love, work, play, and relationships. A person who is experiencing mental health performs meaningful work. He or she enjoys life, has a sense of humor, and is satisfied in his or her interpersonal relationships. The person shows optimism, benefits from rest and sleep, and works well alone and with others. He or she accepts responsibility for actions, reaches sound judgments, and expresses strong feelings, as appropriate.

Elements of mental health that contribute to the above characteristics are as follows:

- *Self-governance.* The person acts independently, dependently, or interdependently as the need arises without permanently losing his or her autonomy.
- *Progress toward growth or self-realization.* The person is willing to move forward to maximize his or her capabilities.
- *Tolerance of uncertainty.* The person faces the uncertainty of life and the certainty of death with faith and hope.
- *Self-esteem.* The person's sense of self-esteem is founded in self-knowledge and awareness of personal abilities and limitations.
- *Reality orientation.* The person distinguishes fact from fantasy and behaves accordingly.
- *Mastery of environment.* The person is competent, effective, and creative in interacting with and influencing his or her environment.
- *Stress management.* The person experiences appropriate emotions in daily life and can tolerate stress, knowing that the feelings are not going to last forever. He or she has several means to cope with stress, including humor, outlets (eg, exercise, meditation), and fulfilling relationships. The person is flexible and can experience failure without thinking of himself or herself as a failure.

Influences on Mental Health

Biologic, psychological, and sociocultural factors influence mental health (Figure 1-1). Biologic influences include prenatal, perinatal, and neonatal events; physical health status; nutrition; history of injuries; neuroanatomy (see Chap. 2); and physiology. Psychological factors include interactions with parents, siblings, peers, and others within the environment; intelligence quotient; self-concept; skills; creativity; and emotional developmental level. Sociocultural factors include family stability, ethnicity, housing, child-rearing patterns, economic level, religion, values, and beliefs. In addition, society and culture greatly influence views of mental health and mental illness, because society largely determines which behaviors are considered acceptable.

Incidence and Prevalence of Mental Illness

Mental illness strikes children, adolescents, adults, and older adults. It knows no racial, ethnic, gender, or socioeconomic barriers. In any given year, more than 48 million people in the United States (one in five or 20%) have a diagnosable mental disorder or illness. Half of all citizens have a mental illness at some time in their lives. Most of these people, however, never seek treatment (U.S. Department of Health and Human Services, 1999).

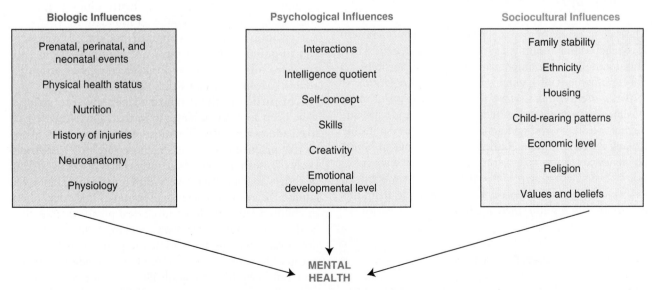

FIGURE 1-1   Influences on mental health include biologic factors, psychological factors, and sociocultural factors.

Mental illness, including suicide, is the leading cause of disability in the United States (heart disease is first). The WHO has listed unipolar depression, alcohol use, bipolar disorder, schizophrenia, and obsessive-compulsive disorder among the 10 leading causes of disability worldwide (Murray & Lopez, 1996). *Mental Health: A Report of the Surgeon General* listed suicide as the ninth leading cause of death in the United States (U.S. Department of Health and Human Services, 1999). About 15% of adults with mental illness also have a co-occurring substance abuse problem (a condition termed **dual diagnosis**), which complicates treatment (U.S. Department of Health and Human Services, 1999).

At least 20% of children in the United States have a diagnosable mental disorder; only 5% of these children have severely impaired functioning. Four to five million U.S. adults (2.1% to 2.6%) have a severe mental illness and live outside institutions. More than 5 million adults experience serious and persistent mental illnesses in any year. In adults aged 18 to 54 years, 14.9% have anxiety disorders, 7.1% have mood disorders, and 1.3% have schizophrenia (U.S. Department of Health and Human Services, 1999).

Depression, a serious mental health problem in any age group, is particularly problematic in older adults. Eight to fifteen percent of older adults have depression, but the condition is often undiagnosed and untreated in this age group because depression is mistakenly thought of as part of "normal aging." People age 65 years or older have the highest suicide rates of any age group. Alzheimer's disease occurs in 8% to 15% of those older than 65 years (U.S. Department of Health and Human Services, 1999). About 1 million people with mental illness live in nursing homes, 50,000 are inmates, 200,000 are homeless, and 50,000 live in mental hospitals (National Institute of Mental Health, 1993).

Etiology of Mental Illness

The specific causes of mental illnesses are largely unknown. It is believed that multiple factors, including genetic, viral, immunologic, environmental, and biologic contribute to the development of mental disorders. *Mental Health: A Report of the Surgeon General* identifies the roots of mental illness as some combination of biologic and environmental factors. "No single gene appears to be responsible for any mental disorder. Rather, small variations in multiple genes contribute to a disruption in healthy brain function" (U.S. Department of Health and Human Services, 1999). Under certain environmental conditions, then, this disruption can result in mental illness.

Diagnosis of Mental Illness

Mental health professionals use the *DSM-IV-TR* (APA, 2000) to diagnose mental illnesses. The *DSM* is a cate-

gorical classification system with diagnostic criteria listed for each mental disorder. It uses a five-axis system to give a more comprehensive picture of the client's functioning. The five axes are as follows:

* Axis I—Clinical disorders
* Axis II—Personality disorders and mental retardation
* Axis III—General medical conditions
* Axis IV—Psychosocial and environmental problems
* Axis V—Global assessment of functioning (GAF), written as numbers (0–100) meaning "current functioning"/"highest level of functioning in past year" (APA, 2000)

Although the *DSM* is universally used as a classification system, it has serious limitations. The categories are descriptions, not explanations. Nurses must guard against the tendency to think that something has been explained when, in fact, it has only been named. In other words, giving a condition a label does not explain or confer any reality to it other than the name itself and the cluster of behaviors subsumed under it. Thus, nurses must avoid explicating a person's behavior based on the diagnostic label given to that person. ("He acts like a schizophrenic because he has schizophrenia.") This logical error in reasoning is known as a **tautology**.

Also, as convenient as the *DSM* system is, its categories imply that sharp dividing lines exist between "normal" and "abnormal" behaviors and among different disorders. The reality, however, is that such categories are not so neat. For example, three clients may suffer from the same disorder; however, manifestations and the personal experience of that disorder will differ for each client. Moreover, the *DSM* diagnostic categories differ somewhat from the taxonomies of other illnesses (eg, hypertension, diabetes mellitus). Although research is available to support most of the major psychiatric illnesses, many of these categories lack an empirical foundation. They were agreed upon by "expert" consensus and therefore are subject to question. Indeed the *DSM* system has been criticized from both within and outside the psychiatric profession (Mohr & Regan-Kubinski, 1999).

In particular, the diagnostic labels given to children have been found troublesome in that they were derived from adult categories. The most problematic issue related to this practice is that the diagnoses are not based on a body of research on children; rather, they are derived from disorders that may have very different manifestations in adults. Depression is one such example, since depression in children has very different clinical manifestations than it does in adults. Moreover, making child categories downward extensions of adult categories is problematic because it assumes that children are little adults and that they can have the same adult illnesses. The reality is that some diagnoses are specific to children, while some are specific to adults (Jensen & Hoagwood, 1997).

Finally, the *DSM* system is not fixed. It is always a "work in progress" and should be thought of in that way. Already there have been six editions of the *DSM;* as knowledge expands, there will be more. New categories will appear, and old ones may be revised, refined, or eliminated altogether. See Appendix B for a complete listing of *DSM-IV-TR* disorders.

An example of how the axes of the *DSM-IV-TR* can be applied to client care is found in Clinical Example 1-1.

▼ Clinical Example 1-1

Judith is a 20-year-old college student living on campus. Three months ago, she broke up with her boyfriend of 2 years. When she calls home, Judith tells her parents that she "feels bad" all the time and cannot stop crying. She says that some days she cannot force herself out of bed to attend class.

Judith's parents decide to visit her at school. Upon arriving at Judith's campus apartment, her parents are troubled by her appearance. Judith looks as though she has not bathed in at least 1 week. When questioned by her parents, she admits that she does not have the energy to shower, wash her hair, or dress in clean clothes. She says that, although she tries to study, she cannot force herself to do much and cannot concentrate or sleep through the night. Judith's interactions with friends have become minimal; she usually feels "too tired" to go out with them. Usually a healthy eater, she has turned to junk food or skips meals because she is too tired to walk to the dining hall. She has lost 10 pounds in the past month. She voices feelings of worthlessness, helplessness, and self-disgust, but she denies thoughts of self-harm.

Although Judith's mother and maternal grandmother had episodes of depression, this is Judith's first depressive experience. When her parents tell her they intend to find medical help and therapy for her, Judith says that she "isn't that bad and doesn't need doctors or therapists." Rather, she says, she just wants to be left alone to sleep. Her father says that, as her parents, they will find the right treatments for her, "whatever it takes."

Judith finally agrees to therapy and begins visiting the practitioner at the university mental health center. After relating symptoms, undergoing a history and physical examination, and performing various tests, the practitioner makes the following diagnoses according to the *DSM-IV-TR* axes:

- **Axis I: Major Depressive Disorder, single episode, moderate 296.22.** Judith qualifies for this diagnosis based on her pervasive feelings of sadness and diminished interest in school, social life, and personal hygiene. She is also complaining of fatigue and has little interest in eating, inability to concentrate, and feelings of worthlessness. She is experiencing trouble sleeping and has lost significant weight. All these symptoms have been present for at least 2 weeks, and she has a family history of depression. According to the *DSM-IV-TR,* the most likely diagnosis based on these criteria is major depression.

- **Axis II: Deferred Axis II.** Axis II is reserved for the diagnoses of personality disorders and mental retardation. Judith is obviously not mentally retarded. The diagnosis of a personality disorder requires an extended history and long-term professional involvement with a client. Judith may have an Axis II diagnosis of a personality disorder, but at this point, the diagnostician has insufficient information on which to make such a judgment. Deferring a diagnosis simply means that the practitioner is reserving judgment until more information is available.

- **Axis III: No diagnosis.** Axis III is reserved for medical conditions (eg, diabetes, chronic obstructive pulmonary disease). If the history and physical examination do not reveal any medical condition, no diagnosis is given on the axis.

- **Axis IV: Recent loss of significant other, problems with social interaction, educational problems.** Axis IV is reserved for reporting psychosocial problems or life stressors that might affect the diagnosis, treatment, or prognosis of the mental illness. A recent stressor for Judith is the breakup with her boyfriend. The subsequent problems of social isolation and school difficulties further complicate the overall diagnostic picture.

- **Axis V: Current GAF—55/Highest GAF in past year—95.** On this axis, the clinician judges the client's overall functioning based on the GAF. The GAF is a hypothetical continuum of mental health and illness arranged from 100 (superior functioning) to 1 (persistent danger of hurting self or others). Judith, based on her present impaired social and school functioning, has a score of 55 on this scale. Her present functioning is compared to her past functioning, which gives the treatment team an idea of her decreased level of functionality and need for treatment.

Judith's therapist prescribes a medication regimen of 20 mg of citalopram (Celexa) each morning. Judith takes the drugs as prescribed. She also starts attending regular counseling sessions with her therapist. Eventually, the depressive symptoms subside, and Judith's functioning increases. At the end of the semester, she feels "almost like herself" and earns satisfactory grades. She continues taking her antidepressant medication and meeting with a therapist.

Points for Reflection and Critical Thinking

- How do the axes reflect different areas of the client's life and functioning?
- What factors seemed to place Judith at risk for a psychiatric disorder? Could anything have been done to help prevent the episode?
- What factors might contribute to a recurrence of depression? Do you think Judith may be at risk for any other problems at this time or in the future?

Prevention and Treatment of Mental Illness

Healthcare has become a national priority, especially in the following areas:

- Health promotion and illness prevention
- Attention to medically underserved populations
- Involvement of managed care in behavioral health
- Quality management, including client outcomes
- Expanded practice of advanced clinical healthcare providers, including nurse practitioners
- Community-based primary care
- Influence of consumer and family advocacy groups
- Decreased benefits through Medicare, Medicaid, and disability programs

As the population continues to age, the incidence of chronic illnesses and disabilities requiring mental healthcare, such as Alzheimer's disease, will also increase. By 2020, predictions are that violence and self-injury will be major disabilities affecting people worldwide (Murray & Lopez, 1996). Violence is a public health problem that will require an integrated approach from families, schools, neighborhoods, communities, and governments. Within this context, the burden of psychiatric illness is immense and expected to grow, requiring more mental health services provided by more mental healthcare professionals. See Historical Capsule 1-1.

The importance of preventing and treating mental illness cannot be underestimated. The following sections discuss problems and goals in treating mental illness and the significant contributions of self-help organizations and advocacy groups for affected clients and their families.

PROBLEMS IN TREATING MENTAL ILLNESS

Given the significant numbers of people with mental illness, why do nearly two-thirds of affected individuals fail to seek treatment? Several factors contribute to the lack of and problems with treatment for mental illness.

Cost-Related Issues

In 1996, the direct costs of medical care and rehabilitation to treat mental illness were $69 billion. Another $17.7 billion was spent to treat Alzheimer's disease, and $12.6 billion was spent to treat drug and alcohol abuse (U.S. Department of Health and Human Services, 1999). Inpatient care is costly, partly because of the number of skilled professionals required to provide it. Other forms of treatment are also costly. Untreated mental illness, however, is prohibitively expensive, in terms of lost productivity and money spent to maintain criminal justice systems and social service agencies.

As it has become increasingly important to provide quality care and to improve access to care, mental health administrators have turned to managed care. A goal of behavioral health managed care has been to reduce hospital

HISTORICAL CAPSULE 1-1

Evolution in Understanding Psychiatric Pathology

In earlier times, healthcare practitioners generally attributed disease to a single pathogenic agent: a toxin, a germ, an endocrine imbalance, a genetic defect, or a nutritional deficiency. This "medical model" of disease and illness failed to recognize that human beings interact reciprocally with their contexts or environments. Historically, practitioners geared treatment to "getting to the root" of difficulties in search of a cure. This approach ignored that individuals cannot possibly remain uninfluenced by their contexts. Gradually, the mental health profession came to realize that even if a pathogenic agent could be identified as the cause of a disease, the reactions of clients to it and the resulting changes in their lives were vitally important to gathering a complete clinical picture.

Scholars in the field of mental health have integrated findings from many diverse disciplines, such as medicine, sociology, psychology, neurophysiology, biochemistry, genetics, anthropology, and nursing, in efforts to understand mental illness. Their work has been incorporated in the service community, where it has become increasingly apparent that a broader understanding, which includes biologic, psychosocial, and sociocultural factors, offers a more comprehensive approach to the complexities of mental illness. Today, clinicians integrate these factors into an overall picture that describes clients' problems, the behavioral context for them, the conditions that might cause added stress, as well as conditions that might help or buffer the effects of stress. Clinicians bring this information together to provide a unique individual assessment on which they base individual treatment.

admissions, which are the most expensive part of psychiatric care. Unfortunately, some managed care "gatekeepers" have denied or restricted access to needed services and, therefore, have added to the discouragement, distress, and even despair of clients and their families. Some programs have actually managed only cost, not care (American Nurses Association, American Psychiatric Nurses Association, and International Society of Psychiatric-Mental Health Nurses, 2000).

An example of the difficulties posed by managed care and cost containment involves psychotropic medications. Many newer psychotropic medications, particularly the antidepressants and atypical antipsychotics, have vastly improved the effectiveness of current treatment. Their results have returned people more rapidly from psychiatric institutions to their families, schools, and jobs. Because many of these newer medications have less severe and more tolerable side effects than drugs used in the past, clients are more likely to adhere to their medication regimens. Moreover, the newer psychotropic medications have demonstrated superior effectiveness and safety profiles (ie, less serious and less frequent side effects). Unfortunately, however, these newer drugs also are more expensive than older drugs, and many managed care plans are unwilling to pay for them, even if they contribute to a higher level of functioning for the client. What those who create such restrictions fail to realize is that these medications may actually save healthcare costs in the long term because they reduce relapses of symptoms and the need for costly hospitalizations.

Stigma

Strong stigma still exists toward people who suffer from mental illness. This stigma is largely related to the public's misunderstanding of, misconceptions about, and fears associated with mental illness. Misconceptions have ranged from attributing mental illnesses to demonic possession to blaming victims for their problems. This stigmatization has led to discrimination and intolerance based on ignorance of mental illness itself. Achievement-oriented cultures like the United States often view mental illness as a moral shortcoming or character flaw as opposed to a natural disease process in the brain. Stereotyping mental illness as a self-induced condition has, over time, effectively discouraged public sympathy for the traumatic life dislocation of people with brain disorders and has prevented public policy from allocating resources (such as medication parity) that would meet their needs. For example, many health plans cover the costs of psychotropic medications at far lower rates than they do for other medications. In the policy arena, research funding for the treatment of mental illnesses is often far lower than funds allocated for funding of other disease states. At an individual level, people with mental illness must deal with a painful level of rejection, isolation, and discrimination that erodes their self-assurance and can systematically undermine their self-confidence. Stigma builds or reinforces interpersonal, financial, employment, and social barriers to accessing care. It even places barriers to obtaining the newer pharmacotherapies. *Mental Health: A Report of the Surgeon General* emphasizes that these attitudes are outmoded and must not be tolerated.

Revolving Door Treatment

The community mental health movement of the 1960s caused many state hospitals and other long-term care facilities to discharge clients with mental illness. The effectiveness of the newer psychotropic medications has reduced the need for hospitalization. Even when hospitalization is necessary, lengths of stay in hospitals have decreased. Managed care companies often mandate certain kinds of treatments. Insurers favor short-term, time-limited, and cognitive-behavioral approaches, even when

a client needs longer, more intensive treatment. For these and other reasons, many clients are being discharged from hospitals and long-term facilities when they lack the skills to survive or "make it" outside institutionalized settings. This "deinstitutionalization" has contributed to people living in communities with inadequate or no programs to serve them. Some deinstitutionalized clients have severe and persistent mental illnesses that require many specialized treatment services. The term "revolving door" has been used to describe those deinstitutionalized clients who enter and leave psychiatric hospitals repeatedly because they cannot effectively manage their care independently or within the community.

New psychotropic medications are not enough to effect positive outcomes for those with mental illness. To recover and become completely well, a client must be reintegrated into his or her community and social group. The money for treatment must follow the client back into his or her community to be used for appropriate and accessible care. Coordination and collaboration among agencies providing services are needed. Many state mental hospitals have closed, increasing the responsibility of local agencies to provide community-based care.

An attempt to tailor services to those individuals with severe and persistent mental illness led to the development of Assertive Community Treatment (ACT) programs. Such programs serve those in greatest need, such as the homeless mentally ill, incarcerated clients, clients with dual diagnoses, and clients who are resistant to usual treatment.

Lack of Parity

Lack of parity means inequality between coverage for mental illnesses and other kinds of illnesses. A gap exists between the most effective treatments available and what people actually receive in practice settings. *Mental Health: A Report of the Surgeon General* states that parity is affordable and should be the objective (U.S. Department of Health and Human Services, 1999).

Limited Access to Services

The fragmented mental healthcare system in the United States often provides inadequate, inappropriate, or no care. It is very difficult for clients and their families to determine what services are needed and where to find them. Healthcare providers often lag behind what researchers know about the effectiveness of various treatments.

GOALS OF CARE AND METHODS OF ACHIEVEMENT

Long-term goals of care in treating mental illness include the following:

- Increase the number of mental health professionals caring for children and adolescents.
- Expand mental health services.
- Understand mental illness through a cultural lens,

and deliver services to racial and ethnic minorities in a culturally congruent and sensitive manner.

- Improve public understanding of mental illness.
- Redesign rehabilitation services to meet clients' physical, mental, cultural, and social needs.
- Ensure that interagency coordination and collaboration become the norm.

These and other goals and strategies for achieving them are discussed in the following paragraphs.

Beyond Response to Recovery

Recovery and quality of life are now important treatment goals for those with mental illness. Commonly, such treatment has aimed at reducing symptoms and teaching the client skills to deal with or diminish his or her distressing symptoms. In recent years, however, it has been discovered that when clients are not fully recovered (as in a partial response to treatment for depression), they are more likely to relapse into acute depression or develop chronic depression (Ferrier, 1999). The aim now is for the client to recover or to experience a remission of his or her illness, that is, to become "well." Full recovery means that the client is restored to his or her premorbid ("pre-illness") psychosocial, educational, and occupational functioning.

Reintegration into Society

The newer psychotropic medications have contributed to clients being able to reclaim aspects of their lives that formerly were lost. Those aspects include family involvement, employment, continued education, social and recreational activities, and community involvement. Drugs alone, however, cannot treat severe and persistent mental illnesses, such as schizophrenia, major depression, bipolar disorder, and obsessive-compulsive disorder. The concept of reintegration is bringing together social programs whose goal is to help individuals with serious mental illness lead meaningful and more self-sufficient lives. This means finding ways to help clients locate safe housing, achieve gainful employment, experience satisfying family and social relationships, and develop a sense of belonging to the community.

Mental Health Parity

Parity legislation is designed to improve coverage for mental healthcare and close the gap between physical and mental healthcare benefits. The federal Mental Health Parity Act went into effect in January 1998. This act requires employers who currently offer coverage for mental healthcare to equalize annual and lifetime spending limits for mental and physical illnesses.

Culturally Competent Care

The majority population of the United States will have shifted to people of color by the middle of the century (American Nurses Association, American Psychiatric Nurses Association, and International Society of Psychiatric-Mental Health Nurses, 2000). As the population needing services changes, so must the delivery of care. A mental health system should value diversity and include the provision of culturally competent care as part of its mission. **Culturally competent care** means that care is provided in a manner acceptable to the person's cultural background, regardless of whether it is provided by a care provider from the same ethnic or minority group as the client. Healthcare professionals must be able to incorporate cultural factors including language, customs, beliefs, and traditions into plans of care.

Medication Adherence

Also called *medication compliance*, **medication adherence** means that clients actually take their medications as they are prescribed for them. To do so, clients need information about the medication and the opportunity to discuss issues that are important to them. Teaching about psychotropic medication should include the following information (Client and Family Education 1-1):

- The medication's generic and brand names
- Dosage, route, frequency, and times to be taken
- Expected common side effects
- Possible toxic or dangerous effects
- How to treat minor and common side effects

Client and Family Education 1-1

MANAGING DRUG THERAPY

Psychiatric-mental health nurses need to fully explain the possible toxic or serious side effects of or allergic responses to psychotropic medications. Following is a sample of information that a nurse must provide to clients who are prescribed Haldol (haloperidol) and their families.

Haldol (haloperidol) is a high-potency neuroleptic that powerfully blocks dopamine to control psychosis. It also blocks dopamine receptors in the "motor strip" of the brain, which controls finely coordinated body movements. This secondary blockade contributes to a group of neurologic movement disorders known as extrapyramidal symptoms (EPS). EPS resemble the symptoms of Parkinson's disease and include akathisia, akinesia, dystonia, and tremors. Akathisia, the most troublesome of these side effects, ranges from an inner feeling of muscular discomfort and restlessness to agitated, desperate, involuntary pacing, "hand-wringing," and weeping. This effect occurs early in treatment, and studies show that it is the one side effect that accounts for most cases of nonadherence to neuroleptic medications. Should EPS occur, notify your healthcare provider immediately, because other medications (atypical antipsychotics) are available.

SELF-HELP MOVEMENTS AND ADVOCACY

The consumer movement has changed the role of family involvement and brought attention to the needs of those with mental illnesses and their loved ones. The influence of mutual support groups, consumer and family education programs, and advocacy services has effected change in treatment services and mental health policy.

National Alliance for the Mentally Ill

The National Alliance for the Mentally Ill (NAMI) is an important self-help group for consumers of mental health services and their social supports. The major thrusts of NAMI are as follows:

- Communicating that mental illnesses are brain disorders
- Advocating for people with mental illness
- Eliminating stigma and discrimination against people with mental illness
- Improving access to treatment services for people with mental illness
- Facilitating accountability to mental health consumers and their families for service delivery
- Integrating mental illness into general health and community life

Family Advocacy Movement

Clients with mental illness and their families bear most of the burden of their condition. The family advocacy movement has made enormous contributions to communicating how families and clients experience mental illness. The healthcare industry once viewed families and clients with mental illness as dysfunctional and their behaviors as pathologic. In fact, it often regarded family members as contributors to the client's illness. In reaction to this "blaming" approach, family advocates conducted research that "normalizes" much of the behavior that families and clients display, explaining it as an adaptive process (Mohr, Lafuze, & Mohr, 2000; Hatfield & Lefley, 1993; Lefley, 1989; NAMI, 1999). The family adaptation model sees families and clients as being challenged by a chronic illness that represents a catastrophic event in their lives. This event is intensely traumatic, and in adapting to it, the client and family progress through a series of difficult stages that their caregivers must understand. These stages, compiled from research conducted by NAMI with families and their mentally ill loved ones, are described briefly in Tables 1-1 and 1-2.

Psychiatric Advanced Directives

Many states are currently enacting psychiatric advanced directives, in which clients formally declare their treatment wishes should they become ill. Such directives may include whether the client wishes the use of psychotropic medication, seclusion and restraint, and electroconvulsive treatment. Advanced directives are not meant to supersede care that is necessary to protect client safety (Vogel-Scibilia, 1998).

TABLE 1-1 ▼ Family Adaptation Model

STAGE	FAMILY'S THOUGHTS AND FEELINGS
1. Dealing with the catastrophic event	
a. Crisis, chaos, shock	Family is overwhelmed, confused, and lost.
b. Denial	Denial provides a protective response that gives time for family to process the catastrophic event.
c. Hoping against hope	Family members think, "I hope that this is not what I think it is. Maybe it will go away."
2. Learning to cope	
a. Anger, guilt, resentment	Family initially blames the client, wants him to her to "snap out of it," and feels guilty for having such thoughts.
b. Recognition	The illness becomes a reality.
c. Grief	Family expresses grief, fear, and sorrow over lost possibilities and the uncertain future.
3. Moving into advocacy	
a. Understanding	Members develop empathy for the client (other family member) and leave fear behind.
b. Acceptance	Family acknowledges and owns the situation as a life circumstance.
c. Advocacy and action	Family focuses anger and grief on empowerment and involvement with support groups. Members confront systems that fail the family and client.

Adapted from the Provider Education Program with permission from the National Alliance for the Mentally Ill.

TABLE 1-2 ▼ **Client Adaptation Model**

EVENT	STAGE	EMOTIONS	NEEDS
1. Crisis (episode of serious mental illness)	1. Recuperation (period of exhaustion and dependence)	Denial, depression, humiliation, resentment, anger	Rest, sleep, someone to take care of client, probably medications
2. Decision (time to begin to heal and move forward)	2. Rebuilding (learning to do things for oneself)	Hope, grief, self-doubt, trust, fear, excitement, frustration, pride	Telling one's story, learning about the illness, having someone believe in the client, learning or relearning skills
3. Awakening (realization that the client is a person of worth with dreams)	3. Recovery/Discovery (healthy interdependence)	Self-acceptance, appreciation of others, confidence, anger at injustice, assertiveness, helpfulness	A personal vision, social acceptance, meaningful work, someone to love, someone to advocate for self and others

Adapted from the Provider Education Program with permission from the National Alliance for the Mentally Ill.

PSYCHIATRIC-MENTAL HEALTH NURSING

The term psychiatric-mental health nursing refers to two aspects of nursing that interact and overlap. **Psychiatric nursing** focuses on the care and rehabilitation of people with identifiable mental illnesses or disorders. **Mental health nursing** focuses on well and at-risk populations to prevent mental illness or provide immediate treatment for those with early signs of a disorder. Thus, the 2000 edition of *Scope and Standards of Psychiatric-Mental Health Nursing Practice* describes **psychiatric-mental health nursing** as the diagnosis and treatment of human responses to actual or potential mental health problems (American Nurses Association, American Psychiatric Nurses Association, and International Society of Psychiatric-Mental Health Nurses, 2000).

Psychiatric-mental health nursing uses the study of human behavior as its science and purposeful use of self as its art. It views people holistically, considering their strengths, needs, and problems. In most ways, psychiatric-mental health nursing is similar to other types of nursing. It is based on the physical and social sciences. It is designed to meet the needs of those with health problems. It is provided by caring and knowledgeable individuals. It relies on a problem-solving approach to plan, deliver, and evaluate care. People with mental health or psychiatric problems need services to recover and return to or improve their previous level of functioning. As in other areas of nursing, services are tailored for primary, secondary, or tertiary care needs.

Psychiatric-mental health nursing has evolved into a unique discipline, combining the knowledge, experience, and skills of nursing and the biologic and behavioral sciences. It offers a wide range of preventive and intervention strategies to promote optimal functioning and health (Historical Capsule 1-2). Box 1-1 lists psychiatric nursing phenomena of concern.

Nursing Process and Standards of Care

The nursing process is the foundation of all clinical nursing decision making (American Nurses Association, American Psychiatric Nurses Association, and International Society of Psychiatric-Mental Health Nurses, 2000). Through this systematic problem-solving approach, nurses provide comprehensive care to individuals, families, groups, and communities. The nursing process in psychiatric-mental health nursing is discussed in extensive detail in Chapter 6. Standards of care describe nursing activities that nurses demonstrate through assessment, diagnosis, planning, outcome identification, implementation of interventions, and evaluation (Box 1-2) (Box 1-3).

Levels of Practice

Psychiatric-mental health nurses are educated and prepared to practice their specialty at both the basic and advanced levels. Nurses who have completed a nursing program and passed their state's licensing examination practice at the basic level. Those who have received at least a master's degree in nursing sciences practice at the advanced level as clinical nurse specialists or nurse practitioners.

At the basic level of practice, psychiatric-mental health nurses promote and encourage the maintenance of health and prevention of disorders, assess biopsychosocial functioning, serve as case managers, design therapeutic en-

BOX 1-1 ▼ *Psychiatric-Mental Health Nursing's Phenomena of Concern*

Actual or potential mental health problems of patients pertaining to:

- The maintenance of optimal health and well-being and the prevention of psychobiologic illness
- Self-care limitations or impaired functioning related to mental, emotional, and physiologic distress
- Deficits in the functioning of significant biologic, emotional, and cognitive systems
- Emotional stress or crisis related to illness, pain, disability, and loss
- Self-concept and body image changes, developmental issues, life process changes, and end-of-life issues
- Problems related to emotions such as anxiety, anger, powerlessness, confusion, fear, sadness, loneliness, and grief
- Physical symptoms that occur along with altered psychological functioning
- Psychological symptoms that occur along with altered physiologic functioning
- Alterations in thinking, perceiving, symbolizing, communicating, and decision making
- Difficulties in relating to others
- Behaviors and mental states that indicate the patient is a danger to self or others or has a severe disability
- Symptom management, side effects, and toxicities associated with psychopharmacologic intervention and other aspects of the treatment regimen
- Interpersonal, organizational, sociocultural, spiritual, or environmental circumstances or events that have an effect on the mental and emotional well-being of the individual, family, or community

From American Nurses Association, American Psychiatric Nurses Association, & International Society of Psychiatric-Mental Health Nurses. (2000). *Scope and standards of psychiatric-mental health nursing practice* (28–41). Washington, DC: American Nurses Publishing.

vironments, and promote self-care activities, including medication and symptom management. They also use psychobiologic interventions such as administering medications and complementary interventions such as teaching relaxation techniques. They educate clients and families about health, illness, and treatment; provide supportive counseling; intervene in crises; and promote psychiatric rehabilitation (American Nurses Association, American Psychiatric Nurses Association, and International Society of Psychiatric-Mental Health Nurses, 2000).

At the advanced level of practice, psychiatric-mental health nurses deliver comprehensive primary mental healthcare services to clients. These functions include teaching about health, screening clients, performing preventive interventions, and evaluating and managing persons with mental illness. Health teaching is important in that many mentally ill clients often have poor health habits and neglect their physical health. Nurses can play a role in teaching them the importance of such things as abstaining from tobacco and alcohol. Teaching is also related to prevention. Preventive interventions might include teaching family and clients about the signs and symptoms of relapse so that treatment can be instituted early and aggressively. Management of mental illnesses includes formulating diagnoses; ordering and interpreting laboratory tests; prescribing and managing psychopharmacologic medications; conducting individual, family, and group therapies; and facilitating psychiatric rehabilitation (American Nurses Association, American Psychiatric Nurses Association, and International Society of Psychiatric-Mental Health Nurses, 2000).

Guiding Principles

Psychiatric-mental health nursing is built on certain principles or beliefs about people and the care they deserve:

- Every person is worthy of dignity and respect.
- Every person has the potential to change and grow.
- All people share basic human needs.
- All behavior is meaningful and can be understood from the person's perspective.
- People have the right to participate in decisions affecting their health and treatment.
- Through the therapeutic use of self, via therapeutic relationships and communication (see Chap. 4), nurses help people adapt, change, and grow.

The Role of the Psychiatric Nurse as a Team Member

In most psychiatric care settings, the nurse is a member of an interdisciplinary team. Recognizing that clients are more than persons with a diagnosis, these teams function collaboratively to provide comprehensive care that may include general medical care, substance abuse services, psychotherapy, medication management, access to entitlements, and other needed therapies or assistance. Each team member brings his or her specialized knowledge to the treatment process, thereby enhancing assessment and treatment. Team members might include psychologists, psychiatrists, psychiatric nurses, social workers, and paraprofessionals such as lay volunteers and former

HISTORICAL CAPSULE 1-2

Time Line of Influences on Psychiatric-Mental Health Nursing

1856 to 1929	Emil Kraeplin differentiated manic-depression from schizophrenia.
1856 to 1939	Sigmund Freud introduced psychoanalytic theory and therapy. He believed that human behavior could be changed.
1857 to 1939	Eugene Bleuler described the psychotic disorder of schizophrenia.
1870 to 1937	Alfred Adler focused on the area of psychosomatic medicine.
1875 to 1961	Carl Jung described the human psyche.
1882	First training school for psychiatric nursing at McLean Asylum.
1913	Euphemia (Jane) Taylor established the first nurse-organized program of study for psychiatric care at Johns Hopkins Phipps Clinic.
1920	Harriet Bailey authored the first psychiatric nursing text, *Nursing Mental Disease*.
1937	Electroconvulsive therapy is developed.
1940 to 1945	World War II veterans received financial support and vocational rehabilitation for psychiatric and physical disabilities.
1947	Helen Render wrote *Nurse-Patient Relationships in Psychiatry*.
1949	The National Institute of Mental Health was established.
1950	Accredited schools are required to offer a psychiatric nursing course.
1952 to 1954	Hildegarde Peplau published *Interpersonal Relations in Nursing* and established the first

	graduate program in psychiatric nursing at Rutgers University.
1955	The Joint Commission on Mental Illness and Health was developed.
1967	The American Nurses Association (ANA) published the *Scope and Standards of Psychiatric-Mental Health Nursing Practice*.
1980	The ANA published *Nursing: A Social Policy Statement*.
1985	The ANA published *Standards of Child and Adolescent Psychiatric and Mental Health Nursing Practice*.
1990s	Insurance companies drastically cut funding in coverage for psychiatric care. The National Alliance for the Mentally Ill (NAMI) is created.
1992	The Center for Mental Health Services is created.
1995	The *Journal of the American Psychiatric Nurses Association (JAPNA)* is published.
1996	The Society for Education and Research in Psychiatric-Mental Health Nursing (SERPN) published guidelines for course content and competencies.
1999	*Mental Health: A Report of the Surgeon General* is published.
2000	The ANA, American Psychiatric Nurses Association, Association of Child and Adolescent Psychiatric Nurses, Inc., and SERPN published a revised *Statement on Psychiatric-Mental Health Nursing Practice*.

BOX 1-2 ▼ *Standards of Care*

Standard I. Assessment

The psychiatric-mental health nurse collects patient health data.

Rationale:
The assessment interview—which requires linguistically and culturally effective communication skills, interviewing, behavioral observation, database record review, and comprehensive assessment of the patient and relevant systems—enables the psychiatric-mental health nurse to make sound clinical judgments and plan appropriate interventions with the client.

Standard II. Diagnosis

The psychiatric-mental health nurse analyzes the assessment data in determining diagnoses.

Rationale:
The basis for providing psychiatric-mental health nursing care is the recognition and identification of patterns

(continued)

BOX 1-2 ▼ *Standards of Care* (Continued)

of response to actual or potential psychiatric illnesses, mental health problems, and potential morbid physical illness.

Standard III. Outcome Identification

The psychiatric-mental health nurse identifies expected outcomes individualized to the patient.

Rationale:
Within the context of providing nursing care, the ultimate goal is to influence health outcomes and improve the patient's health status.

Standard IV. Planning

The psychiatric-mental health nurse develops a plan of care that is negotiated among the patient, nurse, family, and health care team and prescribes evidence-based interventions to attain expected outcomes.

Rationale:
A plan of care is used to guide therapeutic intervention systematically, document progress, and achieve the expected patient outcomes.

Standard V. Implementation

The psychiatric-mental health nurse implements the interventions identified in the plan of care.

Rationale:
In implementing the plan of care, psychiatric-mental health nurses use a wide range of interventions designed to prevent mental and physical illness and promote, maintain, and restore mental and physical health. Psychiatric-mental health nurses select interventions according to their level of practice.

[Note: Va–Vg are basic level interventions. Vh–Vj are advanced practice interventions.]

Standard Va. Counseling

The psychiatric-mental health nurse uses counseling interventions to assist patients in improving or regaining their previous coping abilities, fostering mental health, and preventing mental illness and disability.

Standard Vb. Milieu Therapy

The psychiatric-mental health nurse provides, structures, and maintains a therapeutic environment in collaboration with the patient and other health care clinicians.

Standard Vc. Self-Care Activities

The psychiatric-mental health nurse structures interventions around the patient's activities of daily living to foster self-care and mental and physical well-being.

Standard Vd. Psychobiologic Interventions

The psychiatric-mental health nurse uses knowledge of psychobiologic interventions and applies clinical skills

to restore the patient's health and prevent further disability.

Standard Ve. Health Teaching

The psychiatric-mental health nurse, through health teaching, assists patients in achieving satisfying, productive, and healthy patterns of living.

Standard Vf. Case Management

The psychiatric-mental health nurse provides case management to coordinate comprehensive health services and ensure continuity of care.

Standard Vg. Health Promotion and Health Maintenance

The psychiatric-mental health nurse employs strategies and interventions to promote and maintain mental health and prevent mental illness.

Standard Vh. Psychotherapy

The APRN-PMH uses individual, group, and family psychotherapy, and other therapeutic treatments to assist the patient in preventing mental illness and disability, treating mental health disorders, and improving mental health status and functional abilities.

Standard Vi. Prescription Authority and Treatment Agents

The APRN-PMH uses prescriptive authority, procedures, and treatments in accordance with state and federal laws and regulations, to treat symptoms of psychiatric illness and to improve functional health status.

Standard Vj. Consultation

The APRN-PMH provides consultation to enhance the abilities of other clinicians to provide services for patients and effect change in systems.

Standard VI. Evaluation

The psychiatric-mental health nurse evaluates the patient's progress in attaining expected outcomes.

Rationale:
Nursing care is a dynamic process involving change in the patient's health status over time, giving rise to the need for new data, different diagnoses, and modifications in the plan of care. Therefore, evaluation is a continuous process of appraising the effect of nursing and the treatment regimen on the patient's health status and expected health outcomes.

From American Nurses Association, American Psychiatric Nurses Association & International Society of Psychiatric-Mental Health Nurses. (2000). *Scope and standards of psychiatric-mental health nursing practice* (28–41). Washington, DC: American Nurses Publishing.

| BOX 1-3 ▼ | Canadian Standards of Psychiatric and Mental Health Nursing Practice (2nd ed.) |

Standards Theme

   I. Provides competent professional care through the helping role.

  II. Performs/refines client assessments through the diagnostic and monitoring function.

 III. Administers and monitors therapeutic interventions.

 IV. Effectively manages rapidly changing situations.

  V. Intervenes through the teaching-coaching function.

 VI. Monitors and ensures the quality of health care practices.

VII. Practices within organizational and work-role structures.

Standards Committee of the Canadian Federation of the Mental Health Nurses. (1998). *The Canadian standards of psychiatric and mental health nursing practice* (2nd ed). Ottawa, Ontario: Canadian Nurses Association.

clients (Figure 1-2). The team also includes the client and his or her family. Collaboration among team members implies that they are working toward a common goal and that they share responsibility for the outcomes of care.

LEARNING TO PROVIDE APPROPRIATE CARE

There is no one "right" way to intervene therapeutically for clients who are exhibiting disturbed behavior. Mental healthcare providers must explore their own thoughts and feelings, follow guidelines and standards of care, search for more effective interventions, measure client outcomes, and if needed, redesign interventions.

Nurses who are new to the field of psychiatric-mental health nursing are likely to discover certain feelings, fears, and impressions that, if left unexamined, may hamper their effectiveness with clients and families. Commonly, students facing their first psychiatric nursing clinical experience feel anxious, fearful of clients' actions and possible rejections, fearful of damaging clients through nontherapeutic interventions, or concerned about their own mental health or mental symptoms. If you are a nurse new to this field, consider the following suggestions:

- You may wonder if your attempts at therapeutic intervention will ever produce therapeutic effects. Know that your energy, enthusiasm, and openness to learning and exploring issues with the client are exactly what most clients need and are refreshing to other staff members.

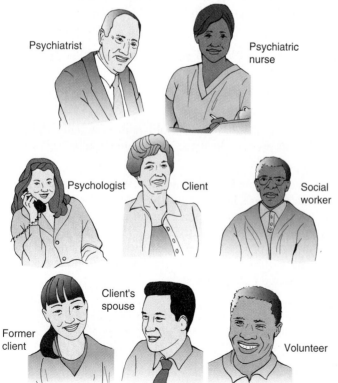

FIGURE 1-2   Team members who care for clients include psychiatrists, psychiatric nurses, psychologists, social workers, other clients, volunteers, and the client and family.

- You may learn from your classes and readings to use certain interventions in certain situations. In real practice, however, things may be done differently. Be open-minded, discuss these differences with your instructor, and realize that clinical practice is not black or white but many shades of gray.
- You may wonder what to discuss with clients. Try to focus on something fairly concrete at first, such as what led the client to seek treatment, what he or she expects to gain from treatment, and what progress the client has made in treatment. These discussions will help the client view various circumstances, gains, and expectations from new perspectives.
- The client may ask you not to repeat some information he or she has revealed to you. Nurses must never promise clients that they will not reveal such information. Rather, they should review with the client the meaning and purposes of confidentiality. Remind clients that you will share pertinent information with other members of the treatment team so that the team can provide optimal care.
- The client may want to become friends with you or maintain a relationship after your clinical experience ends. Personal relationships with clients are never appropriate or wise. Clients must learn the boundaries of relationships and that a professional relationship helps the client learn valuable skills and develop strengths. If a client asks you to be his or her friend or indicates a desire for a personal relationship, discuss this development immediately with your instructor to turn this situation into a professional, therapeutic relationship.
- A client may or may not make progress or get well. Do not take a client's lack of progress personally or feel like a failure. Mental illness has many causes. Clients get better or well through many kinds of treatments—therapy, medications, structured environments, skill development, and social supports. Your participation in a client's care is never a sole determinant in his or her progress or lack of it.

UNDERSTANDING THE CLIENT'S VIEW OF MENTAL HEALTHCARE

Clients seeking mental healthcare are often frightened, relieved, or anxious about what will happen to them. They may fear that treatment will dehumanize them or that providers will overmedicate or not listen to them. They may be suspicious about the process of receiving mental healthcare. They may believe that nurses and other mental health professionals will solve their problems for them and may expect to play a passive role while an "expert" cures them. Nurses and other mental health providers are responsible for clarifying these misconceptions and providing straightforward information about the importance of client participation.

MANAGING STRESS AND BURNOUT

Nurses who enter the psychiatric field are frequently motivated by a sense of **altruism**, that is, they are working with mentally ill persons out of a desire to contribute something valuable to society. Although the work has an innately humanitarian purpose, it also has stressors that induce nurses to feel fearful, anxious, offended, helpless, repulsed, pitying, embarrassed, hopeless, angry, or all of these emotions. The behaviors of clients represent the range of human disturbance—from violent, hostile, or aggressive to bizarre, regressed, or dependent. How nurses deal with these behaviors reflects their personal values and experiences.

If nurses feel ashamed of their reactions to disturbances in clients or feel that their responses are unprofessional, they will often hide or deny their feelings. Learning to acknowledge and deal with feelings is as important for nurses and other mental health professionals as it is for their clients. In fact, nurses model for clients how to cope with feelings in a positive way. See Implications for Nursing Practice 1-1.

⟫⟫ Implications for Nursing Practice 1-1

Managing Work-Related Stress
Staying energized in the face of multiple demands and stressors requires psychiatric-mental health nurses to attend to self-care needs and activities. To do so, they can draw on strategies that promote coping with and managing stress optimally. Some of these strategies are as follows:

- Do physical activity. Engaging in some form of aerobic exercise (eg, walking, running) for 30 minutes three times per week contributes to cardiopulmonary fitness, aids in weight control, improves mood, and fosters a sense of well-being. Strength-training exercises can build endurance, power, and flexibility.
- Eat nutritiously. Follow a diet that contains a variety of foods that are low in fat and saturated fat. Choose plenty of vegetables, fruits, and grains.
- Do not use tobacco, alcohol, and other drugs.
- Explore the use of meditation and other relaxation techniques.
- Learn the value of planning. Anxiety and poor coping can result from feeling overwhelmed. Plan a realistic schedule that includes personal activities and pleasures.
- If necessary, seek help. Never think that because you are a nurse you won't need help from others. Communicate needs to family, friends, and coworkers. If you are feeling especially overwhelmed, obtain assistance from a professional.

The stressors that psychiatric-mental health nurses experience are considerable, exact a heavy toll, and require a great deal of personal and professional resources. Nurses should be alert to the warning signs of increasing job-related stress. Such signs may take the form of **horizontal violence**, which is anger or negativity a nurse directs at another nurse. Or they may take the form of *passive-aggressive behavior,* which undermines the effectiveness of other nurses' work. An example of passive-aggressive behavior can be seen when a nurse resists requests for adequate daily performance but expresses this resistance "indirectly," hence the description as "passive." Such resistance might take the form of procrastination, calling in sick, dawdling, intentional inefficiency, or "forgetfulness" (Cullen, 1995). Other warning signs of burnout are loss of energy and enthusiasm, fatigue, insomnia, and alcohol and drug use. Increasing burnout leads to more severe symptoms: physical illness or exhaustion, withdrawal, mood changes, depression, hopelessness, and increased use of alcohol and drugs.

Some client behaviors are more stressful to deal with than others, including suicidal threats or actions, violence, and passive aggression. Some agencies and institutions are toxic environments that expect nurses to be overinvolved in their work or extremely self-sacrificing in care situations. These unhealthy environments do not promote high quality care. Rather, they drain nurses, leaving them personally and professionally depleted.

Positive coping with job-related stress and burnout requires a concerted effort. Support systems at home and work allow nurses to express feelings and keep situations in perspective. Nurses need to cultivate realistic expectations from the job and from themselves. Frequent, brief vacations have been found to be more relaxing and refreshing than infrequent, longer ones. Paying attention to one's health needs brings great returns in stress reduction and increased satisfaction with life.

In addition, nurses need to honestly evaluate their work environment to determine whether they are forced to lower their standards of care or prevented from providing high-quality care, situations that are likely to result in burnout. To stay healthy and happy, nurses should refuse to accept responsibility for others' problems; manage client care according to priorities; keep priorities for family, friends, and personal goals in order; search for creative ways to express excellence at work; and never stop learning. Lifelong learning is needed to address the changing issues and problems faced by psychiatric-mental health nurses.

▼ CHAPTER SUMMARY

- Mental health and mental illness are imprecisely defined states.
- *Mental Health: A Report of the Surgeon General* analyzes what is known about the causes and treatment of mental illnesses. The overriding message is, "There are effective treatments for mental illness. If you have symptoms, seek help."
- Mental illnesses are diagnosed according to criteria in the *DSM-IV-TR,* a system of classification that is always in development.
- Stigma, costs, changing needs of the population, denial of illness, limited access to services, and lack of parity are some reasons why two thirds of those with symptoms of mental illness do not seek treatment.
- Advances in biological and systems aspects of mental healthcare today offer promising options for treatment and recovery.
- The advocacy movement has contributed to our understanding of the experience of families and clients. Through research of these experiences, a model was conceptualized that describes families and clients as adapting to a catastrophic event in their lives in a way that is pathological.
- Psychiatric-mental health nursing is a unique discipline that contributes to the care of persons with mental illness and to the promotion of mental health in the general population.
- Basic and advanced functions and roles of psychiatric-mental health nurses include advocacy, health promotion and maintenance, case management, screening, milieu therapy, health teaching, psychobiological interventions, and participation in the interdisciplinary mental health team.
- Stress and burnout in the psychiatric nursing workplace can be minimized through early detection of stress symptoms, self-care measures, involvement in nonnursing activities, and setting and maintaining priorities.

▼ REVIEW QUESTIONS

1. Provide definitions for mental disorders and mental illness.

2. What are the elements of mental health?

3. What is the *DSM-IV-TR?* What are some of the limitations of the *DSM-IV-TR?*

4. How have managed care and cost-containment programs influenced the use of psychotropic medications? Explain how this affects clients.

5. Explain the forces behind deinstitutionalization and the "revolving door" phenomenon.

6. Explain the concept of parity and how parity can contribute to achieving the goals of recovery (versus reduction of symptoms) and reintegration into society.

7. Explain how culturally mediated behaviors may be misinterpreted and define culturally competent mental healthcare.

8. Describe the family advocacy movement and contrast it with historical views of the families of clients with mental illness.

9. Consider a scenario in which a client asks you to keep some information confidential because the client considers you a friend. Suggest an approach to the client that will establish the most therapeutic relationship.

10. What is horizontal violence? What is passive-aggressive behavior? Describe other signs of burnout and discuss factors that contribute to stress and burnout in psychiatric mental health nursing. Suggest several strategies for managing stress.

▼ REFERENCES AND SUGGESTED READINGS

*American Nurses Association, American Psychiatric Nurses Association, & International Society of Psychiatric-Mental Health Nurses. (2000). *Scope and standards of psychiatric-mental health nursing practice.* Washington, DC: American Nurses Publishing.

*American Psychiatric Association. (2000). *Diagnostic and statistical manual of mental disorders* (4th ed., text rev.). Washington, DC: Author.

Baier, M., & Murray, R. L. (1999). A descriptive study of insight into illness reported by persons with schizophrenia. *Journal of Psychosocial Nursing, 37*(1), 14–21.

*Cullen, A. (1995). Burnout: Why do we blame the nurse? *American Journal of Nursing, 95*(11), 22–27.

*Ferrier, I. N. (1999). Treatment of major depression: Is improvement enough? *Journal of Clinical Psychiatry, 60*(Suppl. 6), 10–14.

*Hatfield, A., & Lefley, H. (1993). *Surviving mental illness: Stress, coping and adaptation.* New York: The Gilford Press.

*Jensen, P. S., & Hoagwood, K. (1997). The book of names: DSM-IV in context. *Development and Psychopathology, 9*(1), 231–249.

*Lefley, H. P. (1989). Family burden and family stigma in major mental illness. *American Psychologist, 44,* 556–560.

*Mohr, W. K., Lafuze, J. E., & Mohr, B. D. (2000). Opening caregiver minds: NAMI's Provider Education Program. *Archives of Psychiatric Nursing, 14*(60), 285–295.

*Mohr, W. K., & Regan-Kubinski, M. J. (1999). The DSM and child psychiatric nursing: A cautionary reflection. *Scholarly Inquiry for Nursing Practice, 13*(4), 305–318.

*Murray, C. J. L., & Lopez, A. D. Eds. (1996). *The global burden of disease: A comprehensive assessment of mortality and disability from diseases, injuries, and risk factors in 1990 and projected to 2020.* Cambridge, MA: Harvard School of Public Health, on behalf of the World Health Organization and the World Bank.

*National Alliance for the Mentally Ill. (1999). *The provider education program.* Rockville, MD: Author.

*National Institute of Mental Health. (1993). *Mental health statistics.* Rockville, MD: Office of Consumer, Family and Public Information, Center for Mental Health Services.

North American Nursing Diagnosis Association. (2001). *Nursing diagnoses: Definitions and classification, 2001–2002.* Philadelphia: Author.

Selye, H. (1974). *Stress without distress.* New York: New American Library.

*U.S. Department of Health and Human Services. (1999). *Mental health: A report of the surgeon general.* Rockville, MD: U.S. Department of Health and Human Services, Substance Abuse and Mental Health Services Administration, Center for Mental Health Services, National Institutes of Health, National Institute of Mental Health.

*Vogel-Scibilia, S. (1998). Psychiatric advanced directives. *NAMI Advocate, 20*(1), 26–27.

Starred references are cited in text.

For additional information on this chapter, go to *http://connection.lww.com.*

Need more help? See Chapter 1 of the *Study Guide to Accompany Mohr: Johnson's Psychiatric-Mental Health Nursing,* 5th edition.

Neuroscience: Biology and Behavior

WANDA K. MOHR

▼ KEY TERMS

Action potential — The change in electrical potential on the surface of a nerve or muscle cell, often initiated by a change in cellular ionic balance.

Adaptive plasticity — An irreversible change in nervous tissue that usually affects the expression of a genotype into a phenotype.

Axon — A cylindrical neuron structure that relays information away from the cell body.

Blood-brain barrier — A protective system in the lining of blood vessels composed of endothelial cells with tight junctions, thus limiting access of blood constituents to the central nervous system.

Circadian rhythm — A rhythmic activity cycle lasting approximately 24 hours.

Critical periods — Periods during which children should be most exposed to certain stimuli for optimum development to take place. These periods vary according to different domains of functioning.

Concordance rate — The rate at which a trait expressed in one twin is expressed in another.

Dendrites — Branched processes that extend from and relay information to the cell body and receive signals from numerous neurons.

First messengers — Neurotransmitters that are responsible for transmitting impulses between nerve cells.

Glial cells — In the nervous system, non-neural cells that serve supporting and nutritive roles for neurons.

Learning — A process that occurs when organisms take in and store information as a function of experience.

Memory — Information that is stored as a result of learning.

Neurons — Nerve cells, the fundamental units of the nervous system.

Neuropeptides — The newest class of neurotransmitters, which includes endorphins and enkephalins, vasoactive intestinal peptide, cholecystokinin, and substance P.

Neuroplasticity — The ability of nervous tissue to change in its structure and functioning.

Neurotransmitters — Chemical substances that relay messages between presynaptic and postsynaptic cells and are synthesized, stored, and released by neurons.

Psychoneuroimmunology — An emerging field that focuses on the links between a person's emotions, the functioning of his or her immune system, and how both factors alter central nervous system functioning.

Reactive plasticity — A rapid, usually reversible, functional change in nervous tissue.

Receptor — A component of the cell membrane with the capacity to bind to a specific neurotransmitter.

Reuptake — The process of the terminal of a presynaptic nerve cell taking back released neurotransmitter molecules for storage and subsequent release.

Second hit — Environmental factors hypothesized to contribute to the expression and characteristics of a person's illness.

Second messengers — Secondary chemicals produced by the binding of a neurotransmitter to a receptor coupled with a G protein.

Synapse — The area involving the membrane of a presynaptic neuron (sender), the synaptic cleft, and the membrane of the postsynaptic neuron (receiver), across which a nerve impulse passes.

Synaptic cleft — A gap between the cellular membranes of the terminal of the presynaptic neuron and dendritic processes of the postsynaptic neuron.

Transcription — Process whereby a DNA sequence is copied onto RNA.

Translation — Process by which information in RNA produces amino acids (which make up proteins).

▼ LEARNING OBJECTIVES

On completion of this chapter, you should be able to accomplish the following:

- List the major structures of the brain and how they are related to behavior.
- Explain the relationship between the brain, its chemistry, and mental illness.
- Identify the basic structures of a neuron.
- Describe the process of neurotransmission.
- Discuss the concept of neuroplasticity and how it relates to mental health and mental illness.
- Briefly explain the importance of interaction between genes and environment.
- Identify neuroimaging techniques and discuss their relative advantages and disadvantages.

- Discuss how environment can influence the course of the developing brain.
- Explain the different kinds of memory.
- Discuss the relationship between neurotransmitters and mental illness.

Over the past 2 decades, research findings have made it abundantly clear that the brain is the organ of the mind. Just as the lungs exchange gases and the heart pumps blood, the brain influences and is responsible for behavior. This means *all* behaviors of the body, including respiration, locomotion, and sensory activity, as well as cognition or thought. More importantly, the brain, as the major organ of the nervous system, governs all forms of behavior. This includes the behavior of the lungs and heart, as well as the behaviors that constitute conduct, performance, and actions as human persons.

Although these statements are not late-breaking news, they are important for students to internalize completely and make part of a template through which they see and understand everything else in psychiatric-mental health nursing. Too often chapters such as this one are "tacked on" to the rest of the textbook, more or less gratuitously, so that authors and instructors can proceed with the "important" work of describing disorders and interventions for them. The failure to truly integrate the neurosciences into the specialty of psychiatric-mental health nursing impedes students from making the connections between nervous system functioning and behavior.

Perhaps this problem is related to the difficulty in trying to present this material in a meaningful, understandable, and relevant way. Doing so is not easy, but the goals of this chapter are to briefly review the nervous system and summarize theories of higher brain functions as they relate to psychiatric-mental health nursing. One operative word here is "brief," meaning that the neuroanatomical content is *not* presented comprehensively. Knowledge in this area is vast and expanding so rapidly that to do it justice in a single chapter is impossible. Moreover, detailed information on such topics as gray and white matter, membranes, myelin sheaths, and so forth is found in neuroanatomy textbooks written specifically to convey such detailed information. This chapter is limited to "need-to-know" rather than "nice-to-know" material. It is designed to convey fewer microfacts but to give more useful conceptual material. Nurses can use this material to inform themselves on what they see in their clinical settings and to think about their interventions more creatively than generically. As with other textbooks, this chapter briefly describes the nervous system, neurotransmission, and brain structure and function. It also discusses the relationship between the brain, neurotransmission, and psychiatric illness. Going beyond other texts, however, this chapter tries to convey the dynamic nature of nervous system functioning and development by introducing a discussion of how the nervous system changes anatomically throughout the life span and the vital role of and interaction between genetics and environment.

Another operative word for this chapter is "relate." Because it is impossible to be exhaustive, the intention of this chapter is to relate certain nervous system functioning to what students might see in a clinical setting. The hope is to provide an outline that whets students' appetites for further study and "jogs" their memories about relevant material that they learned in their anatomy and physiology classes. For students who want more in-depth information, the chapter's reference list contains current textbooks and articles they may find especially useful. See Historical Capsule 2-1.

NEUROANATOMY AND NEUROPHYSIOLOGY

Neurons

The nervous system contains two broad classes of cells. The first, known as **glial cells**, provide mechanical and metabolic support for the second, known as neurons. **Neurons**, or nerve cells, are the basic units of structure and function in the nervous system (Figure 2-1).

Approximately 100 billion neurons are in the brain alone. Each neuron consists of a cell body, which contains a nucleus and other organelles and has snakelike extensions. These extensions are called **dendrites** and **axons,** and their function is to funnel information in and out of the cell body. Between each neuron are spaces called **synapses**, which serve as points of cellular contact. The estimated number of these contact points in the human nervous system is staggering — from 10 to 100 trillion.

NEUROTRANSMISSION

The job of neurons is to transmit messages across synapses. Every neuron receives information encoded as electrical potentials at its dendritic processes and transmits the information along the axons. In order to transmit this information, the message must cross the gap or synapse between adjacent neurons. The process by which this crossing takes place is complex, involving tiny explosive depolarizations and a release of chemical-transmitting substances called neurotransmitters.

Neurotransmitters are synthesized and stored in the terminal region of the neuron. They are compounds that are released at a synapse and diffuse across the **synaptic cleft** to act on a receptor located on the membrane of a postsynaptic cell (Figure 2-2). This postsynaptic cell may be another neuron, a muscle cell, or a specialized gland cell. Some important neurotransmitters are described in Table 2-1. Nurses need to have a working knowledge of neurotransmitters because many of the medications used in psychiatry work to increase or decrease their levels in the brain.

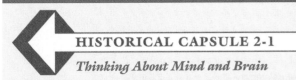

HISTORICAL CAPSULE 2-1
Thinking About Mind and Brain

The brain is the organ of thought and all other mental states. Thus, all functions of the mind reflect activity of the brain. Empirical support for this statement is enormous. *All* mental processes, including the most complex psychological functions, are based on brain activity. What we commonly refer to as "mind" is simply the total functions carried out by the brain. The word "mind" itself has no meaning except as a kind of shorthand reference to "brain activity." Indeed, we would do well to stop referring to states and illnesses as "mental disorders" or "disturbances of the mind." Behavioral disorders or the maladaptive behaviors that characterize psychiatric illnesses are disturbances in brain functioning, even when that disturbance seems to have environmental origins.

The origins of our thinking about the separateness of mind vs. body and psychological factors vs. biologic factors can be traced to the concept of Cartesian dualism. This term refers to the idea espoused by the philosopher René Descartes in the 1600s. Descartes believed that humans had independent material souls (minds) that inhabited and found expression in mechanistically operated bodies.

The problem of mind, body, and their relationship continued to be a pressing concern for philosophers for the next 300 years; debate continued well into the 20th century. One consequence was that the mind became the province of "mind doctors," while the body became the concern of the physician. In fact, there was a time when psychotherapy was thought to be the appropriate treatment for "psychologically based" disorders, while medication was considered the treatment of choice for "biologically based" disorders. Now, however, this distinction is becoming increasingly baseless (Fischbach, 1992).

Unfortunately, the past several decades in psychiatric nursing and psychiatry have perpetuated this dualistic thinking. As progressive as some nursing theorists seemed for their time, their thinking perpetuated this dualism of mind and body. These theories were based on the idea that there were "psychological" factors as well as "biologic" factors operating together, and that these factors contributed to mental illnesses. For example, Roy's Adaptation Model, although stressing unity, nevertheless perpetuated the idea of a physical self, involving sensation and body image, and a personal self, made up of self-consistency, self-ideal, and the moral and ethical self (Roy, 1987). Another example can be seen in the American Psychiatric Association's *Diagnostic and Statistical Manual of Mental Disorders (DSM)* (American Psychiatric Association, 2000). The very word "mental" in its title perpetuates the idea that mental and physical disorders are different and somehow not related.

In the 21st century, increasing evidence from the field of molecular biology shows that "mental states" have their representation in brain neuronal anatomy and functioning. The process of thinking is now considered the mental activity of the brain. Human experience is something that the brain controls, depending on the working of the nervous system and the exposure of individuals to their environments. Adaptive and maladaptive human behaviors are now believed to result from complex and dynamic transactions among individual factors (eg, heredity), environments, and the multiple risk and protective factors inherent in those environments (see Chap. 3) (Fischbach, 1992).

Much has been dixscovered in the last 2 decades about the neurophysiologic processes of the human nervous system, how those processes are mediated, and how they might explain symptoms and signs of mental illnesses. This research promises the discovery of knowledge that should form the scientific bases of psychiatric care practices for the new millennium.

Neurotransmitters are released from nerve endings by nerve impulse activity. Most neurotransmitters are synthesized and stored in the terminal region of neurons, and they are released from the terminal following electrical stimulation (an **action potential**). Each neurotransmitter binds to a **receptor**, which is a protein found in the membrane of the neuron. Receptors are unique to specific neurotransmitters. They can be located either postsynaptically on the next neuron that they excite or inhibit or presynaptically on the neuron that has released the transmitter.

Neurotransmitters are then deactivated in one of two ways. They are either broken down by enzymes, primarily the enzyme monoamine oxidase (MAO), or they are returned back into the neuron — a process known as **reuptake**. To summarize, neurotransmitter molecules cross the synaptic cleft, affect the receptor briefly, and then are eliminated or inactivated.

Neurotransmitters are responsible for transmitting impulses between nerve cells and are referred to as **first messengers**. First messengers are molecules that communicate information or change *from one cell or cell group*

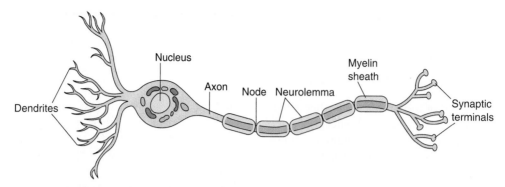

FIGURE 2-1   Structure of a neuron.

to another. Examples include hormones and neurotransmitters. The presence of first messengers in varying quantities at the synaptic site is implicated in many conditions, such as schizophrenia and bipolar disorder. By contrast, **second messengers** are molecules in a cell that communicate information or change *within the cell itself.* An example of a secondary messenger is the calcium ion. Thus, first messengers are outside the cell, whereas secondary messengers are inside the cell. First messengers attach themselves to receptors outside of cell membranes and begin a cascade of events that lead to the release of second messengers inside the cell.

Neurotransmitters can either inhibit the receptor cell or excite it. The inhibitory or excitatory nature of the neurotransmitter makes an axon discharge more or less likely. The nerve cell "decides" whether to send output as a result of the number of inhibitory or excitatory inputs it receives.

Although the specific roles of neurotransmitters in the development of mental illness are not known, recent evidence suggests that no single neurotransmitter is responsible for any single disorder. At one time, students were taught the mantra, "Schizophrenia — too much dopamine; depression — too little serotonin." Today we know that psychiatric illnesses are associated with alterations in several neurotransmitters. Moreover, the difficulties may not be a simple abundance or overabundance but rather ratios of one to another or any number of complex permutations. The chapters in this text reviewing the major disorders will discuss the latest hypotheses concerning neurotransmission and its role in psychiatric illness.

PLASTICITY

In addition to its transmitting properties, the most significant property of nervous tissue is plasticity. Plasticity refers to the remarkable ability of nervous tissue to change its structure and functioning. Neuronal plasticity is a lifelong process. It is responsible for mediating the structural and functional reaction of the central nervous system to new experiences, attrition, and injury. More about neuroplasticity and its importance is presented later in this chapter.

Central Nervous System

The neurons enclosed in the bony coverings of the skull and vertebral column make up the central nervous system

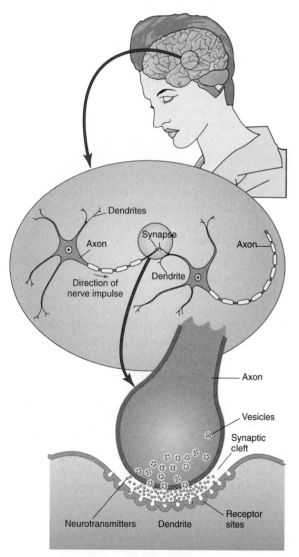

FIGURE 2-2   Neurotransmitter anatomy.

TABLE 2-1 ▼ Neurotransmitters and Their Functions

NEUROTRANSMITTER	FUNCTION AND IMPLICATIONS
Biogenic Amines	
Catecholamines	
Dopamine	Involved in pleasurable feelings and complex motor activities Implicated in schizophrenia
Norepinephrine	Regulates awareness of environment, attention, learning, memory, and arousal Implicated in mood disorders
Epinephrine	Has limited presence in the brain Contributes to the "fight-or-flight" response
Indolamines	
Serotonin	Contributes to temperature regulations Implicated in mood and psychotic disorders; low levels implicated in depression, aggression, suicidality, and impulsivity; high levels implicated in anxiety disorders (fearfulness, avoidance)
Histamine	Involved in allergic responses Role in CNS remains elusive
Cholinergics	
Acetylcholine	Mediates cognitive functioning directly or by modulating another neurotransmitter indirectly Contributes to sleep–wake cycles
Neuropeptides: endorphins and enkephalins, neurotensin, vasoactive intestinal peptide, cholecystokinin, and substance P	Appear to play a secondary messenger role and contribute to modulating the pain response
Amino Acids	
Excitatory: aspartic acid, glutamic acid, cysteic acid, and homocysteic acid	Become toxic when levels are too high; sparse information is available about their role.
Inhibitor: gamma-aminobutyric acid (GABA)	Implicated in dementia, schizophrenia, and anxiety disorders

(*CNS*), which consists of the spinal cord and the brain. Neurons outside the CNS make up the *peripheral nervous system*, which is responsible for carrying information into the CNS. The peripheral nervous system also carries motor impulses outward to muscles and glands of the body.

SPINAL CORD

The spinal cord provides a channel through which sensory information from the body reaches the brain (Figure 2-3). The cord also contains pathways for voluntary control of skeletal muscles and the neural systems that regulate much of the functioning of internal body organs. Also the neural systems of the spinal cord are the bases for the integrated and coordinated movement of the limbs.

THE BRAIN

The adult brain is an exceedingly vital and very complex organ relative to its small size. The brain is composed of neurons and support cells called *neuroglia*. It is encapsu-

lated and protected by three lining membranes or *meninges* (*arachnoid, pia mater,* and *dura mater*), as well as the bony enclosure of the skull. It is also protected by the inner lining of the cerebral blood vessels, which form tight connections that limit the access of blood elements to the CNS (Beatty, 2000). This network of protective connections is known as the **blood-brain barrier**.

Organization and Structure

The brain has a hierarchical organization, from the lower, simpler areas to the more complex higher cortical areas. The "lower" parts of the brain mediate simple regulatory functions, such as respiration, heartbeat, and body temperature. The cortical structures mediate more complex functions, including language and abstract thinking. The major structures of the brain include the cerebrum, thalamus, hypothalamus, cerebellum, brainstem, limbic system, and the ventricles. See Figure 2-4 for an illustration of the structure of the brain and areas responsible for certain functions.

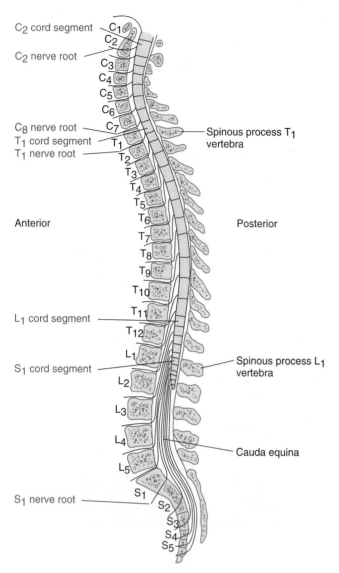

C₂ cord segment
C₂ nerve root
C₈ nerve root
T₁ cord segment
T₁ nerve root
Anterior
L₁ cord segment
S₁ cord segment
S₁ nerve root

Spinous process T₁ vertebra
Posterior
Spinous process L₁ vertebra
Cauda equina

FIGURE 2-3   Structure of the spinal cord.

Brain structures do not operate in isolation from one another. Rather, they operate within systems. Thus, it is usually an oversimplification to say that there is a direct correlation between one area and one function. Table 2-2 illustrates the systems by which the brain is divided, the regions subsumed under those systems, and the functioning of those regions.

Damage to any part of the brain will result in deficits in functioning. For example, damage to two areas in the occipital lobe of the brain (Broca's area and Wernicke's area) will cause certain language deficits specific to that area. Damage to the hippocampus from chronic alcoholism results in *Korsakoff's syndrome,* in which affected individuals cannot form new memories despite their intelligence remaining intact. Destruction of the amygdala causes a decreased aggressive response in animals (Beatty, 2000).

Cerebrum. The *cerebrum,* composed of the frontal, parietal, occipital, and temporal regions, is the brain cen-

ter responsible for intellectual functions, including learning, judgment, reasoning, and memory. It also plays a primary role in processing emotions as well as sensory input from voluntary muscles of the body. The cortex of the cerebrum (*cerebral cortex*) forms the outer layer of the cerebral lobes and plays a very important role in processing sensory information from a person's environment. It can be thought of as a map formation engine that organizes incoming signals from the environment and forms dynamic maps or representations of this input. Depending on the frequency and intensity of such input, these representations change through a complex rewiring of cortical connections. These input-driven changes are called neuroplasticity. Lack of sensory input or severe trauma during crucial periods of a person's life can negatively affect the cerebral cortex and result in future adaptive difficulties. The four lobes of the cerebral cortex are the frontal, parietal, occipital, and temporal. Table 2-3 outlines the basic anatomy and some functions of the cerebral cortex.

Diencephalon. The *diencephalon* consists of the thalamus, hypothalamus, and pineal gland. The thalamus itself acts as a large relay station through which sensory information passes on its way to other cortical regions. Beneath the thalamus is the hypothalamus, which is the control center for endocrine, somatic, and autonomic functioning. Hormones from the hypothalamus are released into the bloodstream and modulate many body functions, including drinking, salt balance, sexual activity, feeding, body temperature, and feelings of rage. The pineal gland secretes melatonin, a hormone that affects the sleep–wake cycle.

Cerebellum. The *cerebellum* is a region that developed early in the evolution of the brain. It is a complex structure that controls and guides movements, as well as maintains muscle tone. Damage to the cerebellum results in characteristic movement disorders. For example, a person with a damaged cerebellum may execute normally delicate movements quite violently. Also, errors in the strength and direction of movements may accompany cerebellar damage. Impaired gait seen with alcohol intoxication is an example of alcohol's toxic effects on cerebellar functioning.

Brainstem. The *brainstem* includes the pons, medulla oblongata, reticular formation, and midbrain. The *pons* contains nerve-fiber pathways that relay information to other areas of the CNS. The *medulla oblongata* controls respiration, gastrointestinal motility, and circulation. The *reticular formation* controls sleep and wakefulness and is the area that directs visual and auditory reflexes. The *midbrain* is vital to life. In some tragic circumstances, it is the only area of the brain maintaining vital functions in an otherwise comatose person with no higher-level functions.

Limbic System. The *limbic system* is located under the cerebral cortex and is composed of the *hippocampus,*

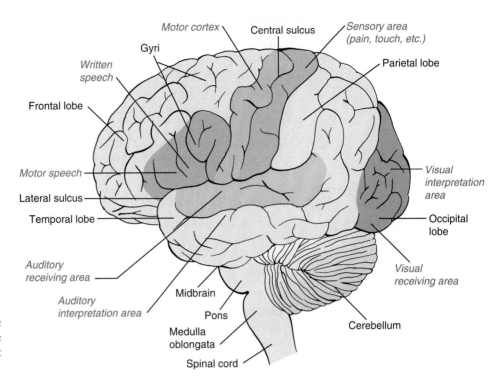

FIGURE 2-4 Structure of the brain. Shaded areas show the region responsible for different functions.

TABLE 2-2 ▼ Structure and Function of the Brain

SYSTEM	FUNCTION
Frontal Lobe	
Motor areas	Initiate movement on opposite side of the body (ie, motor area on right side of brain initiates movement on the left side of the body)
Premotor areas	Control complex motor functions that parallel motor areas and activities such as eating, speaking, and locomotion
Frontal motor eye fields	Act as the center of volitional control over eye movement
Motor speech area	Acts as the center for expressive speech
Prefrontal lobe	Interconnects with sensory areas of the cortex Governs highest intellectual functions (ie, judgment, reasoning, and abstract thinking) Provides motor integration, allowing for appropriate complex responses to environment Initiates psychomotor activity and restraint over emotional impulses
Transitional area	Inhibits contralateral activity
Corticopontocerebellar area	Permits smooth voluntary and automatic skeletal muscle movement
Parietal Lobe	
Primary sensory area	Receives and identifies somatic sensory stimuli (primarily touch and position sensations)
Secondary sensory area	Synthesizes somatic sensory impulses and permits fine perceptions
Posterior parietal cortex	Discriminates among visual signals Connects with motor systems for the purpose of directing responses to targets Performs other complex perceptual functions
Angular and supramarginal gyri	Integrates visual and auditory stimuli with somatic sensations

(continued)

TABLE 2-2 ▼ Structure and Function of the Brain (Continued)

SYSTEM	FUNCTION
Occipital Lobe	
Primary visual receptive area	Receives impulses relayed by retina area
Parareceptive area	Interprets visual responses so that they can be recognized and identified Stores visual memory
Preoccipital area	Connects visual receptive and parareceptive areas with other parts of the cortex Is related to perception, recall, visual association, and orientation
Temporal Lobe	
Auditory receptive area	Receives auditory impulses
Auditory association area	Stores memory patterns for symbolic sounds Differentiates among auditory sounds and interprets them as words May have a vestibular function
Gustatory area	Receives and interprets gustatory (sense of taste) impulses
Olfactory area	Receives and interprets olfactory (sense of smell) impulses
Other areas	Contribute to memory, sexual function, visceral activities, and other complex activities associated with the limbic system
Subcortical Structures	
Thalamus	As part of the diencephalon, acts as a relay center through which all sensory information passes
Hypothalamus	Acts as the central organ of learning
Basal ganglia	Initiate and control motor functions, primarily inhibitory
Subcortical Bundles	
Corpus callosum	Is the pathway that interconnects the two hemispheres of the brain
Limbic system	Is composed of the hippocampus, amygdala, and fornix Controls emotions, memory, and learning Mediates feelings of aggression, sexual impulses, and submissive behavior
Internal Capsule	
Cerebellum	Processes sensory information and projects to the thalamus and brainstem Is part of the motor system involved in equilibrium, postural control, and coordination of motor movements
Brainstem	Connects the spinal cord to the brain Performs life-support functions (ie, breathing and cardiac activity)
Diencephalic area	Is composed of the thalamus, hypothalamus, and pineal gland Performs integration and modulation

amygdala, and *fornix.* The limbic system controls emotions, memory, and learning. It is also thought to mediate feelings of aggression, sexual impulses, and submissive behavior. Damage to the limbic system has been implicated in several conditions. For example, because the hippocampus is the site where new information is consolidated into memories, damage to the hippocampus reduces a person's ability to learn new information.

Basal Ganglia. The *basal ganglia* consist of the *caudate, putamen,* and *globus pallidus.* These functionally related groups of neurons initiate and control activities and muscle tone. They elaborate and integrate complex voluntary motor activities to allow smooth actions. In addition the basal ganglia take over motor skills that have become automatic. Lesions in the basal ganglia cause involuntary movement, slowing of movement, loss of automatic movement, and loss of facial expression.

Brain Development

During infancy and childhood, the human brain develops rapidly, acquiring an entire set of capabilities. This

TABLE 2-3 ▼ Functions of Brain Structures

Brain structure	Cerebrum	Diencephalon	Basal ganglia	Limbic system	Brainstem	Cerebellum
Function	Higher-level thought	Integration, modulation	Motor activity	Emotions	Vital life functions	Muscle synergy
Brain region	Frontal, parietal, occipital, and temporal lobes	Hypothalamus, thalamus, pineal gland	Caudate putamen, globus pallidus	Hippocampus, amygdala, fornix	Midbrain, pons, medulla oblongata, reticular formation	

process of development is sequential, from less complex to more complex capabilities, and is guided by experience. The brain modifies and changes itself in response to new experiences, with neurons and neuronal connections evolving in an "activity-dependent" manner. In other words, the activity to which the neurons are exposed drives their response. For example, new visual learning experiences in children will cause neurons to develop and neuronal connections to take place in the visual pathways. Without such stimuli, however, visual development may not occur. Scientists demonstrated this phenomenon during a study in which they deprived a sample of kittens of light and visual stimuli for several weeks, both before and after the kittens' eyes opened. Despite the fact there were no visible gross anatomical differences between the visually deprived kittens and their littermates, the visually deprived kittens were rendered blind. Their visual neurons were never activated for the job of sight through exposure to the visual stimuli needed for them to grow and network.

Thus, development of the brain is use dependent. As certain neural systems are activated repeatedly, an internal representation of the experience corresponding to the neuronal activity is created in the brain. The use-dependent capacity of the brain to make such internal representations of the internal or external world provides the basis for learning and memory.

The capacity and desire to form emotional relationships is related to the organization and functioning of specific parts of the human brain. The systems in the human brain that allow persons to form and maintain emotional relationships develop during the first years of life. Experiences during this vulnerable period are critical to shaping the capacity to form intimate and emotionally healthy relationships. This capacity is at its peak during childhood, making children far more malleable and receptive to environmental stimuli than adults. By the time that children are 3 years old, the brain is 90% of its adult size, and the emotional, behavioral, cognitive, and social foundation is in place for the rest of life. A child's earlier repertoire of experiences provides an organizing framework or template through which subsequent experiences are filtered.

Human brains are most plastic (ie, most receptive to environmental input) in early childhood. A child's brain organizes in a use-dependent fashion, mirroring the pattern, timing, nature, frequency, and quality of experiences. For brain development to take place, children must be exposed to appropriate sensory experiences. The consequences of sequential development are that as different regions are organizing, they require specific kinds of experiences targeting the region's specific function to develop properly. For example, a child must be exposed to visual input while the visual system is organizing. These developmental times are called **critical periods**. Without a sufficient number and duration of experiences during critical periods, a child will lose some of his or her genetic potential to develop certain skills commensurate with those experiences. Moreover, a disruption in the timing, intensity, quality, or quantity of normal developmental experiences may have devastating consequences (Client and Family Education 2-1).

Neuroplasticity

The brain's ability to develop and alter in response to experience as described previously is known as **neuroplasticity**. This means that the brain adapts to new conditions during its maturation and during its constant interaction with its environment. In a sense, this also means that to some degree, humans can create their own brains by exposing them to certain experiences. Stimuli that arise in the internal or external environment trigger neuroplastic mechanisms. For this reason, as mentioned in the previous section, brain development depends on exposure to certain environmental stimuli and subsequent activation of developing pathways.

Not only is neuroplasticity responsible for the way that our brains develop, but it also says a great deal about how we are not at the mercy of our early learning environments. Our brains continue to grow connections, and exposure to new learning results in new brain changes, even into advanced old age.

Two basic phenomena are involved in neuroplasticity, both of which depend on a structural change in neu-

Client and Family Education 2-1

ENCOURAGING OPTIMAL LEARNING IN CHILDREN

In their teaching role, nurses can educate families about the importance of exposing children to optimal learning experiences. Tips to give parents and adult caregivers of children include the following:

- Because very young brains are more plastic than older ones, interventions are more likely to be successful with younger children than older children. It will take older children longer to develop new behaviors that will override existing ones.

- While optimal and critical periods exist during which children should be exposed to certain activities, parents should not make life stressful for their children by enrolling them in every enrichment program available. Activities as simple as play and reading to children have been shown to positively affect both future prosocial behaviors and language acquisition.

- The interaction of life events and developmental variables, such as genetic characteristics, is important to understanding children's behavior. Behavior comes from somewhere, and it is always meaningful. The meaning of a child's behavior, however, may differ from what parents may think. For example, toddlers may act fussy and difficult during a long religious service. Such behavior is

entirely normal; small children are not "wired" to sit for long periods exposed to things that they perceive as tedium. Exposing children to experiences to which they are not developmentally ready can lead to unintended consequences. In this case, the child may develop an aversion to church. Or a child who normally behaves well during church may simply be hungry or tired. Parents should always look for more than one meaning.

- Children's responses are not "psychological" or "mental" patterns. They are physiologic patterns expressed cognitively and, thereby, behaviorally. The potency of children's behavioral and cognitive responses to like stimuli will correlate strongly with the strength of prior experiences. This is why children like to play the same activity or have the same book read to them over and over. While adults may find such repetition boring, it is essential and comforting to children.

- Children who are exposed to rich sensory experiences and many protective factors, as opposed to risk factors, will experience fewer maladaptive responses than their counterparts. Parents should try to decrease risk factors (eg, exposure to violence) and increase protective factors (eg, stable home life) as much as possible for children to become resilient.

rons. The first type, **reactive plasticity**, is a functional and comparatively rapid type of plasticity that brings about functional changes, which usually are reversible. The second type, **adaptive plasticity**, affects the expression of genotype into phenotype. Adaptive plasticity is not reversible.

The concept of neuroplasticity provides the foundation for learning, memory, and other complex mental processes. It is important to remember that all learning is brain based. Learning is a form of adaptation in response to specific experiences during a person's life. Psychotherapy is nothing more than assisting people to acquire knowledge or develop the ability to perform new behaviors. It is a form of education. Thus, education in the form of psychotherapy is literally an attempt to change the brain's structure so changes in behavior will follow. This would not be possible without neuroplasticity and its role in new learning.

The physiologic effects of psychotherapy are being demonstrated with brain imaging techniques. Research has been conducted on the outcomes of psychotherapy as opposed to psychopharmacotherapy. Using positron emission tomography (PET) in one study, Baxter and col-

leagues (1992; Schwartz, Stoessel, Baxter, Martin, & Phelps, 1996) examined local cerebral metabolic rates for glucose. They found that both behavior therapy and fluoxetine (Prozac) produced similar decreases in cerebral metabolic rates in the head of the right caudate nucleus. This finding suggested that this form of psychotherapy and fluoxetine have similar physiologic effects on the brain.

The Role of Genetics

Genes are segments of deoxyribonucleic acid (DNA). Their organization may be thought of as templates within chromosomes. The *chromosomes* contain the DNA, which in turn contains the instructions for the development and maintenance of the entire human body. Genes are like information bytes, and they carry information for the production of proteins. They have enormous amounts of coding information, which serves as a blueprint for biologic processes. Genes are responsible for transmitting hereditary characteristics.

Cells read genes in two steps: transcription and translation. **Transcription** is the process by which DNA se-

TABLE 3-4 ▼ Behavior Modification Techniques

LEARNING PRINCIPLE	BEHAVIOR MODIFICATION TECHNIQUE	EXAMPLE OF TREATMENT
When an established behavior pattern is no longer reinforced, it tends to extinguish itself.	Withdrawal of reinforcement for undesirable behavior	Parents begin to show less concern for their child's temper tantrums or ignore them altogether.
A specified behavior can gradually be established if successive approximations of that behavior are reinforced.	Shaping of desired behavior	Social reinforcement is provided to develop sustained eye contact in clients with schizophrenia who have social-skills deficits.
Behavior patterns are developed and established through repeated associations with positive reinforcers.	Use of positive reinforcers to establish desired behavior	Token economy is used, in which children exchange tokens, earned for desired behaviors, for toys.

examine the *antecedent condition,* or the cognition that precedes their behaviors and results in self-statements. Clients then examine the consequences related to those antecedents and self-statements. In one cognitive therapy framework called rational emotive therapy (RET), this approach is known as the "ABCD" approach.

- A is the antecedent behavior.
- B is the belief.
- C is the consequence (of the belief).
- D is the disputation of those maladaptive beliefs (Ellis, 1962).

The goals of therapy are for clients to monitor their maladaptive thoughts and beliefs, look for evidence that their beliefs are true, dispute their maladaptive self-statements, substitute more adaptive thoughts, and thus change their pattern of distorted thinking and, consequently, their behavior. This is part of a technique

BOX 3-1 ▼ *Examples of Distorted Beliefs*

- I must do well at everything that I do. Otherwise, I have no worth as a human being.
- People should act better than they do; if they do not, then they should be punished.
- Avoiding life's difficulties is easier than facing them.
- Because I was hurt or traumatized in the past, that past will forever haunt me, and I must be continuously preoccupied with that event.
- If I do not find an instant and perfect solution to my problems, it is a catastrophe.
- I can't stand feeling anxious, frustrated, uncomfortable, guilty, or otherwise emotionally upset.

known as *cognitive restructuring* (Raymond & Corsini, 2000).

Let's consider an example. A woman who has been unemployed for several months is devastated following an unsuccessful job interview. Using cognitive restructuring, a self-help homework exercise might be as follows:

- A (the Antecedent experience or event): I went for a job interview and didn't get the job.
- B (the Beliefs about the experience): How terrible to get rejected! I'm worthless! I'll never get a job.
- C (the Consequences of such negative self-talk): I feel blue and hopeless. I am making myself so anxious that I will do poorly on other job interviews.
- D (the Disputation or debating the original belief): I'll do better next time. Perhaps I can practice with my husband before the next interview.

The client describes his or her thoughts systematically, links those self-defeating thoughts to the present discomfort, and then disputes them. The disputation of what Ellis calls "irrational" beliefs is one way for people to change their self-defeating thoughts, which lead to self-defeating behaviors. Other techniques in the cognitive-behaviorist therapeutic tool kit are briefly described in Table 3-5.

The Humanistic Perspective

The humanistic approach recognizes the importance of learning and other psychological processes that traditionally have been the focus of research. Such psychological processes include creativity, hope, love, self-fulfillment, personal growth, values, and meaning. The humanistic perspective is concerned with human beings, their potentialities, and their personal growth. It represents a positive view of human nature. Humanists believe that psychopathology is the result of blocking or distortion of

TABLE 3-5 ▼ Cognitive-Behavioral Techniques

TECHNIQUE	DESCRIPTION
Cognitive relabeling	The way a person labels something will strongly determine his or her emotional response and behavior. A person who labels things incorrectly will have a maladaptive emotional response and ineffective behavior. This technique involves teaching the client to perceive environmental cues more accurately so that he or she clearly differentiates between realistically dangerous situations and those in which the source of harm is purely imaginary.
Systematic rational restructuring	This technique involves constructing a hierarchy of increasingly difficult situations, with successful coping by the client determining progression to the next, more difficult situation. It is similar to systematic desensitization, except that rational reevaluation replaces relaxation as a coping skill.
Rational problem solving	This technique involves systematic problem-solving training. It consists of five stages: 1) Orientation to the problem 2) Precisely defining the problem 3) Generating alternatives to the problem 4) Making a decision among the alternatives 5) Verifying whether the alternative chosen was useful

personal growth, excessive stress, and unfavorable social conditions.

This perspective has been severely criticized for its lack of scientific grounding. Indeed the humanistic view is less a theory and more a system of values. Its main importance for psychiatric-mental health nurses lies in its optimistic view of human beings and their capacity to become fully functional. Some well-known humanists are Carl Rogers, Abraham Maslow (see Figure 4-1), Thomas Szasz, and Fritz Perls (Carson & Mineka, 1999; Hall, Campbell, & Lindzey, 1997).

The Interpersonal Perspective

Those who adhere to the interpersonal perspective hold the viewpoint that unsatisfactory interpersonal relations are the primary cause for many maladaptive behaviors. At present, no systematic view of human nature and behavior is based entirely on interpersonal relationships or the social context in which people live and function. The closest approximation may be the viewpoint developed by the neo-Freudian psychologist Harry Stack Sullivan (Carson & Mineka, 1999; Hall, Campbell, & Lindzey, 1997). Sullivan believed that poor relationships with others caused a person anxiety, which served as the basis for all emotional problems. Others in the psychiatric field elaborated upon this viewpoint, including Sullivan's student Hildegarde Peplau, the renowned pioneer in psychiatric nursing.

Interpersonal theorists emphasize the interpersonal socialization of human beings throughout their stages of development. Failure to proceed through these stages in a satisfactory way lays the foundation for later maladap-

tive behavior. Within the context of development, this perspective emphasizes the role of early childhood in shaping human beings and their self-concept. Distorted self-concepts can be traced back to early socialization within the framework of the person's family. Two results of distorted self-concept are poor interpersonal functioning and self-defeating "games" that people learn to play (Berne, 1964). The interpersonal perspective is also concerned with the anxiety-arousing aspects of interpersonal relationships.

Interpersonal therapy is concerned with alleviating anxiety and pathogenic or problem-causing relationships. It also focuses on helping clients achieve more satisfactory relationships. Such therapy is concerned with verbal and nonverbal communication, social roles, attributions that people make about themselves and others, and the general interpersonal context of their behavior. It emphasizes remediating the client's interpersonal skills within the therapeutic relationship.

Despite its intuitive appeal and similar to the psychoanalytic and humanistic approaches, incomplete information concerning many aspects of interpersonal functioning handicaps this perspective. As a result, many of its concepts lack adequate scientific grounding.

The Biophysiological Perspective

The biophysiological perspective has slowly gained more influence as continuous efforts to find the causes and treatments of psychiatric illnesses result in promising new findings. Enormous strides have been made in the past 25 years toward understanding the probable biophysiological components of many behavioral disorders. The biophysiological perspective is sometimes called "the medical model," which is misleading. While psychiatrists, who are physicians, direct much of the care of clients with psychiatric disorders, there is nothing inherently "medical" about this model, any more than there is about any of the others. Basically, all the models seek to explain psychopathology, its cause (pathogenesis), and its cure or treatment, regardless of whether that treatment is purely psychotherapy or purely somatic therapy.

The biophysiological perspective proposes that psychopathology results from some physiologic condition, primarily a deviation within the central nervous system (CNS) (Coyle, 1999). The reasons for these deviations are multifaceted, and they involve a complex interplay between genetics, temperament, development, brain circuitry, human biology at the molecular level, and environment (see Chap. 2). While researchers still have a great deal of study to conduct, molecular biologists at the National Institutes of Health and around the globe are making important new discoveries about mental illnesses daily.

Until recently, the therapeutic processes associated with the biophysiological perspective were thought to focus on somatic treatments, such as medications, sleep deprivation and photo (light) therapies, and electroconvulsive therapy. As more research is being conducted on the effects of the environment and psychotherapy on brain circuitry, this perspective will expand its treatment modalities to include more psychosocial therapies.

The Sociocultural Viewpoint

Most theory in early psychology was concerned with the individual. Gradually, however, sociocultural influences, such as family, community, and other environmental factors, have become recognized as having enormous effects on the lives of clients. Many approaches are within the sociocultural perspective, but all of them focus on the role of social and cultural influences on the person.

Culture can be thought of as the "glue" that holds certain groups of people together. It consists of socially acquired and socially transmitted symbols, beliefs, techniques, institutions, customs, and norms. Culture has been found to exert a great influence on the birth, development, and death of human beings. Culture also affects the ways in which the body is treated (Vargas & Koss-Chioino, 1992).

A rapidly growing discipline known as *medical anthropology* deals with the cross-cultural study of medical systems and the influence of ecological, biological, and sociocultural factors on health and disease. Some areas of interest in the field of medical anthropology for psychiatric professionals include the dynamics of health-seeking behaviors, models of mental illness, systems of healing, alcohol drinking patterns, and special mental states, such as trance and spirit possession. Another area of interest includes psychiatric syndromes seen in non-Western cultures but influenced by the social values of those non-Westerns cultures. One such culture-bound syndrome is *koro,* an affliction seen in men of Southeast Asian origin. Koro is characterized by intense anxiety and fear that one's penis is shrinking and receding into one's belly (Dohrenwend & Dohrenwend, 1974; Draguns, 1979). Koro can and has reached epidemic proportions in some countries and is thought to be influenced by the importance and fragility of male sexuality in that culture.

In terms of social influences, a strong association has been shown between social class or socioeconomic position and psychiatric disorders. A classic study by Hollingshead and Redlich found that the lower the social class, the greater the prevalence of psychotic problems (1958). Since that time, research findings in dozens of studies have repeatedly shown that noxious social conditions (eg, poverty) adversely affect human beings. Several explanations have been advanced for these findings. One is that the complex social stressors associated with living in poverty and having few resources inhibit the abilities of poor individuals to cope as effectively as their more affluent counterparts. This ineffective coping leads to a constant cycle of extreme stress and subsequent maladaptation and potential illness. In this view, poverty is seen as a social toxin.

Another sociodemographic factor of interest to sociocultural theorists is marital status. Married people have consistently been found to have better mental health than unmarried people. Race and ethnicity have also been studied in relation to mental health and illness, but race per se has not been found to account for any significant differences in social patterns of mental health. Clients belonging to racial minorities, however, have been found to experience disproportionate amounts of stress because of the prejudices with which they are forced to live and because they are more likely to be poor than whites.

Scholars have recognized the importance of cultural and ethnic factors as they relate to mental health and mental illness. How the client who has a psychiatric disorder is received, understood, and treated has been found to greatly affect the course of his or her treatment. Moreover, solid empirical data support the sociocultural perspective (Vargas & Koss-Chioino, 1992). It is only one perspective, however, and does not fully explain all facets of mental illness.

TOWARD A COMPREHENSIVE, MULTIDISCIPLINARY UNDERSTANDING OF PSYCHOPATHOLOGY

With ongoing research, psychiatric-mental health professionals continue to develop a better understanding of the roles of biologic, psychosocial, and sociocultural factors in the development of psychopathology. It has become increasingly apparent that explanations based on only one of these factors are likely to be incomplete and lacking. Today, the field supports the belief that an interaction of several causal factors produces disorders.

One useful framework was developed by psychologist Dante Cicchetti and his colleagues. This framework incorporates several different theories and perspectives into an all-inclusive conceptual framework (1993, 1984). It was originally developed to explain maladaptation in children, but it is equally valid in its application to adults. Cicchetti's perspective evolved from the work of ecology theorist Uri Bronfenbrenner, who asserted that people's contexts are crucial to understanding their development and behaviors (1989, 1979). Cicchetti's ideas also evolved from the work of various developmental theorists who wrote that, during the course of their development, human beings must achieve *critical competencies* (such as the development of prosocial behaviors) to successfully meet the challenges of later developmental stages. Research has shown that children who do not master competency-specific tasks (eg, prosocial behaviors) are at increased risk for later social maladjustment. For example, studies show that an inability to successfully cope with the implicit social rules and exchanges with peers in play often results in peer rejection and detrimental consequences during later developmental periods (Coie, Dodge, & Kupersmidt, 1990; Denham & Holt, 1993; DeRosier, Kupersmidt, & Patterson, 1994).

This theory addresses both individual and environmental characteristics, simultaneously emphasizing the interactive and reciprocal influences of the individual, his or her family, the community, and the greater sociocultural arena in which he or she develops and lives. It includes the broader contexts of development and functioning, and it is solidly informed by the genetic and neurophysiologic variables inherent within each unique human being (see Chap. 2). In addition, this perspective hypothesizes

that certain contextual characteristics and events may enhance or hinder an individual's development and adaptation (Aber & Cicchetti, 1984). These contextual events can be either risk factors or protective factors. *Risk factors* are those variables that impede development and cause greater hardship. An example would be being born into extreme poverty. *Protective factors* are those variables that constitute buffers and have a helpful effect on individuals. An example would be being born into a supportive family. More risk and protective factors at different levels are described in Table 3-6.

In addition to what they bring by way of their unique ontogenetic characteristics (eg, genetic endowments, temperament) within their contexts, humans continuously are exposed to a multitude of both risk and protective factors across systems that are either proximal or distal to them. *Proximal factors* are those variables that exert the strongest influence on individuals and to which they are more immediately exposed (eg, parents to children). *Distal factors* are less adjacent to individuals and exert less powerful effects (eg, school systems to children). Much of how a child will respond and develop is contingent on this complex web of past experiences.

This ecological and developmental view is based on theories with empirical validation. Scholars are testing this model, which has been advanced as a valuable way in which to frame problems of childhood psychopathology and maladaptation (Dobson & Craig, 1998; National Research Council, 1993). Moreover, it represents the true complexity of people in their contexts. It also serves as a foundation for the kind of interagency collaboration and integration that have been promoted as a holistic and cost-effective way to deliver comprehensive care to persons with serious and persistent mental illnesses and their families (Anderson & Mohr, in press; Walter & Petr, 2000). A schematic of the model is presented in Figure 3-1.

TABLE 3-6   ▼   **Examples of Risk and Protective Factors**

TYPE OF SYSTEM	RISK FACTORS	PROTECTIVE FACTORS
Macrosystem	Violent culture Lack of access to healthcare War	Restricted sales of firearms Governmental support programs (eg, Women, Infants and Children Program, Medicare coverage) Universal lead screening
Exosystem	Violent neighborhood Impoverished neighborhood Paucity of healthcare providers Substandard housing	Strong alliance with community police officers Supportive and strong family and social networks Neighborhood "free" clinics
Microsystem	Domestic violence No affordable child care Chronic illness of a family member	Extended family support Consistent employment Respite care
Ontogenic	Genetic loading for major psychotic illness Low intelligence	High educational attainment Physical health

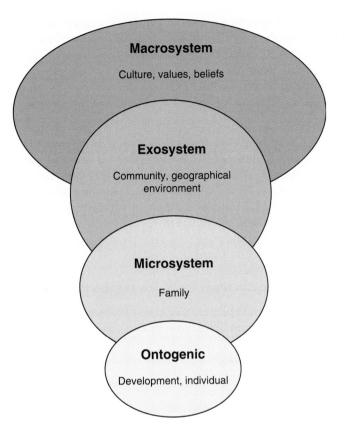

FIGURE 3-1 Developmental ecological model.

The Emergence of Mental Illness

Within Cicchetti's model, the emergence of serious mental illness is seen as disrupting the resolution of a child's developmental tasks. This consideration is important, because many serious mental illnesses manifest themselves in childhood or adolescence. The individual's developmental stage and the particular tasks with which he or she is grappling determine the effects of the illness. In order to understand the potential effects of any intervention, therefore, it is critical to assess and to understand the effects of proximal and distal influences in the individual's environment and how those effects might be manifested in their behavior. This model stresses an appreciation of behavior as being developmentally based. Biophysiologic characteristics interact and transact with environmental events. These important considerations allow the nurse to develop appropriate and individually crafted interventions.

Multidimensionality of Assessment (Assessing Multiple Systems)

The developmental ecological perspective also draws attention to the importance of identifying and attending to the multiple systems that affect child development. This means that the nurse and the multidisciplinary team collect infor-

 Implications for Nursing Practice 3-1

Importance of Assessment in Nursing Care

Nurses must understand that a child's (or adult's) behaviors, while similar in their manifestations, may have very different underlying motivations. For example, three children are displaying aggressive posturing. In the first child, such posturing may be a manifestation of anger. In the second child, it may be a manifestation of fear. The third child may use such behavior to avoid unpleasant or uncomfortable situations. In other circumstances, these same children may use the same behaviors for any of a host of other motivating factors. The point is that nurses must never assume that they know specifically why a client is behaving in a certain way. A careful assessment is key to effective and relevant client care.

mation in accordance with these multiple contexts. Most nurses are aware of how to assess an individual client. Many, however, are less aware of how to consider such factors as the context or environment and what role it might play in how clients are considered and treated (Implications for Nursing Practice 3-1). Let us see what such an assessment might entail in considering the microsystem and exosystem.

FAMILY CHARACTERISTICS (MICROSYSTEM)

The developmental risk literature indicates that multiple risk factors increase a child's risk for maladjustment. This finding suggests that children experiencing a serious mental illness and environmental risk factors are at greater risk for poor outcomes than those who are not living with such concomitant risks (Pellegrini, 1990; Rutter, 1987). Important assessment components include family characteristics and development, because they constitute essential elements of the child's ecology. The structure of the parental unit can be an important indicator of support or stress in a family; for example, the presence or absence of marital conflict within a family can affect a child's development. Other contextual risk factors to consider during an assessment include poverty, employment and family instability, residential instability, child-care burden, parental stress, and social isolation.

COMMUNITY CHARACTERISTICS (EXOSYSTEM)

A second level of ecological characteristics salient to people's lives is the community. Cohesive neighborhoods with strong support services, such as churches or community policing partnerships, can help mitigate the effects of community violence (Marans, 1995). On the other hand, chronic community violence has been shown to be stressful to individuals who are exposed to such events. Furthermore, it can tax family resources and generally impede the performance of daily activities (Garbarino, Bubrow, Kostelny, & Pardo, 1998). Thus, assessing for community-level variables and factors that might mitigate related challenges is crucial for developing well-informed interventions.

▼ CHAPTER SUMMARY

■ Theories and conceptual frameworks are worldviews that provide a way of looking at human behavior as well as a systematic way to frame research studies.

■ Several theories have informed the practice of psychiatric nursing. Such theories include the psychodynamic perspective, behavior theory, cognitive-behavior theory, humanistic theory, interpersonal theory, biophysiological theory, and sociocultural theories.

■ While no one theory has been adequate to explain mental health and mental illness, some theories are more useful than others. Some also have actual empirical evidence to support them.

■ Research indicates that biologic, psychological, interpersonal, and sociocultural factors contribute to mental illnesses. Yet the same circumstance may affect different individuals in different ways.

■ Researchers have constructed models that go beyond the reductionistic ones of the past to view the individual as a complex organism, living, interacting, and transacting with others and negotiating risk and protective factors in their ecologies. This dynamic view of human beings holds great promise for research and for more precise assessment and interventions in the future.

▼ REVIEW QUESTIONS

1. According to the psychoanalytic theory of human behavior, mental illness results from
   a. Excessive stress
   b. Repressed experiences
   c. Learned maladaptive behavior
   d. Distorted self-statements

2. A client in therapy asks the nurse to explain the concept of defense mechanisms. The nurse bases his or her answer on the knowledge that defense mechanisms are
   a. Conscious attempts by people to minimize stress
   b. Unconscious attempts to protect personal stability
   c. Conscious use of denial when confronted with conflict
   d. Unconscious use of hostility when confronted with conflict

3. A 32-year-old man is admitted to an alcohol and drug rehabilitation center. During the interview, he tells the nurse that his family is exaggerating his alcohol use. This is an example of which of the following defense mechanisms?
   a. Regression
   b. Reaction formation
   c. Denial
   d. Sublimation

4. A 16-year-old female client is brought into counseling by her parents because she has been skipping school. The client tells the nurse therapist that her parents are irresponsible and do not care about her feelings. This is an example of which of the following defense mechanisms?
   a. Regression
   b. Reaction formation
   c. Projection
   d. Identification

5. A 35-year-old male client tells his therapist that she reminds him of his mother. The therapist recognizes this as
   a. Projection
   b. Identification
   c. Transference
   d. Countertransference

6. A 32-year-old woman is being treated for agoraphobia. She tells the therapist that she was able to stand near her open front door for 3 minutes. The therapist praises her for this behavior. This is an example of which concept of behavioral therapy?
   a. Shaping
   b. Discrimination
   c. Modeling
   d. Conditioning

7. A 43-year-old male client diagnosed with depression tells the nurse, "I've failed at many things in my life, and I'll probably always be a failure." From the perspective of cognitive-behavior theory, the client is engaging in
   a. Disputation
   b. Rationalization
   c. Regression
   d. Distorted cognition

8. The treatment plan for a client with depression is inpatient care for the therapeutic milieu, antidepressants, weekly 1-hour sessions with the psychiatrist, and a series of electroconvulsive treatments. This treatment approach suggests that the psychiatrist most likely adheres to which of the following models of human behavior?
   a. Humanistic model
   b. Interpersonal model
   c. Biophysiologic model
   d. Sociocultural model

9. The ecological-developmental framework for explaining mental illness posits that
   a. Developmental tasks can overwhelm the person and result in psychopathology.
   b. Distal risk factors have the strongest influence on psychopathology.
   c. Environmental factors have a limited influence on psychopathology.
   d. Biologic, psychosocial, and sociocultural factors influence psychopathology.

10. Using the ecological-developmental framework for assessing a 14-year-old with mental illness, the nurse focuses on
   a. Individual, family, and community characteristics
   b. Individual and family characteristics
   c. Success in individual achievement of higher-level developmental tasks
   d. Biophysiologic characteristics

▼ REFERENCES AND SUGGESTED READINGS

*Aber, J. L., & Cicchetti, D. (1984). The social-emotional development of maltreated children: An empirical and theoretical analysis. In H. Fitzgerald, B. Lester, & M. Yogman (Eds.), *Theory and research in behavioral pediatrics* (pp. 123–145). New York: Plenum.

*Anderson, J. A., & Mohr, W. K. (in press). A developmental ecological perspective in systems of care for children with serious emotional disturbances and their families. *Journal of Child and Family Studies.*

*Axelrod, S., & Van Houten, R. (1993). *Behavior analysis and treatment.* Boulder, CO: Perseus Publishers.

*Berne, E. (1964). *Games people play.* New York: Grove Press.

*Bronfenbrenner, U. (1979). The ecology of human development: Experiments by nature and design. Cambridge, MA: Harvard University Press.

*Bronfenbrenner, U. (1989). Foreword. In A. R. Pence (Ed.), *Ecological research with children and families: From concepts to methodology* (pp. 1–20). New York: Teachers College Press.

Carson, R. C., & Mineka, S. (1999). *Abnormal psychology and modern life* (11th ed.). Reading, MA: Addison-Wesley Longman Publishers.

*Cicchetti, D. (1984). The emergence of developmental psychopathology. *Child Development, 55,* 1–7.

*Cicchetti, D. (1993). Developmental psychopathology: Reactions, reflections, projections. *Developmental Review, 13,* 471–502.

Coie, J. D., Dodge, K. A., & Kupersmidt, J. B. (1990). Peer groups' behavior and social status. In S. R. Aster & J. D. Coie (Eds.), *Peer rejection in childhood* (pp. 17–59). Cambridge, England: Cambridge University Press.

*Coyle, J. T. (1999). The neuroscience revolution and psychiatry. In S. Weissman, M. Sabshin, & H. Eist (Eds.), *Psychiatry in the new millennium* (pp. 7–24). Washington, DC: American Psychiatric Association.

*Crits-Christoph, P. (1998). Training in empirically validated treatments. In K. S. Dobson & K. D. Craig (Eds.), *Empirically supported therapies: Best practices in professional psychology* (pp. 3–25). Thousand Oaks, CA: Sage.

*Denham, S. A., & Holt, R. W. (1993). Preschoolers' likeability as cause or consequence of their social behavior. *Developmental Psychology, 29,* 271–275.

*DeRosier, M., Kupersmidt, J. B., & Patterson, C. J., (1994). Children's academic and behavioral adjustment as a function of the chronicity and proximity of peer rejection. *Child Development, 65,* 1799–1813.

Dobson, K. S., & Craig, K. D. (Eds.). (1998). *Empirically supported therapies: Best practices in professional psychology.* Thousand Oaks, CA: Sage.

*Dohrenwend, B. P., & Dohrenwend, B. P. (1974). Social and cultural influences on psychopathology. *Annual Review of Psychology, 25,* 417–452.

*Draguns, J. G. (1979). Culture and personality. In A. J. Marsella, R. Tharp, & T. Cobwrowski (Eds.), *Perspectives in cross cultural psychology* (pp. 7–28). New York: Academic Press.

*Ellis, A. (1962). *Reason and emotion in psychotherapy.* New York: Lyle Stuart/Citadel Press.

*Esterson, A. (1993). *Seductive mirage: An exploration of the work of Sigmund Freud.* Chicago: Open Court Books.

*Garbarino, J., Bubrow, N., Kostelny, K., & Pardo, C. (1998). *Children in danger: Coping with the consequences of community violence.* San Francisco: Jossey-Bass.

*Goldfried, M. R., & Davison, G. C. (1976). *Clinical behavior therapy.* New York: Holt Rinehart & Winston.

*Hall, C. S., Campbell, G., & Lindzey, G. (1997). *Theories of personality.* New York: John Wiley & Sons.

*Hersen, M. (1985). Overview. In M. Hersen (Ed.), *Practice of inpatient behavior therapy: A clinical guide* (pp. 3–31). New York: Grune & Stratton.

*Hollingshead, A. M., & Redlich, F. C. (1958). *Social class and mental illness.* New York: John Wiley & Sons.

*Kandel, E. R. (1998). A new intellectual framework for psychiatry. *The American Journal of Psychiatry, 155*(4), 457–469.

*Kandel, E. R. (1999). Biology and the future of psychoanalysis: A new intellectual framework for psychiatry revisited. *The American Journal of Psychiatry, 156*(4), 505–524.

*Marans, S. (1995). *The police mental health partnership: A community based response to urban violence.* New Haven, CT: Yale University Press.

*Meichenbaum, D. H. (1977). *Cognitive behavior modification: An integrative approach.* New York: Plenum.

*National Research Council. (1993). *Understanding child abuse and neglect.* Washington, DC: National Academy Press.

*Pellegrini, D. S. (1990). Psychosocial risk and protective factors in childhood. *Developmental and Behavioral Pediatrics, 11,* 201–209.

*Raymond, J. & Corsini, R. J. (2000). *Current psychotherapies.* Itaska, IL: F.E. Peacock Press.

*Rutter, M. (1987). Psychosocial resilience and protective mechanisms. *American Journal of Orthopsychiatry, 57,* 316–331.

*Tallis, R. C. (1996). Burying Freud. *Lancet, 347*(9002), 669–671.

*Vargas, L. A., & Koss-Chioino, J. D. (1992). *Working with culture: Psychotherapeutic interventions with ethnic minority children and adolescents.* San Francisco: Jossey-Bass.

*Walter, U., & Petr, C. (2000). A template for family-centered interagency collaboration. *Families in Society, 81*(5), 494–503.

*Wyden, P. (1997). *Conquering schizophrenia*. New York: Alfred A. Knopf.

Starred references are cited in text.

For additional information on this chapter, go to *http://connection. lww.com.*

Need more help? See Chapter 3 of the *Study Guide to Accompany Mohr: Johnson's Psychiatric-Mental Health Nursing,* 5th edition.

Therapeutic Relationships and Communication

CATHERINE DEERING; JANE FREDERICK

▼ KEY TERMS

Aggressiveness—Communication and behavior that are belittling, threatening, moralizing, coercing, or condescending.

Apathy—A sense of detachment and the belief that nothing a person does makes any difference, leading to a lack of concern about the problem or outcome.

Assertiveness—A technique by which a person communicates what he or she thinks, feels, or wants directly and respectfully.

Caring—A core value of nursing that consists of three primary behaviors: (1) giving of self, (2) meeting the client's needs in a timely manner, and (3) providing comfort measures for clients and family members.

Channel—The route or method a communicator chooses to convey his or her message.

Communication—The process of conveying information through a complex variety of verbal and nonverbal behaviors.

Communicator—A person who simultaneously sends and receives messages through words and nonverbal behaviors.

Confrontation—The skill of pointing out, in a caring way, concern about another person's behavior or discrepancies between what the other person says and what he or she does.

Countertransference—The arousal of uncomfortable, sometimes unprofessional feelings within the nurse while he or she is working with clients who present difficult behaviors and dilemmas.

Decoding—The process by which one communicator discerns or interprets what another communicator is saying.

Empathy—The emotional knowing of another person.

Encoding—The process by which a communicator puts into words or behaviors the ideas or feelings that he or she is trying to convey.

Environment—In communication, the personal experiences and cultural background that a communicator brings to an interaction.

External noise—Any factor outside a communicator that creates distractions.

Feedback—The discernible response that a receiver makes to a sender's message when communicating.

Genuineness—A nursing value that involves being a real person and truly engaged in knowing the client in open, human exchanges.

Listening—The act of focusing on all behaviors exhibited by a person who is communicating.

Maturity—The ability to integrate aspects of life into a whole and find balance in one's outlook and attitudes toward others.

Noise—Any force caused by communicators or in the environment that interferes with effective communication.

Nontherapeutic communication—Interactions in which the nurse uses ineffective responses that result in clients feeing defensive, misunderstood, controlled, minimized, alienated, or discouraged from expressing their thoughts and feelings.

Passive-aggressive communication—Communication that uses indirect aggression through backstabbing, sabotaging, ignoring, or "forgetting" to do something.

Perception check—A confrontational communication technique that uses a three-step formula to clarify another person's behavior. The three steps are to (1) describe the inconsistent or confusing behavior, (2) offer at least two possible interpretations of that behavior, and (3) ask for feedback.

Physiologic noise—Any physical factor within a communicator that detracts from effective communication.

Positive reframing—A communication technique in which the mental healthcare provider specifically states the behavior changes a client should make rather than criticizing the client's negative behavior.

Professional—A person who applies a specific background of knowledge and skills.

Psychological noise—Any emotional or cognitive force within a communicator that interferes with accurately expressing or understanding a message.

Therapeutic communication—A planned process of interaction in which the nurse demonstrates empathy, uses effective communication skills, and responds to the client's thoughts, needs, and concerns.

Transactional analysis—An assertive communication technique by which a person speaks from the adult ego state to others in the adult ego state.

Trust—The risk of sharing oneself with another, knowing that one is opening himself or herself to the possibility of hurt, embarrassment, judgment, and disappointment.

Unconditional positive regard—The ability to give of oneself freely to clients and to see clients as worthy of respect and attention regardless of their behavior, flaws, and setbacks.

▼LEARNING OBJECTIVES

On completion of this chapter, you should be able to accomplish the following:

- List the key ingredients of a therapeutic relationship.
- Identify potential obstacles to the establishment of a therapeutic relationship.
- Describe the three phases of therapeutic relationships.
- Discuss the application of a theoretical model to the components of nurse–client communication.
- Describe effective listening skills to use with clients.
- Contrast effective and ineffective communication techniques with clients.
- Identify techniques for using confrontation and self-assertion with clients.
- Discuss the appropriateness of different levels of self-disclosure with clients.
- Describe the role of the client's family and loved ones in the client's care.
- Analyze case studies that explore specific challenges to establishing therapeutic nurse–client relationships.

▼ Clinical Example 4-1

Mr. Smith is a 38-year-old man with bipolar disorder. He is admitted for his eighth psychiatric hospitalization following an overdose of antidepressant medications. Stressors leading to this hospitalization include stopping his medications about 4 months ago, losing his job, and recently quarreling with his 14-year-old daughter.

Although he has been divorced for 3 years, Mr. Smith's ex-wife continues to provide his emotional and financial support. Before the divorce, the family experienced severe financial difficulties when Mr. Smith went on spending sprees during manic episodes. His erratic behavior, sleeplessness, and sudden disappearances from home for days at a time distressed his wife and children.

Currently, Mr. Smith expresses remorse about the problems he has caused his family. He says he wishes he could reunite with his wife but understands that the relationship seems beyond repair. His greatest worry is that his daughter may never forgive him for the hurtful things he said during their most recent argument. He continues to have suicidal thoughts, but he has no immediate intention to harm himself.

The nurse approaches Mr. Smith to ask him how he is feeling. He replies, "How do you think I'm feeling? I have no family, no job, no future . . . I'm just one big screwup. And here I am, doped up in the hospital. What's the point?"

Points for Reflection and Critical Thinking

- If you were the nurse, how would you initially respond?
- What challenges will the nurse face in building a relationship with Mr. Smith?
- What challenges will the nurse face in communicating with Mr. Smith?
- How can nurses learn to modify their emotions and reactions when dealing with clients?

People who are experiencing mental health problems are vulnerable and usually afraid. Being able to build a relationship and communicate with such people presents challenges for nurses. Meeting these challenges requires skills, knowledge, and perceptiveness to discern what will be most helpful to these clients and their loved ones. At the same time, working with those who are in emotional distress can be highly rewarding for nurses when they know that their clients feel understood, cared about, and better able to cope with their unique situations.

This chapter focuses on how to create a therapeutic relationship and communicate effectively with clients and their families. It explores dimensions of the nurse's attitudes and behaviors that enhance and detract from the development of good working relationships with clients. As these relationships progress over time, several predictable phases occur. This chapter examines the key tasks of each phase, from introduction to termination, and discusses how nurses can facilitate movement toward healthy change and growth. It outlines effective and ineffective listening skills, along with specific guidelines for confrontation, assertiveness, and self-disclosure with clients. The main goal of this chapter is to provide a guide for productive interaction with clients and their families.

THERAPEUTIC RELATIONSHIPS

According to Hildegarde Peplau, the cornerstone of all nursing care is the therapeutic relationship (1952). The *therapeutic relationship* is a close, helping relationship based on trust, which allows the nurse and client to work collaboratively. The purpose of a therapeutic relationship in mental healthcare is to help clients solve problems, cope more effectively, and achieve developmental goals. Despite the significant developments in biotechnology that hold promise for the treatment, and possibly even the cure, of mental disorders, the therapeutic relationship remains the central medium through which all psychiatric care is provided (Krauss, 2000). Without the establishment of meaningful, ongoing communication with clients in an atmosphere of mutual respect, clients will not understand or value mental health services.

Essential Elements

Every human relationship is unique. The nurse and client bring their own backgrounds, beliefs, and personalities to bear on their work together. Certain key elements, however, must exist for a therapeutic relationship to develop. These elements include trust, professionalism, mutual respect, caring, and partnership.

TRUST

In therapeutic relationships, as in all close relationships, the foundation is trust. **Trust** involves choosing to take the risk of sharing oneself with another, knowing that one is exposing himself or herself to the possibility of hurt, embarrassment, judgment, and disappointment. People with mental health problems may be particularly reluctant to trust others because they are in emotional pain and fear being misunderstood. Nurses must earn their clients' trust through their caring presence and sensitive interactions. Some behaviors that foster the development of trust include predictability, consistency, and clear expectations. Nurses need to explain what will happen to clients to prevent feelings of fear, betrayal, and helplessness. For example, hospitalized clients need to know when and if they will be able to have smoking breaks or other privileges. Community mental health nurses who visit families must clearly communicate that nurses are mandated to report cases of child and elder abuse. Nurses must provide clients in outpatient settings with information about how and when they can reach nurses in times of crisis. Through thoughtful, consistent interactions with clients, nurses show that they can be depended on to be honest and available. Even small actions, such as indicating how much time a nurse has available to talk with clients, may help them gauge their level of self-disclosure.

Another important component of trust is *confidentiality*. Mental health providers must reassure clients that they will not share the details of clients' lives outside the professional environment. In this context, confidentiality also includes the right for clients to conceal that they are receiving treatment for a mental health problem. For example, it would be a major breach of trust and a violation of confidentiality for nursing students to mention to their family that they saw someone the family knew on a psychiatric unit and to reveal that person's identity.

Trust is also based on the knowledge that one is accepted without judgment. Mental health problems are often accompanied by shame about socially alienating symptoms (eg, hallucinations, flashbacks, withdrawal) and an inability to manage relationships with others. Clients need to know that nurses will not blame, fear, or look down on them. This means that nurses must gain a level of comfort with psychiatric symptoms so that they can fully accept clients regardless of their level of functioning.

PROFESSIONALISM

In a therapeutic relationship the nurse is acting as a **professional**, a person who applies a specific background of knowledge and skills. The purpose of the professional relationship is to promote the client's mental health. The professional role can be contrasted with a social relationship that is designed to meet the friendship needs of both parties (Table 4-1). Nurses demonstrate professionalism in psychiatric nursing through their knowledge of mental health problems and their ability to intervene effectively. Thus, nurses must learn about their clients' conditions, medications, and treatments so they are ready to provide current information and insight into their clients' symptoms. The foci of the nurse–client relationship are problem solving and identifying community resources to fit each client's needs. In short, nurses must be competent to help their clients on both emotional and pragmatic levels for a relationship to be therapeutic.

MUTUAL RESPECT

A therapeutic relationship is based on mutual respect. Although the stigma surrounding mental illness has decreased with greater awareness of the biologic and genetic factors that contribute to clients' conditions and wider use of mental health services, clients and their families still encounter negative and condescending attitudes. People with mental illness are no less human or deserving of respect than other people. In fact, nurses working with clients who have psychiatric disorders and their families often feel a heightened respect for them when they realize how they have struggled with extraordinary events and disabling symptoms. A sense of reverence for the human spirit and wonder at the uniqueness of each person develops as the nurse truly gets to know people who have overcome mental health problems.

Families of people with mental illnesses often fear being criticized or blamed for causing their loved one's problems. This fear comes from a long history of psychological theories that attributed psychiatric disorders to childhood traumas and family dynamics. Although family difficulties sometimes play a part in the development of mental health problems, experts now know that biologic, genetic, and environmental stressors outside the family unit (eg, poverty, traumatic life events, relationships with peers) also contribute to the equation (see Chap. 3). Mental illness places a great strain on families who cope daily with such problems as withdrawal, unpredictable behavior, dependence, and mood swings. Nurses must show respect for families who are doing the best they can to help their loved ones while also coping with their own, often stressful circumstances.

Nurses must also be sensitive to the family's cultural background and religious beliefs. An awareness of how the client's cultural background influences values, family functioning, and beliefs will help the nurse interact effectively

TABLE 4-1 ▼ Social Relationships Versus Therapeutic Relationships

SOCIAL RELATIONSHIP	THERAPEUTIC RELATIONSHIP
Purpose is to provide companionship, recreation, and support for both parties.	Purpose is to promote health, behavior change, and growth for the client.
Relationship is based on the premise of equal give and take.	Relationship is based on the premise that the nurse is caring for the client; the client is not expected to respond to the nurse's personal needs.
Discussion may sometimes focus on superficial topics, such as the weather or sports.	Superficial discussion blurs boundaries by introducing the nurse's background and personal preferences and distracts from the task of therapeutic change.
Both parties use self-disclosure in an increasingly free exchange as the relationship develops.	The nurse facilitates the client's self-disclosure to promote change and growth. Nurses disclose information about themselves only when it serves the client's needs.
When conflict occurs, both parties may argue freely, with relatively few constraints on their words and emotions.	The nurse uses therapeutic communication skills to listen, confront, and set limits with clients while maintaining a calm, professional, respectful attitude. Even when clients may be out of control, rude, or inappropriate in their behavior, the nurse models appropriate communication.
If dissatisfaction or distance develops, the relationship may gradually fade or abruptly end.	The nurse initiates and encourages discussion of any problems or behaviors that disrupt or inhibit the development of the relationship. Termination of the relationship is expected only when the client resolves the presenting problem or moves to another therapeutic setting. Termination is a planned, deliberate process that has therapeutic value.

and avoid offending clients. For example, in many traditional Hispanic families, acknowledging the father as the head of the family is important. In many African American families, extended family members such as grandparents and aunts are often key figures, viewed as central to the family's everyday life. Nurses should attempt to set aside their own concepts of family structure and learn more about how each client's family relates so that they do not exclude or minimize the importance of people who can influence the client's recovery and assist with planning care in the community. In addition, religious beliefs are an important resource for coping with emotional problems. Sometimes they serve as the most important source of strength from the client's perspective. Clients need to be able to share their beliefs without fear of offending the nurse or provoking judgment. If clients are afraid that their feelings or behavior conflicts with their religious faith or that they have alienated themselves from their religions, a referral to a chaplain may be helpful.

In a therapeutic relationship, respect must be both given and received. Nurses need to set limits when clients are disrespectful so that the boundaries of the relationship remain intact. For example, if a client experiencing a manic phase of bipolar disorder is hypersexual and making seductive remarks to the nurse, the nurse should make it clear that this behavior is unwelcome and needs to stop. Calmly stating, "This is not a time for sexual talk. Tell me about how you are doing, Mr. Jones" should be sufficient. If an intoxicated client insults or swears at a nurse, the nurse should set firm limits on this behavior by saying, "Lower your voice, stop swearing, and let's talk about what you need, Mr. Smith." A calm, nondefensive, and respectful demeanor will eventually help to set the tone for the interaction and reduce the escalation in the client's emotional outbursts. If the problematic behavior persists, the nurse should simply repeat the limit-setting statements calmly and firmly, leave the room to allow for a cooling-off period, or request help if the client appears to be on the edge of losing control. In most cases, the establishment of a therapeutic relationship based on genuine respect, careful listening, responsiveness, and limit setting can prevent escalating patterns of verbal and physical aggression.

CARING

Caring, one of the core values of nursing, consists of three primary behaviors:

1. Giving of the self
2. Meeting the client's needs in a timely manner

3. Providing comfort measures for clients and family members (Chipman 1992; Morse, Havens, & Wilson, 1997)

Creating a therapeutic relationship involves expending time and energy. The nurse must be genuinely invested in the client's welfare and willing to do what it takes to reduce suffering, anxiety, and uncertainty whenever possible. The opposite of caring is **apathy**, a sense of detachment and the belief that nothing one does makes any difference, which leads to a lack of concern about the problem or outcome. Apathy is a feeling that many clients with psychiatric disorders themselves experience when they struggle with chronic symptoms and are tempted to give up trying to cope. Caring means having the energy and optimism to keep trying to help clients, even in the face of discouragement.

Caring also involves showing empathy for clients by listening to their points of view and trying to understand their experiences. Carl Rogers (1952), a psychologist who wrote extensively about the essence of therapeutic relationships, identified three major ingredients of effective helping relationships: empathy, genuineness, and unconditional positive regard.

Empathy can be defined as emotional knowing of another person (van Servellen, 1997). It goes beyond just having data about the client's history; it means feeling what it must be like to be that person (Walker, 2001). Thus, empathy involves listening carefully, being in tune with what clients are saying, and having insight into the meaning of their thoughts, feelings, and behaviors.

Genuineness involves being a real person, truly engaged in knowing and being with the client in an open, human exchange. Obviously, genuineness is not something one can fake. It comes through as an attitude that arises out of deep concern and the ability to let one's guard down and resist trying to impress someone else.

The third key component of helping relationships, **unconditional positive regard**, is the ability to give to the client without strings attached. From this position, clients are worthy of respect and attention regardless of their behavior and despite their flaws and setbacks.

PARTNERSHIP

Historically, relationships between mental health professionals and clients have been unequal. The professional was seen as the healer, and the client was viewed as a relatively passive recipient of treatment. Current approaches, however, emphasize the role of the client and family as active partners in care. Therapies focus on mutual problem solving, planning treatments jointly, and empowering clients to take care of themselves. Families and loved ones are viewed as an invaluable resource for clients, who are now cared for mostly in community settings, often depending on their families for daily support. If the nurse does not view the client's loved ones as partners in care, these important peo-ple may feel alienated, judged, and devalued. Their unparalleled knowledge of the client's situation and insights about how various interventions may work will be lost. See Research in Psychiatric-Mental Health Nursing 4-1.

Obstacles to Establishing a Therapeutic Relationship

Nurses entering psychiatric-mental healthcare settings bring with them values, beliefs, and perspectives that may adversely influence their interactions with clients. At the same time, clients with psychiatric disorders, because of the intensity of their emotional reactions and the complexity of their behavior, pose unique challenges for nurses who must contain their own emotional reactions and check their social biases. The next section of this chapter discusses some potential attitudes and behaviors that may block effective interaction with clients who are experiencing mental health problems. Box 4-1 presents a critical thinking exercise that allows you to explore specific obstacles to establishing therapeutic relationships by examining several clinical examples.

JUDGMENTAL ATTITUDES

Although little research has been done to identify factors that may hinder the development of therapeutic relationships, judgmental attitudes are one obvious problem (Forchuk, 1994; Morse, Havens, & Wilson, 1997). Nurses must examine their own beliefs about mental illness before working in psychiatric settings. They should ask themselves the following questions to assess their own attitudes toward clients with psychiatric disorders:

- Do I believe that mental illness is as real as any physical illness, such as diabetes or asthma?
- Do I suspect that clients are overdramatizing their symptoms or using them as a crutch to avoid work and social responsibility?
- Do I view mental illness as a sign of a weak character?
- Do I find myself asking, "Why doesn't this person just snap out of it, put his or her problems in perspective, or focus on something else?"

If these thoughts run through a nurse's mind when working with clients with psychiatric disorders, he or she requires more education and exposure to the reality of mental illness. Psychiatric symptoms are every bit as real and disabling as any physical disease and often more devastating to the quality of a person's life. Although a nurse may feel critical of a woman who slashes her wrists for the fourth time in what seems to be a bid for attention, the nurse must be aware that anyone who would use this method of coping must feel desperate and see no other alternative. Remembering that clients in psychiatric settings are doing the best they can with the limited coping

Research in Psychiatric-Mental Health Nursing 4-1
POSITIVE CONNECTEDNESS IN THE PSYCHIATRIC NURSE–CLIENT RELATIONSHIP

Purpose: To examine nurses' experience of creating positive connectedness in their therapeutic relationships.

Background: In a connected relationship, while maintaining a professional perspective, the nurse views the client first as a person and second as a client (Morse, 1991).

Method and Sample: Researchers conducted a qualitative study in which they administered structured interviews to a small sample of nurses ($n = 8$) working in acute psychiatric settings with a wide variety of clients. They used grounded theory to identify themes related to positive connectedness.

Findings: Themes related to positive connectedness were as follows:

- *Vulnerability:* The client's willingness to express extreme honesty, share information prompted by guilt or shame, and reveal information never before shared with others
- *Commonality:* The nurse's ability to relate personally in some way to the client's situation, values, or beliefs
- *Reciprocation:* An acknowledgment that not only the client, but also the nurse, benefited from the relationship by feeling better about self and work
- *Investment:* The nurse's willingness to invest time and energy in the relationship

- *Feeling valued by the client:* A special bond with the nurse or recognition of the nurse by name

Application to Nursing Practice: To understand and develop therapeutic relationships, nurses must recognize and apply the essential elements of nurse–client connectedness:

- Nurse makes initial contact with the client.
- Nurse experiences some tension.
- Client shows vulnerability.
- Nurse feels less tension.
- Nurse encourages more disclosure in the vulnerable area.
- Nurse recognizes commonalities that he or she may or may not disclose.
- Nurse experiences a feeling of reciprocity with the client.
- Nurse feels valued by the client.
- Client and nurse invest more in the relationship, each taking risks.
- Connectedness results.

As nurses grow more comfortable with the therapeutic process, they become increasingly helpful to their clients.

From Heifner, C. (1993). Positive connectedness in the psychiatric nurse-patient relationship. *Archives of Psychiatric Nursing, 7,* 11–15.

---

skills they have is helpful. Judgmental attitudes, which clients can easily detect, will halt the therapeutic relationship before it begins.

EXCESSIVE PROBING

Clients in the mental health system typically must tell their stories to many different professionals. Technically, professionals have the right to ask any questions that they deem necessary. They should recognize, however, that the goal of asking questions is to help clients cope with their current situation. Asking clients to relate painful details of their childhood or to recount once again the embarrassing circumstances leading up to their hospitalization (eg, being arrested, going on a manic spending spree, being found in a regressed psychotic state) may place an unfair burden on clients. This is especially true when the relationship is short term.

Nurses must ask themselves whether their questions are designed to satisfy their own curiosity or to meet the client's current needs. Are the nurse and client embarking on a long-term relationship in which the client can fully discuss the details of his or her childhood to bring about some kind of resolution? Or is the nurse unearthing sensitive aspects of the client's history and then proceeding as if nothing happened? Being in a therapeutic relationship does not give nurses unlimited permission to invade a client's privacy (Glen & Jownally, 1995). As the following discussion indicates, communication with clients should follow their lead.

Maslow's hierarchy of needs may provide a useful guide for determining the kinds of questions to ask clients (Figure 4-1). When basic needs such as safety and physical health are not met, it may be irrelevant to probe into the client's history to discover the roots of his or her lowered self-esteem. Concrete help with referrals to social services and education about self-care will be vastly more useful to the client than an exploration of family dynamics, particularly in the brief treatment settings that pervade most of the current healthcare system. Nurses should view their

BOX 4-1 ▼ *Establishing Therapeutic Relationships and Critical Thinking*

This exercise presents several clinical scenarios related to the therapeutic relationship. Compare and contrast each of the following:

Scenario 1

The police bring Mr. Jones to the emergency department for treatment of lacerations after his arrest for drunken and disorderly conduct in a bar. Mr. Jones, an alcoholic, has experienced a relapse after completing three treatment programs in the past 5 years. He has also recently been arrested for driving while intoxicated. His wife and adult daughter are in the waiting room, hoping to take him home. Mr. Jones shouts at the nurse, "You tell those (expletive) women in my family that they can get the hell out of here. While you're at it, you can get lost, too!" He then proceeds to urinate on the floor.

Scenario 2

Mrs. Smith has brought her 8-year-old daughter to the community health center for evaluation of her "impossible behavior." She says that her daughter has been lying, stealing, and talking back to her. Unlike her 9-year-old son who is well behaved and successful in school, this daughter is "good for nothing." When the nurse does a routine blood pressure check, she discovers marks on the daughter's arm that she says are from being "tied up."

Scenario 3

During a home visit, a nurse discovers that Mrs. Bowers, a 55-year-old woman with schizophrenia, has stopped taking her medicine again and is experiencing psychoses. Mrs. Bowers believes that God is telling her to stay in her home and pray for the Second Coming of Christ. She has not eaten or bathed in 2 weeks, and she fears that the nurse is trying to harm her.

Scenario 4

Mr. Washington is a 35-year-old veteran of the Persian Gulf War diagnosed with post-traumatic stress disorder. He served in the U.S. Army in heavy combat as a tank commander. Although he has a college degree in computer science, he has held 12 jobs, each of which have lasted no longer than 2 or 3 months, since returning from combat. He has been abusing alcohol and crack cocaine. While intoxicated, Mr. Washington has beaten his wife and physically attacked a neighbor. He has not been given any jail time because of his mental health problems. During this hospitalization, Mr. Washington is hoping to make a case for receiving 100% psychiatric disability benefits for his condition.

Scenario 5

Ms. Crane is a 22-year-old woman who calls the crisis hot line on a weekly basis. Tonight she is once again threatening suicide because her boyfriend has broken up with her. Last month, she took an overdose of 10 aspirin in front of her boyfriend, forcing him to drive her to the emergency department where her stomach was pumped. Ms. Crane is an attractive, bright woman who is very demanding and needy. She says that she cannot live without her boyfriend, even though he has repeatedly "cheated on her."

Now, for each scenario, ask yourself the following questions:

- What are the potential obstacles to establishing a therapeutic relationship with this client?
- What possible attitudes from the nurse's personal and cultural background may interfere with his or her ability to convey an accepting, nonjudgmental approach to the client?
- What specific actions would be most helpful to establish rapport with the client, define the parameters of the relationship, and reduce anxiety?

---

access to the private thoughts and feelings of clients as a delicate privilege to be handled with the utmost care.

LACK OF SELF-AWARENESS

Interacting with clients who are in emotional pain requires a certain level of maturity and self-awareness (Eckroth-Bucher, 2001). Nurses must be able to monitor and contain their own anxiety when clients discuss frightening incidents or relate tragic events that generate feelings of hopelessness and despair. Being able to listen to clients without mentally or physically fleeing from the situation or offering impersonal platitudes is a key ingredi-

ent to a therapeutic relationship. Clients must feel safe with the nurse. They must be able to sense that the nurse can handle what they are saying without becoming overwhelmed by the nurse's reactions. For this reason, nurses must also appreciate the importance of taking care of their own mental health.

Developing self-awareness is a lifelong process that requires continual work. It necessitates disciplined attention to one's own feelings and needs, as well as insight about how to meet those needs. Nurses go through their own ups and downs in life, rendering them more or less able to respond flexibly and easily to the demands of others. Knowing one's own limits, detecting signs of becom-

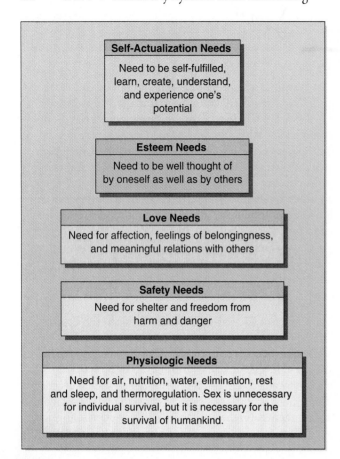

FIGURE 4-1   Maslow's hierarchy of human needs.

ing exhausted or less tolerant, and being able to nourish oneself physically, mentally, and spiritually is essential to becoming a therapeutic agent for others. For some nurses, being critical or defensive with clients is a warning signal that it is time to take a rest or seek support. Other important warning signals include the following:

- Worrying about clients when off duty
- Becoming overinvolved with clients in inappropriate ways (eg, making extra visits when time does not allow for them, calling clients when off duty) (Gallop, 1998)
- Believing that you are the only person who can help a client; that is, having "rescue fantasies"

Both negative, rejecting attitudes and overprotective, rescuing behaviors may be indicators of what are called **countertransference** reactions in nurses and mental health professionals (Ens, 1999) (Research in Psychiatric-Mental Health Nursing 4-2). Determining the appropriate level of involvement with clients that maximizes therapeutic relationships while protecting one's energy and mental health is something most nurses learn with experience (Morse, 1991).

Maturity is another important quality linked with self-awareness. Of course, maturity is not just a function of age. Some middle-aged people behave immaturely,

while some young people are wise beyond their years. **Maturity** involves being able to integrate aspects of life into a whole and find balance in one's outlook and attitudes toward others. This important factor allows nurses to feel empathy for others (Price & Archbold, 1997). Whereas nurses who lack maturity cannot see the similarities between themselves and others, more mature nurses can see and imagine the smallest of similarities because they feel a oneness with all human beings.

Phases of the Therapeutic Relationship

The next section explores the development of the therapeutic relationship. Each phase of the therapeutic relationship has predictable behaviors, dynamics, and challenges. This discussion will enumerate the key tasks of each phase and describe the process of movement through the relationship from introduction to termination.

INTRODUCTORY PHASE

Therapeutic relationships do not occur instantaneously; they take time to develop. The goal of the introductory phase is to establish rapport and build a foundation for further work. During the initial phase of the relationship, the nurse focuses on the following:

- Introducing himself or herself and learning the client's name
- Communicating interest in the client
- Responding to any immediate concerns or needs, such as questions, comfort needs, or emergency issues
- Setting the parameters for the nurse–client interactions
- Gathering data
- Discerning the focal problem, setting goals, and beginning to plan interventions
- Reducing the client's anxieties

Nurses may establish formal or informal *contracts* to determine the parameters of the relationship. Contracts may include such topics as the time and place of meetings, procedures for keeping appointments, limits of confidentiality, types of problems to be addressed, and the process of reevaluating expectations and goals (Arnold, 1999b). Nurses inform the client when the desired goals are beyond their realm of expertise or the duration of the interaction. For example, if a client wants a nurse to help him or her find housing and this is beyond the scope of the nurse's role, the nurse should make an appropriate referral so that the client does not feel frustrated with the nurse's apparent lack of attention to his or her needs.

During the introductory phase of the relationship, clients commonly test the nurse's commitment by acting

Purpose: To explore the question, "What is it like for a nurse working in the area of psychiatric-mental health nursing to experience feelings of countertransference for a client?"

Background: *Countertransference* involves the arousal of uncomfortable, sometimes unprofessional feelings toward clients, which may result in overly protective or rejecting behaviors. While past professionals viewed countertransference in a derogatory, condescending manner, many now see it as a natural outgrowth of working closely with clients who present difficult behaviors and painful emotions. Self-awareness is important for recognizing countertransference reactions and learning to use these feelings to better understand oneself, the client, and the dynamics of the therapeutic interaction.

Method and Sample: This phenomenological study is based on interviews with five experienced psychiatric nurses (two men and three women) who worked on inpatient psychiatric units. The researchers analyzed the data using the seven steps of Colaizzi's procedure for phenomenological data analysis.

Findings:
- As novice psychiatric nurses, the participants recalled experiencing self-doubt when they realized their negative feelings toward clients were contrary to what they had learned in nursing school. They feared openly discussing these feelings and continued to struggle alone unless a peer provided unsolicited guidance. When the anxiety and self-doubt reached intolerable levels, the nurses sought relief by questioning others. An epiphany occurred when the universality of both positive and negative countertransference became obvious and the nurse became aware that complete neutrality was impossible. This led to increased self-awareness

and the ability to recognize the nurse's own reactions as a natural part of the self.
- This learning process was gradual, and it resulted in the nurse's increased ability to accept the client's choices. The nurse could stop reacting to the client in a way that mirrored the reactions of everyone else in the client's social world. A feeling of self-mastery occurred.
- The awareness of countertransference enabled the nurse to monitor his or her tone of voice, body language, and remarks to avoid conveying negative feelings toward the client. It also prevented withdrawal from the client.
- As the nurses developed an understanding of countertransference, they incorporated it into their practice by oscillating their level of attachment to clients so that they could draw back when necessary and avoid inappropriate self-disclosure. They could discriminate between ordinary reactions that anyone might have when faced with a particular behavior and more personal or problematic responses.

Application to Nursing Practice: This study demonstrates the importance of cultivating self-awareness in psychiatric-mental health nursing. Because this learning process is gradual, nurses must encourage open discussion of their countertransference reactions so that they can learn from and support one another along the way. By recognizing positive countertransference reactions, nurses can avoid assuming too much responsibility for clients and pressuring them to behave in ways that conflict with their needs and wishes. Awareness of negative countertransference reactions can prevent nurses and clients from acting out in ways that undermine the therapeutic relationship.

From Ens, I. C. (1999). The lived experience of countertransference in psychiatric/mental health nurses. *Archives of Psychiatric Nursing, 13*(6), 321–329.

out or missing appointments. They may show their worst behavior (eg, challenging, withdrawal) in an attempt to see whether the nurse can handle the intensity of their problems. After all, if a nurse is scared off by the client's symptoms and coping patterns, the relationship may not be safe or there may be no point in investing energy into it. Clients may wonder during this phase whether the nurse is just doing his or her job or if he or she really cares. At this time, the nurse must remain consistently available, caring, and respectful toward clients. Gently confronting or questioning client's acting-out behavior will set the stage for open discussion throughout the rela-

tionship, indicating that the nurse can tolerate conflict and help the client to explore his or her own ambivalence about treatment and behavior change.

In the therapeutic relationship, the nurse exercises a certain amount of power over the client through the use of language and techniques of persuasion and by assuming control of the agenda. The aim, however, should be to create a collaborative and open relationship in which the client feels free to identify needs, desires, and goals. The relationship is under way when the nurse and client progress beyond exchanging information to exploring deeper feelings and issues that are of pressing concern to the client.

Interestingly, one study found that, with the movement toward brief treatment, many clients are discharged or transferred from psychiatric units while they are still in the orientation or introductory phase of the nurse–client relationship (Forchuk, 1995). Whereas negative preconceptions by both clients and nurses have been associated with a lengthening of the orientation or introductory phase, longer interactions with clients (eg, one 30-minute interaction instead of several 10-minute "check-ins") have been found to predict faster movement from the orientation to the working phase (Forchuk, 1994, 1995).

Before moving to the next phase of the relationship, the nurse and client should evaluate whether they have met the following goals of the pivotal initial stage:

- Trust is established, and both parties perceive the relationship as safe.
- The client can verbalize thoughts and feelings.
- Both the nurse and client have identified and agreed upon a focal problem or purpose for the relationship.
- The client's strengths, weaknesses, and priorities for intervention are becoming clear.
- The nurse has explained his or her role.

MIDDLE OR WORKING PHASE

In the working phase of the relationship, the client is actively involved in achieving goals set during the initial phase. He or she makes progress by testing out new behaviors, identifying resources, and discovering new avenues for change. For example, in the working phase of the relationship, a client with schizophrenia may try new cognitive and behavioral strategies for dealing with hallucinations. Success in coping with hallucinations may allow the client to function better in family or community settings, foster a more hopeful attitude toward the illness, and create new opportunities for change, such as supervised employment and friendships. As the client achieves goals, nurses should provide feedback and support. This support is especially important for clients who may not notice or take credit for their own gradual changes. Behaviors do not change easily. It takes energy, practice, and the willingness to risk failure to make any significant change.

Of course, many clients go through periods where they resist change. Implications for Nursing Practice 4-1 discusses how to deal with resistance in clients.

For some clients, the working phase may be a period of major change and life reorganization. An adolescent may stop acting out and find a way to communicate with his or her parents; a homeless individual may find employment; a depressed mother may begin to enjoy her family again. Many clients with chronic conditions revisit their problems throughout their lives, however, focusing on different layers of difficulties and new challenges. For those clients, a consumer-oriented practice model that works in partnership with clients to increase their level of function-

Implications for Nursing Practice 4-1

Dealing With Clients Who Resist Change

Resistance to change is a normal occurrence in the working phase of the therapeutic relationship (Patterson & Welfel, 1994). Change does not usually occur in a linear fashion, but rather in stops and starts, with periods of regression to old patterns. Some clients demonstrate so much resistance to change that it may appear that they are making no progress. Examples include:

- Clients who have repeated episodes of psychosis because they stop taking their medications
- People who make multiple suicide attempts
- Adolescents with anorexia who lose the weight they gained each time they leave the hospital
- Clients recovering from substance abuse problems who resume their use of drugs or alcohol

Such clients may seem unable or unwilling to change.

Nurses must maintain hope and optimism that change will occur when the time is right, when the client has learned what he or she needs to know, when the client has developed new coping skills and adequate support systems are in place, and when circumstances have paved the way for a major shift in thinking. It may be helpful for nurses to reflect on a bad habit or personality trait that they themselves have been trying to change and to note how slow and difficult the process has been for them. When working with clients who are highly resistant to change, mental health professionals may feel so frustrated that they become critical and blaming. Although confrontation and education have a place in the therapeutic relationship, criticism and blame can destroy it. Hoff (2001) refers to this dynamic as the victim-rescuer-persecutor syndrome. In this familiar cycle, the following steps occur:

1. The client is vulnerable and requests help.
2. Mental health professionals offer help.
3. The client has difficulty changing well-established behavior patterns.
4. The professional feels frustrated with the "treatment failure."
5. The professional "persecutes" the client ("victim") for failing to respond.
6. Finally, the victim becomes the persecutor and punishes the professional for well-intended but inappropriate efforts to help.

To avoid this destructive pattern, nurses need to be aware of countertransference reactions (see Research in Psychiatric-Mental Health Nursing 4-2); monitor their levels of patience, empathy, and flexibility in dealing with persistent behavioral patterns that resist change; and seek support and supervision when they become frustrated with clients.

ing and quality of life, while considering their particular symptom patterns, recovery process, cultural background, and overall wellness may be the best paradigm for the working phase (Warren & Lutz, 2000).

The tasks of the working phase of the therapeutic relationship include the following:

- Identify past behaviors that have been ineffective for coping with the focal problem.
- Develop a plan of action, practice implementing it, and evaluate its effectiveness.
- Integrate a new self-concept, worldview, or attitude toward one's illness as a result of changes in behavior and circumstances.
- Increase hopefulness for the future and ability to function independently.

TERMINATION PHASE

Whether the nurse and client work together in a brief or long-term setting, the nurse must pay attention to the termination phase of the relationship. He or she must mention the date of termination well in advance (Carson, 1999). Termination always involves a loss. If substantial work has been done, both the nurse and client may feel the loss of the helping relationship. If goals have not been realized because of time constraints or the limitations of the relationship, the termination may seem less significant.

Clients often regress during the termination phase. Examples of such regression include evidencing the original symptoms or testing the nurse's belief in the client's abilities to function independently. Most likely, the client is afraid or anxious at the loss of the relationship because it has provided him or her with a buffer and source of support. Now the client will have to handle problems on his or her own. Anxiety contributes to reverting to previous bad habits. Considering that loss is a universal aspect of the human experience, the client's historical way of dealing with losses may manifest itself during the termination phase. Some clients feel rejected, others withdraw prematurely to protect themselves from the pain of grieving, and others try to end the relationship angrily and abruptly.

During the termination phase, the nurse's job is to remain consistent, caring, and hopeful about the client's progress. This is the time to review the work that has been done, discuss any remaining questions, clear up misconceptions, and applaud the client's progress in making changes. On a more human level, it is a time for remembering the high points in the relationship (times of laughter or moments of insight), acknowledging and letting go of the low points, and appreciating the time that the nurse and client have spent together. During the termination phase, nurses should feel free to share their positive feelings for clients, admiration, and enjoyment of the relationship.

During the termination phase, nurses need to educate families about the client's condition, advise them of the potential for symptom recurrence, and inform them about signs of relapse (Pillette, Berck, & Archber, 1995). They should make specific recommendations regarding how to help clients maintain their improved level of functioning.

Tasks of the termination phase include the following:

- Spacing contacts with the client further apart or decreasing the length of appointments to allow for increased independence
- Expressing feelings about the loss of the relationship
- Establishing a more relaxed, less intense interaction
- Focusing on the future
- Discouraging cues that lead to new areas of exploration
- Providing necessary referrals and links with community resources

THERAPEUTIC COMMUNICATION

Communication is the process of conveying information through a complex variety of verbal and nonverbal behaviors. This process can be broken down into several components. The **communicators** are those individuals who simultaneously send and receive messages through words and nonverbal behaviors (eg, nodding, eye contact, facial expressions, posture). **Encoding** is the process by which one communicator puts into words or behaviors the ideas or feelings that he or she is trying to convey. Examples of encoding include shouting, crying, looking away, and choosing particular words. **Decoding** means the process by which one communicator discerns or interprets what another communicator is saying. The **channel** is the route or method a communicator chooses to convey his or her message. Channels include writing, talking, looking, e-mailing, and phoning. **Feedback** means the discernible response that a receiver makes to a sender's message. All behaviors, including silence and ignoring, are forms of feedback.

Environment refers to the personal experiences and cultural background that each communicator brings to the interaction. Environmental variables include age, socioeconomic status, race, and life events such as death, divorce, and illness. Whereas similarities in environmental experiences can lead to common understanding, coming from different environments can create communication gaps (Adler & Towne, 2002). Another factor that can influence the effectiveness of communication is **noise**, which consists of any force caused by communicators or in the environment that interferes with effective communication. **External noise** refers to any factor outside a communicator that creates distractions (eg, other people talking, a cold or hot room, background noise). **Physiologic noise** refers to any physical factor within the communicator that detracts from effective communication (eg, hearing loss, tiredness, sedating medication, physical pain). **Psychological noise** refers to any force within a communicator that interferes with accurately expressing or understanding a message (eg, anger, defensiveness, paranoia, apathy, fear).

Therapeutic communication occurs when the nurse demonstrates empathy, uses effective communication skills, and responds to the client's thoughts, needs, and concerns. It is a planned process that allows the nurse and client to build a trusting relationship in which the client is free to express thoughts, feelings, and options without fear of judgment. This communication process is based on specific skills that the nurse learns to implement through careful practice and experience. It does not just arise naturally. Therapeutic (or effective) communication techniques include giving broad openings, paraphrasing, offering general leads, reflecting feelings, focusing, voicing doubt, clarifying, placing events in a time sequence, giving information, encouraging formulation of a plan, and testing discrepancies. The purposes for using these therapeutic communication techniques and examples of them are found in Table 4-2.

Nontherapeutic communication is the process of interaction that develops when the nurse responds in ways that cause clients to feel defensive, misunderstood, controlled, minimized, alienated, or discouraged from expressing their thoughts and feelings. Nontherapeutic techniques include responding socially, using closed-ended questions, changing the subject, belittling, making stereotyped comments, giving false reassurance, moralizing, interpreting, advising, challenging, and defending. While most people have used nontherapeutic responses in their everyday communication with others, it is important to be aware of how these responses deter open discussion and increase the likelihood of withdrawal by clients. Learning the labels for the nontherapeutic approaches will help nurses to recognize and avoid using them. These nontherapeutic approaches, why they are used, and examples of them are found in Table 4-3.

Theoretical Framework and Communication Model

Interactions between any individuals, including the nurse and client, can be understood by using a communication model (Figure 4-2). Looking at communication from the viewpoint of this model, it is apparent that nurse–client communication is made up of many interrelated components, giving rise to highly unique interactions depending on the backgrounds, moods, and circumstances operating in each situation. In this sense, no two interactions are the same, and it is impossible to predict how any encounter may unfold. The wonder of human communi-

cation is that it generates the variety and spontaneity that make nursing challenging and ever-changing work.

External, physical, and physiologic noise can occur at any point in the nurse–client interaction and disrupt the accurate flow of communication. A lack of sufficient overlap in the environments of the communicators (eg, nurses using professional jargon that clients do not understand, clients trying to convey their sense of financial desperation to middle-class nurses who have never known hunger or homelessness) may block the communication process before it begins. The subtle and obvious nonverbal reactions of both the nurse and client continually shape each interaction in a complex way, creating a unique climate or tone for each relationship. Thus, to become effective communicators, nurses must practice the art of carefully observing their clients' messages and consistently monitoring their own words and behaviors. Even the nurses' manner of dress communicates messages that affect others' perceptions (Verderber, 2001).

Listening

Listening, or focusing on all the behaviors expressed by the client, is the foundation of therapeutic communication. Listening requires energy, concentration, and specific skills in asking questions, while allowing the client to determine the content and level of disclosure in the interaction. Listening is an active process that focuses objective, empathic attention on the client. The characteristics of active listening are as follows:

- Maintaining eye contact
- Facilitating close proximity (if this is not threatening to the client)
- Projecting a relaxed physical orientation
- Speaking in a calm voice

The nurse sets the stage for listening by removing distractions from the environment, such as television or the presence of others; preventing interruptions; and attending to the client's physical comfort. Another key component of listening is a nonjudgmental stance that allows for supportive, objective feedback.

The nurse notes congruence (agreement) or incongruence between verbal and nonverbal communication and validates these observations with the client. An example of incongruence would be a client experiencing psychoses who says he is willing to talk but projects nonverbal cues of fear and withdrawal. Nurses must attend to their own feelings and thoughts that may provoke nontherapeutic reactions, such as changing the subject because of anxiety, becoming annoyed or critical, or feeling overwhelmed by sadness or helplessness as a result of the client's situation.

To see how nurses can use effective listening skills in interactions with clients, see Therapeutic Communication 4-1 and Therapeutic Communication 4-2.

(text continues on page 70)

would be most difficult for you to work with and why? How do you think you can cultivate your own self-awareness to become more sensitive to clients, regardless of the setting where you choose to practice?

3. Recall a helping relationship in your life with a teacher, clergy person, counselor, or other community resource person. How did the phases of the therapeutic relationship mirror those described in this chapter? Which tasks were most difficult to achieve? What did the helper do to build an effective therapeutic relationship and to facilitate your movement through the phase?

4. After an interaction with a client, write down a verbatim account of what was said to the best of your recollection. Which therapeutic and nontherapeutic communication techniques did you use? What was the impact of these techniques on the therapeutic relationship? How can you improve your listening skills?

5. Practice the assertiveness, perception-checking, and positive reframing techniques described in this chapter. How difficult were they to use? What was the outcome? How did these techniques differ from your usual mode of communication?

▼ CHAPTER SUMMARY

- Trust, professionalism, mutual respect, caring, and partnership are key elements of a therapeutic nurse–client relationship.
- Obstacles to effective nurse–client relationships in the psychiatric setting include the nurse's judgmental attitudes, excessive probing, and lack of self-awareness.
- The phases of the therapeutic relationship are the introductory phase, working phase, and termination phase.
- Each phase of the therapeutic relationship has a unique set of characteristics and goals.
- A theoretical model of communication can be used to analyze the components of the nurse–client dialogue.
- The nurse uses a specific set of listening skills to facilitate communication with clients, while avoiding ineffective listening techniques.
- Assertiveness and confrontation skills are necessary for communicating effectively and respectfully with psychiatric clients who are in distress.
- The focus of the therapeutic relationship is on the client's needs, and the nurse should follow strict guidelines for using self-disclosure with clients.
- Building a therapeutic relationship with the client's family and loved ones is a key component of effective nursing care.
- Continued self-examination and practice are required to become a skilled, effective, and caring professional nurse.

▼ REVIEW QUESTIONS

1. A client reveals to the nurse that prior to her hospitalization, she had been very promiscuous. The client's revelation suggests she
   a. Respects the nurse
   b. Trusts the nurse
   c. Views the nurse as a professional
   d. Considers the nurse a partner in her recovery

2. The mother of a 17-year-old girl with a history of several hospitalizations for depression seems guarded and defensive during the interview. She tells the nurse, "We really are a loving family." The nurse understands that the mother's defensiveness may be related to
   a. Unspoken blame she has felt by healthcare professionals and others for her daughter's illness
   b. Her own dysfunctional behavior
   c. Her disrespect for the nurse
   d. Her desire to cover up for her own sense of failure

3. When establishing a therapeutic relationship, nurses demonstrate that they can be trusted by
   a. Including the client's family in the recovery process
   b. Being consistent, honest, and sensitive
   c. Being competent and knowledgeable
   d. Honoring cultural traditions

4. A client is telling the nurse about his struggle with schizophrenia. The nurse understands that creating a therapeutic relationship will depend, in part, on her ability to
   a. Provide advice
   b. Be sympathetic
   c. Become emotionally involved
   d. Be empathetic

5. A mental health nurse arranges to meet a depressed client on her weekend off. The nurse is worried that the client will be lonely over the weekend. These actions demonstrate that
   a. The nurse is conscientious and caring.
   b. The nurse has established a therapeutic relationship with the client.
   c. The nurse is overly protective and lacks self-awareness.
   d. The nurse is judgmental.

6. A client has failed to show up for her second appointment with the nurse. She calls later, crying hysterically, saying she's sorry she forgot. The nurse understands that testing behavior is common in the introductory phase of relationship development and responds appropriately by
   a. Gently questioning the client about her acting-out behavior
   b. Firmly establishing boundaries about acceptable and unacceptable behavior

c. Ignoring the behavior and rescheduling the appointment

d. Referring the client to a psychotherapist

7. A client is shouting at the nurse. Which of the following responses by the nurse reflects an assertive statement?

a. "Mr. Smith, I understand that you are upset, but you are acting childishly. Please settle down so we can talk."

b. "Mr. Smith, I understand that you are upset, but I feel threatened by your shouting. I would like you to lower your voice so that we can talk."

c. "Mr. Smith, I feel that you are out of line, so I suggest you lower your voice."

d. "Mr. Smith, please lower your voice. I can only talk with you if you do not shout."

8. A client in the open psychiatric unit tells the nurse he doesn't love his wife and has had many extramarital affairs. After this discussion, the client avoids further talks with the nurse by not meeting scheduled appointments. Which of the following responses would be most helpful to the therapeutic relationship?

a. "I understand that you think you were too open with me, but I feel like you are avoiding me. I would like to schedule a meeting with you to discuss this matter."

b. "You haven't kept our last two appointments. I thought perhaps you were sorry that you revealed your feelings about your wife or that possibly my response was not helpful. Can you tell me more about what your feeling?"

c. "We haven't talked in a few days. Would you like to talk more about your feelings toward your wife?"

d. "When we spoke on Monday, you said that you didn't love your wife. Now it seems as though you are holding back. Is there more going on than you told me?"

9. A client asks the nurse about how she has handled raising her teenagers. The nurse understands that self-disclosure sometimes can be therapeutic. Which of the following statements accurately represents self-disclosure?

a. Self-disclosure can help normalize the client's experience.

b. Self-disclosure about current, painful situations allows the client to see the nurse as a real human being.

c. Self-disclosure can help the client feel like a friend.

d. Self-disclosure should be detailed so the client doesn't feel unimportant or devalued.

10. A nurse is interviewing a family for the first time. He notes that the mother takes charge of introducing

everyone and telling him that they've come to therapy because of the older son's acting-out behavior. The father and the three children nod but do not say anything. The nurse's immediate response is to

a. Acknowledge the older son first, because his behavior has been mentioned as problematic

b. Acknowledge the father first, because he is the other parent

c. Acknowledge the children first, as they may feel left out of the situation

d. Acknowledge the mother first, as she seems to take the lead

▼ REFERENCES AND SUGGESTED READINGS

*Adler, R. A., & Towne, N. (2002). *Looking out/looking in* (10th ed.). Fort Worth: Harcourt.

*Arnold, E. (1999a). Communicating with families. In E. Arnold & K. U. Boggs (Eds.), *Interpersonal relationships: Professional communication skills for nurses* (3rd ed.). Philadelphia: W.B. Saunders.

*Arnold, E. (1999b). Structuring the relationship. In E. Arnold & K. U. Boggs (Eds.), *Interpersonal relationships: Professional communication skills for nurses* (3rd ed.). Philadelphia: W.B. Saunders.

*Bailey, J., & Baillie, L. (1996). Transactional analysis: How to improve communication skills. *Nursing Standard, 35,* 39–42.

*Balzer-Riley, J. (2000). *Communications in nursing* (4th ed.). St. Louis: Mosby.

*Carson, V. B. (1999). The grief experience: Life's losses and endings. In E. Arnold & K. U. Boggs (Eds.), *Interpersonal relationships: Professional communication skills for nurses* (3rd ed.). Philadelphia: W.B. Saunders.

*Chenevert, M. (1994). *Special techniques in assertiveness training* (4th ed.). St. Louis: Mosby.

*Chipman, Y. (1992). Caring: Its meaning and place in the practice of nursing. *Journal of Nursing Education, 30,* 171–175.

*Deering, C. G. (1993). Giving and taking criticism. *American Journal of Nursing, 93,* 56–61.

*Deering, C. G. (1999). To speak or not to speak: Self-disclosure with clients. *American Journal of Nursing, 99,* 34–38.

*Eckroth-Bucher, M. (2001). Philosophical basis and practice of self-awareness in psychiatric nursing. *Journal of Psychosocial Nursing, 39*(2), 33–39.

*Ens, I. C. (1999). The lived experience of countertransference in psychiatric/mental health nurses. *Archives of Psychiatric Nursing, 13*(6), 321–329.

*Forchuk, C. (1994). The orientation phase of the nurse–client relationship: Testing Peplau's theory. *Journal of Advanced Nursing, 20,* 532–537.

*Forchuk, C. (1995). Development of nurse–client relationships: What helps? *Journal of the American Psychiatric Nurses Association, 1,* 146–153.

*Gallop, R. (1998). Postdischarge social contact: A potential area of boundary violation. *Journal of the American Psychiatric Nurses Association, 4*(4), 105–109.

*Glen, S., & Jownally, S. (1995). Privacy: A key nursing concept. *British Journal of Nursing, 4,* 69–72.

*Heifner, C. (1993). Positive connectedness in the psychiatric nurse–patient relationship. *Archives of Psychiatric Nursing, 7,* 11–15.

*Hoff, L. A. (2001). *People in crisis: Understanding and helping* (5th ed.). San Francisco: Jossey-Bass.

*Krauss, J. (2000). Protecting the legacy: The nurse–patient relationship and the therapeutic alliance. *Archives of Psychiatric Nursing, 14*(2), 49–50.

*Morse, J. M. (1991). Negotiating commitment and involvement in the nurse–patient relationship. *Journal of Advanced Nursing, 16,* 455–468.

Morse, J. M., Havens, G. A. D., & Wilson, S. (1997). The comforting interaction: Developing a model of nurse–patient relationship. *Scholarly Inquiry for Nursing Practice: An International Journal, 11,* 321–343.

Palmer-Erbs, V., & Anthony, W. (1995). Incorporating psychiatric rehabilitation principles into mental health nursing: An opportunity to develop full partnership among nurses, consumers, and families. *Journal of Psychosocial Nursing, 33,* 36–44.

*Patterson, L. E., & Welfel, E. R. (1994). *The counseling process* (4th ed.). Pacific Grove: Brooks/Cole.

*Peplau, H. (1952). *Interpersonal relations in nursing.* New York: J.P. Putnam.

*Pillette, P. C., Berck, C. B., & Archber, L. C. (1995). Therapeutic management of helping boundaries. *Journal of Psychosocial Nursing, 33,* 40–47.

*Price, V., & Archbold, J. (1997). What's it all about, empathy? *Nurse Education Today, 17,* 106–110.

*Rogers, C. R. (1952). *Client-centered therapy.* Boston: Houghton Mifflin.

Schafer, P. (1997). When a patient develops an attraction: Successful resolution versus boundary violation. *Journal of Psychiatric and Mental Health Nursing, 4*(3), 203–211.

Shuster, P. M. (2000). *Communication: The key to the therapeutic relationship.* Philadelphia: F.A. Davis.

*van Servellen, G. M. (1997). *Communication skills for the health-care professional: Concepts and techniques.* Gaithersburg, MD: Aspen.

*Verderber, R. F. (2001). *Communicate!* (9th ed.). Belmont, CA: Wadsworth.

*Walker, K. M. (2001). Empathy from a nursing perspective: Moving beyond borrowed theory. *Archives of Psychiatric Nursing, 15,* 140–147.

*Warren, B. J., & Lutz, W. J. (2000). A consumer-oriented practice model for psychiatric nursing. *Archives of Psychiatric Nursing, 14*(3), 117–126.

Starred references are cited in text.

For additional information on this chapter, go to *http://connection. lww.com.*

Need more help? See Chapter 4 of the *Study Guide to Accompany Mohr: Johnson's Psychiatric-Mental Health Nursing, 5th edition.*

Culture

MARY HUGGINS

▼ KEY TERMS

Assimilation—The prevailing expectation during most of the 20th century for immigrants and minority groups in the United States to become like the majority (white) culture.

Cultural competence—The skills, both academic and interpersonal, that allow persons to understand and appreciate cultural differences and similarities within, between, and among groups.

Culture—The integration of human behavior (including thoughts, communications, actions, customs, beliefs, values, and institutions) of a racial, ethnic, religious, or social group.

Culture bound—A term used to describe a person whose understanding of other cultures is limited

because he or she refuses to explore beyond the parameters of his or her personal culture.

Culture care theory—A theory developed by Dr. Madeleine Leininger that emphasizes learning principles related to culture care, culturalogic assessments, the universality of culture care diversity, and the importance of fit between the client's healthcare values and services provided.

Discrimination—Differential treatment based on race, class, gender, or other variables rather than on individual merit.

Ethnocentrism—The belief that one's own cultural practices and values are inherently correct or superior to those of others.

Flexibility—The ability to embrace change by modifying expectations, readjusting old operating norms and stereotypes, and trying new behavior.

Prejudice—Negative preconceived opinions about other people or groups based on hearsay, perception, or emotion.

Stereotyping—Believing that one member of a cultural group will display certain behaviors or hold certain attitudes (usually negative) simply because he or she is a member of that cultural group.

Stigmatization—The attribution of negative characteristics or identity to one person or group, causing the person or group to feel rejected, alienated, and ostracized from society.

▼ LEARNING OBJECTIVES

On completion of this chapter, you should be able to accomplish the following:

- Describe the importance of culture to human behavior and its effect on the provision of effective mental health services.
- Explain how demographic changes in North America are contributing to the importance of cultural awareness.
- Describe the elements of a culturally congruent service system.
- Identify disparities in mental health for clients from minority cultures.
- Explore possible barriers that have led to mental health disparities for clients from minority cultures.
- Discuss biologic variations and various social, psychological, and spiritual perspectives within ethnic groups and across cultures.

- Identify the important aspects of transcultural assessment.
- Describe skills essential to the implementation of culturally competent care.
- Explain nurses' unique position in providing culturally competent care.
- Assess one's own heritage, reference group, and personal and cultural biases.

▼ Clinical Example 5-1

Somalia covers 246,300 square miles on the Horn of Africa. It is a hot, semiarid land. In 1981, clan rivalries, corruption, and abundant weaponry (supplied by the United States and the Soviet Union) combined to spark civil war. By 1992, famine and disease had engulfed Somalia. The United Nations (UN) partly redressed famine; however, many Somalis resented the foreign presence of the UN, which withdrew from Somalia in 1995. Soon after, rival warlords ruled Somalia. A peace pact was forged in 1997; the following year, it fell apart and the fighting resumed.

Somalia is organized into large, extended family clans. These large clans are subdivided into lineage units, which are further subdivided into kinship alliances. Kinship alliances are important to the people of Somalia in terms of how they address one another. Until recently, the language of Somalia was unwritten, with three main dialects spoken. Songs and poetry were the important vehicles for passing oral traditions.

Somali women generally do not touch males when greeting them. These women socialize either at home (in the late afternoon in urban areas) or at the market. Furthermore, women do not eat with men. Most Somalis are Sunni Muslims, who observe the religious practice of praying five times a day. Before prayers, Muslims must cleanse their bodies. They also must abstain from alcohol and pork. Muslims observe Ramadan, the ninth month of the Muslim year, by fasting from sunrise to sunset.

All of this information became important in the case of a 35-year-old Somali woman with schizophrenia who was relocated to a Midwestern city in the United States during the civil war in her homeland. Because Somali women primarily stay at home, the woman had never been diagnosed with mental illness while in her home country. It is difficult to know, therefore, if the stress of war and relocation precipitated her schizophrenia or if she had a prior history of the illness. The client had been attending a Psychosocial Rehabilitation Center for 4 years. She found no one who could understand her dialect, but she could not communicate in English. A Muslim man who spoke Somali participated in a neighboring program and could provide some translation for the client and staff. This situation was uncomfortable for the client, however, because the translator was not from her lineage and was of the opposite sex.

In addition to these problems, several issues were of concern:

- The client had stopped taking her psychotropic medications, and her condition was deteriorating. Rehospitalization appeared imminent.
- She locked herself in the program's only female restroom two or three times a day for long periods. When she was finished, she would leave water all over the floor, creating a hazard for the next person to use the restroom. Other participants would complain of the client's lengthy uses of the bathroom as well as the "mess" she left behind.
- The client refused to eat several of the meals at the program. Because the program served the most substantial meal of the day for its participants, the client's nutritional status was an increasing concern.

The nurse's role was to help create a culturally specific support plan to address these issues and try to stabilize the client in the community. The nurse sought assistance from an interpreter and a Muslim elder in the community. Together, this group worked with the client and determined that the primary issues were the client's religion and the program's ability to meet her needs. The team worked with other healthcare staff to provide the following accommodations:

- The nurse recognized that it was Ramadan, when Muslims are required to fast from sunrise to sunset. During the time the client spent at the Psychosocial Rehabilitation Center, the program served food during lunch and dinner hours only, periods when the client could ingest nothing but water. Because she had no money, the client had nothing at home to eat. Furthermore, because she was supposed to take her medications with meals, she had stopped using them during Ramadan. The nurse found that this client had the same pattern of difficulty and rehospitalization during Ramadan since starting the program 3 years ago. After discussing the situation with a Muslim elder, the nurse created a plan for the client to take her medications and eat meals after sunset and before sunrise. Program staff members made arrangements to send food home with the client to use for meals.
- The team learned that the client was using the restroom for her ritual cleansing and to pray two or three of the required times during the day. The nurse and program staff members arranged to give the client a quiet place for her prayers. They instructed other program participants to allow the client privacy during this time. The nurse also asked the client to remove as much of the water overflow as possible so that it would no longer be a hazard to others after her cleansing.
- The meals that the client was refusing during times other than Ramadan contained pork. Therefore, the nurse arranged to provide an alternative meal when pork was on the menu. The team also arranged for the client to assist in the kitchen with other participants. This decision helped to foster socialization for the client by letting her practice skills within an area of familiarity.
- Finally, the nurse used this opportunity to teach staff members and participants about Somalia. Staff members found speakers originally from Somalia to make presentations discussing their country of origin with program participants. Such presentations helped the client feel accepted and "at home."

As a result of these interventions, this Somali woman was not hospitalized during Ramadan since her immigration to the United States. Furthermore, although she continues to experience stress-related symptoms, she regularly takes her psychotropic medications. She is involved in the program and has not been rehospitalized for 18 months.

Points for Reflection and Critical Thinking

- How do you think cultural stereotyping influences the delivery of psychiatric care? Can you find evidence of stereotyping in the example given here? How might such problems have been prevented?
- What other issues could emerge in the future care of this client?
- What should the role of healthcare providers be when clients do not have a family or community to support them?

Nursing is a reflection of society. U.S. society is, itself, undergoing a transformation. By the middle of the 21st century, predictions are that the average U.S. citizen (as defined by Census Bureau statistics) will trace his or her ancestry to Africa, the Pacific Islands, or Hispanic or Arab lands rather than to European countries. This growing cultural diversity underscores the importance of learning about different cultures and recognizing the various needs of people who come from cultural groups that might be unfamiliar to the nurse.

This chapter assists the nurse to understand how culture influences a client's behavior in health and in illness. When the nurse views clients through a cultural lens, he or she can both expand cultural awareness and provide culturally congruent services for those experiencing psychiatric or emotional stress. Furthermore, the nurse becomes better equipped to promote positive mental health within specific cultural environments. The chapter explores the meaning of culture, the influence of changing demographics on the importance of cultural awareness, and the components of a culturally congruent healthcare system. It discusses disparities found in mental health between minority populations and whites and explores the possible barriers to effective healthcare that have caused such disparities. It examines various beliefs about health and illness that are common to different cultural groups. Finally, the chapter focuses on the nurse's role in providing culturally congruent care.

CULTURE

Culture is the integration of human behaviors (which include thoughts, communications, actions, customs,

beliefs, values, and institutions[...] gious, or social group (Fadiman, [...] vast structure of ideas, attitudes, hab[...] als, ceremonies, and practices peculia[...] group of people. Culture also provides peo[...] eral design for living and with patterns by wh[...] pret reality (Nobles, 1979).

Culture can greatly influence a person's percept[...] health and illness as well as how, when, and why he or [...] would seek treatment for a health problem. This factor[...] becomes especially important in the area of mental health. Many aspects of psychiatric care involve self-perception, roles and relationships, family dynamics and interactions, attitudes toward medications, values, and community supports. Before a mental healthcare provider can administer appropriate and effective treatment, he or she must understand the client's cultural context and how it might influence his or her attitudes toward a particular health concern, its causes, and its treatment. An understanding of the client's cultural context also is necessary to appreciate the client's attitude toward the provider.

Changing Demographics and Cultural Awareness

The ability to view clients through a cultural lens is becoming increasingly important as a consequence of the growing diversity found in the United States and Canada. Although the United States always has been composed of people from various ethnic groups, races, and religions, the majority culture has traditionally been white, English-speaking, Christian, and middle class. Members (mostly men) of this majority culture have held power, and traditions and attitudes in American culture have supported and reinforced the majority ideals.

Recent dramatic shifts in U.S. demographics, however, indicate that the population is becoming incredibly diverse (Lester, 1998). During the 1990s, new arrivals to the United States numbered 12 million. This number exceeded the previous largest wave of immigrants who entered the United States between 1905 and 1914 (approximately 10 million) (Lester, 1998). Unlike the last wave of immigrants, who were predominantly from European countries, recent immigrants have come from Latin America, Asia, the Middle East, and other nonEuropean locations. They are adding to the numbers of people who belong to racial and ethnic groups traditionally considered "minority groups" throughout the United States. They also are increasing the country's cultural diversity.

Another change in U.S. demographics involves the increasing influence of Hispanic Americans. According to the U.S. Census Bureau, the number of Hispanics, currently the second largest minority group in the United States, is projected to more than double over the next 50 years (Bechtel, Davidhizar, & Tiller, 1998). At the same

of a racial, ethnic, reli-
997). It represents the
ts, languages, ritu-
to a particular
le with a gen-
ch to inter-
ons of
she

rrently the major-
proximately 25%,
ns should remain
by the year 2050,
Americans as the
ore, within that
ans will be about
"minority" popu-
important influ-
o be "American"
to examine and
"minority" cul-
S. demographics
over the next half-century.

ASSIMILATION

Throughout most of the 20th century, cultural attitudes were rooted in the idea of **assimilation**, the expectation for immigrants and those of minority groups to become like the majority (white) culture. On settling in the United States, immigrants were expected to abandon their native languages and customs and conform to the norms of the dominant society, including the adoption of Western technology and medicine. Minority groups also were expected to conform to the expectations of the dominant society; in many cases, success for these groups was rooted in achieving a status similar to and accepted by the dominant culture. Unmodifiable characteristics (race, age, sex), however, made assimilation more difficult for nonwhites, the very old and very young, and women. Such groups faced and continue to struggle with significant barriers to full participation in mainstream society. Assimilation also fostered a sense of ethnocentrism throughout the culture. **Ethnocentrism** is the belief that one's own cultural practices and values are inherently correct or superior to those of others. Ethnocentric attitudes can lead to the following problems:

- **Prejudice**—Negative preconceived opinions about other people or groups based on hearsay, perception, or emotion

- **Stereotyping**—Believing that one member of a cultural group will display certain behaviors or hold certain attitudes (usually negative) simply because he or she is a member of that cultural group
- **Discrimination**—Differential treatment based on race, class, gender, or other variables rather than on individual merit
- **Sigmatization**—The attribution of negative characteristics or identity to one person or group, causing the person or group to feel rejected, alienated, and ostracized from society.

IMPLICATIONS FOR HEALTHCARE

Overall, international demographics indicate that the majority populations in most countries are composed of persons of color. Western (European) medicine, which is rooted in a high-technology, intervention-focused approach, however, continues to dominate the thinking of practitioners in many areas. Consequently, practitioners of Western medicine often disregard, supersede, or fail to recognize more traditional healing methods found in nonEuropean cultures (Table 5-2). Western-oriented practitioners often fail to recognize that humankind is a composite of cultural beings with different beliefs, values, and constructs.

Changes in North American ethnic populations will continue to challenge the capabilities of mental healthcare systems. Furthermore, growing numbers of providers who come from nonWestern orientations will increasingly influence the nursing and mental healthcare professions themselves (Historical Capsule 5–1). With more and more people in North America coming from nonWestern cultures, healthcare providers will need to operate in ways that respect different traditions and behaviors while providing optimal care. Therefore, nurses and others who provide mental healthcare must understand cultural diversity and appreciate it as something to celebrate. Practicing and student nurses cannot ignore or be complacent about the cultural needs of their clients. Cultural needs are as real, important, and vital as physical and psychological needs (Glittenberg, 1995).

TABLE 5-1 ▼ **Trends in U.S. Demographics for the Next 50 Years (in Millions)**

GROUP	1996 (%)	2050 (%)
Hispanic	27.8 (10.5)	96.5 (24.5)
African Americans	32.0 (12.1)	53.6 (13.6)
Asian and Pacific Islander	9.1 (3.4)	32.4 (8.2)
American Indian, Eskimo, Aleut	2.0 (0.7)	3.5 (0.9)
White	194.4 (73.3)	207.9 (52.8)
Total	265.3 (100)	393.9 (100)

Data from U.S. Bureau of the Census, 1996.

TABLE 5-2 ▼ **Cultural Variations in Health Concept and Promotion**

CULTURAL GROUP	CONCEPT OF HEALTH	HEALTH PROMOTION
Native American	Traditional health beliefs are holistic and health oriented.	Traditional health practices include physical stamina (running), relaxation (meditation), cleansing (sweats), self-sufficiency, and harmonious living. Participation in religious ceremonies and prayer promotes health of self and family.
African American	Concept focuses on maintaining feelings of well-being, ability to fulfill role expectations, and freedom from pain and excessive stress.	Proper diet, proper behavior, and exercise in fresh air are prescription for maintaining health; protecting against excessive cold is important.
Cambodian	Being healthy is seen as being in equilibrium. Health needs to be individually maintained but is influenced by family and community.	Illness is seen as preventable. Nutrition is important, but not physical activity.
Chinese	Maintaining balance between *yin* and *yang* influences the body and the environment. Harmony is important to maintain body, mind, and spirit.	One should eat a diet balanced with *yin* and *yang* foods and maintain harmony with friends and family.
Gypsies (Roma)	Maintaining moral purity, keeping upper and lower body separate, and practicing good behavior are essential. Good health, prosperity, large families, and good appearance are intertwined.	Staying clean (*wuzho*) and avoiding unclean (*mahrime*) are important.
Mexican	Feeling well and being able to maintain role function are essential.	Orientation to the present and belief that the future is in God's hands mean that health screenings and routine checkup may not be scheduled by traditional Mexican Americans.
Puerto Rican	Absence of mental, spiritual, or physical discomforts as well as *lenities y limipios* (not being too thin and being clean) are perceived as healthy.	Eating well and drinking fruit beverages are important. Multivitamins are commonly used.
Samoan	Culture takes a holistic approach, including aspects of body, mind, and spirit. This includes relationships with family, environment, and spiritual world.	Concept of preventive health is not well established in Samoa.
Vietnamese	Principles of harmony and balance within self matter greatly. Overweight is considered a positive sign of good economic status and contentment.	Health promotion encompasses physical, spiritual, emotional, and social factors. Practices include consuming lots of fresh vegetables, fruit, fish, and meat and keeping clean and warm.

Data from Lipson, J., Dibble, S., & Minarik P. (Eds). (1996). *Culture & nursing care: A pocket guide* (pp. 21, 42, 62–63, 80–81, 136–137, 168, 219–220, 236–237, 262–263, 289). San Francisco: UCSF Nursing Press.

Culturally Competent Healthcare

Cultural competence means having the skills, both academic and interpersonal, that enable a person to understand and appreciate cultural differences and similarities within, between, and among groups. It is a process by which healthcare providers "continuously strive to achieve the ability to effectively work within the cultural context of an individual or community from a diverse cultural or ethnic background" (Campinha-Bacote, 1994, p.1). Skills in cultural competence are relevant for all variables to which differences may apply. Examples include gender, race, ethnic-

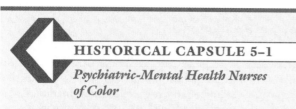

HISTORICAL CAPSULE 5-1

Psychiatric-Mental Health Nurses of Color

Psychiatric nursing is underrepresented by nurses of color; however, the leadership of these nurses has affected not only nursing, but the health of the entire nation.

- Dr. Jeanni Jo was the first Native-American nurse to earn the doctoral degree through the American Nurses Association (ANA) Ethnic Minority Fellowship Program.
- Sojourner Truth worked with the underground railways to free slaves and was known as a nurse and counselor.
- Hilda Richards served as Chancellor at the University of Indiana Northwest.
- In 1956, Elizabeth Lipford Kent was the first African-American nurse to earn the doctoral degree. She provided administrative guidance to the Lafayette Clinic, a state mental health facility in Detroit, Michigan.
- Under the leadership of Dr. Ildaura Murillo-Rohde, the Hispanic Nurses Association was established.
- Through the efforts of Dr. Mary Harper, the National Institute of Mental Health (NIMH) established and funded the ANA Ethnic Minority Fellowship Program in 1974. This outstanding program has helped more than 200 nurses of color—African, Hispanic, Asian, and Native American—to earn doctorate degrees. It continues to be federally funded under the leadership of dynamic nurses such as Dr. Ruth Gordon, Hattie Bessent, and Carla Serlin.
- In 1978, Dr. Rhetaugh Duman became the first psychiatric nurse and the first African American to serve as Deputy Director of the NIMH.

ity, language, country of origin, acculturation, age, religious and spiritual beliefs, sexual orientation, socioeconomic class, and disabilities (Lester, 1998). The culturally competent provider is willing and able to draw on community-based values, traditions, and customs and to work with knowledgeable persons from the community to formulate appropriate interventions and supports for clients according to the different variables mentioned earlier (Parsons & Reiss, 1999; Poss, 1999; U.S. Department of Health and Human Services [DHHS], 1992).

A culturally competent healthcare system is one that acknowledges and incorporates, at all levels, the importance of culture. Such incorporation is evident through the system's assessment of cross-cultural relations, attention to the dynamics that result from cultural differences, growth of cultural knowledge, and adaptation of services to meet culturally unique needs. The system's behaviors, attitudes, and policies are congruent and help others to work effectively in cross-cultural situations (Cross et al., 1989) (Figure 5-1) (Box 5-1).

CULTURAL CONGRUENCE

In a culturally competent healthcare system, care delivery is culturally congruent. This means that clients receive an overall message, conveyed both verbally and nonverbally, of personal and cultural validation. In culturally congruent mental healthcare, providers integrate the client's value system, life experiences, and expectations about treatment into the therapeutic process, even when the client is not fully aware that it is happening. As a result, the full weight of the client's cultural system can help support the healing process.

For mental health services to be culturally congruent, providers from all aspects of the delivery system must respond to diverse cultural values consistent with the client's specific context. Theoretical approaches encompassing such values, while remaining flexible and adaptable to specific contexts, have been long in coming and difficult to define. Since the 1950s, Dr. Madeleine Leininger has consistently urged that, as societies throughout the world become increasingly multicultural, cultural competence in human relationships should be a major concern for nursing and other health disciplines (Wenger, 1995). The health professions, however, traditionally have lacked culture-specific interventions that recognize the unique combinations of disorders found in groups not embraced by Western society. Such disorders (eg, traumatic losses, soul loss, culture shock, cultural isolation, somatoform and anxiety disorders, and unique culture-bound syndromes) require specific culturally oriented treatments (Clarke, 1989).

In focusing on culturally congruent services for African Americans, Hispanic Americans, American Indians and Alaska Natives, and Asian and Pacific Island Americans, the DHHS (1992) has published recommendations for services. These recommendations identify the need for providers to

- Reach consensus regarding terminology (eg, correctly referencing groups as Southeast Asians, Native Americans)
- Distinguish between cultural identification and the culture of poverty
- Distinguish between subgroups within each culture
- Develop skills based on values to develop culturally congruent services

Dr. Jennifer Clarke has identified 20 necessary elements to provide culturally congruent services (Erikson, 1950):

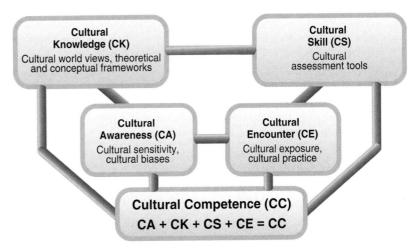

FIGURE 5-1. Culturally competent model of care. (Adapted from Campinha-Bacote, J. [1994]. Cultural competence in psychiatric mental health nursing. *Nursing Clinics of North America, 29*[1], 2.)

1. Theoretical approaches are culturally oriented.
2. Providers understand and incorporate cultural concepts of illness and health into treatment.
3. Diagnostic or classification systems are culturally accurate and acceptable.
4. Providers recognize culture-specific symptom patterns.
5. Client–therapist pairs are culturally similar.
6. Service providers have achieved a positive personal cultural integration.
7. Service is provided in the client's native language.
8. Service settings are easily accessible and culturally familiar to clients.
9. The nature and timing of the intake process reflect cultural priorities and are not offensive to clients.
10. Services are provided at convenient times and in lengths that conform to cultural experiences.
11. The role of extended family in the therapeutic process reflects cultural values.
12. Provider and client are socially related to promote therapeutic rapport.
13. The degree of social involvement or enmeshment of mental health workers with the client is culturally determined.
14. Providers understand, support, and, if culturally appropriate, integrate the client's religious beliefs into the therapeutic process.
15. Providers integrate traditional healing practices and traditional healers into the therapeutic process when culturally appropriate.

BOX 5-1 ▼ *A Culturally Congruent Health Service in Practice*

In Hennepin County, Minnesota, the Mental Health Division launched a 5-year effort to provide culturally congruent services. This plan was based on input from communities of color and native communities. The recommendations were reached after multiple and interacting family, financial, physical, legal, and psychological problems were considered, including chronic mourning, frustration, denial and hopelessness associated with violence, suicide and grief or tragic deaths, abuse, and family breakups.

Hennepin County's Mental Health Plan made many recommendations for cultural congruence within the mental health system. A key factor was the development of cultural assessments and outcome measurements appropriate to specific cultures. To develop these tools, various professionals and community representatives were consulted. Staff developed a job description for a "cultural conscience." The cultural consciences are commissioned with the responsibility of ensuring that every treatment team asks the critical questions regarding culture and ethnicity. They are responsible for seeing that these issues are incorporated into the individual treatment plans.

As a result of direct input from the various ethnic communities represented in the county, funding was made available to make mental health agencies more inviting. Program sites used the funds to purchase appropriate cultural art, music, and reading materials. Brochures were translated into several languages, and a "Welcome" sign for each program greeted clients in eight languages. In addition, structured consultation from various cultural consultants and input from cultural and ethnic communities guided mental health programming.

Critical to any system's ability to move to multiculturalism is the empowerment of the staff to move forward at every level. Therefore, all levels of administration are involved and endorse any initiative where the goal is moving toward a culturally congruent service system.

16. Treatment techniques are culturally comprehensible and acceptable.
17. Therapeutic goals are consistent with the client's cultural biases toward inner or outer control.
18. Therapeutic expectations are consistent with cultural biases toward inner and outer control.
19. Record-keeping systems are minimally intrusive and culturally accurate.
20. Providers obtain the support of appropriate ethnic authorities or institutions.

CULTURE CARE THEORY

Culture care theory, developed by Dr. Madeleine Leininger, emphasizes learning principles related to culture care, culturalogic assessments, the universality of culture care diversity, and the importance of fit between the client's healthcare values and services provided. According to this theory, health professionals are ethically bound to explore their own culture first and then attempt to understand the culture of their clients. Providers must learn how to do culturalogic assessments and then provide culturally congruent care (Wenger, 1995). How to provide care stems from the client's cultural context as part of an extended family, group, and community. Without this vital information, providers are apt to misdiagnose, mismanage, and misunderstand clients.

DISPARITIES IN MENTAL HEALTH AND BARRIERS TO EFFECTIVE TREATMENT

Many studies document major disparities in key health indicators between racial and ethnic minorities and white populations. The Center for Health Economics Research (1993) and Robert Wood Johnson Foundation (1991) report that persons of color, particularly those in inner cities, showed major health disparities in neonatal mortality rates, heart and circulatory problems, and admissions to psychiatric facilities compared with white people. "The high incidence of substance abuse, physical injuries, and deaths from violence greatly distinguish low-income black neighborhoods and communities in terms of potential and actual costs of health care" (Western Interstate Commission For Higher Education, 1998). Such disparities negatively affect health outcomes and explain why minorities are among those most in need of high-quality healthcare (Lester, 1998).

Historically, many members of ethnically and racially diverse populations have avoided the mental healthcare delivery system. This avoidance arose from the fear of being institutionalized or diagnosed or labeled "abnormal" because of culturally ingrained differences. Comas-Diaz and Greene (1994) describe traditional mental health treatment as an institutional vice that invests Euro-

pean-American middle-class values with the legitimacy of psychological normalcy.

Reasons why minority groups may display resistance to, and feel uncomfortable about, seeking mental health services include the following:

- Stress experienced from forced migration, dislocation, or immigration
- Inability to speak or comprehend the dominant language and distrust of culturally inappropriate interpreter services
- Differences in religious beliefs and practices
- Environmental stress as a result of poverty or lack of equal access to education, employment, housing, or medical care
- Culture-specific beliefs about seeking help (eg, history, fear of being labeled or controlled by medications, shame, basic belief about illness)
- Use of traditional healers and alternative medicines for specific culture-bound situations
- Differing values and attitudes
- Misinterpretation of behaviors (eg, lateness, sense of bewilderment, codependence, assimilation, distrust, quietness)

These and other issues are discussed in more detail in the following sections.

Variability and Vulnerability

Variability in the incidence of mental illnesses among different cultural groups may be related to variations in genetic vulnerability (including variances among Native American tribes). For example, Native Americans have increased rates of alcoholism, depression, anxiety, violence, and suicide; they are at higher risk for mental illness than most other ethnic groups in the United States. In addition, many tribes have maintained their sovereign status (adding to the necessity for the practitioner to understand mental health services within the tribe's historical, geographic, and educational context).

Other biologic variations such as body structure, skin color, genetic variations, susceptibility to disease, nutritional preferences and deficiencies, and psychological characteristics may be directly related to race. For example, when doing a physical health examination, providers must remember that it can be difficult to recognize vasodilation or vasoconstriction in darker skinned individuals. Therefore, providers assess for an ashen color rather that a bluish color (Bechtel et al., 1998). Just as providers must remember biologically related variables during physical examinations, they also must consider them when performing psychological examinations.

Unfortunately, many persons of color face issues related to poverty, which providers must consider when assessing for vulnerabilities such as increased rates of illness, homicide, alcohol abuse, and infant mortality. Infant mortality rates, one of the primary indicators of a nation's or culture's health, range from slightly higher for Asian Pacific Island groups to twice as high for African Americans when compared with those of nonminority infants (Office of Minority Health, 1995). The health gap between minority populations and the majority culture is emphasized when reviewing other major causes of death such as cancer, AIDS, diabetes, heart disease, homicide, and suicide.

Accessibility

The Americans With Disabilities Act of 1990 and Title VI of the Civil Rights Act of 1964 mandate accessibility to healthcare services and facilities for all U.S. citizens. Historically, however, mainstream mental health services have failed to adequately meet the needs of persons of color. Populations such as Native Americans, refugees, and illegal immigrants underuse health services, including preventative services, and delay care until conditions become serious. Failure to use such services may be related to cost, language, cultural barriers, fear, or apprehension (Lester, 1998).

Cultural barriers to treatment range from cultural insensitivity to obstacles such as difficulty understanding appointment procedures, lack of public transportation, signs written in a language not understood by the client, and formidable-looking buildings (Lester, 1998). These institutional structures combine to preclude a culturally inviting environment. Cultural barriers also may be related to historical circumstances that have led to a group's economic, social, and political status in the community. Healthcare providers must be aware of the group's underlying history and how it influenced the psychological well-being of its members.

Racial Bias

Clients from nonwhite populations are institutionalized more frequently than are whites. This finding includes admissions to hospitals, involuntary commitments, and incarcerations. Racial bias enters into such decisions as definition of dangerousness, severity of diagnostic labels, and choice of treatment modalities. Data from the National Institute of Mental Health (1987) indicate that African Americans were more frequently diagnosed as having serious and persistent mental illness (SPMI) than any other ethnic or racial population when being admitted to a psychiatric facility. Furthermore, people of African descent

- Drop out of services at a significantly higher rate than do those of white populations
- Use fewer treatment sessions for their mental health problems than those of white populations
- Enter mental health treatment services at a later

stage in the course of their illness than do white populations
- Underuse community mental health services of all kinds
- Overuse inpatient psychiatric care in state hospitals at twice the rate of corresponding white populations
- Are misdiagnosed more often by mental health practitioners than are white populations
- Are diagnosed more often as having a severe mental illness than are whites

To underscore the influence that racial bias has had on mental healthcare delivery to persons of color, Historical Capsule 5-2 discusses the case of Junius Wilson. This case is not an isolated incident, nor is it exclusive to the history of African Americans. Thousands of Native Americans experienced terrible social isolation as the result of the U.S. government's policy of forcibly removing children from their families and placing them in boarding schools to indoctrinate them with Euro-American practices. Forced relocation caused deaths and problems such as dealing with being conquered, shame, forced dependency on the government, and loss of traditional roles. Native Americans dealt with broken treaties, restriction to reservations, poverty, and consequences of not relocating. These issues continue to affect tribes.

HISTORICAL CAPSULE 5-2

Diagnosis and Race: The Case of Junius Wilson

In 1925, Junius Wilson, a 17-year-old black man, was charged with attempted rape in the New Hanover community of Castle Hayne, North Carolina. In court, he was found incompetent to stand trial. The charges were dropped after he arrived at Cherry State Hospital, a state mental institution. Junius was castrated and remained in a locked mental ward for 69 years. In the 1920s, castration was a standard procedure for black men accused of rape. John Badgett, deputy director of the state Division of Mental Health, states that Wilson "has been the victim of social politics that we look back on now and are deeply troubled by." In 1992, after a review of Wilson's medical records, a social worker discovered that Wilson was deaf, not mentally ill. This discovery, with legal assistance, led to the release of Mr. Wilson and compensation by the state for the abuse and years of imprisonment.

Swofford, S. (1995, December 28). *News and Record,* pp. B1–B2.

Religious and Spiritual Influences

Many clients from minority populations interpret symptoms or signs of mental illness as spiritual. Consequently, the may choose to seek help from a trusted spiritual leader for these manifestations. The client, family, and spiritual leader may not identify such signs or symptoms as a mental health problem, or the client may be diagnosed with a mental health problem only after traditional healing methods have failed. For example, folk medicine is an integral part of routine healthcare for many Mexican Americans. Use of traditional healers (Box 5-2) may include *curanderas* (female folk healers believed to be chosen by God), herbalists, *sobadoras* (female healers who use massage and manipulation), *brujos* (male witches), or *brujas* (female witches) (Bechtel et al., 1998). In many cases, clients do not share with Western providers that they are seeing a folk healer.

"Although 44% of Mexican Americans reported the use of alternative practitioners during the past year, 66% of this group indicated they did not tell their healthcare provider" (Bechtel et al., 1998).

Nurses must understand that in many cases, spiritual beliefs provide the structure by which some ethnic groups (eg, Latinos, African Americans, Native Americans, Asian Americans) explain disease. Because Western medicine is technologically focused and emphasizes the biophysical aspects of medicine, Western healthcare providers often consider a group's characteristic response as "abnormal" when it differs from the response of the dominant culture. Awareness of cultural factors that influence client behavior is essential to avoid labeling the client as "being difficult" when the issue is cultural differences. This problem is glaringly evident in a retrospective assessment of a Hmong child named Lia described by Anne Fadiman

---

BOX 5-2 ▼ *Curanderismo*

Curanderismo is the practice of folk healing that evolved from European medical practices of the 15th and 16th centuries. It continues within the Mexican-American community. The Aztecs, Mayas, and other Indian groups left these folk beliefs and curing practices to the Spanish Catholics in Mexico. Curanderismo has persisted as a tradition in Mexican-American culture because of its members' rural background, illiteracy, poverty, and distrust of the modern medical care system.

Curanderas and *curanderos,* or folk healers, usually are women who believe that they are endowed with curing powers from God. The healer comes to hold this belief by being involved in the care of a sick person who recovers. Curanderas are sincere in their belief that they are chosen by God and, therefore, usually do not charge fees for their healing services. They believe that if they expected or demanded payment, their divine gift of healing would be taken away. Recently, however, it has become common for curanderos to institute a fee system, although the charges are minimal.

The diseases treated by the curandera are thought to be the will of God or to result from witchcraft. *Susto,* or fright, is a condition that follows an emotional upset and is characterized by depression, restlessness, loss of strength, and anorexia. If a client experiences susto, the curanderas are the only ones believed to have the power to perform the necessary healing rituals.

Mal ojo, or evil eye, is thought to be caused by envy, covetous expressions, or attention paid by one person to another. For example, a mother may be told that her child, after being complimented, will cast the spell of mal ojo, and the child will become ill with fever. The

person complimenting the child should touch him, thereby breaking the spell of mal ojo.

The belief in mal ojo is widespread. Mexican Americans may take preventative measures such as wearing amulets, gold earrings, snakes' fangs, garlic, or oil crosses on the head to deflect the mal ojo.

Mal ojo and susto are only two of many folk diseases that the nurse might encounter when caring for Mexican-American clients. The nurse should not assume that a client who is educated or acculturated does not hold these beliefs in curanderismo.

For example, when I was pregnant with my son, there was a death in the family. I planned to attend the funeral, but when making arrangements with my mother, she told me that I could not go to the funeral because of my pregnancy. It seemed odd to me that she would say this because she never seemed to hold much faith in some of the Mexican-American cultural beliefs. My grandmother and mother told me that the embalming fluid would be in the air around the body, causing *mal aire,* and this could cause my baby to be born with deformities or make me ill. They further told me that I possibly could miscarry if I came to the funeral. I did go to the funeral, but in respect for their wishes, especially my grandmother's, I sat in the back and did not view the body. (Several months later, I delivered a healthy boy.)

A client's perception of health and illness are influenced strongly by cultural beliefs; providers of healthcare services must understand and acknowledge those cultural beliefs to provide optimal care to Mexican Americans.

Juanta Zapata Flint, MS, RN, FNPC, Dean of Instruction, Brookhaven College, Farmers Branch, Texas.

(1997) in *The Spirit Catches You and You Fall Down: A Hmong Child, Her American Doctors, and the Collision of Two Cultures.*

In this book, Lia had a seizure disorder. Providers asked what caused the disorder, and Lia's family indicated that it was "soul loss," which began when an older sister slammed the door and scared the soul out of the child's body (Fadiman, 1997). When providers attempted to administer traditional healing methods, however, the family expressed reluctance:

> *You should give Lia medicine to take for a week but no longer. After she is well, she should stop taking the medicine. You should not treat her by taking her blood or the fluid from her backbone. Lia should also be treated at home with our Hmong medicines and by satisfying pigs and chickens. We hope Lia will be healthy, but we are not sure we want her to stop shaking forever because it makes her noble in our culture, and when she grows up she might become a shaman. (Fadiman, 1997).*

In this circumstance, everyone involved was concerned for Lia's healthcare, yet no one explored the family's perception of the illness. This exploration of the cultural clash between the medical community and the Laotian refugee family underscores the need to question what a client believes a problem to be to prevent misunderstandings that could result in tragic consequences.

SOCIOCULTURAL VARIATIONS IN RESPONSE TO MENTAL HEALTHCARE

Each person belongs to multiple groups (eg, occupation, community, religion) and as such is influenced by various sets of values, beliefs, and behaviors. Belief systems include concepts such as attitudes toward stress relief (eg, use of drugs, alcohol, yoga), as well as home remedies (eg, use of chicken soup for the common cold), which can shape a client's receptivity to different types of interventions.

Acute symptoms often are masked by related problems such as alcoholism, delinquency, violence, or physical illness. Different cultural values and symptom patterns complicate diagnosis in nonWestern groups. "Overall, there is a pervasiveness of depression and a tendency to experience emotional and psychological problems as either physical illness or as caused by external stress only" (Huggins, 1996). Diagnosis of SPMI is underrepresented or not represented in several nonwhite groups because of reinterpretation of behaviors (as in spiritual issues) or mislabeling the symptom as the disease (as in use of alcohol). For example, the abuse of alcohol is prevalent among Native Americans who are experiencing mental illness, but the Native community often sees the drinking as the cause of

the problem. This interpretation is more acceptable to the community because of the belief that there is a "cure" for drinking. Accurate diagnosis, therefore, is difficult because symptoms are masked by alcohol use or abuse (Huggins, 1996). Treatment approaches must be redefined to provide for co-morbidity to address the mental illness and chemical use simultaneously (Office of Minority Health, 1985).

Mental health programs that provide culturally congruent services integrate prevention and stress reduction through a holistic approach that emphasizes the environment, living arrangements, medical care and healthcare, job availability, and the use of traditional healers and alternative health practices. Effective programs use culturally appropriate assessment tools and develop clinical standards that are culturally and ethnically appropriate. These include terminology that reflects the client's system.

African-American Clients

African Americans are a large, diverse group. Attitudes and beliefs are wide and varied, and are influenced by factors such as occupation, religion, country of origin, social class, and length of time spent in the United States. Attitudes toward mental health problems and treatments depend largely on the individual client. Nevertheless, a common problem faced by African Americans is racial bias, which causes providers to misdiagnose (and subsequently mistreat) their disorders (see earlier discussion).

Native-American Clients

According to Gurnoe and Nelson (1989), successful care of Native American families requires mutual understanding and knowledge between the mental health practitioner and the client. Without the establishment of these factors, poor diagnosis and one-sided assessment are unavoidable. Another factor to consider is the client's particular tribe. Although some North American tribes share common views of the world, other tribes see things differently.

A Native American client demonstrates the need for cultural maintenance or preservation when he or she expresses a desire to use traditional herbs and to participate in a sweat lodge ceremony to aid in the healing process. The healthcare provider whose attitude communicates sensitivity to, interest in, and even rudimentary knowledge about traditional healing practices is more likely to learn from clients about the full range of their health-related beliefs and behaviors. Clients, conversely, are more likely to comply with an approach that allows them to preserve familiar practices. Because belief can play a major part in healing outcomes, it follows that effort should be made to support whatever the client believes will help—unless there is real evidence that a practice is harmful (O'Connor,

1995). Having one's experience discredited or made to seem unimportant is painful.

Hispanic and Latino Clients

Research shows that Latinos are most likely to use formal mental health services primarily during times of crisis. They also are unlikely to turn to such services until all other options (eg, counseling from clergy) have failed.

Healthcare providers working with Hispanic consumers should consider the importance of the Catholic Church, prayers, herbs, and the strong influence of hot-and-cold or good-and-evil imbalances in promoting a sense of well-being. Clients who believe that their psychiatric problems are punishment for their sins may be more likely to follow the medication regimen and recover if their spiritual leader is involved with the treatment.

Asian and Pacific Islander Clients

Asian and Pacific Islanders include more than 30 different ethnic groups with various levels of language proficiency and education. The nurse must distinguish between the various groups. Subjective evidence indicates that Asian and Pacific Islander clients tend to endure distress for long periods before seeking mental health services. When they finally enter the service delivery system, they tend to have more severe disturbances.

Southeast Asian refugees disproportionately experience post-traumatic stress disorder (PTSD) (see Chap. 18). This diagnostic "label" also is found in other dislocated ethnic groups. Many states, however, exclude the diagnosis of PTSD. Thus, access to service is blocked for many of these clients. These factors contribute to the likelihood that Southeast Asian refugees will come to the attention of the mental health system only during periods of acute stress or crisis.

CULTURALLY COMPETENT AND CONGRUENT NURSING CARE

Nurses in mental healthcare settings are critical to the promotion and practice of culturally congruent care. Given that there are hundreds of different cultures, innumerable additional categories of diversity, and as many ways to interpret human experience as there are people, nurses must be reasonable about what they expect themselves to know. It is impossible to know *everything* about cultural beliefs and healthcare. Nevertheless, it is possible to develop and communicate attitudes that express sincere interest, a willingness to learn, and respect for the other person's point of view.

To provide culturally congruent care, nurses must possess knowledge about cultural illnesses and healing practices and intercultural communication skills. They must develop self-awareness, flexibility, and working relationships that cross the lines of differentness (Lester, 1998). Health providers who are not **culture bound** (limited by the parameters of their own culture) are more likely to have a larger worldview and work with clients in a nonjudgmental, accepting way (Bechtel et al., 1998). Nurses also must learn what the client and his or her family identify as "normal" and "abnormal" within the cultural context. Such identification applies not only to defining health problems, but also to outlining expectations for care, cure, or both. In this context, the client's culture and subcultures will influence the expression, presentation, recognition, labeling, explanations for, and distribution of mental illness. See Implications for Nursing Practice 5-1 for an example.

When assessing and intervening with ethnic minorities, the nurse must consider the following (Giger & Davidhizar, 1995):

- Communication, including written and oral language, gestures, facial expressions, and body language
- Personal space, including both the space itself and the items sharing the designated space
- Social organization, including patterns of behavior during life events such as births, puberty, childbearing, illness, and death
- Time, both concrete and abstract
- Environment, including perceptions regarding control of the environment
- Biologic variations among racial groups

Holistic care, however, recognizes and incorporates family care with religious values and cultural beliefs (Leininger, 1995). When determining the client's explanation for the illness, the nurse must listen carefully to the client's story. Several factors, including spiritual beliefs, cultural values, and food preference, are closely related to the healing process.

Within a transcultural focus, the nurse thinks "about differences and similarities among people and their beliefs, practices, and life ways" while learning to "value understanding people regarding their special needs and concerns" (Leininger, 1995). Thus, the nurse develops different, culturally appropriate ways to help by assessing each client's particular cultural orientation. By doing so, the nurse learns from the client how best to provide sensitive, compassionate, and competent care (Box 5-3) (Research in Psychiatric Mental Health Nursing 5-1).

Essential Skills

The nursing profession is rooted in a sense of caring. Nurses are expected to possess the personal characteristics

>>> **Implications for Nursing Practice 5-1**

Working With Clients of Asian Ethnic Origin in Mental Health Settings

Using the criteria for culturally congruent care, a nurse caring for a client of Asian ethnic origin would base care on the following parameters:

- Consider the client's level of acculturation.
- Assess how the client interprets his or her illness.
- Assess the client's concept of the future.
- Don't be intrusive during the first few sessions. Focus on establishing rapport first.
- If a female client seems submissive, be careful not to assume that she has a "psychiatric disorder." Such behavior from women and girls is a cultural expectation in many Asian countries. Be sure to distinguish culturally based psychological phenomena from psychiatric disorders.
- Many Asian cultures expect the healthcare provider to be of the same sex as the client. Therefore, when possible, make sure that the provider is the same sex as the client. If this is not possible, always ensure adequate personal space between male and female clients and providers in seating arrangements.
- Recognize the importance of the family to Asian clients.
- Give clients specific information about prescribed medications, dosages, and side effects. Instruct them not to give their medications to other family members or reduce the prescribed medication dosage.
- Assess, recognize, and accept the influence of religious beliefs on client behavior.
- Consult with Asian or Asian-American practitioners and scholars for advice and recommendations about reading materials, clinical supervision, and staff development.

BOX 5-3 ▼ *Treatment Strategies for Cultural Competence in Mental Healthcare Delivery*

- Determine your own cultural heritage and behavior patterns.
- Recognize coexisting belief systems about mental health and illness.
- Assess client's personal beliefs, concerns, and fears about the illness.
- Assess and consider family history and search for generational patterns.
- Explain, negotiate, and, when indicated, collaborate on a treatment plan that considers the client's cultural beliefs. Discuss the client's expectations of the treatment regimen. Preserve helpful beliefs or repattern acknowledged harmful beliefs or practices.
- Recognize informal caregivers as allies in the treatment process.
- Read documented information about specific cultural groups.
- Determine if the client is seeking Western healthcare in conjunction with, or exclusive of, any personal cultural beliefs about mental illness.
- Collaborate with key informants and others who are adept at interpreting meanings of language and behaviors of specific cultures.
- Demonstrate patience, a nonjudgmental attitude, and genuine respect for the client no matter what behavior he or she exhibits.

of genuineness, empathy, warmth, and objectivity (see Chap. 4). As the nurse develops a transcultural focus, he or she learns to incorporate additional skills in care delivery. Four critical skills that nurses must acquire to provide culturally competent care are as follows (Battaglia, 1992):

1. *Cross-cultural understanding* means knowledge about how and why people of different cultures behave in certain ways. For a nurse to develop cross-cultural understanding, he or she might study the relevant culture or identify a colleague from that culture and learn about the culture's values, norms, and mores. The nurse, however, should not use this strategy in isola-

tion. Doing so may cause the nurse to begin to overgeneralize that he or she should treat all members of a specific group exactly the same.

2. *Intercultural communication* is essential because communication is at the center of cross-cultural psychiatric-mental health nursing. Some differences in communication are readily apparent; others are harder to discern, such as degree of openness, self-disclosure, emotional expression, insight, and even talkativeness. Intercultural communication requires the nurse to develop listening skills, including learning to decipher nonverbal behavior and detect barriers that interfere with communication. The psychiatric-mental health nurse should excel in this area; any unidentified intrapersonal stereotypes and biases would hinder the nurse's communicative skills. If a nurse recognizes that he or she has a different communication style than a client, the nurse should spend additional time with that client to improve understanding and ensure that he or she is providing culturally competent care. If a nurse speaks a different language than the client, he or she

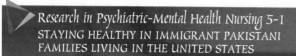

Research in Psychiatric-Mental Health Nursing 5-1
STAYING HEALTHY IN IMMIGRANT PAKISTANI
FAMILIES LIVING IN THE UNITED STATES

Purpose: To determine how immigrant families interpret what it means to "stay healthy."

Background: For care to be culturally competent and congruent, nurses must understand how their clients view health and what causes them to seek health care. With more people from various cultures coming to North America, nurses are likely to see different ideas among clients about what they view as health and illness. This can be especially important for the area of mental health, in which manifestations of illness may not be as apparent or readily accepted as physical illness.

Method and Sample: The researchers collected data from members of four families from Pakistan. Each family had lived in the United States for approximately 15 years and practiced Islam. Although they knew English, they spoke Urdu in the home.

Findings: These Pakistani family members indicated that staying healthy meant feeling understood, being at spiritual peace, and maintaining a strong family.

Application to Nursing Practice: The values mentioned by the Pakistani families may differ from what nurses from U.S. culture might expect for clients to identify as "healthy." These values, however, will direct a client's response to, and, subsequently, the way a nurse should plan and implement interventions. Discussing the meaning of health with clients, including psychiatric health, is essential.

Jan, R., & Smith, C. A. (1998). *Image: The Journal of Nursing Scholarship, 30*(2), 157–159.

1. *Phase I*—Becoming aware of and sensitive to culture care differences and similarities (cultural awareness)
2. *Phase II*—Using theories to discover and explain transcultural nursing phenomena with vague knowledge (use of theories to guide research and explain)
3. *Phase III*—Using transcultural research findings to improve care of people (use of knowledge in practice for congruent care)

Transcultural Assessment

To determine the influences on a client's basic beliefs about illness and wellness, the nurse must ensure that the assessment is transculturally focused. Data from the transcultural assessment can help the nurse to identify cultural factors that are pertinent to the client's health, ranging from religious views to views on the use of folk medicine. Basic beliefs of clients about health and disease vary greatly among cultures in relation to the following (McGoldrick & Giordano, 1996):

- The experience of pain
- What a culture labels as a symptom
- How people of the culture communicate pain or symptoms
- Beliefs about the cause of pain or symptoms
- Attitude toward helpers (doctors and hospitals)
- Desired or expected treatment

Although, some providers believe that assessing a person's cultural perception is too costly and time consuming, when this assessment is not done, the cost is much greater in terms of misperceptions, misdiagnosis, wasted interventions, and delayed treatments. To provide effective cross-cultural services, nurses should ask the following questions, developed by Dr. Arthur Kleinman of Harvard, to elicit the client's explanation of the illness (Fadiman, 1997):

- What is the problem?
- What do you think has caused the problem?
- Why do you think it started when it did?
- What do you think the sickness does? How does it work?
- How severe is the sickness? Will it have a short or long course?
- What kind of treatment do you think the client should receive? What are the most important results you hope he or she receives from this treatment?
- What are chief problems the sickness has caused?
- What do you fear most about the sickness?

should design strategies that will minimize problems during interviews. The nurse and client may need an interpreter to communicate effectively.

3. *Facilitation skills* focus primarily on conflict resolution and the ability to negotiate interactions that may be inconsistent with the value and belief system of a client or family from a culture that differs from that of the nurse.

4. **Flexibility** means the ability to embrace change by modifying expectations, readjusting old operating norms and stereotypes, and trying new behavior.

Phases of Transcultural Nursing Knowledge

Leininger (1995) describes three phases in the development of transcultural nursing knowledge:

Building Cultural Awareness

Nursing's unique advantage is the opportunity to help the client tell his or her story while providing care. Leininger (1995) has developed a conceptual picture of the components of cultural care that can help nurses

Implications for Nursing Practice 5-2

Promoting Cultural Self-Awareness

When nurses or other healthcare providers do not understand, accept, and appreciate their own culture relating to biases influencing treatment, transcultural problems lead to misunderstandings, noncompliance, and resistance to interventions. These influence both satisfaction with services and recovery. Nurses can consider several important issues in their striving to offer unbiased, culturally congruent care:

- What ethnic group, socioeconomic class, and community do I belong to or feel a part of?
- To what extent do I recognize and understand my own racial or ethnic background?
- What are the values of my ethnic group(s)? What do we generally believe about mental health and mental illness?
- What are my earliest images of race and color?
- What are my attitudes toward people who are different from me in appearance and behavior?
- What have been my personal experiences with others' ethnic or racial cultures?
- What do I know about people from ethnic groups that are different from my own?
- Many nurses and clients are descendents of several racial or ethnic cultures. How do different racial or ethnic cultures come together in my own background?

understand the multiple factors influencing an effective transcultural interaction:

- Attend to gender differences, communication modes, special language terms, interpersonal relationships, and use of space and food.
- Show genuine interest in the client while maintaining a learning and respectful attitude.
- Keep alert to whatever the client shares about culture care values, religion, and kinship relationships.
- Discover and remain aware of your own cultural biases and prejudices.
- Be aware of subcultures or special groups to which the client may be a participant (eg, homeless, gay).
- Know the strengths, variabilities, and assets of your own culture.
- Clarify that the purpose is to focus on helping the client.
- Maintain a holistic view of the client's world and environment context.

While listening to the client's story, the nurse maintains the role of active listener and keeps the intervention focused on the client's constructs for health and wellness. Encouraging expressions of culture is important, particularly in the areas of dress and adornment, eating rituals and foods, care activities, sleep rituals, and healing rituals wherever these can be compatible and therapeutic. When nurses display an empathetic and caring attitude, remain flexible, and listen, they are participating in culturally competent care. "It is the natural flow of events that occurs when you put someone else's feelings before your own," no matter where they come from (Lester, 1998).

Cultural Self-Awareness

Erik Erikson (1950) defined the final stage of human development as coming to terms with one's own cultural identity. Looking inward with the culture lens, the nurse can better understand the values associated with belonging to a group and identify with others. The realization of multiple perspectives becomes a reality (Implications for Nursing Practice 5-2). This multicultural approach may cause the nurse to question formerly held "truths" about healthcare delivery. Nurses must identify their own "baggage" to recognize it and leave it at home. This struggle is essential for awareness and elimination of biases, stereotypes, and prejudices. Healthcare providers should learn to change perspectives and view situations based on a specific ethnic or cultural group to modify interventions in ways that are culturally compatible. In this way, providers can ". . . walk in the shoes of others without tripping. They can see the world through many cultural perspectives. Each of us lives in a cultural bubble; a multiculturalist can enter another cultural bubble without bursting it" (Pernell-Arnold, 1995).

Most current mental health treatment modalities have evolved from a Western mindset. The emphasis on technology and distancing usually is incompatible with the traditional beliefs of many cultures. Nurses must examine the belief system of their own culture to ascertain if there is compatibility between their worldview and the client's worldview. Flexibility and adaptability are key to accepting this challenge.

 Reflection and Critical Thinking Questions

1. What roles might be culturally defined for family members? How can such roles hinder or facilitate a client's mental health treatment?
2. How do your own experiences affect your thoughts and feelings toward clients with a cultural frame of reference that differs from your own?

▼ CHAPTER SUMMARY

- Culture is a main ingredient of personality.
- The more stress a person experiences, the greater is the manifestation of his or her culturally based perceptions, beliefs, and behaviors.

■ Self-knowledge facilitates personal comfort and understanding of others when caring for culturally diverse clients in a variety of psychiatric-mental health settings.

■ To provide effective, individualized mental health services, nurses must view consumers with a cultural lens that includes the context of their cultural group and their individual experiences from being a part of that group.

■ Nursing staff development programs are beneficial to improve outcomes of care for culturally diverse psychiatric clients.

■ Although diverse cultural groups may have various responses with respect to the evaluation and treatment of mental illness, culturally competent care is maximized by the nurse's open, honest, and accepting attitude.

■ Recognition of generational patterns within one's own culture can assist the nurse to assess and recognize generational patterns in other cultures.

■ Specific stressors, including war, trauma, violence, migration patterns, economic status, racism, discrimination, cultural values and beliefs, and survival tactics, need to be addressed in providing mental health services.

■ The nurse can ascertain how the above factors relate to the individual and his or her perception of mental health.

■ Nurses' self-knowledge, viewing position, and preparation as culturally competent providers greatly affect the care of diverse clients.

▼ REVIEW QUESTIONS

1. Based on current demographic trends, which of the following cultural groups is expected to rank second by the year 2050?
   a. Asian Americans
   b. Hispanic Americans
   c. American Indians
   d. African Americans

2. When interviewing a client of Polish heritage, he states, "My ancestors used to speak Polish in the house all the time, but then everybody learned to speak English." The nurse would interpret this as indicative of which of the following?
   a. Flexibility
   b. Culture
   c. Assimilation
   d. Cultural competence

3. Which of the following best identifies a rationale for minority groups feeling uncomfortable about seeking mental health services?
   a. Similarities with religious beliefs
   b. Use of traditional healers
   c. Equality in access to housing
   d. Consistent interpretation of behavior

4. When preparing to teach students about persons of African descent and their approach to mental health services compared with that of white populations, which of the following would the instructor discuss?
   a. Entering mental health services at an earlier stage
   b. Using more treatment services at earlier stages
   c. Continuing services at a significantly higher rate
   d. Being more often misdiagnosed by mental health practitioners

5. After continued discussion, the nurse determines that a Mexican-American client sees a female healer who uses massage and manipulation. The nurse understands that this person is called which of the following?
   a. Bruja
   b. Brujo
   c. Subadora
   d. Curandera

6. To provide culturally competent care, which of the following would the nurse consider incorporating into the plan of care for a Native-American client?
   a. Participation in sweat lodge ceremony
   b. Influence of hot-and-cold imbalances
   c. Knowledge of increased incidence of PTSD
   d. Balance of good and evil

7. When intervening with ethnic minorities, which of the following is essential to consider?
   a. Primarily the client's oral language
   b. The client's immediate space
   c. Time limits in concrete terms
   d. Social organization

8. The nurse is explaining cross-cultural understanding to a group of students. Which of the following descriptions would the nurse include?
   a. Conflict resolution with the ability to negotiate
   b. Listening skills with learning how to decipher nonverbal behavior
   c. Ability to embrace change by modifying expectations
   d. Knowledge about how and why people of different cultures behave

9. When developing transcultural nursing knowledge, which of the following would the nurse be involved with during phase I?
   a. Cultural awareness
   b. Theory-guided research
   c. Explanation of nursing phenomena
   d. Improved practice through research

10. When providing culturally competent care, the nurse should do which of the following?
    a. View the client as a single entity
    b. Ignore own cultural biases
    c. Be an active listener
    d. Reject the client's understanding of problem

▼ REFERENCES AND SUGGESTED READINGS

Alacron, R. D., Westermeyer, J., Foulks, E. F., & Ruiz, P. (1999). Clinical relevance of contemporary cultural psychiatry. *Journal of Nervous and Mental Disease, 187*(18), 465–471.

Axelson, J. (1999). *Counseling and development in a multicultural society.* Belmont, CA: Wadsworth/Brooks/Cole.

Baker, F., & Bell, C. (1999). Issues in the psychiatric treatment of African Americans. *Psychiatric Services, 50*(3), 362.

*Battaglia, B. (1992). Skills for managing multicultural teams. *Cultural Diversity at Work, 4*(3), 4.

*Bechtel, G. A., Davidhizar, R., & Tiller, C. M. (1998). Patterns of mental health care among Mexican Americans. *American Journal of Nursing, 36,* 11.

Bhui, K., & Olajide, D. (1999). *Mental health service provision for a multicultural society.* London: W. B. Saunders.

Campinha-Bacote, J. (1999). A model and instrument for addressing cultural competence in health care. *Journal of Nursing Education, 38*(5), 203–207.

*Campinha-Bacote, J. (1994). Cultural competence in psychiatric-mental health nursing: A conceptual model. *Nursing Clinics of North America, 29*(1), 1–8.

Carnevale, F. (1999). Toward a cultural conception of the self. *Journal of Psychosocial Nursing and Mental Health Services, 37*(8), 26.

Comas-Diaz, L., & Greene, B. (1994). *Women of color: Integrating ethnic and gender identities in psychotherapy.* New York: Guilford Press.

Cross, T. L., Bazron, B. J., Dennis, K. W., et al. (1989). *Towards a culturally competent system of care: A monograph on effective services for minority children who are severely emotionally disturbed.* Washington, DC: Child and Adolescent Service System Program Technical Assistance Center, Georgetown University Child Development Center.

*Erikson, E. (1950). *Childhood and society.* New York: WW Norton.

*Fadiman, A. (1997). *The spirit catches you and you fall down: A Hmong child, her American doctors, and the collision of two cultures.* New York: Noonday.

Flaskerud, J. (2000). Ethnicity, culture, and neuropsychiatry. *Issues in Mental Health Nursing, 21*(5).

*Giger, J., & Davidhizar, R. (1995). *Transcultural nursing: Assessment and intervention.* St. Louis: Mosby.

*Glittenberg, J. (1995). Foreword. In M. Leininger (Ed.), *Transcultural nursing concepts, theories, research & practice.* New York: McGraw-Hill.

*Gurnoe, S., & Nelson, J. (1989). Two perspectives on working with American Indian families: A constructivist–systemic approach. In E. Gonzalea-Sautin & A. Lewis (Eds.), *Collaboration, the key: A model curriculum on Indian child welfare* (pp. 63–85). Tempe, AZ: Arizona State University School of Social Work.

Herrick, C., & Brown, H. (1999). Mental disorders and syndromes found among Asians residing in the United States. *Issues in Mental Health Nursing, 20,* 275–296.

*Huggins, M. (1996). *Five year plan.* Minnesota: Hennepin County Adult Services, Department Mental Health Division.

Kim, J., Bramlett, M. H., Wright, L. K., & Pooin, L. W. (1998). Racial differences in health status and health behaviors of older adults. *Nursing Research, 47*(4), 243–250.

*Leininger, M. (1995). *Transcultural nursing concepts, theories, research & practice.* New York: McGraw-Hill.

Lester, N. (1998). Cultural competence—a nursing dialogue: Part one. *American Journal of Nursing, 98*(8), 26–33.

Lester, N. (1998). Cultural competence—a nursing dialogue: Part two. *American Journal of Nursing, 98*(9), 36–42.

Lin, K., & Cheung, F. (1999). Mental health issues for Asian Americans. *Psychiatric Services, 50*(6), 774.

*McGoldrick, M., & Giordano, J. (1996). *Overview: Ethnicity and family therapy.* New York: Guilford Press.

*O'Connor, B. B. (1995). *Healing traditions: Alternative medicine and the health professions.* Philadelphia: University of Pennsylvania Press.

Office of Minority Health. (1995). [On-line.] Available: www.omhrc.gov.

*Parsons, L., & Reiss, P. (1999). Promoting collaborative practice with culturally diverse populations. *Seminars in Nurse Management, 7*(4), 160.

*Pernell-Arnold, A. (1995). *Principles of multicultural rehabilitation services.* Columbia, MD: International Association of Psychosocial Services.

*Poss, J. (1999). Providing culturally competent care: Is there a role for health promoters? *Nursing Outlook, 47*(1), 30.

Spector, R. E. (2000). *Cultural diversity in health and illness* (5th ed.). Upper Saddle River, NJ: Prentice Hall Health.

*U.S. Department of Health and Human Services, Public Health Service Alcohol, Drug Abuse and Mental Health Administration. (1992). *Cultural competence for evaluators: A guide for alcohol and other drug abuse prevention practitioners working with ethnic/racial communities.* Washington, DC: Author.

Wahl, O. F. (1999). Mental health consumers' experience of stigma. *Schizophrenia Bulletin, 25*(3), 467–478.

*Wenger, A. F. (1995). Preface. In M. Leininger (Ed.), *Transcultural nursing concepts, theories, research & practice.* New York: McGraw-Hill.

Western Interstate Commission for Higher Education. (1998). Cultural competency standards in managed mental health care. (On-line.) Available at: *http://wiche.edu.*

* *Starred references are cited in text.*

For additional information on this chapter, go to *http://connection.lww.com.*

Need more help? See Chapter 5 of the *Study Guide to Accompany Mohr: Johnson's Psychiatric-Mental Health Nursing,* 5th ed.

The Nursing Process in Psychiatric-Mental Healthcare

SUZANNE PERRAUD

▼ KEY TERMS

Assessment—The act of gathering, classifying, categorizing, analyzing, and documenting information about a client's health status.

Behavioral statement—A statement in a nursing plan of care in which the verb represents an observable behavior.

Diagnostic and Statistical Manual of Mental Disorders (DSM)—A criteria-based psychiatric diagnostic system that specifies the type, intensity, duration, and effect of the various behaviors and symptoms required for the diagnosis.

Mental status examination—A tool for assessing objective and observational data that yields information about the client's appearance, level of consciousness, motor status and behavior, affect and mood, attitude, intellectual functioning, speech, cognitive status (including attention and concentration), judgment, abstraction, content of thought, and insight.

Nursing diagnosis—A clinical judgment about individual, family, or community responses to actual or potential health problems or life processes; it is the product of the analysis of data collected during the assessment step of the nursing process.

Nursing process—A problem-solving method of five steps (assessment, nursing diagnosis, planning, intervention, and evaluation) that nurses systematically apply to the care of clients.

Objective data—Phenomena that a person other than the client observes to be present.

Psychosocial assessment—The assessment of psychological, sociological, developmental, spiritual, and cultural data commonly derived from interviews with a client.

Subjective data—Data that the nurse gathers by interviewing the client.

Taxonomy—A classification system that uses a hierarchical structure.

Variance—Anything that alters the client's progress through a normal critical pathway; examples include an unexpected complication or an unusual occurrence in the care delivery system.

▼ LEARNING OBJECTIVES

On completion of this chapter, you should be able to accomplish the following:

- Apply the nursing process to the practice of psychiatric-mental health nursing.
- Explain the components of a psychosocial assessment.
- Describe the importance of the interview in the assessment process.
- Explain a focused assessment approach used to structure a psychosocial assessment.
- List several nursing diagnoses that may apply to the care of clients with psychiatric disorders.
- Explain the use of the multiaxial diagnostic system in the American Psychiatric Association's *Diagnostic and Statistical Manual of Mental Disorders,* 4th edition, text revision (2000).
- Discuss how to organize and use psychosocial assessment data in formulating nursing care plans.
- Explain the use of standardized nursing care plans and clinical pathways in mental healthcare.
- Describe the critical thinking process that shapes moment-to-moment interventions with clients.
- Explain how evaluation relates to the other phases of the nursing process.

▼ Clinical Example 6-1

"I'm going to hurt someone if you don't watch out!" exclaimed Vincent, a 68-year-old nursing home resident with a history of bipolar disorder. Vincent was admitted earlier in the day to an open psychiatric unit because he had become increasingly manic at the nursing home where he lived. The unit staff, after hearing his statement, discussed the possibility that Vincent would need to be placed in seclusion. His threats and posturing were scaring other clients as well as staff members.

The charge nurse decided that further assessment was necessary. She asked Vincent if they could meet in his room to talk. During the conversation, Vincent began to calm down, stating that "finally" someone was listening to him. He told the charge nurse of his experience with a young staff member who had frightened him. The psychiatric technician had apparently told Vincent he would be "sorry" if he didn't stop pacing and talking so much. The technician didn't explain what "sorry" meant, and Vincent thought it meant he would be hurt. Vincent felt that no one listened to him when he tried to tell others that the staff member had threatened him. Vincent saw no alternative but to become aggressive to protect himself.

The nurse listened carefully throughout the interview. She then spoke with the technician who stated that Vincent had been bothering the other clients and that they had asked him to intervene. He acknowledged that he had told Vincent he would be sorry if he didn't stop, meaning that clients who cannot exercise some control over their behaviors are often transferred to a more secure environment.

The nurse considered both sides of the story and determined that the primary problems were a breakdown in communication and a lack of understanding about what constituted acceptable behavior. She felt that both the client and the staff member could learn more effective means of communicating. At a meeting, the nurse guided both the client and the young staff member through an exploration of their feelings of being intimidated and helped them work out alternate methods of expressing needs. Together, they identified clear guidelines for appropriate behavior on the unit and acceptable ways to communicate when enforcing behavioral limits (for the staff) or expressing dissatisfaction with those limits (for Vincent). Both Vincent and the staff member related feeling more understood and better able to handle a similar situation in the future. They scheduled a follow-up meeting to evaluate the long-term effectiveness of their behavioral plan.

In Clinical Example 6-1, the charge nurse used the nursing process to address a problem. The nurse took the following steps:

- Assessed the situation
- Identified the problem based on assessment data
- Developed a plan for addressing the problem
- Implemented the plan
- Evaluated the outcomes

This problem-solving procedure is also known as the scientific method and is a key component of critical thinking activities. It requires gathering data, analyzing and interpreting data, making judgments, setting goals, establishing priorities, selecting appropriate interventions, implementing the interventions, and evaluating the outcomes to determine if the plan has been effective. When applied to the practice of nursing, the process helps nurses solve clin-

ical problems. Nurses systematically apply the nursing process to plan the care of all clients.

This chapter will discuss the steps of the nursing process and provide a framework for applying the nursing process to the care of persons with psychiatric and mental health problems. As you read the chapter, consider the case of Vincent in Clinical Example 6-1. You will learn more about the progression of Vincent's care in Nursing Care Plan 6-1. You will also have the opportunity to apply your understanding of this client and how nurses use the nursing process when caring for clients in the Reflection and Critical Thinking section at the end of this chapter.

STEPS OF THE NURSING PROCESS

The steps of the **nursing process** supply an organized approach for providing quality psychiatric-mental health nursing care. These five steps are the same as those used in other nursing specialties (eg, maternity nursing, medical-surgical nursing). Differences for this nursing specialty, however, exist in terms of the manner and focus of the nurse's observations, the particulars of interviewing during data collection, and the types of interventions used for identified problems.

The five steps of the nursing process are:

1. *Assessment,* or gathering data
2. *Diagnosis,* or identifying a problem
3. *Planning,* or creating a plan that will achieve desired outcomes
4. *Implementation,* or enacting the plan
5. *Evaluation,* or determining the effectiveness of the plan

The steps in the nursing process provide a convenient way to organize and implement nursing practice in a variety of settings, circumstances, and time frames. It is useful to envision each part of the nursing process as a step, because doing so implies sequencing, or passage through time. Each step in the nursing process, however, depends on and is related to the others. For example, an accurate diagnosis is impossible without assessment, and effective interventions are equally impossible to enact without a diagnosis and plan for guidance.

In addition, the nurse may return to a step in the nursing process at any time in a client's care. In other words, assessment becomes reassessment with the revelation of new data or information. For example, a client may reveal new data as his or her trust in the nurse–client relationship increases. Or a change in the client's status may necessitate reassessment. The information obtained from reassessment may be significant enough to change the focus of care or nursing diagnosis. Similarly, information that the nurse obtains during evaluation of a plan may lead to an adjustment in a nursing action to achieve the desired outcome.

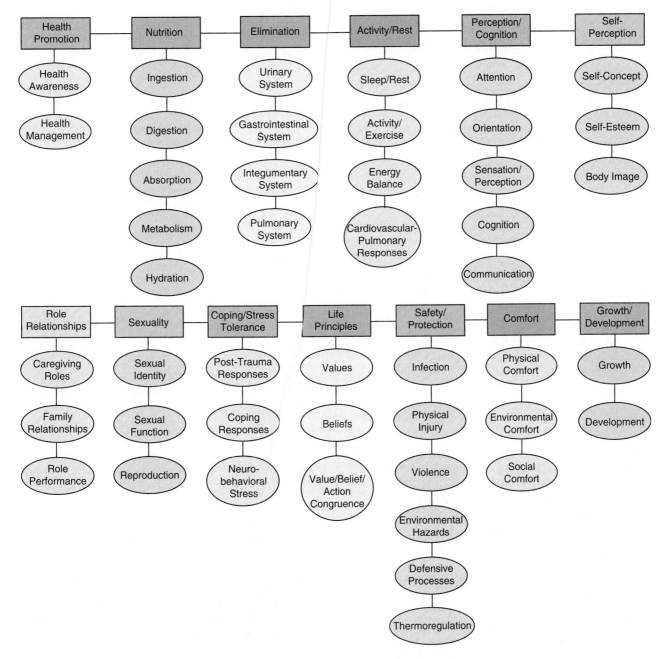

FIGURE 6-1   NANDA Taxonomy II Domains and Classes. (With permission from NANDA).

NURSING DIAGNOSIS AND PSYCHIATRIC DIAGNOSIS

The taxonomy used to make the *psychiatric* diagnosis is provided in the ***Diagnostic and Statistical Manual of Mental Disorders,*** 4th edition, text revision (*DSM-IV-TR*) (APA, 2000). The *DSM-IV-TR* is a criteria-based diagnostic system that specifies the type, intensity, duration, and effect of the various behaviors and symptoms required for the diagnosis. Guidelines represent the clinical judgments of experts in the field of psychiatry. The nurse assists in this process by sharing important infor-mation about the client from the nursing history, MSE, and daily observations. Thus, a working knowledge of the *DSM-IV-TR* is important in maximizing the team effort to help the client. Knowledge of the criteria for deciding on a particular psychiatric diagnosis from the *DSM-IV-TR* may help the nurse in making a clinical decision about a nursing diagnosis.

For example, nurses cannot cure schizophrenia within their nursing role, but they can design interventions for problems within the domain of nursing practice related to schizophrenia. Such problems would include anxiety, self-care deficits, and disturbances in thought processes. The

TABLE 6-2 ▼	Writing the Diagnostic Statement: Examples of Incorrect and Correct Diagnoses	
INCORRECT	**CORRECT**	**RATIONALE**
Depression related to loss of spouse	Dysfunctional Grieving related to lack of adequate support secondary to death of spouse, as evidenced by the statement "I have nothing to live for" and weepy affect	Depression is a psychiatric diagnosis, not a nursing diagnosis. The complete nursing diagnosis includes an etiology that, in most cases, nursing can change through appropriate interventions. Interventions will focus on development of support. Defining characteristics are usually included from the assessment data ("as evidenced by") to justify the diagnosis from the client's behavior.
Ineffective Coping related to lack of adequate ability to cope	Ineffective Coping related to overuse of denial, rationalization, and projection secondary to alcoholism, as evidenced by euphoric affect and blaming of problems on wife	Etiology ("related to") should not repeat the main idea of the nursing diagnosis.
Disturbed Sleep Pattern related to noise on the unit and lack of adequate supervision	Disturbed Sleep Pattern related to oversensitivity to environmental stimuli	Avoid any statements implying poor nursing judgment or poor staffing that may have legal implications.

chapters in Unit IV of this book include foci of care or nursing diagnoses associated with specific *DSM-IV-TR* diagnoses, along with nursing care plans designed to address those problems.

Planning

The third step of the nursing process is *planning,* which involves outcome identification and intervention selection. Planning requires use of evidence-based interventions to attain expected outcomes (American Nurses Association, American Psychiatric Nurses Association, International Society of Psychiatric-Mental Health Nurses, 2000). The plan of care is a result of the collaboration of the client, family, nurse, and other healthcare team members.

IDENTIFYING OUTCOMES

During *outcome identification,* the nurse both identifies realistic, measurable outcomes that are expected as a result of care and establishes a realistic time line for their accomplishment. Identifying expected client outcomes creates a link between the nursing diagnosis and the selection of appropriate nursing interventions (McFarland & McFarlane, 1997, p. 9). Specific outcomes also serve as the basis for evaluating the effectiveness of nursing interventions.

Client outcomes should logically flow from the nursing diagnoses. Outcomes are typically stated in behav-

ioral terms. A **behavioral statement** means that the verb used in the statement represents a behavior that may be observed (Sundeen, Stuart, Rankin, & Cohen, 1998). Examples of behavioral statements linked with client outcomes in psychiatric nursing are as follows:

- The client will bathe daily and wash hair without needing reminders from staff.
- The client will describe situations that trigger increased anxiety.
- The client will demonstrate respect for authority and obey school rules.
- The client will refrain from binge eating and purging.

Client outcomes should be realistic, meaning that the client should have a good chance of achieving them. To assess if an outcome is realistic, the nurse considers the nature of the problem, the efficacy of the treatment approach, the client's contextual resources, and any barriers to treatment. For example, attending therapy at the community health clinic may not be an appropriate outcome for a client with obsessive-compulsive disorder (OCD) if his or her ritualistic behaviors prevent him or her from dressing completely before leaving his or her apartment (see Chap. 18). A more realistic outcome may be to reduce the frequency or intensity of ritualistic behavior.

Another aid to the development of realistic outcomes is the establishment of short-term outcomes that are incremental steps toward a long-term outcome. Nurses

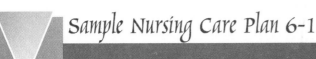

Sample Nursing Care Plan 6-1

During Vincent's first day on the unit, he continues exhibiting manic behaviors such as hyperactivity and excessive talking; however, he is no longer threatening anyone with "getting hurt." His conversation jumps illogically from topic to topic (flight of ideas) and often concerns his plans for "making millions." He can't stay still long enough to eat or drink, and his transfer sheet from the nursing home indicates that he hasn't eaten in 2 days.

When the nurse takes his vital signs, she finds that Vincent is tachycardic and mildly hypertensive. His weight is 5 lb less than the last recorded weight from the nursing home. His laboratory values are consistent with mild dehydration. The nurse obtains more information during the interview, including the fact that Vincent stopped taking his lithium carbonate several weeks ago and doesn't want to take it now because he "feels great!" Rather than answer the nurse's interview questions, Vincent outlines his plans for getting rich and says he has many important phone calls to make. He then terminates the interview, saying, "You're no fun" when the nurse declines to sing and joke with him. Based on these data, the nurse identifies several diagnoses and prioritizes them, formulates realistic desired outcomes, and chooses interventions that will help the client achieve those outcomes.

Nursing Diagnosis: Deficient Fluid Volume related to insufficient intake of oral fluids

Goal: Vincent will maintain optimal hydration.

Interventions	Rationales
Promote intake of fluids by offering appealing drinks between meals and providing fresh water, Popsicles, or fruits with a high water content. Obtain a sports–drink-type bottle that the client can carry. Check it throughout the day or remind the client to replenish it. Frequently give the client specific instructions to drink.	Clients with mania often do not attend to their bodies' needs for fluids. Making beverages available "on the run" enhances the likelihood that Vincent will remember to ingest liquids. Vincent is easily distracted and will need reminders and specific instructions.
Monitor the client's intake and engage him in keeping a record of fluid intake.	Vincent will require supervision to ensure that fluid intake goals are met. Engaging him in the process will help him remember to drink appropriately.
Assess the client daily for signs of dehydration such as dry mucous membranes and weight loss.	Ongoing assessment is required to prevent dehydration, which can result in confusion, electrolyte imbalance, hypotension, and dysrhythmias.

Evaluation: The intake record should reflect that Vincent is drinking 2 to 3 L per day. Moist mucous membranes, modest weight gain, normal laboratory values, and heart rate and blood pressure at Vincent's preadmission baseline are clinical indicators of optimal hydration.

Nursing Diagnosis: Imbalanced Nutrition: Less than Body Requirements related to manic state and inability to sit still to eat

Goal: Vincent will maintain sufficient caloric intake to meet energy requirements.

Interventions	Rationales
Ask for the client's food preferences and offer finger foods throughout the day. Sit with the client during meals. Encourage the client to eat foods high in nutritive value.	Arranging for Vincent to have his favorite foods will increase the likelihood that he will eat, as will offering finger foods that he can carry around during the day. Sitting with Vincent will remind him of the importance placed on his nutrition. When dietary intake is insufficient, highly nutritive and densely caloric foods are preferred over empty calories.

(continued)

Sample Nursing Care Plan 6-1 (Continued)

Interventions	Rationales
Monitor the client's food intake and engage him in keeping track of foods eaten.	Vincent will require supervision to ensure that caloric and nutritive goals are met. Engaging him in the process will help him remember to eat appropriately.
Assess the client daily for weight loss and signs of a catabolic metabolic state such as fruity breath and urinary ketosis.	Rapid weight loss, urinary ketosis, and fruity breath suggest that Vincent's body is breaking down proteins to convert to carbohydrates to meet energy needs. This undesirable metabolic state can lead to complications.

Evaluation: Vincent's weight loss should stop, and his weight should gradually return to normal. Simple observation of the client ingesting sufficient amounts of nutritive food is evidence that the interventions are effective.

Nursing Diagnosis: Noncompliance related to mood disorder-induced euphoria and denial

Goal: Vincent will take his medication, as prescribed.

Interventions	Rationales
Help the client acknowledge that his euphoric state is the result of chemical imbalances and that medication balances his mood, preventing highs as well as lows. Help the client identify inappropriate behaviors that may lead to unpleasant or regrettable circumstances.	Cognitive restructuring can help Vincent alter his distorted beliefs and manic thought patterns and help him to see his situation more realistically.
Observe the client swallow the medication and inspect the mouth after the medication has been taken.	Vincent may require direct supervision and observation until he becomes compliant with the medication regimen.

Evaluation: Therapeutic lithium levels are the best indicator that Vincent is taking his medication as prescribed. Changes in behavior attributable to the lithium may not be seen for 1 to 2 weeks.

Nursing Diagnosis: Disturbed Thought Processes related to mood disorder and manic state

Goal: Vincent will interact appropriately with others and exhibit logical, realistic thought processes.

Interventions	Rationales
Use a firm, calm, neutral approach with the client and provide direction using short, clear statements. Make your expectations clear about appropriate behavior.	This approach provides structure and a sense of security to Vincent. Communicating clearly with him will help him understand his environment and reinforce appropriate behavior.
Do not support acting-out behaviors or the client's delusional or irrational behaviors.	Supporting acting-out behaviors or participating in the client's jokes or irrational conversations encourages the manic behavior and subjects the nurse to manipulation.
When possible, help the client channel energies into productive activities.	Doing so will help Vincent regain behavioral control and limit the progression of manic behaviors.
Provide a calm environment; steer the client away from highly stimulating activities.	A stimulating environment can lead to increased manic behaviors, including excessive activity and aggressiveness.

Evaluation: Improvements in Vincent's thought processes can be evaluated by observing his interactions with other clients and staff. The content of his conversation can be evaluated for increasing logic, realism, and cohesiveness.

accomplish this by identifying the terminal outcome and then determining the steps leading to that outcome (Sundeen, Stuart, Rankin, & Cohen, 1998). For example, a long-term outcome for a person with agoraphobia and panic disorder would be the ability to function outside the home without panic. A short-term component or step toward this outcome might be the ability to stand outside the front door without panic. Once the client successfully achieves the first short-term outcome, then the nurse can plan another short-term outcome, such as walking to the end of the driveway (see Chap. 18). Table 6-3 contains examples of long-term and short-term goals and illustrates how they are typically defined.

A related aspect of care planning that the nurse should address as early as possible in the episode of care is *discharge planning* or posttreatment follow-up care. Once the treatment team members define the expected outcomes for their phase of treatment, referrals should begin that target issues relevant to the continuity of care. Discharge planning helps ensure that when leaving a specific treatment environment, the client has a treatment plan in place that matches the intensity of follow-up services with the intensity of the client's needs and will aid in the achievement of the desired outcomes.

SELECTING INTERVENTIONS

After establishing behavioral outcomes, the nurse *identifies the interventions* needed to help the client achieve these outcomes (Duldt, 1995). A wide scope of nursing interventions exist, and psychiatric-mental health nurses select interventions according to their levels of practice. Box 6-2 contains categories of nursing interventions appropriate to the basic-level psychiatric-mental health nurse. Advanced practice nursing interventions, appropriate for clinical nurse specialists and psychiatric nurse practitioners, include psychotherapy, consultation, and prescriptive authority and treatment (American Nurses Association, American Psychiatric Nurses Association, International Society of Psychiatric-Mental Health Nurses, 2000).

Examples of psychiatric-mental health nursing interventions include the following:

- Assisting a client with depression to make decisions about what to wear
- Providing finger foods and a water bottle to a client with mania who cannot slow down to eat or drink
- Offering to listen to an angry, defiant adolescent
- Suggesting alternative ways to handle problems to a suicidal client

TABLE 6-3 ▼ Long-Term and Short-Term Goals

Changes require goal setting. Goals must be observable and measurable by others. Long-term goals are oriented toward the future, whereas short-term goals are the markers of achievement that one attains along the way toward a goal.

Examples of both types of goals are listed below.

LONG-TERM GOALS	SHORT-TERM GOALS
To achieve independence through employment	To graduate from high school or pass an equivalency examination To graduate from an appropriate vocational or collegiate program To apply for and attain a job
To increase ability to cope with stress, as demonstrated by decreased angry outbursts	To seek counseling or a self-help group and attend meetings regularly To identify one coping strategy and try that coping method for 1 month
To improve organization and promptness	To organize and list responsibilities of home, work, school, children To prepare general schedules based on prioritization of responsibilities To prepare individual daily schedules with daily tasks and appointments
To increase self-esteem by altering body image	To achieve ideal body weight To improve body tone through daily exercise To assess and redo wardrobe

• Removing an aggressive client from a group setting in which he or she has threatened others

When planning interventions for clients, nurses can refer to resource materials, such as standardized care plans and clinical pathways.

Standardized Care Plans

Standardized care plans list nursing actions and interventions. They are organized according to the problem areas of a specific diagnostic category or nursing diagnosis. Standardized care plans provide nurses with a documented standard of practice for each diagnostic category (Doenges, Moorhouse, & Burley, 1995). The purpose of standardized care plans is to achieve consistent care of specific clients within an organization. In other words, a standardized care plan reflects the facility's goal that all clients with a specific health problem, regardless of context of care (such as shift, nursing skill, or day of the week), will receive the same care. Standardized care plans for a wide range of diagnostic categories can be found in reference texts.

Clinical or Critical Pathways

Clinical pathways are similar to standardized nursing care plans, but they are designed for the entire treatment team. Clinical pathways, also known as critical pathways, care maps, clinical maps, and clinical trajectories, have been developed as a way to ensure that the healthcare team meets a standard of quality in providing care during this time of scarce health resources. Clinical pathways also provide a map for the treatment team members to follow when they deliver essential clinical services to clients with a particular condition. Box 6-3 contains common components of a clinical pathway.

A **variance** is anything that alters the client's progress through the normal critical pathway. Examples of variances include an unexpected complication or an unusual occurrence in the care delivery system, such as lost requisitions for laboratory tests (Komplin, 1995). Significant variances signal the need for a change in the plan. Although their use is controversial in psychiatric care where similar conditions have such different consequences for different people, clinical pathways have been developed for the treatment of major depression, cognitive mental disorder, schizophrenia, chemical dependency, and bipolar disorder (Barry, 1998).

Implementation

Implementation is the fourth step in the nursing process and occurs when nurses perform planned nursing actions. All identified interventions are performed by all nursing shifts. Continuity in carrying out specific interventions is critical to achieving the desired outcomes. In most institutions, nurses are expected to document that the interventions were carried out, followed by the client's response to the intervention. Quality care only occurs through careful and ongoing observation of the effects of the care. For the client with a psychiatric disorder or mental health problem, as for clients with medical problems, the incremental responses to each intervention and nurse–client interaction serve as the building blocks for the full achievement of desired outcomes.

For the nursing student, interactions with clients may be awkward and anxiety provoking. Although students will have communicated with many clients through various clinical experiences, they confront an important difference in psychiatric-mental health nursing. When mentally preparing for a planned interchange with a client, the focus is no longer on performing a psychomotor skill correctly, but rather on verbal and nonverbal behavior. The therapeutic intent of words and actions takes center stage.

In a typical interaction, the client makes a statement or exhibits a behavior, and the nursing student understands that a response is required. The student has read the client's chart and plan of care. Now the student must combine this knowledge of the client's history with what is happening at the moment to formulate a therapeutic response.

Consider, as an example, the therapeutic principle of empathy (see Chap. 4). It is not enough to understand the concept of empathy and its use in supporting the client and recognizing the human meaning of illness. During face-to-face discussion with a client who is in distress or facing a stressful recovery, nurses must use words to forge a mutual understanding of that experience.

The first few attempts at conveying empathy, combining a natural act like talking with intent, may be awkward. Students are aware of the pressure to frame a statement so that the client experiences the nurse understanding and responding to him or her. After some practice with the technique, however, demonstrating empathy with a client will probably come naturally.

The same internalization of principles to frame statements with intent must occur with psychiatric-mental health nursing interventions. Internalizing intervention principles is more complicated, however, because the process demands that nurses keep several considerations in focus while crafting the response.

INTERVENTION STRATEGIES FOR BEGINNING PRACTITIONERS

Intervention strategies for the beginning practitioner include counseling interventions: problem solving, crisis intervention, stress management, and behavior modification (see Box 6-2). A problem-solving approach might focus on reinforcing some thought-stopping techniques the client learned in a cognitive therapy group. Using a behavioral approach, the nurse might suggest that when negative thoughts are overwhelming, the client should initiate a distracting pleasant activity. The nurse and client might compose a list of useful activities for this situation. With a psychoeducational approach, the nurse would focus on teaching the client about his depression, perhaps discussing how negative thoughts often accompany depression. A biological approach might point toward the use of psychotropic medication. This book details the conceptual framework for a variety of intervention strategies specific to various mental disorders.

Which one of these basic approaches the nurse uses in a moment-to-moment interaction depends on the care plan and the particulars of the client situation. For instance, if it were late in the day and the client were about to travel home, the nurse might talk about behavioral techniques the client could use in the evening hours to cope with negative thoughts. There is no one "right" approach. It is crucial that the nurse has a clear theoretical rationale for an intervention and that the intervention is consistent with assessment and nursing care plan data.

SUPERVISION

Supervision is the process by which psychiatric-mental health nurses obtain feedback about their interventions and analyze the emotions particular clients generated in them. This process helps nurses and other mental health professionals learn to be objective about their reactions and to "bracket off" emotions. In subsequent interactions, these emotions are then less likely to interfere with moment-to-moment interventions.

This skill develops during interventions with clients when professionals learn to maintain at least a partial awareness of their own reactions and emotions. This awareness should not interfere with the nurse's focus on what the client is communicating. On the contrary, this self-awareness is essential so that the nurse's own emotional reactions do not intrude on processing and understanding the client's communication.

A particular challenge for beginning nurses is to control their own anxiety during initial client interactions. In postclinical conferences, nursing students should recall the feelings and reactions that arose while talking with clients, because training oneself to recall interactions and accompanying emotions is the essence of supervision, which, in turn, is central to the work of psychiatric nursing.

Evaluation

Evaluation is the process of determining the value of each intervention or the attainment of desired outcomes. Evaluation of practice is essential because of professional accountability and the nursing profession's commitment to clients and families. This commitment demands that nurses continually monitor interventions to determine if they are effective and if they serve the needs of individuals and families. The nursing process is cyclical, so evaluation is the catalyst for modifying the other components of the care plan.

Evaluation of a client's care is twofold. It centers on the changes experienced by the client and the quality or the effectiveness of the nursing care itself. For example, the nurse may assess a withdrawn client as disoriented and specify as an outcome of nursing care, "The client will verbalize awareness of time and place." Nursing interventions to achieve that goal might include visual cues placed in the client's environment (calendars and clocks) and verbal reinforcement of time and place.

The nurse evaluates the effects of these interventions by observing client behaviors. The nurse may ask the following questions: Is the client present at activities that he or she is expected to attend? How did the client respond to periodic mental status checks of orientation to time, person, and place? If the client's behavior does not change, the nurse must review and modify the care plan by modifying the outcomes or devising new intervention strategies (Figure 6-2).

The review of the care plan also provides information relevant to evaluating nursing care. Was the initial assessment of the client complete? Were the client goals realistic, specific, and measurable? Did other nurses who intervened with the client follow the care plan consistently? Did care plan modifications sufficiently address unanticipated complications in the client's response to interventions? Seeking the answers to these and related questions engages nurses in problem solving, which is essential to the evaluation and improvement of nursing care.

▼ Reflection and Critical Thinking Questions

1. How would different treatment settings influence the prioritization of the client's needs?
2. Describe how you would explain "nursing diagnosis" to someone from a social work background.
3. Plan three nursing interventions for a client with depression.

▼ CHAPTER SUMMARY

■ Nursing assessment involves gathering client data and exploring the needs, problems, and adaptive resources of the individual.

■ Through the holistic approach to assessment, the nurse–interviewer explores client functioning in psychological, social, biological, behavioral, cognitive, cultural, and spiritual areas of life.

■ The nurse's communication and relationship skills are essential in conducting an assessment interview.

■ Analysis of client assessment data results in determination of important, clearly written, definitive nursing diagnoses.

■ The nursing diagnosis is a statement of a client's response pattern to a health disruption and guides the planning and intervention phases of the nursing process.

■ The *DSM-IV-TR* contains a multiaxial classification system that fosters a holistic approach to the client; it includes specific behavioral criteria for each psychiatric diagnosis.

■ The current NANDA taxonomy contains nursing diagnoses useful for psychiatric nursing.

■ Nursing care plans define the goals or outcomes of care and the methods to achieve them.

■ Standardized care plans provide nurses with documented standards of practice for clients with particular conditions.

■ Intervention requires nurses to combine data from plans of care with information from what is occurring at the

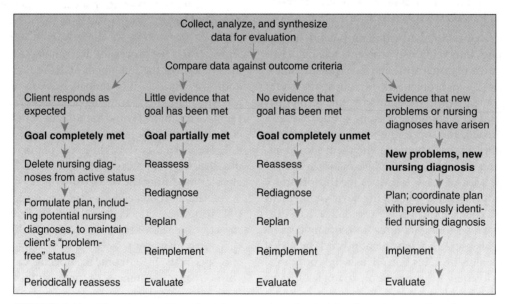

FIGURE 6-2   Flowchart to identify actions to take after judging how interventions have affected achievement of client goals.

moment, prioritize client needs, and then match this information with an appropriate therapeutic strategy.

■ Evaluation is the final phase of the nursing process in which nurses determine the effectiveness of an intervention or the attainment of a preset goal.

▼ REVIEW QUESTIONS

1. The nursing process is a
   a. Framework for documenting the multidisciplinary plan of care
   b. Standardized care plan
   c. Procedure for solving clinical problems
   d. Method for developing nursing diagnoses

2. A client is admitted for severe depression and is brought to the inpatient unit. The nurse, adhering to the nursing process, begins by
   a. Developing relevant diagnoses
   b. Assessing the client's mental and physical health status
   c. Establishing outcomes such as, "The client will not express suicidal thoughts"
   d. Offering to teach the client stress management techniques

3. In the nursing diagnosis Risk for Violence: Self-Directed or Directed at Others, the "related to" factors would be
   a. A list of actual risk factors
   b. Behaviors indicating the presence of the problem
   c. Another nursing diagnosis
   d. The medical diagnosis

4. A nursing diagnosis is defined as
   a. A clinical judgment about individual responses to medical or psychiatric conditions or life processes
   b. A clinical judgment about family systems and individual responses to health problems
   c. A clinical judgment about individual, family, or community responses to actual health problems or life processes
   d. A way of prioritizing nursing interventions.

5. The NANDA taxonomy was developed to
   a. Teach clinicians how to create nursing diagnoses
   b. Group related diagnoses in a logical way
   c. Match nursing diagnoses with medical or psychiatric diagnoses
   d. Define nursing's unique knowledge base

6. A 44-year-old woman is being seen in the outpatient mental health clinic for treatment of anorexia nervosa. The nurse performs a thorough psychosocial and physical assessment, which reveals, among other things, that the 5′6″ client weighs 100 lb. The client also describes her severely ritualistic behaviors around food, such as cutting food into 1/2-inch size pieces and eating only certain foods on certain days. When planning the client's care, the nurse and the client identify goals. Which of the following represents a well-thought-out goal for this client?
   a. The client will gain 4 lb per week until she reaches her goal weight of 130 lb.
   b. The client will eliminate ritualistic behaviors within 1 month of initiating therapy.
   c. The client will learn to identify situations that trigger anxiety.
   d. The client will acknowledge that she is emaciated and looks very ill.

7. Bill, a 70-year-old client, has been referred to the mental health clinic by his primary care provider. Bill's wife died suddenly 3 months ago, and Bill has been severely depressed since then. He states that he cries all the time and can't sleep or eat well. Based on these data, which of the following diagnoses is most appropriate?
   a. Hopelessness
   b. Dysfunctional grieving
   c. Spiritual distress
   d. Ineffective coping

8. A nurse diagnoses her client with Impaired Social Interaction related to self-concept disturbance, as evidenced by client's verbalized inability to experience satisfying relationships with peers or family. When choosing interventions to address this problem, the nurse seeks to design interventions that will
   a. Improve the client's social environment
   b. Help the family cope with the client
   c. Address the client's self-concept
   d. Help the client make new friends

9. The nurse is evaluating a client's plan of care 5 days after his admission to a closed unit. The client, a 15-year-old boy, has a history of inflicting daily self-injury by cutting himself. The plan included the goal that the client would stop injuring himself. The nurse contracted with the client that he would seek out a staff member whenever he felt like hurting himself and would gain privileges for doing so. Of the following, which is the best indicator that the plan is effective and the goal is being met?
   a. The client reports that he has not cut himself in 3 days.
   b. There are no fresh cuts on the client's body, and staff members report that the client has been seeking them out for help.
   c. The client has only one new cut in 3 days and has been able to refrain from cutting without the staff's help.
   d. The client reports that when he feels like hurting himself, he begins exercising instead.

10. During the evaluation process, the nurse notes that the goals have not been met. What is the nurse's next step?

   a. Begin assessing the client's current status and developing new goals and diagnoses.

   b. Revise the interventions.

   c. Revise the goals.

   d. Continue the plan and reevaluate it in 2 days.

▼ REFERENCES AND SUGGESTED READINGS

*American Nurses Association, American Psychiatric Nurses Association, & International Society of Psychiatric-Mental Health Nurses. (2000). *Scope and standards of psychiatric-mental health nursing practice.* Washington, DC: American Nurses Publishing.

*American Psychiatric Association. (2000). *Diagnostic and statistical manual of mental disorders* (4th ed., text rev.). Washington, DC: Author.

*Barry, P. D. (1998). *Mental health and mental illness* (6th ed.). Philadelphia: Lippincott.

Brown, W. W., Griepp, A. Z., Buckley, S., James, A., & VanderMolen, N. (1998). Process-oriented critical pathways in inpatient psychiatry: Our first year. *Journal of Psychosocial Nursing, 36*(6), 31–36.

DePalma, J. (1999). Measuring outcomes related to nursing. *Home Health Care Management & Practice, 11*(4), 67–68.

*Doenges, M. E., Moorhouse, M. F., & Burley, J. T. (1995). *Application of nursing process and nursing diagnosis* (2nd ed.). Philadelphia: F.A. Davis Company.

*Duldt, B. W. (1995). Nursing process: The science of nursing in the curriculum. *Nurse Educator, 20,* 24–30.

Dyer, J. G., Sparks, S. M., & Taylor, C. M. (1995). *Psychiatric nursing diagnoses: A comprehensive manual of mental health care.* Springhouse, PA: Springhouse.

Fortinash, K. M., & Holoday-Worret, P. A. (1995). *Psychiatric nursing care plans.* St. Louis: CV Mosby.

Jones, A. (1997). Managed care strategy for mental health services. *British Journal of Nursing, 6*(10), 564–568.

*Komplin, J. (1995). Care delivery systems. In P. S. Yoder-Wise (Ed.), *Leading and managing in nursing.* St. Louis: Mosby.

*McFarland, G. K., & McFarlane, E. A. (1997). *Nursing diagnosis and intervention* (3rd ed.). St. Louis: Mosby.

*North American Nursing Diagnosis Association. (2001). *Nursing diagnoses: Definitions and classification* (*2001–2002*). Philadelphia: Author.

Smith, G. B. (1999). Practice guidelines and outcome evaluation. *Outcome Management for Nursing Practice, 2*(3), 24–29.

Souder, E., & O'Sullivan, P. S. (2000). Nursing documentation versus standardized assessment of cognitive status in hospitalized medical patients. *Applying Nursing Research, 13*(1), 29–36.

Sparks, S. M., & Taylor, C. M. (1998). *Nursing diagnosis reference manual* (4th ed.). Springhouse, PA: Springhouse.

*Sundeen, S. J., Stuart, G. W., Rankin, E. A., & Cohen, S. A. (1998). *Nurse–client interaction: Implementing the nursing process* (6th ed.). St. Louis: Mosby.

Worley, N. K. (1997). *Mental health nursing in the community.* St. Louis: Mosby.

*Starred references are cited in text.

For additional information on this chapter, go to *http://connection.lww.com*.

Need more help? See Chapter 6 of the *Study Guide to Accompany Mohr: Johnson's Psychiatric-Mental Health Nursing, 5th edition.* For a complete list of current NANDA diagnoses, refer to Appendix C. For a list of commonly used NIC/NOC labels associated with psychiatric disorders, refer to Appendix F.

Legal and Ethical Aspects of Psychiatric-Mental Health Nursing

ROBIN S. DIAMOND; GWEN LARSEN

▼ KEY TERMS

Autonomy—The right to make decisions for oneself.

Battery—The act of touching another person without his or her permission.

Beneficence—The principle of doing good, not harm.

Emergency admission—Admission to a psychiatric hospital that occurs when a client acts in a way that indicates that he or she is mentally ill and, as a consequence of the particular illness, is likely to harm self or others. State statutes define the exact procedure for the initial evaluation and the possible length of detainment.

Ethical dilemma—A situation in which there are conflicting moral claims or in which two ethical principles conflict.

Ethics—Principles that serve as a code of conduct about right and wrong behavior to guide the actions of individuals.

Fidelity—Faithfulness to duties, obligations, and promises.

Informed consent—Consent that a recipient of healthcare gives to treating providers that enables the recipient to understand a proposed treatment, including its administration, prognosis after treatment, side effects, risks, possible consequences of refusal, and other alternatives.

Involuntary admission—Admission to a psychiatric hospital that occurs when a person with mental illness who refuses psychiatric hospitalization or treatment poses a danger to self or others and cannot safely be cared for in a less restrictive setting.

Malpractice—A tort action that a consumer plaintiff brings against a defendant professional from whom the plaintiff believes that he or she has received injury during the course of the professional–consumer relationship; professional negligence.

Paternalism—An ethical principle by which the intent is to do good; however, professionals determine what is considered "good" and may override a client's wishes and self-determination.

Reasonable person test—A legal concept that refers to how a reasonable and prudent healthcare professional is expected to perform with regard to his or her professional role in a practice situation.

Respondeat superior—A Latin term meaning that acts of employees are attributable to their employer, whom the court also will find responsible for damages to injured third parties.

Substituted consent—Authorization that another person gives on behalf of a client who needs a procedure or treatment but cannot provide consent for it independently.

Veracity—A systematic display of honesty and truthfulness in speech.

Voluntary admission—An admission to a psychiatric hospital that occurs (1) through a client's direct request by coming to the hospital or (2) following evaluation of a client who is determined to be dangerous to self or others or unable to adequately meet his or her own needs in the community but is willing to submit to treatment and is competent to do so.

▼ LEARNING OBJECTIVES

On completion of this chapter, you should be able to accomplish the following:

■ Identify basic legal issues related to psychiatric-mental health nursing care.

■ Explain the role of nursing practice acts in terms of legal concerns.

■ Discuss issues related to malpractice and measures that healthcare professionals can take to protect themselves from litigation.

■ Discuss the basic rights of people with mental illness.

■ Describe different types of commitments and states of competency.

■ Describe the term *standard of care* as a concept in practice.

■ Discuss everyday ethics as they apply to psychiatric-mental health nursing practice.

■ Explain the American Nurses Association's code for nurses.

■ Analyze the ethical principles of autonomy, beneficence, paternalism, veracity, and fidelity in relation to care of the client with a psychiatric disorder.

■ Describe the role of ethics in community practice settings.

■ Discuss situations in which there is a conflict between two or more ethical principles.

Probably no other nursing specialty area demands as great a need for knowledge of the law and ethics as does psychiatric-mental health nursing. Clients are becoming increasingly informed about legal and ethical issues related to healthcare and have improved access to legal counsel through legal clinics, the American Civil Liberties Union, and other advocacy groups (Historical Capsule 7-1). Psychiatric-mental health nurses are increasingly responsible and accountable for the services they perform and may fail to perform. They must conduct accurate assessments, plan carefully, implement competent interventions, identify measurable outcomes, and work within the interdisciplinary process. While doing so, psychiatric-mental health nurses also must ensure that their practices meet professional standards, legal mandates, and ethical guidelines.

The major goal of this chapter is to prepare nurses to include legal and ethical principles in their practice. By doing so, nurses can benefit and protect themselves and their clients and enhance the quality of their care. This chapter discusses the legal authority of professional nursing practice and acknowledges the expansion of nursing's scope of practice. It addresses basic and evolving rights of clients and the importance of acknowledging and protecting these rights. It clarifies some differences related to important legal and ethical concepts that may seem similar on the surface. It addresses different types of commitment as well as significant legal issues that apply to special client populations.

The chapter also introduces ethics as basic and obvious moral truths that guide deliberation and action when providing care to those with psychiatric disorders ("everyday ethics"). It reviews familiar bioethical principles of autonomy, beneficence, nonmaleficence, veracity, and fidelity and discusses ethical considerations for the community psychiatric nurse. Finally, the chapter discusses the importance of professional boundaries when working in therapeutic relationships with clients.

▼ Clinical Example 7-1

Lillian, an 82-year-old client with schizophrenia, lives alone in her two-story home. She is not experiencing delusions or hallucinations. She is oriented and generally can engage in lucid conversation. A psychiatric nurse from a Visiting Nurse Association (VNA) calls on Lillian once a week to assess her mental and physical status and to refill her medications. A home health aide provides Lillian with assistance with activities of daily living (ADLs) three times a week; during these visits, the aide usually cleans Lillian's house. Lillian also receives Meals on Wheels several times a week. She has no other support systems.

During the last few weeks, Lillian's physical health has deteriorated. She has fallen several times; twice the home health aide found Lillian on the floor upon arrival. The nurse has attempted to explore alternative living arrangements for Lillian, but the client is adamant about staying in her own home. Lillian does not seem to understand the seriousness of her situation. She states that the VNA should provide her with daily visits so she can continue to live at home.

The VNA's mission is to provide intermittent care; it is not sanctioned to provide the continuous care that Lillian seems to require. When the nurse conveys this information, Lillian remains unyielding. The nurse contacts Adult Protective Services (APS) twice to inform them of Lillian's situation. APS assigns a case manager to investigate the situation; however, APS does not consider Lillian's case a high priority compared to many of their other cases. Thus, the APS manager cannot visit Lillian immediately or confirm when he will be able to do so.

The psychiatric nurse feels obligated to continue to visit Lillian. She even tries to increase her visits from one to two or three times per week, though she realizes that by doing so, she is disobeying agency procedure. The nurse and the home health aide believe that abandoning Lillian in her current situation would be unethical. They find themselves torn: Should they follow the procedures outlined by the VNA and the client's insurance, which would mean discontinuing the visits and possibly forcing APS to take action? Would doing so further compromise Lillian's health? Should the nurse continue to visit, citing the need to fill the client's medication as the rationale for care, even though doing so would mean using government funding in an unauthorized way?

Points for Reflection and Critical Thinking

- What are some possible legal concerns if the nurse continues to make extra visits to Lillian? What are some possible legal concerns if the nurse stops making visits?
- What are the responsibilities of and risks to the VNA? What are the responsibilities and risks for APS?
- What would you do if you were the nurse in this situation? Defend your actions.

LEGAL ISSUES IN PSYCHIATRIC-MENTAL HEALTH NURSING CARE

Nurses must learn to value, respect, and seek out knowledge about laws, legislation, and the legal processes that regulate, impede, and facilitate professional nursing practice. By being aware of such standards, staying informed

HISTORICAL CAPSULE 7-1
Past and Present Legal Trends in Mental Healthcare

For the last few hundred years, society has dealt with people who have mental disorders in various ways. Until recently, the principal method was segregation from the general population. This isolation from society is reported in K. Jones' *Lunacy, Law, and Conscience* (1955):

- Sixteenth century: The deranged were expelled, shipped off, or executed.
- Seventeenth century: The insane were locked in jails and houses of correction.
- Eighteenth century: Madmen were confined in madhouses.
- Nineteenth century: Lunatics were sent to asylums.
- Twentieth century: The mentally ill were committed to hospitals.

Current laws regarding treatment of the mentally ill evolved from the Common Law of England. During the 11th century, the king of England was responsible for the care of the insane if no kinsmen could provide it. By the beginning of the 14th century, the church and the lord of the manor were responsible for the mentally ill. At that time, Edward II proclaimed the king's responsibility toward the mentally ill and extended the national law of guardianships to the mentally ill, who were again made the duty of the crown. W. Blackstone used the term *parens patriae* to refer to the power and the responsibility of the state to care for the disabled members of society.

In the British colonies, settlers dealt informally with the mentally disabled who came to the New World. Families locked up their mentally ill relatives in back rooms or outhouses. Others, who had nowhere to go, wandered or were confined in jails with criminals, drunkards, and other social outcasts. Eventually, however, the states assumed the *parens patriae* power of the king.

In 1752, Philadelphia Hospital, the nation's first general hospital, provided treatment to the mentally ill. During this period, Pinel's and Luke's work in France and London regarding the "moral treatment" of the mentally ill implied a mental condition that was curable in an appropriate psychological and social environment.

By the middle of the 19th century, it was obvious that the hospitals could not meet the needs of the mentally disabled. Social crusaders, such as Dorothea Dix, assisted with funding, building, and enlarging public mental hospitals. Despite their humanistic purposes, these hospitals actually allowed for an era of custodial treatment through the unwarranted commitment of thousands of homeless people in overcrowded hospitals. Little regard was given toward any legal protective processes.

To combat these increasingly unacceptable conditions, the clients' rights movement developed. It supported the concept of deinstitutionalization of the mentally ill. During the last several decades, the deinstitutionalization concept and its implementation have been at the forefront of mental healthcare delivery. Community mental health centers have opened their doors to provide necessary psychiatric treatment to people who do not require inpatient hospitalization. From the late 1980s to the present, social and economic initiatives have encouraged mental health services that help the mentally ill live outside hospitals and in the least restrictive setting possible. Community mental health centers send crisis teams into the client's home to provide services. Home behavioral health services assist clients to meet their needs while living in the community. As a result of this community approach, inpatient psychiatric numbers have decreased dramatically since the early 1950s, and the criteria for judicial commitment have narrowed considerably.

Deinstitutionalization mandated the development of more than 2000 public mental health centers to provide care for the mentally ill for whom inpatient care is not necessary, leaving hospital facilities to care for those who are not functioning safely in society because of mental illness. The integration of the mentally ill into the general population has engendered a great deal of political and social controversy and conflict. An increased understanding of mental health and illness by society is slowly replacing the stigma attached to mental illness. The health delivery system must continue to develop community support services, such as housing, employment, and accessible aftercare to facilitate social integration of the mentally ill population.

Legal rights and remedies for the mentally ill have been evolving. Over the last 20 years, new statutes resulting from judicial decisions regarding the right to refuse psychotropic medications have had a major impact on the care and treatment of the mentally ill. The passage of the Americans With Disabilities Act of 1990 provides broad civil rights protection for people with mental illnesses. Dramatic changes in healthcare financing following the failure of the passage of healthcare reform are complicating the availability and the accessibility of mental health services. Managed care companies are

(continued)

HISTORICAL CAPSULE 7-1
Past and Present Legal Trends in Mental Healthcare (Continued)

revolutionizing the way individuals gain access to and providers deliver behavioral healthcare services. Currently, some states now require insurance companies, including health maintenance organizations (HMOs), to provide at least the same amount of lifetime coverage for psychiatric illnesses as they provide for major medical coverage.

(Source: Jones, K. [1955]. *Lunacy, Law, and Conscience.* London: Routledge and Kegan Paul; Kaimowitz v. Michigan Department of Mental Hygiene, 2 P. L. 433 [1979]; Parham, Commissioner, Department of Human Resources of Georgia et al. v. J. R., et al., 442 U. S. 584, [1979]).

about new and changing legislation that affects clinical practice, and understanding proposed and past legislation affecting mental healthcare, psychiatric mental-health nurses can provide quality care that safeguards the rights and safety of clients. Furthermore, such behavior can only improve the influence of nurses as peers within the interdisciplinary healthcare team.

Nurse Practice Acts and the Expanding Role of Nursing

Standards of nursing practice are written documents that outline minimum expectations for safe nursing care. They are used to guide and evaluate nursing care, and courts look to standards of practice for guidance when malpractice cases are deliberated. The nurse practice act in each state defines nursing, describes its scope, and identifies its limits within that state. Although nurse practice acts differ according to state, the definition of professional nursing in the Texas Code is similar to that in most states:

> *"Professional nursing" shall be defined as the performance for compensation of any nursing act (a) in the observation, assessment, intervention, evaluation, rehabilitation, care and counsel and health teachings of persons who are ill, injured or infirm or experiencing changes in normal health processes; (b) in the maintenance of health or prevention of illness; (c) in the administration of medications or treatments as ordered by a licensed physician, including a podiatric physician . . ., or dentist; (d) in the supervision or teaching of nursing; (e) in the administration, supervision, and evaluation of nursing practices, policies, and procedures; (f) in the requesting, receiving, signing for, and distributing of prescription drug samples to patients at sites at which a registered nurse is authorized to sign prescription drug orders . . .; or (g) in the performing of acts delegated by a physician . . .(Vernon's Civil Statutes of the State of Texas, 1995)*

Nursing is expanding its scope and roles as a result of increasing nursing education, health access needs in com-

munities, and the strong political activities of nursing organizations. With this broadened scope come new challenges, responsibilities, and opportunities. Advanced nurse practitioners have prescriptive authority in 48 states and receive third-party reimbursement from private insurers and Medicaid reimbursement in many states. Nurses are increasing access to the quality and cost-effectiveness of care consumers need.

Malpractice

Malpractice is a particular kind of tort action that a consumer plaintiff brings against a defendant professional from whom the plaintiff feels that he or she has received injury during the professional–consumer relationship. Malpractice is professional negligence (Historical Capsule 7-2). For a plaintiff to receive monetary damages by successfully suing a professional nurse for malpractice, he or she must prove the following five elements of nursing negligence:

1. The nurse professional had a duty of due care toward the plaintiff.
2. The nurse professional's performance fell below the standard of care and was, therefore, a breach of that duty.
3. As a result of the failure to meet the standard of care, the plaintiff consumer was injured, and the nurse's action was the proximate cause of the injury.
4. The act in which the nurse engaged could foreseeably have caused an injury.
5. The plaintiff consumer must prove his or her injuries.

To decrease their chances of liability for malpractice, psychiatric nurses must ensure that their professional practice is within the bounds of statutory and professional standards. In a malpractice action against a nurse, proof of the "standard of care" becomes essential. Both sides usually present expert witness testimony to give the jury perspectives about what are considered professional practices and standards. The appropriate expert witness for psychiatric-mental health nursing practice is another psychiatric nurse who knows about the standard of care in same or similar situations. Both sides present include such expert testimony

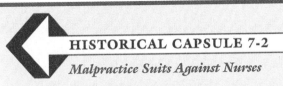

HISTORICAL CAPSULE 7-2
Malpractice Suits Against Nurses

In the history of malpractice litigation, nurses were largely protected from direct suits from clients. One contributing factor was the public perception that nurses were dependent on either physicians or authorities within a healthcare facility for orders. Attorneys, using the "deep pocket" theory of recovery, tended to bring most suits against well-insured physicians or the employer–healthcare facility rather than against nurses. With growing consumer knowledge and increasing recognition of professional nursing as an independent discipline, however, the trend to sue individual nurses as codefendants along with physicians and healthcare facilities is becoming more common.

This trend has many implications for the nursing profession. As nurses are held increasingly responsible and monetarily liable for practice and malpractice, the nursing profession must strive to control such issues as staffing, productivity, educational qualifications and competencies, and the nurse's role within the healthcare team.

and submit it with all other testimony and evidence to the jury for a decision. The issue of negligence refers to a peer standard for reasonableness of action, not a standard for excellence of action. Thus, when making legal decisions, the court asks the jury to apply the reasonable person test to the facts of the case at hand. The **reasonable person test**, as applied to the nurse defendant, is what a reasonably prudent nurse would have done under similar circumstances if that nurse came from the same or a similar community.

When nurses are found liable in malpractice cases, their employers are usually also found liable to the plaintiff under the legal theory of respondeat superior. **Respondeat superior** is a Latin term meaning that acts of employees are attributable to the employer, whom the court will also find responsible for damages to injured third parties (Prosser, 1991). If a nurse acted outside the scope of nursing practice, however, the doctrine of respondeat superior may not apply. In such cases, the nurse's employer also may withdraw any legal assistance it would otherwise have provided. The court may then find the nurse liable, or the healthcare facility may file an indemnity action against the nurse.

Obtaining Legal Counsel

Psychiatric-mental health professionals must know how and when to obtain appropriate legal consultation on an ongoing basis. First, the attorney they consult must be aware of the issues in mental health law to evaluate the institution's policies and procedures and to provide a review for the staff in a problem-solving manner. Second, healthcare facilities and programs should make arrangements to have an attorney offer continuing and regular education programs to review, with the staff, updates on court decisions and recent legislation that affect care in the psychiatric setting. Also, having legal consultation readily available on a case (client) consultation basis when the staff is endeavoring to ensure legal accountability is extremely valuable. Many institutions provide this kind of legal consultation, if requested, for the benefit of their clients and to protect the institution from potential liability. Moreover, individual malpractice insurance carriers provide legal representation in the event that a nurse is sued. Although nurses are not sued as often as other healthcare professionals, especially in psychiatric nursing, it is prudent for nurses to carry individual malpractice policies as litigation climates change.

Basic Rights of Clients Receiving Psychiatric Nursing Care

An important issue in psychiatric-mental health nursing care is recognizing the basic rights of clients (Box 7-1). This issue is particularly relevant because treatment of clients with mental illness tends to be more coercive, less voluntary, and less open to public awareness and scrutiny than are the treatment and hospitalization of clients with other types of disorders.

When clients with psychiatric disorders enter a hospital, they may lose their freedom to come and go, schedule their time, and choose and control activities of daily living (ADLs). If also adjudicated incompetent, they lose the freedom to manage financial and legal affairs and make many important decisions. Because of the loss of these important freedoms, the courts and advocates of clients with psychiatric disorders closely guard and value the rights that these clients retain. Some of these rights include the right to communicate with an attorney, the right to send and receive mail without censorship, the right to have visitors, the right to the basic necessities of life, and the right to safety from harm during hospitalization.

Certainly, treatment issues sometimes arise that call for limitations on visitors. Clients may participate in a behavior modification treatment program that requires the earning of tokens to secure certain privileges or articles. Despite such limitations, clients still retain the right to challenge such restrictions, and treatment facilities may have to prove the value or necessity of such abridgments to rights.

The application of restraints and the use of seclusion are considered high-risk treatment modalities because they are dangerous interventions that can result in injury or even death (Mohr & Mohr, 2000). From a legal standpoint they are also high risk because clients may perceive such methods as a form of punishment, and these modalities greatly

BOX 7-1 ▼ *Universal Bill of Rights for Mental Health Patients*

1. The right to appropriate treatment and related services in a setting and under conditions that are the most supportive of such person's personal liberty, and restrict such liberty only to the extent necessary and consistent with such person's treatment needs, applicable requirement of law, and applicable judicial orders.

2. The right to an individualized, written treatment or service plan (such plan to be developed promptly after admission of such person), the right to treatment based on such plan, the right to periodic review and reassessment of treatment and related service needs, and the right to appropriate revision of such plan, including any revision necessary to provide a description of mental health services that may be needed after such person is discharged from such program or facility.

3. The right to ongoing participation, in a manner appropriate to a person's capabilities, in the planning of mental health services to be provided (including the right to participate in the development and periodic revision of the plan).

*4. The right to be provided with a reasonable explanation, in terms and language appropriate to a person's condition and ability to understand the person's general mental and physical (if appropriate) condition, the objectives of treatment, the nature and significant possible adverse effects of recommended treatment, the reasons why a particular treatment is considered, the reasons why access to certain visitors may not be appropriate, and any appropriate and available alternative treatments, services, and types of providers of mental health services.

5. The right not to receive a mode or course of treatment in the absence of informed, voluntary, written consent to treatment except during an emergency situation.

6. The right not to participate in experimentation in the absence of informed, voluntary, written consent (includes human subject protection).

7. The right to freedom from restraint or seclusion, other than as a mode or course of treatment or restraint or seclusion during an emergency situation with a written order by a responsible mental health professional.

*8. The right to a humane treatment environment that affords reasonable protection from harm and appropriate privacy with regard to personal needs.

9. The right to access, on request, to such person's mental health care records.

10. The right, in the case of a person admitted on a residential or inpatient care basis, to converse with others privately, to have convenient and reasonable access to the telephone and mails, and to see visitors during regularly scheduled hours. (For treatment purposes, specific individuals may be excluded.)

11. The right to be informed promptly and in writing at the time of admission of these rights.

12. The right to assert grievances with respect to infringement of these rights.

13. The right to exercise these rights without reprisal.

14. The right of referral to other providers.

Title II, Public Law 99-319, *Restatement of Bill of Rights for Mental Health Patients,* Title II—Restatement of Bill of Rights for Mental Health Patients established by Mental Health Systems Act of 1988.

inhibit the client's right to freedom. Therefore, accrediting agencies and governmental entities require policies and procedures to govern these practices. Many states have developed statutes to define the use of restraints and seclusion within psychiatric facilities, and the federal government (Health Care Financing Agency) has issued strict guidelines for their use in facilities that receive federal funds as third-party reimbursement. The Joint Commission on the Accreditation of Healthcare Organizations (JCAHO) has revised the standards guiding the use of restraints and seclusion several times since 1996. These standards guide the application of restraints or initiation of seclusion, monitoring of the client while these methods are imposed, and assessment for continuing need of the restraints or seclusion. The standards also specifically require the leaders of the organization to limit the use of restraints and seclusion to clinically justified situations (JCAHO, 2000).

Clients have limited rights to be paid for work within long-term residential institutions. Forced or even voluntary labor by clients without payment violates the principles of law in our society.

Nursing has long espoused that one of its important roles in the healthcare system is to act as a client advocate. Discussing rights within treatment teams, including these rights in the nursing care plan, and ensuring that methodologies for rights protection are included in facility and unit policies and procedures are nursing activities that fulfill the client advocate role (Table 7-1). One important resource that should be accessible to nursing is ongoing legal advice and consultation in the area of client rights.

INFORMED CONSENT

Informed consent means consent that a recipient of healthcare gives to treating providers in an interaction (or series of interactions) that enables him or her to understand a proposed treatment or procedure, including the following:

TABLE 7-1 ▼ Nursing Care Guidelines to Maintain Legal Rights of Clients

Expected Outcome: Client feedback will reflect satisfaction with nursing care.

INTERVENTIONS	RATIONALES
Provide at least a "reasonable person" standard of care when using the nursing process to delivery client care.	Breach of guidelines for safe practice and standards of care can provide the basis for negligence and malpractice suits.
Attend periodic workshops that review standards and legal and ethical issues.	The responsibility to update one's knowledge base continually is essential to the practice of safe nursing care.

Expected Outcome: The client's right to informed consent will be maintained.

INTERVENTIONS	RATIONALES
Apply the elements of informed consent, including the following: • The person must be competent. • The person must have the ability to refuse consent. • The person must have adequate information to give consent, including information about risks, benefits, and alternatives. • The person must give consent voluntarily.	A basic client right is control over his or her body. The physician has the legal obligation to ensure that clients are giving informed consent, considering the nurse's observation and assessment of the client.
Observe and document client behavior indicating consent is valid.	The client record must reflect specific nursing assessment of current behaviors, and the nurse needs to take appropriate action if consent is questioned or invalidated.
Record and report any discrepancies in consent or behavior, revocation of consent, or other issues to the client's physician.	The nurse acts as a client advocate and has the interdependent role of assessment of consent, compliance, and consent revocation with the physician.

Expected Outcome: The client's right to confidentiality of health data will be protected.

INTERVENTIONS	RATIONALES
Protect the client's record and chart and share data only with client authorization.	The client's written authorization is necessary before the nurse can share information in records or charts.
Maintain communication about the client and client care among treatment team members.	The nurse can share information about client care with treatment team members to provide continuity.
Use policies and procedures that reflect the nurse's duty to protect himself or herself or others in cases of threats to harm the nurse or other people.	The nurse has a responsibility to breach confidentiality to protect the client and others from harm.

Expected Outcome: The clients' rights will be protected.

INTERVENTIONS	RATIONALES
Review the policies and procedures of the unit to ensure they are in accordance with client rights.	Policies and procedures need to be in place to support protection of clients' rights.
Attend training on legal issues, such as voluntary or involuntary commitment and treatment consequences.	As a member of the psychiatric treatment team, the nurse has a responsibility to ensure that client care is compliant with legislation and statutory laws dealing with commitment and treatment issues.
Suggest that legal consultation be obtained for legal updates, review of policies and procedures, and case consultation.	A legal consultant should be available to staff.
Participate in ongoing performance monitoring.	The nurse must develop or participate in performance improvement strategies to ensure quality care.

- The way the treatment or procedure will be administered
- The prognosis if the treatment or procedure is given
- Side effects
- Risks
- Possible consequences of refusing the treatment or procedure
- Other alternatives (Rossoff, 1981)

All clients have the right to give informed consent before healthcare professionals perform interventions. The administration of healthcare treatments or procedures without a client's informed consent can result in legal action on the client's part against the primary provider and the healthcare agency. The client will prevail in such a lawsuit, alleging **battery** (touching another without permission) if it can be proven that he or she did not consent to the procedure (Prosser, 1991).

Consent is an absolute defense against battery, which is why informed consent is so necessary in healthcare situations. In the case of *Canterbury v. Spence* (1972), the court said that the client could truly be informed only if the primary provider shared with the client all things that the client "would find significant" in deciding whether to permit or participate in a particular treatment regimen. Informed consent requires that healthcare professionals give clients adequate and accurate knowledge and information. It mandates for the client to have the legal capacity to give consent and give it voluntarily.

As a broad mandate for informed consent, Congress passed the Patient Self-Determination Act (PSDA), which went into effect on December 1, 1991. The PSDA requires healthcare facilities to provide clear written information for every client concerning his or her legal rights to make healthcare decisions, including the right to accept or refuse treatment.

Informed consent also protects clients from being subjected to experimental treatments and research projects without their knowledge and agreement. Because of the complexity of informed consent issues with clients who have psychiatric disorders, institutions with programs that involve research or experimental treatment approaches must have institutional review boards to evaluate such projects and programs and to approve or disapprove them based on strict client protection criteria. Human subjects committees usually view favorably research approaches that entail no undue risks to clients, have strong expectations of benefit, and allow clients to withdraw from the project at any time, provided that clients give voluntary consent to participate.

Special Considerations in Psychiatric Settings

A major problem with consent related to clients who have psychiatric disorders involves the validity of their competence to agree to procedures. Many clients with mental illness certainly are capable of giving informed con-

sent. They are aware of their surroundings, understand what is being said, make their decisions based on what they think is best for them, and agree to treatments or procedures without coercion. Nevertheless, some clients with psychiatric disorders are incapable of giving informed consent. It may be questionable whether clients whom the court has already determined to be incompetent for the purposes of handling civil and business affairs possess the ability to make treatment decisions. Likewise, some clients who have not been so adjudicated are so clearly impaired by their psychiatric illnesses that they cannot truly understand what healthcare professionals are communicating. They therefore cannot give valid consent.

Because of this unreliability, major nursing considerations for informed consent in psychiatric-mental health practice are the constant monitoring and observing of clients for the following:

- A state of legal capacity or competence when they are asked to give informed consent
- Continuing understanding of the information they have been given
- Power and opportunities to revoke consent at any time during a course of treatment

Ensuring legally adequate informed consent before treatment is an important part of the psychiatric nursing care plan. The nurse serves as the client's advocate, the team's colleague, and the facility's excellent employee by continually evaluating the client's ability to give informed consent and his or her willingness to participate and continue with a treatment modality. Unless serving as the primary provider, the nurse is not responsible for obtaining informed consent—that is the role of the primary provider. It is the nurse's prerogative, however, to actively pursue the observations previously outlined to protect the client's rights during treatment.

Every agency should clearly define the nurse's role in assisting with obtaining a client's signature on a consent form. A joint signing between the primary provider and the client at the time of the decision is a preferred method of documenting consent; many agency policies and consent forms reflect this preference.

Substituted Consent

When a client cannot give informed consent, healthcare providers must obtain substituted consent for necessary treatments or procedures. **Substituted consent** is authorization that another person gives on behalf of a client who needs a procedure or treatment but cannot provide such consent independently. The appointment of a healthcare proxy is one example of the concept of substituted consent.

Substituted consent can come from a court-appointed guardian or in some instances from the client's next of kin. If the client has not previously been adjudicated incompetent and if the law so permits and no next of kin are available to give substituted consent, the healthcare agency may initiate a court proceeding to appoint a guardian so that treatment professionals can carry out the procedure or treatment. In an emergency, the client who is in danger of harming self or others can be given medication or be restrained or secluded without consent.

Nurses and other healthcare providers must know the statutory requirements for obtaining substituted consent. In their role as client advocates, nurses also must know whether a client has been adjudicated incompetent and whether consent from a next of kin or guardian is a legally acceptable substitution.

CONFIDENTIALITY

It is a professional and an ethical duty to use knowledge gained about clients only for the enhancement of their care and not for other purposes, such as gossip, personal gain, or curiosity. Nurses must maintain the confidentiality of verbal and written information.

Preserving confidentiality is especially important in the care of clients with mental illness. Despite some advances, society still attaches a tremendous stigma to anyone with a diagnosis of psychiatric illness. Any breach of confidentiality of data about clients, their diagnoses, symptoms, behaviors, and the outcomes of treatment can certainly affect the rest of their lives in terms of employment, promotions, marriage, insurance benefits, and so forth. The healthcare practitioner, however, must maintain a delicate balance. With managed care companies being the payers for behavioral health services in many cases, providers (hospitals, nurses, social workers, physicians) must provide clinical information to the managed care company case manager to justify admission and continued treatment of clients. Thus, healthcare providers must obtain "fiscal informed consent" from the client or family (Dasco & Dasco, 1995). It is the provider's responsibility to know the legal requirements regarding clinical confidentiality and the requirements of managed care companies to be informed of the client's clinical condition for reimbursement.

Responsible Record Keeping

According to *A Patient's Bill of Rights* of the American Hospital Association, each client has a right to a written record that enhances care (American Hospital Association, 1994). Accrediting agencies such as JCAHO also require each client to have a medical record (JCAHO, 2000). Documentation may be in the form of narrative notes, SOAP notes (recording information by subjective data, objective data, assessment, and plan), or clinical pathways. Records may be kept manually or electronically. Records are legal documents that can be used in court; therefore, all nursing notes and progress records should reflect descriptive, nonjudgmental, and objective statements. Examples of significant data include here-and-now observations of the client through the use of the nurse's

critical assessment, an accurate report of verbal exchanges with clients, and a description of the client outcomes of the care provided. The medical record is the best source of legal protection in a malpractice suit (Parham, 1979).

Verbal communication should be straightforward, forthright, descriptive, without opinion, and limited to those involved in the client's care and treatment. It is wise to have an established methodology of reminding staff members about their professional and legal responsibilities for confidentiality, such as an annual requirement to sign a form certifying the nurse's understanding and commitment to maintaining confidentiality.

Privileged Communication

Privileged communication is provided by statute in each state. These statutes delineate which categories of professionals are given the legal privilege to withhold conversations and communications. Although statutes differ among states, they customarily provide this privilege to physicians, attorneys, clergymen, and in some states, psychologists, nurses, and other healthcare providers. Psychiatric nurses should be aware of statutorily privileged communication, and if the nursing privilege is limited or nonexistent, they should know what boundaries to set in therapeutic interviews. In the absence of statutory privileges for nurses, the nurse may be required to repeat communications between the nurse and client in court through the subpoena process. Therefore, the nurse should not encourage the client to share sensitive or incriminating data. He or she should limit therapeutic communication to that required by the treatment plan.

Some cases have involved the issue of the identification of the appropriate circumstances that warrant breach of the confidential relationship with a client. A leading case in this area is *Tarasoff v. Board of Regents of University of California* (1974), which held that therapists might have a duty to protect a person who is threatened by a client. Subsequent decisions discuss the issues of foreseeable violence and the amount of control that the therapist could reasonably use to prevent the harm (Beck, 1987). In these types of cases, courts have said that the mandate on therapists to hold clients' verbalizations in confidence is cut off when those confidences include threats against the lives of others.

Courts have held that, although the duty of confidentiality between client and therapist should be recognized, a higher duty to protect the public safety intervenes and supersedes the duty of confidentiality. There are no nursing cases per se on this point, but nurses must be aware that threats against other people cannot be ignored or unattended, especially when there is some reasonable opportunity for the client to follow through on these threats.

Other types of situations in which a breach of confidentiality may be required by law include allegations of child abuse, threats of suicide, and allegations of sexual misconduct made against a therapist.

Evolving Legal Rights

U.S. laws constitute the system of binding rules of action or conduct that governs the behavior of people with respect to their relationships with their government and with others. In general, laws are meant to reflect the moral values and beliefs of a given population and are intended to reflect the popular belief about the "rightness" or "wrongness" of particular acts. Although guided by ethical principles, which are foundational, laws change and evolve to reflect the changing values and beliefs of society (Kapp, 1998). Examples of areas affected by recent changes in the law include fetal tissue use, abortion, confidentiality for clients with AIDS, the expanded role of nurses and prescriptive privileges, and others. Nurses need to familiarize themselves with the law and legal system to make informed choices and to ensure that their practices are consistent under the legal system.

RIGHT TO TREATMENT

The idea that clients with psychiatric illnesses have a legally actionable right to psychiatric treatment began to develop in the late 1960s and culminated in the early 1970s in the circuit court case of *Wyatt v. Stickney* (1971). The case provided innovative statements about the rights of civilly committed clients with mental illnesses in state hospitals. The court stated that such clients do have certain treatment rights, which include the following:

- Treatment must give some realistic opportunity for improvement or cure.
- Custodial care is insufficient to meet treatment requirements.
- A lack of funding does not excuse the state from treatment responsibilities.
- Commitment without treatment violates the due process rights of clients.

Perhaps the most important pronouncement in this case concerns the three determinants for the adequacy of treatment: (1) a humane environment, (2) a qualified staff in adequate numbers, and (3) individualized treatment plans. This case gave the nation guidance about treatment rights; however, the Supreme Court did not review it. The Supreme Court decision on *O'Connor v. Donaldson* (1975) is commonly thought to be the leading case for the right to treatment. The decision states, however, that no state can confine a person with mental illness who is not a threat to self or others in a state hospital if he or she can survive safely in the community alone or with the help of willing, responsible family members or friends.

RIGHT TO TREATMENT IN THE LEAST RESTRICTIVE ENVIRONMENT

Courts have given guidance to the mental health system on many matters, including standards about the settings in which treatment should occur. As early as 1969, in *Covington v. Harris,* the court held that a person treated involuntarily should receive such treatment in a setting that is least restrictive to liberty but will still meet treatment needs. Least restrictive environments can be community resources instead of hospitalization, open units instead of locked units, or outpatient or home care instead of inpatient care (*Covington v. Harris,* 1969). Nurses must constantly assess a client's condition and status so that healthcare professionals can initiate more or less restrictive treatment alternatives based on the client's evolving needs.

RIGHT TO REFUSE TREATMENT

The doctrine of informed consent implies that clients have the right to choose or refuse medical and health treatment. Certainly, healthcare providers, through interpersonal relationships and client education, may try to convince clients about the need for certain treatments. Only in rare or life-threatening instances, however, will courts intervene in treatment decisions.

RIGHT TO AFTERCARE

Care in the community following psychiatric hospitalization is needed to prevent readmission and to ensure the rehabilitation of former inpatients. There is no absolute legal right at this time to aftercare programs unless state statutes provide such a right. It is conceivable that case laws may evolve to mandate aftercare services as a right of clients with mental disorders.

In conjunction with other members of the interdisciplinary team, nurses plan for aftercare treatment. As knowledgeable and responsible citizens, they voice their concerns at all levels of the political system to see that clients with psychiatric illnesses have access to adequate aftercare services. These services include outpatient counseling, home care, medication follow-up, vocational placement, and sheltered living environments.

Client Status and Specific Legal Issues

When clients with psychiatric disorders are hospitalized, the type of admission determines the treatment plan. Civil commitment admissions include the following:

- Voluntary admissions
- Emergency admissions
- Involuntary commitments (indefinite duration)

Each state has specific statutory regulations pertaining to each admission status that mandate procedures for admission, discharge, and commitment for treatment.

VOLUNTARY ADMISSIONS

Clients who present themselves at psychiatric facilities and request hospitalization are considered **voluntary**

*Jackson v. Indiana, 46 U.S. 715 (1972).

*Joint Commission on the Accreditation of Healthcare Organizations. (2000). *Comprehensive accreditation manual for hospitals.* Oakbrook Terrace, IL: Author.

*Jones, K. (1955). Lunacy, law, and conscience. London: Routledge and Kegam Paul.

*Kaimowitz v. Michigan Department of Mental Hygiene, 2 P.L. 433 (1979).

*Kapp, M. B. (1998). *Our hands are tied: Legal tensions and medical ethics.* Westburn, CT: Auburn House Press.

*Kelly, B. (1990). In M. Leininger (Ed.), *Respect and caring: Ethics and essence of nursing in ethical and moral dimensions of care.* Detroit: Wayne State University Press.

*Mohr, W. K., & Mohr, B. D. (2000). Mechanisms of injury and death proximal to restraint use. *Archives of Psychiatric Nursing, 14*(6), 285–295.

*O'Connor v. Donaldson, 422 U.S. 563 (1975).

*Olson, L. (1998). Hospital nurses' perceptions of the ethical climate of their work setting. *Image: Journal of Nursing Scholarship, 30*(4).

*Parham, Commissioner, Department of Human Resources of Georgia et al. v. J. R. et al., 442 U.S. 584 (1979).

*Parker, J. (1995). Chemical restraints and children: Autonomy or veracity. *Perspectives in Psychiatric Care, 31*(2), 25–29.

*Patient Self-Determination Act. Omnibus Budget Reconciliation Act of 1990, Pub. L. No. 101–508, § 4206, 104 Stat. 1388–115 (codified at 42 U.S.C.A. § 1395cc[f]).

*Prosser, W. (1991). *Cases and materials on torts.* New York: Foundation Press.

*Rennie v. Klein, 653 F.2d 836 (1981).

Roberts, L., et al. (2000). Perspectives of patients with schizophrenia and psychiatrists regarding ethically important aspects of research participation. *American Journal of Psychiatry, 157*(1), 67.

*Rossoff, A. J. (1981). *Informed consent: A guide for health care remedies.* Rockville, MD: Aspen Systems.

Srebnik, D., & La Fond, J. (1999). Advance directives for mental health treatment. *Psychiatric Services, 50*(7), 919.

*Tarasoff v. Board of Regents of University of California, 592 P.S. 553 (1974).

Thomasa, D. C., & Kissell, J. L. (2000). *The health care professional as friend and healer.* Washington, DC: Georgetown University Press.

*Vernon's Civil Statutes of the State of Texas, Chapter 7, Title 71, Article 4518, 1995.

Weiner, B., & Wettstein, R. (1993). Legal issues in mental health care. New York & London: Plenum Press.

*Wyatt v. Stickney, 325 F. Supp. 781 (1971).

Starred references are cited in text.

For additional information on this chapter, go to *http://connection. ww.com.*

Need more help? See Chapter 7 of the *Study Guide to Accompany Mohr: Johnson's Psychiatric-Mental Health Nursing, 5th edition.*

UNIT II

Conceptual Bases of Treatment

Working With Individuals

JEANNEANE L. CLINE

Cognitions—Beliefs and thoughts that color a person's construction of his or her world.

Countertransference—The way that a therapist responds to a client because of feelings the that client triggers from the therapist's past; a nontherapeutic event that can be resolved with consultation, supervision, or both.

Free association—A technique in which a client says the first thing that comes to his or her mind, without restrictions, in response to something said by the therapist.

Negative reinforcement—Removal of an aversive stimulus that results in an increase in behavior or response.

Positive reinforcement—The addition of something that increases the probability of a behavior or response.

Punishment—Presentation of a negative or aversive stimulus or event that results in a decrease in a response or behavior.

Reinforcer—A stimulus that strengthens a new response (behavior) by its repeated association with that response.

Schema or core beliefs—An accumulation of the person's learning and experience within the family, religion, ethnicity, gender, regional subgroups, and broader society.

Structural and functional analysis—An assessment of the functional relationships between various purported motivational variables and the rate of occurrence of certain behaviors.

Transference—The unconscious reenactment of relationship patterns and feelings from the client's past in which there is a distorting of the therapist's behaviors and then an unconscious placing of positive or negative feelings about the situation or person on the therapist.

On completion of this chapter, you should be able to accomplish the following:

- Define psychotherapy.
- Discuss the collaborative goals of individual therapy.
- Describe various methods or techniques of psychotherapy.
- Compare and contrast the roles of the basic and advanced nurse in individual psychiatric care.
- Discuss therapeutic interventions in nursing.

Fundamental to working with individuals in the psychiatric arena are the concepts of individual psychotherapy. Psychotherapy is a treatment modality based on a trusting relationship between a client and a therapist. Its goals are a change in a particular problem behavior or behaviors, a change in the client's self-perceptions, a change in the client's subjective emotional comfort (including anxiety or tension), and insight or clear rational and emotional understanding of the client's problems. Roughly 400 types of "psychotherapies" have been described at one time or another in the literature, but the general types practiced by most clinicians include dynamic, behavioral, cognitive, family, humanistic, and Rogerian approaches (Crits-Christoph, 1998). Psychotherapy, despite sounding mystical, is only a systematic process of interpersonal influence entailing the use of certain skills on the therapist's part (Carson & Mineka, 1999). Examples are coaching, giving feedback, and engaging clients in corrective learning techniques.

In general, most psychotherapy can be conceptualized as oriented toward having clients acquire or increase behavior deficits or decrease or eliminate behavioral excesses. Approaches to such changes vary within the schema of the various therapeutic approaches, but techniques with the greatest empirical support are predominantly cognitive and behavioral treatments, both of which identify discrete behaviors as units of analysis and outcome (Dobson & Craig, 1998).

This chapter explores cognitive and behavioral treatments and several additional therapeutic approaches used in individual psychotherapy. It also explores the psychotherapeutic nursing role in working with individuals, including basic psychological interventions that the nurse can use when working with individuals. The primary intervention is "listening," which entails the following components:

1. Focusing on what the client is saying (not what the nurse thinks the client is going to say)
2. Waiting until the client has finished before replying (not formulating a response while the client still is talking)
3. Seeking more clarification to ensure maximum understanding (rather than trying to "fix" problems for the client)
4. Encouraging self-determined action (not action that the nurse thinks the client should take)

This is one of the big differences between psychiatric nursing and medical–surgical nursing. Psychiatric nurses facilitate and encourage clients to identify and use their own resources, which sometimes are hidden, rather than "doing" things for clients.

COLLABORATIVE GOALS OF INDIVIDUAL THERAPY

In both inpatient and outpatient settings, the client often works with a team consisting of nurses, a social worker, a psychologist, adjunctive therapists, and a psychiatrist who follow one or more psychological theories or methods as a basis for their treatment. The overall goals of individual therapy are to empower the client to experience more satisfying relationships, to have increased self-esteem and self-worth, to feel integrated with self-chosen work activities, and to find greater meaning in life.

Positive outcomes result from the therapeutic relationship, which facilitates the client's learning of new ways of thinking and new behaviors (Haley, 1993; Rogers, 1961; Schofield, 1998; Wilshaw, 1997). Psychiatric nurses foster a client's positive change through teaching and developing coping strategies, using communication skills, and encouraging healthy lifestyles that encourage self-determination and participation. A therapeutic relationship should begin with the belief that the client is competent and capable and that the client and therapist will identify solutions jointly. Perhaps Milton Erickson said it best when he noted, "individuals have a reservoir of wisdom learned and forgotten but still available" (Haley, 1993).

TYPES OF INDIVIDUAL PSYCHOTHERAPY

Individual psychotherapy has moved from the traditional long-term finding of "why" to the more contemporary short-term focus of understanding "how," changing thoughts, feelings, and behaviors and identifying successes

(Historical Capsule 8-1). The psychotherapy of Freud was long term and primarily insight oriented. In the current environment of managed care with limited inpatient stays (3 to 5 days) and outpatient therapy sessions (4 to 10 sessions for 6 to 12 months), the focus of psychotherapy with individuals includes an educational arm along with a psychotherapeutic arm (Schofield, 1998). The contemporary psychotherapies typically are of shorter duration and have the goals of improved functioning and practical results.

This section discusses seven approaches to psychotherapy including the classic, insight-oriented psychoanalysis of Freud and the more contemporary cognitive, behavioral, cognitive-behavioral, rational emotive behavioral, choice, and brief solution-focused therapies (Table 8-1).

HISTORICAL CAPSULE 8-1

The Changing Focus of Psychotherapy

Early theorists believed that lunar cycles and other astrologic bodies controlled the emotions (hence the term *lunacy* for mental illness). Others believed that magical fluids in the body (eg, black bile) and spirits or devils controlled the mind. Departing from popular magical thinking, St. Augustine, a 5th-century Christian monk, thought psychological self-understanding would help change inner values and behaviors. St. Augustine worked to reverse the inhumane treatment of the mentally ill that endured for centuries.

Sigmund Freud (19th to 20th centuries) revolutionized psychiatry by focusing on faulty relationships (primarily, poor mothering) and the ways in which the person's early mother–child experiences influenced adult behaviors and problems. In the 1960s, Abraham Maslow began to emphasize the person's strengths and capabilities. Jay Haley and Thomas Szasz believed that when others treat a person as normal, that person will act in more socially acceptable ways. Szasz and Glasser rejected the biochemical model of mental illness. They emphasized the importance of personal responsibility for behavior.

Milton Erickson (1901–1980) contributed significantly to the idea that the person is capable of making positive changes. Erickson believed that the client, not the therapist, is capable of determining "unusual interventions." The therapist's role is that of a facilitator of the client's ideas. Erickson's focus was changing unacceptable behaviors, not understanding the underlying cause for the behavior.

TABLE 8-1 ▼ Selected Approaches to Psychotherapy

THERAPY APPROACH	FOCUS	KEY INTERVENTIONS AND TECHNIQUES	OUTCOME
Psychoanalysis	Client's conscious and unconscious conflicts Past coping patterns	Free association Transference Therapeutic alliance (development of a relationship to allow client to progress and change)	Insight into repressed conflicts Restructuring of the personality based on integration of repressed conflicts
Cognitive therapy	"Hows" rather than "whys" Client's perception of self, experiences, world and future (cognitive triad) Positive or negative distortions Basic rules of life (schema or core beliefs)	Trust building Active listening Empathy Development of problem lists Session agendas Homework Evaluation of successes and failures	Recognition of irrational thinking patterns Enhancement of functional responses
Behavior therapy	Promotion of desirable behaviors with alterations of undesirable behaviors	Formal token economy systems Positive and negative reinforcement	Reshaping of behavior with elimination of negative behaviors
Cognitive-behavioral therapy	Promotion of client's current thinking and actions	Participatory relationship between client and therapist Therapist acting as coach and teacher assisting in identification of situations involving undesirable thoughts and actions Development of alternatives Homework assignments to change behavior with precise monitoring of progress to goals	Results oriented Client learning new skills
Rational emotive behavior therapy	Client's view of things and events Past having nothing to do with present Changing of situations to ones involving what client would like to occur	Identification of activating situation and unhealthy negative emotions leading to irrational beliefs Definition of new constructive thoughts or a healthy negative emotion	Client control of behavior and thinking Assumption of responsibility and blame for irrational beliefs
Choice therapy	Client's choice to change and how to deal with information "Doing" rather than "feeling"	Problem identification with orientation to the present Assumption of responsibility for complaints Belief in choice about feeling back to belief that client can do something about it	Direct control over acting and thinking based on self-responsibility and self-discipline

(continued)

TABLE 8-1 ▼ **Selected Approaches to Psychotherapy (Continued)**			
THERAPY APPROACH	**FOCUS**	**KEY INTERVENTIONS AND TECHNIQUES**	**OUTCOME**
Brief, solution-focused therapy	Problems resulting from the mishandling of life events	Joint partnership between therapist and client to facilitate alternate views. Client development of alternate views of situation of past successes and factors maintaining the problem. Validation of client's perception of the situation	Satisfactory life adjustments and ability to change, interact, and reach goals through solutions

Classic Psychoanalysis

Sigmund Freud (1856–1939) pioneered psychoanalysis, a form of psychodynamic therapy in which the client and therapist explore the client's conscious and unconscious conflicts and coping patterns from the past. Psychoanalysis is a long-term treatment (four to five sessions per week for 3 to 5 years) that promotes insight into and then integration of repressed conflicts into the reconstructed personality. Currently, it is seldom practiced because of its cost and because there is no empirical evidence for its efficacy.

The primary techniques of psychoanalysis are free association, transference, and therapeutic alliance. **Free association,** the core of psychoanalytical treatment, is a technique in which the client says the first thing that comes to mind, without restrictions, in response to something said by the therapist. **Transference** is the unconscious reenactment of relationship patterns and feelings from the client's past in which there is a distorting of the therapist's behaviors and then an unconscious placing of positive or negative feelings about the situation or person on the therapist. The client needs to identify and resolve transference for change and growth; transference feelings may include adoration, esteem, love or hate, anger, and rage.

Countertransference is when the therapist responds to the client because of feelings that the client triggers from the therapist's past. It is a nontherapeutic event that can be resolved with consultation, supervision, or both (Freud, 1960). Nurses and nursing students in particular also must be aware of possible countertransference responses. Freud's therapeutic alliance is similar to the nurse–client relationship that must be established for the client to progress and make changes (see Chap. 4).

Cognitive Therapy

Cognitive therapy (CT) is both a psychoeducational and a coping model of therapy. It is based on the premise that the way a person perceives an event, rather than the event itself, determines its relevance and the emotional response to it. CT helps clients recognize the process of their thinking and its results. CT is a way for the therapist to help clients alter their basic life schema (the plan and rules). It is a short-term, active, directive, collaborative psychoeducation model with the goal of behavioral change. The psychiatric nurse can apply the principles of CT to education and therapy (Freeman & Yates, 1998).

CT is rooted in the early work of Aaron Beck's treatment of depression (Beck 1979, 1993; Beck, Rush, Shaw, & Emery, 1979; Beck, Wright, Newman, & Liese, 1993). It helps people to examine their beliefs and relationships about whatever is going on with their beliefs about values, meanings, and their ability to impact or have power and influence in defined situations. Because it focuses on process (how) rather than content (what), therapists may use CT with any client, problem, or therapeutic context. For example, it is applicable for persons of all ages and cultures; it is used to treat anxiety, eating disorders, personality disorders, suicidal thoughts or attempts, schizophrenia, and sexual disorders; and it is used in individual, family, and group settings. CT is about understanding the client's construction of his or her world (the **cognitions**) and experimenting with new ways of responding to situations (the behaviors). By understanding the idiosyncratic ways that people perceive themselves, their experiences, the world, and the future, therapists can help clients to alter negative emotions, change their view of life experiences, and behave more adaptively.

CT teaches new skills in responding to depressive or anxious thoughts, recognizing the beginnings of panic attacks, and coping socially. Its overall goal is to increase the client's self-efficacy or proficiency and sense of control over life. The client must be an active participant and committed to the decision for change. The client–therapist interaction is a goal-oriented, collaborative partnership with a beginning, middle, and an end.

ISSUES IDENTIFIED BY COGNITIVE THERAPY

Cognitive therapy defines three issues that result in the formation and maintenance of common psychological disorders: cognitive triad, cognitive distortion, and schema or core beliefs.

Cognitive Triad

In his work with depression, Beck (1979) developed the triad to help understand the interaction of the client's negative view of self, the world, and the future. All issues and problems can be subsumed under one or a combination of these three areas. These issues vary in intensity for each client; one client may be more concerned about self ("Can I do this?"), whereas another may be concerned about the future ("Will there be a job for me?"). In anxiety, this triad represents the client's concern about a threat to the self from the world or an experience in the future.

Cognitive Distortion

The client may distort in either a positive or negative direction. The client exhibiting positive distortions may take chances that most would avoid (ie, risky stock deals or risky relationships) or may be unrealistically positive about health-threatening conditions (ie, ignoring chest pains or an unusual lump with "I'm too healthy for a heart attack," or "It's just a cyst."). Negative distortions include "I always do it wrong," "Nobody likes me," or "It's all his fault!" It usually is the negative distortions that are maladaptive and become the focus of treatment. Treatment involves the identification and effects of the distortion on the client's life. "I'd look stupid!" is a strong reaction about a behavior whose underlying unspoken part says, "That would be terrible," "I won't survive," or "They'll send me away." Clients may apply distortions to self, experiences, or behavior expectations of others (eg, family, friends, religious and gender groups). Examples of cognitive distortions are found in Table 8-2.

Schema or Core Beliefs (Basic Rules of Life)

Core beliefs begin to be established at birth and are well fixed by middle childhood. **Schema** or **core beliefs** are an accumulation of the individual's learning and experience within the family, religion, ethnicity, gender, regional subgroups, and broader society. The client's ability to change these core beliefs depends on the following:

- Whether there is a powerfully associated belief that something cannot be changed, no matter what (eg, "My father said this is the *only* way.")
- Whether significant others (ie, parents, teachers, religious leaders) have reinforced the belief continuously
- Whether there has been reinforcement for a positive contrary belief (an ignoring of one's sense of self-worth); parents or significant others often offer opposition to the developing positive image by saying, "It's not nice to brag," instead of "I'm glad you're feeling better about yourself."
- Having clients say "up until now," which lets them give themselves the option of seeing and saying it differently, which is a beginning break in the old patterns

COGNITIVE THERAPY TREATMENT APPROACH

A general CT treatment approach includes the following:

1. Building trust, active listening, and having empathy (see Chap. 4)
2. Turning data into goals or a working problem list to know where the client is going and when to assess his or her progress
3. Reviewing the past week and successes and problems that the client had with homework assigned by the therapist
4. Deciding on an agenda for each session (may include previous problem, dysfunctional thinking, or a new desired skill)
5. Working on an agenda (Box 8-1)
6. Reviewing the session. Three to 5 minutes before the end of a session, the client should review the session, state feelings about it, and explain what he or she has gained from the session. The therapist then can clarify, note accomplishments, and assign homework for the next session.

The therapist questions the thinking distortions and the underlying schema to help the client respond in more functional ways and recognize irrational thinking patterns. Sometimes, the client may seem to be noncompliant during a session or with assigned homework. There could be many reasons, including headache, poor nutrition, new family difficulties, or just not wanting to do it, all of which may indicate the need to make a change in assignments or goals. The therapist must recognize the client's anxiety and concerns as well as the progress that he or she has made. The client defines progress; current goals may no longer fit and may need to be reset. The therapist must find some way to complement the client, even if only recognizing that the client is "surviving a terrible situation."

Behavioral Therapy

Behavioral therapy is defined as interventions that reinforce or promote desirable behaviors or alter undesirable ones. Behavior modification often is used with children and adolescents and also is used to eliminate negative behaviors (eg, smoking).

TABLE 8-2 ▼ **Examples of Cognitive Distortions**

COGNITIVE/THOUGHT DISTORTIONS	EXTREME AND COMMON IN CLINICAL DIAGNOSES
All-or-nothing thinking: "I'm either a success or a failure." "The world is either black or white."	Borderline and obsessive-compulsive personality disorders
Mind reading: "They probably think that I'm incompetent." "I just know that he disapproves."	Avoidant and paranoid personality disorders
Emotional reasoning: "Because I feel inadequate, I am inadequate." "Because I feel uncomfortable, the world is dangerous."	Anxiety disorders
Overgeneralization: "Everything I do turns out wrong." "Whatever my choices, they are always wrong."	Depression
Catastrophizing: "If I ____, there will be terrible consequences." "If I _____, it always fails."	Social anxiety, social phobia, panic disorders
Control fallacies: "If I'm not in complete control all the time, I will go out of control." "I must control all things in my life."	Obsessive-compulsive and obsessive-compulsive personality disorders
Disqualifying the positive: "This success was only a fluke."	Depression
Perfectionism: "I must do everything perfectly or I will be criticized and a failure."	Anxiety disorders
Selective abstraction: "The rest of the information doesn't matter." "I must focus on negative details and ignore all the positive aspects of this."	Depression
Externalization of self-worth: "My worth is dependent on what others think of me." "They think/believe _____; therefore, I am _____."	Depression and low self-esteem
Should/shouldn't/must/ought statements: "I should visit my family every time they want me to." "You should do whatever I say because it is right."	Obsessive-compulsive disorders
Jumping to conclusions: "I know they will not let me join."	Low self-esteem
Fallacy of change: "You should change your behavior because I want you to." "They should act differently because I expect it."	Narcissistic personality disorder
Fallacy of worrying: "If I worry about it enough, it will be resolved." "One cannot be too concerned."	Anxiety disorders
Fallacy of ignoring: "If I ignore it, maybe it'll go away." "If I don't pay attention, I won't be responsible."	Depression and anxiety disorders
Fallacy of fairness: "Life should be fair." "People should be fair."	Avoidant personality disorder and social anxiety
Fallacy of attachment: "I can't live without a man." "If I was in a relationship, all of my problems would be gone."	Depression and anxiety disorders
Being right: "I must prove that I am right because being wrong is unthinkable." "To be wrong is to be a bad person."	Obsessive-compulsive and narcissistic personality disorders

BOX 8-1 ▼ *Therapeutic Techniques of Cognitive Therapy*

1. **Look for idiosyncratic meaning**. Ask the client directly about what words and thoughts mean to him or her. "What does that mean to you?" "Give me an example."

2. **Question the evidence**. Examine the source of data and recognize that the client may be overlooking parts. "That sounds like what your mother would say." "It seems to me that it also might mean ____." "What evidence do you have that that is true?"

3. **Reattribute**. Distribute responsibility among all relevant parties, not just the client. "Your brother and sister were also part of that." "At that age you could not know ____."

4. **De-catastrophize**. Recognize that the client is overestimating the catastrophic nature of the situation. "What is the worst that can happen?" or "If it does occur, what would be so terrible?" "What might be the effects in 10 years?"

5. **Fantasize consequences**. Ask the client to describe the situation. Often, he or she can see the irrationality of his or her ideas. If the problem remains real, then help the client develop coping strategies.

6. **Weigh advantages and disadvantages**. Ask the client to look at all sides of the issue before defining a reasonable course of action. Writing helps concretize thoughts.

7. **Examine options and alternatives**. Ask the client to generate additional options; this is especially difficult for the suicidal client. Don't discount his or her feelings: "You may be right, something may be wrong with you. What other conclusion might there be?"

8. **Turn adversity to advantage**. Looking for the advantages in disasters. "Losing this job may be an entry point to a new job or career."

9. **Use thought stopping**. Stopping dysfunctional thoughts is best at the beginning, not the middle. Dysfunctional thoughts can have a snowball effect. Ways to stop thoughts include hearing a bell, seeing a stop sign, snapping your fingers, popping a rubber band around the wrist, or tapping on your knee.

10. **Use distraction**. Distraction is especially helpful with anxiety problems because it is difficult to maintain two thoughts at the same time, and anxiogenic thoughts generally preclude more adaptive thinking. A focused thought distracts the anxiogenic thought. For example, have the client count to 200 by 13s (not by 2, 5, 10 or 11); count people wearing yellow or count only small trucks. The therapist also can have the client do a physical activity such as walking, focusing on the in and out of breathing, or counting every other step; it works best when using a complex activity.

BEHAVIORAL THEORY

Behavior therapy has its roots in psychology and attempts to explain how people learn and act. It is based on the early stimulus–response research of Ivan P. Pavlov (1849–1936) in Russia and John B. Watson (1878–1958) at the Johns Hopkins University. Pavlov noticed that the sight and smell of food, not just the food reaching the stomach, stimulated stomach secretions in dogs. The meat was the unconditioned stimulus (not dependent on previous training) that elicited an unconditioned response (the salivation, a specific response). Pavlov became interested and paired the food with a bell, a ticking metronome, and a triangle drawn on a large cue card as the conditioned stimulus given just before the meat. Eventually, only the conditioned stimulus elicited salivation. The phenomenon of recurring responses after a specific stimulus was called *classical conditioning* (pavlovian).

Watson believed that all learning was classical conditioning and that people are born with certain stimulus–response behaviors called reflexes. He rejected the distinction between mind and body, focused on the study of objective behavior, and developed a learning model with the two principles of frequency and recency. The principle of frequency states that the more frequently a

response is made to a given stimulus, the more likely it is that the response will be repeated. The principle of recency states that the more recently a specific response to a particular stimulus is made, the more likely it is to be repeated.

Stimulus–response theory was followed by the reinforcement theories of E. L. Thorndike (1874–1949) and B. F. Skinner (1904–1990). Thorndike believed in the importance of the effects that followed the response–reinforcement of the behavior and developed an understanding of the importance of reinforcement through his experiments with cats. He was the first reinforcement theorist, and his view of learning became a dominant theme in American learning theory.

Skinner received a doctorate in psychology from Harvard in 1931 and did most of his research there. He recognized two different kinds of learning, each with a separate kind of behavior. Respondent behavior, the end result of classical conditioning, is elicited automatically by specific stimuli. The other kind of learning is operant behavior, by which the consequence of a particular behavioral response is of importance. If a behavior occurs and is followed by reinforcement, it is probable that the behavior will recur. Skinner also developed the concept of shaping behavior, in which complex tasks are learned through a series of reinforcements for successive approximations to the desired behavior.

Reinforcement *always* refers to an increase in the likelihood or probability of a response when that response is immediately followed by a consequence. A **reinforcer** is a stimulus that strengthens a new response (behavior) by its repeated association with that response. The stimulus may be either pleasant (positive) or aversive (negative). Therefore, the person may learn a certain response either to receive a reward or to avoid a punishment. In both positive and negative reinforcement, the person is rewarded for making an appropriate response. When **positive reinforcement** is used, the response happens by adding or introducing something to increase the probability of the response. It can be a reward but is not necessarily a reward. One example of a positive reinforcer might be allowing a child to watch television for finishing homework on time. Another type of positive reinforcement, however, could be yelling at a child who is whining. The child may feel ignored and whine to get a response from the parent. The parent's yelling will likely result in more whining to get attention; thus, the whining has been reinforced. The idea is that the yelling, although seemingly aversive, constitutes parental attention and therefore is a positive reinforcer.

Negative reinforcement refers to the increase in the likelihood or probability of a response by removing an aversive event immediately after the person has performed the response. For example, a parent is nagging his teenaged son. The son leaves the room and no longer hears the nagging. The outcome is that, in the future, the likelihood of the teenager leaving the room increases. The removal of the source of nagging is a negative reinforcer.

In learning theory, the words "negative" or "positive" do not have anything to do with the value (or valence) of the stimulus. They both increase behaviors. The negative and positive designations merely refer to the removal of something in the first case and the introduction of something in the second.

Many people often confuse negative reinforcement and punishment, but they are different. **Punishment** presents or introduces an unpleasant stimulus, event, or circumstance. This unpleasant stimulus happens after a behavior and may be of two types: introducing an aversive event, such as spanking, or removing a cherished privilege. Punishing stimuli presented after a behavior most likely will result in decreasing that behavior. The effects of punishment, however, do not have a sustained response. When the punishment stops, the unwanted behavior for which it was imposed gradually resumes. An additional problem is that punishment may have negative emotional effects.

Reinforcers can be set up on variable schedules. Continuous reinforcement, in which reinforcement is given for every response, is the simplest. This is used at the start of training. When the response is learned, the schedule may be changed to intermittent reinforcement, where only some of the responses are reinforced. There also may be a fixed ratio (when the reinforcer is presented after a certain number of responses), a fixed variable schedule (reinforcers given after a variable number of responses), a fixed interval (reinforcers given after a set amount of time, regardless of the number of responses), and a variable interval (where time of reinforcers is varied). Decisions regarding the type of schedule are based on the desired behaviors. For example, homework turned in on time receives one reward, no reward if late, or an unexpected bonus reward for excellence.

THE PROCESS OF BEHAVIORAL THERAPY

The process of behavioral therapy involves assessing and formulating a specific treatment plan for each client individually. This concept is not new; what is new is that this assessment must contain a **structural and functional analysis**, which includes an assessment of the functional relationships between various purported motivational variables and the rate of occurrence of certain behaviors. Because behaviors do not *always* occur, the focus is on what influences the occurrence of these behaviors (Olson & Mohr, in press).

The functional analysis of an identified behavior must contain contextual variables and their effect on whether a certain behavior occurs. These things are called "triggers" and are people, events, situations, and things (food, smells, colors, or music) that frequently lead to the undesirable behaviors. The new or target behaviors identified to extinguish or reinforce will be observable and measurable, and have no prefix with descriptive adjectives or adverbs that usually have a vague, judgmental aspect and user-specific meaning (eg, better, adequate, proper, improved, more, or less). In addition, rather than stating that the client will "not" do something, the plan should state what the client will do instead—*instead* being the key word. An example is that the client will "sit quietly for 10 minutes when Aunt Pat is here," rather than "not yell and run around the room." Simply stated, the overall goal is to increase or decrease a particular behavior when confronted with similar situations in the future.

After identifying target behaviors and the operant variables that maintain them, behavioral therapy involves the formulation and practice of certain corrective learning techniques to reinforce desirable behaviors and eliminate noxious behavior. Techniques may include desensitization, flooding, extinction and fading (the ignoring of behaviors rather than commenting on or reacting to them) (Wolpe & Lazarus, 1966), behavioral rehearsal, and assertiveness training (McFall & Twentyman, 1973). An example of a behavioral therapy program is the implementation of a "token economy," the giving of tokens for the performance of specific behaviors; the tokens then can be exchanged for reinforcers of the client's choice. Structure has reference as to how the treatment program is implemented. The therapist must not instigate treatment in a level-system program where points are awarded for designated behaviors. Level systems are provided for a group of clients (often adolescents) and contain elements that apply to all clients with limited room for individualization. Instead, it is recommended that in addition to overall unit rules that apply to all clients, the focus and reward for progress should be determined individually. This involves general staff training with a specific focus to provide consistency for a particular client. It also consists of identifying "triggers" on the unit for the behavior being extinguished. The plan may include having staff accompany the client to an activity; this may ward off anxiety, prevent the occurrence of an undesirable behavior (ie, improper dress, bringing or using a restricted object), and provide more consistent reinforcement of the desired behaviors (Olson & Mohr, in press).

After devising and implementing the behavioral therapy treatment program, data needs to be collected about the frequency, duration, or magnitude of the target behaviors. This will determine whether the treatment intervention is having the desired outcome. If the treatment goals are not met, the healthcare provider modifies the treatment program with a new set of hypotheses about the conditions necessary to obtain the treatment goal. Thus, a functional analysis enables the healthcare provider to set specific treatment goals so that it is possible to determine whether the treatment goals are being attained (Olson & Mohr, in press).

Cognitive-Behavioral Therapy

As discussed earlier, CT focuses on how clients think about themselves and their world; behavioral therapy is based on the assumption that human behaviors, or responses, are learned and therefore may be unlearned. Cognitive-behavioral therapy is a fusion of cognitive and behavioral techniques. It does not focus on how a person got to be a certain way; instead, it focuses on making changes in current ways of thinking and behavior. It is results oriented and defines goals so that progress toward them can be monitored. The therapist is a coach and teacher for the client who is learning new skills. The therapist may help the client identify situations in which undesired thoughts and actions occur and then assist with the development of alternatives. The behavioral part comes when the therapist gives the client homework assignments to work on before the next appointment (McCrone, 1998; Montgomery & Webster, 1994; Wolpe, 1973).

Rational Emotive Behavior Therapy

After becoming dissatisfied with psychoanalysis in 1955, Albert Ellis developed rational emotive behavior therapy (REBT) from cognitive-behavior therapy. He posited that people are disturbed not by things or events but by their view of those things and events. The theory of REBT incorporates the following ideas:

- The sin is condemned, but the sinner is forgiven.
- Humans are at the center of their universe (but not of the universe) and have the power of choice of emotions.
- Emotional processes depend on human thought, which is greatly affected by the language used.
- Humans are happiest when they establish life goals and pursue them.
- "Rational" beliefs promote goal achievement; "irrational" beliefs often prevent goal achievement.
- Humans, even bright people, often adopt new irrationalities after giving up previous ones.
- Humans can see that they make themselves disturbed by the irrational views they bring to situations.
- Humans can change their thinking and actively work toward new thinking and behaving by applying cognitive, emotive, and behavioral methods.

Rational beliefs, as differentiated from irrational beliefs, are evaluative cognitions that are preferential (not demanding) and are nonabsolute. They are expressed as wishes, likes, and dislikes that may or may not be attained. For example, they can lead to pleasure and satisfaction or sadness, concern, or regret. Irrational beliefs tend to be dogmatic and are expressed in the form of rigid "musts," "shoulds," "oughts," or "have-tos." They lead to negative emotions (eg, depression, anxiety, guilt, anger) that interfere with goal pursuit and attainment.

Healthy beliefs underlie functional behaviors, whereas unhealthy beliefs underlie dysfunctional behaviors (ie, withdrawal, procrastination, alcoholism, and substance abuse). Cognitive distortions also occur with REBT (see Table 8-1).

The foundation for REBT rests on the client's realization that he or she is the creator of the psychological disturbance along with the recognition that he or she can change these disturbances. Crucial to this realization and recognition is the understanding that these disturbances are primarily the result of irrational beliefs. Once identified, they can be disputed and philosophically restructured, ultimately leading to changes. These changes mean moving from the musts, shoulds, and oughts to "preferences" (ie, what the client would like to happen). Making a change in focus can facilitate these thoughts. Clients must remove the blame and responsibility from other people and place it on themselves. For the rest of the client's life, he or she must continue to challenge irrational beliefs and use multiple methods of change by doing the following (Ellis & Dryden, 1997):

- Identifying the activating event; describing the aspect of the situation that is most disturbing (eg, "The teacher told the other students that I made a B!")
- Identifying the unhealthy negative emotion: anger, shame or embarrassment, hurt, anxiety, jealousy (eg, likely shame because "I usually make As.").
- Looking for the irrational belief (eg, "They think I'm stupid.")

- Disputing the belief (eg "Is that true? Probably not. Is it logical? No. Is it helpful? No.")
- Defining a new healthy negative emotion or constructive thought (eg, "I have sadness, annoyance, remorse, disappointment, regret, or concern about the relationship, the event, or what was said."; "I'm still somewhat embarrassed, but I no longer believe that the world is going to come to an end, and maybe they'll like me better now.")

Choice Therapy

Glasser (1998) developed his model of reality therapy in 1965 and further refined it into *choice therapy* in 1998. This pragmatic model focuses on the here and now, with the present as the only reality to consider. Glasser does not subscribe to the theory that biochemical imbalances lead to mental illness. Therefore, reality theory sometimes is seen as harsh and unnurturing. The basic premise of choice therapy is that a person can choose to change what he or she wants others to do or can choose to change how he or she deals with a person, situation, or both. According to this model, a person can control only his or her own behavior. He or she is free to choose to do or not to do what someone else wants. A person can give or get information from others, but ultimately it is the person's own choice as to how to deal with that information. Glasser believes that there is no way to rewrite a person's past; therefore, considering the past is fruitless. It is not acceptable to blame unhappiness or personal failures on external circumstances, lack of opportunity, poor family relationships, or anything else. In this model, the therapist encourages the client to rewrite his or her life script for a different outcome by making plans based on self-responsibility and self-discipline. The focus is on "doing" rather than "feeling."

According to choice therapy, a person is driven by five genetic needs: survival, love and belonging, power, freedom, and fun. These needs must be satisfied, and only the person can decide when this has occurred. In addition, behaving is all one does from birth to death. All behavior is total and is made up of four inseparable components: acting, thinking, feeling, and physiologic makeup (eg, heart, lungs, and muscles). The person chooses all total behavior and has direct control over only the acting and thinking components. He or she has only indirect control of feelings and physiologic makeup through how the individual chooses to act and think. Glasser believes that unsatisfying relationships are the source of most crime, addictions, mental illness, and marital, family, and academic failures (Glasser, 1998).

Implementing choice therapy includes the following components:

1. Identifying the problem or unsatisfying relationship (eg, "My spouse left me.").
2. Leaving the past alone because the person cannot change it and focusing on building a more effective present (eg, "I'll join a group to meet more people.").
3. Changing all complaints about symptoms or people from adjectives and nouns to verbs. Doing so teaches that the person is actively choosing what he or she is complaining about and can learn to make better choices (eg, change "I am depressed," to "I am depressing.")
4. Beginning to identify one's own part in the situation.

Brief, Solution-Focused Therapy

Traditional psychotherapeutic philosophy identifies the person as the problem and asks, "What is the cause of the problem?" This suggests that there is a relationship between the cause and the solution to the problem—in other words, effecting change by eliminating the problem. In the 1950s, the view changed from "What is the cause of the problem?" to "What maintains the problem?" primarily within interactional patterns. Recently, the question has become, "How do we construct solutions?"

Brief, solution-focused therapy is based on concepts of family therapy and the work of Milton Erickson, who helped people make satisfactory life adjustments while ignoring the causative underlying maladjustments (De-Shazer, 1994). Brief, solution-focused therapy does not deal with insight but focuses on the behaviors and thoughts that are maintaining the symptoms. Also, solution-focused therapy does not focus on the client's past. Instead, it focuses on identifying past successes as well as what behaviors are maintaining the complaint. Such behaviors are the inadvertent facilitators of the undesirable behaviors or feelings. The primary focus is on the relativistic and constructivist view with a future orientation. Solution-focused therapists also use the word "we" (client and therapist), suggesting a joint experience.

Solution-focused therapy is not a collection of techniques but reflects ideas about change, interaction, and reaching (not just setting) goals. It does not see problems as coming from inside the person, character flaws, or mental illness. Rather, it promotes the idea that problems come from mishandling life's difficulties. It is based on the belief that the subject of therapy is the way people make sense of themselves and their interactions, and it is people's view of their situation that stands in the way of their finding "solutions." The therapist is not the expert but the co-discoverer whose task is to facilitate the client's construction of an alternate view of his or her situation, one that allows for different responses, behaviors, and outcomes. It is more important for the therapist to validate the client's perception of the situation than to provide a diagnosis or label. The process of solution-focused therapy is described in Box 8-2.

BOX 8-2 ▼ *Process of Solution-Focused Therapy*

1. **Setting the agenda:** What brings you here today? What would be helpful for us to talk about? What would be helpful for me to know about you and your situation? What would be more helpful? Tell me why this is more helpful?

2. **Understanding effects of the problem:** What effect has this problem had on you and your life? In what way(s) is the problem still affecting you? In what way(s) has this problem kept you from moving forward in the way you would like? In what way(s) has this problem gotten in the way of your life? How would your best friend, teacher, mother, or spouse say this problem has had an effect on your life? Would you agree? What are your feelings about that?

3. **Identifying exceptions:** Are there times when you would expect the problem to happen, but it does not? How do you get that to happen? (A focus on client competency.) What are you doing differently when you're standing up to the problem? Tell me about a time when you were even a little successful in standing up to the problem. Would your family or friends say there are times when the problem is less of a problem? What's going on when they say that?

4. **Making sense of the exceptions:** How do you account for your ability to do this (the exception)? Is this something that surprised you about yourself? What about you helped you to be able to do this? Did you know before you did ____ that you would be able to do it? If yes: How did you know this about yourself? What was different about this situation compared with a situation when the problem was more in charge? What was different about you? What would your family, friends, mate, teacher, or boss say if I were to ask them how they think you did this?

5. **Using future orientation:** Create the expectation of noticeable change. Expecting change implies that the client has the power to change.

6. **Asking the "miracle question":** If a miracle happened tonight while you were asleep and tomorrow morning you awoke to find that this problem no longer existed, what would be different? How would you know the miracle had taken place? How would others know without you telling them? What would your feelings be when _____ is not controlling your behavior or thinking? (Keep increasing the level and amount of details.)

7. **Asking for a "video description":** If I had two videotapes, one of you when you are standing up to the influence of the problem and another when the problem is getting the best of you, what would I notice about the one where you are in charge? What's different? If one tape is in the past and one is in the future, what's most noticeable in the future tape of you that tells us that things are better for you?

8. **Reinforcing small steps:** What will be a small sign, something you'll likely notice in the next day or so, that will tell you that things are better for you? What will indicate to you there's reason to be hopeful?

9. **Scaling questions:** On a scale from 1 to 10, with 1 being "pretty bad" and 10 being "pretty good," how would you rate how you are doing now? When you're able to move one or two points toward 10, what will be happening differently? What's the highest you've ever been? When was that? How were you able to do that?

10. **Continuing to working toward solutions:** Client is to
    - Observe and take note of things that go well in the next week; look for examples of exceptions.
    - Pretend that the solution has occurred, the miracle has happened, or the client has attained a higher point on the scale. This may involve picking particular days to pretend or a daily coin tossing with the pretending to be done on "heads" days. If others are involved in the therapy, they may be asked to pretend also or to try to "guess" when the client is pretending.
    - "Practice" particular steps and behaviors that have been identified, such as making a phone call to say ____, or talking out loud to yourself in the mirror. What is the most far-fetched explanation for this problem you can think of?

THE NURSE'S ROLE

Levels of Clinical Nursing Practice

There are two basic levels of psychiatric nursing: the generalist and the advanced practice registered nurse in psychiatric-mental health. Generalists in psychiatric nursing receive initial education in a basic nursing program, work in the psychiatric-mental health area, receive additional on-the-job training, and often engage in continuing education activities to further their knowledge and skill level. They function in both inpatient and outpatient settings within the community. When working with the individual client, the generalist assesses behaviors, assists in formulating individual care plans, administers medication, monitors side effects, educates clients and families, evaluates progress, discharges clients, provides facility-specific follow-up contact as indicated, and always communicates therapeutically (Burgess, 1998).

The basic-level nurse (with a bachelor of science in nursing) can become certified (registered nurse [RN], certified) as a psychiatric-mental health nurse after working in the field and continuing his or her education. Achieving certification "demonstrates that the basic level nurse has met the profession's standards of knowledge and experience in the specialty, exceeding those of a beginning RN or a novice in the specialty (American Nurses Association [ANA], American Psychiatric Nurses Association [APNA], & International Society of Psychiatric-Mental Health Nurses [ISPMHN], 2000)."

An advanced practice nurse (APN) has education at the graduate level as a clinical nurse specialist or nurse practitioner. In addition to the previously listed activities and responsibilities, the APN usually is a primary healthcare provider, functions autonomously, often works in a semi-isolated situation, has limited medication prescription privileges (as determined by individual state laws), manages the overall care of people with emotional and psychiatric problems, and usually has a consultative arrangement with a psychiatrist. The level of decision making and responsibility is higher than that of the generalist (Burgess, 1998).

Therapeutic Interventions in Nursing

When working with individuals, the nurse tries to understand the client's life experience and uses this understanding to support and promote learning related to health and personal development. The key here is "understanding the client's life experience," again, not what the nurse believes, but what the client believes. This teaching–coaching function includes the concepts of disease process, medication, emotional content, and effective management of rapidly changing situations. The additional word "coaching" implies teamwork and improvement and thus is a concept that can facilitate client acceptance of treatment.

No matter which type of intervention used by the nurse, to be therapeutic, the nurse must have no predetermined agenda, be present with the client as the possibility for transformation emerges, and support the client as he or she makes decisions and choices (Marchione, 1993). The emphasis is on listening, unconditionally accepting, and supporting the direction chosen by the client. It means accepting the client's model of the world and respecting the desired outcome (Montgomery & Webster, 1994). Implementing these concepts reinforces the nonjudgmental nature of nursing and recognizes the effects that people can have on one another, in this case, the nurse with the client and the client with the nurse.

Nurses at the basic level may incorporate principles from different psychotherapeutic techniques into their general interactions with clients, but they do not function as individual therapists. For example, nurses can learn and incorporate solution-focused therapy into most nursing interactions. Nurses who use techniques from this ther-apy have to consciously change their orientation from the "whys" of the past to focus on previous successes and then define specific behaviors and goals for the future. Practicing the questions and techniques increases the nurse's comfort level and effectiveness when working with a client. Basic-level nurses need to define and use techniques that seem to make the most sense to them. A particular treatment program may have a defined focus, however, and the nurse should use techniques that are compatible with the basic philosophy of the treatment program.

The primary focus of psychiatric nursing at the basic level is implementing nursing interventions that "promote and foster health, assess dysfunction, assist patients to regain or improve abilities, and prevent further disability" (ANA et al., 2000, p. 12). According to the *Scope and Standards of Psychiatric-Mental Health Clinical Nursing Practice* (ANA et al., 2000), basic nursing interventions include health promotion and health maintenance, intake screening and evaluation, case management, provision of a therapeutic environment (milieu), tracking clients and assisting them with self-care activities, administering and monitoring psychobiological treatment regimens, health teaching, counseling and crisis intervention, psychiatric rehabilitation, community-based care, outreach activities, and advocacy (see Box 8-1). These interventions are discussed briefly in the following section and within other chapters in the text. These basic psychiatric-mental health nursing interventions are compatible with therapeutic interventions in nursing, which were pioneered in the 1950s by Hildegard Peplau with her interpersonal theory and its emphasis on the nurse–client relationship. Development of the therapeutic relationship is primary, requires intensive work, and includes skillful application of learned information and activities. It also is objective, goal directed, and client centered and must include the development of boundaries, trust, and safety (see Chap. 4).

HEALTH PROMOTION AND HEALTH MAINTENANCE

The goals of health promotion and health maintenance are to help the client understand and accept the suggested changes in lifestyle, usual activities, and interpersonal interactions and how this will lead to a more functional life. Interventions include the following:

- Scheduling routine follow-up with healthcare providers
- Instructing about early identification of problematic signs and symptoms
- Teaching stress reduction techniques
- Implementing, or referring the client to, substance abuse awareness programs
- Helping the client recognize that positive mental health is a direct function of choices; the client may not want to use the "crutch," but that may be the only way to achieve a desired goal

INTAKE SCREENING AND EVALUATION

Intake screening and evaluation may include the following (ANA et al., 2000):

- Assessing the client's physical and psychosocial state
- Making diagnostic judgments
- Facilitating the client's movement into appropriate services
- Considering biophysical, psychological, social, cultural, economic, and environmental aspects of the client's life to understand his or her experience of the problem and the type of assistance that he or she requires
- Referring the client for additional testing

CASE MANAGEMENT

The goal of nurses functioning as case managers is to help clients achieve their highest level of functioning so that they may be more self-sufficient and make progress toward optimal health (ANA et al., 2000). Interventions that may help nurses meet this goal (and thus assist their clients) include the following:

- Assessing risk
- Counseling
- Problem solving
- Teaching
- Monitoring medication and health status
- Providing care planning
- Identifying and coordinating with other health-care services

ASSISTING WITH SELF-CARE ACTIVITIES

When working with individuals in the therapeutic milieu, assisting with self-care activities is a significant dimension of direct nursing care. Examples of interventions within this category include the following (ANA et al., 2000):

- Developing recreational activities
- Helping the client improve practical life skills including cooking, hygiene measures, shopping, and using public transportation
- Teaching medication and symptom management

IMPLEMENTING PSYCHOBIOLOGICAL INTERVENTIONS

Nurses play a key role in implementing psychobiological interventions because of their ability to assess the client holistically and treat the clients' responses to actual and potential health problems (ANA et al., 2000). Interventions may include (but are not limited to) the following:

- Relaxation techniques
- Nutrition and diet management
- Exercise and rest schedules

HEALTH TEACHING

The nurse incorporates basic health teaching into the specific care of each individual client. It includes the following concepts:

- Assisting clients to achieve more satisfying, productive, and healthy patterns of living (eg, how increased levels of stress can affect the client's health condition)
- Aiming health teaching at the client, family, and other involved individuals
- Focusing health teaching on the following:
  - Psychobiologic effects
  - Effects of medication
  - Overall effect of the particular mental health diagnosis on interactions within the identified family, work, and school situation
  - How to deal with stress and anxiety
  - Relaxation techniques and imagery
- Individualizing teaching for the client; examples include the following:
  - Educating the client with major depression about antidepressant agents, maintenance of adequate nutrition, sleep measures, ways to enhance self-care management, goal setting effective problem solving, and social interaction skills
  - Educating the client with obsessive-compulsive disorder about psychopharmacologic therapy, skin care measures, appropriate alternative activities for ritualistic behaviors, thought-stopping and relaxation techniques, and appropriate follow-up and available community resources

COUNSELING AND CRISIS INTERVENTION

The nurse uses counseling interventions to assist clients with improving or regaining their previous coping abilities, fostering mental health, and preventing mental illness and disability. This also may include crisis management for clients who have faced traumatic personal situations (eg, loss of job, bodily function, family member, role status), natural or national disasters (eg, fires, floods, terrorist attack of September 11th), or both. When providing crisis management for clients, it is essential that nurses

- Understand that the person's experience of the crisis situation is his or hers alone (not the nurse's experience)
- Become self-aware (eg, knowledgeable of their own anxiety levels during crisis situations and how they demonstrate these signs)
- Recognize and respond to the person's experience with compassion and understanding
- Actively listen, provide empathy, and develop therapeutic communication techniques such as acceptance, reflection, validation, and use of open-ended statements

PSYCHIATRIC REHABILITATION

The focus of psychiatric rehabilitation is strengthening self-care and promoting and improving the quality of an individual's life through relapse prevention. Areas of focus within psychiatric rehabilitation include the following (ANA et al., 2000):

- Consumer empowerment
- Recognition of the role of the family and larger social network
- Focus on accountable programming, cost effectiveness, and outcomes
- Stronger collaborative relationships with treatment services
- Emphasis on recovery of hope and development of functional competencies

▼ *Reflection and Critical Thinking Questions*

1. Smoking cessation programs often use behavior modification. Explore how such programs apply this technique of behavioral therapy.

2. Describe how you would incorporate the techniques for solution-focused therapy into your nursing interactions with clients.

3. Discuss how the basic-level nurse should prepare before providing counseling to a client and how this will influence the effectiveness of the nursing interventions.

4. Develop a health teaching plan detailing the types of information you would want to include for a client and his or her family about ways to deal with stress and anxiety.

▼ CHAPTER SUMMARY

- The client in individual therapy often works with a team consisting of nurses, a social worker, a psychologist, adjunctive therapists, and a psychiatrist. All members of the team, including the client, have the same overall goals: to empower the client to experience more satisfying relationships with a resultant increase in self-esteem and self-worth, to enable clients to integrate themselves with self-chosen work activities, and to enable the client to find greater meaning in his or her life.

- Psychotherapy is the treatment of mental and emotional disorders using the psychoeducational methods of support, suggestion, persuasion, reeducation, reassurance, and insight to alter maladaptive patterns of coping and to encourage personality growth. It has moved from long-term analysis of the causes of dysfunction to short-term focus on changing thoughts, feelings, and behaviors.

- There are many different types of individual psychotherapy. Cognitive therapy, behavioral therapy, cognitive-behavioral therapy, REBT, choice therapy, and solution-focused therapy are some of the most common types.

- There are basically two types of psychiatric nurses: basic-level nurses and advanced practice nurses. Basic-level nurses work with individuals, families, groups, and communities to assess mental health needs, develop diagnoses, and plan, implement, and evaluate nursing care. Advanced practice nurses have all the basic-level knowledge as well as expertise in psychotherapy and psychobiologic interventions.

- In addition to listening and observing nonjudgmentally to understand the client's life experience, therapeutic nursing interventions in individual psychiatric nursing care at the basic level include health promotion and health maintenance, intake screening and evaluation, case management, provision of a therapeutic environment (milieu), tracking clients and assisting them with self-care activities, administering and monitoring psychobiological treatment regimens, health teaching, counseling and crisis intervention, psychiatric rehabilitation, community-based care, outreach activities, and advocacy.

▼ REVIEW QUESTIONS

1. When beginning a therapeutic relationship with a client, the nurse would assume which of the following about the client?
   a. The client assumes a passive, dependent role.
   b. The client is incompetent.
   c. The client has necessary capabilities.
   d. Clients develop solutions on their own.

2. A therapist says the following, "Fence." The client replies with the first thing that comes to his mind, saying, "Gate." This is an example of which of the following?
   a. Free association
   b. Countertransference
   c. Cognitive thread
   d. Schema

3. During an interview, the client states, "Whatever I do, it always comes out wrong." The nurse interprets this statement as which of the following?
   a. Catastrophizing
   b. All-or-nothing thinking
   c. Perfectionism
   d. Overgeneralization

4. A nurse is implementing a token economy system for a client. The nurse understands that this system is a component of which of the following?
   a. Choice therapy
   b. Behavioral therapy

c. Rational emotive behavioral therapy
d. Brief solution-focused therapy

5. The goals of NAMI are based on the work of which of the following theorists?
   a. Sigmund Freud
   b. Abraham Maslow
   c. Thomas Szasz
   d. Milton Erickson

6. Which of the following descriptions characterizes irrational beliefs?
   a. Expression of dislikes that may or may not be attained
   b. Views that foster the attainment of goals
   c. The foundation for functional behavior
   d. Rigid, absolute views and experiences

7. When caring for the client receiving choice therapy, the nurse understands that the focus of this therapy is on which of the following?
   a. Exploring the person's conscious and unconscious conflicts of the past
   b. Building a more effective present by doing and taking responsibility
   c. Using positive and negative reinforcers to modify behaviors
   d. Developing alternatives by learning new skills

8. Which of the following questions would be most appropriate to use when setting the agenda for a client who is to undergo solution-focused therapy?
   a. "In what ways is the problem still interfering with your life?"
   b. "Are there times when you expect the problem to happen and it doesn't?"
   c. "What would be helpful for me to know about you and your situation?"
   d. "What does your spouse say about the way this problem is affecting your life?"

9. Which of the following correctly identifies the roles and functions of a psychiatric nurse practicing at the basic level?
   a. Acts as a primary mental healthcare provider
   b. Possesses expertise in psychobiologic interventions
   c. Can function as an individual therapist
   d. Has a baccalaureate degree in nursing

▼ REFERENCES AND SUGGESTED READINGS

*American Nurses Association, American Psychiatric Nurses Association, & International Society of Psychiatric-Mental Health Nurses. (2000). *Scope and standards of psychiatric-mental health clinical nursing practice.* Washington, DC: Author.

*Beck, A. T. (1979). *Cognitive therapy and the emotional disor-ders.* New York: Penguin Books, International Universities Press.

*Beck, A. T. (1993). Cognitive therapy: Past, present, and future. *Journal of Consultant Clinical Psychology, 61*(2), 194–198.

*Beck, A. T., Rush, A. J., Shaw, B. F., & Emery, G. (1979). *Cognitive therapy of depression.* New York: Guilford Press.

*Beck, A. T., Wright, F. D., Newman, C. F., & Liese, B. S. (1993). *Cognitive therapy of substance abuse.* New York: Guilford Press.

*Berg, I. K. (1990). *Solution-focused approach to family based services.* Milwaukee: Brief Family Therapy Center.

*Brief Intervention for Alcohol Problems. (1999). NIAAA alcohol alert (No. 43). *The Counselor, 17*(5), 32–35.

*Burgess, A. W. (1998). *Advanced practice psychiatric nursing.* Stamford, CT: Appleton & Lange.

*Cade, B., & O'Hanlon, W. H. (1993). *A brief guide to brief therapy.* New York: W. W. Norton.

*Canadian Nurses Association. (1995). *Canadian Federation of the Mental Health Nurses: Canadian standards of psychiatric and mental health nursing practice.* Ottawa, Ontario: Author.

*Carson, R. C., & Mineka, S. (1999). *Abnormal psychology and modern life* (11th ed.). Reading, MA: Addison-Wesley Longman Publishers.

*Crits-Christoph, P. (1998). Training in empirically validated treatments. In K. S. Dobson, & K. D. Craig (Eds.), *Empirically supported therapies: Best practices in professional psychology* (pp. 3–25). Thousand Oaks, CA: Sage.

*DeShazer, S. (1985). *Keys to solution in brief therapy.* New York: W. W. Norton.

*DeShazer, S. (1994). *Words were originally magic.* New York: W. W. Norton.

*Dobson, K. S., & Craig, K. D. (Eds.). (1998). *Empirically supported therapies: Best practices in professional psychology.* Thousand Oaks, CA: Sage.

*Ellis, A., & Dryden, W. (1997). The practice of rational emotive behavior therapy (2nd ed.). New York: Springer Publishing Co.

*Freed, P. E. (1998). Perseverance: The meaning of patient education in psychiatric nursing. *Archives of Psychiatric Nursing, 11*(2), 107–113.

*Freeman, A., & Yates, M. J. (1998). Cognitive therapy. In A. W. Burgess (Ed.), *Advanced practice psychiatric nursing* (pp. 213–238). Stamford, CT: Appleton & Lange.

*Freud, S. (1960). The complete introductory lectures on psychoanalysis. In J. Stachey (Ed. & Trans.), *The standard edition of the complete psychological works of Sigmund Freud* (Vols. 15–17). New York: Norton.

*Freud, S. (1960). The ego and the id. In J. Stachey (Ed. & Trans.), *The standard edition of the complete psychological works of Sigmund Freud* (Vols. 15–17). New York: Norton.

*Glasser, W. (1998). *Choice theory: A new psychology of personal freedom.* New York: Harper Collins Publisher, Inc.

*Haley, J. (1993). *Uncommon therapy: The psychiatric techniques of Milton H. Erickson, MD.* New York: W.W. Norton.

*Havens, R. A. (1992). *The wisdom of Milton H. Erickson: Human behavior & psychotherapy* (Vol. 2). New York: Irvington Publishing Co.

*Marchione, J. (1993). *Margaret Neuman: Health as expanding consciousness.* Newbury Park: Sage Publications.

*Maslow, A. H. (1968). *Toward a psychology of being* (2nd ed.). New York: Van Nostrand Reinhold.

*Matthews, W. J. (1999). Brief therapy: A problem solving model of change. *The Counselor, 17*(4), 29–32.

*McCrone, S. H. (1998). Brief individual psychotherapies. In A. W. Burgess (Ed.), *Advanced practice psychiatric nursing* (pp. 187–201). Stamford, CT: Appleton & Lange.

McFall, R. M., & Twentyman, C. T. (1973). Four experiments on the relative contributions of rehearsal, modeling, and coaching to assertion training. *Journal of Abnormal Psychology, 81,* 199–218.

*Medcalf, L. (1992). *Solution-oriented brief therapy.* Inservice presentation at CPC Oak Bend Hospital, Ft. Worth, TX.

*Montgomery, C. L., & Webster, D. (1994). Caring, curing, and brief therapy: A model for nurse-psychotherapy. *Archives of Psychiatric Nursing, 8*(5), 291–297.

*Neimeyer, G. J. (Ed.). (1993). *Constructivist assessment: A case book.* Newbury Park, CA: Sage Publications.

*O'Hanlon, W. H., & Weiner-Davis, M. (1989). *In search of solutions.* New York: Norton & Company.

*Olson, J. N., & Mohr, W. K. (in press). *The lost art of accuracy: A contextual approach to assessment.* Newark, NJ: Rutgers College of Nursing.

*Peplau, H. E. (1988). *Interpersonal relations in nursing.* New York: Springer.

*Rogers, C. (1961). *On becoming a person.* Boston: Houghton-Mifflin.

*Rogers, M. E. (1970). An introduction to the theoretical basis of nursing. Philadelphia: F. A. Davis.

*Schofield, R. (1998). Empowerment education for individuals with serious mental illness. *Journal of Psychosocial Nursing, 36*(11), 35–40.

*Szasz, T. (1974). *The myth of mental illness.* New York: Harper & Row.

*U.S. Department of Agriculture, & U.S. Department of Health and Human Services. (1995). *Nutrition and your health: Dietary guidelines for Americans.* Washington, DC: Author.

*Walter, J. L., & Peller, J. E. (1992). Becoming solution-focused in brief therapy. New York: Brunner-Mazel.

*Wilshaw, G. (1997). Integration of therapeutic approaches: A new direction for mental health nurses? *Journal of Advanced Nursing, 26*(1), 15–19.

*Wolpe, J. (1973). *The practice of behavior therapy* (2nd ed.). New York: Pergamon Press.

*Wolpe, J., & Lazarus, A. A. (1966). *Behavior therapy techniques.* New York: Pergamon Press.

Starred references are cited in text.

For additional information on this chapter, go to *http://connection. lww.com.*

Need more help? See Chapter 8 of the *Study Guide to Accompany Mohr: Johnson's Psychiatric- Mental Health Nursing,* 5th ed.

Working With Groups

BARBARA G. TUNLEY CRENSHAW

▼KEY TERMS

Autocratic leader—A leader who exercises significant authority and control over group members, rarely, if ever, seeks or uses input from the group, and does not encourage participation or interaction from the group.

Democratic leader—A leader who encourages group interaction and participation in group problem solving and decision making, values the input and feedback of each group member, seeks spontaneous and honest interaction among group members, creates an atmosphere that rewards members for their contributions, solicits the group's opinions,

and tailors the group's work to their common goals.

Formal group—A group with structure and authority, which usually emanates from above; interaction in the group usually is limited.

Group—Three or more people with related goals.

Group norm—The development over time of a pattern of interaction within a group to which certain behavioral expectations are attached.

Informal group—A group that provides much of a person's education and contributes greatly to his or her cultural values; members do not depend on one another.

Laissez-faire leader—A leader who allows group members to operate as they choose.

Power—The perceived ability to control appropriate reward, therefore lending influence.

Primary group—A group that has face-to-face contact, boundaries, norms, and explicit and implicit interdependent roles.

Secondary group—A group that usually is larger and more impersonal than primary groups; members do not have the relationship bonds or emotional ties of members of a primary group.

▼LEARNING OBJECTIVES

On completion of this chapter, you should be able to accomplish the following:

- Identify the characteristics of a group.
- Explain group norms.
- Compare styles of group leadership.
- Define three major categories of group roles.
- Identify communication processes within groups.
- Describe the stages of group development.
- Discuss the advantages of group therapy.
- Discuss the therapeutic factors of group therapy.
- Compare the various types of group therapy.
- Discuss the nurse's role in working with groups.

We live and work in groups. Each of us is born into a family; we attend school with groups of peers, enter into friendships and work-related groups, and establish our

own groups of family or significant others. In psychiatric-mental health nursing and other areas of healthcare, nurses interact with groups of students, faculty, professional colleagues, clients, and clients' families. An understanding of group dynamics and their application is essential to effective functioning for nurses in their personal and professional lives.

This chapter is organized into three major sections: group process, group therapy, and nurses and group process and therapy. The group process section presents foundational group information, including a definition of group, group characteristics, types of groups, group norms, group leadership, group roles, group communication, and stages of group development. The group therapy section presents the purposes, advantages and disadvantages, therapeutic factors, and approaches of this type of therapy. Finally, the nurses and group process and therapy section discusses the nurse's role in working with groups.

GROUP PROCESS

What Is a Group?

A **group** is three or more people with related goals. Many factors influence these goals, including interpersonal and intrapersonal needs, the physical environment, and the unique interaction of the group. For example, the physical environment or climate in some countries is so severe that the survival of the individual depends on his or her relationships with other individuals. The individuals form relationship bonds that develop into groups (Kelly & Vanderslott, 1995). These groups develop structures, characteristics, and roles. The further creation of systems and subsystems leads to the development of more complex societies that display certain characteristics called culture (see Chap. 5).

Characteristics of Groups

The following are characteristics of groups:

- Size of the group
- Homogeneity or heterogeneity of group members
- Stability of the group
- Degree of cohesiveness, or bonding power, between members
- Climate of the group (eg, warm, friendly, cold, aloof)
- Conformity to group norms
- Degree of agreement with the leader's and the group's norms
- Ability to deal with members' infractions
- Goal directedness and task orientation of the group's work

Types of Groups

Groups may be primary or secondary, formal or informal. Members of **primary groups** have face-to-face contact. They have boundaries, norms, and explicit and implicit interdependent roles. An example of a primary group is a family.

Secondary groups usually are larger and more impersonal than primary groups. Members of secondary groups do not have the relationship bonds or emotional ties of members of a primary group. An example of a secondary group is a political party or a business.

A **formal group** has structure and authority. Authority in a formal group usually emanates from above, and interaction in the group usually is limited. A faculty meeting is an example of a formal group. **Informal groups** provide much of a person's education and contribute greatly to his or her cultural values. In an informal group, such as a friendship or hobby group, the members do not depend on each other.

Group Norms

A **group norm** is the development, over time, of a pattern of interaction within a group to which certain behavioral expectations are attached. Group norms affect the scope and functioning of a group. Norms also help to structure role expectations and provide sanctions, taboos, and reference power to the group.

To explain group norms, consider the example of a nursing team meeting designed to discuss client care planning and communication among the nursing staff. A role expectation norm is that the team leader will chair the meeting. A membership norm is that the members will be on time and possibly will sit in certain places. There may be a formalized norm called an agenda of the meeting, which states that communication among nursing staff members will occur before the discussion to plan client care. Other group norms may be universal with regard to the task role of one member, such as the role of the secretary who records the minutes of the meeting. Group members who present their clients' history and assessment accurately, clearly, and with organization receive sanction. A group taboo is to fall asleep and snore while another member is talking. When a group member falls asleep and snores during meetings, especially if this occurs numerous times, the member is viewed as a deviant.

Norms exert a controlling element over groups by setting the boundaries of group activities. To promote the growth and stimulation of group members, groups must learn to change their norms when they no longer function for the group. A group is more creative if each member becomes a so-called change agent for norms no longer needed.

Group Leadership

To become an effective group leader, the nurse must understand the concepts of leadership and their accompanying forces, scope, and limitations. The three concepts of power, influence, and authority have an impact on leadership. **Power** is the perceived ability to control appropriate reward, therefore lending influence to the leader. The nurse leader gains authority through influence, power, and knowledge or expertise. The leader also understands that there are effective ways of using authority and decides to what extent he or she will expand or limit this authority.

The effective leader also decides to what extent the authority will be autocratic (centralized) or democratic (decentralized). The leader reaches this decision, in part, according to the type of group. For example, the leader may readily relinquish authority in a training group (T group). The purpose of the T group is to improve the group members' ability to communicate or relate to others in the group. The members, however, generally possess a certain degree of knowledge and experience in relating to others and therefore are capable of imparting their skills to other group members.

In groups where members are likely to exhibit high degrees of personality disorganization and faulty communication and interpersonal skills, the leader may exercise centralized authority. In other types of therapy groups, such as gestalt groups, which deal with the here and now and whose members generally are healthy, the distribution of power within the group may depend on the age and emotional maturity of the group members.

STYLES OF GROUP LEADERSHIP

Leadership styles are influenced by several factors, including the philosophy of treatment; personality of the leader; traits, characteristics, and purpose of the group; and degree of mental, emotional, or cognitive impairment of the group members. The nurse group leader alters the style of group leadership according to the demands of the therapeutic situation. The three basic styles of group leadership are autocratic, democratic, and laissez-faire.

An **autocratic leader** is one who exercises significant authority and control over group members, rarely seeks or uses input from the group, and does not encourage participation or interaction from the group. In some circumstances, such as in emergencies, the autocratic style of leadership may be the most effective; it conserves time and energy and dictates roles and responsibilities to members. Conversely, constant use of an autocratic leadership style may cause hostility, scapegoating behavior, dependence on the leader, and limitation of growth potential for group members.

The **democratic leader** encourages group interaction and participation in group problem solving and decision making. A democratic group leader values the input and feedback of each group member, seeks spontaneous and honest interaction among members of the group, and creates an atmosphere in which members are rewarded for their contributions. The group's opinions are solicited, and the group's work is tailored to common goals. A group with a democratic leadership style may require more time and effort than an autocratic group to accomplish its goals; however, the group's efforts are more productive and cohesive and instill in members a sense of participation in decision making.

In a **laissez-faire** style of leadership, group members are free to operate as they choose. This style of group leadership may be effective if the members are highly knowledgeable, task oriented, and motivated. Conversely, the laissez-faire approach is time consuming and often inefficient in the accomplishment of group tasks.

DECISION MAKING

Decision making is a necessary component of leadership, power, influence, authority, and delegation of authority. In formal groups, specific guidelines determine which decisions will be made by the leader and which decisions will be decentralized; that is, delegated to group members.

The ability to make effective decisions depends on the group's knowledge of the subject, its ability to choose appropriate methods to solve problems, its ability to test and evaluate problem solving and decision making after a decision has been put to the test, and its maturity and ability to reverse or modify a decision that has proven to be unwise, unfair, or otherwise unacceptable.

Decisions may be made by consensus, majority vote, or minority decision. In a *consensus,* all members of the group agree on a decision. Although consensus may prove to be time consuming and costly, especially in a large group, it gives more satisfaction to the total group. The democratic leader uses consensus whenever possible. *Majority vote* is a form of decision making in which the issue is decided by the larger number of group members. This method often is used by democratic leadership when it is not possible to reach a consensus. A *minority decision* may be formulated by a self-delegated subgroup or a group appointed as a subcommittee to explore the situation in greater depth and reach a decision.

STRUCTURING THE GROUP

The group leader is instrumental in establishing and maintaining cohesiveness in the group. The leader also selects and orients new group members in beginning and continuing groups. An effective leader ensures that the structuring process for the group defines group norms, clarifies expectations, sets standards for group performance, and maintains cohesiveness as new members are introduced into the group. The leader discusses some of these issues with new members before introducing them to the group. An example of such a discussion follows:

Leader: Jane, welcome. I am Ms. C., the group leader. I always meet with new members to share with them the goals and expectations of the group. (pause) The group will have eight members, including you. We will meet from 1 to 2 PM each day in the blue room. Members will enter and leave the group as their behavior and needs change. (pause)

Jane: What are we expected to do?

Leader: Group members are expected to share their problems and their feelings about those problems with other members of the group.

Jane: Is that all?

Leader: No. It is also my expectation that group members will discover techniques of problem solving through exploring these problems and feelings and that, eventually, when members learn to relate more effectively to each other, they will transfer these newly acquired skills to other relationships.

Jane: That sounds difficult and frightening.

Leader: Changing and growing involves a certain amount of pain.

The leader structures the group by determining its size, homogeneity of group members, and leadership style.

The group's purpose and goals define its scope, limitations, and desired accomplishments. The group leader's responsibilities to members include ensuring the psychological safety of group members, establishing and maintaining group norms, role-modeling relationship skills, and commenting on group process. To receive gratification from group membership, members must participate by introspecting, self-disclosing, nurturing others, expressing feelings, and contributing to the maintenance of the group.

Group Roles

The functions of group leaders and members are interdependent. Member roles can enhance the effectiveness of a group leader and vice versa. Roles observed in groups are categorized as group task roles, group building and maintenance roles, and individual roles. All of these roles are observed in group behavior. Individually oriented behavior, which often grows from anxiety, distracts from and temporarily stymies the group and its progress, whereas task, maintenance, and building roles promote group growth and productivity.

GROUP TASK ROLES

Group task roles identify group problems and select methods to solve those problems. Problem solving helps the group to reach its goal or mission. Examples of group task roles include the following:

Initiator–contributor, who suggests or proposes to the group new ideas or different ways of regarding the group problem or goal

Information seeker, who asks for clarification

Information giver, who offers facts or generalizations that are considered authoritative or who shares personal experiences in relation to the group problems

Coordinator, who shows or clarifies how ideas can work

Orienteer, who keeps the group on target by defining where the group is in relation to its goal

Recorder, who is the group's memory and writes down productive discussion and group decisions

GROUP BUILDING AND MAINTENANCE ROLES

Group building and maintenance roles are oriented toward the functioning of the group as a whole. They alter or maintain the group's way of working to strengthen, regulate, and perpetuate the group. Examples of group building and maintenance roles include the following:

Encourager, who gives acceptance to the contributions of others

Harmonizer, who reconciles differences between group members

Gatekeeper, who facilitates the contributions of oth-

ers, thereby keeping communication open by encouraging remarks about these contributions

Group observer, who notes what is occurring in the group and feeds it back to the group with an evaluation or interpretation of the group's procedure

Follower, who goes along with the ideas of other members, assuming more of an audience role

INDIVIDUAL ROLES

Individual roles are those that meet only the needs of the group member, not of the group. They hamper rather than enhance group functioning. They support individual needs and goals not group needs and goals. Examples of individual roles include the following:

Aggressor, who deflates the status of individual and group accomplishment

Blocker, who resists progress by arguing or disagreeing beyond reason

Recognition seeker, who calls attention to himself or herself through boasting and pointing out achievements

Play person, who horses around, demonstrating lack of involvement

Dominator, who asserts authority and superiority in manipulating the group or certain members of the group

Group Communication

Nurses use various therapeutic communication techniques with clients. Examples of techniques are included in Table 9-1.

LATENT AND MANIFEST COMMUNICATION

Groups use latent and manifest communication. Latent content is content that is not discussed, occurs on an emotional level, and seldom is verbalized, such as hidden agendas. Manifest content involves spoken words. Groups are most effective when their latent and manifest content are similar. The further apart these levels of communication are, the more the group experiences communication problems.

A group may not solve its problems readily because of the interference of latent content. Hidden agendas hinder group communication. For example, if a group member believes that he or she would be punished if he or she verbalizes an opinion in the group, especially if it disagrees with that of the leader, his or her latent communication would influence overt behavior and interfere with group growth.

CONTENT AND PROCESS COMMUNICATION

Content and process are important concepts of group communication. What is being said during discussion is

TABLE 9-1 ▼ Examples of Group Communication Techniques

TECHNIQUE	DESCRIPTION	EXAMPLE
Approval	Condoning or encouraging an attitude, feeling, or action	Frank: "I decided to move to a new apartment." Nurse: "You made a wise decision."
Acceptance	Conveying an attitude or a relationship that recognizes an individual's worth without implying approval of behaviors or personal affection	Marty: "Nurse, I was angry at you for not cancelling the session." Nurse: "It's all right for you to get angry at me, Marty."
Clarification	Restating of the substance of what the client has said	Abel: "I feel hopeless, no way out." Nurse: "You feel you have no way out?"
Exploration	Shifting from considering one aspect of a situation to considering another	Frank: "My son decided to leave the business." Nurse: "Tell me how that came about."
Identification	Delineating specific factors for the purposes of understanding or clarifying	Frank: "I often do favors for others, like my father did. He said it is rewarding and makes us better people." Nurse: "Sounds like you had respect for your father's opinions and judgment."
Interpretation	Finding or explaining the meaning or significance of the information	Mr. B: "All this talking is really a pain in the neck." Nurse: "Mr. B., you seem annoyed at all the talking," or Abel: "I feel hopeless, no way out." Nurse: "You sound suicidal."
Information giving	Stating facts about a problem	Marty: "All the staff write notes in the charts after the group meeting and put their own interpretation on what we say, don't they?" Nurse: "I can only speak for myself. I write notes in the chart, but I try hard not to misinterpret what members state in the group."
Encouraging expression of feelings or ideas	Indicating in some way that it is permissible or desirable to talk about feelings or ideas	Mr. W.: "It takes me 10 or 15 minutes to get oriented in the morning and then I'm all right." Nurse: "Are there others who feel this way?" Ms. S: "I always get up to eat and have some coffee. Then I feel more like facing others."
Reassurance	Offering the client confidence about a favorable outcome through suggestion, persuasive arguments, or comparing similar situations	Frank: "I was afraid to move at first." Nurse: "Frank, we are always here to listen to your fears and try and help you work them out."
Support	Giving comfort, approval, or acceptance	Marty: "My busted arm has played heck with me. Getting anything for it has been a federal case. And I'm not one who shows pain easily." Nurse: "This must be pretty infuriating." Marty: "Well, it really bugs me."

(continued)

TABLE 9-1 ▼	**Examples of Group Communication Techniques (Continued)**	
TECHNIQUE	**DESCRIPTION**	**EXAMPLE**
Intervention	Performing an action that directs or influences the client's behavior	Nurse: "Frank, you've been silent, inattentive, and haven't shared with the group since your weekend pass. Will you tell us what is going on with you?" Frank: "I had a horrible weekend. I don't know how to share what happened, but I'll try."
Understanding	Indicating verbally or nonverbally that the feelings being communicated by the client are comprehended	Marty: "Nurse, I feel frightened about discharge." Nurse: "I can understand your feeling frightened. Leaving the hospital is not always easy."
Reflection	Repeating to clients what they said; mirroring their statement	Mr. B.: "All this talking is really a pain in the neck." Nurse: "This talking is a pain in the neck."
Listening	Concentrating on the client's communication without interrupting	Nurse listens and attends to client.
Teaching	Helping the client learn specifics in relation to events and behavior	Abel (to the nurse): "You were irritated at me, weren't you, but we were able to talk about it and work it out." Nurse: "Yes, we did. I was irritated because I felt you were not listening, and we did talk about it."
Silence	Using no verbal or spoken words	Nurse is silent while attending to client.
Structuring	Shaping the content of the group meeting	Frank: "I'm going home soon." Mrs. C.: "Really?" Nurse: "Maybe you would like to talk about it?"
Limit setting	Deciding how far group members and the group may go before the therapist ceases or restricts to a point the behavior, activity, or verbal expression of members	Marty: "I feel we need to cancel our therapy session next week because the next day is a holiday and we need a long weekend to travel." Nurse: "Holiday weekends are difficult; however, we will not cancel our group session."

the content. How the group is handling its communication is process. Who talks to whom, what is said, and what is left unspoken are examples of process.

Examples of content and process communication follow:

- *Content:* Discussing how a mother does not take care of her children
- *Process:* May mean that the leader or therapist is not meeting the dependency needs of the group
- *Content:* Talking about the fighting of sisters and brothers at home

- *Process:* May mean that there is a lot of conflict and fighting in the therapy group

TRANSFERENCE AND COUNTERTRANSFERENCE

Transference occurs when a client attributes characteristics and behavior of a family member or significant other to the therapist, thereby responding to the therapist in a certain manner. The clarification of this distortion with the client helps to create a therapeutic process of learning. Countertransference occurs when the therapist responds in a negative manner to the client's transference, further complicating communication.

COMMUNICATION THEMES

The group leader observes for themes in the group's communication that relate one group session to another and then explores the meanings of these themes. Through therapeutic communication, the leader may help the group uncover and solve the problem. Group functioning also is evaluated by observing changes in members' behavior, such as their ability to apply these new techniques to solving future problems. Box 9-1 illustrates how communication themes are used.

Higher functioning groups or those with less overt psychopathologic symptomatology will work through problems with minimal hidden agendas and symbolic language. The therapist can encourage the group to deal with here-and-now material and can manage anxiety more readily than in a group that communicates on a symbolic level. The co-therapist in Box 9-1 listened for latent and manifest content to identify the group theme and used communication techniques (see Chap. 4) to help the group solve the problem.

Stages of Group Development

INITIAL STAGE

The initial stage of group development is likely to involve superficial, rather than open and trusting, communication. The members are becoming acquainted with each other and are searching for similarity between themselves and other group members. Members may be unclear about the purposes or goals of the group. A certain amount of structuring of group norms, roles, and responsibilities takes place during this stage (Table 9-2).

WORKING STAGE

During the working stage of group development, the real work of the group is accomplished. Because members are already familiar with each other, the group leader, and the group's rules, they are free to approach and attempt to solve their problems. Conflict and cooperation surface during the group's work.

MATURE STAGE

The mature group demonstrates its maturity through such positive characteristics as empathy, effective communication skills, and a definite, inclusive group culture. Its characteristics are described in detail in Table 9-2. Even if a group reaches a mature stage in its development, its members can regress as individuals. This change may be precipitated by the addition of a new group member, loss of a member, or a group problem that introduces stress. All of these can cause some degree of return to an earlier stage of functioning, and the more serious the disturbance, the greater the potential regression. The more experience the group has in applying problem-solving skills, the more able it is to be resilient in the face of difficulties and return to its former stage of mature functioning. If the group "image" is one of a "problem solver," this also facilitates group functioning. Leadership also is important in sustaining the group and returning it to a mature level of functioning after crisis or change.

TERMINATION STAGE

During termination, the group evaluates the experience and explores members' feelings about it and the impending separation. The termination of the group may be an opportunity for group members who have difficulty saying goodbye to learn to deal more realistically and comfortably with this normal part of human experience, separation.

BOX 9-1 ▼ *A Group Case*

Theme

The group theme is authority or, more pointedly, transference. "Our therapist is punitive to the group, like our mothers, if we disagree."

Countertransference

Therapist I, Mrs. A. (angry): You are rebellious and won't listen to reason. I am particularly angry at Marty because she started this.

Resistance

Three fourths of the group did not attend the next meeting.

Interpretation

Therapist II, Mr. B. (at a later session): Marty, when you stated we were like your mother, it sounded as if you were angry.

Acceptance

Marty: Yes, and afraid.

Exploration

Therapist I, Mrs. A. Marty, I wonder if you felt that your weekend pass being canceled was related to you disagreeing with me in group?

Acknowledgment

Marty: Yes.

Consensual Validation

Group: You know, Mrs. A., we all thought that.

TABLE 9-2 ▼ **Stages of Group Development**	
STAGE	**CHARACTERISTICS**
Initial	1. Works on getting acquainted with group leader and members 2. Depends on the leader for direction 3. Searches for meaning and purpose of the group 4. Restricts content and communication style 5. Searches for similarity among members 6. Gives advice
Working	1. Solves selected problems of working together 2. Handles conflicts between members or between members and leader 3. Works on issues of dominance, control, and power within group 4. Cooperates to accomplish the group's work
Mature	1. Develops workable norms and a group culture 2. Resolves conflict when it occurs; conflict arises from issues of importance, not emotional issues 3. Evaluates own work and individuals assume responsibility for their work 4. Accepts each others' differences without placing value judgments on them 5. Sanctions role assignment by members of the group 6. Discusses topics and makes decisions by means of rational behavior, such as sharing information and open discussion 7. Provides a feeling of "we" for the leader and members 8. Demonstrates cohesion 9. Validates itself; has a group image
Termination	1. Evaluates and summarizes the group experience 2. Explores positive and negative feelings about the group experience

GROUP THERAPY

Purposes

One of the purposes of group psychotherapy is to intervene in mentally disordered behavior, thinking, and feeling. Group therapy offers multiple stimuli to reveal, examine, and resolve distortions in interpersonal relationships. The purpose of a group is related to its goals and expected outcomes. For example, a T group's purpose is to help members improve their present styles of relating to others. An individual needing to develop or heighten these skills would join a T group instead of a psychotherapy group.

Advantages and Disadvantages

Group therapy as a form of treatment for psychiatric-mental health clients has advantages and disadvantages. The advantages of group therapy include the following:

- More clients can be treated in group therapy, making the method cost-effective.
- Members profit by hearing other members discuss their problems; feelings of isolation, alienation, and uniqueness often are decreased, encouraging members to share feelings and problems.
- Group therapy provides an opportunity for clients to explore their specific styles of communication in

a safe atmosphere where they can receive feedback and undergo change.

- Members learn multiple ways of solving a problem from other group members, and group exploration may help them discover new ways of solving a problem.
- Members learn about the functional roles of individuals in a group. Sometimes, a member shares the responsibility as the co-therapist. Members become culture carriers.
- The group provides for its members' understanding, confrontation, and identification with more than one individual. The member gains a reference group.

There also are disadvantages of group therapy, as follows:

- An individual's privacy may be violated, for example, when a conversation shared within the group is repeated outside of the group. This behavior obstructs confidentiality and hampers complete and honest participation in a group.
- Clients may experience difficulty in exposing themselves to a group or believe that they lack the skills to communicate effectively in a group. Some clients may use these factors as resistance; others may be reluctant to expose themselves to the group because they do not want to change (Table 9-3).
- Group therapy is not a helpful form of therapy if

TABLE 9-3 ▼ Common Problems Affecting Group Therapy and Process

GROUP PROBLEM	GOAL	NURSING INTERVENTION	RATIONALE
Fear of authority resulting in timid, hostile, aggressive, or withdrawn behavior	Group members will deal with authority directly and openly discuss their views and feelings about authority.	Use nonverbal and verbal communication techniques; listen to and encourage client to share and explore feelings. Respond in an understanding manner when the client expresses feelings (even when they are hostile). Reassure client that the nurse–therapist will not respond punitively to the expression of feelings.	The nurse–therapist functions as a role model of healthy communication. Acceptance of feelings allows group members to acknowledge and own their feelings.
Initial anxiety in a group, displayed by silence, fidgeting, nervous movement, and selective hearing	Group members' anxiety will be lessened so they can function more effectively in a group. Group members will respond to leader and other members in a productive manner.	Give "strokes" for positive interaction. Help client establish a role in the group, one related to the client's skills. Share with client that discomfort in the initial state of group development is common. Meet client's dependency needs.	Reinforcing group members' interaction increases their continuing interaction and promotes the development of group roles. Reassurance and meeting group members' dependency needs allows them to feel safe in the group.
Hidden agenda	Group members will communicate and act openly. Group members will express their feelings about the issues being discussed.	Identify the source of individual and group anxiety causing the hidden agenda. Explore the hidden agenda with the group and its meaning and effect on the group's functioning.	Hidden agendas sabotage the group's progress, create anxiety in members, and may cause members to form subgroups or leave the group.
Subgrouping	Unproductive subgroups will be eliminated. Members will discuss content related to group topics in the group.	Establish clarifying goals and purpose of the group (thereby lessening the group's anxiety and aiding in elimination of subgroups). Direct subgroup interest toward the goals of the group, thereby lessening subgroup preoccupation with outside themes.	Clarification allows group members to establish their group roles, which aids in problem solving. A sense of belonging to the group increases members' participation and furthers their comfort in role taking.
Deviant behavior— behavior that meets personal needs and undermines the group	Members' deviant behavior will be modified. Group members will function comfortably and effectively in an independent fashion; group will not disintegrate in leader's absence.	Identify deviant behavior and discuss it with the client. Identify sources of discomfort in the environment that affect the client. Explore with the client whether he or she identifies the behavior as deviant.	Dealing directly with deviant behavior helps the group learn effective ways to problem-solve.

(continued)

TABLE 9-3 ▼ Common Problems Affecting Group Therapy and Process (Continued)			
GROUP PROBLEM	**GOAL**	**NURSING INTERVENTION**	**RATIONALE**
		Help members of the group identify deviant behavior. Help the client explore how this behavior affects his or her relationship in the group. Use group pressure to help the deviant member change or conform to group norms.	Giving the client an independent role in the group allows the client to explore, achieve, and receive reinforcement.
Resistance to therapy (eg, grunting, moaning, staring into space, overresponding to situations, changing the subject, absence from group	Members will demonstrate increased acceptance of, and participation in, therapy. Members will discuss problems and feelings in place of acting out.	Explore resistance behavior with client. Confront the client with his or her actions and behavior, using an understanding approach.	Some degree of resistance is common in every group. To promote individual and group progress, resistance must be confronted.
Termination of the group, resulting in increased anxiety and self-defeating behavior	Members will accept group termination and learn from termination experience. Members will explore achievements accomplished in the group and feelings related to termination.	Help the client identify what he or she has accomplished while a member of the group. Help the client work through feelings of loss during termination (ie, feelings of anger, depression, euphoria, rejection). Help the client express both positive and negative feelings about the group and evaluate the group experience realistically. Plan a termination activity that allows expression of group members' feelings. Lessen intensity of group interaction as group nears termination.	Learning process in the group depends on the ability to express feelings and evaluate members' achievements at termination.

the therapist conducts the group as if it is individual therapy. Such a therapist may see dynamics and group processes as incidental or antagonistic to the therapeutic process. The effective group leader must be skilled in techniques and interventions that foster group interaction and shape group behavior and growth.

Therapeutic Factors of Group Therapy

Various authors, such as R. Corsini, B. Rosenberg, and, recently, I.D. Yalom, have researched and described the therapeutic factors in group therapy. Therapeutic factors are interdependent; they do not operate separately. Different factors are more functional and helpful to group process at different stages of the group. Although the same therapeutic factors operate in all types of therapy groups, their emphasis and importance vary according to the type of the group.

Every therapy group emphasizes various therapeutic factors according to the group's purpose and goals. Group therapists focus on the process of interpersonal learning and change. Yalom (1995) describes 11 therapeutic factors of group therapy:

1. Instillation of hope
2. Universality
3. Imparting of information
4. Altruism
5. Corrective recapitulation of the primary family group
6. Development of socializing techniques
7. Imitative behavior
8. Interpersonal learning
9. Group cohesiveness
10. Catharsis
11. Existential factors

INSTILLATION OF HOPE

Instillation of hope helps the client to maintain faith in the therapeutic modality. The client is optimistic and believes that he or she will get better. Instillation of hope is important in pre-therapy and can be correlated with a positive therapy outcome. Inpatient groups have selected the instillation of hope as a therapeutic factor, affecting outcome more than outpatient groups.

UNIVERSALITY

Universality prevents the client from feeling unique and different. Within the group, the client begins to feel less isolated and more like other people. This feeling is strengthened by the client's learning that others in the group have similar problems, thoughts, and feelings. Universality limits the fears that clients have about being alone in having unacceptable thoughts, impulses, and fantasies, and provides more consensual validation than individual therapy (Yalom, 1995).

IMPARTING OF INFORMATION

Imparting of information is the use of information in a planned, structured manner, such as didactic instruction given in a lecture format. These lectures may be accompanied by audiovisual and other teaching aids. The topic of the didactic presentation is clear (Yalom, 1995).

GROUP COHESIVENESS

Group cohesiveness relates to bonding and solidarity, the feeling of "we" instead of "I." Cohesiveness is demonstrated through group attendance and the ability of the group to communicate positive and negative expressions without the group disintegrating. In cohesive groups, members try hard to impress one another, are accepting, and enter and leave the group with minimal disruption of the process. There is a protection of group norms and low tolerance of members who deviate from the norms. The client's role in a cohesive group greatly influences his or her self-esteem. Cohesive groups produce positive client outcomes (Yalom, 1995).

CATHARSIS

Catharsis is the expression of feelings, especially those that involve deep emotions. Expression of feelings is a particularly important therapeutic factor. Catharsis is effective in group therapy when it is followed by insight and cognitive learning (Yalom, 1995).

EXISTENTIAL FACTORS

Existential factors emphasize the quality, content, subjective awareness, freedom of choice, and state of being. They are important in boundary situations as clients work through impending death and inevitable developmental life experiences, such as retirement and aging; that is, things that "are." Existential factors, such as responsibility, capriciousness of existence, and recognition of mortality, are factors with therapeutic value that are explored in group therapy (Yalom, 1995).

Types of Therapy Groups

Most types of group therapy can be categorized as psychotherapeutic or growth oriented. Factors that determine the maximal therapeutic benefit of a psychotherapy or growth group include the following:

- Extent of personality disorganization of the participant
- Effect of personality disorganization on interpersonal functioning as a family member, provider, and productive citizen
- Degree of functional ability and role success or failure of the participant
- The participant's ability to harness impulses in stressful group situations
- The member's purpose or goals in joining a group, including both articulated goals and hidden agendas
- The participant's ability to share and support others in problem-solving tasks
- The participant's ability to use the material produced in a group to solve problems in his or her own situation

PSYCHOTHERAPEUTIC GROUPS

There are many different theoretical approaches to group psychotherapy, including psychoanalysis, transactional analysis, rational–emotive theory, rogerian theory, gestalt theory, and interpersonal theory (see Chaps. 3 and 9). In addition, psychodrama can be used as a form of group psychotherapy that explores the truth through dramatic methods.

The leader of the psychotherapy group assumes more responsibility for the group than does the leader of a growth group. In the psychotherapy group, the members or clients may have limiting or maladaptive-to-severe emotional disorders. The members may be referred to the group from individual therapy, where they were seen in an initial crisis state but later are able to tolerate the group setting. Clients in a therapy group do not become the therapist, and the therapist never assumes the client's role in the group. The leader also provides more support for members of a therapy group who may have less tolerance for stress.

GROWTH GROUPS

In the last three decades, numerous forms of growth groups, including self-help groups and group counseling, have been developed. In a growth or self-help group, such as a T group, the leader and members have attained a certain degree of emotional stability, and there is not a great discrepancy between their functioning by the end of the growth group experience. The group initially uses the leader to provide guidance and clarification. However, toward the end of the group experience, the leader becomes a part of the group, and the group members may perform several leadership functions. In a growth group, the members may receive less support from the leader while dealing with their anxiety, but there is conflict resolution by the end of the group. Three types of growth groups include encounter groups, T groups, and community support groups, which are described as follows.

Encounter Groups

The purpose of an encounter group is personal change, often as a result of deeply felt experiences. The differences between marathon and encounter groups are minimal, and the theoretical orientations of group leaders are diverse. Marathon group refers to the amount of concentrated time the participants spend together as a group. Examples of themes of encounter groups are "The Challenge of Change, Danger, and Fulfillment," "Closeness: Can It Hurt?" and "Marriage: How to Survive It."

Training Groups

The T group is the oldest and best-known therapeutic method coming out of the sensitivity T-group movement. The first T-group conference was held in Bethel, Maine, in 1946. The goal of each T-group conference is to verify experimentally the T-group method. This involves the study of group norms, roles, communication distortions, and the effects of authority on behavior patterns, personality, and coping mechanisms. Group members receive feedback by exposing their inner selves to others in the group, and they experiment with new and more productive behavior.

Community Support Groups

Numerous support groups have emerged under the category of community mental health psychiatry. Some were founded to lend continued or added support to previously hospitalized psychiatric clients. Other groups have been formed as a result of the needs of individuals in the community. Self-help groups have been developed by lay people to address specific needs shared by group members. Community support groups, of which there are more than 500 examples, may be classified in various ways (Table 9-4).

The main purpose of community support groups is to provide identification, clarification, understanding, role-modeling, feelings of togetherness, and group cohesion. They help prevent the individual from feeling lonely and isolated. Some groups evolve into educational models that enhance communication, self-image, body image, problem solving, decision making, and growth processes.

Most community support groups help their members to decrease levels of stress and increase levels of self-acceptance. With the help of the group, the member is better able to deal with the problems that he or she brought to the group. The outcome of this process is rewarding; the member develops new or more effective patterns of behavior.

Although community support groups have structures similar to those of other groups, they may be larger than therapy groups. Leadership in community support groups may be shared among the members; that is, leadership is a process. Senior members are expected to provide direction and structure and help establish norms.

NURSES AND GROUP PROCESS AND THERAPY

Nurses have used groups and group process in hospitals and other healthcare settings. As nursing progressed from functional assignments to the team approach, many studies were undertaken to discover ways to enhance the team's tasks and maintenance roles. Nurses have collaborated with colleagues in examining group theory, group dynamics, and group functioning in various healthcare delivery systems. Psychiatric-mental health nurses have specifically explored the use of groups as a teaching method and as a therapeutic tool with clients.

Group Process and Therapy in Nursing Education

Nurse educators use group seminars as part of the teaching–learning process to enable nursing students to participate in

TABLE 9-4 ▼ Community Support Groups

TYPE OF GROUP	TARGET MEMBERS	EXAMPLES
Community support groups for victims of violence	Individuals and families who have been physically or emotionally abused	Safe house, rape trauma, battered children
Birth anomaly support groups	Individuals and families with birth defects and congenital anomalies	Down syndrome, cerebral palsy
Acquired diseases support groups	Individuals and families coping with, and adjusting to, diseases originating after birth that are not inherited or innate	Leukemia, AIDS, diabetes
Chronic illness support groups	Individuals and families in which there is an illness of long-term duration, slow progression, and, often, little change in the symptomatology	Chronic obstructive pulmonary disease, cancer, arthritis
Developmental adjustment groups	Individuals and families with physical or emotional development that deviates from the norm	Autistic children, runaway teens
Grief education and resolution groups	Individuals and families with physical and emotional loss	Loss because of death of a significant person, sudden infant death syndrome
Interracial and biracial support groups	Individuals and families of interracial siblings, children, spouses, parents, and neighborhoods	Asian American families
Self-help and improvement support groups	Perspectives on behavior and attitude change	Assertiveness, Weight Watchers, Alcoholics Anonymous
Family structure support groups	Individuals and families of non-traditional (non-nuclear) family structure	Step-parenting, Parents without Partners, Lucky Mother's Club
Work-related support groups	Workers who experience job-related stress	Burnout groups, Friday evening groups

groups, learn group roles, and learn the function and dynamics of the student–participator role. Instructors delegate a certain amount of authority to the nursing students, yet serve as democratic leaders who structure the course and define expectations of the class. This experiential learning sparks an exciting way to learn group theory, enabling students to transfer their knowledge of, and experience in, group dynamics to other arenas of therapy such as milieu, client groups, and supervision groups. Often, these seminars are prerequisites for advanced courses in group therapy in graduate nursing programs.

In addition to group seminars, the use of groups in nursing education has increased in the form of study groups, special project groups, and testing groups. The following example is the Front Range Community College nursing program, which formed student groups to help their students learn about groups and group theory. With increased challenges, the nursing faculty formed additional groups with the following objectives:

- Initiate brainstorming among the members to enhance critical thinking.
- Foster "bonding" of group members.
- Help students increase their survival skills.
- Help students learn conflict resolution and assertiveness and become change agents.
- Practice collaboration in the student role to apply this process on the job after graduation and thus prevent unhealthy competition.
- Build self-esteem.
- Learn how to teach clients and families by teaching each other.
- Learn decision making and the responsibility that accompanies this process.
- Foster achievement of peers, for example, an "A" student helping students with lower grades.

Study groups developed their own operational rules and norms. They established tolerance, limit setting, and group problem solving. Student group members learned group dynamics and how to reach out for help through the group. Groups sponsored individual growth through imitative behavior. Students learned about the change process by developing these skills in their groups and discovered that diversity of group members fosters strength.

Evaluation of these nursing student groups revealed that the experience was positive. Members gained knowledge about group functioning through their participation and expressed individual growth. Identified problems were group meeting times that conflicted with family schedule and finding a mutually convenient meeting time for all group members.

Group Process and Therapy in Nursing Practice

HISTORICAL PERSPECTIVE

In the past, psychiatric-mental health nurses learned group therapist and co-therapist roles and responsibilities. Dr. Hildegard Peplau, an early authority on psychiatric nursing specialist programs, augmented nurses' involvement in group therapy through what is known as experiential learning. Nurses developed increasing skills in the techniques of group therapy; psychiatric nursing clinical specialists became highly skilled in group intervention.

The mental health revolution, sponsored by President John F. Kennedy, demanded that more health professionals administer formal and informal group therapy in community mental health centers. Responding to this need, psychiatric clinical nurse specialists have become more active in group leader or co-leader roles in many formal and informal psychotherapeutic and growth group therapies within therapeutic communities, outpatient settings, and private therapy settings. They also have become more active as liaison psychiatric nursing consultants in general hospital settings.

CONTEMPORARY NURSING GROUPS

Reassessing the need for change in individuals, groups, and environments has led nurses to seek alternative ways to improve communication. Economics and nurses' expanded collaborative and cooperative practice have encouraged nursing toward innovation in group work. Because computer networks are interactive media, computer groups have been established to diminish the problems of distance, time, and need for speedy feedback. Economics also has fostered short-lived crisis groups with a solution-focused framework. It has encouraged the use of more "open–open" groups (members can enter or leave the group at any time), which also provides a richer medium of information that can lead to problem solving.

Contemporary nursing groups are influenced by social and societal needs. An important role of the nurse in relation to group therapy is referral of clients to various community-based support groups, including National Alliance for the Mentally Ill, Alcoholics Anonymous, Narcotics Anonymous, Overeaters Anonymous, and other eating-disorder groups (see Community Support Groups discussed earlier). These types of support groups are inexpensive or free and are more effective long term for clients compared with ongoing psychotherapy.

Nurses use various methods and approaches when working with groups. Some of the methods and approaches include the following: (1) didactic and experiential learning, (2) cognitive behavioral training (panic disorder and agoraphobia), (3) solution-focused group therapy, (4) directive therapist approach (in clinical gerontology), and (5) validation therapy (for those with dementia). Examples of contemporary nursing groups are as follows:

- Groups that emphasize intergenerational relationships (seniors with youths)
- Groups at risk (incarcerated women and men's groups)
- Victims of violence (gangs, school violence)
- Medication noncompliance group (clients whose noncompliance may lead to acts of socially deviant behavior)
- Alzheimer groups where members (1) bond with each other, emphasizing what they remember and supporting each other in their loss, and (2) learn what they have lost and accept their losses
- Disability groups (caused by work or industrial injury and other trauma)
- Senior counseling groups to help prevent and work with depression
- Behavior pattern groups, which are feelings-oriented programs that teach children, in a school setting, how to manage their emotions
- Creativity group in which psychiatric nurses lead groups with a focus on creative expression rather than psychotherapy; these activities promote acceptance of self and acceptance by the group
- Coping skills group in which clients with a chronic disability or disabling disease learn to deal with fear, live with chronic pain, and cope with loss, anger, and depression

▼ Reflection and Critical Thinking Questions

1. How does a client in a therapy group become a culture carrier?

2. How does a leader affect the initial stage of a group? Give an example.

3. What are the stages of a group? List a characteristic of each stage.

4. Discuss six characteristics of a mature group.

5. What are the six advantages of group therapy?

6. Discuss five therapeutic factors observed in a group therapy.

▼ CHAPTER SUMMARY

- A group is three or more people with related goals; groups vary according to their size, homogeneity of membership, climate, norms, and goal directedness.

- Group norms are the patterns of interaction that develop within a group.

- Three styles of group leadership are autocratic, democratic, and laissez-faire.

- Roles in groups are task building, maintenance, and individual roles.

- Important concepts of group communication include latent and manifest communication, content and process communication, transference and countertransference, and communication themes.

- The three stages of group development are the initial, working, and termination stages.

- The advantages of group therapy include its effectiveness and efficiency in time and cost.

- There are at least 11 therapeutic factors observed in group therapy, including instillation of hope, universality, imparting of information, altruism, corrective recapitulation of the primary family group, development of socializing techniques, imitative behavior, interpersonal learning, group cohesiveness, catharsis, and existential factors.

- Most therapeutic group experiences can be categorized as psychotherapy or growth groups.

- Nurses participate as leaders and co-leaders in multiple formal and informal groups; contemporary nursing groups are influenced by social and societal needs. Examples include intergenerational groups, medication noncompliance groups, and coping skills groups.

▼ REVIEW QUESTIONS

1. Which of the following best describes a primary group?
   a. Primary groups have a great deal of structure and authority.
   b. Primary groups have explicit and implicit interdependent roles, boundaries, and group norms.
   c. Primary groups tend to be large and impersonal.
   d. Primary groups provide education and cultural values.

2. Which of the following is true about group norms?
   a. Group norms do not influence role expectations in the group.
   b. They influence patterns of interaction and behavioral expectations in the group.

   c. They are developed over a short period of time.
   d. Group norms are not connected to sanctions, taboos, or the reference power of the group.

3. The nursing department of a psychiatric hospital has organized a group of nurses to develop a continuing education program in psychiatric-mental health nursing research and ethics. The group leader develops a list of tasks and assigns a task to each group member. Which of the following describes this nurse's leadership style?
   a. Laissez-faire
   b. Democratic
   c. Autocratic
   d. Egalitarian

4. Which of the following are the three major group roles assumed by various group members?
   a. Group building and maintenance roles, group task roles, and individual roles
   b. Harmonizer, gatekeeper, follower
   c. Aggressor, recognition seeker, blocker
   d. Information giver, coordinator, information seeker

5. A group is meeting to develop a plan for a rural community outreach program. The group learns that funding for the program has been cut by 40%. Of the following responses, which one suggests that the group is in the mature stage of development?
   a. Group members are unsure how to proceed and look to the leader for direction.
   b. Group members suggest solutions. There is a great deal of conflict, but the group tries to cooperate.
   c. Group members are upset but supportive of each other. After a period of disorganization, the group begins problem solving.
   d. Group members are supportive of each other and begin trying to solve the problem. The group cannot reach a decision about how to proceed and informs the group leader.

6. A group of women recovering from alcoholism meets weekly. One member has been sharing about how her in-laws have been aloof and distant from her since she started treatment. She feels ashamed and tongue-tied around them. Which of the following responses by the group suggests a highly functioning, therapeutic group?
   a. The group can share their experiences with their in-laws.
   b. A member of the group can accompany her to the next family function to provide support.
   c. The group can give her feedback about developing effective communication with her in-laws.
   d. The group can confront her about her passive personality and offer advice.

7. The main difference between growth groups and psychotherapeutic groups is

a. Members' functional level
b. The leader's educational preparation
c. Members' ability to tolerate the group setting
d. The leader's willingness to share leadership with a co-therapist group member

8. Alcoholics Anonymous is an example of a (an)
a. Psychotherapeutic group
b. T group
c. Encounter group
d. Community support group

9. Group therapy has advantages and disadvantages. Which of the following is a disadvantage?
a. Group members can be confronted with negative feedback.
b. Group therapy can work as individual therapy.
c. Group members may be expected to function as a co-therapist.
d. Group members are exposed to the problems of others.

10. Existential factors explored in groups refers to
a. Topics such as responsibility, mortality, and freedom of choice
b. Expression of deep emotions
c. Lessening of feelings of isolation
d. Bonding and solidarity

▼ REFERENCES AND SUGGESTED READINGS

*Antoni, M. H. (1997). Intervention for persons with HIV. In J. Spira (Ed.). *Group therapy for medically ill patients.* New York: Guilford Press.

*Applegate, M. (1996). Outpatient group therapy for dissociative trauma survivor. *Journal of the American Psychiatric Nurses Association, 2*(2), 37–45.

Bender, A., & Ewashen, C. (2000). Group work is political work: A feminist perspective of interpersonal group psychotherapy. *Issues in Mental Health Nursing, 21,* 297.

Cudney, S., & Weinert, C. (2000). Computer-based support groups: Nursing in cyberspace. *Computer Nurse, 18,* 1.

*Davis-Berman, J. (1995). Let the process unfold: A lesson learned by a directive therapist. *Clinical Gerontologist, 16*(1), 66–67.

*Farkas-Cameron, M. M. (1998). Inpatient group therapy in a managed health care environment: Application to clinical nursing practice. *Journal of the American Psychiatric Nurses Association, 4*(5), 145–153.

*Fawzy, F. I., Fawzy, N. W., Hyun, C. A., & Wheeler, J. G. (1997). Brief, coping-oriented therapy for patients with malignant melanoma. In J. Spira (Ed.). *Group therapy for medically ill patients.* New York: Guilford Press.

Gorski, T. T. (2000). Making group therapy work in the age of cost containment. *Treatment today, 1,* 16.

*Holkup, P. A. (1998). Our parents, our children, ourselves: A therapy group to facilitate understanding of intergenerational behavior patterns and to promote family healing. *Journal of Psychosocial Nursing and Mental Health Services, 36*(2), 20–26, 36–37.

*Kelly, J. S., & Vanderslott, J. (1995). Efficacy of validation therapy is unproven. *Professional Nurse, 10*(7), 408.

*Lantz, M. S., Buchalter, E. N., & McBee, L. (1997). Practice concepts. The wellness group: A novel intervention for coping with disruptive behavior in elderly nursing home residents. *Gerontologist, 37*(4), 551–556.

*Lanza, M. L. (1998). A multidisciplinary course to teach staff to conduct psychodynamic group psychotherapy for assaultive men. *Perspective in Psychiatric Care: The Journal for Nurse Psychotherapists, 34*(1), 28–35.

*Matano, R. A., Yalom, I. D., & Schwartz, K. (1997). Interactive group therapy for substance abuser. In J. Spira (Ed.). *Group therapy for medically ill patients.* New York: Guilford Press.

*McDougall, G. J. (1995). Existential psychotherapy with older adults. *Journal of the American Psychiatric Nurses Association 1*(1), 16–20.

*McGarry, T. J., & Prince, M. (1998). Implementation of groups for creative expression on a psychiatric inpatient unit. *Journal of Psychosocial Nursing and Mental Health Services, 36*(3), 19–24, 404.

*Nickersen, P. R. (1995). Solution-focused group therapy: Social work. *Journal of the National Association of Social Workers, 40*(1), 132–133.

Paleg, K., & Jongsma, A. E., Jr. (2000). *The group therapy treatment planner.* New York: John Wiley & Sons.

*Puskar, K. R., Lamb, J., & Tusaie-Mumford, K. (1997). Teaching kids to cope: A preventive mental health nursing strategy for adolescents. *Journal of Child and Adolescent Psychiatric Nursing, 10*(3), 18–28.

*Ripich, S., Moore, S., & Brennan, P. (1992). A new nursing medium: Computer network for group intervention. *Journal of Psychosocial Nursing, 30*(7), 15–19.

*Rissane, D. W., Bloch, S., Mrach, P., Smith, G. C., Seddon, A., & Kes, N. (1997). Cognitive–existential group therapy for patients with primary breast cancer: Techniques and themes. *Psycho-Oncology, 6*(1), 25–33.

Rokke, P. D., Tomhave, J. A., & Zefjko, J. (2000). Self-management therapy and educational group therapy for depressed elders. *Cognitive Therapy and Research, February* (24), 99–119.

Salvendy, J. T. (1999). Ethnocultural considerations in group psychotherapy. *International Journal of Group Psychotherapy, 49*(4), 429–464.

*Spira, J. (Ed.). (1997). Understanding and developing psychotherapy groups for medically ill patients. In *Group therapy for medically ill patients.* New York: Guilford Press.

*Spira, J. (Ed.). (1997). Existential group psychotherapy for advanced breast cancer and other life-threatening illnesses. In *Group therapy for medically ill patients.* New York: Guilford Press.

*Thoresen, C. E., & Bracke, P. (1997). Reducing coronary and coronary-prone behavior: A structured group treatment approach. In *Group therapy for medically ill patients.* New York: Guilford Press.

*Wifley, D. E., Grilo, C. M., & Rodin, J. (1997). Group psychotherapy for the treatment of bulimia nervosa and binge eating disorder: Research and clinical methods. In *Group therapy for medically ill patients*. New York: Guilford Press.

*Yalom, I. D. (1995). *Theory and practice of group psychotherapy* (4th ed.). New York: Basic Books.

Starred references are cited in text.

For additional information on this chapter, go to *http://connection. lww.com*.

Need more help? See Chapter 9 of the *Study Guide to Accompany Mohr: Johnson's Psychiatric-Mental Health Nursing,* 5th ed.

Working With Families

VICTORIA CONN

▼ KEY TERMS

Deinstitutionalization—The massive discharge of clients from state hospitals that began in the 1950s, accelerated in the 1960s and 1970s, and continues today as psychiatric treatment continues to move from inpatient to outpatient settings.

Depressive/Manic Depressive Association (DMDA)—A national support and advocacy association with regional chapters for people with depressive and bipolar disorders and their families.

Families—In this chapter, used to mean families with a relative who has a serious mental illness.

Family burden—The effects of serious mental illness on the family (see the key terms *iatrogenic burden, objective burden,* and *subjective burden*).

Family consultation—A professional service offered to families to reduce family burden; it is a type of secondary prevention, originally called *supportive counseling.*

Family education—Educational programs of varying duration to increase family members' knowledge about mental illness, caregiving, and self-care, with the objective of improving the entire family's quality of life.

Family member—In this chapter, used to mean the parent, sibling, offspring, or spouse of a person with a serious mental illness.

Family psychoeducation—A lengthy educational program for families (including the client) that is taught by a team of professionals and includes, in addition to didactic content about mental illness, extensive training in behavioral skills intended to create a home environment conducive to reducing relapse and recidivism.

Family support services—Opportunities for mutual support available without cost to families through groups organized by family organizations (eg, DMDA).

Iatrogenic burden—Family burden exacerbated by the mental health system or mental health professionals; *iatro* is derived from the Greek word *iatros* (physician) and *iasthai* means *to heal.*

NAMI, The Nation's Voice on Mental Illness—Formerly known as the National Alliance for the Mentally Ill, a national advocacy organization with state and local affiliates dedicated to improving the lives of persons with serious mental illness and their families.

Objective burden—The practical problems associated with caregiving (eg, employment issues, financial drain).

Resilient families—Family members who are able to rebound from the effects of mental illness.

Secondary prevention—An intervention to prevent further damage after a traumatic event; in this context, it consists of interventions to prevent families subjected to the trauma of mental illness from experiencing further adverse consequences (eg, caregiver burnout, disrupted interpersonal relationships, psychiatric and medical health problems).

Serious mental illness—A term given to a psychiatric disorder that meets the criteria for duration (at least 1 year), disability (relatively severe functional impairment), and diagnosis (including schizophrenia, bipolar disorder, and major depression) (National Advisory Mental Health Council, 1993).

Subjective burden—The emotional response that the client and family have to mental illness and caregiving (eg, grief, fear, guilt, anger). (*Note:* Some researchers define subjective burden differently, as *perceived* objective burden.)

▼ LEARNING OBJECTIVES

On completion of this chapter, you should be able to accomplish the following:

- Trace the history of family caregiving in the United States from 1850 to 2000.
- Explain the rationale for involving families in client treatment.
- Define *family burden*.
- Differentiate among objective, subjective, and iatrogenic burden.
- Define *family resilience.*
- Describe a resilient family.
- Explain secondary prevention and its relevance to working with families who have a relative with a serious mental illness.
- Explain *family consultation* and how it differs from family therapy.

- Provide examples of how nurses can function as family consultants.
- Differentiate between family psychoeducation and family education.
- Refer families to local support, educational, and advocacy services available from NAMI and DMDA.

This chapter teaches students how nurses work with families struggling with a member who has a serious mental illness to help reduce their burden and involve them collaboratively in their relative's treatment. Students will begin to recognize family consultation as a primary service for families and learn new roles for nurses as family consultants. But first, they will trace the history of a mental health system that now makes families the primary caregivers of relatives with mental illness, thus putting them at risk for stress-related disorders and in need of preventative services.

FAMILY CAREGIVING FROM 1850 TO 2000

Before state asylums were established in the mid-19th century, people with mental illness in the United States lived where vast numbers of them live now: on the streets, in homes for the poor or ailing, in jails, and *with their families*. It is true that during the past 150 years, Americans with **serious mental illness** have journeyed to the asylum and back! In an address to Congress in 1848, Dorothea Dix claimed to have seen "more than nine thousand idiots, epileptics, and insane in these United States, destitute of appropriate care and protection; and of this vast and most miserable company, sought out in jails, in poorhouses, and in private dwellings, there have been hundreds—nay, thousands, bound with galling chains, bowed beneath fetters and heavy iron balls, attached to drag chains, terrified by storms of profanity and cruel blows" (Geller, 2000). After the federal government turned down Dix's pleas to provide humane care and moral instruction to this "vast and most miserable company," she turned to the states. There she succeeded. Eventually, state-operated "asylums," designed to protect vulnerable people from the stress of society, provided the services she recommended. Beginning in the mid-1800s, state governments encouraged families to turn over the care of their ill relatives to the state. Until the 1950s, family caregiving became obsolete.

In the 1950s, in a dramatic reversal of previous trends, clients by the thousands were discharged from asylums under a policy called **deinstitutionalization**. For some families, the assumption of the caregiving role came as a shock. As one caregiver recounts, "The social worker said my brother was coming home, and I said, 'What brother?' My parents had never told me that I had an older brother in the state hospital" (Tolbert, 1980). See Historical Capsule 10-1.

FAMILY BURDEN

Unquestionably, psychiatric disorders have always been dreadful experiences for those suffering from them. Today, however, most affected people live within the community, much as in the pre-asylum days. The stresses for their **families** are tremendous (Hatfield & Lefley, 1987). Researchers have conceptualized these stresses as **family burden**, or the effects of serious mental illness on the family. **Family members** express this concept succinctly:

> *Researcher: What have you missed most as a result of your son's illness?*
> *Parent: My life*
>
> *(Terkelsen, 1987).*

Another parent related a prophetic experience:

> *When I was 52 years old I went back to college to finish a degree I had begun 34 years earlier. One of the plays I studied was The Trojan Women by Euripides. There was a line in the play that puzzled me. The Trojan queen announced her daughter's arrival by saying, "This is my daughter, Cassandra. She is mad." I didn't realize that in four years I would share with Cassandra's mother experiences that would make a matter-of-fact statement high drama.*
>
> *(Marlatt, 1989)*

Just as people of a certain age remember December 7, 1941, some families recall the exact moment they became aware that something was wrong with their relative:

> *"We were sitting down to Thanksgiving dinner when we noticed our son wasn't at the table. He said the food was poisoned."*
>
> *"We answered the doorbell, and there stood our daughter with a police officer, who said, 'This young lady says her father wants to kill her.'"*

Other families take years to identify the warning signs, and in the meantime, they try to normalize puzzling behaviors. This is called *denial*, but it is more appropriate to call it *disbelief*, because no one should be expected to leap to the conclusion that a family member has a psychiatric disorder. Such problems are the last thing most people expect. As the sister of a man with schizophrenia recalls, "*When he quit Harvard to travel cross country, we thought he was 'finding himself.'*" A father says, "*When our daughter started to send hundred dollar bills to television evangelists, we didn't think 'manic'; we thought 'born again Christian.'*"

When the relative finally begins treatment, the family learns the painful lesson that psychiatry is not an exact science. Many families expect a speedy recovery, only to find that their family member never fully recovers or that the recovery process is quite lengthy. Moreover, the first diagnosis is not always the correct diagnosis and can be the first

HISTORICAL CAPSULE 10-1
Deinstitutionalization and Beyond

- By the mid-1950s, there emerged a consensus, based on reports of conscientious objectors who served as psychiatric aides during World War II and on the findings of investigative journalists, that most state hospitals were run-down, poorly managed "snake pits," as Mary Jane Ward's novel of that name so vividly described them. Consequently, advocates began calling for the "liberation" of clients from settings that a social scientist describe as "causing" rather than "curing" mental illness.

- The introduction of antipsychotic drugs in the 1950s made it possible for many clients to leave the hospitals. Armed with Thorazine and public indignation about the condition of the hospitals, state mental health administrators began discharging clients and closing down wards. In 1955, about 560,000 clients were in state asylums. By 1985, there were 109,039, an 80% decline (Torrey, 1989). By the 1990s, well under 100,000 clients were institutionalized (Bachrach, 1996).

- Following World War II, the federal government finally assumed responsibility for its citizens with mental illness as Dix had urged a century previously. The Community Mental Health Center Act of 1963 created local community mental health centers. Once this plan was announced, the states became increasingly motivated to discharge clients from state hospitals (where states paid for care) to community settings (where the federal government paid.)

- Unfortunately, the political rhetoric that heralded deinstitutionalization in terms of "replacing the cold mercy of custodial care in hospitals with the warmth of community concern and capability" (Kennedy, 1962) became hollow words. For multiple reasons, people with serious mental illness fell through the cracks in the new community system.

- The failures of deinstitutionalization ushered in a new era in treatment, the era of "revolving door" hospitalization, where by clients are discharged only to relapse and be readmitted in a repetitive cycle. The treatment and rehabilitation services required to keep persons with serious mental illness living well in the community are still not available for all who need them in 2002. This is true in spite of two interim innovations in healthcare policy that were intended to improve the nation's mental health services and health services generally. These innovations were the Community Support Program (CSP), 1979 to the present, and managed care, 1999 to the present.

For additional information, read the following:

Isaac, R. J., & Armat, V. C. (1990). *Madness in the streets: How psychiatry and the law abandoned the mentally ill.* New York: The Free Press, MacMillan.

Torrey, E. F. (1989). *Nowhere to go: The tragic odyssey of the homeless mentally ill.* New York: Harper and Row.

Torrey, E. F. (1997). *Out of the shadows: Confronting America's mental illness crisis.* New York: John Wiley and Sons.

of many. A survey of the membership of DMDA revealed that members with bipolar disorder had consulted with professionals for an average of 10 years before receiving an accurate diagnosis and appropriate treatment. Families also have reported that finding a doctor with combined skills in psychotherapy and psychopharmacology is as difficult as finding the proverbial needle in a haystack (R. Berman, personal communication, February 11, 2001). To learn about how family burden affects family members differently according to their role within the family, see Box 10-1.

Objective Burden

Objective burden refers to the practical problems family members encounter while caring for ill relatives. Examples include the following:

- Housing
- Food and laundry
- Transportation
- Medication management
- Money and money management
- Companionship and recreation
- Crisis intervention
- Mediation with the police (Tessler & Gamache, 2000)

Today, these services often are the responsibility of case managers employed by the mental health system. Because of high caseloads and the high rate of employee turnover for poorly compensated case managers, however, families also continue to serve in these roles. As a parent recalls, "My daughter's mental illness pushed us back into parenting of the most demanding kind, probably for the rest of our lives" (Marsh, 1998).

BOX 10-1 ▼ *The Meaning of Mental Illness to Family Members*

Parents

When a child develops a psychiatric disorder, parents generally experience a range of intense losses, both real and symbolic. Moreover, they are the people most likely to assume responsibilities as primary caregivers or informal case managers, sometimes for a lifetime. They are also prone to feelings of guilt and responsibility, which may be intensified by professionals who espouse earlier conceptual models that incorporate unsupported assumptions of family pathogenesis or dysfunction.

Spouses

Spouses often experience emotional, social, and financial losses similar to those that accompany the death of a spouse. Husbands and wives may face increased responsibility for parenting and other aspects of family life as well as substantial conflict if they consider separation or divorce. For example, "He says I didn't live up to my marriage vows because we married 'for better, for worse, in sickness and in health.'"

Young Siblings and Offspring

Because of their developmental status, young siblings and offspring are especially vulnerable to family burden. The mental illness of a close relative might undermine the acquisition of basic trust during infancy, the development of peer relationships and academic skills during childhood, and the establishment of a secure sense of identity during adolescence. For example, "Very much of my young life was affected. I had trouble concentrating in

school, was afraid Dad would appear on the school grounds when he was sick. I could not bring any school friends home for fear they would not understand. Mom was busy working full time to make ends meet. Not much time was spent helping me to get prepared for school."

Older Siblings

Siblings may experience the dual losses of their brother or sister and of their parents, whose energy may be consumed by mental illness. The siblings may feel their needs are neglected or may try to compensate for their siblings problems by being "model children" (the replacement child syndrome).

Older Offspring

Offspring also have unique issues. Because of the significance of the parent–child bond, the losses of these family members may be profound. Especially if the offspring are exposed to mental illness when they are very young, they may become enveloped in the psychotic system, with adverse effects on their own lives. They may find it hard to interpret which experiences are "normal" and which are not. They may move into a parent-like role before they have finished being children or may attempt to become "perfect children" to spare their beleaguered family additional problems.

Marsh, D., & Johnson, D. (1997). The family experience of mental illness. *Professional Psychology, Research, and Practice,* 25(2), 232–233.

Caregiving, even if construed as a labor of love, remains demanding. Families cope with behaviors that are embarrassing (eg, asking neighbors for sanctuary), irresponsible (eg, spending money like water), disturbing (eg, playing loud music at night), bizarre (eg, seeing demons), and sometimes dangerous (eg, refusing to eat from fear of being poisoned) (Francell, Conn, & Gray, 1988). Although violence is rarely a problem when a client is receiving treatment, a family member is the usual target when it does occur. Families are also painfully aware of the elevated suicide risk in clients with schizophrenia or bipolar disorder.

▼ Clinical Example 10-1

I was in my office when I received a call informing me that the child of one of our members had committed suicide the night before. My first thought was "Oh, My God, how horrible!" Then came my next thought, "Thank God, it wasn't my son."

The next morning at the graveside, it was extremely hot and humid. Carrying my sport coat over my arm, I got under the canopy just to escape the direct sunlight. From that vantage point, I looked at the people who had assembled to pay their last respects.

A dozen or so immediate family members, including a twin sister, sat closest to the coffin. A group of about 15 people stood at the rear. They were from the community residential unit where Tommy lived and included several well-dressed professional staff members as well as the residents. The residents wore ill-fitting clothes and kept their eyes lowered toward the ground.

None of Tommy's friends from high school, college, or the Army was present. Many of us take for granted the ability to make and keep friends, but doing so is hard for people with psychiatric disorders. Their "inappropriate behavior," as we euphemistically call it, and their frequent "decompensations" often preclude lasting friendships.

The largest contingent was from our NAMI chapter, of which Tommy's mother is the secretary. Although the rest of us had never met Tommy, we could all empathize with the family's tragedy. Perhaps they have a sense of relief, knowing they no longer have to care for an adult who could not care for himself. Or they may be thinking, "If only we had visited him last weekend" or "If only we had him over to dinner more often." There will probably be no end to the "If onlys" the family thinks of. There is a definite limit, however, to the time and energy a family can devote to one member and still carry on somewhat normal lives.

Why Tommy took his life will never be fully known. Did he decide life was no longer worth living? Did a voice tell him to do it? What makes this tragedy even sadder is that only 2 days ago, I received a flyer from our state NAMI informing us that two new drugs for schizophrenia will soon be available. They might have improved Tommy's condition.

Since his discharge from the U.S. Army, Tommy had been a prisoner of a semi-functional mind that kept him from holding a job, maintaining friendships, managing his money, or even grocery shopping by himself. Tommy is now free of the mind that made him an outcast. He no longer has to grieve internally while watching his former friends do many things he could not. He no longer has to watch people self-righteously turning away from him or hear people whispering about him behind his back. In the words of an old Negro spiritual, He's free at last! Thank God Almighty, Tommy's free at last! All we can do now is extend our deepest sympathy to the family and continue to advocate for other people like Tommy.

Points for Reflection and Critical Thinking

- Why do you think a 24-year-old college graduate and Army veteran with schizophrenia would commit suicide?
- What do you imagine Tommy's twin sister was thinking and feeling at the funeral?
- Would you predict that Tommy's family would continue to advocate for an improved mental health system?
- What kinds of thoughts were going through the minds of the residents of the mental health center?

Ron Schwarz, DVD, NAMI Georgia.

Nurse researchers have described the seemingly endless effects of mental illness as a story with a beginning and middle—but no end. "The beginning is knowing that something is wrong. The middle is the family's everyday life, with the caregiving experience described as having no end" (Tuck, duMont, Evans, & Shupe, 1997). Even when the relative's condition improves, a crisis can recall the caregiver to active duty. Parental concern about "what will happen when I am gone" is so widespread that more than 10 years ago, it acquired its own acronym, WIAG (Lefley, 1987a). Siblings, the successor candidates, entertain mixed feelings about inheriting the caregiver mantle. In the words of a member of a sibling support group, "I am not looking forward to being in charge of my sister. I love her, but she is a very high maintenance person."

Subjective Burden

Subjective burden refers to the grief, fear, guilt, anger, and other negative emotions that family members experience in response to a loved one's mental illness. Because the grief seems interminable, many family members experience a sense of *mourning without end* (Willick, 1994). Many family members must deal with professionals who misconstrue their signs of grief:

> "In all the therapy we participated in and in all our communications with the professionals who worked with our son, it was never suggested to us that our responses (of fright, anxiety, guilt, and self-doubt) were an expression of normal grief, and indeed we as well as our son had lost something precious. Why is it that a discipline whose major focus is on feelings, thoughts, and relationships has so little to say about grief and loss?"
> (MacGregor, 1994).

Another common problem is *fear* (Lewis, 1989). Many grieving family members have experienced the same fearlike feeling: fluttering in the stomach and restlessness. But they also notice explicit fear, asking such questions as, "Is this illness going to put us in the poorhouse?" and "It costs $10,000 per month to keep him in the hospital. How can we afford that?" (Eakes, 1995). Many family members with mentally ill relatives feel as if they are walking along a precipice, afraid to make a wrong move. As one family member recalls, "I just panicked. I would cry, and I'd have to go to work, and I just spent all my energy trying to figure out what to do. I was so scared" (Mohr & Regan-Kubinski, 2001).

Guilt, a common response when a family member succumbs to any serious illness, is exaggerated in psychiatric illness because of the unfounded beliefs related to parental causation. Siblings, too, often irrationally torture themselves with feeling of guilt over being well and living a "normal" life while their brothers or sisters must contend with mental problems.

Family members direct *anger* irrationally at themselves, one another, the ill relative, God, or treating professionals. Kayla Bernheim and Anthony Lehman, coauthors of the first book on mental health professionals working with families, attributed family hostility to guilt and fear about the illness, resistance to acceptance of chronic disability and its implications for their lives, and previous, negative experiences with the treatment system. These authors urged families to use anger constructively to change the system and called advocacy sublimation of the healthiest, most adaptive kind (Bernheim & Lehman, 1985). Box 10-2 recounts the story of a family of five in

BOX 10-2 ▼ *A Love Story*

My husband and I will celebrate 25 years of married life this April. Twenty-five years ago, I did not know how our marriage would go. He was diagnosed with schizophrenia, and I knew next to nothing about mental illness. I only knew that I loved him, and I had to try to make marriage work. He was a doctoral candidate then, and now is retired from 30 years in state service, working with the most seriously mentally ill as a clinical psychologist.

Initially I had hoped that the schizophrenia would go away, but I learned that mental illnesses are long-term, even lifetime conditions. When he would become symptomatic, I would get very anxious; torturing myself with all kinds of "what ifs . . . " . Eventually, I learned the pattern: excitement leading to expansive thinking; a rush of activity and self-absorption (living in his head); increased medication followed by a period of crashing; and then back to normal. These episodes occurred every year to 18 months; and with each passing episode they became less worrisome to me.

I also had to learn what the illness meant on a daily basis. Some activities are more difficult for him than others, such as those requiring attention to details or high degrees of organization. Gradually, a division of labor evolved that worked for us. I picked up those responsibilities that were problematic for him, and he supported me in taking care of things that were hard for me to attend to while teaching at the university. He was very successful with his work and was always able to provide for us, and we were very fortunate that insurance always covered our mental health expenses.

Although these illnesses have a genetic component, we had hoped that our children would escape them. One by one, however, as they entered puberty, they began to exhibit symptoms. I later discovered that depression runs in my side of the family, so our children were getting genes from both sides. Because by this time we were active in the family movement, and Fred was a Board member of NAMI, we had a broad circle of friends who could support us with good advice. Getting help for our children was not easy, as childhood mental illnesses were only beginning to appear on the radar screen, and we had some scary times with children whose lives were rapidly deteriorating—but once again Providence carried us. We decided to be very open about mental illness in our family, treating it as one would any other medical disorder.

Mental health providers and the children's school systems really worked with us to help bring them through the onset of their illnesses.

When the worst was over and our children's lives were stabilized, we all dedicated ourselves more diligently to increasing understanding of mental illness in the general public. We accepted speaking engagements as a family, and eventually produced a video on childhood depression. This advocacy work increased our children's self esteem while educating them about their illness. As it turned out it also gave them wonderful resumes for college. Their advocacy was admired at school, and they were even called on to talk with other students who were experiencing difficulties.

With everyone in the family diagnosed with a mental illness and taking medication, except me, sensitivity and compassion among family members increased. We learned to recognize the heightened sensitivity that comes with these disorders and to soften our interactions with one another. It was OK to back off from tasks that were overwhelming and return to them later when we felt better equipped to deal with them. It was OK to sleep at just about anytime. In fact, in our house, you could probably find someone asleep and someone awake at almost any time of the day or night.

A zany, delightful sense of humor prevailed; the kind that happens with people who go through difficult times together. And in the dark times, faith saw us through. Today we are doing well, aware that there are still difficult times ahead, but having enough successes behind us to give us confidence that we will be able to meet the hard times when they come.

Points for Reflection and Critical Thinking

- What signs did Penny Frese learn to recognize as signaling the return of her husband's symptoms?
- What accommodations in their daily routine did the couple make to cope with the illness?
- To what mission did the family members dedicate themselves after everyone's conditions were stabilized?
- Name three factors that contributed to this family's resiliency. (Hint: One of them is love.)

Penny Frese, PhD.

which the mother is the only one not receiving treatment for a psychiatric disorder. The parents in this story are NAMI family member professionals.

Iatrogenic Burden

Iatrogenic burden is attributable to a dysfunctional mental health system and to the attitudes and behaviors of some mental health professionals who cling to outmoded theories about families. If the mental health system were truly equipped to meet the needs of clients for treatment and rehabilitation, most adults with serious mental illness could function without family caregivers. Unfortunately, this system is not yet in place. In exposés of community treatment reminiscent of those of Dorothea Dix, investigative journalists are now calling the U.S. treatment system flawed and U.S. jails the asylums of the 21st century (Washington Post, 2001). In the mid-1990s, a landmark report on treatment outcomes revealed that thousands of Americans with schizophrenia are receiving substandard care despite the availability of treatments that work (Lehman, Thompson, Dixon, & Scott, 1995).

The lag between availability and use prompted the surgeon general of the U.S. Public Health Service to challenge our nation's health and social service agencies to translate research-based knowledge about the brain and behavior into practice (see Chap. 1). Underused services include comprehensive treatment packages that combine the judicious use of medications, psychotherapy, client and family education, rehabilitative services, and (for clients at greatest risk of relapse) community treatment teams with nurse members to provide around-the-clock assistance.

In addition to generalized system failure, families identify confidentiality laws, involuntary treatment laws, and discrimination in insurance, treatment, housing, and employment as specific sources of burden.

CONFIDENTIALITY ISSUES

With respect to confidentiality, nurses have cited data showing that families have a legitimate need for information related to diagnosis, current treatment, medications, community resources, and effective strategies for managing the illness (Jones, 1993; Krauss, 1992). To learn how nurses should handle issues related to confidentiality and still involve families in their relatives' treatment, see Therapeutic Communication 10-1.

When family caregivers are not involved, the client's progress is likely to be slower. In worst-case scenarios, the results can be tragic. In the well-publicized case of Andrea Yates, the Texas woman who murdered her five children while suffering from severe depression, her husband testified that her professional caregivers never told him that she had fantasies of violence and voiced fears of harming others (People Magazine, 2002). A woman in Florida never knew that her alcohol-abusing husband had been diag-

nosed with bipolar disorder. Following his suicide, she found a bottle of unused lithium in his sock drawer. "It might not have made a difference. But I think if I had known, I could have helped" (Darling, 1995).

INVOLUNTARY TREATMENT STATUTES

Involuntary treatment statutes originally intended to protect citizens from being "put away" by unconcerned or conniving families now prevent *caring families* from getting loved ones into treatment before their symptoms escalate dangerously. Families point to people with psychiatric disorders eating out of garbage cans and cite media accounts of violent acts committed by untreated persons. They contend that the *right to treatment* should outweigh the *right to refuse treatment* when a person does not recognize that he or she is ill simply because he or she is ill. In such cases, the illness blocks the ability to objectively evaluate one's health (see Chap. 7).

DISCRIMINATION

Discriminatory practices persist in insurance coverage despite advocacy for parity with nonpsychiatric disorders, and they occur in housing and employment despite statutes that forbid it. Managed care companies discriminate by limiting access to rehabilitation strategies on the grounds that they are not a medical necessity.

BURDEN ATTRIBUTABLE TO PROFESSIONALS

Burden attributable to professionals is decreasing as professionals schooled in theories that lead to the misunderstanding of families retire from academia or practice settings. Unfortunately, old attitudes—even as they fade away—leave a legacy in terms of disinterest in the needs of families and failure to provide family services. For example, mothers have been prevented from visiting their ill children in psychiatric hospitals because they were believed to have caused the illness (ie, "schizophrenogenic mothers") (Johnson, 2001). Spouses thought to be deriving secondary gain from their partner's illness heard subtle indictments: "I guess your wife's depression makes your role in the family very important" (Appleton, 1974). Family therapy based on the premise that the client's symptoms were a function of marital discord left families feeling not only misunderstood but also shortchanged. As one parent states, "We paid $150 an hour to find out that we caused our son's illness" (McCory, 1986).

A survey of textbooks used by undergraduate nursing students in Nebraska in 1990 revealed that 100% taught psychoanalytic or family systems theories attributing mental illness to family etiology. They also taught biological theories but often with the disclaimer that the evidence was inconclusive (Moller et al., 1991). As Susan McCabe has discussed, the editors of these texts added new content without eliminating old, possibly outdated material (McCabe, 2000).

THERAPEUTIC COMMUNICATION 10-1
Involving Families in the Client's Treatment

This scenario was written by Mary D. Moller, ARPN, to illustrate how nurses involve family caregivers in the client's treatment. The scene opens as the nurse opens the door from her office and speaks to the client's parents who are waiting outside.

Ineffective Dialogue

Nurse: Hello, Mr. and Mrs. Williams. I would like to invite you into the remainder of my session with Matthew. Won't you come in?

Father: This is strange. No one has ever invited us in before.

Mother: Matthew has never wanted us to speak to his mental health professionals.

Nurse: Treatment won't be successful unless all the people involved in symptom management share their observations with one another. Later on, you two and Matthew will take a 12-session class I teach. Let's go into my office. *(Enters the office)* Matthew, your parents are a little nervous about us being together in my office. Tell them about some of the things we've already discussed.

Matthew: I told the nurse that you get mad at me because I can't do the things my brother does. I feel bad because I'm a disappointment to you.

Mother: Matthew, I'm sorry we've come across like that. I don't know what to say.

Father: We didn't come here to listen to this kind of crap. Come on, Ann, let's get out of here.

Nurse: *(Frowns and sighs)* Mr. Williams, no one is trying to upset you. You have to remember that this is Matthew's problem. All of you should realize that your feelings are normal. You just haven't had all the information and tools you need to be as successful as you would like.

Mother: *(Looks at Mr. Williams, who rolls his eyes at her) (To nurse)* What can you tell us?

Nurse: Let me just say that people with the kind of symptoms that Matthew has have a very hard time completing tasks, especially the first time they try. They get overwhelmed and just give up. He can change his pattern. Won't you both sit down?

Father: I'm sorry, but I don't buy any of this. I'll wait outside. *(Walks out)*

Mother: *(Looks dismayed)* I'm sorry. Maybe the class would work out better.

Nurse: *(Looks at Mrs. Williams with pity)* I appreciate your willingness to try. We can start now by talking about all the different meds that Matthew has been on.

Mother: I tried my best to write them all down like you asked. Here is the list.

Nurse: Matthew, let's look at the list together. Can you remember what each of these pills made you feel like?

Effective Dialogue

Nurse: Hello, Mr. and Mrs. Williams. I would like to invite you into the remainder of my session with Matthew. Won't you come in?

Father: This is strange. No one has ever invited us in before.

Mother: Matthew has never wanted us to speak to his mental health professionals.

Nurse: I hope we can change that. I learned a long time ago that treatment isn't successful unless all the people involved in symptom management share their observations with one another. Later on, I'll be asking you two and Matthew to take a 12-session class I teach. Now, let's go into my office. Matthew, your parents are a little nervous about all of us being together in my office. Tell them about some of the things we've already discussed.

Matthew: I told the nurse that you get mad at me because I can't do the things my brother does. I feel bad because I'm a disappointment to you.

Mother: Matthew, I'm sorry we've come across like that. I don't know what to say.

Father: We didn't come here to listen to this kind of crap. Come on, Ann, let's get out of here.

Nurse: Mr. Williams, I can tell you're pretty upset by what Matthew just said. I need to tell you that most parents feel the same way when sensitive topics like this come up. And Mrs. Williams, you don't have to say anything. It's enough to be open to Matthew's feelings. All three of you should realize that your feelings are normal. You have had your lives turned upside down, and under the circumstances, you've all done a wonderful job. You just haven't had all the information and tools you need to be as successful as you would like.

Mother: *(Aside to Mr. Williams)* Please, Jim! *(To nurse)* Well, what can you tell us?

Nurse: Let me just say that people with the kind of symptoms that Matthew has have a very hard time completing tasks, especially the first time they try. They get overwhelmed and just give up. I want to reassure all three of you that we can change this pattern. Now, won't you both sit down?

Father: Well, all right. As long as you don't expect me to talk.

Mother: I would love for all of us to get involved. That class sounds like just what we need.

(continued)

THERAPEUTIC COMMUNICATION 10-1 (CONTINUED)
Involving Families in the Client's Treatment

Ineffective Dialogue	*Effective Dialogue*

Ineffective Dialogue

Matthew: I can't remember them all, but I remember that one made me feel real stiff and that one stopped me from being able—you know. I can't say it in front of my mother.

Nurse: You mean it affected your sexual functioning. Did you have pain at night?

Matthew: Yes, how did you know that?

Nurse: Matthew, it is very common and in fact is one of the main reasons men stop taking this medication. There is no reason to be embarrassed. You are all going to do very well.

Mother: *(Sighs)* I just wish your father could be involved as well.

Nurse: *(Shrugs)* Maybe next time. Here is the information about our class. I'll see you next week.

Effective Dialogue

Nurse: Good! Mr. Williams, I totally respect how difficult this is for you, and I really appreciate your willingness to give this approach a try. Let's start now by talking about all the different meds that Matthew has been on.

Mother: I tried my best to write them all down like you asked. Here is the list.

Nurse: Matthew, let's look at the list together. Can you remember what each of these pills made you feel like?

Matthew: I can't remember them all, but I remember that one made me feel real stiff, and that one stopped me from being able—you know. I can't say it in front of my parents.

Nurse: You mean it affected your sexual functioning. Did you have pain at night?

Matthew: Yes, how did you know that?

Nurse: Matthew, it is very common and in fact is one of the main reasons men stop taking this medication. There is no reason to be embarrassed.

Mother: You really make it easy to discuss these very personal matters.

Nurse: Psychiatry is a branch of medicine. We have to consider all body systems and how medications affect each one. Then we have to teach everyone concerned about the kinds of problems people have that make them want to stop taking their medications.

Matthew: Mom and Dad, I think this is going to work.

Nurse: Yes, I am sure that you are all going to do very well. Mr. Williams, here is the information about our class. I'll see all three of you next week.

Reflection and Critical Thinking

- Did the issue of confidentiality apply here?
- The differences in the two dialogues are subtle. Even though both nurses included the client's family in care, what measures did the second nurse take to ensure that all participants remained open to the discussion? How did she avoid alienating Mr. Williams?
- Why do you think the parents were never invited into their son's session before?
- In the more effective scenario, what was the nurse's point when she called psychiatry a branch of medicine? How might this have influenced the client's parents?

In nursing textbooks examined by family member professionals in NAMI during the 1990s (the designated Decade of the Brain), the concept of working with families existed only in the context of family therapy. Families were routinely described in terms derived from psychoanalytic or family systems theories, and students were instructed to observe parents for marital skew, communication deviance, or other behaviors believed to contribute to the client's symptoms (Rosenthal, 1990). It followed that students were not taught about family burden, nor instructed in ways of supporting families or involving them in their relatives' treatment.

NAMI family member professionals have been advocating for change in the preservice training programs of their respective disciplines since 1980. The goal was always to *make the training of mental health professionals more rel-*

evant to the needs of persons with serious mental illness and their families (NAMI, 1980). The first objective in nursing education was to produce graduates prepared to respond to the needs of the most vulnerable populations. Echoing the distinguished nursing leader who questioned whether nursing would ever respond to the unmet needs of the chronically mentally ill (Aiken, 1987), NAMI advocated for nurses prepared to work "in the trenches" with the community residents who, in years past, would have been in state hospitals. The second objective was to dispel the delusion that families cause mental illness and to cast them in new roles as treatment allies (NAMI Training Matters, 1985).

Advocacy for change in academia encountered strong resistance from tenured faculty who not only "knew" that families caused mental illness but "knew" three or four theories explaining how they did it. A nursing leader editorializing about resistance to change cited her own reluctance (later overcome) to abandon explanations that were easy to grasp in favor of biological theories that required a background in neuroscience to understand (Taylor, 1996). The message of this chapter is that change is welcome. Families are allies to be consulted, not pathologized and excluded from treatment.

FAMILY RESILIENCE

While studying family burden, researchers found families who appeared to have found a "silver lining" in the clouds cast by mental illness. In these so-called **resilient families,** mental illness apparently acts as a catalyst for positive change (Marsh, 2001). For instance, some families are quicker than others to accept the illness, are more adaptive about sharing caregiving responsibilities among several family members, are better able to change their expectations for the future, and in general, find it easier to make peace with mental illness. This should not be interpreted to mean that resilient families do not need supportive services like other families. It only suggests that some families have assets that give them an advantage over similarly challenged families, and it raises the interesting question as to what these assets are. Are the marriages in these families stronger? Do they have a larger pool of relatives and friends? Greater access to peer support? More spirituality? Higher education? More creativity? These are some of the hypotheses that could be tested to learn more about the source of resiliency and how to build upon family strengths.

Twenty years ago, a mother in California captured the essence of resiliency in a family story called *And They Lived Happily Ever After.* Contacted again when this chapter was in process, Helen Gardner Teisher brought the story up to date:

> *My husband and I are in our eighties now, and we have healthy grandchildren and great-grandchildren. Our*

> *son with schizophrenia is doing well, although his life is not what we once envisioned. We made our peace with mental illness long ago, and really did live happily ever after.*

For further discussion, see Box 10-3.

NEEDS OF FAMILIES FOR SECONDARY PREVENTION

Secondary prevention is provided to prevent further damage after a traumatic event. For example, after the events of September 11, 2001, many of the survivors and families of victims received counseling to allay post-traumatic stress disorder (see Chap. 18). A relative's mental illness is also a traumatic event (albeit less acknowledged) that leaves families at risk for further damage.

Families as a Population at Risk

According to Burland (1997), those in the family movement contend that "the impact of mental illness is a shattering, traumatic event in the life of a family. We believe that the families of people with serious mental illness can certainly qualify as a population under emotional siege and are ideal candidates for secondary prevention strategies." Although secondary prevention is mentioned in psychiatric nursing textbooks with respect to other types of trauma, it has not often been mentioned in relation to mental illness. This may be one of the first nursing texts to discuss family risks, such as caregiver burnout (which then puts clients at risk of homelessness); damaged interpersonal relationships, including broken marriages; developmental delay in younger family members; and stress-related health problems for all family members. In addition, there are known genetic risks for mental illness that vary according to the family member's relationship to the ill person (Torrey, Bower, Taylor & Gottesman, 1994).

Inasmuch as risk attributable to living in proximity to mental illness has received less attention than genetic risk, the Institute of Medicine has called for research on the possible consequences of family burden in relation to depression, sleep deprivation, irritability, drug and alcohol abuse, and marital discord (Mrazek & Haggerty, 1994). Other stress-related health problems could be added to the list (eg, stroke, cardiac conditions, asthma, smoking).

Two studies conducted in the 1980s were possibly the first to examine the relationship between family burden and poor health. Florida researchers found significantly higher levels of anxiety and depression in family caregivers in comparison to a control sample (Arey & Warheit, 1980), and 38% of mental health professionals who were caregivers for relatives with mental illness reported a negative effect on their health (Lefley, 1987). More recently, a

BOX 10-3 ▼ A Resilient Family: And They Lived Happily Ever After!

There we were on a Sunday afternoon, Mom and Dad, our son and daughter-in-law, and two grandchildren. Over the din of the football game on television, we shared our news as the children ran to and fro. Our youngest son was enjoying his new position as an electronic engineer. His older brother and our pregnant daughter-in-law were taking Lamaze classes in preparation for the birth of our third grandchild. A beautiful second-grader displayed her new school clothes. The 3-year-old begged for a horsie ride from an accommodating grandpa.

All of us were nervously aware of the third son lying on the couch, legs drawn up and mouth agape, even in sleep exhibiting the marks of deep unhappiness.

The hours sped along, the conversation never pausing. The good-byes were affectionate, full of concern and thanks for the feast, good cooking, and care packages doled out in the kitchen. Then came the laments from the son who stayed behind. "I don't know how to act with the rest of the family. Why can't I have a kid, too? How come they have so much and I have nothing?" Paranoia soon took over, and he hid his medication under the soggy towels in the laundry basket. "Someone around here wants to poison me." He began gesturing wildly, his eyes darting from side to side, feet shuffling in uncontrolled frenetic motion. To his father, he said, "How, Geronimo! How are you, Great Tribesman?" In my direction, he hailed Helen of Troy. "Is this the face that launched a thousand ships?"

The scenario was familiar to us. We played our parts and showed our love with great hugs, reassuring words, and hot chocolate accompanied by Benadryl. There we were: Geronimo, Helen of Troy, and John the Baptist, all together on the couch, our warm bodies conveying the message, "Fear not. We are with you." Gradually, the identities faded, and we were again an ordinary family.

Later that evening, I looked in on my son sleeping peacefully in his bed. The years vanished, and it was I who hallucinated. I saw a little boy tired from play, resting before the next day's adventures. I saw images of the good high school years when he always ended his day on the golf course near his school. I would arrive to pick him up when he reached the fifteenth hole from where he could see the parking lot. How I loved to watch his beautifully coordinated swing and his purposeful walk from stroke to ball. Precious moments! He would lift his club in greeting, and I would answer with a soft beep of the horn.

Standing by his bed that Sunday evening, I filled my mind with memories. There was one special day when we went for a ride in San Diego's back country. The hills were aflame with orange poppies. Green grass grew about the great gray granite outcroppings. Great white billows decorated the indigo sky arching above the brilliant landscape. We walked together on the hillside, becoming part of the whole magnificent scene. Pausing, my son slipped an arm over my shoulder and I heard his reverent prayer, "The Lord is my shepherd. I shall not want."

Thinking back on that moment, I knew the ecstasy of true perspective. We were indeed so very small a part of the Great Scheme of Things Entire that our problems, too, were entirely inconsequential. Peace enveloped me.

Points for Reflection and Critical Thinking

- What family strengths are evident from this account?
- What coping strategies did the parents use when their son exhibited psychotic symptoms?
- How did the mother cope with grief?
- What part does spirituality play in this family's resilience?

Helen Gardner Teisher, NAMI California.

research team that included a psychiatric nurse found a significant relationship between subjective family burden and self-reports of poor maternal health (Greenberg, Greenly, McKee, Brown, & Griffin-Francell, 1993).

Family Consultation

Family consultation is a secondary prevention strategy based on the assumption that the model family dealing with mental illness is healthy and competent but lacks sufficient knowledge and skills. In the role of family consultant, nurses *mentor* families to expand their experientially based knowledge and to help them access NAMI, DMDA, or other family organizations. They also *support* families with empathic understanding, help them set priorities and problem-solve, and refer them to clinical services for psychotherapy, grief counseling, marital counseling, or medications. Ultimately, it is up to the family members to select the interventions they want to receive, and the choice is likely to vary with their evolving needs and circumstances.

FAMILY CONSULTATION VERSUS FAMILY THERAPY

Family consultation is not to be confused with *family therapy.* The latter, which was introduced into graduate nursing education in the 1970s, was based on "a new way of viewing mental illness." Proponents of family therapy viewed it as both a signal and a function of a disturbance in an ongoing system (Peplau, 1975). According to this view, the family member with symptoms was not sick; he or she was the "symptom bearer" for a disturbed family system. This view of mental illness remained the basis for family therapy as described in nursing textbooks throughout the 1990s. The premise of family therapy is that the member with the presenting symptoms signals pain in the whole family. This pain may arise from the disappointment of the marital partners with one another (Hogarth & Weeks, 1997).

Family therapy was introduced as a treatment for schizophrenia that required the participation of the entire family. In contrast, family consultation (originally called supported family counseling) was introduced as a service to families, not as a treatment for schizophrenia. Family consultation is based on the premise that the client's symptoms, instead of *signaling* distress in the family, *spread* distress through the family by a ripple effect (Wasow, 1995).

COMPONENTS OF FAMILY CONSULTATION

The standard dictionary definition of *consultation* indicates how family consultation works. Just as families consult with an attorney to obtain legal advice, they consult with a mental health professional for advice about mental illness. In a typical situation, the family consultant makes a "secondary prevention scan" by asking how family members are getting along and how he or she can help them. The format for family consultation is flexible, but Edie Mannion, director of the Training, Education and Consultation (TEC) Family Center in Philadelphia, recommends the "Three F" approach: feeling, focus, and finding (Marsh, 1998).

In the *feeling stage,* the consultant acknowledges the feelings of all family members and tries to normalize them with statements such as, "If that happened to me, I'd be angry, too." In the *focus stage,* the consultant helps family members set priorities, a process that may depend upon finding the common denominator in competing issues. If the mother of a daughter with bipolar disorder is concerned because the daughter is a messy housekeeper, the father worries because she runs up the telephone bill, and the sister is tired of lending her clothes, the common denominator is "setting limits." *Finding the solution* is the final stage. As the expert on mental illness, the consultant takes the lead in finding solutions, but the family also contributes their own experientially based expertise. Clinical Example 10-2 provides a glimpse of family consultation in practice.

▼ *Clinical Example 10-2*

A nurse is talking with Mr. and Mrs. Connor, the parents of Stuart, who has schizophrenia. The following dialogue takes place after the nurse and parents have identified the priority problem as "possible medication noncompliance."

Nurse: Mrs. Connor, what made you think your son is not taking his medication as prescribed?

Mrs. Connor: I counted the pills in the bottle, and there were too many left.

Mr. Connor: I'm not so sure my wife should have done that, but I have to admit I'm also worried about what might happen if Stuart cuts back on his meds.

Nurse: Tell me, have either of you noticed whether Stuart is hearing voices again?

Parents: (Together) No, we haven't noticed anything. Of course, Stuart might not be letting on that he's hearing voices. He doesn't talk about things like that with us.

Nurse: Well, I'll try to find out when I meet with Stuart this afternoon. I'll ask him about side effects, too, and try to find out if he has some reason to want to reduce his dosage.

Mrs. Connor: I hope you won't tell him that I checked the pill bottle. I know he would think I was interfering.

Nurse: No, I don't have to tell him. I understand your dilemma—wanting to be sure he's getting the benefit of his treatment but also wanting him to take the responsibility of managing his own medications. This is a common dilemma, and it's addressed in an educational course that is being offered by your local NAMI. Here is the brochure. I'll highlight the telephone number of the contact person. I really advise both of you to enroll if you possibly can. It's an excellent course, and it's free!

Mrs. Connor: Thank you so much. We really appreciate your understanding and help.

Nurse: Well, your son is fortunate to have parents who are interested and willing to become better informed about his illness. You have important roles to play in his treatment. I have to tell you that family caregivers are usually the first to notice signs of relapse, before the client and before the doctor or nurse. If we all work together as a team, Stuart's chances of recovering soon are much better.

Before Mr. and Mrs. Connor leave, the nurse shows them a pocket-sized booklet called *My Portable Medication Record* (PMR). The nurse explains how she will teach their son to use it to communicate with her, his doctor, and them about his medications and their effects and side effects. She explains that copies of the PMR are available free of charge from the Pennsylvania state affiliate of NAMI (Conn & Edwards, 1999). The parents are glad to see that the PMR contains a section called "Ways To Make Your Meds Work Better" based on information provided by an advanced practice psychiatric nurse.

THE NURSE AS FAMILY CONSULTANT

Family consultation can take place in family sessions called specifically for this purpose, on an impromptu basis whenever the nurse and family members happen to meet, and even by telephone. For examples of nurses functioning as family consultants, see Research in Psychiatric-Mental Health Nursing 10-1.

The knowledge base required by nurses functioning as family consultants includes thorough knowledge about serious mental illness and treatment, an empathic understanding of family burden, and a grasp of caregiving skills, as well as an awareness of government entitlement programs and community resources including those offered by family advocacy organizations. Consultants also need teaching skills and the ability to communicate with family members with clarity and respect.

The need for *clarity* is not based on the belief that family members experience *communication deviance,* as was once assumed, but is because they are under stress and

likely to be preoccupied and anxious. Furthermore, some family members share (to a lesser degree) the same problems with concentration and memory that trouble their ill relatives (Green, 2002). In the examples of family consultation given in this chapter, the consultants tried to compensate for possible cognitive problems by repeating information and writing down key points. Some consultants advise family members to use a tape recorder.

Respect is an indispensable component of effective communication. To be respectful means to recognize the expertise that family caregivers have acquired through experience and to assume until proved otherwise that they are doing the best they can and have the best interests of their relatives at heart. In family language, the concepts of *enabling* and *codependency* translate into *adding insult to injury.* Family members are especially affronted

---

> **Research in Psychiatric-Mental Health Nursing 10–1**
> **TIME-LIMITED FAMILY CONSULTATION WITH FAMILIES BEFORE AND AFTER CLIENT DISCHARGE**

Principal Investigator and Research Support: Rose Marie Friedrich, MA, RN, The Nellie Ball Trust Fund

Purpose: To study the outcomes of time-limited family consultation provided to families immediately before and for 3 months after client discharge from inpatient treatment

Expected Outcomes: For families, (1) increased knowledge about schizophrenia, (2) more positive mood, (3) decreased family burden, (4) increased coping abilities, (5) and satisfaction with the program; for clients, (1) increased medication compliance and (2) decreased hospitalization

Background: Because of a shift in social policy, more people with schizophrenia now live in the community. A NAMI survey found that 42% lived at home (Torrey, 1995). Family caregivers are challenged to meet the needs of their ill relatives despite a lack of adequate community services. In Iowa (the site of this study), 67 of 99 counties have no psychiatrists; only 16 certified psychiatric-mental health nurse practitioners work in the entire state. A study of 181 clients and 130 family members in Iowa found that caregivers lacking in knowledge and resources experience high levels of family burden (Friedrich et al., 1999).

Research Base: Psychoeducational programs designed to offer support and education to families, although effective, are costly because of staff involvement with families from 9 to 12 months. The present study seeks to evaluate a time-limited, low-cost method whereby one 3-hour educational session is followed by monthly consultation by telephone twice a month for 3 months. A precedent for this approach exists in

the fields of pediatrics, cardiology, and gerontology, where advanced practice nurses have used this same strategy with significantly improved client outcomes (Brooten et al., 1986; Keeling & Dennison, 1995; Naylor, 1994).

Method and Sample: The participants are families of clients hospitalized at the University of Iowa. A total of 32 families will be randomly assigned to the intervention or control group. Family members in both groups will complete self-reports of demographic information, knowledge of schizophrenia, and levels of family objective and subjective burden. The intervention group (only) will receive a 3-hour educational session with the nurse plus a take-home packet including information about the illness, the protocol for telephone conversations, a community resource guide (including crisis services) for Iowa counties, a journal for recording questions or comments during the telephone consultations, and a copy of Dr. E. Fuller Torrey's *Surviving Schizophrenia: A Manual for Families, Consumers, and Providers* (1995). During the calls, the nurse and family caregiver(s) will discuss symptoms, medication management, and related health problems, including medical illnesses and substance abuse. They also will discuss the caregivers' emotional responses to caregiving and practical problems related to access of services. The nurse will model a problem-solving approach and encourage family caregivers to collaborate in the client's care.

Results: Because the study is not yet complete, results are pending. The potential exists, however, to significantly improve client and family outcomes through this type of intervention.

when these labels are used stereotypically, without taking time to get to know the people. In Therapeutic Communication 10-2, the nurse in the ineffective dialogue not only fails to respond to Mr. Silverman's distress when he enters the office, but she also assumes that he and his wife had something to do with the son's explosive behavior. This assumption strikes the father as both irrelevant and disrespectful, and he turns defensive. The nurse actually intended no disrespect; she was simply pursuing a line of reasoning suggested to her by family systems theory (ie, the putative association between marital discord and the client's symptoms). Nevertheless, her comment angered the father and ended the session before the real reason for Eric's behavior became apparent.

In the effective dialogue, the nurse responded with empathy to Mr. Silverman before they even began to talk

---

THERAPEUTIC COMMUNICATION 10-2
Family Consultation

Mr. Silverman, the father of a 30-year-old man with schizophrenia, enters the community mental health center office of the nurse who sees his son for weekly blood work to ensure that his treatment with Clozaril is not affecting his white cell count.

Ineffective Dialogue	*Effective Dialogue*
Nurse: Is Eric with you?	*Nurse:* Good morning, Mr. Silverman. Is Eric with you?
Mr. S.: No, he refused to come.	*Mr. S.:* No, he refused to come.
Nurse: Mr. Silverman, it's very important that Eric gets his blood work done. What is wrong?	*Nurse:* Why? What's wrong?
Mr. S.: Eric threw a chair though the living room wall. That's what's wrong!	*Mr. S.:* Eric threw a chair through the living room wall.
Nurse: (Thinking) Hmmm. Mr. Silverman, what is going on at home?	*Nurse:* That's terrible! You must be very upset.
Mr. S.: (Baffled) I just told you. Eric got mad and threw a chair through the wall.	*Mr. S.:* To tell the truth, I am. I just can't figure out what got into Eric.
Nurse: I heard what you said, Mr. Silverman. But, I mean, have you and Mrs. Silverman been having any problems lately? Arguments perhaps?	*Nurse:* Maybe we can figure it out together. Tell me more about it.
Mr. S.: (Defensively) What's that got to do with anything? It's Eric we're talking about!	*Mr. S.:* Well, for one thing, I suspect he hasn't been taking medicine the way he's supposed to. His mother keeps tabs on that, and she's been away since Friday.
	Nurse: Where did she go?
	Mr. S.: She went to Ohio to see her mother, and while she was there, her mother had a slight stroke.
	Nurse: I am so sorry to hear that. Eric has mentioned his grandmother to me, and I know he's very fond of her. How did he take the news?
	Mr. S.: You know that's a funny thing. Eric didn't seem bothered at all when his mother called about the stroke. He just went into his room for a real long time, and when he came out, that's when he threw the chair through the wall.
	Nurse: Mr. Silverman, I can see you're having a rough time. What can I do to help?

Reflection and Critical Thinking

- How do you think Mr. Silverman was feeling when he entered the office? How did he feel as a result of the nurse's responses in the ineffective dialogue? The effective dialogue?
- What was the nurse's hypothesis about the cause of Eric's behavior in the ineffective dialogue? Was she on the right track or the wrong track?
- What did the nurse in the effective dialogue accomplish when she said, "Tell me more about it." What did she accomplish when she said, "What can I do to help?"

about Eric. With his feelings validated, the father relaxed and, with the nurse's prompting, related the events that turned out to be the probable cause of Eric's behavior. The information can be useful in terms of Eric's vulnerability to relapse, but in the meantime, the nurse again empathized with the father, who truly was "having a rough time."

Family Empowerment

All communication, regardless of its specific purpose in terms of conveying information or teaching skills to family members, must support the family members' sense of self-worth. In the vocabulary of the Community Support Program (CSP) movement, this is called family empowerment, the companion piece to *client empowerment*.

Currently, family empowerment is more of a dream than a reality. As this chapter is being written, a nurse researcher has just published data about the lack of professionally provided **family support services** for family caregivers despite the evidence of their value for clients and caregivers (Doornbos, 2002). Family advocacy organizations have tried to address this shortage by starting support groups for caregivers in all parts of the country. Peer support groups can be beneficial in terms of reducing family burden and increasing coping and adaptation (Solomon & Draine, 1995b). NAMI affiliates offer a wide range of support and educational services, as is evident from the January 2002 events calendar of NAMI Chester County, Pennsylvania:

- Enroll in the Hand to Hand Educational Course—eight sessions for families with children or adolescents with mental illness or emotional disorders
- Enroll in Family to Family, a 12-session, 36-hour course for families of adults with serious mental illness
- Welcome to NAMI-Can, a monthly support group for families of children and adolescents with mental illness
- Welcome to NAMI Rap Session, a monthly group for families of adults with serious mental illness
- Join NAMI-CARE, support groups for adult clients
- Welcome to the Grief and Loss Group, monthly support meetings with a nurse in attendance
- Come to the Depression and Manic/Depression group, a monthly support group
- Welcome to the January Educational Forum: *Understanding Borderline Personality Disorder: The Dialectical Approach* by Marsha Linehan, PhD, on tape; Jean Froy, RN, MN, discussant.

Family Education

Although family education has been included in the nurse's role since the days of Florence Nightingale, the families of persons with medical illnesses, such as diabetes or heart disease, have been the primary beneficiaries. In contrast, the families of psychiatric clients seldom receive educational services from any mental health professional. The report by the Schizophrenia Patient Outcomes Research Team (PORT), cited previously for its reference to system failure in the treatment of people with schizophrenia, confirmed that only 10% of the family caregivers of these persons received any kind of education (Lehman & Steinwachs, 1998). The 10% included caregivers who were merely handed a brochure or a package insert from a pharmaceutical company. In the mid-1980s, a number of practicing family therapists began modifying family therapy (the primary intervention for families at the time) to produce a new modality they called family psychoeducation.

FAMILY EDUCATION VERSUS FAMILY PSYCHOEDUCATION

Just as the first automobiles were built to resemble "horseless carriages," the first educational programs for the families of clients with psychiatric disorders resembled family therapy in format, timing, goals, and outcome measures. The family sessions included all members of the family and the ill member, lasted over an extended period, and were aimed at changing family behaviors and communication styles. The outcome measure, just as in family therapy, was symptom reduction in the client.

There were also major differences between family therapy and family psychoeducation. The family therapists who developed **family psychoeducation** put aside theories about family causation and substituted the proposition that with proper training, the family could exert a positive effect on treatment. An early form of psychoeducation aimed at lowering the family's level of expressed emotion (EE), as measured by a quantitative analysis of critical remarks directed by family members toward clients in a test situation. This model proved effective when combined with medication in reducing relapse and recidivism. Family advocates criticized it, however, for attributing treatment failure to the family's "high EE" in a manner reminiscent of the "schizophrenogenic mother" hypothesis.

Most psychoeducation programs today begin with a process of "joining with the family," followed by extensive training in communication and behavioral skills. The aim is to create a low-stress home environment that is therapeutic for the client and incidentally benefits the entire family.

COMPONENTS OF FAMILY EDUCATION

Family education was introduced independently of family therapy by Agnes Hatfield, a professor of education at the University of Maryland and a founding member of NAMI. Hatfield asked NAMI families what they wanted from family therapists and found that they wanted education, not therapy (Hatfield, 1983). Using her training in the principles of adult education, her personal experience as a caregiver for an ill son, and extensive interviews with other caregivers, Hatfield wrote a manual called *Coping With Mental Illness in the Family* for family use and to train providers in community mental health centers to offer family education. Since then, Hatfield has written extensively on family education and acquired an international reputation as a specialist in this area.

The successful outcome measures for family education are reduced family burden and improvement in the family's quality of life. Client improvement often accompanies this outcome but (in contrast to family psychoeducation) is not a primary goal.

THE NURSE AS FAMILY EDUCATOR

Mary Moller and Jo Ann Wer pioneered family education by nurses but referred to it as *simultaneous family/patient education* because they taught families and clients in the same classes (Moller & Wer, 1989). Moller made a series of videos on preventing relapse and communicating with persons who were hallucinating or delusional and made them available to both families and professional caregivers. Currently, she teaches a course to clients and families that is an integral part of treatment at the Suncrest Wellness Center in Nine Mile Falls, Washington. See Box 10-4.

PEER-TAUGHT FAMILY EDUCATION

Peer-taught family education was introduced in 1987 by social workers in collaboration with the NAMI Kansas, using a curriculum written by Richard T. Wintersteen, PhD. The first program to reach families throughout the entire country was The NAMI Family to Family Education Program, a 12-session, 36-hour curriculum based on a trauma-recovery model. The course is by a team of trained family members, using a curriculum written by Joyce Burland, PhD, a NAMI family member psychologist. To qualify for training as teachers, applicants must have a relative

---

BOX 10-4 ▼ *NAMI Family to Family Education Program*

NAMI's Family to Family Education Program (FFEP) is a free, 12-session, 30-hour, peer-taught course that orients families to the world of mental illness. It teaches the following:

> *Everyone needs to understand that when a family member has a mental illness, you and your loved one are, like Alice in Wonderland, going to fall down the rabbit hole. The world you are entering is overwhelmed by the demand for services and ill equipped to meet your needs. You are up against centuries of bias against you, against the illnesses, against getting organized to do anything about them. What is important here is to recognize system failure and stigma as part of the reality we must deal with. It is also essential to realize how difficult this makes it for our ill relatives to get the help they deserve and to "rejoin" society.*
> (Burland, 2002)

The curriculum casts a wide lens, integrating the biological, psychological, and social aspects of brain disorders that present as mental illnesses. It teaches a "feast of facts" about the symptoms and treatments of schizophrenia and schizoaffective disorder; major depression; and bipolar, panic, obsessive-compulsive borderline personality, and co-occurring addictive disorders. Families learn more than facts; they learn new coping skills based on a deeper understanding of mental illness and the client's inner world.

Four sessions cover medical aspects (eg, brain function, diagnosis and prognosis, symptoms, and medication management); another four teach psychological aspects (eg, normative responses to trauma and defensive coping strategies) by means of skills training workshops on understanding psychosis, problem solving, communicating, and empathic listening. The remaining four classes are on recovery, rehabilitation, and advocacy.

The class isn't over when it's over. Families retain for future reference a crisis file and a 250-page syllabus and are linked to a local NAMI affiliate for support and advocacy. Because NAMI regards advocacy as the final step in a family's rehabilitation, all graduates of the course are commanded to "charge!".

A psychiatrist whose mother has a mental illness wrote, "Your course turned out to be a treasure that I fervently wish had been presented to me during my training instead of ten years into my practice. It was the first course that taught me concise, empathetic communication with a patient. When I used my new skills with my mother, her joy and relief that someone actually understood how she felt almost reduced me to tears (Miller, 2000).

FFEP is sponsored by NAMI's Center for Research, Education, and Practice. NAMI also offers a peer-taught educational program for clients and a provider education program taught by clients, family members, and a family member professional.

For further information, contact Dr. Joyce Burland at NAMI.

Burland, J. (1998). *NAMI family to family education program* (p. 2.5).

Miller, M., letter to Marcia and Paul Garret, Family to Family teachers, May 16, 2000.

with a serious mental illness and be recommended by a local NAMI affiliate. Many course teachers are nurses.

NAMI's Family to Family Education course reduces subjective family burden and increases the family's sense of empowerment with respect to the mental health system, the community, and the family (Dixon, 2001). A study directed by a psychiatric nurse researcher is now underway to determine whether the course has a parallel effect on the ill relative.

The family-to-family course is one of several programs offered free of charge through NAMI state affiliates. Other educational programs include a peer-taught course for clients, a course for the families of children and adolescents with mental illness, and the NAMI Provider Education Course that is taught to providers by two clients, two family members, and a family member professional.

For information about specific family education programs in use throughout the country, refer to Diane Marsh's publication *Serious Mental Illness and the Family: The Practitioners' Guide* (1998).

Psychotherapy and Medication

Although the nonclinical services described earlier in the chapter will meet the needs of most families, an important minority will choose to receive more extensive services. For example, some family members will choose psychotherapy, medication, or both. Some couples will want to receive counseling to help them work together constructively as caregivers.

In a study of siblings and offspring, 77% of the participants reported that they had received psychotherapy as adults; among those who were younger than 10 years of age when their relative became ill, the percentage rose to 90% (Marsh, 1998). Many of these siblings and offspring regretted that no one had offered them supportive or therapeutic services when they were children. Optimally, support services should be provided to pregnant women who have a mental illness to help them have the best start possible in child rearing (Mowbray, 2002).

In an educational group for spouses, 50% of the "well" spouses were receiving psychotherapy, antidepressant medications, or both to help them manage their difficult lives (E. Mannion, personal communication, March 5, 2002). Some were convinced that mental illness (depression in particular) was contagious and that they had contracted it from their ill spouses. A husband and wife, after seeking a second opinion about the husband's diagnosis, were told that both partners had post-traumatic stress disorder. The husband's illness was attributed to an early trauma rekindled by the events of September 11, 2001, and the wife's condition was attributed to living with her husband. Both partners are now receiving psychotherapy (Anonymous, 2002).

Spouses who enroll in educational classes are the most likely of all family members to drop out prematurely, citing their mental state: "I know I need this class, but I'm too upset to concentrate." Some seek individual therapy to help them resolve their guilt about wanting to leave the marriage. Some seek a therapist with whom to discuss their spouse's symptoms because the spouse's therapist refuses to communicate.

Parents' marital problems, not uncommon in a culture with a high divorce rate, can seriously hinder joint caregiving for ill children and can also lead to a broken marriage. Marital counseling can sometimes enable the parents to survive as a couple and also become more effective caregivers for an ill son or daughter.

Another factor creating the need for clinical services for caregivers is that in many families, more than one member has a psychiatric diagnosis. Instead of a "well spouse" caring for an "ill spouse," two ill spouses may be serving as one another's caregivers. This situation is more common today because clients living in the community have opportunities to meet one another, date, and marry. It is also not unusual for mental illness to span two generations, as was reported by a client member of the NAMI Provider Education Course teaching team:

> *Because my mother had schizophrenia, my father left us when we were small. My grandparents helped raise us, but they both died before I got through college. I took off on a trip around the world, but in Crete I thought I saw my grandparents rising from their graves. The authorities decided I had schizophrenia and sent me home. My mother and my brother—who by then was also diagnosed with schizophrenia— met me at the airport. I have now been taking Clozaril for 10 years. My mother and my brother and I try to help one another. (Anonymous member of NAMI provider course teaching team, personal communication, March 24, 2002).*

▼ Reflection and Critical Thinking

1. What aspects of family burden do siblings and offspring have in common? What option does a spouse have that other family members lack? What prevents this option from being a good one?

2. Which family member is likely to help out when one parent is ill and the other one has to earn a living?

3. What is likely to be an aging parent's primary concern about an ill child?

▼ CHAPTER SUMMARY

■ In the past 150 years, Americans with mental illness have been "to the asylum and back." The result is that their families are again their primary caregivers.

- Nurses work with families of those with psychiatric disorders for two purposes: to help them cope with the traumatic effects of mental illness and caregiving and to involve them as allies in their ill relatives' treatments.
- The stress associated with caregiving is conceptualized as family burden, further divided into objective (the practical aspects of caregiving) and subjective (the emotional response).
- A large part of family burden is iatrogenic, meaning it stems from a dysfunctional mental health system or from the attitudes and behaviors of mental health professionals who generalize about families on the basis of outdated theories.
- Stigma and discrimination in housing, employment, and insurance coverage, as well as confidentiality laws and involuntary commitment laws, are additional sources of burden.
- Some families, known as resilient families, can see better than others the silver lining in the clouds cast by mental illness. Resiliency is a promising area for research.
- The family members of persons with a serious mental illness are a population at risk for genetically linked mental illnesses, stress-related medical disorders and social problems, or both.
- Family consultation designed to reduce family burden is a prime example of a needed secondary prevention strategy.
- Nurses functioning as family consultants mentor families, meaning they provide information and advice about mental illness and caregiving; support families with empathy, grief counseling, and conflict mediation; and provide access to psychotherapy, marriage counseling, and medication, as needed.
- Effective communication with families is clear and respectful and based on the assumption (unless proven otherwise) that families are doing their best and have the client's best interests at heart.
- Members of the family subsystem (parents, children, siblings, spouses) experience burden in different ways.
- Although most family members' needs are met by nonclinical services (support and education), a minority (including caregivers who are also clients) needs clinical services (psychotherapy, marriage counseling, and medication prescription).
- Family advocacy organizations such as NAMI and DMDA are excellent resources for families and professional caregivers.

▾ REVIEW QUESTIONS

1. Mrs. Owens is the 81-year-old mother of Jonathan, who is 54 years old. Jonathan has had schizophrenia since he was 16 years old. Which of Mrs. Owens's concerns is likely to predominate?
   a. Will my retirement funds outlast me?
   b. Who will handle my funeral arrangements?
   c. What will become of Jonathan when I am gone?
   d. How can I get Jonathan's doctor to talk to me?

2. Which of the following services is not part of family consultation?
   a. Assisting with vocational rehabilitation
   b. Providing information about the illness
   c. Teaching effective communication
   d. Helping families problem-solve

3. Which of the following is an example of subjective burden?
   a. Financial drain
   b. Grief
   c. Daily hassles
   d. Conflict with the police

4. Which of the following is an example of iatrogenic burden?
   a. A nurse calling a client's spouse an enabler
   b. A flawed mental health system
   c. A mother feeling guilty
   d. Both a and b

5. According to a survey of DMDA, what is the average time lapse before members receive the correct diagnosis?
   a. 4 years
   b. 2 years
   c. 6 months
   d. 10 years

6. What is the primary goal of family education?
   a. Symptom reduction
   b. Improved quality of life
   c. Increased knowledge about mental illness
   d. Improved caregiving skills

7. Families receiving family consultation, unless proven otherwise, are considered
   a. To be healthy and competent
   b. To lack knowledge and skills
   c. To have the client's best interests at heart
   d. All of the above

8. In a study of siblings and offspring conducted by Marsh, how many respondents said they had participated in therapy?
   a. 50%
   b. 77%
   c. None
   d. Only the females

9. When a person with serious mental illness becomes violent, who is the most likely target?
   a. A mental health professional
   b. A police officer

c. A stranger

d. A family caregiver

10. Why is it necessary for the family consultant to be clear in communicating with family members?

a. Some families do not speak English.

b. Family members may be preoccupied.

c. Family members may be experiencing communication deviance.

d. Otherwise, the consultant may not remember what was said.

▼ REFERENCES AND SUGGESTED READINGS

*Aiken, H. L. (1987). Unmet needs of the chronically mentally ill: Will nursing respond? *Image: Journal of Nursing Scholarship, 19*(3), 121–125.

Amenson, C. (1993). *Education, consultation and treatment of families with a mentally ill member: A guide for effective professional intervention.* Pasadena, CA: Pacific Clinics Institute.

Anonymous participant in Spouse Coping Skills Workshop. (2002, March 26). TEC Family Center, Mental Health Association of SE Pennsylvania.

*Appleton, W. S. (1974). Mistreatment of patients' families by psychiatrists. *American Journal of Psychiatry, 131*(5), 655–657.

*Arey, S., & Warheit, G. J. (1980). Psychosocial costs of living with psychologically disturbed family members. In L. N. Robins, P. J. Clayton, & J. K. Wing (Eds.), *The social consequences of psychiatric illness* (pp. 158–175), New York: Brunner/Mazel.

Backlar, P. (1994). *The family face of schizophrenia.* New York: Tarcher/Putnam.

*Bernheim, K. F., & Lehman, A. F. (1985). *Working with families of the mentally ill.* New York: Norton.

Bisbee, C. (1991). *Educating patients and families about mental illness: A practical guide.* Gaithersburg, MD: Aspen.

*Burland, J. C. (1997). *The family education course for professional providers.* Arlington, VA: NAMI Press.

*Community Mental Health Center Act of 1963, Pub. L. No. 88–164.

Conn, V. (1999). Nurses as providers of prevention services for relatives of patients with serious mental illness. *The Journal of NAMI California, 10*(5), 28–30.

*Conn, V., & Edwards, N. (1999). *My portable medication record.* Glenside, PA: NAMI Montgomery County, PA.

Deveson, A. (1992). *Tell me I'm here: One family's experience of schizophrenia.* New York: Penguin Books.

Dixon, L., Lyles, A., Scott, J., Lehman, A. K., Pastrado, L., Goldman, H., & McGlunn, E. (1999). Services to families of adults with schizophrenia: From treatment recommendations to dissemination. *Psychiatric Services, 50*(2), 233–238.

*Doornbos, M. M. (2002). Family caregivers and the mental health system: Reality and dreams. *Archives of Psychiatric Nursing, 16*(1), 39–46.

*Eakes, G. G. (1995). Chronic sorrow: The lived experience of parents of chronically mentally ill individuals. *Archives of Psychiatric Nursing, 11*(2), 77–84.

Flach, F. (1988). *Resilience: Discovering a new strength at times of stress.* New York: Fawcett Columbine.

*Francell, C. G., Conn, V. S., & Gray, D. P. (1988). Families' perceptions of burden of care for chronic mentally ill relatives. *Hospital and Community Psychiatry, 39*(12), 1296–1300.

*Frese, F. J., & Frese, P. (1991). *Part 1: Schizophrenia: Surviving in a world of normals. Part 2: A love story: Living with someone with schizophrenia.* Beachwood, OH: Wellness Reproductions.

Frese, P. (1996a). Family life and mental illness: Making it work. *The Journal of the California Alliance for the Mentally Ill, 7*(3), 52–54.

Frese, P. (1996b). When Daddy gets sick: Helping kids cope. *The Journal of the California Alliance for the Mentally Ill, 7*(3), 54–55.

*Geller, J. L. (2000). Excluding institutions for mental illness from federal reimbursement for services: Strategy or tragedy? *Psychiatric Services, 51*(11), 1397–1403.

Gerace, L. M., Camilleri, D., & Ayres, L. (1993). Sibling perspectives on schizophrenia and the family. *Schizophrenia Bulletin, 19*(3), 637–647.

Goffman, E. (1961). *Asylums: Essays on the social situation of mental patients and other inmates.* New York: Anchor Books.

*Green, M. F. (1998). *Schizophrenia from a neurocognitive perspective: Probing the impenetrable darkness.* Boston: Allyn and Bacon.

*Greenberg, J. S., Greenly, J. R., McKee, D., Brown, R., & Griffin-Francell, C. (1993). Mothers caring for an adult child with schizophrenia. *Family Relations, 42*, 205–221.

*Hatfield, A. B. (1983). What families want from family therapists. In W. R. McFarlane (Ed.), *Family therapy of schizophrenia* (pp. 41–65). New York: Guilford Press.

Hatfield, A. B. (1990). *Family education in mental illness.* New York: Guilford Press.

*Hatfield, A. B., & Lefley, H. P. (Eds.). (1987). *Families of the mentally ill: Coping and adaptation.* New York: Guilford Press.

*Hogarth, C. R., & Weeks, M. W. (1997). *Families and family therapy.* In B. S. Johnson (Ed.), *Psychiatric-mental health nursing: Adaptation and growth* (4th ed., pp. 277–298). Philadelphia: Lippincott Williams & Wilkins.

*Johnson, D. (2001, First Quarter). Psychoeducation or family education: What's it all about? *Newsletter of the World Fellowship for Schizophrenia and Allied Disorders, 12*, 3–4.

*Jones, S. (1993). More on confidentiality [Editorial]. *Archives of Psychiatric Nursing, 7*(3), 123–124.

*Krauss, J. (1992). Confidentiality [Editorial]. *Archives of Psychiatric Nursing, 6*(5), 255–256.

Lefley, H. P. (1987a). Aging parents as caregivers of mentally ill adult children: An emerging social problem. *Hospital and Community Psychiatry, 38*(10), 1063–1070.

Lefley, H. P. (1987b). An adaptation framework: Its meaning for research and practice. In A. Hatfield & H. P. Lefley (Eds.), *Families of the mentally ill: Coping and adaptation* (pp. 309–327). New York: Guilford Press.

Lefley, H. P. (1987c). Impact of mental illness in families of mental health professionals. *Journal of Nervous and Mental Disease,* 613–619.

*Lefley, H. P. (1996). *Family caregiving in mental illness.* Thousand Oaks, CA: Sage Publications.

*Lehman, A. F., & Steinwachs, D. M. (1998). At issue: Translating research into practice: The Schizophrenia Patient Outcomes Research Team (PORT) treatment recommendations. *Schizophrenia Bulletin, 24*(1), 10.

*Lehman, A. F., Thompson, J. W., Dixon, L. B., & Scott, J. E. (1995). Schizophrenia: Treatment outcomes research. *Schizophrenia Bulletin, 21*(4), 516–566.

*L'Engle, M. (1989). Forward. In C. S. Lewis, *A grief observed*. New York: Harper Collins.

Lyden, J. (1997). *Daughter of the queen of Sheba*. Boston: Houghton Mifflin.

*MacGregor, P. (1994). Grief: The unrecognized parental response to mental illness in a child. *Social Work, 39*(2), 160–166.

*Marlatt, J. (1987, November). *Reflections on the parental role in rehabilitation*. Paper presented at the annual conference of the National Rehabilitation Association, New Orleans, LA.

*Marsh, D. T. (1998). *Serious mental illness and the family: The practitioner's guide*. New York: John Wiley & Sons.

*Marsh, D. T. (2001). *A family-focused approach to serious mental illness: Empirically supported interventions*. Sarasota, FL: Professional Resource Press.

*McCabe, S. (2000). Bringing psychiatric nursing into the twenty-first century. *Archives of Psychiatric Nursing, 14*(3), 109–116.

*McCory, T. (1986). History of NAMI. *Ways, 1*, 16–18.

*Mohr, W. K., & Regan-Kubinski, M. J. (2001). Living in the fallout: Parent's experiences when their child becomes mentally ill. *Archives of Psychiatric Nursing, 15*(2), 69–77.

*Moller, M. D., et al. (1991). Psychiatric nursing education in Nebraska: 1989–1990. *Issues in Mental Health Nursing, 12*(4), 343–357.

*Moller, M. D., & Wer, J. (1989). Simultaneous patient/family education regarding schizophrenia: The Nebraska model. *Archives of Psychiatric Nursing, 3*(6), 332–337.

Moorman, M. (1992). *My sister's keeper: Learning to cope with a sibling's mental illness*. New York: Norton.

*Mowbray, C. T. (2002, March). *Seriously mentally ill women coping with parenting: Recent findings on diagnosis, living arrangements and the meaning of motherhood*. Presentation at the 2001–2002 Center for Mental Health Policy and Services Research Seminar Series, Philadelphia, PA.

*Mrazek, P. J., & Haggerty, R. J. (Eds.). (1994). *Reducing risks for mental disorders: Frontiers for preventive intervention research*. Washington, DC: National Academy Press.

*National Advisory Mental Health Council. (1993). Health care reform for Americans with serious mental illness. *American Journal of Psychiatry, 150*, 1447–1465.

*National Alliance for the Mentally Ill. (1992). *The role of professionals in NAMI*. Arlington, VA: NAMI Press.

*National Alliance for the Mentally Ill. (1998). *Consumer and family guide to schizophrenia treatment: Treatment works*. Arlington, VA: NAMI Press.

**People Magazine*. (2002, March 4).

*Peplau, H. E. (1975). Forward. In S. Smoyak (Ed.), *The psychiatric nurse as a family therapist* (p. 1x). New York: John Wiley.

Rosenfeld, E. (1990, Spring). Stigma in professional education. *Training Matters: Newsletter of NAMI Curriculum and Training Network, 5*, 2–3.

Sacher, D. (1994). *Mental health: A report of the Surgeon General*. Rockville, MD: U.S. Department of Human Services, Substance Abuse, and Mental Health Services Administration, Center for Mental Health Services, National Institutes of Health, National Institutes of Mental Health.

Secunda, V. (1997). *When madness comes home: Help and hope for the children, siblings, and partners of the mentally ill*. New York: Hyperion.

Solomon, P., & Draine, J. (1995a). Adaptive coping among family members of persons with serious mental illness. *Psychiatric Services, 46*(11), 1156–1159.

*Solomon, P., & Draine, J. (1995b). Subjective burden among family members of mentally ill adults: Relations to stress, coping and adaptation. *American Journal of Orthopsychiatry, 65*, 419–427.

Tarbutton, L. (personal communication, July 12, 2001).

*Taylor, C. M. (1996). Change [Editorial]. *Archives of Psychiatric Nursing, 10*(3), 127–128.

Teisher, H. G. (February 12, 2002) personal communication.

*Terkelsen, K. (1987). The meaning of mental illness to the family. In A. Hatfield & H. Lefley (Eds.), *Families of the mentally ill: Coping and adaptation* (p. 128). New York: Guilford Press.

*Tessler, R., & Gamache, G. (2000). *Family experiences with mental illness*. Westport, CT: Auburn House.

*Tolbert, E. (1980). *The mentally ill are coming back to town*. Unpublished manuscript.

*Torrey, E. F. (1989). *Nowhere to go: The tragic odyssey of the homeless mentally ill*. New York: Harper & Row.

*Torrey, E. F. (1995). *Surviving schizophrenia: A manual for families, consumers, and providers* (3rd ed.). New York: Harper & Row.

*Tuck, I., duMont, P., Evans, G., & Shupe, J. (1997). The experience of caring for an adult child with schizophrenia. *Archives of Psychiatric Nursing, 11*(3), 118–125.

Walsh, M. (1985). *Schizophrenia: Straight talk for family and friends*. New York: Warner Books.

**The Washington Post*. [Editorial]. (2001, December 18).

*Wasow, M. (1995). *The skipping stone: Ripple effects of mental illness on the family*. Palo Alto, CA: Science and Behavior Books.

*Willick, M. S. (1994). Schizophrenia: A parent's perspective—mourning without end. In N. C. Andreasen (Ed.), *Schizophrenia: From mind to molecule* (pp. 5–18). Washington, DC: American Psychiatric Press.

**Starred references are cited in text.*

▼ RESOURCES

Depressive/Manic Depressive Association (DMDA), 730 N. Franklin Street, Suite 501, Chicago, IL; telephone: 1-800-826-3632. The mission of DMDA is to educate clients, families, professionals, and the public concerning the nature of depressive and manic-depressive illnesses as treatable medical diseases; to foster self-help for patients and families; to eliminate discrimination and stigma; to improve access to care; and to advocate for research toward the elimination of these illnesses.

The Nation's Voice on Mental Illness (NAMI), formerly the National Alliance for the Mentally Ill, Colonial Place Three, 2107 Wilson Blvd., Suite 300, Arlington, VA

22201-3042; telephone: 703-524-7600. NAMI's mission is to eradicate mental illness and to improve the lives of persons with serious mental illnesses (brain disorders) and their families.

For additional information on this chapter, go to *http://connection. lww.com.*

Need more help? See Chapter 10 of the *Study Guide to Accompany Mohr: Johnson's Psychiatric-Mental Health Nursing,* 5th edition.

Working With Special Environments: Forensic Clients, Crisis Intervention, and the Homeless

CINDY A. PETERNELJ-TAYLOR, ANITA G. HUFFT, PHYLLIS M. CONNOLLY, AND KAY PETERSON

▼ KEY TERMS

Adventitious crisis—A crisis precipitated by an unexpected event (eg, natural disasters, bombings, mass shootings).

Crisis intervention—Methods and techniques used to assist a person in distress to resolve the immediate problem and regain emotional equilibrium.

Expressive violence—Interpersonal violence, usually between people known to one another and of similar age, ethnicity, and cultural background.

Gang violence—Violence associated with group membership and committed for retaliation or revenge (Labecki, 1994; Sigler, 1995).

Instrumental violence—Violent acts that usually are premeditated and motive driven (frequently, economic gain), usually involving people unknown to one another.

Maturational or developmental crisis—A crisis precipitated by the normal stress of development.

Situational crisis—A crisis precipitated by a sudden traumatic event (eg, job loss).

▼ LEARNING OBJECTIVES

On completion of this chapter, you should be able to accomplish the following:

- Describe the nurse's role in the forensic milieu.
- Describe characteristics of and health concerns specific to the forensic population, addressing implications for nursing care.
- Apply the nursing process to care of clients in forensic settings.
- Discuss the development phases of crisis theory.
- Differentiate maturational, situational, and adventitious crises.
- Discuss the goals and methods of crisis intervention.
- Apply the nursing process to a client or family in crisis.
- Discuss crisis intervention as a component of case management, psychosocial rehabilitation, and managed care.
- Identify current trends in the homeless population.
- Discuss factors that contribute to homelessness in the mentally ill population.
- Discuss barriers that prevent homeless mentally ill persons from receiving care and measures to promote their access.
- Describe specific healthcare concerns of homeless mentally ill people.
- Apply the nursing process to the care of homeless mentally ill clients.

This chapter describes how nurses provide psychiatric-mental healthcare in special contexts: within the criminal justice system, to clients in the midst of various crises, and to clients who are homeless. The needs of these clients are special, but the goal of quality and effective nursing care always remains the same. Clients in these situations have extraordinarily varied and complex mental health needs; assisting them to reach their potential is a challenging and rewarding nursing experience. Discussions focus on descriptions of the populations served, influential social and cultural factors, particular needs, and application of the nursing process.

FORENSIC NURSING

Forensic psychiatric nursing is an exciting, challenging, and developing specialty area of nursing practice. Influenced in part by the public's growing awareness of the overlap between the criminal justice and mental health systems, forensic psychiatric nursing is a rapidly growing field in Britain, Canada, and the United States. Nurses working with offenders share distinct and common concerns about legal, ethical, political, administrative, and professional issues. These concerns, and the professional nursing response dictated by them, have strengthened the designation of forensic nursing as a specialty (Hufft, 2000; Mercer, Mason, McKeown, & McCann, 2000; Peternelj-Taylor, 2000).

The terminology used to describe nursing with forensic populations has varied over the years and generally is linked to the setting in which the nurse is employed. *Forensic nursing, jail nursing, prison nursing, correctional nursing,* and *forensic psychiatric nursing* all have been used (sometimes interchangeably). To clarify the scope of forensic nursing practice, the International Association of Forensic Nurses (IAFN), founded in 1992, has defined the role of the forensic nurse more globally to include nurses working with victims, perpetrators, and their families (IAFN & American Nurses Association [ANA], 1997). Clarification of the forensic nursing role depends not only on what the nurse does (role expectations) but also on where the nurse works (role setting) (Hufft, 2000). Subspecialties identified by the IAFN are identified in Box 11-1.

In this chapter, forensic psychiatric nurses integrate psychiatric-mental health nursing philosophy and practice within a sociocultural context that includes the criminal justice system to provide comprehensive care to clients, their families, and communities. How the nurse's role is defined may restrict or enlarge his or her image and potential influence within the forensic setting and the community at large.

As crime and violence continue to escalate, all psychiatric nurses, regardless of setting, will need forensic knowledge and skills. Crime transcends individual and family boundaries and must be viewed as a societal problem (see Chaps. 17 and 26). Therefore, principles of psychiatric nursing are applicable to any setting in which criminal behavior and mental health problems occur (Burrow, 1995; Hufft & Peternelj-Taylor, 2000; Lynch & Burgess, 1998).

Forensic Settings

The care and management of the criminal offender with a psychiatric disorder challenges the collective wisdom of both the criminal justice system and the mental health system. Enduring contradictions about how to best meet the needs of the forensic population prevail. Today's settings for forensic psychiatric nursing are many and varied. This diversity includes a continuum of controlled environments that may be part of the mental health system, criminal justice system, or both. Osborne reminds us "that in these times of radical capitalism and individualism, there is a blurring of the mission of corrections and mental health facilities" (1995, p.5).

Forensic settings include those based in the community, secure units within general hospitals, state psychiatric hospitals, hospitals for the "criminally insane," and custodial-type settings such as young offender facilities, jails, and prisons (ANA, 1995; Goldkuhle, 1999; Peternelj-Taylor & Johnson, 1995; Scheela, 1999). It is common for nurses practicing in different jurisdictions to experience differences in roles, expectations, physical resources, and clinical and professional boundaries (Hufft, 2000).

Factors Contributing to Incarceration

Currently, the United States has the highest rate of incarceration in the Western world. In 1997, 1.7 million men and women were in U.S. jails and prisons (Vitucci, 1999c). Many factors contribute to the burgeoning forensic population, including increased illegal drug-related activities, increased interpersonal and urban violence, anticrime legislation, poor economic conditions and associated homelessness (discussed later in this chapter), and, perhaps most tragically, the "criminalization of the mentally ill" (Hufft & Fawkes, 1994). This criminalization is a direct result of the deinstitutionalization movement that began in the 1960s, reached its peak in the 1970s, and continues today (see Chaps. 1 and 10). Unfortunately, the ongoing lack of community-based services for the needs of chronically mentally ill clients has resulted in a fragmented mental healthcare system. Many people cannot access appropriate treatment and ultimately experience a "revolving door syndrome" that includes courts, jails, and prisons (Milestone, 1995; Peternelj-Taylor, 2000). Currently, U.S. correctional facilities house more mentally ill people than do hospitals and mental institutions; 210,000 severely mentally ill people are in jails or prisons, whereas approximately 70,000 are

---

BOX 11-1 ▼ IAFN *Subspecialties of Forensic Nursing*

- Forensic nursing educators/consultants
- Nurse coroners
- Death investigators
- Legal nurse consultants
- Nurse attorneys
- Clinical nursing specialists in trauma, transplant, and critical care
- Forensic pediatric nurses
- Forensic gerontological nurses
- Forensic psychiatric nurses
- Forensic correctional nurses

From the International Association of Forensic Nurses (IAFN), & the American Nurses Association. (1997). *Scope and standards of forensic nursing practice*. Washington, DC: American Nurses Association.

receiving treatment in public psychiatric facilities. Of those in public facilities, almost 30% are forensic clients (Hufft, 2000; Vitucci, 1999b). It is not surprising that Reeder and Meldman conclude that "the jail has become the mental hospital that can't say no" (1991, p. 41).

Characteristics of the Forensic Population

Forensic clients present with complex and multifaceted issues that are further complicated by environmental and social factors unique to the forensic milieu. Love and Hunter conclude that "the commingling of severe and persistent mental illness with criminality poses vexing clinical challenges and complex moral dilemmas not faced in either general psychiatric or correctional environments" (1999, p. 35). Factors to consider when working with forensic populations include prevalence of mental disorder, cultural and demographic variations, and the needs of special at-risk groups.

Generally, forensic clients demonstrate poor judgment, limited reasoning abilities, and a history of not learning from past mistakes (Hufft & Peternelj-Taylor, 2000). They also report an exceptionally high level of substance abuse. Estimates are that drug offenders represent 60% of the federal prison population (Vitucci, 1999a). People addicted to drugs or alcohol are at increased risk for mental illness (see Chap. 27). Accompanying behavior patterns include depression, suicidal ideation, aggressiveness, and irritability (Sowers, Thompson, & Mullins, 1999).

The inaccurate caricature of the mentally ill offender as a crazed psychotic killer, however, has adversely influenced effective treatment planning for the forensic population. Depending on the setting, jurisdiction, location, and facilities available, the population may include suspects or those convicted of crimes, those who are sentenced or unsentenced, those who are not guilty by reason of insanity or are incompetent to stand trial, and those not criminally responsible as a result of a mental disorder. Because of this wide variation, nurses must be aware of the laws and legal provisions governing the jurisdiction in which they work.

MENTALLY ILL OFFENDERS

In forensic psychiatric nursing, the predominant client group is composed of those with psychiatric disorders. The research suggests that, in any prison or jail population, up to 20% of those incarcerated will be designated as having a mental disorder, requiring the services usually associated with severe or chronic mental illness (Peternelj-Taylor, 2000; Peternelj-Taylor & Johnson, 1995; Sowers et al., 1999; Vitucci, 1999b). As a rule, schizophrenia, mood disorders, and organic syndromes with psychotic features are common. Psychotic presentations often are complicated by

the coexistence of personality disorders, substance abuse, or both; many clients self-medicate with drugs and alcohol (Peternelj-Taylor & Johnson, 1995).

The young age of most mentally ill clients in prisons presents a set of characteristics distinct from other settings and contributes to the special nature of forensic psychiatric nursing. This subgroup is characterized by illicit drug use, a history of dropping out of treatment, violence, and resistance to viewing themselves as mentally ill. In addition to those with mental disorders, many offenders present with mental health problems associated with a criminalized lifestyle: substance abuse, violence, and aggression (manifested in domestic and sexual violence) are among the most common (Kent-Wilkinson, 1999; Schafer, 1999; Schafer & Peternelj-Taylor, 2000; Scheela, 1999) (see Chaps. 26 and 27).

▼ Clinical Example 11-1

Edmond, 42 years old, has had a long history of antisocial behavior, coupled with long-standing difficulties getting along with others. His father was an alcoholic who often was verbally and physically abusive. Edmond had many difficulties with schoolwork and had to repeat fourth grade. When Edmond was 11 years of age, the courts ordered him to spend time in a closed-custody facility for juveniles because his parents could not provide the supervision he required. Feelings of anger and hatred quickly replaced initial feelings of loss. Reports indicate that Edmond had a "short fuse" and responded to others with physical aggression.

On release from the juvenile facility, Edmond cut off all communication with family members and felt some satisfaction that he was inflicting his pain and loss on them. He moved from foster home to foster home, primarily because of his acting-out behavior. His problems with school continued; eventually, he ran away to a large city far from his home. With no education or job skills, he quickly became involved in robbery, drugs, and prostitution. He blamed the world for his problems, lashing out at those who tried to get close to him. He experienced a great sadness, but could not cry.

In his late teens, Edmond found himself in an experimental treatment group after an involuntary admission to a psychiatric facility. The material presented in this group was far beyond his level of comprehension. A controlling coping style soon replaced his feelings of powerlessness. After treatment, Edmond further isolated himself from others. He began to drink heavily and take drugs to numb and self-medicate his depressive symptoms. His thoughts became increasingly irrational, and he believed that the only way to deal with his feelings of vulnerability was to hurt others before they could hurt him.

By 20 years of age, Edmond's interpersonal difficulties, coupled with a serious substance abuse problem, culminated in an indefinite sentence for a murder of which he had no recollection. Initially, he had no feelings about serving time. Two years passed before he began to question his future and despise his situation. He made numerous suicide and self-mutilation attempts of which his scarred body constantly reminds him. He lived one day at a time; his formula for success was morphine and opiates. Drugs gave Edmond a sense of power and control. He sold drugs to make money in prison, which, in turn, gave him a sense of power. He usually was "high" on something, which gave him a temporary sense of control over his emotions and environment. He began to realize that he had feelings of depression and turned to the healthcare center for prescribed antidepressants. When medication failed to "solve all his problems," he turned to illicit substances for a temporary fix. He was in a vicious cycle of drugs, depression, and detoxification.

After 20 years in prison, Edmond states he has matured and is ready to lead a more prosocial lifestyle. He has entered a specialized treatment program designed to deal with dual diagnosis and is beginning to deal with some of the feelings he has ignored for most of his life. He states that he will never be able to forgive himself for what he has done to himself and those around him, particularly the victim of his crime.

Points for Reflection and Critical Thinking

- What do you think is Edmond's most immediate problem?
- In counseling Edmond, what issues or problems might the therapist encounter?
- What factors make the care of this client different from other clients with depression?

Tracy Edmonds, RN, Staff Nurse, Regional Psychiatric Centre, Correctional Service of Canada, Saskatoon, Saskatchewan.

VIOLENT OFFENDERS

Studies of violence in prison populations reveal two major categories of violent offenders: those with expressive violence and those with instrumental violence. **Expressive violence** involves interpersonal altercations, usually with people known to the assailant and of similar age, ethnicity, and cultural background. **Instrumental violence** involves acts that usually are premeditated and motive driven (frequently, economic gain). It usually involves people unknown to one another. A third type of emerging violence is **gang violence**, which is associated with group membership and is committed for retaliation or revenge (Labecki, 1994; Sigler, 1995). Group alliances lead to gang violence; typical victims are sexual offenders, those who have hurt children, and those with mental illness and or physical and mental handicaps.

In forensic settings, nurses work with clients with a proven capacity for violence. Although staff injuries generally are rare, violence is considered an occupational

hazard (Hufft & Fawkes, 1994; Peternelj-Taylor & Johnson, 1995). Safety is a frequent topic of discussion with forensic clients, whether it be the preservation of personal safety, institutional safety (including clients), or community safety. Atascadero State Hospital, a 1000-bed, all-male maximum-security institution has maintained a novel violence-prevention alliance between clinical staff and the client government for several years. Since implementing the project, the number of aggressive special incident reports and staff injuries from inpatient violence has been reduced by more than 50%. This is partly the result of the involvement of the client government in violence-prevention programs (and subsequent understanding of the client's perspective) and the commitment to a norm of nonviolence that both staff and clients support (Love & Hunter, 1999).

SPECIAL POPULATIONS

In general, populations with special needs include juveniles, women, older adults, ethnic and racial minorities, clients with HIV, AIDS, and hepatitis A and B. When working with these clients, mental health professionals must relate to the population's unique needs and concerns in addition to the facility's mission or mandate.

Juvenile Offenders

Increasing numbers of juvenile offenders are being retained in jails and prisons, requiring special services to meet their needs related to growth and development, education, and special health concerns. The overcrowding in the prison system, along with the increased number of violent teen offenders, has resulted in the detainment of many young people in facilities designed only for adults. Referral to mental health services is high among this population (Kemph, Braley, & Ciotola, 1998).

Female Offenders

One of the most dramatic changes in the forensic population in the last few decades is the increased number of incarcerated women. Trends among female offenders indicate increased incidences of personality disorders, substance abuse, and post-traumatic stress disorder (Research in Psychiatric-Mental Health Nursing 11-1). Often, these offenders are both victims and perpetrators of crime, having experienced physical, emotional, and sexual abuse (Hufft, 2000; Maeve, 1997).

Older Adult Offenders

The increased "graying population" in many facilities has resulted in the need for special adaptations to accommodate these older adults. Smyer, Gragert, and LaMere (1997) report that the aging population is special in terms of criminal patterns, healthcare needs, problems in adjustment to institutional life, and problems related to family relationships. These factors pose special difficulties to the prison system, particularly related to custody, rehabilita-

Research in Psychiatric-Mental Health Nursing 11-1
LIFE EVENTS AND PSYCHOSOCIAL WELL-BEING IN WOMEN SENTENCED TO PRISON

Purpose: To identify stressful life events experienced by women in the 12 months before incarceration and to examine the relationship between life events and their effects on psychological well-being (indicated by the absence of anxiety and depression)

Background: Historically, little research has been done to define the characteristics and special circumstances of women in prison. Little is known about their lives before imprisonment. Moreover, empirical evidence of the psychological well-being of women who have been convicted of felonies, are housed in general population, and have not been preselected for psychiatric care is lacking. Recidivism rates in female offenders are estimated to be one in every three offenders, thus supporting the significance of this study.

Method and Sample: The researchers conducted a descriptive correlational study in a large correctional facility for female offenders. A convenience sample of 62 sentenced women, who were imprisoned for at least 1 week, participated. The researchers obtained informed consent. Several instruments were used: (1) the Coping Resource Questionnaire designed to collect descriptive data on each woman's demographic profile, social support systems, and financial support; (2) the Social Readjustment Scale, which addresses the occurrence and frequency of 43 life events in the 12 months preceding incarceration; (3) the State-Trait Anxiety Inventory, which measures current feelings of anxiety; and (4) the Center for Epidemiological Studies Depression Scale, which addresses components of affective distress and is useful as an initial screening tool for depression.

Findings: Most women in the study were young (average age, 32 years), white, and single. They had limited education, were unemployed, and were receiving financial assistance. The findings indicate that the women experienced multiple life events characterized by loss in the 12 months preceding incarceration (family-related events, health-related events, and work-related events) that affected their psychological well-being. Nearly 90% of the participants had seriously high levels of anxiety and depressive symptomatology, a rate significantly higher than nonincarcerated women. A positive correlation between the number of life events and depression was identified ($r = .24$, $P < .05$).

Application to Nursing Practice: When the client is admitted, nurses should incorporate assessments that address the major and minor life events that clients experience in the year before incarceration. The high level of depression found in this population is particularly noteworthy. The researchers recommend that nurses direct interventions (focusing on individual strengths) at reducing psychological distress at the time of admission because this may reduce the feelings of loss, inadequacy, and powerlessness that the women might otherwise have to endure.

From Keaveny, M. E., & Zauszniewski, J. A. (1999). Life events and psychological well-being in women sentenced to prison. *Issues in Mental Health Nursing, 20,* 73–89.

tion, and parole. In many ways, older clients in forensic settings are no different from their counterparts in the general public and have many life issues (complicated by the correctional milieu) to address (see Chap. 30). In addition to problems with mental health, they also are more prone to the debilitating effects of chronic illness and often require more services for physical illnesses.

Minority Offenders

Clients from ethnic and racial minorities are disproportionately represented in most North American forensic facilities. Specific ethnic groups may predominate, and traditional psychiatric practices often are incompatible with cultural beliefs. Healthcare providers must consider cultural implications when providing mental healthcare. The failure by client and staff to recognize and respond appropriately to differences creates tension, with the potential to disrupt therapeutic relationships, cultivate stressful environments, and instigate violence (duPont & Halasz, 1998).

In many ways, the nature of client concerns in the forensic milieu is no different than those in more traditional healthcare settings. The effects of the controlled environment, however, can create many barriers to care. Nurses must be cognizant of the problems unique to the clients with whom they work (see Chap. 5).

Offenders With HIV, AIDS, or Hepatitis

Issues related to HIV and AIDS are not only controversial, but also challenging to the administrative and clinical management in forensic settings. The incidence of HIV, AIDS, and hepatitis B and C are higher in the forensic population than in the general population, primarily as a result of the high-risk behaviors demonstrated by many in the forensic population, such as tattooing, ear and body piercing, risky sexual activity, and using intravenous (IV) drugs (Goldkuhle, 1999). Increasing the availability of condoms, bleach, and needle exchange programs are recommended harm-reduction strategies; unfortunately, policies vary greatly regarding these recommendations and are not the norm in many jurisdictions. Palliative care for clients with HIV and AIDS in prison settings is a growing trend, particularly in areas that prohibit early release for compassionate reasons.

Effects of Incarceration on Mental Health

In addition to offenders who enter the correctional system with a mental disorder, forensic psychiatric nurses care for people who become mentally ill while incarcerated. All forensic clients are affected by the conditions in which they live every day. Creating a healing therapeutic environment in a forensic setting is a challenge. The physical setting, client population, and authoritarian interpersonal environment result in forensic settings being identified as the most extreme and stressful known to society (Doyle, 1998; Hufft & Fawkes, 1994; Peternelj-Taylor & Johnson, 1995). Box 11-2 summarizes stressors in the forensic setting.

Clients with chronic mental illnesses, mental retardation, brain injuries, or decreased social skills or physical strength often are cruelly abused by other offenders (especially among the male population) and endure torment, beatings, and sexual assault. The safety of those belonging to these vulnerable populations presents ongoing dilemmas

---

BOX 11-2 ▼ *Common Stressors to Mental Health in Secure Environments*

Stressors That Affect the Client

- Overcrowding
- Double stigmatization
- Grief, isolation, loneliness
- Gang violence
- Institutional violence: stabbing, beating, sexual assault
- Deteriorating living conditions
- Lack of privacy
- Protective custody
- Segregation

Stressors That Affect the Nurse

- Actual or implied threats of violence
- Constant barrage of swearing
- Need to be constantly on guard against manipulation
- Dual responsibility of providing custody and caring
- Role confusion and ambiguity
- Professional isolation
- Stigma of "second class nurse"
- Institutionalization

---

for administrators, who often find it necessary to confine them to protective custody units. Unfortunately, this can be counterproductive, leading to further decompensation of the client's mental illness (Peternelj-Taylor & Johnson, 1995).

Characteristics of Forensic Psychiatric Nurses

Regardless of the practice setting, nurses who specialize in forensic psychiatric nursing have dual obligations: one of social necessity and social good, and one of custody and caring. This debate is framed by doing what is beneficial for the community versus advocating for what is most therapeutic for the client. Comprehending and confronting this paradox is essential to the provision of good care in settings devoted to social necessity (custody). The ramifications of this paradox are at best perplexing, if not disconcerting, and forensic psychiatric nurses often feel torn between the needs of society and the needs of their clients. This is not surprising since the distinction between social necessity and social good is not always easy to discern (Osborne, 1995; Peternelj-Taylor, 1999).

Forensic psychiatric nurses frequently experience role ambiguity and role confusion, often because of these overlapping and conflicting expectations. They must maintain security standards to provide a safe working environment for staff and clients. Thus, they spend much time attending to issues related to the therapeutic milieu and security. This dual responsibility can lead to increased self-esteem and accomplishment for nurses who master the inherent dilemmas between the two philosophies and achieve professional resolution and personal understanding. More commonly, however, nurses perceive this as a source of stress and role conflict (Hufft, 2000; Hufft & Fawkes, 1994; Peternelj-Taylor & Johnson, 1995).

In response to the growing number of nurses working in correctional settings and to guide professional nursing practice, the ANA first published *Standards of Nursing Practice in Correctional Facilities* in 1985. Revised 10 years later (ANA, 1995), these standards clearly delineate the nurse's role within the realm of healthcare. The biggest challenge to nurses working within the forensic setting is to remain true to the nursing role and to avoid the seduction of institutionalization and the pull toward the custodial role, where expectations and responsibilities may be more clearly defined (Maeve, 1997; Peternelj-Taylor & Johnson, 1995).

ATTITUDES

Forensic psychiatric nurses care for a frequently stigmatized and stereotyped population. Negative attitudes that nurses hold toward offenders inhibit the entire nurse–client relationship. Psychiatric mental health nurses traditionally have based their practice on the concept of caring. This commitment does not change when those receiving care are in correctional settings (Anonymous, 1995; Maeve, 1997).

When the client is in a forensic setting, the nurse's affective response may be intensified and can be influenced by the client's mental health background and criminal history. Mercer, Mason, and Richman (1999) studied the structural and linguistic contradictions of treatment and punishment as they affect those on the secure psychiatric ward. Results support the notion that a caregiver response is more likely when caregivers perceive forensic clients to be mentally ill (psychotic) versus evil (psychopaths). Assessing and exploring common preconceptions, beliefs, and stereotypes (eg, "criminally insane") help forensic psychiatric nurses to decrease potential fears, anxieties, and negative attitudes. Participating in a tour, interacting with a client, or observing an experienced nurse in practice are ways to confront thoughts and feelings, verify reality, and overcome natural apprehension to working with incarcerated clients (Hufft & Peternelj-Taylor, 2000; Peternelj-Taylor & Johnson, 1996).

Ongoing self-reflection and self-awareness are essential to successful adaptation (Peternelj-Taylor, 1998; Peternelj-Taylor & Johnson, 1995). Being able to adopt the therapeutic role requires the nurse to "transcend judgmental and prejudicial attitudes toward those who have committed crimes against society" (Hufft & Fawkes, 1994, p. 39). Nurses should reflect on the following questions:

- What has motivated my decision to work in forensic psychiatric nursing?
- What are my feelings about heinous violent crimes such as murder and sexual assault? Can I put my feelings aside, see beyond the crime, and care for the person who has committed such crimes?
- How would I respond to questions like "How can you care for them?" "Why don't you just lock the door and throw away the key?"
- Can I work in an area where professional roles and responsibilities are not clearly defined, particularly as this relates to balancing the custodial and caring roles?

SKILLS

Not all nurses are suited for the forensic environment, nor is it appropriate to place all student nurses in such a setting. Those working in forensic institutions must have good communication skills, be able to work within a team structure, and possess physical and psychological assessment skills. Furthermore, social maturity, adaptability, professionalism, and analytical skills are critical. Other essential attributes include confidence, nonjudgmental attitudes, ability to work independently, decisiveness, and ability to work in a secure environment while applying nursing knowledge to decisions about client care. Educa-

tional facilities and forensic agencies favorably view personal characteristics such as stability, integrity, assertiveness, maturity, and friendliness (Hufft & Peternelj-Taylor, 2000; Peternelj-Taylor & Johnson, 1996).

Unfortunately, not all people believe that forensic clients have the potential for change and the right to treatment. Nurses who are most successful in mastering the complexities of the forensic psychiatric nursing role are those who view clients as people who deserve respect and professional care, believe that people can be rehabilitated, and see their role as caregiving (Hufft & Peternelj-Taylor, 2000; Schafer, 1999; Schafer & Peternelj-Taylor, 2000). See Box 11-3.

APPLICATION OF THE NURSING PROCESS TO THE FORENSIC CLIENT

In forensic settings, the effects of the distinctive environment modify the essence of nursing. Special adaptations

---

BOX 11-3 ▼ *Levels of Prevention in Forensic Settings*

Primary Prevention

Mental health promotion
Classification of stressors
Political involvement
Appropriate referrals
Provision of education and information
Advocacy

Secondary Prevention

Assessment, evaluation, diagnosis
Crisis intervention
Program planning and implementation
Substance abuse treatment
Sex offender treatment
Aggressive behavior control
Life and social skills training
Acute inpatient psychiatric nursing
Suicide prevention and management
Short-term therapy
Counseling, psychotherapy

Tertiary Intervention

Case management
After-care services
Rehabilitation
Vocational training
Relapse prevention

are necessary to achieve professional standards and personal goals.

Assessment

All forensic psychiatric nurses, regardless of setting, have a significant role to play in the observation and assessment of the forensic client. The context of care can facilitate or hamper the nurse's ability to provide the necessary services for mentally ill offenders. Marx (1995) reports problems related to assessing clients in isolation of their support systems, home environments, and daily routines because in the forensic setting, the client is closely supervised, and institutional policies restrict and mandate his or her behavior. The physical environment and lack of privacy further complicate assessment and diagnosis. Security concerns affect every aspect of forensic psychiatric nursing practice and can complicate the creation of a therapeutic relationship. Often, interview rooms are completely glassed in to allow for maximum observation of the nurse who is conducting the assessment. These rooms are soundproof, but all can see inside, violating the right to privacy and confidentiality that is common to the psychiatric nurse–client relationship (yet vital to security). Many clients may not want to be identified with the forensic psychiatric nurse because of the stigma associated with mental illness (Peternelj-Taylor & Johnson, 1995). At times, correctional personnel are required to be present, and this further complicates the assessment process because clients are reluctant to disclose information to security personnel.

CONTENT

Correctional facilities include mental health questions as part of receiving, screening, and conducting follow-up for every offender. Comprehensive assessments help to identify the client's needs, particularly those requiring immediate attention. Additionally, a separate mental health screening and evaluation process is performed on all admissions to mental health facilities or treatment centers to identify level of functioning and to uncover less obvious mental conditions (Vitucci, 1999a, 1999b; Welch & Ogloff, 1998).

Critical information needed to plan nursing care with forensic clients often includes police reports, correctional files, and previous mental health records. Crime histories and history of aggression also are essential (Schafer & Peternelj-Taylor, 2000). Assessments should include a history of psychiatric illness, hospitalization and outpatient treatment, current psychotropic medication, suicidal ideation, self-mutilating behavior, risk assessment, and drug and alcohol use. Nurses need to be alert to assessing substance use because many clients continue to abuse substances while hospitalized or incarcerated. Focused in-depth assessments are conducted on clients admitted for special programming, for example, sexual offenders, psychopathic

offenders, and clients with anger management disorders or intermittent explosive disorder (Schafer, 1999; Schafer & Peternelj-Taylor, 2000; Welch & Ogloff, 1998).

RISK OF SUICIDE

The incidence of self-violence and suicide in forensic settings is higher than that in the general population, with the suicide rate for people in custody at least six times that of the general population. Strict guidelines for accurate and timely assessment of suicide risk are imperative. Unrestricted access to psychiatric care must be available for any offender presenting with suicidal ideation or at-risk behaviors (Burrow, 1995).

Factors contributing to the significantly higher rate of suicide in the forensic population include history of a psychiatric illness, substance abuse, difficulties facing the crime and the length of the sentence, actual or perceived victimization by other offenders, inability to cope within a confined environment, and lack of communication with family (Burrow, 1995). Green, Andre, Kendall, Looman, and Polvi (1992) observe that, regardless of the length of the sentence, the first 6 months after sentencing represents a particularly high-risk period.

Suicide (or attempted suicide) in the forensic setting must be followed by a full debriefing. Forensic psychiatric nurses have a role to play as facilitators and can provide leadership for group processing of the event. They use critical incident stress management to minimize adverse effects of stressful or traumatic events such as inmate disorders, riots, and suicide by teaming mental health professionals and trained lay persons to debrief and manage incidents. The National Correctional Health Care Commission (1998) has added this successful process to its accreditation standards for postsuicide care.

Nursing Diagnosis

The common North American Nursing Diagnosis Association diagnoses relevant to the forensic population include Ineffective Coping, Fear, Dysfunctional Grieving, Noncompliance, Chronic Low Self-Esteem, Risk for Self-Mutilation, Disturbed Sleep Pattern, Impaired Social Interaction, Social Isolation, and Risk for Violence: Self-Directed or Directed at Others. As with all clients, however, the nurse uses the assessment data to formulate nursing diagnoses and a plan of care that meet each client's particular needs.

Planning

In planning any treatment program with a forensic client, the nurse considers the realities and limitations of the setting. Working knowledge of the inmate subculture and the operation and culture of secure or controlled environments is essential (Peternelj-Taylor & Johnson, 1995).

Planning short-term goals, which frequently involve completion of tasks and practice of selected communication or self-care skills, must revolve around the mandatory regimens set up for the offender. In many settings, therapy is in conflict with the realities of the structured environment, which includes work details, lock-ups, formal counting of offenders, and endless security procedures. Nevertheless, manageable, feasible goals must be set up to achieve outcomes that bring the offender to a higher level of functioning, regardless of the environment. The challenge to the forensic nurse is to be sensitive to scheduled assignments that can be changed and those that cannot. Planning also requires attention to the processes that allow for continuity. It is typical for clients to be transferred from facility to facility, often without their health records. When possible, planning should include the client's active participation in the identification of realistic and attainable goals.

Long-term goals must be consistent with the reality of the client's circumstances. It is unrealistic to plan for reentry to the community for a client at the beginning of a life sentence. Often, it is important to acknowledge that long-term goals, such as developing trusting relationships with peers and staff, may be unrealistic.

Implementation

The ability to establish a therapeutic relationship with a forensic client is one of the most important competencies needed by nurses working in forensic settings. Therapy issues can be stressful and complicated, and the effects of the forensic milieu on both nurses and clients cannot be ignored. Cultural and ideological variations among correctional personnel, forensic clients, and helping professionals must be considered when navigating the counseling role in the forensic milieu (Peternelj-Taylor & Johnson, 1995).

Recurring themes of power and control, negotiation, and trust building dominate therapeutic interventions in this setting; clients have, in varying degrees, learned to adapt to an environment that rewards distrust, manipulation, and deceit (Allen & Bosta, 1993; Peternelj-Taylor & Johnson, 1995; Peternelj-Taylor, 1990). The criminal history, the frequent diagnoses of antisocial and borderline personality disorder, and the aggressive interpersonal style of many forensic clients can evoke strong emotional responses, and countertransference and splitting reactions are common. Most would agree that diverse opinions make for a resource-rich team; however, when emotional reactions mix with sound clinical judgment, team members may become polarized, which negatively affects the overall integrity of therapeutic interventions (Schafer, 1999; Schafer & Peternelj-Taylor, 2000).

Establishing and maintaining boundaries of the professional nurse–client relationship clearly are an issue. The familiarity and trust that develops over time, coupled with the seductive pull of helping, can contribute to nurses becoming overly involved in their work, which also may erode therapeutic boundaries. Nurses have been known to transgress the boundaries of the professional relationship and become intimately involved with their clients, a phenomenon that Peternelj-Taylor (1998) refers to as forbidden love. The intensity of the forensic environment contributes to this immediate risk because institutions are considered "hotbeds" for potential problems. Sexual dilemmas must be considered an occupational hazard and not a social and professional taboo (Peternelj-Taylor, 1998; Peternelj-Taylor & Johnson, 1995).

Often, students and novice nurses have a hard time dealing with sexually explicit remarks or compliments made by forensic clients. Instead of acknowledging the compliment or confronting the behavior, they withdraw. This is particularly problematic because most forensic clients interpret silence as approval, which can lead to more brazen compliments and behaviors. Allen and Bosta (1993) observe that a simple "thank you" (generally accompanied by a blush) is not sufficient to get the message across to a client. A more appropriate response is recommended: "Thank you for the compliment, but I would appreciate that from this point on you keep your comments to yourself. Your remarks are irrelevant to my purpose with working with you." The nurse must confront any inappropriate responses verbally (eg, "I'm not here to discuss my eyes, hair, or body") followed by documentation in the client's chart. Strategies for boundary maintenance are presented in Implications for Nursing Practice 11-1.

PROMOTING HEALTH

Forensic nursing includes health promotion. Unfortunately, fiscal constraints cause nurses to be increasingly preoccupied with acute care. Defining and delineating the problems experienced by many clients in the forensic setting is one way to target resources while providing a comprehensive health-promotion program (Goldkuhle, 1999). Women offenders, in particular, are interested in their own health, and a discussion about contraception and birth control can be an opportunity to express feelings related to abuse, powerlessness, or social awkwardness (Sowers et al., 1999).

Nurses in forensic settings also are responsible for mental health and wellness promotion. Stress management is not just a health-promotion strategy in the forensic setting, it is a real life skill. Programs that promote adaptation and coping in selected situations may translate into life skills that allow for more effective rehabilitation. Nevertheless, nurses must be aware that improving opportunities for the highest level of physical, psychosocial, and social functioning puts clients in a "catch 22" position because the skills

Implications for Nursing Practice 11-1

Personal Boundary Maintenance Strategies

Be aware of red flags such as:

- "You are such a good nurse."
- "You are the only one who understands me."
- "I would never have gotten into trouble if I had someone like you in my life."

Clients may use such comments to split an individual member apart from the rest of the team, hoping that the nurse will regard the relationship as special or unique. Proceed with caution.

Do not seek to satisfy social needs. Do not seek friendships with or become dependent on clients to meet your social needs. Have a good, intact, and separate social life.

Avoid inappropriate self-disclosure. Therapeutic self-disclosure requires thoughtful consideration. A therapeutic goal should be kept in mind. Self-disclosure frequently meets the needs of the nurse, not the client, and often leads to a role reversal.

Confront feelings of attraction. Sexual attraction is common to the human experience and is not the same as sexual exploitation. Ask yourself the following self-awareness questions:

- "What do I do when I am sexually attracted to a client, or when a client is attracted to me? How do I set the boundaries?"
- "Am I having my intimacy needs met through my relationship with clients?"
- "Would I say or do this in front of my supervisor? Colleagues? Other clients?"

Talk to trusted colleagues. Be honest with yourself regarding your feelings about clients. Talking to trusted colleagues and supervisors will assist in effective boundary maintenance. Clinical supervision is an effective way to manage feelings related to the nurse–client relationship.

to survive in prison are not the same as those required to survive on the street (Hufft, 2000; Hufft & Fawkes, 1994).

MAINTAINING AN INTERDISCIPLINARY APPROACH TO CARE

Teamwork is essential to working in forensic environments. Communication among nurses, other healthcare professionals, and the correctional personnel is vital to safe and professional practice. The cross-training required of an interdisciplinary approach to forensic health treatment requires sharing knowledge of therapeutic modalities while incorporating professional standards of practice (Hufft & Peternelj-Taylor, 2000).

Many different healthcare providers are involved in the provision of forensic mental health services, and all need to work collaboratively to deliver high-quality care consistent with the community standard. In correctional settings, the security personnel also are a part of the team, and information sharing is vital. Correctional personnel need to be informed when suicidal, homicidal, or out-of-control behavior is suspected or is of concern (Peternelj-Taylor & Johnson, 1995). Although the potential for territoriality is a reality, narrow partisan views of the role of the various team members are counterproductive to the promotion of quality care. The most successful client outcomes are achieved when team members share a common philosophy: professionalism in providing security and quality healthcare to those in custody (Doyle, 1998; Hufft, 2000; Mercer et al., 2000).

FOCUSING ON THE FAMILY

Working with forensic clients most frequently occurs apart from family and the community. Goldkuhle (1999) observes that family members, children, and friends of offenders comprise a hidden forensic population. They are seldom accounted for or discussed, yet they are linked to the total health profile of the forensic population and represent a significant portion of at-risk society. Current trends in healthcare are calling for increased access to mental health services, more emphasis on prevention, and community partnerships. To be effective, a collaborative community-based partnership model is recommended.

ENSURING CONTINUITY OF CARE

Continuity of care is nonexistent for offenders once they leave the correctional or treatment setting. Many mentally ill offenders experience high rates of recidivism, high symptom levels, and poor quality of life. Little opportunity exists for long-term case management or discharge planning for clients eventually released from prison. The life skills learned to survive in prison may conflict with therapeutic goals. It is difficult to evaluate the progress of a client with a view of returning to the community if there are no opportunities to interact with that community (Hufft & Fawkes, 1994).

Dvoskin and Broaddus (1993) propose a mental healthcare model for the efficient and systematic treatment of the mentally ill offender. This approach advocates a seamless continuum of services that includes the prison setting and satellite services within the community, linking correctional and parole staff with community mental healthcare providers. The underlying premise is that forensic settings are communities in which people live and work together under the influence of various stressors. This program, designed to address stressors as challenges to community living, provides a framework that bridges the forensic and nonforensic setting. Components include screening and referral, crisis beds, intermediate care (residential care), outpatient services, predischarge planning services, and postrelease services including mental health, probation, and parole services. Such a system would be ideal; unfortunately, funding and service restrictions make its implementation unlikely.

ACTING AS AN ADVOCATE

Traditional principles of advocacy involve informing clients of their choices and rights and then supporting their decision. In any psychiatric setting, this standard is controversial; in the forensic setting, it is inflammatory. Client actions and communications are not privileged information. Advocacy standards demand that nurses be honest with clients, informing them that disclosure of medical records is a reality and that nurse testimony may be required in any court proceeding against the client.

The advocacy role in forensic psychiatric nursing is different from the role in other settings or specialties because the nurse embraces the destigmatization and decriminalization of the client group. Rehabilitation into the public arena is difficult, particularly because of public and political antipathy toward offenders.

From a public health perspective, the state of health or illness of the correctional population is a reflection of the state of health or illness of the community at large. Nurses need to acquaint themselves with policies that affect the forensic population and the society as a whole. Multisectoral collaboration is seen as one avenue to meet the complex needs of the forensic client and includes not only health and justice, but also the social and economic sectors (Goldkuhle, 1999; Milestone, 1995; Peternelj-Taylor, 2000). Furthermore, supporting the implementation of policies that are based on well-designed research and questioning those that are based on convenience or "conventional wisdom" are appropriate political roles.

Evaluation

To assess the effectiveness of the nursing process in the forensic setting, the nurse must measure client behaviors that indicate resolution or change in the diagnostic criteria, specifically the signs and symptoms that indicated a psychiatric problem. Depending on the client's diagnosis and prognosis, the nurse learns to evaluate the client's outcome in terms of small successes, which often are "giant steps" for many clients. Change that leads the client to solve problems, to demonstrate the ability to reason and show good judgment, or to comply with the rules of the institution is a form of success (Schafer & Peternelj-Taylor, 2000).

Greenwood (1995) observes that when measuring effectiveness of treatment outcomes in the forensic setting, the healthcare professional needs to be cognizant of the definition of the forensic mental health treatment being used. The goal of mental health treatment is to address a mental disorder, whereas the goal of correctional treatment is to decrease the likelihood of recidivism. These terms are not mutually exclusive and do not always work in tandem. An individual may deal well with a mental health problem but continue to break the law.

▼ *Clinical Example* 11-2

Tanya, a 19-year-old college student living in the freshmen dormitory, has become increasingly concerned about feeling overwhelmed, is having difficulty concentrating, is confused, is not able to sleep, and deals with problems poorly. This is the second month of the semester, and a teacher recently returned her assignment as "not meeting expected academic standards." Tanya is beginning to doubt herself and her abilities to cope with college studies and college life. She cannot prioritize assignments and frequently feels confused about course assignments and due dates.

Tanya graduated in the top 10% of her high school class and always was on the honor roll. Although she looked forward to going away to college, this is her first time away from a close family. None of her classmates were accepted to the college she is attending, and she has been so busy trying to meet her academic assignments that she has not formed any close relationships on campus. Her roommate is not friendly.

Tanya phones her mother. After talking with her mother, she feels some relief. Her mother suggests that Tanya ask about counseling services on campus. Tanya does so and receives an emergency appointment at the student services counseling center.

Points for Reflection and Critical Thinking

- What might be some potential problems for Tanya if she does not seek help?
- Do you think Tanya's experience is common for people in her circumstances? What can be done to help students adjust?

NURSING CARE FOR THE CLIENT IN CRISIS

Crisis means a turning point, whether in a disease or another condition. In Chinese, two symbols communicate crisis: "danger" and "opportunity." Crisis and stress commonly are used interchangeably; however, they are not synonyms. Everyone experiences stressful life events: a new job, prematurely gray hair, the loss of a friend, the acquisition of dentures. As long as a person can cope and is not overwhelmed by stress, it is not considered a crisis. Conversely, any stressful event can precipitate a crisis, depending on the person's perceptions, coping skills, and available support systems.

During a crisis, a person is unsure what to do. Usual methods of problem solving are ineffective or unavailable. As anxiety and pain increase, the person may become more willing to try new ways of problem solving. In this willingness lies the opportunity for growth. Good mental health is thought to be predominantly the result of a life history of successful crisis resolution (Erikson, 1963). Intervention during crisis has been found to reduce the incidence and severity of mental disorders such as post-traumatic stress syndrome. There is little argument over the demand and increased need for cost-effective and well-organized crisis services the world over.

Crisis Theory

Crisis has been an issue of serious study only for the last 55 years (Historical Capsule 11-1). Caplan (1964) defines crisis as a threat to homeostasis. During crisis, an imbalance exists between the magnitude of the problem and the immediate resources available to deal with it. This imbalance causes confusion and disorganization (Caplan, 1964). The active crisis state is relatively short, approximately 4 to 6 weeks. No person can tolerate this level of anxiety and imbalance, however, for long. Quick, appropriate intervention is crucial to help the person in crisis return to an optimal state of functioning.

According to crisis theory, a person strives to maintain a constant state of emotional equilibrium. If a person is confronted with an overwhelming threat and cannot cope, crisis ensues. Crisis response is a normal, not pathologic, life experience. Because high anxiety accompanies the crisis state, the person will adapt and return to the previous state of mental heath, develop more constructive coping skills, or decompensate to a lower level of functioning.

Factors that influence the outcome of a crisis include the following:

- Previous problem-solving experience
- Perception or view of the problem
- Amount of help or hindrance from significant others
- Number and types of past crises
- Time elapsed since the last crisis (Aguilera, 1998; Hoff, 1995)

Maladaptive crisis resolution increases the probability of unsuccessful resolution of future crises. During a crisis, a person is open to receiving professional help and learning new ways of problem solving and is likely to change attitudes and behaviors quickly. Crisis intervention focuses on the problem or stressor that precipitated the crisis state rather than on personality traits. It views the person in crisis as normal and capable of problem solving and growth with assistance from others (Aguilera, 1998; Hoff, 1995).

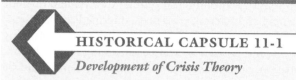

HISTORICAL CAPSULE 11-1
Development of Crisis Theory

Numerous researchers have contributed to the development of crisis theory. Lindeman (1994) studied the survivors and families of victims of the disastrous Coconut Grove nightclub fire in Boston in which many people died. Based on his observations and study of other families who had lost family members, Lindeman described the commonalties of the experience of crisis and bereavement (1994). From this classic study, he developed some basic tenets of crisis theory. Caplan (1964), who has done the most extensive work on crisis theory, was influenced by the research and writings of Lindeman, Parad, Rapaport, and Erikson. Crisis theory is derived from the psychoanalytic theory and ego psychology that stresses the human ability to learn and grow throughout life (Aguilera, 1998; Hoff, 1995).

Crisis theory emerged in an era of increased social consciousness. President John F. Kennedy passionately addressed the Congress and the nation about the need for a national health program with a new approach to mental illness, the promotion of mental health. Congress directed the establishment of a Joint Commission on Mental Illness and Health, which led to funding for a nationwide system of community mental health centers that emphasizes prevention of emotional disorders. The recent tragedies of violence committed by children as well as adults and the anti-stigma campaign of the NAMI were some factors that led to the first White House Conference on Mental Health held June 7, 1999. Another historical event in December 1999 was the first Surgeon General's Report on Mental Health. It provides a comprehensive historical perspective, current practices and research, and a vision of the future that is hopeful. It supports the need for crisis intervention across the life span.

PHASES OF A CRISIS

When a person experiences a traumatic or overwhelming event, he or she moves through phases or steps that determine the level of the crisis state. The first phase is increased anxiety in response to trauma (Caplan, 1964). A person tries to use familiar coping mechanisms to resolve the feeling of increased anxiety. If coping mechanisms are effective, there is no crisis; if they are not effective, a person enters the second phase of crisis, which is marked by further increased anxiety from the failure of usual coping mechanisms. In the third phase, anxiety continues to escalate; the person usually feels compelled to reach out for assistance. A person who is emotionally isolated before experiencing a traumatic event usually will experience a crisis.

In the fourth phase, the active state of crisis, the person's inner resources and support systems are inadequate. The precipitating event is not resolved, and stress and anxiety mount to an intolerable level. The person in an active state of crisis demonstrates a short attention span, ruminates, and looks inward for possible reasons for the trauma and how he or she might have changed or avoided it. Anguish, apprehension, and distress accompany this rumination. Behavior becomes increasingly impulsive and unproductive. Relationships with others usually suffer. The person becomes less aware of the environment and begins to view others in terms of their ability to help solve the problem.

The high anxiety level may make people feel like they are "losing their mind" or "going crazy" (Hoff, 1995). Although anxiety greatly affects perceptive ability, this is not the same as psychosis. People in crisis often need this explanation and to be reassured that when they feel less anxious, they will be able to think clearly again.

Hoff (1995) describes the responses to crisis related to illness, hospitalization, or both in the following areas: (1) biophysical, (2) feelings, (3) thoughts and perceptions, and (4) behavior. An understanding of these responses, particularly the role of cultural differences, assists the nurse to provide culturally competent interventions. Hoff emphasizes that hospitalized clients need to be able to express their feelings, gain an understanding of the illness, and have staff understand their behavior.

TYPES OF CRISES

There are three types of crises:

1. **Maturational or developmental crisis**, precipitated by the normal stress of development (eg, adolescence)
2. **Situational crisis**, precipitated by a sudden traumatic event (eg, job loss)
3. **Adventitious crisis**, precipitated by an unexpected event (eg, natural disasters, bombings, mass shootings)

Maturational Crisis

Erik Erikson (1963) identified specific periods in normal development when anxiety or stress increases and could precipitate a maturational crisis. Some common examples within various developmental stages include mastering control of body functions, starting school, experiencing puberty, leaving home, getting married, becoming a parent, losing physical youthfulness, and entering retirement.

A maturational or developmental crisis may occur at any transitional period in normal growth and development. Because each developmental stage depends on the previous stage, according to Erikson, the inability to master the tasks of one stage is thought to prevent growth and development in subsequent stages.

Why are these times considered a crisis for some and not for others? One explanation is that some people cannot make the role changes necessary for the new maturational level. For instance, the birth of the first child brings numerous role changes for parents. Some can adapt; others, because of emotional immaturity, marital discord, or financial stress, may not be able to adapt readily to the new roles.

There are three main reasons why people may not be able to prevent a maturational crisis. First, they may not be able to visualize themselves in the new role because of inadequate role models. For example, a male child reared without a father's love and guidance may have difficulty assuming the role of a loving, guiding, involved parent. Second, people may lack the interpersonal resources to make the appropriate and necessary changes. For example, a person may lack the flexibility to alter life goals to avoid a midlife crisis or may lack the communication skills needed to maintain a long-term relationship. Third, others may refuse to recognize the person's maturational role change. For instance, parents may fail to acknowledge their adolescent's movement toward adulthood and attempt to preserve the role of the child, precipitating a crisis for the adolescent.

In each stage of development, a person needs nurturance and resources from others to work through the risks of that stage and to obtain the necessary skills for the next stage (Erikson, 1963). Maturational crises are predictable and occur gradually; therefore, it is possible to prepare for them and prevent a crisis. Premarital counseling, preparation for parenting, and planning for retirement are examples of anticipatory guidance in crisis prevention.

Situational Crisis

A situational crisis is a response to a traumatic event that usually is sudden and unavoidable. When a stressful event threatens a person's physical, emotional, or social integrity, crisis is likely to result.

A situational crisis usually follows the loss of an established support. The usual ways of presenting the self are disrupted, threatening the way people view themselves. The threat to a person's self-image or loss of a role that maintains self-image usually leads to a crisis state. The loss of a spouse or job, academic failure, birth of a child with a disability, or diagnosis with a chronic or terminal illness affects the way people perceive themselves (Aguilera, 1998; Hoff, 1995). The most common response to loss or deprivation is depression. The difficulty of dealing with a situational crisis is compounded when it occurs while the person is struggling with a developmental or maturational crisis.

Adventitious Crisis

An adventitious crisis is one that occurs outside the individual. Examples include natural disasters, hurricanes, fires, floods, earthquakes, riots, kidnappings, war, and bombings. These crises affect many people who experience both acute and post-traumatic stress reactions.

Crisis Prevention

Based on research related to maturational and situational crises, healthcare professionals can help clients and families prepare for possible crises. Although not all teens have difficulties during adolescence, many do. Providers can prepare families and assist them to deal with the conflicts and challenges presented by adolescence with parenting classes, support groups, and school programs. Childbirth classes are another example of a way to prepare parents for both the physical aspects of birth and the demands of the parenting role. Preparation for the role changes of retirement may prevent a crisis. People considering divorce can seek counseling to ease their own responses and those of their children. Recognizing symptoms of relapse and seeking early interventions often prevent a crisis for those with chronic physical and mental illness. Encouraging people to establish balance in their lives and manage stress are effective approaches to crisis prevention.

Eating a healthy diet, exercising, playing and having fun, and meeting spiritual needs are means to maximize wellness and prevent crisis. Visualization, meditation, massage, acupressure, progressive relaxation, and water exercise may help. Added possibilities for people who tend to be susceptible to stress include therapeutic touch, biofeedback, acupuncture, and hypnosis. Clients may benefit from taking formal courses in assertiveness training, stress management, or tai chi or using self-help books or tapes. Groups such as the National Alliance for the Mentally Ill (NAMI) provide support, information, advice, and strategies for preventing and dealing with crises for family members and caregivers (see Chaps. 1 and 10).

Teaching or coaching the client may be a primary strategy used for crisis prevention. Psychoeducational classes for consumers, families, and care providers can help them learn to recognize symptoms of relapse and triggers to symptoms and to develop a crisis plan.

Crisis prevention is an ongoing role for staff members on any psychiatric unit. As the push for more cost-effective care continues, clients are more acutely ill and have shorter stays within inpatient units. Their behaviors are more likely to put them and others at risk for injury. Most facilities require staff to be trained; many use the intervention techniques of the National Crisis Prevention Institute (CPI). Box 11-4 lists 10 tips for crisis prevention developed by the CPI.

Crisis Intervention and Stabilization

The goal of **crisis intervention** is to assist the person in distress to resolve the immediate problem and regain emo-

---

BOX 11-4 ▼ *Ten Tips for Crisis Prevention*

1. **Be empathic.** Try not to be judgmental of your client's feelings. They are real, even if not based on reality, and you need to attend to them.
2. **Clarify messages.** Listen to what really is being said. Ask reflective questions and use both silence and restatement.
3. **Respect personal space.** Stand at least 1½ to 3 ft from the acting-out person. Encroaching on personal space tends to arouse an individual and escalate the situation.
4. **Be aware of body position.** Standing eye to eye and toe to toe with the client sends a challenge message. Standing one leg length away, at an angle off to the side, is less likely to incite an individual.
5. **Permit verbal expression when possible.** Allow the individual to release as much energy as possible by venting verbally. If this cannot be allowed, state directives and reasonable limits during lulls in the venting process.
6. **Set and enforce reasonable limits.** If the individual becomes belligerent, defensive, or disruptive, state limits and directives clearly and concisely.
7. **Avoid overreacting.** Remain calm, rational, and professional. How you, the staff person, respond directly affects the individual.
8. **Use physical techniques as a last resort.** Use the least restrictive method of intervention possible. Using physical techniques on an individual who is only acting out verbally can escalate the situation.
9. **Ignore challenge questions.** When the client challenges your authority, such as your position, training, or policy, redirect the individual's attention to the issue at hand. Answering these questions often fuels a power struggle.
10. **Keep your nonverbal cues nonthreatening.** Be aware of your body language, movement, and tone of voice. The more an individual loses control, the less he listens to your actual words. More attention is given to your nonverbal cues.

---

tional equilibrium. This problem solving hopefully leads to enhanced coping to deal with future stressful events.

The role of the intervener is one of active participation with the person in solving the current problem. The crisis state is not an illness; the intervener does not take over and make decisions for the person unless the person is suicidal or homicidal (Aguilera, 1998; Hoff, 1995). The underlying philosophy of crisis intervention is that, with varying degrees of assistance, people can help themselves. To maximize the opportunity for growth, the person must be actively involved in resolving the problem. Crisis intervention is a partnership.

The intervener helps the person in crisis to:

- Analyze the stressful event.
- Express feelings.
- Explore ways to deal with stress and anxiety.
- Seek support from family, friends, and community resource groups.
- Avert possible future crises through anticipatory guidance.

The intervener affirms the person's right to his or her feelings (whatever they may be) and reinforces the person's strengths and abilities.

CRISIS INTERVENTION VERSUS TRADITIONAL THERAPIES

Crisis intervention assists clients to resolve immediate problems that they perceive as overwhelming. Sometimes, the crisis stirs up unresolved past issues. The intervener does not explore or confront these issues. He or she may encourage the client to do so, however, after the crisis resolves and generally with another therapist.

Crisis intervention emphasizes the healthy, not the unhealthy, aspects of the personality. There is no diagnosis of mental illness in crisis work. The intervener evaluates the client in terms of coping skills, strengths and potential, and problem-solving ability. The focus of the therapeutic approach is the client's social structures rather than personality dynamics (Aguilera, 1998; Hoff, 1995). The intervener assumes that the client will make appropriate decisions when given the necessary information and support. Crisis intervention requires a more directive approach than traditional therapies.

CRISIS INTERVENTION ACROSS CONTEXTS

The need for crisis prevention, intervention, and stabilization arises across all contexts: emergency departments, acute care settings, community and public health settings, schools, work settings, homes, jails, psychiatric inpatient units and day programs, primary care settings, nursing homes, and clinics. Nurses need to be prepared and competent to perform such work.

CHARACTERISTICS AND SKILLS OF THE CRISIS INTERVENER

To intervene in a crisis effectively, a provider must demonstrate calmness, caring, and empathy. Because the person in crisis often is confused, the intervener must be able to identify the facts in a situation and think clearly to plan solutions. He or she must make the person in crisis feel safe. The healthcare provider may be a nurse at the basic or advanced practice level, or he or she may be from other mental health disciplines (eg, social work, occupational therapy, psychology, counseling, therapeutic recreation). The intervener must possess courage, self-confidence, and assertiveness.

The pain involved in a crisis is never pleasant. Listening to accounts of personal tragedies is difficult; however, these people need others to commit to working with them until the crisis resolves. This may include tolerating anguish, sadness, and anger.

The skills needed for crisis work include communication, active listening, assessment, collaboration, advocacy, documentation, consultation, teaching, and coaching (Aguilera, 1998; Hoff, 1995; Palmer-Erbs, Connolly, Bianchi, & Hoff, 1996). The intervener must quickly establish trust and build a therapeutic relationship.

The intervener also must be nonjudgmental and appreciate different cultural values. Various cultures have different established patterns of response to death, illness, divorce, and pregnancy (Aguilera, 1998; Hoff, 1995; Palmer-Erbs et al., 1996). Interveners should never impose their own value systems on the client. Crisis intervention, with its focus on immediate problem solving, direct approach, avoidance of psychiatric diagnoses, time limitation, and emphasis on healthy personal strengths, may be more acceptable to people from some ethnic groups and cultures than others. See Chapter 5 for more information.

CRISIS INTERVENTION VARIATIONS

Team Approach

Short-term inpatient psychiatric treatment facilities, as well as many emergency mental health services, use a crisis team approach. The team may be composed of a psychiatrist, psychiatric-mental health nurse, psychologist, social worker, psychiatric aide, minister, and students in the mental health field. In an inpatient facility, one clinician assumes the role of the primary person responsible for the management of a client; however, continuity of care must be built into the system because so many people are involved with the client. The crisis team meets daily to discuss the client's progress and make decisions about care. A case manager or primary therapist outlines goals for the client; the other team members implement the plan and decide on time of discharge and method and frequency of follow-up. These time lines also may be subject to specific protocol from third-party payers, including managed care contracts. As in any crisis-intervention mode, the team must keep the goals clearly in mind. As soon as the client reaches his or her goals, he or she is discharged, even if it is the same day as admission.

Crisis Groups

The goal of a crisis group is the same as that of individual crisis intervention. A crisis group helps members regain or improve on their pre-crisis functioning and ability to problem solve.

Some clients find a crisis group more beneficial than one-to-one therapy, particularly those who have difficulty with interpersonal relationships. Crisis groups also benefit those who have few support systems or difficulty accepting information from psychiatric professionals. Members may feel less isolated (Aguilera, 1998; Yalom, 1995). By observing other people express their feelings, members realize that others have similar feelings and problems. Often, reticent clients can more easily express opinions and feelings after observing others do so. Members offer suggestions to one another for coping and solving problems, which helps bolster members' self-esteem.

Crisis groups also have some disadvantages. It is difficult to keep each client's crisis in focus in a group setting. Group members may suggest a destructive form of coping or maladaptive problem. These problems underscore the need for a trained and experienced crisis group leader.

Crisis groups usually are scheduled for $1\frac{1}{2}$ to 2 hours once a week for 6 to 8 weeks. A group of 8 to 10 members is considered as having an ideal size. Some crisis groups are homogeneous, with every member having a similar problem. For example, successful groups have been formed for people experiencing divorce, Alzheimer's disease, incest, cancer, and AIDS. Peer groups organized by lay people, rather than professionals, may be effective and supportive. Among the best known of these groups are Alcoholics Anonymous and the Caring and Sharing groups of NAMI. In a heterogeneous group, all members are in crisis but have different problems. The group may be an open one, in which new members come in and others work through their problems and leave the group. This gives members an opportunity to deal with feelings about intrusion and separation. A closed group does not accept new members after it is formed and continues for a specified time.

Families in Crisis

Seldom does a person live in total isolation. Usually, a crisis occurs within a family and affects all those in close contact with the client. It is common for parents to struggle with midlife crisis at the same time their adolescent is struggling to establish a separate identity (Aguilera, 1998; Erikson, 1963; Hoff, 1995). People in crisis are either helped or hindered by those in their social network: friends, family, doctors, teachers, employers, and everyone else with whom the client routinely interacts (Aguilera, 1998; Hoff, 1995). The issues of crisis can be viewed within a social framework; the crisis is unresolved until severed social relationships are reestablished (Aguilera, 1998; Hoff, 1995).

While working with families in crisis, the intervener determines which family member is exhibiting crisis symptoms. Next, he or she attempts to identify what the client needs to ensure safety and security for all members of the family. In collaboration with the client and family, the intervener identifies strategies to reduce the most severe symptoms. He or she also assesses the family's resources

and additional social resources. The intervener teaches about crisis and its resolution to the person in crisis and supportive others. Often, respite for the client or family member is needed during a crisis.

The intervener is directive in bringing together the client in crisis and all members of his or her social system for a meeting. During the meeting, all those involved in the crisis analyze the problem and its effect on each family member. Everyone is given an opportunity to voice comments or concerns. Available resources and possible solutions are discussed. By the end of the meeting, the participants should develop a definite plan of action, including exactly who is to do what and when. The nurse should set up a follow-up meeting and help the group decide the time, place, participants, and purpose. The social system approach is effective in dealing with many-faceted crisis situations such as family crisis (Hoff, 1995; Palmer-Erbs et al., 1996).

Telephone Counseling

With growing demands for healthcare services to be more responsive and cost-effective, telephone counseling is increasing. Medical advice "hotlines" operate all over the country with more than 1 million calls per month (Dale, Williams, & Crouch, 1995). Estimates are that 12% to 18% of primary medical care in the United States is conducted over the telephone.

During suicide crisis calls, the crisis worker should keep the caller talking to allow time for the call to be traced, contact relatives or police if necessary, and develop a relationship with the caller (Porter, Marcial, & Sobong, 1997). Telephone advice lines also have been incorporated into emergency departments with specially trained staff to answer the calls (Dale et al., 1995). Although less common, video conferencing for crisis intervention has been used in rural areas with equipment installed in client's homes, at remote service centers, or both. The benefit of video conferencing is obvious in that the practitioner can see the client and assess nonverbal behaviors.

APPLICATION OF THE NURSING PROCESS TO THE CLIENT IN CRISIS

Assessment

Assessment of the person in crisis is the most important, and often most difficult, step of crisis intervention. First, the nurse determines whether the psychiatric symptoms are related to a physical problem. One in five persons with a brain disorder have a medical problem that is causing or exacerbating their psychiatric condition (Liefland, Carporale, Wellington, & Barber, 1997). The assessment includes a physical examination and a history of substance use (caffeine, nicotine, street drugs, alcohol), which might cause psychiatric symptoms. An assessment also includes current intake of any prescribed or over-the-counter medications, vitamins, supplements, or even herbal teas. Side effects, interactions, and reactions to medications or other substances frequently explain symptoms.

Tears or anger do not automatically mean that a person is overwhelmed (Aguilera, 1998; Jeste, Gladsjo Akiko, & Lindamer, 1996). If the client is experiencing great anxiety, having difficulty thinking clearly, or cannot identify solutions to the problem, and if medical or substance-induced causes have been ruled out, then encouraging the client to talk about the events that immediately preceded the distress is helpful. This verbalization frequently calms the client and helps the nurse and client establish rapport. The nurse focuses on the client's immediate problem, not on history. With improved data management systems access, however, medical history and past treatment are available for crisis workers' review. Usually, when people in crisis reach out for help, the precipitating event has occurred within the previous 14 days, sometimes within the last 24 hours (Aguilera, 1998; Hoff, 1995).

EVALUATING FEELINGS

Feelings may be so overwhelming that the client has difficulty describing them. Some clients have little experience in identifying or describing feelings before the crisis. The nurse encourages the client to describe his or her feelings and accepts them without judgment, thus helping the client to accept feelings as well. The nurse naturally may feel some discomfort in the presence of a person in pain. The human inclination is to stop the person from crying or talking about what is horrible and upsetting. By avoiding the topic of distress, the client may appear to be in less pain. Nevertheless, it is beneficial for the person in crisis to express feelings and experience the pain and frustration. Therefore, the nurse must learn to tolerate these feelings of discomfort as part of crisis intervention training.

Usually, the nurse's increased anxiety stems from fear of "saying the wrong thing" or feeling inadequate to deal with the situation. The nurse must understand cognitively and emotionally that ultimately clients make their own decisions. In fact, it is not expedient for the nurse to have all the answers to a client's problems. For clients to grow, the work of problem solving must come from them.

DETERMINING PERCEPTION OF THE EVENT

The nurse first determines the client's perception of the stressful event. How threatened is the client? Is the client realistic or distorting the meaning of the event?

ASSESSING SUPPORT SYSTEMS

After determining the client's perception of the event, the nurse focuses on who is available to support the client.

Questions that can help identify the client's support systems include the following: "Whom do you trust?" "Who is your best friend?" "Are you particularly close with any member of your family?" Children in a crisis usually can cope better if they are with their parents. The nurse also inquires about the client's religious beliefs. For many religious families, God is a source of comfort and strength. The religious affiliation of the client or family may be an excellent source of support.

It is best to have several supportive people involved with the client. Because a crisis lasts for a brief time and the nurse will be involved only temporarily, the client needs others on whom to rely for continued support.

ASSESSING COPING SKILLS

To assess coping skills, the nurse asks what the client does when a problem is difficult to resolve or how the client deals with anxiety or depression (Aguilera, 1998; Hoff, 1995; Palmer-Erbs et al., 1996). The nurse encourages the client to describe specific coping methods and then determines whether the coping mechanisms are adaptive or maladaptive. For example, clients may use alcohol or street drugs—maladaptive coping mechanisms. Is the client still functioning in a job? Is the client still attending school and fulfilling other roles, such as wife and mother? How are the client's significant others affected? Are they also upset? They may need crisis counseling as well.

DETERMINING POTENTIAL FOR SELF-HARM

The nurse asks clients in crisis if they are having thoughts of hurting themselves. Most clients will not volunteer this information but, when asked, will readily talk about suicidal thoughts (Aguilera, 1998; Hoff, 1995; Palmer-Erbs et al., 1996). In fact, many people who commit suicide have seen a healthcare provider shortly before their death (Repper, 1999). Therefore, when clients appear in any healthcare setting—emergency departments, primary care centers, hotlines—nurses must ask about suicidal ideation (Repper, 1999). Clients who have attempted suicide before or have decided how, when, and where to kill themselves need protection. They should not be left alone.

Nursing Diagnosis

A crisis or pre-crisis state is neither a psychiatric illness nor a prolonged, disabling condition. While gathering data from the client and family members, the nurse begins to conceptualize the appropriate descriptions of the client's responses to health problems in terms of nursing diagnoses. Responses particularly evident in crisis are Ineffective Coping, Anxiety, Disturbed Thought Processes, Situational Low Self-Esteem, Social Isolation, and Impaired Social Interaction.

Planning

A crisis plan is necessary no matter how critical the time. After collecting data, the nurse obtains a specific statement of the problem from the client. The client's active involvement in planning solutions to the problem will ensure the plan's success.

The nurse conveys that the client will be able to work through the crisis and take charge of life again. A basic principle is not to do things for clients when they can do them for themselves. The more distraught and confused the client is, the more directive the nurse needs to be. Together, the nurse, client, and other available support people define goals and a time frame for crisis resolution.

It is helpful for the nurse to outline the problem and available resources using Aguilera's paradigm (Figure 11-1) of the balancing factors in a stressful event (1998). By using the decision counseling approach, the intervener can clarify with the client the boundaries of the problem:

What are the tentative solutions? Where will the client try the solutions? What is the time frame? Who will do what? Follow-up is critical and should be part of the initial plan.

The overall goal of crisis intervention is to help the client to reestablish equilibrium. To reach that end, the supporting goals include the following:

- Client will establish a working relationship with the nurse.
- Client will identify the specific problem.
- Client will reduce the distortion of his or her perception of the event.
- Client's self-esteem will improve.
- Anxiety will decrease.
- Family and friends will provide support.
- Client will use healthy coping mechanisms.

It may be difficult, but essential, for the nurse to accept that the goals of crisis intervention are different from the goals of other therapies. It is not the crisis inter-

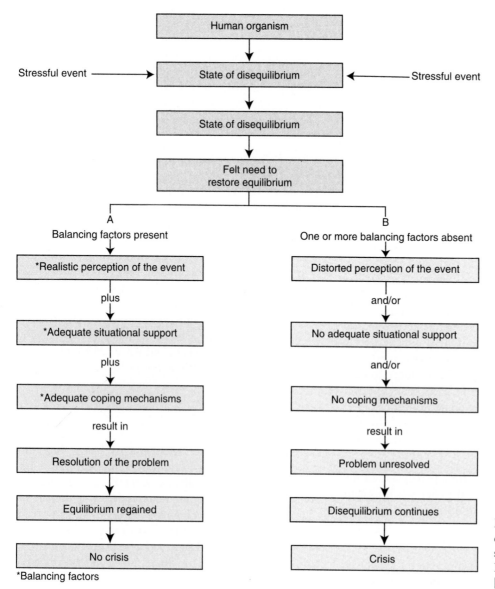

FIGURE 11-1   Paradigm: The effect of balancing factors in a stressful event. (From Aguilera, D.C. [1998]. *Crisis interventions* [8th ed.]. St. Louis: CV Mosby.)

vener's task to deal with all the client's problems or to orchestrate major changes in his or her life (Aguilera, 1998). Crisis intervention assists the client to solve immediate problems that are so overwhelming that the client cannot cope. Once the client has regained emotional equilibrium and can cope again, the work of crisis intervention has been accomplished.

Implementation

REALIZING THE POTENTIAL FOR GROWTH

Nurturing, caring, listening, and being willing to help are powerful and saving forces for clients in crisis. In any crisis, the client facing an overwhelming stressor has the potential to improve coping skills. Whether he or she realizes this possibility for growth depends partly on the effectiveness of crisis intervention. Hoff's crisis paradigm (Figure 11-2) emphasizes the positive crisis resolution as growth and development (Hoff, 1995).

The nurse and client reexamine any feelings that might interfere with adaptive coping. If a client has extremely negative feelings, it is particularly difficult to face these circumstances. This client must deal with those feelings to cope adequately with the crisis.

LEARNING TO ASK FOR HELP

In a crisis, it is natural to withdraw and feel isolated. Therefore, the nurse helps the client to communicate directly with significant others. Clients who place high value on independence may need particular assistance to recognize interdependence as a healthy balance. Often, the nurse must teach such clients how to ask for help. The nurse can demonstrate this skill to the client through role-playing.

USING ADAPTIVE COPING

The nurse also helps the client develop healthier coping skills. Helpful strategies include openly expressing feelings, using positive self-talk, engaging in progressive relaxation, exercising, and drinking warm milk or herbal tea to aid relaxation and sleep.

FOCUSING ON PROBLEM RESOLUTION

As the crisis intervener, the nurse keeps the client focused on the problem and specific goals leading to its resolution. The client's high anxiety may make it difficult for him or her to focus on one issue. Therefore, he or she may need direction to avoid fragmentation. After the client has attempted some of the alternative solutions to the problem, the client and nurse evaluate their effectiveness and decide whether additional plans are needed. The nurse reinforces the client's abilities by reviewing the crisis event, coping skills, and the newly acquired methods of problem solving or coping.

USING INFORMATION TECHNOLOGY

Using internet resources may be an intervention to reduce anxiety by quickly accessing needed information. For example, receiving a medical diagnosis may be a trigger for a crisis response. Providing clients with current informa-

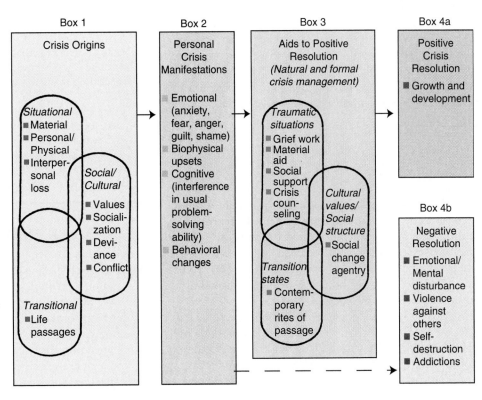

FIGURE 11-2 A crisis paradigm. Crisis origins, manifestations and outcomes, and the respective functions of crisis management have an interactional relationship. The intertwined circles representing distinct yet interrelated origins of crisis and aids to positive resolution, even though personal manifestations are often similar. The arrows pointing from origins to positive resolution illustrate the opportunity for growth and development through crisis; the broken line at the bottom depicts the potential for danger of crisis in the absence of appropriate aids (From Hoff, L. [1995] *People in crisis: Understanding and helping* [4th ed.]. Menlo Park, CA: Addison-Wesley.

tion about options, research, outcomes, and resources for more information and treatment is one way to reduce anxiety and, ultimately, a crisis response. Furthermore, clients themselves may access the internet and will need assistance in evaluating information.

Evaluation

In the evaluation process, the nurse and client together evaluate whether the crisis response has been resolved. Has the client regained equilibrium and usual level of functioning? The nurse must recognize when the client is ready for discharge. Before dissolving the partnership, the nurse and client engage in anticipatory planning to maximize the client's ability to avoid crisis responses in the future (Aguilera, 1998; Hoff, 1995). The client may need additional information about community services or community resources. After working through the crisis response, some clients are motivated to seek additional mental health services to resolve earlier issues or prior trauma; therefore, the nurse may make referrals (Aguilera, 1998; Hoff, 1995).

NURSING CARE OF HOMELESS CLIENTS

Before identifying the homeless, some of the problems associated with studying homelessness must be considered. For example, studies have different operational definitions of homelessness. Most studies focus on people in shelters. As a result, many homeless people are uncounted, such as families who live with other families in single-family dwellings, people displaced by domestic violence, street youth, and "invisible" homeless people who live on the streets, under bridges, or in homeless camps. Even in the shelters, difficulties in interviewing make the accuracy of data suspect.

Demographics

The homeless population in shelters primarily is white. African Americans and Hispanics are overrepresented, although actual racial composition depends on whether the area being considered is urban or rural. Most are long-term residents of the area in which they are homeless. The percentage of homeless women is increasing in many cities (Smith & North, 1994).

Most homeless populations include persons with mental illness, veterans, victims of domestic violence, families, and people with addictions (National Coalition for the Homeless, 1999a, 1999b). Families are the fastest growing subpopulation among the ranks of the homeless.

Frequently, homeless families consist of a single mother with children. Homeless children commonly experience developmental delays, depression, anxiety, and learning difficulties. Their homelessness may be a source of shame. They also may demonstrate a resiliency to their multiple stressors (Conrad, 1998). Because of the lack of policies and programs that target prevention, homelessness is becoming intergenerational as more children grow up in a climate of poverty.

The homeless population encompasses a diverse array of people. Examples include the disabled or chronically ill whose benefits do not allow them permanent housing; people on fixed incomes who cannot afford the housing market; Vietnam veterans estranged from their support systems; street youth whose families have rejected them; immigrants, both documented and undocumented; those connected with the criminal justice system; and unemployed and underemployed persons who work but do not earn enough to pay the ongoing cost of housing (Historical Capsule 11-2).

▼ Clinical Example 11-3

The police have asked the mental health outreach team to make contact with a woman about whom they have received multiple calls from people in the community, who have noticed the woman sleeping on a bench outside the supermarket. When the team arrives, they notice that the woman has a cart overloaded with bags and a soiled sleeping roll. Observable sores are on her legs. She is reluctant to speak with the nurse on the team, although she does accept clean socks. The team is able to persuade the woman to accompany them to a shelter, where she receives soup, blankets, and clothing.

At the shelter, the woman reveals that her name is Louise. She relates that she recently spent time in a hospital where she believes that she was poisoned with Haldol, adding that she was poisoned several other times in other cities. She believes that Haldol caused the ulcers on her legs. She left the city where she had been hospitalized because "the police chief bugged the sewer system" to follow her. Louise has a son in another state but hasn't spoken to him in years. She was getting a Social Security check until 2 months ago when she left the city where she was hospitalized. She has no identification.

Homeless Mentally Ill People

Most research findings agree that the homeless mentally ill account for 25% to 33% of the homeless population, and that 50% of the total homeless population demonstrates symptoms of depression. Compared with the general population, the homeless are more likely to have experienced psychiatric hospitalization.

Schizophrenia is the most common chronic mental illness affecting homeless people. This disorder is the most

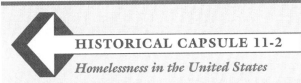

HISTORICAL CAPSULE 11-2

Homelessness in the United States

During the Great Depression, the number of homeless surged as young men left their homes seeking employment throughout the country. After World War II, so-called "skid rows" developed in major urban areas, populated primarily by middle-aged, unemployed, or underemployed white men. Many of them struggled with alcoholism; some were disabled as a result of mental or physical problems.

State hospitals found themselves increasingly unable to provide adequate care for the growing number of chronically mentally ill clients. Institutional care began to deteriorate, and the care of the mentally ill became known as "warehousing." Nurses attempted to provide care with fewer resources than those available in the private sector. In the 1940s, media exposure increased public awareness of deplorable conditions in mental hospitals.

Treatment changed significantly with the introduction of the first major tranquilizers in 1953. During the Civil Rights Movement of the 1950s and 1960s, the rights of the chronically mentally ill also came to the forefront, giving rise to the community mental health movement (Torrez, 1988). As social reform responded to deplorable hospital conditions, the movement toward deinstitutionalization began. The widespread transfer of formerly institutionalized clients to community-based care culminated in the Community Mental Health Act of 1963, which gave communities the primary responsibility for providing mental health treatment. During this time, the treatment community acknowledged a breakdown syndrome associated with institutional living, marked by withdrawal, excessive dependency, and lack

of initiative (Lamb, 1984). By the late 1960s, clients were being discharged to nursing homes, single-room occupancy dwellings, hotels, boarding houses, and low-income housing units (Torrez, 1988). By the 1980s, many deinstitutionalized people were counted among the ranks of the homeless.

The early 1980s brought a new type of homeless population who were no longer concentrated in skid rows but were scattered throughout urban areas. These homeless people were younger and more economically destitute than before and included more women and children. Although the homeless population still was predominantly white, African Americans and Hispanics were overrepresented.

Throughout the 1980s and early 1990s, the federal government significantly decreased funding for low-income housing and reduced federal entitlements to the disabled, many of whom were mentally ill. The nation also faced a rising unemployment rate, rising inflation, and the consequences of persistent poverty and widespread family breakdown. In earlier times, extended families were likely to take in disenfranchised members; traveler's aid was prevalent in many communities. However, a climate had developed of decreased tolerance of persons on the social margins and outside the cultural mainstream. One consequence of such attitudes has been that chronically mentally ill persons again have become casualties of a well-intended system. Unfortunately, the criminal justice system and homeless shelters often are the primary providers for homeless mentally ill persons.

---

distressing to the person without support who is too symptomatic to negotiate a bureaucratic mental health system. The incidence of major affective disorders and substance abuse disorders also is higher in the homeless than in the general population. Box 11-5 delineates frequently observed *DSM-IV-TR* diagnoses (*Diagnostic and Statistical Manual of Mental Disorders*, 4th edition, text revision) among the homeless mentally ill population.

Because of changes in treatment, mental health laws, and the effects of managed care, many younger mentally ill adults are joining the ranks of the homeless. Treatment of this younger population usually demonstrates a common pattern. They are referred to community treatment yet often do not follow through and thus decompensate, perhaps resulting in hospitalization. Frequently, they are discharged from the hospital without a full stabilization of their symptoms and return to a stressful environment with-

out needed structure and support, thus starting the pattern over again. Many may complicate their illness by using drugs or alcohol to self-medicate their psychiatric symptoms. They may perceive taking medication as an acknowledgement that their lives are no longer "normal." Homeless adolescents and young adults may be observed by the clinician to be experiencing symptoms of their first psychotic break. In this population, it is common to see depressive symptoms with a high risk for suicide.

Clearly, homelessness adversely affects mental health. People who become homeless because of economic stressors, loss of job, domestic violence, or eviction are more prone to mental illness, substance abuse problems, and other health concerns. These homeless people, who are not necessarily chronically mentally ill, may be brought to the attention of nurses by shelter staff because of behavioral characteristics associated with stress reactions, impaired

BOX 11-5 ▼ *Common DSM-IV-TR Diagnoses Observed in the Homeless Mentally Ill Population*

Schizophrenia (paranoid, disorganized, undifferentiated, residual)
Schizoaffective disorder
Delusional disorder
Psychotic disorder NOS
Major depressive disorder
Bipolar I disorder
Bipolar II disorder
Obsessive-compulsive disorder
Post-traumatic stress disorder

Antisocial personality disorder
Borderline personality disorder
Personality disorder NOS
Alcohol dependence
Alcohol-related disorder
Amphetamine abuse
Hallucinogen-related disorder
Nicotine dependence
Polysubstance dependence

intellectual functioning, or personality disorders. Addressing such dependent, demanding, manipulative, or aggressive behaviors poses special challenges to the nurse who also is caring for the acutely psychotic or suicidal client.

FACTORS CONTRIBUTING TO HOMELESSNESS IN THE MENTALLY ILL

Homelessness in mentally ill people has many different causes. Common contributing factors include the lack of a comprehensive and effective mental healthcare system, the disabling functional deficits of chronic mental illness, the effects of substance abuse or dependency, the effects of poverty, inadequate housing, and mobility.

Lack of Prevention

Failure to address risk factors that contribute to homelessness has caused the number of homeless mentally ill people to increase. Examples of such risk factors are comorbidity of mental illness and substance abuse disorders, inadequate discharge planning, lack of crisis services, insufficient disability benefits, inadequate supported housing, and the stigma and discrimination associated with mental illness (Lezak & Edgar, 1988).

Creative and innovative measures to decrease risk factors are needed. Each community must decide what is best and most realistic according to their resources. Examples of interventions that may decrease homelessness include intensive case management, housing supports (including landlord mediation), respite and crisis stabilization facilities, and a wider range of subsidized housing.

Functional Abilities and Deficits

Functional characteristics of chronic mental illness often are exaggerated in homeless mentally ill clients. These clients are considered to be in a constant state of transition. Thus, their distorted perceptual abilities, lack of situational supports, and poor symptom control may cause them to be unable to face the crisis of homelessness.

Some of the most influential functional characteristics include difficulties with basic activities of daily living (eg, personal hygiene, cooking, housekeeping). Other significant deficits include difficulty relating to others, lack of self-confidence and self-esteem, dependency needs, difficulty with self-direction, and limited motor capacity from side effects of medications.

Poverty

In the United States, the gap between rich and poor continues to widen. For many, the margin between poverty and homelessness is narrow. The most seriously affected are people of color, children, and older adults. High unemployment rates, cuts in funding for public assistance, inadequate insurance for debilitating illnesses including mental illness, and increased domestic violence all contribute to a cycle of poverty that promotes despair, poor self-esteem, and feelings of alienation. Homelessness is one visible consequence of this cycle. Even employed Americans are not immune from this cycle. Many Americans are only one missed paycheck away from homelessness.

Inadequate Housing

In general, people with low incomes are paying more for housing. In many areas, those receiving entitlements pay a certain percentage of their income for subsidized housing. The reality for people with mental illness who are living in such housing situations is that incidence of eviction is high and support for maintaining housing is lacking. The mentally ill person, particularly one who has been homeless for a long time, experiences a difficult process in establishing residential stability. They may be evicted from their housing because of their psychiatric symptoms. For example, a person may be responding loudly in the middle of the night to auditory hallucinations that they are experiencing. Often, the nurse as a community provider needs to advocate for the client in the process of eviction prevention. To accommodate the diverse functioning levels of the chronically mentally ill, a wide array of community housing and support is needed.

Substance Abuse

Many mentally ill people, particularly young adults, misguidedly attempt to self-medicate psychiatric symptoms with street drugs or alcohol. Whereas the rate of alcoholism in the general population is high, the drinking and drug abuse habits of homeless people are more visible. In general, health problems for most disorders and diseases, particularly liver disease, trauma, seizure disorders, and nutritional deficiencies, occur more often among alcohol-abusing homeless people (Blakeney, 1992).

Crack cocaine has changed the economic status of many people, including the homeless mentally ill. Many spend their limited funds on this highly potent and rapidly addictive drug instead of on housing or food. Many new drugs appear on the street each year, and others reemerge, such as LSD. Marketing of such drugs often targets such vulnerable populations as the homeless mentally ill. In the late 1990s, the street use of heroin and methamphetamines has created a higher incidence of crime, death by overdose, and unpredictability in criminal behavior.

Common psychosocial characteristics of homeless persons with dual diagnoses (those with a mental illness and a substance-abuse disorder) may include greater levels of denial of illness, psychiatric symptoms, housing instability, lack of family support, involvement with the criminal justice system, and a greater risk for suicide. Specialized programs are needed that provide communication among the mental health, drug and alcohol treatment, and criminal justice systems and coordinate treatment planning (Oakley & Dennis, 1996).

High Mobility

A phenomenon of restlessness affects many homeless mentally ill people. Their homelessness may be episodic in that they move in and out of homelessness or between residential and outpatient treatment facilities. The mobility of the homeless mentally ill person may be seasonal; for example, a person may move from city to city within a certain geographic area because of impaired thought processes, "voices" that tell them what to do, or simply frustration with their symptoms. Chronically mentally ill young adults struggling with the desire to obtain independence from their families may find a sense of autonomy in being homeless. However, this independence is complicated by lack of treatment, use of street drugs, and inability to cope with mental illness. Homeless mentally ill people who are frequently mobile may become disconnected from their disability entitlements, complicating their ability to obtain housing, food, and healthcare.

CRITICAL ISSUES AFFECTING THE HOMELESS MENTALLY ILL

A homeless person incurs losses far greater than simply losing a house; he or she also loses a sense of belonging and a psychological sense of home. If newly homeless, a mentally ill person finds himself or herself in a culture filled with fears. He or she is a stranger in a system difficult to negotiate. Other losses may involve family ties, friends, work, health, and community support. If a client cannot turn this process around, he or she is at risk for chronic homelessness. When attempting to cope with such losses, the client is likely to disaffiliate from conventional society and identify with homeless culture. In this sense, he or she uses acculturation to survive.

A Changing Mental Health System

In the 1960s and 1970s, deinstitutionalization began as a positive process in support of the civil rights of clients with psychiatric disorders. The negative effects of deinstitutionalization came not from its intentions, but rather from minimal community support, fragmented services, and few housing alternatives in the community. The current homeless mentally ill population includes not only clients who have been deinstitutionalized, but also those who no longer meet criteria for hospitalization because of changes in the commitment laws. These laws vary in each state, but shared issues include the right to receive treatment, the right to refuse treatment, and the right to be treated in the least restrictive environment. The troublesome question arises, however, as to whether the least restrictive setting also is the most therapeutic setting. Involuntary commitment now occurs only if a client is judged to be a danger to self or others.

Often, those with financial resources do not experience the negative effects as harshly as those without such resources. Most people receiving mental healthcare must do so in a managed care environment that limits coverage. In the current system, a client is likely to receive limited hospitalization and to experience inadequate remission of symptoms. At times, a client may be followed under an outpatient commitment or trial visit; this process can be difficult when a client is homeless.

Barriers to Care

One of the first steps in promoting access to care for homeless mentally ill people is to identify the barriers to care, which include the following:

- Lack of insurance
- Lack of transportation
- Eligibility criteria, which may require an address
- Loss of identification (a frequent requirement for accessing services)
- Lack of knowledge of available services
- Fear of having to leave, and possibly lose, possessions by attending clinic appointments

- Concern over missing meals or a place in line for a shelter bed
- Fear of scrutiny by caregivers

Because of their inability to meet admission criteria or the need for an address, homeless mentally ill people may be excluded from other homeless and community mental health programs. Also, clinician bias toward clients who respond more favorably to treatment may be an internal barrier to accessing care within the system. Chronically mentally ill people routinely experience inconsistent treatment approaches, frequent medication changes, overmedication, and poor coordination of care, which leaves them feeling justifiably distrustful of the system.

The process of withdrawal by the nurse from the therapeutic relationship may cause an internal psychological barrier to care. When professional expectations do not balance with practice realities, the nurse may withdraw psychologically from the client. The effects of poverty and alienation may promote a client's threatening and abusive behavior, further alienating the client from care providers. The nurse should be cautious regarding the frustration that may develop and should not allow this to interfere with the treatment plan (Chafetz, 1990).

The traditional healthcare delivery system usually does not reach the homeless population. Services that can improve access to healthcare include shelter-based clinics, clinical day programs, freestanding clinics specific to the needs of homeless people, respite care services, mobile outreach units, and street outreach teams. Nurses manage some of these services; multidisciplinary teams manage others. Providing such services can be challenging in a managed care environment (Fisk, Rakfeldt, Hefferman, & Rowe, 1999; Morse, 1999).

Other access-to-care issues are specific to homeless families. A family may have difficulty negotiating an unfamiliar healthcare system; because of constraints of the shelter, families may have difficulty maintaining records. Clinicians may be critical of parents for losing their child's immunization records. Sometimes, because of their homelessness, parents fear being reported to protective agencies for child neglect or abuse (Berne, Dato, Mason, & Rafferty, 1990).

The Shelter System

Shelters are a necessary stopgap to the problem of homelessness; however, they are not the solution. They have been given the impossible task of replacing the mental institutions in many urban settings. Shelters vary in capacity and services offered. Some provide cots or beds; others offer only floor space. Common-services shelters provide meals, reading materials, laundry facilities, and clothing. Some shelters provide support services for recovery from substance abuse disorders as well as psychiatric and medical services.

Shelters commonly are staffed by paid personnel as well as by volunteers, both professional and nonprofes-

sional. These staff members may need instruction in the areas of communicable disease, conflict resolution, seizure management, mental illness, substance abuse, and medication management (Blakeney, 1992). These situations give nurses valuable opportunities to provide health education.

Health Concerns

Compared with the general population, clients with chronic mental illness have higher disease morbidity rates. Homeless mentally ill clients have even higher rates. Chronic physical disorders commonly affecting homeless people include hypertension, diabetes, pulmonary disorders, liver disease, seizure disorders, and peripheral vascular disease. Having these chronic disorders lowers life expectancy significantly. Health problems specific to urban homeless people are related to exposure, high population density, poor ventilation, and dependent positioning because frequently they are on their feet most of the day. The crowded conditions of shelters have contributed to the rise in tuberculosis (Chafetz, 1990). The risk of illness, whether airborne or through bodily fluids, increases in a shelter. The nurse may be asked to assist with the management of various illnesses, which may include medication management. Implications for Nursing Practice 11-2 provides medication management suggestions for assisting homeless clients.

Thermoregulatory disorders, such as heat stroke and frostbite, are common. Secondary infections from infes-

---

 Implications for Nursing Practice 11-2

Medication Management Suggestions for the Homeless Person

- When possible, simplify the dosage and times of administration.
- Assist in locating a secure place to keep medications (refrigeration if needed).
- Assist client to locate screening clinics to evaluate ongoing therapeutic effectiveness of medications.
- Provide a telephone call service for shelters or agency providers to answer their questions and concerns about medications.
- Show clients how to carry medications on their person (if necessary) so that they don't make noise. (Rattling noises may identify homeless people as "targets" for drug theft.)
- Provide written and verbal education to the client and providers on medication, side effects, and measures to control side effects.
- Assist clients in obtaining adequate fluids, dietary needs, and sun protection; the nurse frequently needs to be creative in mobilizing volunteer services.

tation by lice, scabies, or insect bites occur in all seasons (Blakeney, 1992). Underlying every acute and chronic illness is the poor nutritional state of most homeless people. Special challenges exist in the management of diabetes in an environment where dietary factors are mostly out of the person's control. Seizure disorders may result in bodily injuries from falls. Trauma is a significant problem for urban homeless people. Sexual assaults, stabbings, fractures, and contusions secondary to assaults are common in most downtown areas. Because of their anonymity, homeless people often are victims of senseless crimes. In fact, the homeless mentally ill are the victims more often than the perpetrators of such crimes.

Another significant health concern is the increased risk of exposure to disease of younger homeless mentally ill people. Because of certain aspects of their illnesses, such as sexual acting out, poor impulse control, or hypersexuality associated with mania, they may participate in unprotected sexual practices. Substance abuse may involve the sharing of needles for IV drug use, thus increasing exposure to infectious agents such as hepatitis and HIV.

The Criminal Justice System

More people detained in jails and prisons have a chronic mental illness (see earlier discussion). Crimes leading to incarceration may result from symptoms of mental illness, such as command hallucinations or diminished capacity to make clear judgments. If mental illness is associated with drug and alcohol use, the likelihood of arrests increases. Other criminal behavior may be an attempt to maintain daily needs such as sleeping in an abandoned building and being charged with criminal trespassing.

The growing number of homeless mentally ill people in jails underscores the need for outreach and mental health practitioner services within jails and discharge planning for treatment, which may include coordination with corrections officers. Because homeless mentally ill clients more often are the victims of crimes than the perpetrators, mental health providers also must support and advocate for clients within the criminal justice system.

APPLICATION OF THE NURSING PROCESS TO THE HOMELESS CLIENT

Assessment

In assessing homeless clients with or without mental illness, the nurse must consider how the conditions in which they live each day affect them. Box 11-6 lists common stressors that may influence a homeless person's mental health.

Assessment of a homeless client with mental illness that takes place in a shelter presents special challenges

---

BOX 11-6 ▼ *Stressors of Homelessness That Influence Mental Health*

- The effect of constant vigilance for safety, resulting in lack of sound sleep, fearfulness, suspicion, and insecurity
- Social isolation, being shunned by others, or feelings of "invisibility"
- Use of drugs or alcohol in a futile attempt to create comfort or a sense of community
- Poor diet, which may contribute to biochemical imbalances and mood changes
- Susceptibility to physical illness
- Constant uncertainty and disruptions
- Lack of medical, psychiatric, or other needed assistance
- Pervasive sense of hopelessness and uncertainty

From Haus, A. (1988). *Working with homeless people*. New York: Columbia University Press.

---

because of the lack of privacy and noise level. Outside the shelter, distractions may inhibit adequate assessment. The client may not want to be identified with a psychiatric care provider and may agree to meet with the nurse only under pressure from shelter staff. The nurse must consider and appreciate the effects a nursing assessment might have on the client.

Conducting a thorough mental status examination can be difficult because of shelter conditions and lack of client cooperation; however, the nurse should proceed with the examination as much as possible. The nurse also should assess neurologic signs, including a careful history for head trauma or other organic damage. If possible, he or she should make contact with family or other healthcare agencies to provide collateral information. Other screening may be indicated; for example, most shelters require tuberculosis screening before admittance.

The assessment process may involve a sensitive questioning process, particularly with a client with a mental illness. Implications for Nursing Practice 11-3 suggests measures that may facilitate communication with the homeless mentally ill client.

Nursing Diagnosis

The nurse formulates nursing diagnoses cautiously. He or she first becomes familiar with the norms and necessities of street life because some unusual behaviors may be adaptive mechanisms. For example, clients may wear excessive clothing to prevent theft or to keep others from disturbing them. Likewise, clients may consciously exhibit bizarre behaviors to keep others away. Nursing diagnosis

Implications for Nursing Practice 11-3

Communication Suggestions with Homeless Mentally Ill Clients

- Be aware of your own feelings, fears, and even your breathing.
- Create physical space so that both you and the client can leave the room if either of you decide to do so; it creates a safety zone.
- Involve significant others in communication if it facilitates a client's sense of security; don't involve others until you have asked the client's permission to do so.
- Discuss basic needs—it may be the best starting place for communication.
- Promote the client's sense of control and choice within the current environment; it may simply involve giving the client a choice of placement for his or her bedroll or whether you should give an injection in the left or right side.
- Be mindful and respectful of confidentiality issues.
- Be sensitive to possible feelings of not wanting to be identified with a psychiatric nurse or program.
- Be concrete in your interactions, avoiding metaphors, until you understand the client's cognitive functioning.
- For clients experiencing psychotic symptoms, let them know that you are not afraid of them and that your presence is not intrusive or demanding.
- For clients responding to internal stimuli, it may be helpful to ask if you could have their attention for a little while.
- For clients with delusions, let them experience that you have some sensitivity and understanding of the situation (or desire understanding); attempt to connect with the symbolism of the delusion.
- For clients with paranoia, it may be helpful to sit side by side rather than in front of them; it is possible to identify with the feeling more than the content of the paranoia and let clients know you understand that feeling.
- For clients who are suicidal, be direct in your concern and your questions in assessing for suicidality.
- Be aware of clients' varying insights into their illness.
- It may be helpful to summarize with clients, expressing your observations of their situation, then assessing with them if your observations are congruent with theirs.

addresses clients in relation to their illness, family, and community. Possible nursing diagnoses for a homeless mentally ill client include the following:

- **Interrupted Family Processes** related to recent displacement
- **Social Isolation** related to new onset of homelessness
- **Ineffective Coping** related to family disruption
- **Powerlessness** related to lack of personal control over environment
- **Chronic Low Self-Esteem** related to onset of psychotic illness
- **Social Isolation** related to mistrust of others and lack of social support system
- **Risk for Infection** related to congested environment and poorly ventilated shelter setting
- **Risk for Injury** related to inability to maintain personal boundaries

Planning

In planning any treatment program, the nurse recognizes the realities of available local resources, the client's perception of needs, the conditions under which the client must function, and the nature and symptomatology of the client's mental illness. Another important consideration is that over time, the shelter lifestyle may have become the most important organizing factor in the client's life, providing needed structure and support. Preparing for a new life typically produces anxiety and may cause decompensation. Despite reality-based and reasonable goals, the nurse may have to function without a tangible treatment outcome.

Major goals for a homeless mentally ill person are as follows:

- Client will satisfy physical needs and remain safe.
- Client will understand the symptoms of his or her mental illness.
- Client will build a therapeutic alliance with providers.
- Client will identify and use psychosocial supports.

Outcome criteria should be reasonable and attainable. For example, an outcome criterion for a client with paranoid schizophrenia might be that he or she will control paranoid thoughts long enough to spend a complete night in a shelter. Other examples might include that the client will demonstrate increased appropriate independent functioning, increased contact with case management services, or increased use of clinic services. The nurse must be willing to evaluate outcomes in terms of small and client-focused successes. The nurse should not necessarily designate the end of homelessness as an outcome criterion; he or she also should not view the client's episodic homelessness as a failure. The chronically mentally ill client may move in and out of homelessness as part of a lengthy adjustment process to residential stability.

Implementation

FORMING A THERAPEUTIC ALLIANCE

A homeless mentally ill client may distrust anyone who represents the mental health system. Thus, the nurse initiates the helping relationship in a nonthreatening manner, giving the client as much control as possible. The nurse avoids attitudes of wanting to "fix" the client's problems. Nurses advocate for their clients while knowing their own limits. They avoid making quick referrals before building trust with clients.

The nurse may need to postpone interventions (or even discussions of them) for the most disturbing symptoms to avoid creating a negative therapeutic experience for the client. Discussing medical conditions before psychiatric problems may help build the client's trust in the nurse and improve the nurse–client relationship. An alliance can develop as the client experiences a consistent and nonjudgmental attitude from the nurse.

MANAGING MEDICATIONS

A homeless mentally ill client has special medication management needs. Many medications have sedating effects that place clients in danger. Because homeless persons must stay consistently vigilant for safety reasons, they cannot afford drowsiness. Carrying medications also increases the risk of assault and robbery because most medications have street value. The nurse also must caution clients against combining medications with alcohol and drugs.

The nurse provides specific instructions to a client taking certain medications. For instance, he or she instructs the client taking lithium to maintain an adequate fluid intake, which may be difficult, depending on the availability of water in the client's environment. A client taking certain neuroleptic medications must know the importance of skin protection to prevent sunburn, which may be difficult during summer. Nurses should involve clients in medication management. The clients alone can determine when they have access to their medication, how they can carry the medication safely, and the particular risk factors in daily life.

TEACHING CLIENTS

A homeless client needs information to promote health and to access and use pertinent healthcare resources. Client education may include topics such as personal hygiene, infestation, thermoregulatory disorders, cancer risks, respiratory problems, sexually transmitted diseases, and substance abuse issues (Blakeney, 1992). The nurse also educates clients about the nature of mental illness; symptoms to expect; side effects, risks, and benefits of prescribed medications; and the complexities of the mental health system.

PERFORMING CASE MANAGEMENT

Case management is the key intervention that connects the client with the community. The nurse–case manager coordinates services to ensure that the client receives the structure and support he or she needs to achieve and maintain optimal functioning. Case management encompasses health teaching, crisis intervention, symptom monitoring, providing assistance with federal entitlements, assisting with transportation, teaching about money management, and consumer advocacy. For some homeless clients, the case management relationship may extend for years, long after the client has a home. In a managed care environment, transfer of case management may be difficult because of waiting lists, increased case loads, and fear that the client will become lost in the system. For a client who already has experienced multiple decompensation, the anxiety produced by such a change can be challenging for both the nurse and client.

BECOMING POLITICALLY INVOLVED

Wherever a nurse practices, responsibilities involve interventions in the lives of homeless mentally ill clients as well as in the community. Hospital nurses will have homeless clients; nursing administrators will set policies for caring for homeless clients; nursing educators will devise curriculums regarding homeless issues. Nurses should be knowledgeable of governmental influences on healthcare and willing to testify from their knowledge base and experience on the effects of homelessness. They must influence policies regarding healthcare, employment, housing, and the effects of poverty on the health status of all citizens. Nurses can stay informed on such policies by using informational resources.

Evaluation

Reviewing the effects of the nursing care plan is an integral part of the nursing process. Without this evaluative process, there is no learning or improvement. To measure the effects, nurses define behavioral criteria. For example, such measures might include how often a client accomplished target activities, how much time he or she spent on a target activity, the degree of insight gained by the client, or the number of symptoms relieved by the treatment given in accordance with the care plan. Also, care plans need to be reevaluated in terms of new barriers to care that may have arisen or to further clarify nursing diagnoses.

In qualitatively evaluating services, the nurse performs an overall review of the program's characteristics. Such evaluative criteria address the quality of the continuum of care provided; they measure a program's ability to be comprehensive, individualized, flexible, and meaningful to the client.

▼ *Reflection and Critical Thinking Questions*

1. Correctional institutions have been described as among the most extreme living environments. Can this environment lead to healing and personal growth, or does it reinforce the client as a criminal, an inmate? How might the forensic psychiatric nurse create a healing therapeutic environment within the forensic milieu?

2. What aspects of crisis intervention might be needed in forensic settings? What about for homeless clients?

3. If you were to lose your income and residence today, immediately becoming homeless, what three belongings would you take with you to a shelter? Remember that you must carry these items with you and be accountable for them 24 hours a day.

4. If you could rewrite history, would you change the deinstitutionalization movement? How and why?

▼ CHAPTER SUMMARY

- Forensic psychiatric nursing helps to bridge the gap between the criminal justice system and the mental healthcare system.

- Deinstitutionalization, homelessness, increased rates of incarceration for drug-related activities, interpersonal and domestic violence, and anticrime legislation have been attributed to the soaring forensic population.

- Forensic clients are young and old, male and female, and often are victims and perpetrators of crime.

- Forensic settings include forensic psychiatric facilities, locked units of general hospitals, and state hospitals. The common practice sites, however, are the jail and prison.

- Legal and ethical issues related to the forensic client are pertinent to forensic psychiatric nursing, and nurses need to be familiar with relevant legislation governing the settings in which they are employed.

- Crisis intervention differs from traditional psychotherapy primarily because it focuses on the here and now and immediate problem solving.

- A crisis occurs when a client cannot solve a problem that he or she perceives as overwhelming, when usual coping mechanisms fail to solve the problem, when perception of the event is distorted, or when others do not supply necessary support.

- The client in crisis has the potential to develop more adaptive coping and healthier functioning capabilities after the crisis experience.

- A crisis may be maturational, situational, or adventitious.

- Nurses often are the first healthcare professionals in contact with the client in crisis; therefore, they are uniquely positioned to intervene in crisis.

- The homeless population is heterogeneous and encompasses the young, older adults, families with children, victims of domestic violence, street youth, veterans, those released from jails, immigrants, and the mentally ill.

- Homelessness is a result of personal crises, lack of community and family support, symptoms of chronic illness, and pervasive effects of poverty.

- Homeless mentally ill people are at increased risk for both acute and chronic illnesses. Their access to healthcare may be limited by attitudes of care providers, symptoms of mental illness, and the complexities of a bureaucratic mental health system.

- Shelters and programs for the homeless are crucial, but they do not offer the solution to the deeper structural problems of poverty, inadequate housing, and prejudice toward the mentally ill. The process of returning from homelessness to the community is a complex and anxiety-producing experience for the chronically mentally ill person who has been on the street for any length of time.

- The role of the nurse is crucial in identifying and removing barriers to care, providing fair and thorough assessments, and providing quality care to those who are so alienated in the margins of society that they are incapable of using the traditional mental health system.

▼ REVIEW QUESTIONS

1. A universal characteristic of forensic institutions is that they reflect
   a. The latest developments in healthcare technology
   b. The treatment needs of the population being served
   c. The social and political convictions of society
   d. The holistic needs of clients and their families

2. One of the largest changes in the composition of the forensic population that has required special adaptations within institutional settings is associated with
   a. Increased elderly offenders
   b. The number of juvenile offenders
   c. Decreased female offenders
   d. Increased offenders charged with drug offenses

3. A nurse is caring for a verbally aggressive forensic client who reminds her of her ex-boyfriend. At the end of the interview, she seeks out an experienced nurse colleague to explore her feelings about this client. The nurse's actions indicate
   a. Inability to cope with the forensic milieu
   b. The need for psychotherapy
   c. Boundary exploitation
   d. Appropriate self-awareness

4. An example of the forensic psychiatric nurse's role in primary prevention is

a. Conducting a relapse prevention program for sexual offenders

b. Applying principles of crisis management after a suicide attempt

c. Developing a medication management program for an offender with schizophrenia

d. Participating in a multidisciplinary committee focusing on domestic violence

5. Which of the following risk factors contribute to a higher rate of suicide in forensic populations?

a. History of psychiatric illness, difficulties facing the crime, perceived victimization by other offenders

b. Actual victimization by other offenders, lack of observation by nursing staff, ability to cope with a confined environment

c. Substance abuse, difficulties facing the length of the sentence, open communication with family members

d. Men older than 45 years, previous suicide attempts, acceptance of the crime

6. During the first phase of a crisis, the nurse is likely to observe which of the following in the client?

a. Increased levels of anxiety

b. Effective problem solving

c. Reaching out for help

d. Short attention span and rumination

7. The nurse recognizes that the goal for crisis intervention is which of the following?

a. Resolution of long-term problems

b. Gaining insight into past problems

c. Reestablishment of pre-crisis level of functioning

d. Resolving the crisis within 24 hours

8. The crisis that occurs as one grows older is called

a. Situational crisis

b. Maturational crisis

c. Crisis of values

d. Crisis of spirit

9. The nurse may evaluate the positive outcome for the nursing diagnosis of **Disturbed Thought Process** related to impaired ability to make decisions by which of the following:

a. The client's report of a decrease in feelings of anxiety

b. The client's use of the agreed-on coping (problem-solving) strategies

c. The client's ability to give a realistic interpretation of the crisis event

d. The client's recognition of personal capabilities

10. The rise in the number of mentally ill living outside the hospital setting has significantly increased because of all of the following except

a. The introduction of major tranquilizers

b. The reduction of low-income housing

c. An increase in U.S. immigration

d. The civil rights movement

11. Over the last two decades, the most rapidly increasing percentage of the homeless population is

a. Veterans

b. Families

c. Street youth

d. The mentally ill

12. The homeless population differs from the general population by having a

a. Higher incidence of schizophrenia

b. Greater likelihood of having an addictive disorder

c. Higher incidence of major affective disorders

d. All of the above

13. Which of the following would most likely be a barrier preventing a homeless mentally ill person from seeking services?

a. Type of symptoms they experience

b. Family history of disease

c. Clinic eligibility criteria

d. Length of time of homelessness

14. Which of the following general factors would most contribute of healthcare concerns among the homeless population?

a. Dependent positioning, exposure, population density, poor ventilation

b. Dependent positioning, exposure, inadequate hygiene, poor ventilation

c. Exposure, poor ventilation, drug abuse, irregular eating habits

d. Dependent positioning, exposure, anonymity, shelter rules

15. As a therapist who is communicating with a homeless mentally ill client in a shelter setting, you should

a. Identify yourself as a mental health nurse.

b. Avoid metaphors and use short, concrete sentences.

c. Discuss the symptoms you perceive the client to be experiencing.

d. Be gently indirect in expressing concerns regarding suicidal thoughts.

▼ REFERENCES AND SUGGESTED READINGS

*Aguilera, D. C. (1998). *Crisis intervention: Theory and methodology* (8th ed.). St. Louis: Mosby-Year Book.

*Allen, B., & Bosta, D. (1993). *Games criminals play*. Sacramento: Rae John Publishers.

*American Nurses Association. (1995). *Scope and standards of nursing practice in correctional facilities*. Washington, DC: Author.

*American Psychiatric Nurses Association. (1998). *Psychiatric-*

mental health nurse roles in outcomes evaluation and management [Position statement]. Washington, DC: Author.

*Anonymous. (1995). *Life goes on.* The John Howard Society of Saskatchewan Newsletter 3.

*Bardadell, J. (1994). Cost effectiveness and quality of care provided by clinical nurse specialists. *Journal of Psychosocial Nursing, 32*(3), 21–24.

*Berne, A. S., Dato, C., Mason, D. J., & Rafferty, M. (1990). A nursing model of addressing the health needs of homeless families. *Image Journal of Nursing Scholarship, 22*(3), 8–13.

*Blakeney, B. A. (1992). Health care and homeless people. In R. K. Schutt, & G. R. Garrett (Eds.), *Responding to the homeless: Policy and practice* (pp. 163–190). New York: Plenum Press.

*Burrow, S. (1995). Suicide: The crisis in the prison service. *British Journal of Nursing, 4*(4), 215–218.

*Caplan, G. (1964). *Principles of preventive psychiatry.* New York: Basic Books.

*Chafetz, L. (1990). Withdrawal from the homeless mentally ill. *Community Mental Health Journal, 26*(5), 449–461.

*Connolly, P. M. (1992). What does a nurse need to know and do to maintain an effective case management? *Journal of Psychosocial Nursing, 30*(3), 35–39.

*Conrad, B. S. (1998). Maternal depressive symptoms and homeless children's mental health: Risk and resiliency. *Archives of Psychiatric Nursing, 12*(1), 50–58.

*Dale, J., Williams, S., & Crouch, R. (1995). Development of telephone advice in A & E: Establishing the views of staff. *Nursing Standard, 9*(21), 28–31.

*Doyle, J. (1998). Prisoners as patients: The experience of delivering mental health nursing care in an Australian prison. *Journal of Psychosocial Nursing, 36*(12), 25–29.

*Duffey, J., Miller, M., & Parlocha, P. (1993). Psychiatric home care: A framework for assessment and intervention. *Home Health Nurse, 11*(2), 22–28.

*duPont, K., & Halasz, I. M. (1998). *Diversity: Communicating effectively.* Landam, MD: American Correctional Association.

*Dvoskin, J. A., & Broaddus, R. (1993). Creating a mental health care model. *Corrections Today, 55*(7), 114–115.

*Eppard, J., & Anderson, J. (1995). Emergency psychiatric assessment: The nurse, psychiatrist, and counselor roles during the process. *Journal of Psychosocial Nursing, 33*(10), 17–23.

*Erikson, E. (1963). *Childhood and society* (2nd ed.). New York: WW Norton.

*Fisk, D., Rakfeldt, J., Heffernan, K., & Rowe, M. (1999). Outreach workers' experiences in a homeless outreach project: Issues of boundaries, ethics and staff safety. *Psychiatric Quarterly, 70*(3), 231–246.

*Goldkuhle, U. (1999). Professional education for correctional nurses: A community based partnership model. *Journal of Psychosocial Nursing, 37*(9), 38–44.

*Green, C., Andre, G., Kendall, K., Looman, T., & Polvi, N. (1992). A study of 133 suicides among Canadian federal prisoners. *Forum on Corrections Research, 4*(3), 17–19.

*Greenwood, A. (1995). Forensic mental health treatment: Do we really know what we are talking about? *Forum on Correctional Research, 7*(3), 27–29.

*Hancock, P. (1998). CCHP's convene seminar on managing stress in correctional health environments. *CorrectCare, 12*(2), 4.

*Haus, A. (Ed.). (1988). *Working with homeless people.* New York: Columbia University.

*Hoff, L. (1995). *People in crisis: Understanding and helping* (4th ed.). Menlo Park, CA: Addison-Wesley.

*Hufft, A.G. (1999). Girl scouts beyond bars: A unique opportunity for forensic psychiatric nursing. *Journal of Psychosocial Nursing, 37*(9), 45–51.

*Hufft, A.G. (2000). The role of the forensic nurse in the USA. In D. Robinson, & A. Kettles (Eds.), *Forensic nursing and multidisciplinary care of the mentally disordered offender* (pp. 213–239). London: Jessica Kingsley Publishers.

*Hufft, A. G., & Fawkes, L. S. (1994). Federal inmates: A unique psychiatric nursing challenge. *Nursing Clinics of North America, 29*(1), 35–42.

*Hufft, A.G., & Peternelj-Taylor, C. (2000). Forensic nursing: An emerging specialty. In J. T. Catalano (Ed.), *Nursing now! Today's issues, tomorrow's trends* (pp. 427–444). Philadelphia: F.A. Davis Company.

*International Association of Forensic Nurses & the American Nurses Association. (1997). *Scope and standards of forensic nursing practice.* Washington, DC: American Nurses Association.

*Jambunathan, J., & Bellaire, K. (1999). Evaluating staff crisis prevention intervention techniques: A pilot study. *Issues in Mental Health Nursing, 17*(6), 541–558.

*Jeste, D. V., Gladsjo Akiko, J., Lindamer, L., & Lacro, J. (1996). Medical comorbidity in schizophrenia. *Schizophrenia Bulletin, 22,* 413–430.

*Kemph, J. P., Braley, R. O., & Ciotola, P. V. (1998). A comparison of youthful inmates who have committed violent vs. nonviolent crimes. *Journal of the American Academy of Psychiatry and Law, 26*(1), 67–74.

*Kent-Wilkinson, A. (1999). Forensic family genogram: An assessment and intervention tool. *Journal of Psychosocial Nursing, 32*(9), 52–56.

*Kline, M., Schonfeld, D. J., & Lichtenstein, R. (1995). Benefits and challenges of school-based crisis response. *Journal of School Health, 65*(7), 245–249.

*Labecki, L. A. S. (1994). Monitoring hostility: Avoiding prison disturbances through environmental scanning. *Corrections Today, 56*(5), 104–106.

*Lamb, H. R. (1984). Deinstitutionalization in the homeless mentally ill. In H. R. Lamb (Ed.), *The homeless mentally ill.* Washington, DC: American Psychiatric Association.

*Lezak, A. D., & Edgar, E. (1988). *Preventing homelessness among people with serious mental illnesses: A guide for states.* New York: Policy Research Associates, Inc.

*Liefland, L., Carporale, E. M., Wellington, T., & Barber, L. (1997). A crisis intervention program: Staff go the extra mile for client improvement. *Journal of Psychosocial Nursing and Mental Health Services, 35*(2), 32–35, 40–41.

*Lindeman, E. (1994). Symptomology and management of acute grief. *American Journal of Psychiatry, 101,* 141–148.

*Love, C. C., & Hunter, M. (1999). The Atascadero state hospital experience: Engaging patients in violence prevention. *Journal of Psychosocial Nursing, 37*(9), 32–36.

*Lynch, V. A., & Burgess, A. W. (1998). Forensic nursing. In A.W. Burgess (Ed.), *Advanced practice psychiatric nursing* (pp. 473–490). Stamford, CT: Appleton & Lange.

*Maeve, M. K. (1997). Nursing practice with incarcerated women: Caring within mandated (sic) alienation. *Issues in Mental Health Nursing, 18,* 495–510.

*Martin, K., & Scheet, N. (1992). *The Omaha system: A pocket guide for community health nursing.* Philadelphia: W. B. Saunders.

*Marx, G. (1995). Prisons try new therapies to treat sex offenders. *CorrectCare, 9*(1), 6.

*Meehan, T., & Boateng, A. (1997). Crisis intervention workers in New South Wales: Knowledge, skills, qualities, and preparation. *Australian New Zealand Journal of Mental Health Nursing, 6*(3), 122–128.

*Mercer, D., Mason, T., & Richman, J. (1999). Good and evil in the crusade of care: Social constructions of mental disorders. *Journal of Psychosocial Nursing, 37*(9), 13–17.

*Mercer, D., Mason, T., McKeown, M., & McCann, G. (2000). *Forensic mental health care.* Edinburgh: Churchill Livingstone.

*Milestone, C. (1995). *The mentally ill and the criminal justice system: Innovative community-based programs.* Ottawa: Minister of Supply and Services, Canada.

*Mitchell, J. T. (1983). When disaster strikes: The critical incident stress debriefing process. *Journal of Emergency Medical Services, 8,* 36–39.

*Morse, G. (1999). *Reaching out to homeless people with serious mental illnesses under managed care.* Delmar, NY: Policy Research Associates, Inc.

*National Coalition for the Homeless (1999a). *Who is homeless?* (NCH Fact Sheet No. 3). Washington, DC: Author.

*National Coalition for the Homeless. (1999b). *Why are people homeless?* (NCH Fact Sheet No. 1). Washington, DC: Author.

*Neely, K. W. (1997). A model for a statewide critical incident stress (CIS) debriefing program for emergency services personnel. *Prehospital & Disaster Medicine, 12*(2), 43–48.

*Norris, M. P., & May, M. C. (1998). Screening for malingering in a correctional setting. *Law and Human Behavior, 22*(3), 315–323.

*Oakley, D. A., & Dennis, D. L. (1996). Responding to the needs of homeless people with alcohol, drug and/or mental disorders. In J. Baumohl (Ed.), *Homelessness in America* (pp. 179–186). Phoenix, AZ: Oryx Press.

*Osborne, O. (1995). Public sector psychosocial nursing. *Journal of Psychosocial Nursing, 33*(8), 4–6.

*Palmer-Erbs, V., Connolly, P. M., Bianchi, R., & Hoff, L. (1996). Nursing perspectives on disability and rehabilitation. In K. Anchor (Ed.), *Disability analysis handbook: Tools for independent practice* (pp. 173–201). Dubuque, IA: Kendall/Hunt.

*Peternelj-Taylor, C. (1998). Forbidden love: Sexual exploitation in the forensic milieu. *Journal of Psychosocial Nursing, 36*(6), 17–23.

*Peternelj-Taylor, C. (1999). Forensic psychiatric nursing: The paradox of custody and caring. *Journal of Psychosocial Nursing, 37*(9), 9–11.

*Peternelj-Taylor, C. A. (2000). The role of the forensic nurse in Canada: An evolving specialty. In D. Robinson & A. Kettles (Eds.), *Forensic nursing and multidisciplinary care of the mentally disordered offender* (pp. 192–212). London: Jessica Kingsley Publishers.

*Peternelj-Taylor, C. A., & Johnson, R. L. (1995). Serving time: Psychiatric mental health nursing in corrections. *Journal of Psychosocial Nursing, 33*(8), 12–19.

*Peternelj-Taylor, C. A., & Johnson, R. L. (1996). Custody and caring: A unique partnership in psychiatric nursing education. *Perspectives in Psychiatric Care, 32*(4), 23–29.

*Pollack, P. H., Quigley, B., Worley, K. O., & Bashford, C. (1997). Feigned mental disorder in prisoners referred to forensic mental health services. *Journal of Psychiatric and Mental Health Nursing, 4*(1), 9–15.

*Porter, L. S., Marcial, A., & Sobong, L. (1997). Telephone hotline assessment and counseling of suicidal military veterans in the USA. *Journal of Advanced Nursing, 26*(4), 716–722.

*Project Respond, Mental Health Services West, Portland, Oregon (1997). Gold award: Linking mentally ill persons with services through crisis intervention, mobile outreach, and community education. *Psychiatric Services, 48*(11), 1450–1453.

*Ragaisis, K. M. (1994). Critical incident stress debriefing: A family nursing intervention. *Archives of Psychiatric Nursing, 8*(1), 38–43.

*Reeder, D., & Meldman, L. (1991). Conceptualizing psychosocial nursing in the jail setting. *Journal of Psychosocial Nursing, 29*(8), 40–44.

*Repper, J. (1999). A review of the literature on the prevention of suicide through intervention in accident and emergency departments. *Journal of Clinical Nursing, 8*(1), 3–12.

*Rowe, M., Hoge, M. A., & Fisk, D. (1996). Critical issues in serving people who are homeless and mentally ill. *Administration and Policy in Mental Health, 23*(6), 555–565.

*San Blise, M. L. (1994). Crisis intervention: Aftershocks in the quake zone. *Journal of Psychosocial Nursing, 32*(5), 29–30.

*Schafer, P. (1999). Working with Dave: Application of Peplau's interpersonal nursing theory in the correctional environment. *Journal of Psychosocial Nursing, 37*(9), 18–24.

*Schafer, P., & Peternelj-Taylor, C. (2000). Anger management. In D. Mercer, T. Mason, M. McKeown, & G. McCann (Eds.), *Forensic mental health care: A case study approach* (pp. 129–137). Edinburgh: Churchill Livingstone.

*Scheela, R. (1999). A nurse's experiences working with sex offenders. *Journal of Psychosocial Nursing, 37*(9), 25–31.

*Sigler, R. T. (1995). Gang violence. *Journal of Health Care for the Poor and Underserved, 6*(2), 198–203.

*Smith, E. M., & North, C. S. (1994). Not all homeless women are alike: Effects of motherhood and the presence of children. *Community Mental Health Journal, 30,* 601–610.

*Smyer, T., Gragert, M. D., & LaMere, S. (1997). Stay safe! Stay healthy! Surviving old age in prison. *Journal of Psychosocial Nursing, 35*(9), 10–17.

*Sowers, W., Thompson, K., & Mullins, S. (1999). *Mental health in corrections: An overview for correctional staff.* Landam, MD: American Correctional Association.

*Torrez, E. F. (1988). *Nowhere to go: The tragic odyssey of the homeless mentally ill.* New York: Harper & Row.

*Vitucci, N. (1999a). Corrections challenged with treating mentally ill inmates. *CorrectCare, 13*(3), 1, 14, 17–18.

*Vitucci, N. (1999b). Drug offenders represent 60% of the federal prison population in 1997. *CorrectCare, 13*(1), 8.

*Vitucci, N. (1999c). National prison population increases by five percent during 1997. *CorrectCare, 13*(1), 19.

*Vitucci, N. (1999d). New mental health publication to be offered. *CorrectCare, 13*(2), 14.

*Welch, A., & Ogloff, J. (1998). Mentally ill offenders in jails and prisons: Advances in service planning and delivery. *Current Opinion in Psychiatry, 11*(6), 683–687.

*Yalom, I. (1995). *The theory and practice of group psychotherapy* (4th ed.). New York: Basic Books.

**Starred references are cited in text.*

For additional information on this chapter, go to *http://connection. lww.com.*

Need more help? See Chapter 11 of the *Study Guide to Accompany Mohr: Johnson's Psychiatric Mental-Health Nursing, 5th ed.*

Psychopharmacology

GERALDINE PEARSON

Adherence—A client's willingness to receive recommended drug treatment as prescribed by a caregiver.

Affinity—A drug's tendency to be found at a given receptor site.

Agonist—A drug that initiates a therapeutic effect by binding to a receptor.

Antagonist—A drug that binds to receptors without causing any regulatory effect; its action is to block the binding of an endogenous agonist.

Efficacy—The information encoded in a drug's chemical structure that causes the receptor to change accordingly when the drug is bound.

Loss of efficacy—The loss of a drug's ability to achieve its maximum benefit.

Maximal efficacy—The maximal effect a drug can produce.

Neuroleptic malignant syndrome—A serious and potentially fatal side effect that accompanies use of certain antipsychotic agents. Characteristics include severe muscular rigidity, altered consciousness, stupor, catatonia, hyperpyrexia, and labile pulse and blood pressure.

Polypharmacy—Use of two or more psychotropic drugs, two or more drugs of the same chemical class, or two more drugs with the same or similar pharmacologic actions to treat different conditions.

Potency—The concentration of a drug in plasma.

Psychopharmacology—The study of the chemistry, disposition, actions, and clinical pharmacology of drugs used to treat psychiatric disorders.

Refractoriness—A state of desensitization in which a drug's effect diminishes with repeated or subsequent use of the same concentration.

Refractory mania—Bipolar disorder with mania that is completely unresponsive or marginally responsive to drug therapy with conventional mood-stabilizing agents.

Side effects—Dysfunctions and discomforts that a client experiences directly as a result of taking a medication.

Tardive dyskinesia—The most serious side effect of long-term use of neuroleptics, often with irreversible and severely disabling symptoms that include involuntary choreoathetotic movements affecting the face, tongue, perioral, buccal, and masticatory muscles.

Target symptoms—The specific symptoms that a medication aims to change.

On completion of this chapter, you should be able to accomplish the following:

- Describe principles of psychopharmacology and why they are important to the course of a client's treatment.
- Identify important classes and subclasses of psychotherapeutic drugs and the disorders for which they are commonly used.
- List the actions, mechanisms of action, therapeutic dosages, uses, side effects, potential toxicity, administration, contraindications, and nursing implications of various psychotropic medications.
- Explain how developments in psychopharmacology have changed the provision of and settings for psychiatric healthcare.
- Describe important components of the nursing process as they relate to medication management.
- Formulate a nursing care plan for a client whose treatment involves the use of psychotropic medication.

This chapter describes **psychopharmacology**, the study of drugs used to treat psychiatric disorders. It discusses many psychoactive medications that alter synaptic transmission in certain ways. For example, antidepressants called selective serotonin reuptake inhibitors (SSRIs) affect the serotonergic system by preventing the reuptake of serotonin at the synapse. An example of an SSRI is fluoxetine (Prozac). Likewise, antiseizure medications, such as valproic acid (Depakote), may increase the regulation of γ-aminobutyric acid (GABA).

Psychoactive medications, however, are *not* "silver bullets." They do not target *only* those neurotransmitters thought to control the symptomatic problem, they affect other neurotransmitters as well, which can lead to adverse effects or new problems. Psychopharmacology is not an exact science. Psychoactive medications are more like "buckshot": they have a wide "strike zone" (NAMI Provider Education Program, 2001). Not only do they hit the target, but they also affect everything around the target to a degree. They may shut down other neurotransmitter systems, or they may affect the same target receptors in other parts of the brain that control other vital functions. Thus, whereas psychotherapeutic drugs may improve a client's symptoms in one area, the client may experience unpleasant dysfunctions and discomforts in entirely new areas. These dysfunctions and discomforts are called **side effects**. The nurse, client, and family must understand the inexactitude of current psychopharmacologic treatment. Furthermore, nurses must avoid judging clients who fail to adhere to medication regimens. They also must keep an open mind to the mixed blessings of the medications that clients must take to function on a daily basis.

This chapter begins with a detailed discussion of important principles of psychopharmacotherapeutics, which can greatly influence the course of a client's treatment. The chapter discusses the actions, therapeutic dosages, uses, side effects, potential toxicity, administration, contraindications, and implications of the most important psychotropic medications used currently. It explores the influence of psychopharmacology on nursing care and each step of the nursing process as it relates to the client using psychotherapeutic drugs. Finally, the chapter presents special issues related to the use of psychotherapeutic drugs, such as life span considerations and concomitant use with alternative therapies.

IMPORTANT PRINCIPLES OF PSYCHOPHARMACO-THERAPEUTICS

Regardless of treatment setting, nurses assume an invaluable role in assisting clients and families as they deal with psychotropic medications. For example, the nurse who coordinates an outpatient medication group for clients with schizophrenia monitors symptoms, general functioning, and health needs of group members throughout treatment. A nurse practicing in a home healthcare agency discusses medication issues with clients and families in their home environment. Nurses in inpatient settings provide the health teaching about medications needed by clients and families in preparation for discharge to the community. All nurses should view multiple aspects of a client's life while he or she is undergoing psychopharmacotherapeutic treatment, monitor response to medication, and continually assess the client's needs to maximize functioning.

This section discusses the principles of psychopharmacotherapeutics that are especially important for nurses to understand. Concepts include agonists and antago-nists, affinity, efficacy, potency, target symptoms, refractoriness, and polypharmacy.

Agonists

Drug interactions with the human body are complex and involve biochemical and physiologic responses. Understanding these responses and what they mean for the client—the relief of target symptoms or the development of side effects—is essential for nurses.

Most drug effects result from the medication's interaction with "macromolecular components of the organism" (Ross & Kenakin, 2001, p. 31). The drug alters the function of the physiologic component, which results in biochemical changes that become the response to the drug.

An **agonist** is a drug that initiates a therapeutic effect by binding to a receptor (Aschenbrenner, Cleveland, & Venable, 2002). It is essential to understand the following:

> *The statement that the receptor for a drug can be any functional macromolecular component of the organism has several fundamental corollaries. One is that a drug potentially is capable of altering the rate at which any bodily function proceeds. Another is that drugs do not create effects, but instead, modulate intrinsic physiological functions.*
>
> —*(Ross & Kenakin, 2001, p. 31)*

Thus, drugs used to treat a particular psychiatric illness can significantly affect other body functions. An example is the use of lithium carbonate to treat bipolar disorder. Whereas lithium can relieve the symptoms of bipolar disorder, it can adversely affect thyroid and kidney function.

Partial agonists are drugs that are only partially effective as agonists; *inverse agonists* are agonists that stabilize the receptor in an inactive state (Ross & Kenakin, 2001).

Antagonists

Drug **antagonists**, in contrast to agonists, bind receptors without causing any regulatory effect. Their binding, in turn, blocks the binding of the endogenous agonist. These drugs are useful because of their inhibitory action. As antagonists, they compete for agonist binding sites.

Affinity

Drugs generally affect receptors in two ways: they may bind to them, or may change their behavior towards the host cell system (Ross & Kenakin, 2001). Binding is influenced by the chemical property of **affinity**, which means the tendency of a drug to be found at a given receptor site. The chemical forces that make the drug associate with receptors govern affinity.

Efficacy

The second way that drugs affect receptors involves **efficacy**, which is the information encoded in a drug's chemical structure that causes the receptor to change accordingly when the drug is bound (Ross & Kenakin, 2001). **Maximal efficacy**, or the maximal effect that a drug can produce, is different. The properties of the drug and its receptor–effector system principally determine maximal efficacy, which is reflected in the plateau of the concentration effect curve (Nies, 2001).

Understanding efficacy is essential because some psychoactive medications lose their effectiveness over time, even when clients have been using them successfully for years. Often, a client presents to a clinician with a complaint that "my medication just 'pooped out.'" This is a result of loss of efficacy. This principle of efficacy also suggests that the healthcare team may need to limit or change the dose of a given drug according to its undesirable side effects or adverse effects. The maximal efficacy of a given drug may not be achievable for certain clients. For example, a client with schizophrenia might have a favorable clinical response (ie, improvement in symptoms of schizophrenia) to clozapine (Clozaril); however, he or she will need to discontinue the drug if blood studies reveal agranulocytosis.

Potency

Potency is related to the concentration of a drug in plasma. Although the dose of a drug required is thought to produce an effect, Nies (2001) cites it as "relatively unimportant in the clinical use of drugs as long as the required dose can be given conveniently and there is not toxicity related to the chemical structure of the drug rather than to its mechanism" (Nies, 2001, p. 50).

Target Symptoms

Target symptoms are the specific symptoms that a medication aims at changing. The healthcare team must identify and understand the client's target symptoms before starting the client on a medication regimen. Certain drugs target particular symptoms. The client also must understand his or her target symptoms and participate in identifying and monitoring changes in symptoms.

Instruments, such as the Brief Psychiatric Rating Scale (BPRS), are available to systematically rate symptoms before and after drug administration (Lachar et al., 2001) (Figure 12-1). The BPRS can be used in con-

junction with the opinions of interdisciplinary treatment team members, including nurses.

Refractoriness

Refractoriness, also called *down-regulation*, generally occurs when agonists continually stimulate cells. As a result, the cells are repeatedly exposed to the same concentration of the drug, which causes the cells to become desensitized and the drug to have diminished effectiveness (Ross & Kenakin, 2001).

The phenomenon of refractoriness is important in psychiatric nursing. Many clients with psychiatric disorders must take the same medication for months to years. Over time, the effectiveness or efficacy of a medication may diminish, causing the symptoms that first required treatment to reappear. Thirty percent of people taking psychoactive medications do not respond to or cannot tolerate them. Early identification of refractoriness and the resulting changes in medication type or dose could prevent a relapse of symptoms.

Polypharmacy

Polypharmacy is defined as the use of two or more psychotropic drugs, the use of two or more drugs of the same chemical class, or the use of two more drugs with the same or similar pharmacologic actions to treat different conditions (Kingsbury, Yi, & Simpson, 2001). The frequency of polypharmacy tends to be high, especially in the treatment of clients with serious psychiatric disorders (Frye et al., 2000). While polypharmacy can be critical in the treatment of psychiatric disorders, it can increase the chance of adverse effects, drug interactions, client nonadherence, and medication errors (Kingsbury et al., 2001). It also can result in symptom amelioration in clients with severe psychosis (Stahl, 1999), resistant schizophrenia (Lemer, Chudakova, Kravets, & Polyakova, 2000), and depression (Mischoulon, Nierenberg, Kizilbash, Rosenbaum, & Fava, 2000).

Nurses must question the use of several agents to treat a disorder and should understand the rationale behind polypharmacy. They must explore specific target symptoms, drug-to-drug interactions, and the client's understanding of medication management. Taking more than one agent can confuse a client, especially if dosing times for each drug differ. Health education can assist clients to understand the purpose, side effects, and efficacy. The goal of medication management always should be optimal treatment with the fewest medications possible.

Nurses should understand the philosophy regarding polypharmacy held by the treatment setting where they practice. Although not appropriate for all clients, with careful management, the practice can provide symptom relief to clients with refractory disorders.

DIRECTIONS: Place an X in the appropriate box to represent level of severity of each symptom.

	Not Present	Very Mild	Mild	Moderate	Mod. Severe	Severe	Extremely Severe
SOMATIC CONCERN—preoccupation with physical health, fear of physical illness, hypochondriasis.	☐	☐	☐	☐	☐	☐	☐
ANXIETY—worry, fear, overconcern for present or future, uneasiness.	☐	☐	☐	☐	☐	☐	☐
EMOTIONAL WITHDRAWAL—lack of spontaneous interaction, isolation deficiency in relating to others.	☐	☐	☐	☐	☐	☐	☐
CONCEPTUAL DISORGANIZATION—thought processes confused, disconnected, disorganized, disrupted.	☐	☐	☐	☐	☐	☐	☐
GUILT FEELINGS—self-blame, shame, remorse for past behavior.	☐	☐	☐	☐	☐	☐	☐
TENSION—physical and motor manifestations of nervousness, over-activation.	☐	☐	☐	☐	☐	☐	☐
MANNERISMS AND POSTURING—peculiar, bizarre unnatural motor behavior (not including tic).	☐	☐	☐	☐	☐	☐	☐
GRANDIOSITY—exaggerated self-opinion, arrogance, conviction of unusual power or abilities.	☐	☐	☐	☐	☐	☐	☐
DEPRESSIVE MOOD—sorrow, sadness, despondency, pessimism.	☐	☐	☐	☐	☐	☐	☐
HOSTILITY—animosity, contempt, belligerence, disdain for others.	☐	☐	☐	☐	☐	☐	☐
SUSPICIOUSNESS—mistrust, belief others harbour malicious or discriminatory intent.	☐	☐	☐	☐	☐	☐	☐
HALLUCINATORY BEHAVIOR—perceptions without normal external stimulus correspondence.	☐	☐	☐	☐	☐	☐	☐
MOTOR RETARDATION—slowed weakened movements or speech, reduced body tone.	☐	☐	☐	☐	☐	☐	☐
UNCOOPERATIVENESS—resistance, guardedness, rejection of authority.	☐	☐	☐	☐	☐	☐	☐
UNUSUAL THOUGHT CONTENT—unusual, odd, strange, bizarre thought content.	☐	☐	☐	☐	☐	☐	☐
BLUNTED AFFECT—reduced emotional tone, reduction in formal intensity of feelings, flatness.	☐	☐	☐	☐	☐	☐	☐
EXCITEMENT—heightened emotional tone, agitation, increased reactivity.	☐	☐	☐	☐	☐	☐	☐
DISORIENTATION—confusion or lack of proper association for person, place, or time.	☐	☐	☐	☐	☐	☐	☐

Global Assessment Scale (Range 1–100)

FIGURE 12-1   Brief Psychiatric Rating Scale. (Reprinted with permission from Overall, J. E. [1998]. The Brief Psychiatric Rating Scale [BRPS]: Recent developments in ascertainment and scaling. *Psychopharmacology Bulletin, 24,* 97–99.)

IMPORTANT PSYCHOTHERAPEUTIC DRUGS

This section explores the most important psychotherapeutic drugs in current use: antidepressants, mood stabilizers, anxiolytics, antipsychotics (neuroleptics), and stimulants. The reader will find more information throughout Unit IV of the text about these and other drugs as they relate to specific disorders. All nurses working in psychiatric-mental healthcare, however, must be familiar with the particulars of the drugs discussed here.

Medications for Mood Disorders

In the fourth edition of the *Diagnostic and Statistical Manual of Mental Disorders,* text revision, the American Psychiatric Association (APA, 2000) divides mood disorders into depressive disorders (unipolar depression) and bipolar disorders. Both types can occur in children and adults; the APA does not differentiate between adults and children with regard to symptom manifestation of mood disorders. Chapter 24 describes in detail mood disorders and their treatment. The two major subclasses of medications for mood disorders are antidepressants and mood stabilizers.

ANTIDEPRESSANTS

Both unipolar depressive and bipolar disorders respond to antidepressant medications; antidepressants are used regularly to treat major depressive disorders and the symptoms of depression not associated with major depressive disorders (Table 12-1). These symptoms are as follows:

- Dysphoric mood
- Change in appetite and energy level
- *Anhedonia,* or lack of interest in routine activities
- Difficulty concentrating
- Feelings of hopelessness
- Suicidality

Antidepressants also have been used to treat obsessive-compulsive disorder (OCD) and other anxiety disorders (see Chap. 18).

Whereas antidepressants are considered appropriate treatment for major depression, they should be used with caution in clients with a history of cardiac or seizure disorders (Baldessarini, 2001). A thorough physical examination of the client is required to determine cardiovascular irregularities before the provider initiates medication. A baseline electrocardiogram usually is recommended as well.

The ingestion of large amounts of antidepressant medications is potentially life threatening; therefore, providers must use caution when dispensing all categories of antidepressant medication to clients who are at risk for suicide or self-injury. Outpatient providers frequently give only a few days' to 1 week's worth of medication, requiring the client to return for evaluation before dispensing more medication.

Antidepressant medications are divided into three categories (Baldessarini, 2001) (Box 12-1):

- Tricyclic antidepressants (TCAs) and atypical agents
- Monoamine oxidase inhibitors (MAOIs)
- Selective serotonin reuptake inhibitors (SSRIs), selective reuptake inhibitors (SRIs), and selective norepinephrine reuptake inhibitors (SNRIs)

Tricyclic Antidepressants

The TCAs, including desipramine (Norpramin), imipramine (Tofranil), doxepin (Sinequan), and amitriptyline (Elavil), inhibit neuronal uptake of both serotonin and norepinephrine. They are anticholinergic at central nervous system (CNS) and peripheral receptors and act as sedatives. Developed in the 1960s, these drugs were the medications first used to combat major depressive disorders, and they were the early precursors to the newer SSRIs. All TCAs have a three-ring molecular core; most of them share pharmacologic and clinical (antidepressant and anxiolytic) properties (Baldessarini, 2001). Currently, TCAs are used most often for cases of severe melancholia. The typical symptom pattern in clinical depression (early morning wakening, feeling worse in the morning, anxiety, and weight loss) is predictive of a good response to TCAs.

TCAs are used to relieve depression and, in some cases, panic disorder and OCD (see Chap. 18). They are thought to inhibit the reuptake of norepinephrine and serotonin in the synapse. Because TCAs are medications with the "buckshot" approach discussed earlier, they also block another neurotransmitter, acetylcholine, which controls the cholinergic system. Blockage of acetylcholine leads to the predominant side effects of TCAs: sedation and the anticholinergic effects of dry mouth, blurred vision, urinary retention, delayed micturition, dizziness, and fainting. Other side effects include confusion, disturbed concentration, and constipation. Nausea, headache, and vertigo can result if the medication is withdrawn abruptly. Nurses should watch for orthostatic hypotension in clients beginning to take TCAs.

As a rule, the more sedating the TCA, the more anticholinergic properties it will have. The tetracyclic antidepressant mirtazapine (Remeron) (see discussion later) has been developed to reduce the discomfort of these side effects. Other ways to control side effects from TCAs include starting the client with low doses and raising doses slowly or changing to another antidepressant with less problematic side effects. Because clients taking TCAs frequently do not experience clinical effects for 2 to 6 weeks, they require support and encouragement to get through this time of adjustment.

Administration is oral. TCAs should be carefully distributed to suicidal clients, given the high risk and lethality of overdose. The most drastic consequence of this class of medications is the danger that they pose as lethal agents of suicide. Taken together, a 10-day supply of these medications may cause cardiac and cerebral toxicity. With clients beginning antidepressant medication therapy, a good rule of thumb is for practitioners to limit the amount of medication prescribed at any one time. Moreover, clients beginning these medications should be carefully monitored because research indicates that risk for suicide increases when clients begin to "feel better" or energized.

When TCAs are given in conjunction with oral anticoagulants, the client may be at risk for bleeding. Administration with clonidine may cause severe hypertension. Although MAOIs and TCAs can be used together to successfully treat refractory depression, severe adverse reactions (including hyperpyretic crises and hypertensive episodes) may occur. Nurses must observe and document adverse reactions to TCAs, especially if administration

text continues on page 232

TABLE 12-1 ▼ Antidepressants

GENERIC AND BRAND NAMES	USUAL DOSE	SEDATION LEVEL/ HALF-LIFE	SIDE EFFECTS	RELIEF OF SYMPTOMS
Tricyclic Antidepressants (TCAs)				
desipramine (Norpramin, Pertofrane)	100–350 mg/day	Less sedating than other TCAs	Dry mouth, tremors, blurred vision, bloating and weight gain, urinary retention	2–4 wk; side effects may be discouraging
imipramine (Tofranil)	100–150 mg/day PO in divided doses; gradually increase to 200 mg/day; if no response after 2 wk, may be increased to 250–300 mg/day	May be sedating, at least initially; half-life is 8–16 hr	Sedation, anticholinergic effects, confusions, disturbed concentration, dry mouth, constipation, orthostatic hypotension	Decreased anxiety immediately evident; antidepressant response may require 2–3 wk
nortriptyline (Aventyl, Pamelor)	75–150 mg/day PO	May be sedating	Dry mouth, tremors, blurred vision, bloating and weight gain, urinary retention	2 to 4 wk; side effects may be discouraging
doxepin (Sinequan)	25 mg PO TID for mild to moderate anxiety and depression; 50 mg PO TID (up to 300 mg/day) for more severe anxiety and depression	May be sedating; half-life is 8–25 hr	Sedation and anticholinergic effects, confusion, disturbed concentration, dry mouth, constipation, orthostatic hypotension	2–4 wk
amitriptyline (Elavil)	Initially, 75–100 mg/day PO in divided doses; gradually increase to 200–300 mg/day PO	May be sedating; half-life is 10–50 hr	Sedation and anticholinergic effects, confusion, disturbed concentration, dry mouth, constipation, orthostatic hypotension	Beginning relief of symptoms may take 2–4 wk
protriptiline (Vivactil)	15–40 mg/day PO	Moderately sedating	Decreased sexual function, dry mouth, tremors, blurred vision, bloating and weight gain, urinary retention	2–4 wk; side effects may be discouraging
amoxapine (Ascendin)	150–300 mg/day PO	Sedating	Too high a dose can cause irregularities in heartbeat; dry mouth, tremors, blurred vision, bloating and weight gain, urinary retention	Can be lethal in a suicide attempt; 2–4 wk; side effects may be discouraging

(continued)

TABLE 12-1 ▼ **Antidepressants (Continued)**

GENERIC AND BRAND NAMES	USUAL DOSE	SEDATION LEVEL/ HALF-LIFE	SIDE EFFECTS	RELIEF OF SYMPTOMS
trimipramine (Surmontil)	100–250mg/day PO	Sedating	Cognitive impairment, memory loss, confusion, dry mouth, tremors, blurred vision, bloating and weight gain, urinary retention	Can be lethal in a suicide attempt; 2–4 wk; side effects may be discouraging
clomipramine (Anafranil)	75–250 mg/day PO	Sedating	Cognitive impairment, memory loss, confusion, dry mouth, tremors, blurred vision, bloating and weight gain, urinary retention	Can be lethal in a suicide attempt; 2–4 wk; side effects may be discouraging
Tetracyclic Antidepressants				
maprotiline (Ludiomil)	25 to 75 mg/day PO	High sedation	Increased likelihood of seizure; sedation and anticholinergic effects, confusion, disturbed concentration, dry mouth, constipation, nausea, agranulocytosis, neutropenia	Clinical response in 3–7 days or up to 2–3 wk
mirtazapine (Remeron)	Initial dose of 15 mg/day PO as a single evening dose; may be increased up to 45 mg/day PO as needed	May be sedating; half-life is 20–40 hr	Sedation and anticholinergic effects, confusion, disturbed concentration, dry mouth, constipation, nausea, agranulocytosis, neutropenia	Clinical response in 3–7 days or up to 2–3 wk
Monoamine Oxidase Inhibitors (MAOIs)				
phenelzine sulfate (Nardil)	Initially, 15 mg PO TID; increase dose to at least 60 mg/day at rapid pace according to client tolerance; some may require 90 mg/day	Likely to energize; half-life is unknown	Dizziness, vertigo, headache, overactivity, hyperreflexia, tremors, muscle twitching, mania, hypomania, jitteriness, confusion, memory impairment, insomnia, weakness, fatigue, drowsiness, restlessness, overstimulation, in-	Up to 4 wk for maximum response

(continued)

TABLE 12-1 ▼ **Antidepressants** (Continued)

GENERIC AND BRAND NAMES	USUAL DOSE	SEDATION LEVEL/ HALF-LIFE	SIDE EFFECTS	RELIEF OF SYMPTOMS
			creased anxiety, agitation, blurred vision, sweating, constipation, diarrhea, nausea, abdominal pain, edema, dry mouth, anorexia, weight changes, hypertensive crisis, orthostatic hypotension, disturbed cardiac rate and rhythm	
tranylcypromine (Parnate)	Most effective dose usually is 30 mg/ day PO in divided doses; if no improvement within 2 wk, increase dosage in 10-mg/ day increments to a maximum of 60 mg/day	May be stimulating, especially to clients with agitation or schizophrenia; half-life is unknown	Dizziness, vertigo, headache, overactivity, hyperreflexia, tremors, muscle twitching, mania, hypomania, jitteriness, confusion, memory impairment, insomnia, weakness, fatigue, drowsiness, restlessness, overstimulation, increased anxiety, agitation, blurred vision, sweating, constipation, diarrhea, nausea, abdominal pain, edema, dry mouth, anorexia, weight changes, hypertensive crises, orthostatic hypotension, disturbed cardiac rate and rhythm	Improvement within 48 hr to 3 wk
Selective Reuptake Inhibitors (SRIs)				
nefazodone (Serzone)	200 mg/day PO in two divided doses; increase at 1-wk intervals to 100–200 mg/day; usual range is 300–600 mg/day	May cause nervousness or insomnia *or* be slightly sedating; half-life is 2–3 days	Headache, nervousness, insomnia, drowsiness, anxiety, tremor, dizziness, light-headedness, nausea, vomiting, diarrhea, dry mouth, anorexia,	Beginning relief of symptoms may take 2–4 wk

(continued)

TABLE 12-1 ▼ Antidepressants (Continued)

GENERIC AND BRAND NAMES	USUAL DOSE	SEDATION LEVEL/ HALF-LIFE	SIDE EFFECTS	RELIEF OF SYMPTOMS
			dyspepsia, constipation, taste changes, sweating, rash, pruritus	
trazodone (Desyrel)	Initially, 150 mg/day PO with increase of 50 mg/day every 3–4 days; maximum dose should not exceed 600 mg/day in divided doses for severely depressed clients	May cause drowsiness *or* agitation; half-life is 3–6 hr and then 5–9 hr	Anger, hostility, agitation, nightmares/vivid dreams, hallucinations, delusions, hypomania, confusion, disorientation, decreased concentration, impaired memory, impaired speech, dizziness, lack of coordination, drowsiness, fatigue, gastric disorder, decreased/increased appetite, dry mouth, bad taste in mouth, nausea, vomiting, diarrhea, flatulence, constipation, hypertension, hypotension, shortness of breath, syncope, tachycardia, palpitations, decreased libido, allergic skin conditions, edema	10–14 days and up to 2–4 wk
bupropion (Wellbutrin)	300–450 mg/day	Low; if anything, energizing; half-life is 8–24 hr	Weight loss, agitation, risk of seizures, relative absence of sexual dysfunction	10–14 days
Selective Serotonin Reuptake Inhibitors (SSRIs)				
citalopram (Celexa)	Initially 20 mg/day PO as a single dose; may be increased to 40 mg/day if needed	May be energizing; half-life is 35 hr	Nausea, dry mouth, sweating, somnolence, dizziness, insomnia, ejaculatory disorders	4–6 wk
fluoxetine (Prozac)	Initial dose of 20 mg/day PO in AM; if no improvement after several weeks, increase dose on a BID	May be energizing; half-life is 2–9 days	Headache, nervousness, insomnia, drowsiness, anxiety, tremor, dizziness, lightheadedness	Up to 4 wk

(continued)

TABLE 12-1 ▼ **Antidepressants** (Continued)

GENERIC AND BRAND NAMES	USUAL DOSE	SEDATION LEVEL/ HALF-LIFE	SIDE EFFECTS	RELIEF OF SYMPTOMS
	schedule up to 80 mg/day PO		nausea, vomiting, diarrhea, dry mouth, anorexia, dyspepsia, constipation, taste changes, upper respiratory infections, pharyngitis, painful menstruation, sexual dysfunction, urinary frequency, sweating, rash, pruritus, weight loss, asthenia, fever	
paroxetine (Paxil)	20 mg/day PO as a single dose; may be increased up to 50 mg/day	May be energizing; half-life is 21 hr	Somnolence, dizziness, insomnia, tremor, nervousness, headache, nausea, dry mouth, constipation, diarrhea, ejaculatory disorders, male genital disorders, sweating, headache, asthenia	1–4 wk
sertraline (Zoloft)	Administer daily, AM or PM, 50 mg/day PO; may be increased up to 200 mg/day; increases occur at 1-wk intervals	May be energizing; half-life is 26 hr	Headache, nervousness, drowsiness, anxiety, tremor, dizziness, insomnia, nausea, diarrhea, dry mouth, rhinitis, painful menstruation, sweating	Beginning relief of symptoms may take 2–4 wk

occurs in conjunction with other psychotropic medications (Karch, 2002).

Atypical Antidepressants

Atypical antidepressants affect both noradrenergic and serotonergic neurotransmission. They include drugs such as bupropion, mirtazapine, nefazodone (Serzone), and trazodone (Desyrel) (Baldessarini, 2001). Administration and clinical management of clients taking these medications is the same as for clients taking TCAs. Side effects are similar: headache, nervousness, nausea, vomiting, and postural hypotension (Karch, 2002).

Monoamine Oxidase Inhibitors

The MAOIs were first derived from hydrazone, a potent hepatotoxic substance (Baldessarini, 2001). Drugs in this class, including phenelzine sulfate (Nardil) and tranylcypromine (Parnate), inhibit monamine oxidase (MAO), an enzyme that breaks down amines (epinephrine, norepinephrine, and serotonin). Amines thus are able to accumulate in neuronal storage sites, resulting in the clinical efficacy of MAOIs as antidepressants (Karch 2002). MAOIs are used to treat atypical forms of depression or are prescribed for clients who are unresponsive to other antidepressant regimens. Their use has been replaced largely by the SSRIs.

Therapeutic doses of phenelzine sulfate range from 45 to 60 mg daily. The most serious risk of MAOI use involves hypertensive crises. Other side effects include dizziness, vertigo, headache, overactivity, manic-like behavior, constipation, diarrhea, and nausea.

Clients taking MAOIs must avoid ingesting foods that contain tyramine. Examples include dairy products (especi-

Clients with refractory mania often take several different medications (Stahl, 2000). A growing body of data supports the use of other atypical antipsychotics (eg, olanzapine [Zyprexa], risperidone [Risperdal]) for stabilization of bipolar disorder because these medications are proving to be effective antimanic and antidepressant agents.

Similarly, primidone (Mysoline), traditionally used to treat epilepsy, has been shown, in a drug study, to have a positive therapeutic effect in 31% of the 26 clients experiencing refractory mania (Schaffer, Schaffer, & Caretto, 1999). The authors acknowledge that a 31% response rate may appear modest; however, given the refractory nature of the psychopathology, this response is worth noting.

Other drugs that may be used to treat refractory mania include pramipexole (Mirapex), a direct dopamine agonist used to treat Parkinson's disease (Goldberg, Frye, & Dunn, 1999); gabapentin, an antiepileptic agent; and nimodipine, a calcium channel blocker. Gabapentin inhibits polysynaptic responses and posttetanic potentiation. Its mechanism as an antiepileptic agent is unknown (Karch, 2002). Available for oral administration in capsule form, adult doses range from 900 to 1800 mg/day in three divided doses. Predominant side effects include dizziness, insomnia, somnolence, and ataxia. Gabapentin has decreased effectiveness when given with antacids and should not be used during pregnancy or lactation. It should be given with food to prevent gastrointestinal upset (Karch, 2002). Lamotrigine (Lamictal), an anticonvulsant, also has been suggested as treatment; it has shown effectiveness in both monotherapy and adjunctive therapy in treating refractory mania (Calabrese et al., 1999). Although effective in decreasing manic symptoms in 74% of clients studied, it caused a rash in 15% of clients. Co-administration of valproic acid or exceeding the recommended dose of the drug appears to increase the risk of rash (Calabrese et al., 1999).

Nurses working with clients with refractory mania need to maintain awareness of several clinical issues. They must carefully monitor side effects of atypical agents used for this disorder. Teaching clients about medications, doses, and side effects is especially important if more than one agent is being used to treat the disorder. Given the lethality of overdose with many of these drugs, nurses must maintain an awareness of a client's suicide risk and intervene if this becomes a clinical issue.

Anxiolytics

Anxiolytic or antianxiety medications are used to treat generalized anxiety disorder and may provide relief for acute anxiety states, social phobia, performance anxiety, and simple phobias (see Chap. 18) (Table 12-3). They also are used for short-term relief of insomnia. Anxiolytic medications include buspirone (BuSpar) and the benzodiazepines. Benzodiazepines are used to treat alcohol withdrawal and control symptoms such as anxiety and

agitation. They also may prevent seizures and progression to delirium tremens (Arana & Rosenbaum, 2000). Benzodiazepines also are useful in treating clients with mania or acute psychoses when safe and rapid sedation with relatively few side effects is desired.

BUSPIRONE

Buspirone is a novel anxiolytic that binds serotonin receptors. Its mechanism of action is not known; however, it lacks anticonvulsant, sedative, or muscle relaxant properties (Karch, 2002).

Buspirone generally is administered orally in tablet form. Adults usually begin with 15 mg daily in three divided doses. Increases of 5 mg/day are made every 2 to 3 days, with the maximum dose not to exceed 60 mg daily.

Buspirone is contraindicated in clients with marked renal or liver impairment and in lactating women. Adverse effects include dizziness, headache, nervousness, insomnia, light-headedness, nausea, dry mouth, and gastrointestinal distress. Buspirone must be used cautiously in clients who use alcohol or other CNS depressants; fluoxetine decreases the drug's effects. If taken with erythromycin, itraconazole, or nefazodone, serum levels of buspirone may increase and must be monitored (Karch, 2002).

BENZODIAZEPINES

In contrast to buspirone, benzodiazepines have the pharmacologic effects of anxiolysis, sedation, centrally mediated muscle relaxation, and elevation of the seizure threshold (Karch, 2002). Benzodiazepines act directly on GABA receptors and are thought to increase the amount of GABA available to dampen neural overstimulation. These medications generally are considered safe and effective, and their adverse side effects are extensions of their central actions. They may be excessively sedating. Concurrent use with narcotics or alcohol can potentiate the effects of benzodiazepines. In addition to these effects and the side effects also found with buspirone, benzodiazepines can stimulate a mild paradoxical excitatory reaction at the beginning of treatment.

Benzodiazepines have the potential to lose their efficacy. Clients may begin increasing their doses to achieve the previous response and discover that the medications are causing dependence. Dependence means that when the client stops taking the medication, he or she experiences pathologic symptoms and signs. In the past, a distinction was made between *physical* and *psychological* dependence, with physical withdrawal syndromes being the key indicator of "addiction." Moreover, stigma was attached to the idea of being "physically dependent" or "addicted" to these drugs. As stressed in Chapter 2, however, there is no psychology without physiology, and the concept of dependence (or addiction) is understood to

TABLE 12-3 ▼ **Anxiolytics**

GENERIC AND BRAND NAMES	USUAL DOSE	SEDATION LEVEL/ HALF-LIFE	SIDE EFFECTS	RELIEF OF SYMPTOMS
buspirone (BuSpar)	Initially 15 mg/day PO (5 mg TID); increase dose 5 mg/day at intervals of 2–3 days to achieve maximum therapeutic response; do not exceed 60 mg/day	Energizing; half-life of 3–11 hr	Dizziness, headache, nervousness, insomnia, light-headedness, nausea, dry mouth, vomiting, abdominal/gastric distress, diarrhea	Maximum benefit after reaching therapeutic dose
Benzodiazepines				
diazepam (Valium)	For anxiety disorder: 2–10 mg two to four times a day	Transient, mild drowsiness; half-life of 20–50 hr	Transient, mild drowsiness initially, sedation, depression, lethargy, apathy, fatigue, light-headedness, disorientation, restlessness, confusion, possible mild paradoxical excitatory reactions during first 2 wk of treatment, constipation, diarrhea, bradycardia, tachycardia, incontinence, urinary retention, changes in libido, drug dependence with a withdrawal syndrome	Immediately effective at therapeutic dose
lorazepam (Ativan)	Oral: 2–6 mg/day IM: 0.05 mg/kg	Transient, mild drowsiness; half-life 10–20 hr	Depression, lethargy, apathy, fatigue, light-headedness, disorientation, restlessness, constipation, dry mouth, nausea	Intermediate
alprazolam (Xanax)	Oral: 0.25–1 mg TID	Transient, mild drowsiness; half-life 6–20 hr	Depression, lethargy, apathy, fatigue, light-headedness, disorientation, restlessness, constipation, dry mouth, nausea	Intermediate
chlordiazepoxide (Librium)	Oral: 5–10 mg three to four times a day IM/IV: 50–100 mg/ day	Transient, mild drowsiness; half-life 30–100 hr	Depression, lethargy, apathy, fatigue, light-headedness, disorientation, restlessness, constipation, diarrhea,	Intermediate

(continued)

TABLE 12-3 ▼ Anxiolytics (Continued)

GENERIC AND BRAND NAMES	USUAL DOSE	SEDATION LEVEL/ HALF-LIFE	SIDE EFFECTS	RELIEF OF SYMPTOMS
			bradycardia, tachycardia, urinary retention, incontinence, changes in libido	
flurazepam (Dalmane)	10–30 mg/day	Transient, mild drowsiness; half-life 50–160 hr	Depression, lethargy, apathy, fatigue, light-headedness, disorientation, restlessness, asthenia, constipation, diarrhea, dyspepsia, bradycardia, tachycardia, urinary retention, incontinence, changes in libido	Rapid

be a cluster of cognitive, behavioral, affective, and physiologic signs that indicate compulsive use of a substance. Thus, the distinction between psychological and physiologic dependence is not useful.

Benzodiazepines should be used cautiously with older adults, debilitated clients, depressed or suicidal clients, and clients with a history of substance abuse. Withdrawal syndrome is possible on discontinuation of the medication and is most common with high doses of medication used for more than 4 months (Karch, 2002). Withdrawal symptoms include anxiety, irritability, tremulousness, sweating, lethargy, diarrhea, insomnia, depression, abdominal and muscle cramps, vomiting, and, at its most severe, convulsions. Benzodiazepines should be discontinued gradually with careful monitoring of client symptoms during the process. Onset of symptoms related to withdrawal or discontinuation generally reflects the half-life of the medication (1 to 2 days for short-acting drugs and 2 to 5 days for longer-acting drugs). Withdrawal symptoms, however, have been known to occur as late as 7 to 10 days after discontinuation. Symptoms generally peak several days after onset and disappear slowly over 1 to 3 weeks (Arana & Rosenbaum, 2000; Stahl, 2000). Clients must be cautioned not to abruptly discontinue taking these medications.

Diazepam is a commonly prescribed benzodiazepine. Although its mechanism of action is not understood, it acts mainly at the limbic system and reticular formation and may act at spinal cord sites to produce skeletal muscle relation. It also can be used in acute alcohol withdrawal and to control seizures.

Diazepam is available in several forms including oral tablets, intramuscular injection, and intravenous drip.

For anxiety disorders, the usual oral dose is 15 to 30 mg/day. In alcohol withdrawal, doses of 10 mg three times a day can be administered. If given intramuscularly or intravenously, a dose of 10 mg usually is prescribed (Karch, 2002).

Side effects of diazepam include transient, mild drowsiness; sedation; lethargy; fatigue; confusion; and depression. Clients may experience a mild paradoxical excitatory reaction during the first 2 weeks of therapy. Other side effects include constipation, diarrhea, bradycardia and tachycardia, incontinence, urinary retention, and changes in libido. Clients can develop drug dependence; discontinuation of the drug should be gradual if it has been prescribed for longer than 4 months (Karch, 2002).

Alcohol use and concurrent administration with cimetidine, disulfiram, and oral contraceptives increase the effects of diazepam. Use with theophyllines and ranitidine decreases the effects. Use of this drug is contraindicated in clients with sensitivity to benzodiazepines, psychoses, acute alcoholic intoxication, or acute narrow-angle glaucoma. It is contraindicated in pregnant and lactating women. Diazepam should be used cautiously in debilitated clients, older adults, and clients with impaired liver or kidney function.

Other benzodiazepines include lorazepam (Ativan), alprazolam (Xanax), chlordiazepoxide (Librium), and flurazepam (Dalmane) (see Table 12-3).

Antipsychotic (Neuroleptic) Agents

Antipsychotic medications, also known as neuroleptics, are used to treat severe psychiatric disorders such as schizophrenia (see Chap. 25). They also are used for acute and chronic thought disorders and confusion that commonly accompanies psychotic disorders, extreme aggressive behaviors, and dementia that accompanies conditions such as Alzheimer's disease (see Chap. 28). Target symptoms for these drugs include disorganized speech and behavior, flat or inappropriate affect, delusions, hallucinations, and catatonic behavior. Antipsychotic medications are subdivided into typical or traditional antipsychotic drugs and atypical antipsychotic drugs (Table 12-4).

TYPICAL OR TRADITIONAL ANTIPSYCHOTICS

For many years, traditional antipsychotic agents (neuroleptics) were the only class of medications to treat psychosis. Typical or traditional antipsychotic agents block dopamine receptors in the brain, thus altering the release and turnover of dopamine. Antipsychotic drugs are lipophilic and are metabolized by hepatic mechanisms (Baldessarini & Tarazi, 2001). All clients taking antipsychotic medications must be followed closely for adverse side effects. Unlike other medications such as antidepressants, the risk of overdose is low, even with large doses of the medication. The incidence of lethality also is low (Baldessarini & Tarazi, 2001).

The greatest hazard involves the development of adverse side effects, such as extrapyramidal reactions and tardive dyskinesia (TD). This risk of extrapyramidal symptoms and other movement disorders is highest for clients who use older, high-potency neuroleptic medications, such as haloperidol or perphenazine, for long periods. These neuroleptics set up a powerful dopamine blockade to control psychosis, but they also block dopamine receptors in the "motor strip" of the brain, which controls finely coordinated movements of the body. This "secondary blockade" gives rise to a group of neurologic movement disorders. Table 12-5 summarizes all the potential motor side effects of antipsychotic medications.

Monitoring the development of movement disorders is a complex process that should involve the client and family. Before initiating any neuroleptic medication, the client must understand the risks and hazards of taking the drug. If the client cannot participate in the process because of acute psychiatric symptoms, healthcare providers must involve the family or significant supports. Early diagnosis of beginning symptoms may result in prompt withdrawal of the neuroleptic or a change in medication. A thorough understanding of the symptoms and their cause will alleviate client and family anxiety if a movement disorder emerges.

Movement disorders occur most often with low-dose, high-potency phenothiazine medications such as fluphenazine. The most serious and potentially fatal side effect is **neuroleptic malignant syndrome**, which is characterized by severe muscular rigidity, altered consciousness, stupor, catatonia, hyperpyrexia, and labile pulse and blood pressure. This life-threatening condition can occur after a

single dose of a neuroleptic drug; however, it is more common in the first 2 weeks of administration or with an increase in dose (Baldessarini & Tarazi, 2001). This syndrome can continue for up to 2 weeks after the discontinuation of medication; treatment involves immediate cessation of the medication and hospitalization to stabilize acute symptoms.

Tardive dyskinesia (TD) is the most serious side effect of long-term use of neuroleptics because of its often irreversible and severely disabling symptoms, which include involuntary choreoathetotic movements affecting the face, tongue, perioral, bucca, and masticatory muscles. TD also may involve the neck, torso, and extremities. The risk of developing irreversible TD increases with cumulative dose and duration of neuroleptic treatment. Fine wormlike movements of the tongue may be the first signs of TD; discontinuing the medication when this occurs may prevent development of the full-blown syndrome (Baldessarini & Tarazi, 2001). Whereas decreasing or discontinuing neuroleptic medication is the best treatment for TD, it also can precipitate the development of withdrawal dyskinesia. These symptoms are the same as those of TD, but they tend to resolve within a few weeks. Clients need help in understanding that it may take time for the symptoms to resolve even if the medication has been discontinued.

Low-Potency Typical Antipsychotics

Two examples of low-potency typical antipsychotics include chlorpromazine (Thorazine) and thioridazine (Mellaril). Chlorpromazine, developed in the early 1950s, was found to decrease arousal and motility in clients experiencing psychotic symptoms (Baldessarini & Tarazi, 2001). Thioridazine was developed soon after; like chlorpromazine, it depresses the parts of the brain involved with wakefulness and emesis and is an anticholinergic, antihistaminic, and alpha-adrenergic blocker (Karch, 2002).

Chlorpromazine is a phenothiazine used for psychotic disorders. It is available in tablets, sustained-release capsules, liquid concentrate, suppositories, and as an injection. Up to 2000 mg/day can be given to inpatients. The usual dose is 200 to 800 mg/day for the management of psychotic symptoms. Its use is contraindicated in clients with severely depressed or comatose states, bone marrow suppression, and cerebral or arterial arteriosclerosis. Adverse effects include drowsiness, insomnia, vertigo, dry mouth, salivation, nausea, vomiting, and constipation. Other side effects include hypotension, anemia, urinary retention, blurred vision, and photosensitivity (Karch, 2002). Risk of tachycardia or hypotension is increased if chlorpromazine is taken with epinephrine or norepinephrine. An additive effect might occur for both drugs if taken with beta blockers. CNS depression and hypotension can occur if given with barbiturate anesthetics, alcohol, or meperidine. Chlorpromazine is contraindicated in clients with bone marrow suppression, respiratory disorders, or liver disorders (Karch, 2002).

TABLE 12-4 ▼ Antipsychotics/Neuroleptics

GENERIC AND BRAND NAMES	USUAL DOSE	SEDATION LEVEL/ HALF-LIFE	SIDE EFFECTS	RELIEF OF SYMPTOMS
Typical (Traditional) Antipsychotics				
fluphenazine (Prolixin)	Oral: 0.5–10.0 mg/ day in divided doses every 6–8 hr; give doses of 20 mg/day with caution IM: initial dose of 12.5–25 mg; determine subsequent doses based on client response; dose not to exceed 100 mg	Initially causes drowsiness; half-life: Oral, 4.5–15.3 hr IM, 6.8–9.6 days	Drowsiness, pseudo-parkinsonism, dystonia, akathisia, autonomic disturbances, refractory dysrhythmias; sudden death related to asphyxia or cardiac arrest has been reported	Full therapeutic effects may require 6 wk to 6 mo of treatment
chlorpromazine (Thorazine)	May be given IM— 25 mg, repeated in 1 hr; dose can be increased to 400 mg every 4–6 hr with move to oral administration; 25–50 mg PO TID up to 800 mg, increase oral dose by 20–50 mg semi-weekly until optimum dose achieved	Sedating; half-life is 2 hr, then 30 hr	Drowsiness, insomnia, vertigo, extrapyramidal syndromes, dry mouth, salivation, nausea, vomiting, anorexia, constipation, hypotension, orthostatic hypotension, anemia, urinary retention, photophobia, blurred vision, urticaria, photosensitivity	Immediate relief of agitation from psychiatric symptoms
thioridizine (Mellaril)	50–100 mg PO TID with gradual increase to maximum of 800 mg/ day if needed to control symptoms	Sedating; half-life is 10–20 hr	Drowsiness, pseudo-parkinsonism, dystonia, akathisia, neuroleptic malignant syndrome, refractory dysrhythmias, photophobia, blurred vision, dry mouth, salivation, nasal congestion, nausea, urine discolored pink to red–brown	Relief of symptoms at most effective dose
trifluoperazine (Stelazine)	Oral: 2–5 mg BID with optimum response at 15–20 mg/day IM: for prompt relief of severe symptoms, 1–2 mg by deep IM injection every 4–6 hr (should not need to exceed 6 mg/ day)	Sedating; half-life is 47–100 hr	Drowsiness, pseudo-parkinsonism, dystonia, akathisia, refractory dysrhythmias, photophobia, blurred vision, dry mouth, salivation, nasal congestion, nausea, urine discolored pink to red–brown	Relief of symptoms at optimum dosage in 2–3 wk if orally administered

(continued)

TABLE 12-4 ▼ Antipsychotics/Neuroleptics (Continued)

GENERIC AND BRAND NAMES	USUAL DOSE	SEDATION LEVEL/ HALF-LIFE	SIDE EFFECTS	RELIEF OF SYMPTOMS
haloperidol (Haldol)	Oral: 0.5–2.0 mg two to three times a day PO; daily doses up to 100 mg have been used, but safety not demonstrated IM: 2–5 mg and up to 10–30 mg every 30–60 minutes or every 4–8 hr IM as necessary for relief of acute agitation and severe symptoms Decanoate: initial dose is 10–15 times the daily oral dose; repeat at 4-wk intervals	Sedating; half-life is 21–34 hr for oral administration and 3 wk for decanoate	Drowsiness, pseudo-parkinsonism, dystonia, akathisia, neuroleptic malignant syndrome, refractory dysrhythmias, suppression of cough reflex and potential for aspiration, anaphylactoid reactions	Relief of symptoms at optimum oral dose; immediate relief of acute symptoms with IM
thiothixene (Navane)	Oral: Initially 2 mg two or three times a day or 5 mg BID; increase dose as needed to optimum dose of 20–30 mg/day; may increase to 60 mg/day but few benefits reported IM: usual dose is 4 mg two or four times a day with most clients controlled on 16–20 mg/day; maximum IM dose is 60 mg/day	Sedating; half-life is 34 hr	Drowsiness, pseudo-parkinsonism, dystonia, akathisia, autonomic disturbances, refractory dysrhythmias, photophobia, blurred vision, dry mouth, salivation, nasal congestion, nausea, urine discolored pink to red–brown	Immediate relief especially with IM administration
Atypical Antipsychotics				
clozapine (Clozaril)	25 mg BID; gradually increase to a maximum of 900 mg	Initially sedating	Weight gain, sedation, salivation, seizures, danger of agranylocytosis, sexual dysfunction	Takes 6 mo or more to show effectiveness
risperidone (Risperdal)	1 to 9 mg/day	Low—may be energizing	Insomnia, agitation, anxiety, headache, nausea, vomiting, neuroleptic malignant syndrome	Some relief immediately; more at peak dose
olanzapine (Zyprexa)	Initially 5–10 mg orally QID, increase to 10 mg	May be sedating, at least initially; half-life is 30 hr	Somnolence, dizziness, neuroleptic malignant syn-	Relief of symptoms when therapeutic dose achieved

(continued)

TABLE 12-4 ▼ Antipsychotics/Neuroleptics (Continued)

GENERIC AND BRAND NAMES	USUAL DOSE	SEDATION LEVEL/ HALF-LIFE	SIDE EFFECTS	RELIEF OF SYMPTOMS
	PO QID within several days; may be increased by 5 mg/day at 1-wk intervals; do not exceed 20 mg/day		drome, constipation, postural hypotension, fever	
quetiapine (dibenzothiazine, Seroquel)	Initial dose of 25 mg PO twice a day; increase in increments of 25–50 mg two to three times a day to reach a therapeutic level	May be sedating, at least initially; half-life is 6 hr	Drowsiness, neuroleptic malignant syndrome, orthostatic hypotension	Relief of symptoms when therapeutic dose achieved

When administering chlorpromazine, nurses should caution clients to take the medication exactly as it is prescribed and to avoid getting the oral concentrates on skin or clothes because it can be an irritant. Clients need to avoid operating machinery or driving because the drug may cause drowsiness. Clients should avoid alcohol and must wear sunscreen because chlorpromazine precipitates photosensitivity (Karch, 2002).

Low-potency neuroleptics have the same anticholinergic properties as TCAs, causing the same bothersome

TABLE 12-5 ▼ Motor Side Effects of Antipsychotic Medications

SYMPTOMS	AS EVIDENCED BY	TREATMENT
Extrapyramidal Side Effects		
Acute dystonic reactions	Tonic contractions of muscles in the mouth and torso that can last from minutes to hours; often associated with high-potency neuroleptics (eg, haloperidol)	Intramuscular administration of diphenhydramine, 25 mg, *or* benztropine, 0.5–1.0 mg
Parkinsonian reactions	Rigid, masklike facial expressions; shuffling gait; drooling; finger and hand tremors; or muscular rigidity (cogwheel phenomenon)	Intramuscular or intravenous administration of diphenhydramine or benzotropine
Akathisia	Restlessness or an inability to sit still, excitement, or agitation Usually develops in first 5 wk of treatment; may appear as motoric hyperactivity Should be carefully noted by nurse	Changing to a different neuroleptic or decreasing the dose
Tardive Dyskinesia	Results from prolonged use of neuroleptics Early signs: tongue movement or increased blinking Later signs: tongue protrusion and unusual mouth movements such as sucking, smacking lips, or chewing jaw movements (rabbit syndrome)	Prevention (ie, regular re-evaluation of drug dose and assessment for beginning side effects) along with maintenance on lowest dose of medication

From Pearson, G. S. (1995). Psychopharmacology. In B. S. Johnson (Ed.), *Child, adolescent, and family psychiatric nursing* (pp. 410–423). Philadelphia: J.B. Lippincott.

symptoms of dry mouth, constipation, blurred vision, and drowsiness.

High-Potency Typical Antipsychotics

Drugs such as fluphenazine, trifluoperazine, haloperidol, and thiothixene are examples of typical high-potency antipsychotics. Like other typical antipsychotics, they cause a higher risk of side effects such as TD or dystonia. All of these drugs are dopaminergic blocking agents.

Haloperidol continues to be widely used despite the advent of atypical antipsychotics. The mechanism of action is not fully understood; it blocks postsynaptic dopamine receptors in the brain, but this action may not be necessary for antipsychotic activity (Karch, 2002).

Haloperidol is administered in several forms, including orally as capsules or liquid concentrate and through intramuscular injection. Initial dose of oral medication usually is 2 mg three times daily or 5 mg three times daily, with the usual optimum dose being 20 to 30 mg/day. Doses may go as high as 60 mg/day but dose increases beyond this rarely yield sufficient clinical benefit (Karch, 2002).

The predominant side effects of haloperidol include drowsiness, pseudoparkinsonism, dystonia, akathisia, and more serious, albeit rare, autonomic disturbances. Other side effects include refractory dysrhythmia, photophobia, dry mouth, salivation, nasal congestion, and nausea (Karch, 2002).

Haloperidol is contraindicated in clients with severe CNS depression, blood dyscrasia, Parkinson's disease, liver disease, or compromised renal function. Nurses should advise clients to take the medication exactly as prescribed and to avoid driving if CNS or vision changes result from the drug. Clients must maintain fluid intake and avoid overly warm situations that could precipitate heatstroke (Karch, 2002).

ATYPICAL ANTIPSYCHOTICS

While revolutionary in their time, typical or traditional antipsychotic agents had another serious drawback. They did not improve the negative symptoms of schizophrenia. Atypical antipsychotic drugs differ from traditional antipsychotic agents in their ability to act as dopamine receptor and serotonin receptor blockers. This simultaneous blocking may account for the increased efficacy of these drugs in improving the negative symptoms of schizophrenia with fewer extrapyramidal side effects (Baldessarini & Tarazi, 2001).

Many healthcare providers choose to use atypical antipsychotic agents rather than traditional drugs because of the markedly decreased risk of long-term, irreversible side effects, such as TD, carried by typical antipsychotic agents. Although use of these atypical agents has increased, many clients remain on the traditional agents that they have taken for many years. All require careful monitoring of side effects. Whereas the incidence of extrapyramidal symptoms is decreased compared with traditional

antipsychotic medications, clients may experience these side effects. Neuroleptic malignant syndrome also can occur in clients receiving these medications. Other negative side effects include orthostatic hypotension, dizziness, tachycardia, weight gain, sleep disturbance, constipation, and rhinitis. Despite the reduced extrapyramidal side effects, atypical antipsychotics also can cause adverse effects such as seizures, weight gain, diabetes, and hyperprolactinemia (Baldessarini & Tarazi, 2002).

In severely disturbed clients with long-term psychiatric illness, self-induced water intoxication, or hypernatremia, may occur. More common in men than women, it can cause psychological and physiologic symptoms that may lead to death (May, 1995). It is most common in clients with psychoses and can lead to medical complications including dilated and hypotonic bowel and bladder, hydronephrosis, renal failure, congestive heart failure, mild confusion, acute delirium, seizures, coma, and death (Cosgray, Davidhizar, Giger, & Kreisl, 1993). Self-induced water intoxication often is accompanied by extreme anxiety and cognitive difficulties; clients may report a lessening of anxiety after consuming large amounts of water.

Behaviors can include drinking from the shower or toilet, as well as drinking one's own urine. Nursing management in an inpatient psychiatric setting involves keeping clients away from sources of water. Management of symptoms through the use of neuroleptics also is recommended. Unfortunately, many chronically ill clients do not respond to neuroleptic treatment and need behavioral skills to manage their anxiety and psychosis. This disorder is a complex problem, requiring evaluation and intervention at many levels. Fluid control is one part of a larger treatment plan that involves multiple interventions (May, 1995).

With the arrival of clozapine, the treatment of schizophrenia improved dramatically. More than 30% of people with schizophrenia never responded to traditional neuroleptics. For many of these clients, the atypical antipsychotics have given them a degree of functioning that they never would have thought possible. Many experts in the treatment of schizophrenia recommend the use of atypical antipsychotic medications as first-line treatment.

Clozapine

Before the advent of agents such as clozapine, the only option for treating TD was discontinuing antipsychotic medication and making attempts at behavioral management of psychotic symptoms. Clozapine produces little or no TD and may significantly decrease or eliminate existing TD while the client takes the medication (Yovtcheva, Stanley-Tilt, & Moles, 2000). The symptoms of TD tend to return once clozapine is discontinued.

Use of clozapine requires weekly monitoring of white blood cell (WBC) counts to assess for agranulocytosis. Clozapine suppresses the development of WBCs in 1% to 2% of all clients who receive it. If WBC levels decrease significantly from baseline blood levels, immediate discontinuation of the medication is recommended. Clients never should use clozapine with other agents that suppress WBC production, such as carbamazepine.

The increased risk of potentially life-threatening blood disorders makes clozapine most appropriate for clients with severe schizophrenia who have not responded favorably to other antipsychotic medications or are at risk for worsening TD. Risperidone and quetiapine should be considered for any client needing medication for disordered thinking or psychotic symptoms. There are markedly fewer side effects compared with more traditional agents such as haloperidol or chlorpromazine.

Risperidone

Risperidone is an atypical antipsychotic whose mechanism of action is not fully understood. It blocks dopamine and serotonin receptors in the brain and has anticholinergic, antihistaminic, and alpha-adrenergic blocking activity that may contribute to both its therapeutic and adverse actions (Karch, 2002).

Risperidone is administered in tablets or in an oral solution. The initial adult dose is 1 mg orally twice a day with gradual increases to a target dose of 3 mg orally twice a day. When changing antipsychotic medications, providers must minimize the overlap period before beginning therapy with risperidone. Side effects include insomnia, anxiety, agitation, headache, nausea, vomiting, constipation, and, rarely, neuroleptic malignant syndrome. There is a risk of increased therapeutic and toxic effects if given with clozapine and a decreased clinical effect if administered with carbamazepine (Karch, 2002).

Risperidone is contraindicated during pregnancy, and clients should maintain the use of contraception while taking the drug. Clients should not stop taking this medication abruptly and should gradually decrease the dose to avoid side effects. Clients must be monitored for underlying signs of infection such as fever or malaise and should be observed carefully to rule out a drug reaction (Karch, 2002).

Olanzapine

Olanzapine is an antipsychotic dopaminergic-blocking agent that also blocks serotonin receptor sites. It is anticholinergic and antihistaminic. It produces fewer extrapyramidal effects than do traditional antipsychotic drugs.

Olanzapine is prescribed in tablet form in doses ranging from 2.5 to 20 mg per tablet. It usually is prescribed initially as 5 to 10 mg given orally four times a day, with increases to 10 mg orally four times a day within several days. Maximum dose is not to exceed 20 mg/day (Karch, 2002).

Side effects of olanzapine include somnolence, dizziness, neuroleptic malignant syndrome (rare), constipation, fever, and postural hypotension. Risk of orthostatic hypotension is increased with antihypertensives, alcohol, and benzodiazepines. Clients should avoid using alcohol when taking this drug. Risk of seizures is increased with this medication, and olanzapine may have decreased effectiveness with rifampin, omeprazole, carbamazepine, and smoking. There is an increased risk of toxicity if co-administered with fluvoxamine (Karch, 2002).

Nurses must monitor for the side effect of orthostatic hypotension, instruct clients to take the medication exactly as prescribed, and observe for signs of fever, lethargy, weakness, or sore throat. Olanzapine is not safe for use during pregnancy.

Quetiapine

Quetiapine is a dibenzothiazine antipsychotic drug that blocks dopamine and serotonin receptors in the brain. It also is an antagonist at histamine and adrenergic receptor sites. This action likely contributes to its adverse effects, which include somnolence and orthostatic hypotension (Karch, 2002).

Quetiapine is administered in tablets in 25-, 100-, and 200-mg doses. The initial adult dose usually is 25 mg orally twice a day, with increasing increments of 25 to 50 mg two or three times each day. The maximum dose per day is 800 mg (Karch, 2002).

When taking this drug, alcohol or other CNS depressants potentiate the drug's CNS effects. Phenytoin, thioridazine, carbamazepine, phenobarbital, rifampin, and glucocorticoids decrease the effects of quetiapine. Effects are increased when quetiapine is given with antihypertensives or lorazepam; effects are decreased when quetiapine is given with levodopa and dopamine antagonists. Clients must be watched carefully for side effects and taught to report unusual symptoms (Karch, 2002).

Quetiapine should be given to suicidal clients in small quantities. Clients exposed to extreme heat should be monitored carefully. Administration is not safe during pregnancy. Clients should monitor their own physical health for sore throat, fever, unusual bleeding or bruising, rash, weakness, and tremors, reporting any such findings to their provider (Karch, 2002).

Stimulants

Stimulants are a class of drugs commonly used to treat attention-deficit hyperactivity disorder (ADHD) (see Chap. 29). Adult clients with diagnosed childhood-onset ADHD may benefit from a trial of methylphenidate (Ritalin) or other stimulants. Research findings suggest that robust doses of methylphenidate, used to treat ADHD in children, were effective in treating ADHD in adults (Kinsbourne, DeQuiros, & Rufo, 2001) (Table 12-6).

Methylphenidate is a CNS stimulant with actions similar to those of amphetamines. It is used to treat ADHD and narcolepsy. It is contraindicated in clients with glaucoma and motor tics, and in those in severely

TABLE 12-6 ▼ Stimulants

GENERIC AND BRAND NAMES	USUAL DOSE	SEDATION LEVEL/ HALF-LIFE	SIDE EFFECTS	RELIEF OF SYMPTOMS
methylphenidate (Ritalin, Ritalin-SR, Concerta, Metadate-ER)	Tablets: 5, 10, 20 mg SR tablets: 20 mg ER tablets: 18, 36 mg Doses range from 10–60 mg/day orally	None, may be energizing; half-life 1–3 hr	Nervousness, insomnia, increased or decreased pulse or blood pressure, tachycardia	Immediate response if dosing is correct
dextroamphetamine sulfate (Dexedrine, Dexedrine Spansules, Dextrostat)	Tablets: 5, 10 mg SR capsules: 5, 10, 15 mg Usual dose: 5 to 60 mg/day orally	None, may be energizing; half-life 10–30 hr	Overstimulation, restlessness, dizziness, insomnia, dry mouth, unpleasant taste, diarrhea, palpitations, tachycardia, hypertension	Immediate response if dosing is correct

depressed states. It should be used cautiously in clients with seizure disorders (Karch, 2002).

Methylphenidate is available in tablets ranging from 5 to 20 mg and in sustained-release tablets in 18- and 36-mg doses. It usually is given in divided doses two or three times during the day, 30 minutes before meals. Doses range from 10 to 60 mg/day administered orally. Sustained-release tablets generally are given at a starting oral dose of 18 mg in the morning; doses are increased at 1-week intervals from 18 mg/day to a maximum of 54 mg/day.

Side effects include nervousness, insomnia, anorexia, nausea, increased or decreased pulse and blood pressure, and tachycardia. Effects and toxicity are increased if methylphenidate is given with MAOIs; phenytoin, TCAs, oral anticoagulants, and SSRIs show increased serum levels if administered with methylphenidate. The effects of guanethidine are decreased.

Children on long-term methylphenidate therapy should have their growth carefully monitored. If insomnia occurs, the last dose should be given before 6 PM. The nurse emphasizes that timed-release tablets must be swallowed whole and not chewed. Methylphenidate should be taken exactly as prescribed (Karch, 2002). Methylphenidate should be kept in a secure place; as a street drug, it has high value for individuals using it for illicit purposes.

Use of stimulants requires careful diagnosis of the disorder, the lowest possible effective dose, and careful monitoring of response. Stimulants, when used for illicit purposes, are considered valuable for resale. Like all controlled substances, they are prescribed in smaller amounts than are other psychotropic medications.

APPLICATION OF THE NURSING PROCESS TO CLIENTS RECEIVING PSYCHOPHARMACOLOGIC AGENTS

The use of psychotropic medications to treat psychiatric disorders marked the beginning of a new era in the management of mental health problems. Before the development of these medications, clients were destined to long hospital stays with little hope of symptom amelioration. This new era changed many aspects of psychiatric-mental health nursing and moved the management of clients with psychiatric disorders primarily from hospitals into the community. Historical Capsule 12-1 shows important milestones in the evolution of psychopharmacology, including when several important classes of drugs were first introduced.

Nurses manage and monitor the medication regimens of clients and assume a primary role in assisting them with these issues. They frequently are the link between the client's family and other caregivers. In most states, nurse practitioners are licensed with prescriptive authority, meaning that they prescribe and manage the administration and monitoring of medications.

Nurses are likely to encounter clients with mental health problems in all aspects of care. Many of these clients may benefit from psychopharmacology as part of their treatment regimen. Nurses must understand the importance of brain-based psychiatric illness within the

HISTORICAL CAPSULE 12-1

Development of Psychopharmacology

Late 19th century	Synthetic compounds such as bromides, chloral hydrate, and morphine are used successfully in the treatment of psychiatric illness.
1940s	Barbiturates and amphetamines are created.
1950s	Lithium is created for manic agitation. Chlorpromazine is developed as a tranquilizer and is used to treat schizophrenia in the United States.
1960s	Benzodiazepines are created to treat anxiety disorders. Tricyclic antidepressants are used to treat depression.
1970s	Phenothiazines are used predominantly to treat institutionalized clients with psychiatric disorders.
1990s	New medications proliferate, including selective serotonin reuptake inhibitors and atypical antipsychotic agents such as clozapine.

broader context of client-centered nursing care. They need to focus on the aspects of client care ignored by traditional medical models: health education, case management, family issues, client management, and advocacy.

The proliferation of available medication to treat psychiatric problems makes it imperative that nurses understand the medication, its actions, and side effects. Also essential to professional nursing care is a thorough understanding of the client for whom the medication is prescribed. For many clients, medication is an adjunct therapy to other interventions that the nurse coordinates, including family counseling or individual therapy. Medications can enhance the effectiveness of other nursing interventions by alleviating symptoms and making the client more emotionally available to change. They can help clients avoid psychiatric hospitalization and allow them to remain in communities. Medications alone, however, do not magically facilitate family communication, help clients get jobs, or cause chronic, long-term problems to disappear.

Assessment

Assessment of the client receiving medications for psychiatric disorders involves reviewing his or her health history, experience with psychotropic medications, past side effects, and efficacy of past treatments. The setting in which the nurse provides care influences the type and extent of assessment conducted as part of medication management. For example, is the client experiencing a psychiatric crisis requiring hospitalization? Is the request for services part of routine psychiatric care in an outpatient clinic? Is the need for psychotropic medication part of a long-term treatment strategy that involves few medication changes? Clients with more acute disorders usually take medication for a prescribed time, and the crisis may be traceable to a specific life event. These clients also are more likely to experience brief psychiatric hospitalizations for their problems. Thus, the nurse would need to tailor assessment questions to focus on the events leading up to the episode and on dealing with the immediate problems. Clients with chronic difficulties may have longer and more frequent need for inpatient care. A client's place along a continuum of care can change according to the acuity of his or her psychiatric symptoms and varying need for different types of services.

Regardless of setting, the nurse must assess the following in all clients:

- Life history, including history of psychiatric illness, past hospitalizations, and past use of medication
- Target symptoms requiring need for medication
- Client's perception of the problem
- Presence or absence of established community and family supports
- Need for adjunct care such as group, individual, or family treatment

Nurses should encourage clients to carry a list of medications with doses and times of administration and the prescribing mental health professional for each. The client then can show this list to other caregivers who provide emergency or routine medical care. Family members also could provide supplemental knowledge of medication if a client chooses to use their support in obtaining medical care.

Understanding the psychosocial needs of clients who potentially benefit from psychotropic medications implies an awareness of their basic needs for food, shelter, family, and kinship. It also involves appreciating the personal meanings of their psychiatric disorders. Nurses must be willing to consider the prejudices and biases that often are leveled on individuals with chronic psychiatric problems; understand the role of gender, culture, and ethnicity in provision of psychiatric care; and consider whether psychotropic medication is in the client's best interests (Lin, Smith, & Ortiz, 2001).

The nurse needs to summarize and document assessment findings in the client record in a clear, readable format useful to other providers. He or she also should develop a nursing care plan from these findings (see Chap. 6).

Nursing Diagnosis

Nursing diagnoses for clients taking psychotherapeutic drugs will be as varied and specific to the client's needs as the drugs themselves and the disorders being treated. A list of common nursing diagnoses related to the effects of pharmacotherapy is found in Box 12-2. Additionally, a few diagnoses are common for most clients requiring psychopharmacotherapy. For example, most clients just starting their medication regimens will meet the criteria for **Deficient Knowledge**. Clients who have problems with following their drug regimens may qualify for a diagnosis of **Ineffective Therapeutic Regimen Management** or **Ineffective Coping**. These are just a few examples; nurses must keep in mind that all diagnoses must be individualized to meet the client's particular assessment data and desired outcomes (Aschenbrenner et al., 2002).

Planning

Planning for care involves ascertaining the length of the medication trial, the client's need for follow-up, and monitoring of side effects. Ensuring client safety is the most important aspect of planning medication administration. To do so, the nurse must know the following:

- Method of administration
- Expected drug action

BOX 12-2 ▼ *Selected Nursing Diagnoses Pertaining to Drug Effects*

- Constipation
- Diarrhea
- Acute Pain
- Chronic Pain
- Fatigue
- Risk for Infection
- Risk for Injury
- Disturbed Sensory Perception
- Ineffective Sexuality Patterns
- Disturbed Sleep Pattern
- Disturbed Thought Processes
- Interrupted Breast-feeding
- Acute Confusion
- Deficient Fluid Volume
- Excess Fluid Volume
- Imbalanced Nutrition: More than Body Requirements
- Imbalanced Nutrition: Less than Body Requirements
- Impaired Urinary Elimination
- Urinary Retention

- Side effects
- Adverse effects (short and long term)
- Nursing implications

PRESCRIBED AND MAXIMUM DOSE

Nurses are responsible for knowing essential information about a prescribed drug before administering it to a client. This information includes the class of drug, target symptoms for which it is prescribed, the route of administration, dosing information, adverse effects, contraindications, and nursing implications. This information should be clearly communicated to clients and families (if appropriate) as part of client–family education.

Nurses carefully monitor drug administration, noting if the correct drug is being given in the correct manner, prescribed dose, and at the correct time to the client for whom it is intended (Karch, 2002). The nurse needs to be aware of storage issues for particular medications, whether this involves refrigeration or protection from light. Nurses must maintain an awareness of other nursing interventions associated with a drug such as monitoring vital signs, administration with food, or other physical parameters.

If a prescribed dose of a drug appears outside of normal dosing standards, it is the nurse's responsibility to contact the prescribing physician or nurse practitioner for clarification. It is imperative that all questions about a medication are clarified, whether these involve confusion about spelling, dose, or administration. When the nurse administers a medication, he or she is taking responsibility, under a nursing license, for giving this medication to a specific client. For example, clonidine and clozapine are two different psychotropic medications but have similar-sounding names. Clarification of confusion is essential when administering medication.

METHOD OF ADMINISTRATION

Determining the best mode of medication administration is important when tailoring a plan of care to suit a client's particular needs. For example, many clients with schizophrenia prefer oral tables or capsules. Some who take neuroleptics for long periods find that taking decanoate injectables of fluphenazine or haloperidol is more convenient and eliminates the need to remember to take oral medications (Implications for Nursing Practice 12-1). Some clients prefer liquid forms of their medication. Disadvantages to this method of administration include difficulties obtaining an accurate dose, risk of overdose, and need for juice or other liquid to mix with the medication. Many elderly clients receiving haloperidol or chlorpromazine in long-term care settings and nursing homes are given their liquid medication in juice for ease of administration. Most of these clients do not independently pour their medication, so the nurse performs this function. These examples illustrate ways that nurses must consider method of administration when planning care.

Implications for Nursing Practice 12-1

Decanoate Injections

- Antipsychotics are the only medications currently available in decanoate form. Such injections generally are given every 4 to 6 weeks. Clients receiving them require close monitoring for side effects after the first few administrations of the drug.
- Some researchers question the practice of using decanoate injections to treat clients with schizophrenia (Marland & Sharkey, 1999). They note that research data supporting the use of decanoates are inconclusive. An increasing body of knowledge suggests that nursing approaches to drug therapy that empower clients might be as effective. Examples of this empowerment include encouraging the client to make an informed choice about medication and the effects on lifestyle and functioning. Further research is needed.

EXPECTED DRUG ACTION

Before administration of a drug, the nurse must understand the client's physical and psychiatric functioning. This gives a baseline from which to gauge medication response after drug therapy begins. It also can assist the client and nurse to ascertain side effects that may come specifically from a psychotropic medication versus another source. Drug action is influenced by other drugs taken by the client, allergies, past pattern of healthcare, and general physical health. The nurse must have a picture of the client's health history and current health strengths and weaknesses to manage the effects of psychotropic medication. "Because the nurse has the greatest direct and continual contact with the patient, the nurse has the best opportunity to detect the minute changes that will determine the course of drug therapy and therapeutic success or discontinuation because of adverse or unacceptable responses." (Karch, 2002, p. 3).

SIDE EFFECTS

Most medications given to treat psychiatric conditions have some side effects. These effects can be common and well known for a particular drug or rare and idiosyncratic, affecting only a few clients. Clients must be educated about the side effects of the drugs they take. Based on ability, they need to understand all information about the medications they are taking. They have a right to know about all side effects and the changes that they might encounter when taking a particular medication.

Side effects are best monitored through a combination of techniques. For example, visual observation of the client will illuminate the overt presence of TD or other side effects of neuroleptics. The use of the Abnormal Involuntary Movement Scale is a more definite and precise way of evaluating abnormal movements (National Institute of Mental Health, 1995) (Figure 12-2). The most important monitoring comes from the client's perceptions of response to medication. An improvement in psychiatric symptoms (a positive response) might be accompanied by adverse side effects (negative). Careful processing with the client may need to occur to ensure that he or she continues with the medication. A careful review of the consequences of discontinuing medication also is essential.

Nurses can plan interventions to decrease anticipated effects of particular drugs while promoting client safety (Karch, 2002). Such planning might include education about sensitivity to light or heat, use of sunscreen, avoiding driving, maintaining skin care to avoid dryness, dietary considerations, and prevention of constipation. For example, clients taking lithium carbonate must take special care to hydrate regularly in environmentally hot situations. Dehydration can precipitate lithium toxicity and severe illness. Instructing a client to carry a water bottle might be a nursing intervention in this situation. Planning for side effects must be geared to the client's ability to understand, lifestyle needs, and psychiatric status.

ADVERSE EFFECTS

A client may respond well to a drug (eg, show decreased depression and suicidality), but may experience negative side effects (eg, inability to perform sexually, dry mouth, nausea). The nurse must work with the client to provide support in the early stage of drug therapy, ascertain if side effects will become less prominent over time, and determine if adverse effects are annoying or a genuine threat to health.

Since the introduction of phenothiazines, various psychotropic medications have been associated with cases of sudden death. The possible association between such deaths and medication with antipsychotics remains controversial, with the role played by these drugs in such deaths difficult to determine. Despite various confounding factors, such as intense emotional states or substance abuse, treatment with phenothiazines is an over-represented finding among clients with psychiatric disorders who die suddenly. Moreover, the cardiotoxicity of antipsychotics, especially at high doses, cannot be ignored. Indeed, major cardiac effects have been well documented for several commonly prescribed psychotropics.

The onset of a lethal dysrhythmia is one change contributing to sudden death and cardiac arrest. Prolongation of the heart's QT interval, or the time required for cardiac depolarization, repolarization, or both, can precipitate a dysrhythmia called the prolonged QT interval syndrome. Two forms of prolonged QT syndrome exist, one hereditary and the other acquired. The hereditary form appears to be related to an imbalance in the sympa-

	None	Minimal	Mild	Moderate	Severe
Facial and Oral Movements					
1: Muscles of Facial Expression eg, movements of forehead, eyebrows, periorbital area, cheeks; include frowning, blinking, smiling, grimacing	0	1	2	3	4
2: Lips and Perioral Area eg, puckering, pouting, smacking	0	1	2	3	4
3: Jaw eg, biting, clenching, chewing, mouth opening, lateral movement	0	1	2	3	4
4: Tongue Rate only increase in movement both in and out of mouth, NOT inability to sustain movement	0	1	2	3	4
Extremity Movements					
5: Upper (arms, wrists, hands, fingers) Include choreic movements (ie, rapid, objectively purpose-less, irregular, spontaneous), athetoid movements (ie, slow, irregular, complex, serpentine). Do NOT include tremor (ie, repetitive, regular, rhythmic).	0	1	2	3	4
6: Lower (legs, knees, ankles, toes) eg, lateral knee movement, foot tapping, heel dropping, foot squirming, inversion and ever-sion of foot	0	1	2	3	4
Trunk Movements					
7: Neck, shoulders, hips eg, rocking, twisting, squirming, pelvic gyrations	0	1	2	3	4
8: Severity of abnormal movements	0	1	2	3	4
Global Judgment					
9: Incapacitation due to abnormal movements	0	1	2	3	4
10: Patient's awareness of abnor-mal movements Rate only patient's report	No awareness — 0 Aware, no distress — 1 Aware, mild distress — 2 Aware, moderate distress — 3 Aware, severe distress — 4				

FIGURE 12-2   Abnormal Involuntary Movement Scale. (Reprinted from Guy, W. [1976]. *ECDEU: Assessment manual for psychopharmacology* [DHEW Publ. No. 76–338]. Washington, DC: Department of Health, Education, and Welfare. Psychopharmacology Research Branch.) (*continued*)

		None	Minimal	Mild	Moderate	Severe

Global
Judgment

11: Current problems with teeth
and/or dentures

| | | No | | | 0 | |
| | | Yes | | | 1 | |

12: Does patient usually wear
dentures?

| | | No | | | 0 | |
| | | Yes | | | 1 | |

Examination
Procedures for
AIMS

Either before or after completing the Examination Procedure, observe the patient unobtrusively, at rest (eg, in waiting room). The chair to be used in this examination should be a hard, firm one without arms.

1: Ask patient whether there is anything in his/her mouth (ie, gum, candy, etc.) and if there is, to remove it.

2: Ask patient about the *current* condition of his/her teeth. Ask patient if he/she wears dentures. Do teeth or dentures bother patient *now?*

3: Ask patient whether he/she notices any movements in mouth, face, hands, or feet. If yes, ask to describe and to what extent they *currently* bother patient or interfere with his/her activities.

4: Have patient sit in chair with hands on knees, legs slightly apart, and feet flat on floor. (Look at entire body for movements while in this position.)

5: Ask patient to sit with hands hanging unsupported. If male, between legs, if female and wearing a dress, hanging over knees. (Observe hands and other body areas.)

6: Ask patient to open mouth. (Observe tongue at rest within mouth.) Do this twice.

7: Ask patient to protrude tongue. (Observe tongue at rest within mouth.) Do this twice.

*8: Ask patient to tap thumb with each finger, as rapidly as possible for 10–15 seconds; separately with right hand, then with left hand. (Observe facial and leg movements.)

9: Flex and extend patient's left and right arms (one at a time). (Note any rigidity and rate on NOTES.)

10: Ask patient to stand up. (Observe in profile. Observe all body areas again, hips included.)

*11: Ask patient to extend both arms outstretched in front with palms down. (Observe trunk, legs, and mouth.)

*12: Have patient walk a few paces, turn, and walk back to chair. (Observe hand and gait.) Do this twice.

*Activated movements.

FIGURE 12-2 (*Continued*)

thetic nervous system. The acquired form may develop as a complication of drugs that prolong the QT interval by blocking potassium channels or interfering with the inward sodium and calcium currents. More than 40 marketed drugs and an equal number of drugs under development have been found to block potassium channels, prolong the QT interval, and induce, in some individuals, torsades de pointes. Torsades de pointes is a polymorphic ventricular tachycardia in which QRS complexes vary from beat to beat. Heart rates range from 150 to 250 bpm, with a significant potential for the development of lethal ventricular fibrillation and subsequent death.

Drug-induced torsades de pointes is rare, but its incidence can be as high as 2% to 3% with some drugs. Little is known about the drug-induced syndrome because of the infrequent and sporadic nature of the dysrhythmia, the absence of a comprehensive data base, and the fact that only 1% of serious adverse reactions to drugs are reported to the Food and Drug Administration.

Lithium carbonate is another psychotropic medication that may precipitate this syndrome by prolonging the QT interval. Thus, it is associated with increased incidence of sudden death Additionally, TCAs also increase the QT and PR intervals and also have been associated with sudden deaths. Some other common psychotropic medications known to prolong the QT interval are nortriptyline, imipramine, clomipramine, doxepin, thioridazine, haloperidol, chlorpromazine, mesoridazine, risperidone, olanzapine, quetiapine, and ziprasidone. Given that certain psychotropic medications alone or in combination can precipitate a lethal cardiac process in clients, the process is that much more lethal when it happens in conjunction with highly charged events in the presence of an unknown hereditary form of QT prolongation syndrome. Recent reports suggest significant QT prolongation in clients taking psychotropic medications who had no history or manifestation of cardiac disease. Scholars have voiced concern over this finding, especially in view of low levels of awareness of this phenomenon and the lack of overall cognizance that QT prolongation and the appearance of a torsade de pointes on electrocardiogram is a lethal marker of cardiotoxicity.

In that same vein, compounds with anticholinergic properties, such as many of the psychoactive agents used in psychiatric settings, are potentially toxic. These compounds act by inhibiting the action of acetylcholine at autonomic effector sites innervated by postganglionic cholinergic nerves, and at presynaptic and postsynaptic muscarinic receptors on neurons and ganglia. Antihistaminic agents—phenothiazines, tricyclic antidepressants, and some anti-Parkinsonian medications—also possess muscarinic receptor blocking activity. Children in particular are more susceptible to the adverse effects of anticholinergic drugs, which range from dryness of skin and mucous membranes to mild tachycardia, confusion, myoclonus, delirium, fever, and seizures.

All nursing interventions require a careful, thoughtful relationship with clients where they feel free to discuss adverse effects and are included in planning for management. Clients need to understand that different drugs in the same class can have varying effects on individuals. If one medication is not tolerated well by a client, another may have fewer adverse effects and will better treat symptoms. The nurse–client relationship is essential to assisting clients as they manage all effects of a drug. This is key in promoting adherence to a drug regimen aimed at positive amelioration of a symptom.

Implementation

Often, clients receive medicine without understanding its purpose, risks, or benefits. It is essential for nurses to make client and family education an integral part of psychiatric-mental health nursing practice, particularly when administering psychotropic medications. Implications for Nursing Practice 12-2 provides principles, using steps of the nursing process, for nurses to follow when providing client education. Other aspects of intervention involve the following:

- Assessing where and how the client will receive medication
- Arranging follow-up appointments and prescription renewal
- Understanding the client's financial resources
- Educating about safe storage of medication if young children live in or visit the home frequently

Implications for Nursing Practice 12-2

Developing and Implementing a Teaching Plan for Clients Using Psychotropic Drugs

Assess the information needs of the client and family.

- Are the client and family able to fully comprehend information?
- What do the client and family think about taking medication regularly?
- Do the client and family have any cultural or other biases about use of medication?
- Has the client had past problems with medication adherence? If so, were these issues resolved? How?
- Are the client and family willing to adhere to a medication schedule?

Plan education.

- Do handouts provide clear, useful information about medication, intended effects, side effects, treatment implications, and self-care?
- Is educational material appropriate to the language needs and developmental levels of client and family?
- Does the educational presentation meet the client and family's learning needs?

Implement medication teaching.

- Would individual or joint client–family teaching be more effective?
- Has the nurse carried out follow-up teaching several times to determine information gaps and the need for further education?
- What issues has the client or family expressed about adherence, especially regarding medication side effects and taking medication regularly?

Evaluate effectiveness of medication teaching.

- Is the nurse frequently monitoring the client and family to elicit their perceptions of medication, efficacy, and adherence?
- Do others who work with client and family have access to this medication information?

PROMOTING ADHERENCE TO THE MEDICATION REGIMEN

One of the most difficult aspects of treatment with psychotropic medications involves the client's adherence with recommended drug therapies. **Adherence** is defined as the client's willingness to receive recommended drug treatment as a caregiver prescribes. It involves the client's right to know and understand all aspects of the medication, including potential side effects, benefits, and dangers.

Some healthcare providers believe that complete knowledge of the drug may cause a client to refuse to follow the medication regimen. For example, if a client knows that a likely side effect of a certain drug is significant weight gain, he or she may refuse to start the medication or stop taking it once weight gain begins. Providers must be aware, however, that the client has the right to refuse all treatments unless he or she is judged legally incompetent to make treatment decisions (see Chap. 7). Nurses have a responsibility to understand the specifics of legal competence and adherence to treatment regimens within their geographic area of practice. Legalities differ among states.

Factors Contributing to Nonadherence

Clients may have many reasons for failing to adhere to their medication regimens. The most frequent reason is adverse side effects, many of which are debilitating and difficult to manage. Some clients with chronic psychiatric disturbances believe that they have little control over their lives or environment; these clients may refuse to take medication as a way to exert control over some aspect of their situation.

Unfortunately, many clients experience social stigma associated with having a long-term psychiatric condition. For some, the need for psychotropic medication means that they can no longer deny their symptoms or problems. Others perceive that taking psychotropic medications means that they agree with the label of "crazy" or "psychotic," regardless of whether they experience symptom relief and improved functioning as a result.

Other clients fear becoming addicted to medications, especially if they or a family member have a history of drug or alcohol abuse and have received treatment for it. Clients may be influenced by their experiences with medications, including memories from childhood when they witnessed family members receive more primitive forms of psychiatric treatment. Some clients had difficult experiences as children and adolescents in the mental health system, when long stays in state psychiatric hospitals meant custodial care and high doses of medication often used as chemical restraints.

The deinstitutionalization movement has dramatically altered the controlled living situations where clients received structured care. Clients who live in the community or on the streets are less likely to adhere to prescribed medication regimens. In one study, clients admitted to an acute care hospital system who refused medication were found to have more previous admissions than did nonrefusers. They more often were admitted involuntarily, and their refusal to adhere to a medication regimen generally led to a poorer clinical outcome, measured by length of hospitalization and incidence and duration of restraints episodes (Littrell, Mainous, Karem, Coyle, & Reynolds, 1994).

Perkins (1999) found that among clients who took traditional antipsychotics, approximately 40% stopped taking their medication within 1 year, and about 75% stopped within 2 years. Clients cited adverse side effects as the predominant reason for discontinuance. Perkins recommended using a health belief model in which healthcare providers determine a client's adherence to treatment through assessment of the client's perceived benefits of treatment and risk of illness versus cost of treatment, including adverse side effects. In Perkins's study, clients who believed that the risks of treatment were worth the benefits were more likely to adhere to prescribed medication regimen.

Implications for Practice

Nurses must treat clients who are having difficulty adhering to their medication regimens with compassion and understanding. For clients who are stopping use because of side effects, titration of the dose or a change in medication usually can solve this problem. Continuing discussion with the client and family and regular monitoring of the client's treatment plan are useful interventions.

Families want medication to "cure" or "fix" their psychiatrically ill relative. When the symptoms abate and the client is no longer posing a problem, he or she may decide to stop taking the medication because the "cure" has occurred. With many chronic disorders, however, the client's need for medication is long term. It is essential for clients and their families to understand this aspect of the disorder and its management (Czuchta & McCay, 2001). Nurses must assist both client and family to realize that the client's condition is no different from other chronic physical conditions that require medication (eg, diabetes, hypertension).

Caregiver sensitivity to each client and his or her specific issues can positively influence adherence (Verdoux et al., 2000). Psychiatric nurses should adopt nonadversarial approaches that combine psychoeducation and brief motivational interviewing to assist clients in adherence.

Others methods to assist clients in adhering to medication regimens include the following:

- Keep in close contact with the client, including performing careful follow-up.
- Respond immediately to client complaints and change dose, time of administration, and medication if it helps alleviate the difficulty.
- Develop a strong therapeutic alliance with the client.

- Understand community and family supports available to the client.

▼ *Clinical Example* 12-1

Michelle, a 20-year-old white woman, presents to the community mental health clinic with complaints of depression and weight gain. She states, "My medicines aren't working anymore, and I'm getting fat." She mentions that she recently spent 2 weeks at her parents' home during spring break from college. Michelle appears agitated and annoyed that she had to stay in the waiting room for a few minutes before seeing the intake nurse.

The nurse notes that Michelle presents as an overweight, somewhat unkempt young woman with dirty hair. She is dressed in a skirt and sandals with no coat or socks, even though the weather is cold and rainy. During the interview Michelle alternately sits across from the nurse and stands up, pacing in front of the office window.

Michelle states that she started taking desipramine during the fall semester because she was feeling "depressed" and "sad." She indicates that she has gained 30 lb since beginning the medication. The physician in her college's health clinic had prescribed the initial medication and provided regular follow-up through the fall and winter.

Michelle angrily states that the physician did not listen to her when she complained about gaining weight and that she wanted to stop the medicine and take "something else." She denies suicidality or homicidality but notes that, at times, she feels "revved up and hyper," with periods of extreme depression following. She says that the desipramine helped in the beginning but "not anymore."

At one point in the interview, Michelle stands up and says, "If you don't help me with these pills, I'll find someone who will." She responds to a firm, supportive request from the nurse to "work together to figure out the best plan of action" by crying and sitting huddled in her chair in the office.

Points for Reflection and Critical Thinking

- Although she denies suicidality or homicidality, Michelle's behavior suggests some impulsivity that might make her a danger to herself. What should the nurse do about this? Should the nurse involve Michelle's parents or a supportive friend? Is it safe for Michelle to leave the clinic? Should the nurse consider the possibility of psychiatric hospitalization?
- What information about Michelle's family history should the nurse gather?
- Should the nurse contact Michelle's physician at the college health clinic? Is a release of information from Michelle necessary to do this?

WORKING WITH THE FAMILY

Family members play an essential role in medication management. Many adult clients depend on parents and siblings for housing support, monetary assistance, and emotional guidance. The movement toward deinstitutionalization has required increased dependence of clients on families and community-based models of care (Lamb & Bachrach, 2001). Furthermore, the families of clients with persistent mental illness are caring for the most disabled and underserved populations in society. Informal and formal networks of care available to the aging parents of chronically disturbed adults often are inadequate.

Medication management usually is a part of a care network and requires the nurse to approach case management with the client and family from a collaborative perspective, including the family in a partnership of caring (Pejiert, 2001). Pejiert found that parents of chronically ill adults often felt that they were in conflict with caregivers, mostly involving their adult child's issues of autonomy and integrity in managing self-care. She emphasizes the need to view families as a resource and to avoid adversarial relationships, given that families provide intense support to their chronically disturbed offspring. Families can assist and support medication adherence and management of adverse side effects.

"Family" can be defined broadly for clients with psychiatric illness and may include a significant other who is not a spouse, a caring neighbor, or a good friend. The client must identify a person as a support, and this person must agree to provide assistance in medication and illness management.

Families may positively influence adherence to medication regimens, act as the first line of assessment for adverse side effects, and supervise administration of the medication and refill of prescriptions. The nurse must help to resolve any conflicts between the client's confidentiality and the family's need for information (National Board of Health and Welfare, 1999). Family education about mental illness and the medications used to treat it should focus on family coping skills rather than family problems. Pejiert (2001) notes that social support is a resource that nurses must cultivate and use. "In nursing it may be a mission of special importance to provide opportunities for family members to meet one another" (Pejiert, 2001, p. 202).

Although many adult clients may prefer not to have family members involved in medication management, parents usually are available as support for their offspring with mental illness (Pejiert, 2001). Including them in decision making regarding medication management, especially when they are actively assisting a psychiatrically ill family member, can only enhance the benefits of psychotropic medication and the client's positive response to this treatment.

PERFORMING SELF-CLARIFICATION

Nurses must clarify their own values about the benefit of psychotropic medication to treat psychiatric disorders.

This clarification will influence the care they provide to clients who may refuse medication. Should nurses support a client's decision to refuse medication, even if refusal lowers quality of life or increases the risk of psychiatric hospitalization or incarceration? Nurses must understand the multiple factors influencing their attitudes, including legal rights, institutional values of their working environment, and personal value system about client care.

Evaluation

Evaluation of a client's medication regimen involves the following:

- Reviewing the drug's efficacy in improving functioning
- Discussing client's subjective perception of response to medication
- Regularly monitoring perceived response, feelings about the medication, and potential difficulties

Clients may spontaneously discontinue medication without consulting caregivers. When this happens, the best treatment strategy is to avoid criticism, rejection, or ultimatums. Nevertheless, the treatment team, including the nurse, needs to decide, after carefully considering all factors, whether care can continue should the individual choose not to take psychiatric medication.

IMPORTANT ISSUES RELATED TO PSYCHOPHARMACOLOGY AND NURSING MANAGEMENT

Certain client-related variables are especially important to consider during drug administration. Two especially important considerations in psychopharmacology are the client's age and his or her use of complementary or alternative remedies.

Life Span Considerations

PREGNANT AND LACTATING WOMEN

Pregnant women with psychiatric problems present special problems when they require psychotropic medications to stabilize their symptoms. Whereas evidence of teratogenic effects of psychotropic medications has been mixed, a pregnant woman's use of many drugs, such as lithium, valproic acid, and carbamazepine, can expose the fetus to an increased risk of congenital malformation (Baldessarini & Tarazi, 2001).

Unfortunately, the first trimester is the time when a woman is most likely to be unaware that she is pregnant.

Nurses must thoroughly assess women of childbearing age who may be pregnant or planning to conceive and are starting drug therapy. Doing so, however, can be especially difficult if a client is in an acute psychotic state and cannot give an adequate or a reliable sexual history.

At any time during pregnancy, the major concern involves the transfer of medications across the placenta, given that the placenta is not an absolute barrier to drugs taken by the mother. The fetus cannot metabolize the medication or its byproducts safely. After delivery, the placenta is no longer available to assist with secretion, and drug toxicity may result (Wilkinson, 2001).

When it is imperative for a pregnant woman to receive psychotropic medication, the prescriber should use the lowest possible dose. Careful monitoring of the fetus should be part of the nursing care plan. Hypervigilance to potential pregnancy also assists in planning and managing medications.

Breast-feeding also poses dilemmas when nursing mothers take psychotropic medications. The postnatal period is a time of increased onset and relapse of mental illness (Austin & Mitchell, 1998). All major classes of psychotropic medication pass into maternal breast milk, transferring undetermined amounts of medication to the infant.

Llewellyn and Stowe (1998) reviewed the literature on the use of psychotropic medications during lactation and found that the issue had not been investigated in a controlled or systematic fashion. They noted the prevalence of case reports and the surprising lack of reported adverse effects on nursing infants exposed to psychotropic medications in breast milk. They conclude that the goal of treatment should be minimizing infant exposure while maintaining maternal emotional health.

▼ Clinical Example 12-2

Teresa, a 24-year-old woman of Italian descent, presents to the outpatient crisis service with complaints of hearing voices and "seeing things on the television set that aren't really there." Her husband, 26 years old, accompanies her. He reports that his wife's behavior has become increasingly bizarre and frightening to him. She is not sleeping and is starting to believe that someone is poisoning her food. He urged her to come to the clinic.

The couple has been married for 2 years; they have no children, although the client's husband reports that they were trying to start a family right before the client's recent symptoms developed. They live in the urban neighborhood where they both grew up. Extended family on both sides lives nearby.

Teresa reports a history of psychiatric problems that began at age 18 during her first semester living at college. She states that she had her "first breakdown," came home, was hospitalized, and did not return to school. She believes that she did recover from what she calls "my psychosis," but was continually plagued with auditory and visual hallucinations.

After the first breakdown, Teresa began working with a private psychiatrist (her parents paid for the treatment). Over the 6 years of care, the psychiatrist attempted several drug trials to deal with the hallucinations. Teresa reports that her psychiatrist had begun a clozapine (Clozaril) trial approximately 1 year ago. She believes that she was "much better" on clozapine and had even started taking college courses again. She adds, however, that her psychiatrist retired 2 months ago. This development, coupled with a 45-lb weight gain, caused her to stop taking the medication.

Healthcare team members note Teresa's increasing paranoia and vague threats toward her husband. They recommend a brief inpatient stay at a psychiatric hospital. Teresa reluctantly agrees to the hospitalization and a re-evaluation of her medication.

While hospitalized for 7 days, the psychiatrist restarts Teresa on clozapine. At discharge, the client agrees to visit the clinic nurse for help in managing her medication. Teresa also begins to attend a therapy group for women and resumes college classes.

Points for Reflection and Critical Thinking

- Can you think of any teaching or concerns that the nurse will need to address with Teresa's husband or other members of her extended family?
- What steps should the nurse take to develop an ongoing relationship with Teresa that allows the client to discuss her worries and concerns about medication rather than abruptly discontinue it in the future?
- What teaching points should a nurse consider for this client, a woman of childbearing age with severe psychiatric problems?

CHILDREN AND ADOLESCENTS

Psychotropic medications have been administered to children for several decades. Whereas the standard of care for most practitioners makes such use acceptable, controversy and questioning surround the need for these medications in the pediatric population. Researchers have identified issues regarding efficacy, side effects, and long-term effects on development. Nurses must clarify their personal attitudes about the use of psychotropic medication with children and adolescents (Pearson, 1995).

The same principles of medication administration and management with adult clients apply to children and adolescents with psychiatric disturbances. Additionally, nurses must be aware of the legal, physical, and emotional dependence that children younger than the age of consent have on their parents or guardians. Nurses must explain the principles of informed consent and health education to youthful clients and their family members. They must ensure that health teaching is developmentally based and gear it to the level of the client's understanding.

Medication management becomes more complicated with the involvement of school personnel, pediatric care providers, and after-school or day care providers. Supervision of medication administration, assessment of efficacy through parent and school reports, and careful monitoring of family response to the pediatric client's difficulties are greater issues than they are with adult clients.

Several psychotropic medications are useful when treating psychiatric disorders of children and adolescents (see Chap. 29) (Kutcher, 2000). They include TCAs, SSRIs, lithium, and clozapine. Kutcher (2000) notes that "many compounds have not yet undergone the sophisticated critical evaluation necessary to establish their efficacy, tolerability and safety in various mental disorders of children and adolescents" (p. 245). Yet, the clinical usefulness of using psychotropic medication with children and adolescents must be approached rationally and in a balanced way that considers the clinical needs of pediatric clients.

Issues particular to psychotropic treatment of children and adolescents include diagnosis and assessment, measurement of change, education, and the role of the family in supporting and managing treatment (Kutcher, 2000). An understanding that medication management in youthful populations is more complicated than with adults is essential and requires a developmental perspective for maximum clinical effectiveness (see Chap. 29).

OLDER ADULTS

The pharmacologic actions of psychotropic medications change dramatically for persons older than 60 years. These changes may result from differences in drug absorption secondary to diminished gastrointestinal motility, decreased plasma proteins, decreased kidney function, or congestive heart failure. Other explanations include normal age-related changes in body composition, lean body mass, and muscle mass or increased fatty tissue (Zubenko & Sunderland, 2000).

Regardless of the reasons, nurses must be aware that older adults may respond differently than their younger counterparts to psychotropic medications. Because many older clients take several medications simultaneously for various physical ailments, the need for hypervigilance concerning side effects from polypharmacy is increased. Coordination between medical and psychiatric providers is essential.

Psychiatric syndromes in older adults produce suffering, disability, and a loss of independence (Zubenko & Sunderland, 2000). These problems also increase burdens for caregivers. Nevertheless, psychotropic medications can dramatically improve functioning in older clients when the drugs are administered cautiously. Atypical antipsychotic medications have increased safety and efficacy. Older clients still present particular challenges to caregivers because of their propensity for chronic medical conditions.

Use of Alternative Agents to Treat Psychiatric Illness

The concept of alternative medicine is becoming increasingly important in U.S. healthcare. Eisenberg et al. (1998) estimate that more than 42% of Americans used complimentary and alternative medicine (CAM) in 1997. Types of CAM include herbal medicine, massage, megavitamins, acupuncture, chiropractic manipulation, fields of mind–body medicine, and self-help groups (Straus & Engel, 2000).

In 1991, Congress established the Office of Alternative Medicine at the National Institutes of Health. The status, mandate, and authority of this office were expanded in 1998 to create the National Center for Complementary and Alternative Medicine (NCCAM). The task of the NCCAM is to conduct and support basic and applied research regarding the identification, investigation, and validation of CAM treatments; diagnostic and prevention modalities; disciplines; and systems (Straus & Engel, 2000).

The most common alternative agent used to treat depression is St. John's wort. Its chemical composition has been well studied, and pharmacologic benefits include antidepressant, antiviral, and antibacterial effects (Barnes, Anderson, & Phillipson, 2001). Several studies using meta-analysis confirm the benefit of St. John's wort in treating mild to moderately severe depression (Linde & Mulrow, 2001; Kim, Streltzer, & Goebert, 1999). Nevertheless, several difficulties accompany the use of St. John's wort in treating depression. For example, the client who takes an antidepressant drug along with St. John's wort is at risk for serotonin syndrome (discussed earlier). Because agents like St. John's wort are available in health food stores and over the counter, they are unregulated in terms of content and manufacturing. If a client chooses to self-medicate, health professionals have had little opportunity to evaluate the client's total health status and identify other metabolic or health-related causes for depression. The provider also has not been able to evaluate other substances used by the client or factors that may contraindicate the use of St. John's wort or other alternative remedies.

Omega-3 polyunsaturated fatty acids found in fish, fish oil, and flaxseed have been found to ameliorate the symptoms of psychiatric disorders such as bipolar disorder and schizophrenia (Kaplan, 1999). Several studies show that fish oil might possess elements that assist in stabilizing mood. Stoll et al. (1999) recommend using omega-3 polyunsaturated fatty acids as an adjunct therapy rather than a first-line monotherapy. The predominant adverse effect of taking omega-3 polyunsaturated fatty acids was cited as mild gastrointestinal distress.

For nurses, the most important consideration in treating a client with mental illness who is taking psychotherapeutic drugs is to carefully assess what other agents he or she may be using to alleviate symptoms.

Nurses should contact a pharmacist or homeopathic physician familiar with alternative therapies if they have any doubt about a vitamin or other substance a client is taking concurrently with a psychotropic medication.

NURSING RESEARCH

Nurses frequently are an adjunct (although essential) part of research efforts initiated by physicians or pharmaceutical companies. They usually play specific roles in monitoring the adherence of clients to medication regimens and noting specific side effects. They also should integrate into practice nursing research that studies and evaluates outcomes of health teaching or case management. Nursing research questions might include the following:

- Does a medication control symptoms more effectively if a particular type of nursing care also is delivered?
- What aspects of community management facilitate client adherence to medication regimens?
- What biases and prejudices exist in clients regarding the use of psychotropic medication?

Puskar, McAdam, Burkhart-Morgan, and Isadore (1990) describe the management of clients with acute psychosis on a clinical research unit without the use of psychotropic medication. They evaluated the effectiveness of multiple nursing interventions in assisting clients to manage psychotic symptoms. Their work points to the need for nurses to consider both pharmacologic and nonpharmacologic aspects of the treatment of clients with psychiatric disorders in several different inpatient, outpatient, and community settings.

▼ *Reflection and Critical Thinking Questions*

1. What aspects of a biopsychosocial evaluation must the nurse consider before the client begins psychotropic medication?
2. What are some possible legal, ethical, and social issues involved when a client who has a chronic psychiatric illness refuses to adhere to a medication regimen?
3. How can a nurse's personal attitudes about psychiatric medications influence (positively or negatively) the care that he or she provides to clients?

▼ CHAPTER SUMMARY

- The development of psychopharmacology has paralleled the increasingly important role of the nurse in medication management.
- The administration of psychotropic medication involves specific nursing responsibilities.

- Principles of medication management are applicable to psychiatric clients.
- Particular psychotropic medications are characterized by side effects and administration guidelines. Medications should be used to treat psychiatric target symptoms for a specified period.
- Specific client populations who may require psychotropic medication include pregnant and lactating women, older adults, and children and adolescents.
- Families provide essential support to clients receiving psychotropic medication.
- Nurses must be aware of the specific management issues inherent in polypharmacy in client use of alternative substances to treat mental health disorders.
- Nurses can blend an understanding of psychosocial needs with specific symptoms to provide optimal nursing care.
- Nurses must engage in a research process that evaluates multiple effects of medication on a client's life and functioning.

▼ REVIEW QUESTIONS

1. After teaching a client and family about the use of psychoactive medications, which of the following statements from family members indicates successful teaching?
   a. "The drugs act primarily on specific target sites."
   b. "The drugs help the symptom but may lead to other problems."
   c. "The effects of drugs on other body systems usually is minimal."
   d. "Drug therapy is highly effective in treating psychiatric problems."

2. A client diagnosed with major depression has been taking a TCA for several months. She comes to the clinic with decreased appetite and energy level, lack of interest in daily activities, and feelings of hopelessness. She states, "I feel like I felt before I started taking the medicines." The nurse would interpret this as a possible indication of which of the following?
   a. Affinity
   b. Refractoriness
   c. Potency
   d. Polypharmacy

3. Which of the following would be most important for the nurse to do for a client who is beginning therapy with a TCA?
   a. Have the client change positions slowly.
   b. Assess for prompt elevation in mood.
   c. Monitor for hypertensive crisis.
   d. Anticipate the need for an antidiarrheal agent.

4. After teaching a client who is prescribed phenelzine sulfate (Nardil) about dietary restrictions, which of the following client statements indicates the need for additional teaching?
   a. "I'll have to stop using blue cheese salad dressing."
   b. "I'll have a turkey sandwich instead of a salami sandwich for lunch."
   c. "I'm going to have tacos with sour cream and guacamole tonight."
   d. "I'll switch to drinking orange juice in the mornings with breakfast."

5. Which of the following side effects would most likely pose the greatest risk for client adherence to therapy with an SSRI?
   a. Nausea
   b. Agitation
   c. Drowsiness
   d. Sexual dysfunction

6. Which of the following instructions would the nurse include in a teaching plan for a client who is receiving lithium?
   a. "Avoid getting overheated when you're outside."
   b. "Have your blood levels checked every 6 months."
   c. "Limit your intake to two to three glasses per day."
   d. "Expect to experience some weight loss with this drug."

7. Which of the following would the nurse expect to assess in a client who is being maintained on lithium therapy and has a blood level of 1.6 mEq/L?
   a. Ataxia
   b. Stupor
   c. Coarse hand tremors
   d. Slurred speech

8. The nurse develops a plan of care for a client receiving diazepam (Valium) based on the understanding that this drug acts on which of the following?
   a. Serotonin
   b. Norepinephrine
   c. Dopamine
   d. GABA

9. A client who has been receiving haloperidol (Haldol) for a long time exhibits fine worm-like movements of the tongue. Analysis of this finding would lead the nurse to suspect which of the following?
   a. TD
   b. Akathisia
   c. Extrapyramidal syndrome
   d. Pseudoparkinsonism

10. Which of the following would the nurse expect to assess in a client who is receiving fluphenazine (Prolixin) and is admitted to the hospital with neuroleptic malignant syndrome?
    a. Muscle flaccidity

b. Hyperpyrexia
c. Bradycardia
d. Hyperalertness

11. Which of the following would be most important for the nurse to monitor for in a client receiving clozapine (Clozaril)?
    a. Signs of TD
    b. Refractory dysrhythmia
    c. Decreased WBC count
    d. Orthostatic hypotension

12. The mother of a child diagnosed with ADHD receiving methylphenidate (Ritalin) three times per day states, "He hasn't been able to sleep since he started taking this medication." Which of the following would the nurse instruct the mother to do?
    a. Give the drug 30 minutes after eating.
    b. Administer the last dose before 6 PM.
    c. Switch to the sustained-release form.
    d. Continue the same regimen; insomnia is temporary.

13. When planning medication administration, which of the following areas would be most important for the nurse to keep in mind?
    a. Community or family supports
    b. Client's perception of the problem
    c. Previous history of psychiatric illness
    d. Prescribed and maximum dosage

14. Which of the following is the most frequent reason for a client not adhering to the medication regimen?
    a. Social stigma of long-term illness
    b. Loss of control over life
    c. Debilitating or difficult side effects
    d. Fear of addiction to the medication

15. Which of the following would the nurse identify as contributing to changes in drug absorption when planning the care for a 70-year-old client who is receiving psychotropic medication?
    a. Increased gastrointestinal motility
    b. Reduced kidney function
    c. Decreased fatty tissue
    d. Increased plasma protein levels

▼ REFERENCES AND SUGGESTED READINGS

Allison, D. B., Mentore, J. L., & Heo, M. (1999). Antipsychotic-induced weight gain: A comprehensive research synthesis. *American Journal of Psychiatry, 156,* 1686–1696.

*American Psychiatric Association. (2000). *Diagnostic and statistical manual of mental disorders* (4th ed., text rev.). Washington, DC: Author.

*Arana, G. W., & Rosenbaum, J. F. (2000). *Handbook of psychiatric drug therapy* (4th ed.). Philadelphia: Lippincott Williams & Wilkins.

Arana, G. W. (2000). An overview of side effects caused by typical antipsychotics. *Journal of Clinical Psychiatry, 61* (Suppl 8), 5–13.

*Aschenbrenner, D. S., Cleveland, L. W., & Venable, S. J. (2002). *Drug therapy in nursing.* Philadelphia: Lippincott Williams & Wilkins.

*Austin, M. P., & Mitchell, P. B. (1998). Use of psychotropic medications in breast-feeding women: Acute and prophylactic treatment. *Australia and New Zealand Journal of Psychiatry, 32,* 778–784.

*Baldessarini, R. J., & Tarazi, F. I. (2001). Drugs and the treatment of psychiatric disorders: Psychosis and mania. In J. G. Hardman, L. E. Limbard, & A. G. Gilman (Eds.), *Goodman & Gillman's the pharmacological basis of therapeutics* (10th ed., pp. 485–520). New York: McGraw-Hill Medical Publishing Division.

*Baldessarini, R. J. (2001). Drugs and the treatment of psychiatric disorders: Depression and anxiety disorders. In J. G. Hardman, L. E. Limbard, & A. G. Gilman (Eds.), *Goodman & Gillman's the pharmacological basis of therapeutics* (10th ed., pp. 447–483). New York: McGraw-Hill Medical Publishing Division.

*Barnes, J., Anderson, L. A., & Phillipson, J. D. (2001). St. John's wort (*Hypericum perforatum*): A review of its chemistry, pharmacology, and clinical properties. *Journal of Pharmacy and Pharmacology, 53,* 583–600.

*Calabrese, J. R., Bowden, C. L., McElroy, S. L., Cookson, J., Andersen, J., Keck, P. E., et al. (1999). Spectrum of activity of lamotrigine in treatment-refractory bipolar disorder. *American Journal of Psychiatry, 156,* 1019–1023.

*Cosgray, R., Davidhizar, R., Giger, J. N., & Kreisl, R. (1993). A program for water-intoxicated clients at a state hospital. *Clinical Nurse Specialist, 7,* 55–61.

*Czuchta, D. M., & McCay, E. (2001). Help-seeking for parents of individuals experiencing a first episode of schizophrenia. *Archives of Psychiatric Nursing, 15,* 159–170.

*Eisenberg, D. M., Davis, R. B., Ettner, S., Appel, S., Wilkey, S., Van Rompay, M., et al. (1998). Trends in alternative medicine use in the United States, 1990–1997. *Journal of the American Medical Association, 280,* 1569–1575.

*Frye, M. A., Ketter, T. A., Levevich, G. S., Huggins, T., Lantz, C., Denicoff, K. D., et al. (2000). The increasing use of polypharmacotherapy for refractory mood disorders: 22 years. *Journal of Clinical Psychiatry, 61,* 9–15.

Glazer, W. M. (2000). Extrapyramidal side effects, tardive dyskinesia, and the concept of atypicality. *Journal of Clinical Psychiatry, 61,* 16–21.

*Goldberg, J. F., Frye, M. A., & Dunn, R. T. (1999). Pramipexole in refractory bipolar depression. *American Journal of Psychiatry, 156,* 798.

*Green, A. I., Tohen, M., Patel, J. K., Banov, J., DuRand, C., Berman, I., et al. (2000). Clozapine in the treatment of refractory psychotic mania. *American Journal of Psychiatry, 157,* 982–986.

Goodwin, F. K., & Ghaemi, S. N. (2000). The impact of mood stabilizers on suicide in bipolar disorder: A comparative analysis. *CNS Spectrums, 5*(2), 12–19.

*Himmelhoch, J. M. (1994). On the failure to recognize lithium failure. *Psychiatric Annals, 24*(5), 241–249.

*Kaplan, A. (1999). Omega-3 fatty acids evaluated for bipolar disorder. *Psychiatric Times XVI.*

*Karch, A. M. (2002). *2002 Lippincott's nursing drug guide.* Philadelphia: Lippincott Williams & Wilkins.

*Kim, H. L., Streltzer, J., & Goebert, D. (1999). St. John's wort for depression: A meta-analysis of well-defined clinical trials. *Journal of Nervous and Mental Disorders, 187,* 532–539.

*Kingsbury, S. J., Yi, D., & Simpson, G. M. (2001). Psychopharmacology: Rational and irrational polypharmacy. *Psychiatric Services, 52,* 1033–1036.

*Kinsbourne, M., DeQuiros, G. B., & Rufo, T. (2001). Adult ADHD: Controlled medication assessment. *Annals of the New York Academy of Science, 931,* 287–296.

*Kutcher, S. (2000). Practical clinical issues regarding child and adolescent psychopharmacology. *Child and Adolescent Psychiatric Clinics of North America, 9,* 245–260.

*Lachar, D., Bailley, S. E., Rhoades, H. M., Espadas, A., Aponte, M., Cowan, K. A., et al. (2001). New subscales for an anchored version of the Brief Psychiatric Rating Scale: Construction, reliability, and validity in acute psychiatric admission. *Psychological Assessment, 13,* 384–395.

*Lamb, H. R., & Bachrach, L. L. (2001). Some perspectives on deinstitutionalization. *Psychiatric Services, 52,* 1039–1045.

*Lemer, V., Chudakova, B., Kravets, S., & Polyakova, J. (2000). Combined use of risperidone and olanzapine in the treatment of clients with resistant schizophrenia: A preliminary case series report. *Clinical Neuropharmacology, 23,* 284–286.

*Lin, K. M., Smith, M. W., & Ortiz, V. (2001). Culture and psychopharmacology. *The Psychiatric Clinics of North America, 24,* 523–538.

*Linde, K., & Mulrow, C. D. (2001). St. John's wort for depression (Cochrane Review). In *The Cochrane Library,* Issue 1, Oxford Update Software.

*Littrell, R. A., Mainous, A. G., Karem, F., Coyle, W. E., & Reynolds, C. M. (1994). Clinical sequelae of overt noncompliance with psychotropic agents. *Psychopharmacology Bulletin, 30,* 239–244.

*Llewellyn, A., & Stowe, Z. N. (1998). Psychotropic medications in lactation. *Journal of Clinical Psychiatry, 59* (Suppl 2), 41–52.

Madhusoodanan, S., Brenner, R., & Cohen, C. I. (2000). Risperidone for elderly patients with schizophrenia or schizoaffective disorder. *Psychiatric Annals, 30*(3), 175–180.

*Marland, G. R., & Sharkey, V. (1999). Depot neuroleptics, schizophrenia and the role of the nurse: Is practice evidence based? A review of the literature. *Journal of Advanced Nursing, 30,* 1255–1262.

*May, D. L. (1995). Patient perceptions of self-induced water intoxication. *Archives of Psychiatric Nursing, 9,* 295–304.

*McNamara, J. O. (2001). Drugs effective in the therapy of the epilepsies. In J. G. Hardman, L. E. Limbard, & A. G. Gilman (Eds.), *Goodman & Gillman's the pharmacological basis of therapeutics* (10th ed., pp. 521–547). New York: McGraw-Hill Medical Publishing Division.

*Mischoulon, D., Nierenberg, A. A., Kizilbash, L., Rosenbaum, J. F., & Fava, M. (2000). Strategies for managing depression refractory to selective serotonin reuptake inhibitor treatment: A survey of clinicians. *Canadian Journal of Psychiatry, 45,* 476–481.

*Mohr, W. K. (in press). The use of calcium channel blockers as adjunct medications for the treatment of refractory mania. *Journal of Psychosocial Nursing and Mental Health Services.*

*NAMI Provider Education Program. (2001). [On-line.] Available: www.nami.org.

*National Board of Health and Welfare. (1999). The Psychiatric Care Reform: Final report of the 1995 Psychiatric Care Reform. *National Board of Health and Welfare:* Vol. 1. Stockholm: Author.

*National Institute of Mental Health. (1995). *Abnormal involuntary movement scale (AIMS).* [On-line.] Available: www.NIMH.nih.gov.

*Neis, A. S. (2001). Principles of therapeutics. In J. G. Hardman, L. E. Limbard, & A. G. Gilman (Eds.), *Goodman & Gillman's the pharmacological basis of therapeutics* (10th ed., pp. 45–66). New York: McGraw-Hill Medical Publishing Division.

*Pearson, G. S. (1995). Psychopharmacology. In B. S. Johnson (Ed.), *Child, adolescent and family psychiatric nursing* (pp. 410–423). Philadelphia: J. B. Lippincott.

*Pejiert, A. (2001). Being a parent of an adult son or daughter with severe mental illness receiving professional care: Parents' narratives. *Health and Social Care in the Community, 9,* 194–204.

*Perkins, D. O. (1999). Adherence to antipsychotic medications. *Journal of Clinical Psychiatry, 60,* 25–30.

*Pi, E. H. (2001). Ethnicity and psychopharmacology. *Ethnicity and Disease, 11,* 166–167.

*Puskar, K. R., McAdam, D., Burkhart-Morgan, C. E., & Isadore, R. B. (1990). Psychiatric nursing management of medication-free psychotic patients. *Archives of Psychiatric Nursing, 4,* 78–86.

*Ross, E. M., & Kenakin, T. P. (2001). Pharmacodynamics: Mechanisms of drug action and the relationship between drug concentration and effect. In J. G. Hardman, L. E. Limbard, & A. G. Gilman (Eds.), *Goodman & Gillman's the pharmacological basis of therapeutics* (10th ed., pp. 32–43). New York: McGraw-Hill Medical Publishing Division.

Sajatovic, M. (2000). Clozapine for elderly patients. *Psychiatric Annals, 30*(3), 170–174.

*Sampson, S. M. (2001). Treating depression with selective serotonin reuptake inhibitors: A practical approach. *Mayo Clinic Proceedings, 76,* 739–744.

*Schaffer, L. C., Schaffer, C. B., & Caretto, J. (1999). The use of primidone in the treatment of refractory bipolar disorder. *Annals of Clinical Psychiatry, 11,* 61–66.

*Stahl, S. M. (2000). *Essential psychopharmacology: Neuroscientific basis and practical applications* (2nd ed.). Cambridge: Cambridge University Press.

*Stahl, S. M. (1999). Antipsychotic polypharmacy: 1. Therapeutic option or dirty little secret? *Journal of Clinical Psychiatry, 60,* 425–426.

*Stoll, A. L., Severus, W. E., Freeman, M. P., et al. (1999). Omega 3 fatty acids in bipolar disorder: A preliminary double-blind, placebo-controlled trial. *Archives of General Psychiatry, 56,* 407–412.

*Strakowski, S. M., McElroy, S. L., Keck, P. E., & West, S. A. (1996). Suicidality among patients with mixed and manic bipolar disorder. *American Journal of Psychiatry, 153,* 674–676.

*Straus, S. E., & Engel, L. W. (2000). Psychopharmacology: An essential discipline for the critical investigation of complementary and alternative medicines. *Journal of Clinical Psychopharmacology, 20,* 497–499.

*Verdoux, H., Lengronne, J., Liraud, F., Gonzales, B., Assens, F., Abalan, F., et al. (2000). Medication adherence in psychosis: Predictors and impact of outcome. A 2-year follow-up of first-admitted subjects. *Acta Psychiatrica Scandinavia, 102,* 203–210.

*Wilkinson, G. R. (2001). Pharmacokinetics: the dynamics of drug absorption, distribution, and elimination. In J. G. Hardman, L. E. Limbard, & A. G. Gilman (Eds.), *Goodman & Gillman's the pharmacological basis of therapeutics* (10th ed., pp. 3–29). New York: McGraw-Hill Medical Publishing Division.

*Yovtcheva, S. P., Stanley-Tile, C., & Moles, J. K. (2000).

Reemergence of tardive dyskinesia after discontinuation of clozapine treatment. *Schizophrenia Research, 46,* 107–109.

*Zubenko, G. S., & Sunderland, T. (2000). Geriatric psychopharmacology: Why does age matter. *Harvard Review of Psychiatry, 7,* 311–333.

**Starred references are cited in text.*

For additional information on this chapter, go to *http://connection. lww.com.*

Need more help? See Chapter 12 of the *Study Guide to Accompany Mohr: Johnson's Psychiatric-Mental Health Nursing,* 5th ed.

can provide needed support to clinicians by providing a history and a welcome insight into clients' lives and worldviews. Many clients turn to their clergy for help, and they often consider their clergy to be their primary mental healthcare providers (Larson, Milano, Weaver, & McCullough, 2000). Moreover, many are satisfied with the quality of the care that they receive. Studies show that clergy are frontline mental health resources not just for people having adjustment problems, but also for those with more serious mental disorders. Currently, clinicians are not well prepared to deal with psychiatric clients' spiritual concerns. Little content is devoted to the issue of spirituality in psychiatric nursing curricula and texts. Yet, clients clearly want this aspect of their lives to be considered in their care. Nurses are encouraged to build collaborative relationships with clients' clergy and chaplains to learn more about spiritual interventions and the rich diversity of spiritual and religious views. They are encouraged to invite them to consult and to be members of the clients' treatment team. As clients express a desire for greater attention to spiritual issues in their care, structured collaborations can provide those with mental health problems the balanced and holistic approach that they seek, but which is not always available to them.

The Role of the Nurse in Mental Healthcare

The nursing literature contains many different views on the topic of spiritual assessment and intervention. Nursing theorists such as Watson (1985) and Roy (1984) clearly identify spiritual care as a nursing responsibility (Reed, 1992; Ross, 1994) and state that the provision for clients' spiritual needs are part of the nursing role (Carson, 1989). As mentioned earlier, however, the research literature on the benefits of spiritual and religious involvement are inconclusive, and nursing studies substantiating benefits of nursing interventions is sparse in the psychiatric literature (Stuart, 2001). With respect to nursing interventions in the spiritual domain, they do not exist at all despite the fact that the North American Nursing Diagnosis Association recognizes spiritual distress and the potential for enhanced spiritual well-being as two nursing diagnoses.

Therefore, what should nurses do? They certainly should approach clients holistically as beings that are more than the sum of their parts. They should acknowledge and respect the spiritual lives of clients and always keep interventions client centered.

▼ Clinical Example 13-1

Marilyn is a 64-year-old female who is brought to the community mental health center by her daughter because she seems "so depressed." Her daughter states, "All she wants to do is stay in bed and sleep all day, and she isn't eating or taking care of herself like she should."

Marilyn is sitting in the chair, somewhat withdrawn and distant. She is dressed neatly but her hair is uncombed. Further inquiry reveals that Marilyn's husband died about 1 year ago after a lengthy illness. During her husband's illness, Marilyn was the primary caretaker. Before her husband's illness and death, they would get up early every morning and go to church. They also were active in helping at church-sponsored activities. The daughter states, "They did everything together, and the church was a big part of their lives. Now she won't even go out to the grocery store, let alone to church."

Points for Reflection and Critical Thinking

- What additional information would you consider exploring with Marilyn and her daughter? Explain your answer.
- How would you assess the spiritual aspects of Marilyn's life? What types of questions would you ask?
- How would you determine if spiritual interventions would be an appropriate component of Marilyn's plan of care? What ethical issues might arise from these interventions? Explain why they might arise.

SPIRITUAL ASSESSMENT

Acknowledging the spiritual lives of clients may involve asking about that aspect of their lives when taking a history. A spiritual history is not appropriate for every client. Some practitioners suggest four simple questions that might be asked of seriously ill clients:

1. Is faith (religion, spirituality) important to you in this illness?
2. Has faith been important to you at other times in your life?
3. Do you have someone to talk to about religious matters?
4. Would you like to explore religious matters with someone?

The nurse can preface these questions by explaining that such information is important in planning for support services in the event that the client develops a serious health problem (Astrow et al., 2001).

In addition, open-ended questions that allow clients to tell nurses about how they view relationships, the meaning of their illness, or what kinds of coping have helped them in the past can yield information about spiritual concerns and practices that may help nurses with plans of care (Burkhardt & Nathaniel, 1998). Clients who are less comfortable talking about this private and personal aspect of their lives also may drop hints about their spirituality. Therefore, attention to their interactions and conversation with their families, other clients, and staff members are vital. Conducting a brief spiritual assessment can help nurses better understand their clients' worldviews and help determine whether clients' religious and spiritual beliefs and community could be used as a resource to help them better cope, heal, and grow.

SPIRITUAL COPING PRACTICES AND INTERVENTIONS

The nursing literature on spiritual coping strategies used by clients in illness is limited (Baldacchino & Draper, 2001) and focuses mostly on religious coping mechanisms. Knowledge of spiritual and religious coping practices can inform client intervention. Richards and Bergin (1997) differentiate between religious and spiritual interventions on the basis of structure. Religious interventions are more structured, denominational, external, cognitive, ritualistic, and public, whereas spiritual interventions are more ecumenical, crosscultural, internal, affective, transcendent, and experiential. However, because religion and spirituality are interrelated so closely in the healthcare literature, no distinction between the two is made in this section. Moreover, all strategies discussed later can be either ecumenical or denominational. Interventions should be agreed on in partnership with clients. They should be tailored to clients' worldviews and unique personal coping mechanisms, in particular, those reported by clients to have helped them in the past during times of illness or crisis.

There are several situations in which spiritual interventions are contraindicated. They are contraindicated when clients are psychotic or delusional, when they have made it clear that they do not want to participate in these interventions, and when they involve minors whose parents are unaware that their child may be participating in an activity that is contrary to their denomination and faith. The latter can result in unwanted legal repercussions.

Prayer

People report that prayer is a powerful form of coping that helps them physically and mentally. Fifty-seven percent of Americans report praying on a daily basis (Boehnlein, 2000). **Prayer** is a kind of communication or conversation with a power that is recognized as divine. Prayer is practiced by all Western theistic religions and several of the Eastern traditions (eg, Hinduism, Buddhism, Shinto, and Tao). Prayer may differ in form and content from religion to religion. Different kinds of prayer seem to have different effects on well-being and satisfaction, with group prayer being associated with greater well-being and happiness and solitary prayer being associated with depression and loneliness (Poloma & Pendleton, 1991). One national poll found that 48% of clients want their physician to pray with them, and 64% of Americans think that physicians should join in prayer with clients if asked (Yankelovich Partners, 1996).

Whether nurses should join their clients in prayer if they ask is a personal choice. The nursing literature has addressed the subject of nurses praying with their client with respect to its ethical or legal implications. However, one ethicist caution that the prayer should be led by an "identified religious leader distinct from the medical team whenever possible so as to avoid even an appearance of religious coercion (Dagi, 1995). Moreover, Kaufmann (2000) counsels that prayer as an adjunct to appropriate treatment might seem innocuous at first blush but that praying with vulnerable clients could create a new source of liability if clients see themselves as being influenced unduly by practitioners.

Bibliotherapy With Sacred Writings

Bibliotherapy involves the use of literature to help clients gain insight into feelings and behavior and learn new ways to cope with difficult situations. It has been identified as a process of interaction between the personality of the reader and the literature, which may be used for personality assessment, adjustment, or growth (Alpers, 1995; Finnegan & McNally, 1995). All major world religious traditions have some type of text or writing that their followers view as holy and that they use as a source of comfort, insight, wisdom, and guidance (Nigosian, 1994). Western theistic religious traditions generally teach that God has revealed Himself and His word to humanity through these writings. Major Eastern religious view their sacred writings as a source of wisdom but not one necessarily revealed by a deity. The stories and narratives in these writings can be a solace and inspiration for clients. Spiritual reading is a significant part of 12-step programs (Finnegan & McNally, 1995). Before recommending any literature to clients, nurses should consult with the treatment team, as well as with the clients' family and clergy.

Contemplation and Meditation

Contemplation and meditation are types of mental exercises that involve calmly limiting thought and attention. There are several meditative traditions, for example, Zen, vipassans, visualization, transcendental, and devotional (Benson, 1997; Borysenko & Borysenko, 1994). Many forms of contemplation and meditation have their origins in Eastern religious traditions, most notably Hinduism and Buddhism. All forms involve isolation from distracting environmental noise, active focusing or repetition of thoughts or a word (mantra), muscle relaxation, release, and a surrender of control. Guided imagery is a popular form of meditation that uses visualization and can be augmented by music and voice on cassette tapes. Caution is urged in using contemplation and meditation as an intervention without knowledge of a client's denomination. Some forms of Eastern meditation may be viewed negatively with Christian clients (McLemore, 1982). Moreover, contemplation and meditation may not be appropriate as interventions in clients with disorders that have paranoid ideation who may believe that their minds are being controlled.

Repentance and Forgiveness

All major theistic world religions teach that people should forgive those who have harmed them and seek forgiveness from those whom they have harmed (Richards & Bergin, 1997). From a religious perspective, repentance and forgiveness are viewed as acts with important spiritual consequences associated with admitting one's shortcomings and failings and making restitution. The weight of the past can be lifted, which may release spiritual, emotional, and psychological pain. Forgiveness and repentance are integral parts of the 12-step program (steps 4 and 5) practiced in Alcoholic Anonymous in public "confessions" and recounting of wrongdoing. The process of repentance can be intensely painful for clients. Forgiveness and repentance in psychiatric settings should be interventions that are within the purview of a pastoral counselor or clergyperson (Latovich, 1995).

Worship and Rituals

All major religious traditions encourage their followers to engage in private and public acts of worship. **Worship** is the devotion accorded to a higher power or deity, and **rituals** are the ceremonies, rites, or acts such as prayer, singing hymns, fasting or abstaining from food, water, or sexual relations, and partaking of sacramental emblems. Acts of worship and ritual express peoples' devotion to a deity. They facilitate their commitment or recommitment to a spiritual or moral life, offer penitence, offer settings and opportunities for solidarity with others, and provide spiritual enlightenment (Smart, 1983). Benson (1997) suggests that worship services are full of "potentially therapeutic elements such as music, aesthetic surroundings, familiar rituals, distraction from everyday tension, prayer and contemplation, and opportunities for socializing and fellowship with others" (p. 176). Nurses should make certain that clients who wish to worship are given the opportunity to do so. Richards and Bergin (1997) caution that professional service providers should be careful about participating with clients in worship or ritual because of potential role boundary confusion.

Fellowship and Altruistic Service

The basic need for mutual support and connection with others is universal among humans. All world religions encourage fellowship and provide opportunities for expression and fulfillment of this need (Richards & Bergin, 1997). Altruistic service can take many forms, such as providing emotional support to people who are discouraged, taking clothes or food to the needy, or visiting the sick. Fellowship and altruistic service provide a way of helping reduce client isolation and self-preoccupation, and may be particularly helpful with clients who are socially isolated, lonely, depressed, suicidal, or who are experiencing major life crises (Richards & Bergin, 1997).

Journal Writing

Nurses can encourage clients to keep journals concerning their spiritual struggles, insights, and experiences.

ETHICAL CONCERNS

Despite the promotion of spiritual interventions and the incorporation of clients' religious beliefs in their treatment by several enthusiasts and devout practitioners (Richards & Bergin, 1997; Tan, 1994), some have raised ethical concerns.

All professionals have a privileged status with respect to individuals outside that profession. This status is privileged by virtue of the professionals possessing what those outside the profession do not have—specialized knowledge (Freidson, 1986; Kultgen, 1988; Sokolowski, 1990). Thus, health professionals are in positions of great influence with respect to clients by virtue of their specialized knowledge or expertise. When they depart from areas of established expertise to promote a personal agenda or go into an area in which they are not expert, they abuse their status as professionals. Inquiries into a client's spiritual life with the intent of making recommendations that link religious practice with better health outcomes may represent such a departure (Sloan et al., 1999).

A second ethical consideration involves the limits of the current research in this area. As previously mentioned, religious or spiritual factors have not been shown convincingly to be related to health outcomes (Kaufman, 2000). The nurse must take care that he or she does not misrepresent the state of the research, lest suggestible clients abandon allopathic treatment in favor of spiritual interventions to the detriment of their health.

A third ethical consideration has to do with the danger of imposing one's own values on clients. Devout nurses may view their work as an extension of their religious beliefs. Whereas there is no moral objection to discussing faith issues, preaching, teaching, or otherwise attempting to persuade clients to the nurse's religious or spiritual viewpoint is intrusive and unethical (Richards & Bergin, 1997). It is clearly a violation of boundaries and roles and may harm vulnerable clients. Such harm might happen if, for example, the nurse conveys to the client that he or she is spiritually deficient or immoral because of a choice (eg, abortion) with which the nurse may not agree. By the same token, it also is a clear violation of boundaries to engage in religious proselytizing. Examples of proselytizing are giving clients literature about nurses' spiritual tradition or denomination or teaching clients about one's religious beliefs when such information has not been requested or is irrelevant to client treatment goals.

Another ethical consideration is raised by Richards and Bergin (1997) who note that clinicians should pursue religious or spiritual goals and interventions only when clients have explicitly expressed their desire to do so. They also recommend that clinicians using spiritual or religious interventions should obtain informed consent from their clients and clients' parents where appropriate.

A final ethical pitfall has to do with the possibility of violating work setting (church–state) boundaries. Richards and Bergin (1997) advise professionals who work in civic settings to make certain that they understand and adhere to work-setting policies regarding the separation of church and state. In light of legal rulings about school prayer and devotional scriptural readings (Staver, 1995), they specifically urge caution about the use of spiritual interventions in the case of children and adolescents because there may be the potential of perceived governmental influence. Indeed, they advise clinicians working with children in schools or other civic settings not to pray with clients, read Scriptures with them, or pass out religious bibliotherapy literature.

▼ Reflection and Critical Thinking Questions

1. What ethical considerations or principles should guide nurses whose clients request the nurse to pray with them?
2. What actions should a nurse take in the event that a client is actively trying to convert other clients to his religious beliefs on the hospital unit?
3. Do you believe that it is ever appropriate to discuss your religious beliefs with psychiatric clients who are experiencing religious delusions or hallucinations?

▼ CHAPTER SUMMARY

- Spirituality has been described as a person's experience of, or a belief in, a power apart from his or her own existence. It also has been described as an individual search for meaning. Religion is the outward practice of a spiritual system of beliefs, values, codes of conduct, and rituals. It is an organized system of practices and beliefs in which people engage.
- There has been a resurgence of interest in spiritual and religious matters, and research has been conducted to document their beneficial effects on people's health. This research has both strengths and weaknesses.
- Religious and spiritual themes may be manifested as psychopathologic distortions of normative religious beliefs in clients with schizophrenia or bipolar disorder. In addition, a client with normal religious beliefs who experiences a stressful event may become excessively preoccupied with self-blame or guilt over real or imagined transgressions.
- Various reasons are given for a resurgence of interest in spiritual aspects of healthcare, including the health benefits of a spiritual life, acknowledgement of the limits of medical care, discoveries in physics, and research in religion and mental health.
- Nurses and other healthcare providers must become aware of their own personal values, their client's values, and the differences between them. This helps them to act from their own perspectives without imposing their values on others.
- Clergy can play a large role in mental healthcare. They can provide needed support to clinicians by giving a history and a welcome insight into clients' lives and worldviews. In addition, clients often turn to clergy for help and often consider their clergy to be their primary mental healthcare provider.
- The role of the nurse with respect to spirituality and religion is fraught with ethical concerns. Nurses can conduct a brief spiritual assessment, but in the absence of special training, spiritual interventions are best implemented with the aid of clergy or spiritual healers of the clients' choice.

▼ REVIEW QUESTIONS

1. During assessment a client states, "I believe in a power that is bigger than all of us." The nurse interprets this statement as indicative of which of the following?
   a. Religion
   b. Spirituality
   c. Values
   d. Worship

2. In which of the following conditions would spiritual interventions be contraindicated?
   a. Depression
   b. Self-esteem disturbance
   c. Psychosis
   d. Moderate anxiety

3. Which of the following statements reflects current research findings associated with spirituality and health?
   a. Definitions of religious variables are highly specific.
   b. Research performed has demonstrated consistent associations.
   c. Confounding variables have been tightly controlled.
   d. Research suggests the positive benefits of spirituality.

4. Which of the following factors have contributed to changes in attitudes and philosophies associated with spiritual care?
   a. Acknowledgement that medical care is unlimited
   b. Increased awareness of complimentary health practices
   c. Research demonstrating minimal health benefits of spiritual life
   d. Increase in scientific and technologic advances

5. While interviewing a client, the nurse asks, "What is important to you?" The nurse is attempting to do which of the following?
   a. Clarify the client's values
   b. Determine client rituals
   c. Assist with meditation
   d. Use bibliotherapy

6. Which of the following questions would be most helpful to use when eliciting information about a client's spiritual concerns?
   a. "Do you go to church regularly?"
   b. "What religion do you practice?"
   c. "What does being ill mean to you?"
   d. "Do you participate in any special rituals?"

7. After teaching a group of students about significant spiritual interventions used in 12-step programs for substance abuse, which of the following, if stated by a student as a type used, indicates the need for further teaching?
   a. Bibliotherapy
   b. Repentance
   c. Forgiveness
   d. Meditation

8. Which of the following would the nurse identify as the major goal for clients engaging in altruistic service?
   a. Gain insight into own (client's) feelings
   b. Reduce client isolation and self-preoccupation
   c. Learn new ways to cope with difficult situations
   d. Provide a means to surrender control

9. Which of the following is an example of a ritual?
   a. Fasting on the eve of a holiday
   b. Providing food to the needy in a soup kitchen
   c. Practicing guided imagery
   d. Reading Bible stories for insight

10. Which of the following would be most important for the nurse to keep in mind when planning spiritual interventions?
    a. Religious practice is highly and positively correlated with better health outcomes.
    b. Giving clients literature about the nurse's religion is an appropriate teaching strategy.
    c. Obtaining informed consent is essential before implementing any spiritual intervention.
    d. Spiritual interventions are appropriate for use with any client, regardless of age.

▼ REFERENCES AND SUGGESTED READINGS

*Alpers, R. J. (1995). Spiritual reading as bibliotherapy. *Journal of Chemical Dependency, 5*(2), 49–63.

*Astrow, A. B., Puchalski, C. M., & Sulmasy, D. P. (2001). Religion, spirituality, and health care: Social, ethical, and practical considerations. *The American Journal of Medicine, 110*(4), 283–287.

*Baldacchino, D., & Draper, P. (2001). Spiritual coping strategies: A review of the nursing literature. *Journal of Advanced Nursing, 34*(6), 833–841.

*Benson, H. (1997). *Timeless healing: The power and biology of belief.* New York: The Gale Group.

*Bergin, A. E., & Jensen, J. P. (1990). Religiosity and psychotherapists: A national survey. *Psychotherapy, 27*, 3–7.

*Black, W. A. (1991). An existential approach to self-control in the addictive behaviors. In N. Healther, W. R. Miller, & J. Greeley (Eds.), *Self control and the addictive behaviors* (pp. 262–279). Sydney, Australia: Maxwell-McMillan Publishing.

*Boehnlein, J. K. (2000). *Psychiatry and religion: The convergence of mind and spirit.* Washington, DC: American Psychiatric Press.

*Booth, L. (1995). A new understanding of spirituality. In R. J. Kus (Ed.), *Spirituality and chemical dependency* (pp. 5–18). Binghamton, NY: Haworth Press.

*Borysenko, J., & Borysenko, M. (1994). *The power of the mind to heal: Renewing body, mind, and spirit.* Carson, CA: Hay House.

*Bown, J., & Williams, S. (1993). Spirituality in nursing: A review of the literature. *Journal of Advances in Health and Nursing Care, 2*(4), 41–66.

*Brown, D. G., & Lowe, W. L. (1951). Religious beliefs and personality characteristics of college students. *Journal of Social Psychology, 33*, 103–129.

*Burkhardt, M. A., & Nathaniel, A. K. (1998). *Ethics and issues in contemporary nursing.* Albany, NY: Delmar Publishers.

*Carson, V. (1989). *Spiritual dimensions of nursing practice.* Philadelphia: W. B. Saunders.

Cassell, E. (1991). *The nature of suffering and the goals of medicine.* New York: Oxford University Press.

*Dagi, T. F. (1995). Prayer, piety, and professional propriety: Limits on religious expression in hospitals. *Journal of Clinical Ethics, 6*, 274–279.

Dyson, J., Cobb, M., & Forman, D. (1997). The meaning of spirituality: A literature review. *Journal of Advanced Nursing, 26*(6), 1183–1188.

*Emmons, R. A. (1999). *The psychology of ultimate concerns: motivation and spirituality in personality.* New York: Simon & Schuster.

*Fadiman, A. (1999). *The spirit catches you and you fall down.* New York: Strauss & Groux.

*Fenwick, P. (1996). Neurophysiology of religious experience. In D. Bhugra (Ed.), *Psychiatry and religion: Context, consensus and controversies* (pp. 167–177). London: Routledge.

*Finnegan, D. G., & McNally, E. B. (1995). Defining God or a higher power: The spiritual center of recover. In R. J. Kus (Ed.), *Spirituality and chemical dependency* (pp. 39–48). Binghamton, NY: The Haworth Press.

*Fulford, K. W. M. (1996). Religion and psychiatry: Extending the limits of tolerance. In D. Bhugra (Ed.), *Psychiatry and religion: Context, consensus and controversies* (pp. 5–22). London: Routledge.

*Freidson, E. (1986). *Professional powers: A study of the institutionalization of formal knowledge.* Chicago: University of Chicago Press.

*Gartner, J., Larson, D. B., & Vacher-Mayberry, C. D. (1990). A systematic review of the quantity and quality of empirical research published in four pastoral counseling journals: 1975–1984. *Journal of Pastoral Care, 44*, 115–129.

*Gallup, G. (1990). *Religion in America: 1990.* Princeton, NJ: Princeton Religious Research Center.

Gallup, G., & Bezilla, R. (1992). *The religious life of young Americans.* Princeton, NJ: Gallup International Institute.

*Hatch, R. L., Burg, M. A., Naberhaus, D. S., & Hellmich, L. K. (1998). The spiritual and beliefs scale: Development and testing of a new instrument. *Journal of Family Practice, 46,* 476–486.

*House, J. S., Robbins, C., & Metzner, H. L. (1982). The association of social relationships and activities with mortality: Prospective evidence from the Tecumseh Community Health Study. *American Journal of Epidemiology, 116,* 123–40.

*Hummer, R., Rogers, R., Nam, C., & Ellison, C. (1999). Religious involvement and U.S. adult mortality. *Demography, 36,* 273–285.

*Jackson, M., & Fulford, K. W. M. (1997). Spiritual experience and psychopathology. *Philosophy Psychiatry and Psychology, 4,* 41–65.

*Idler, E. L., & Kasl, S. V. (1992). Religion, disability, depression, and the timing of death. *American Journal of Sociology, 97,* 1052–1079.

*Kaufman, A. (2000). Medicine and religion. *New England Journal of Medicine, 343*(18), 1339–1342.

Koenig, H. G. (1997). *Is religion good for you?* Binghamton, NY: Haworth Pastoral Press.

*Koenig, H. G., McCullough, M., & Larson, D. (2000). *Handbook of religion and health.* New York: Oxford University Press.

*Koenig, H. G., Cohen, H., Blazer, D., Pieper, C., Meador, K., Shelp, F., et al. (1992). Religious coping and depression in elderly hospitalized medically ill men. *American Journal of Psychiatry, 149,* 1693–1700.

*Koenig, H. G., George, L., & Peterson, B. (1998). Religiosity and remission from depression in medically ill older patients. *American Journal of Psychiatry, 155,* 536–542.

*Kultgen, J. (1988). *Ethics and professionalism.* Philadelphia: University of Pennsylvania Press.

*Larson, D. B., Milano, M. G., Weaver, A. J., & McCullough, M. E. (2000). The role of clergy in mental health care. In J. K. Boehnlein (Ed.), *Psychiatry & religion: The convergence of mind and spirit* (pp. 125–144). Washington, DC: American Psychiatric Press.

*Latovich, M. A. (1995). The clergyperson and the fifth step. In R. J. Kus (Ed.), *Spirituality and chemical dependency* (pp. 79–89). Binghamton, NY: Haworth Press.

*Littlewood, R. (1997). Commentary on "spiritual experience and psychopathology." *Philosophy Psychiatry and Psychology, 4,* 66–77.

*Mayo, C. C., Puryear, H. P., & Richeck, H. G. (1969). MMPI correlates of religiousness in late adolescent college students. *Journal of Nervous and Mental Disorders, 149,* 381–385.

*McClure, R. F., & Loden, M. (1982). Religious activity, denomination membership, and life satisfaction. *Quarterly Journal of Psychology and Human Behavior, 19,* 13–17.

*McIntosh, D. N., Silver, R. C., & Wortman, C. B. (1993). Religious role in adjustment to a negative life event. *Journal of Personality and Social Psychology, 6,* 812–821.

*McLemore, C. (1982). *The scandal of psychotherapy.* Wheaton, IL: Tyndale House.

*Nigosian, S. A. (1994). *World faiths* (2nd ed.). New York: St. Martin's Press.

*O'Connell, L. J. (2000). The worlds of psychiatry and religion: Bioethics as an arbiter of mutual respect. In J. K. Boehnlein (Ed.), *Psychiatry and religion: The convergence of mind and spirit* (pp. 145–157). Washington, DC: American Psychiatric Press.

*Payne, I. E., Begin, A. E., Bielema, K. A., & Jenkins, P. H. (1991). Review of religion and mental health: Prevention and enhancement of psychosocial functioning. *Prevention in Human Services, 9,* 11–40.

*Payne, I. E., Begin, A. E., Bielema, K. A., Jenkins, P. H., Levin, J. S., & Vanderpool, H. Y. (1991). Religious factors in physical health and the prevention of illness. *Prevention in Human Services, 9,* 41–64.

*Poloma, M. M., & Pendleton, B. F. (1991). The effects of prayer and prayer experiences on measures of well being. *Journal of Psychology and Theology, 19,* 71–83.

Post, S. G., Puchalski, C. M., & Larson, D. B. (2000). Physicians and patient spirituality: Professional boundaries, competency, and ethics. *Annals of Internal Medicine, 132*(7), 578–583.

*Pressman, P., Lyons, J. S., Larson, D. B., & Strain, J. J. (1990). Religious belief, depression, and ambulation status in elderly women with broken hips. *American Journal of Psychiatry, 147,* 758–760.

*Princeton Religious Research Center. (1994). *Religion in America, 1993–1994.* Princeton, NJ: Author.

*Reed, P. (1992). An emerging paradigm for the investigation of spirituality in nursing. *Research in Nursing and Health, 15,* 349–357.

*Richards, P. S., & Bergin, A. E. (1997). *A spiritual strategy for counseling and psychotherapy.* Washington, DC: American Psychological Association Press.

*Rogers, C. R. (1957). The necessary and sufficient conditions of therapeutic personality change. *Journal of Consulting Psychology, 21,* 95–103.

*Roy, C. (1984). *Introduction to nursing: An adaptation model.* Englewood Cliffs, NJ: Prentice Hall.

*Ross, L. (1994). Spiritual aspects of nursing. *Journal of Advanced Nursing, 19,* 439–447.

*Sadock, B. J., & Sadock, V. A. (2000). *Kaplan & Sadock's comprehensive textbook of psychiatry* (7th ed.). Philadelphia: Lippincott Williams & Wilkins.

*Shorto, R. (1999). *Saints and madmen: Psychiatry opens itself to religion.* New York: Henry Holt & Co.

*Smart, N. (1983). *Worldviews: Cross-cultural explorations of human beliefs.* New York: Scribners.

*Sloan, R. P., Bagiella, E., & Powell, T. (1999). *Lancet, 353* (9153), 664–667.

*Sokolowski, R. (1990). The fiduciary relationship and the nature of professions. In E. D. Pellegrino, R. M. Veatch, & J. P. Langan (Eds.), *Ethics, trust, and the professions: Philosophical and cultural aspects* (pp. 23–45). Washington, DC: Georgetown University Press.

*Speck, P. (1998). The meaning of spirituality in illness. In M. Cobb & V. Robshaw (Eds.), *The spiritual challenge of healthcare* (pp. 21–33). London: Churchill Livingstone.

*Staver, M. D. (1995). *Faith and freedom.* Wheaton, IL: Crossway Books.

*Strawbridge, W. J., Cohen, R. D., Shema, S. J., & Kaplan, G. A. (1997). Frequent attendance at religious services and mortality over 28 years. *American Journal of Public Health, 87,* 957–961.

*Stuart, G. W. (2001). Evidence based psychiatric nursing practice: Rhetoric or reality. *Journal of the American Psychiatric Nursing Association, 7,* 103–111.

*Tan, S. Y. (1994). Ethical considerations in religious psychotherapy: Potential pitfalls and unique resources. *Journal of Psychology and Theology, 22,* 389–394.

*Thomason, C. L., & Brody, H. (1999). Inclusive spirituality. *The Journal of Family Practice, 48*(2), 96–98.

*Watson, J. (1985). *Nursing: The philosophy and science of caring.* Boulder, CO: University of Colorado Press.

*Williams, D. R., Larson, D. B., Buckler, R. E., Hechman, R. C., & Pyle C. M. (1991). Religion and psychological distress in a community sample. *Social Science & Medicine, 32,* 1257–1262.

*Wuthnow R. (1998). *After heaven: Spirituality in America since the 1950s.* Berkeley, CA: University of California Press.

*Yankelovich Partners Inc. (1996, June). Time/CNN poll.

* *Starred references are cited in text.*

For additional information on this chapter, go to *http://connection. lww.com.*

Need more help? See Chapter 13 of the *Study Guide to Accompany Mohr: Johnson's Psychiatric-Mental Health Nursing,* 5th ed.

Complementary and Alternative Medicine

JEANNEANE CLINE

▼ KEY TERMS

Aromatherapy—The use of essential oils to treat symptoms for physiological and psychological benefits.

Healing touch and **therapeutic touch**—Two methods of energetic healing that incorporate the therapist's intention to heal, through either actual touch or nontouch repatterning, energy fields around the person.

Licensure—A nonvoluntary process through which a government agency regulates a profession.

Mantras—Sounds, short words, or phrases repeated in the mind.

Meditation—A state of consciousness and an experience of the mind in which one tries to achieve awareness without thought.

Naturopathy—An umbrella term used in most Western countries to cover a range of therapies, referred to as *natural medicine;* it is also a way of life wherein the body innately knows how to maintain health and heal itself.

Professional certification—A voluntary process that grants recognition to people for having met certain qualifications.

T'ai chi—A Chinese blend of exercise and energy work with a series of choreographed, continuous slow movements performed with mental concentration and coordinated breathing.

Yoga—A manipulative and body-based method that teaches basic principles of spiritual, mental, and physical energies to promote health and wellness.

▼ LEARNING OBJECTIVES

On completion of this chapter, you should be able to accomplish the following:

- Define *complementary and alternative medicine (CAM).*
- Describe the current state of research of CAM therapies for psychiatric-mental healthcare.
- Discuss legal and ethical considerations for CAM.
- List the domains of CAM therapy.
- Provide examples of therapies within each domain.
- Understand the nurse's role in CAM therapy.

The field of complementary and alternative medicine (CAM) has multiplied exponentially since the topic was introduced in previous editions of this book. What was new and relatively unknown then has become almost commonplace in the healthcare field, the market, and information sources (journals, newspapers, and the Internet). This chapter will define CAM, discuss different groups and specific types of CAM and healthcare practices, and describe the nurse's role regarding CAM. The information in this chapter is selected for the mental health field and thus is not a comprehensive discussion of CAM.

OVERVIEW OF COMPLEMENTARY AND ALTERNATIVE MEDICINE

CAM generally refers to practices that are not considered "conventional" in Western medical practice, that is, not taught widely in medical schools, not typically used in hospitals, and not generally reimbursed by medical insurance companies (NCCAM Report, 2002). CAM practices often are not readily integrated into the dominant healthcare model because they pose challenges to diverse societal beliefs and practices. CAM practices are used instead of (alternative) or in addition to (complementary) mainstream medical practices. A term sometimes used instead of complementary is *integrative,* which is more comprehensive and implies the use of complementary practices in conjunction with traditional healthcare practices in the care of individuals.

In 1999, Eliopoulos identified five basic principles underlying CAM:

1. The body has the ability to heal itself.
2. Health and healing are related to a harmony of mind, body, and spirit.

3. Basic, good health practices build the foundation for healing.
4. Healing practices are individualized.
5. People are responsible for their own healing.

National Center for Complementary and Alternative Medicine and CAM Expansion

The Office of Alternative Medicine (OAM), a department within the National Institutes of Health (NIH), was created by congressional mandate in June 1992 and allotted a $2 million budget. In 1996, the OAM budget was increased to $7.5 million. In January 1999, OAM became one of 25 freestanding centers within the NIH and changed its name to the National Center for Complementary and Alternative Medicine (NCCAM). By the year 2002, NCCAM's budget had been increased to more than $104.6 million dollars (NCCAM Report, 2002). NCCAM has three goals:

- To gain recognition for and provide validation of the existing "unconventional" methods and treatments through research
- To assist with licensure concerns
- To increase reimbursement for various services

In the last 2 to 3 decades, people have begun to seek other systems of healthcare because of dissatisfaction with increasing costs, managed care, low personal interactions, and focus on symptoms rather than the cause (Fetrow & Avila, 2001). Holistic concepts and practices have continued to increase with the establishment of the American Holistic Medical Association (AHMA) in 1978 and the American Holistic Nurses Association (AHNA) in 1981. Furthermore, a study in 1998 indicated that almost two thirds of mainstream medical schools have integrated CAM into their curricula.

Prevalence of Complementary and Alternative Medicine

In 1997, four out of 10 adults in the United States used at least one method of CAM. For people between 35 and 49 years of age, the numbers increased to one out of two. Visits to alternative healthcare providers increased from 427 million in 1990 to an estimated 629 million in 1997; these visits to CAM providers exceeded visits to primary care physicians by approximately 243 million, and an estimated $12.2 billion was paid out of pocket.

The therapies used most frequently are relaxation techniques, herbal medicine, massage, and chiropractic manipulation (Eisenburg et al., 1998). Neck and back problems are the most often cited (42%) medical problems for which CAM is used. CAM also is used for anxiety and depression, fatigue, insomnia, headaches, arthritis, gastrointestinal problems, sprains and strains, allergies, lung problems, and hypertension. One of three people using a medical physician also consulted a CAM provider for the same condition; most did not discuss their CAM treatment with their medical physician. The people most likely to use CAM have a higher level of education, poorer health status, interest in spirituality and personal growth psychology, interest with groups committed to environmentalism or feminism, and a history of a transformational experience that altered the individual's world view.

Research Studies

Sixty-two percent of NCCAM's fiscal year 2001 budget (about $86 million) was spent on clinical research, investment in centers, and basic science research (NCCAM Report, 2002). Current CAM research includes eight new health science research studies and five grants to integrate CAM in medical and nursing curricula. CAM research focusing on psychiatric and mental health is limited. A study on treatment of major depression using hypericum (St. John's wort) has been completed and submitted for publication, and a trial using ginkgo biloba to prevent dementia is in progress (NCCAM Report, 2002). The Stanley Medical Research Institute has announced the availability of funds to support clinical trials for treatment of schizophrenia or bipolar disorder with herbals and other indigenous treatments (NCCAM Report, 2002). Funding for research for these high-profile, costly disorders should be a priority, along with continued focus on treatment of addictions, attention-deficit hyperactivity disorder, and child–adolescent behavior disorders.

Ethical and Legal Considerations

The ethical and legal considerations for CAM are manifold. Many considerations are related to herbal therapy. For example, the Food and Drug Administration (FDA) has no authority over herbals, even though 25% of prescription drugs are still derived from trees, shrubs, or herbs and 80% of the world uses herbals for primary treatment. In addition, drug companies do not want to spend the money to research the validity of different herbals because their production cannot be patented.

Of the 600 botanicals sold in the United States, less than a dozen have been tested in controlled clinical trials that determine their safety and effectiveness, and there is sketchy clinical trial information for approximately 50 other botanicals. The United States Pharmacopoeia (USP), a private nonprofit organization, set legal recognized standards for medications, including purity, quality, and strength. The USP has 18 standards for vitamins and minerals and is working on standards for 30 herbs. At this time, however, it is "Buyer beware!" with herbal products (Kuhn, 1999, pp. 19–37).

Because the FDA does not regulate herbals, they are considered nutritional and dietary supplements and their packaging cannot claim prevention or treatment of disease. The FDA has judged at least 16 herbs to be safe and effective, thus allowing them to carry health claims and be sold as over-the-counter drugs. Examples of herbals deemed safe by the FDA include slippery elm bark (Throat Coat tea) and the laxatives senna (Senokot) and psyllium seeds (Metamucil).

Another ethical consideration relates to the practitioner's need to know all vitamins, herbs, or energy treatments that a client is receiving, along with standard medical treatment and medications. This is critical to prevent a lethal combination at the worst or to alter the effectiveness (either increased or decreased) of a particular drug or treatment at the least. At first clients were hesitant to discuss the "other things they were doing" with their current medical practitioner because of feared ridicule and "really not believing that it would make any difference." Western nurses and physicians have gotten better at obtaining the information as they have become more tolerant and understanding. There is now a focus on helping to integrate the "other" treatment with the one being considered currently.

Legal considerations include required education or training with designated actions for licensure or certification. For example, 27 states and the District of Columbia require licensure for a massage therapist, but all of the states have different requirements. **Licensure** is a nonvoluntary process through which a government agency regulates a profession. **Professional certification** is a voluntary process that grants recognition to people for having met certain qualifications. Again, these requirements may vary by state. For example, one of the State Boards of Nursing considered requiring certain education for various CAM methodologies but because of the complexity and confusion eventually came up with the statement that "a registered professional nurse choosing to provide services including, but not limited to, midwifery, scleral therapy, and the use of alternative/complementary therapies, must comply with the Nurse Practice Act (NPA) and Board's rules" (Texas State Board of Nurse Examiners, 1998). Professional nurses are "to practice to the level of their knowledge and skills." This implies that to use massage, healing touch, or Reiki, one must be credentialed, licensed, or both as required by the particular modality or related organization.

CLASSIFICATION OF COMPLEMENTARY AND ALTERNATIVE MEDICINE

The NCCAM created a classification system that groups all CAM therapies into five major domains (NCCAM Report, 2002):

- Alternative systems of medical practice
- Mind-body interventions
- Biologically based therapies
- Manipulative and body-based methods
- Energy therapies

Alternative Systems of Medical Practice

Alternative systems of medical practice are complete systems of theory and practice that have evolved independently from, and often before, conventional medicine (Table 14-1). Examples discussed in the following section include traditional Chinese medicine, acupuncture, Ayurvedic medicine, homeopathy, and naturopathy.

TRADITIONAL CHINESE MEDICINE

The earliest Chinese medical text, "Yellow Emperor's Canon of Internal Medicine," is thought to have been written between 500 and 300 BC and is still used today. Chinese medicine is based on the principle of internal balance and harmony; that one has health when the interdependent forces of yin and yang are balanced. According to Chinese medicine, the body is made up of five basic elements: wind, water, earth, fire, and metal, which must exist in balance. If there is an unbalance, disease will result (Shealy, 1996). The concept of universal energy or "life force" is Qi (pronounced chee), which is the basis of all life. Yin and yang regulate Qi. Eastern medicine notes that the Qi energy is focused in the chakras and flows along meridians that run throughout the body. The meridians connect the acupressure points and are close to, but do not precisely follow, the somatic nervous system and anatomical boundaries. Chinese medical practitioners use treatment measures such as acupuncture, moxibustion, exercise, advice on diet and lifestyle, and herbal medicines to restore Qi.

ACUPUNCTURE

Acupuncture dates back to 3000 BC in China when stone needles, animal bones, or bamboo were used to treat specific illness at identified points. These locations were mapped as the meridian system of the body that roughly follows the current circulatory system. The meridians, though they cannot be seen or detected with any current equipment, have some 2000 identified acupoints and connect 12 organs. Acupuncture is based on the belief that health is determined by a balance of energy flow or Qi that puts one in harmony with the universe. Disease occurs with an imbalance of these forces and manifests as excesses or deficiencies of basic life energy in the particular organs. If the energy balance is not restored, then physical changes occur and disease becomes present in the body. Acupuncture helps correct and rebalance the energy flow and consequently relieves pain and restores health. The needles draw energy away from organs with excess and redirect it to organs with deficiency (Kuhn, 1999).

TABLE 14-1 ▼ Differences Between Alternative and Conventional Medical Systems

ALTERNATIVE MEDICAL SYSTEMS	CONVENTIONAL MEDICAL SYSTEMS
Originated approximately 1500 BC or earlier	Originated with Hippocrates in about 5 BC
Believe that health results from harmony between the person, his or her environment (nature, universe), and energy force	Believe that health results from normal physiologic function
Focus on maintaining a healthy state	Focus on treating illness or injury
Do not correlate symptoms of disease with any specific organ or anatomic location	Correlate symptoms with the organ or location of the person's disorder
Identify with and are sensitive to cultural traditions	Recognize cultural differences but may not incorporate the client's beliefs in the treatment regimen
Incorporate religious principles	Do not reject spirituality, but do not apply any religious significance to a person's illness or recovery
Rely heavily on medicinal plants	Rely on manufactured pharmaceuticals
Accept the efficacy of treatment approaches based not on specific scientific explanation but rather on traditional use	Demand scientific evidence for the mechanisms of treatment and replication of results through unbiased research
Do not have established educational standards for practitioners	Require practitioners to have formal education beyond college
Do not regulate practice	Require formal licensure for practice

From Timby, B., & Smith, N. E. (2003). *Introductory medical-surgical nursing* (8th ed.). Philadelphia: Lippincott Williams & Wilkins.

Mental health conditions treated by acupuncture include food, alcohol, and tobacco addictions. Other health conditions that may benefit from acupuncture include acute and chronic pain, migraines, psoriasis and eczema (if combined with a psychological component), and HIV symptoms. Thirty-eight states require licensing; some states limit the practice to physicians and chiropractors, and some health insurance companies pay for acupuncture (Kuhn, 1999).

Treatment consists of the practitioner inserting stainless steel needles into acupoints just under the skin and leaving them in place from a few minutes to more than an hour; twenty minutes is the average. The needles are used to "even" the flow—neither reduce nor enforce the energy level. The benefits of acupuncture include the following:

- Improvement of microcirculation
- Relaxation of muscles
- Release of endorphins, enkephalins, serotonin, and adrenocorticotropic hormone (ACTH)
- Activation of B and T lymphocytes
- Improvement in the complete blood cell (CBC) count (begins to change in 4 hours and becomes significant 24 hours after treatment)

AYURVEDIC MEDICINE

Ayurveda, a Sanskrit word that means "the science of life and longevity," is the 5000-year-old medical system of India. Ayurveda is a comprehensive approach to health that encompasses all areas of life and focuses on daily liv-

ing in harmony with the laws of nature to achieve a clear mind, sturdy body, and peaceful spirit. Ayurvedic medicine is similar to Chinese medicine in the belief that the life force, called *prana* (similar to Qi in Chinese medicine), moves through chakras. Ayurvedic practitioners prescribe treatment such as meditation, herbal therapy, yoga, and massage to maintain health or heal disease.

NATUROPATHY

Naturopathy is an umbrella term used in most Western countries to cover a range of therapies, referred to as *natural medicine*. It often includes acupuncture, herbalism, homeopathy, osteopathy, hydrotherapy, massage, nutrition, and diet. It is a way of life wherein the body innately knows how to maintain health and heal itself. The term was coined by Dr. John Scheel in 1895 and formalized by Benedict Lust, a German who immigrated to the United States in the early 20th century. Health is promoted through a diet that is high in fiber and low in red meat, similar to the diet recommended by the NIH in the 1990s. Faith, hope, and beliefs are significant in the treatment; the primary focus is teaching healthy living with an emphasis on people assuming responsibility for themselves. Drugs and hospitalizations are rarely used.

HOMEOPATHY

Founded by 18th-century German doctor Samuel Hahnemann (1755–1843), *homeopathy* means to "treat like with like." The name comes from the Greek word *homios,* meaning "like," and *pathos,* meaning "suffering." This means that a substance that causes symptoms of illness in a healthy person may, in minute doses, also be used to cure similar symptoms resulting from an illness. It augments the person's own immune and defense systems.

Homeopathy is used for prevention and to treat acute and chronic illnesses. In addition, current immunizations and allergy treatments are based on the homeopathic principle of similars. Homeopathy was successful therapeutically during the major epidemics of cholera and typhus. Because of much criticism, however, it almost disappeared from the United States. During the last 150 years, it has been able to secure a solid base in Europe and South America and is offered as part of the National Health Service in Great Britain.

Mind-Body Interventions

This domain includes various techniques designed to harness the mind's capacity to affect bodily function and symptoms. Not all mind-body interventions are considered CAM; many mind-body interventions are used in mainstream medical practice (eg, imagery, relaxation therapy, biofeedback). Examples of mind-body interventions that are still considered CAM include meditation, music therapy, and spiritual healing and prayer. Meditation, imagery, music therapy, and spiritual healing and prayer are discussed in the following sections.

MEDITATION

Meditation was used routinely in ancient Syria, India, Japan, and the monasteries of Europe. **Meditation** is a state of consciousness and an experience of the mind in which one tries to achieve awareness without thought. It also entails paying nonjudgmental, moment-to-moment attention to bringing about changes in perception and cognition. Transcendental Meditation (TM) uses **mantras**, sounds, short words, or phrases repeated in the mind to help subdue the many thought processes of the mind. It is not a withdrawing from the world but rather a way of being more fully present in the moment. The focus on breathing is effective because one cannot think about breathing and other things at the same time. Varying states of consciousness include waking time (active thinking and doing), sleeping time (conscious mind not aware), dreaming time (a middle state of which people are sometimes aware), and *pure awareness* (a moving of the mind from activity into the relaxed, alert silence of the meditative state) (Fugh-Berman, 1997; Kahn, 1996; Strehlow & Hertzka, 1988).

IMAGERY

Imagery, often combined with meditation, also has an ancient lineage in the healing arts and is currently accepted into healthcare in general as well as mind-body medicine.

It is known that holding negative thoughts and images can lead to illness; likewise, changing negative images to positive images can reverse the process. Regular use of imagery can increase relaxation, decrease pain, decrease side effects of chemotherapy, and increase the speed of healing. Imagery also can be used to increase skills in interpersonal activities and sports (Achterberg, 1999).

Because imagery is symbolic, images have no boundaries; they may be realistic, logical, illogical, humorous, or magical. Images can be whatever seems to have the most meaning and be the most powerful for the individual. Imagery is not a one-time miracle activity; like taking medication, this technique must be done at prescribed frequencies and lengths of time (eg, for 15 minutes, three times a day).

MUSIC THERAPY

Music therapy is the use of music to alter behavior, emotions, or physiology. Musical vibrations can help restore regulatory function to a body "out of tune" and help maintain and enhance regulatory functions to a body "in tune." Music therapy helps clients develop self-awareness and creativity, improve learning, clarify personal values, and cope with a variety of psychophysiologic dysfunctions. It can help the mind to slow down to achieve inner quietness and relaxation, or it can be stimulating. The immediate effects are on the mind state, which in turn influences the body state with a psychophysiologic response and then the balance of body, mind, and spirit (Guzzetta, 1997).

SPIRITUAL HEALING AND PRAYER

For centuries there was no division between the sacred and the secular. The presence of God(s) was felt as part of everyday life, the healer and the spiritual leader were often the same person, and prayer was an inseparable part of that experience. Spirituality and religion were separated from the healing profession in the 19th century. There was a particular intent to restrict religion in the psychiatric setting as it was thought to be detrimental for the clients. The field has now come full circle, and the positive aspects of spirituality in healthcare and healing are being recognized (Ameling, 2000).

Dossey (2000) has written much about the change in healthcare (in Western medicine) from Era I with the "mechanical, material mindless medicine" or "brain-body" (1860 to 1945) to Era II and the recognition of psychosomatic disease and "mind-body" medicine (1945 to 1990). Era III (1990 to present) brings in the concept of "*nonlocality,*" unlimited in space and time, and the ability of human intervention, and "intention," the use of the mind to not only improve the health status of the self but also of others. Dossey refers to these distant healing practices as prayer.

Another physician designed an eight-segment Prayer Wheel for clients to use by themselves. The clients were asked to use their own favorite inspirational stories, poems, songs, or prayers at each of the segments for about 5 minutes each. The segments included count your blessings, sing of love, request protection, forgive self and others, ask for needs for self and others (record and date these requests), fill self and others with love and inspirations, and *listen* with pen in hand and write what comes to mind (5 minutes are mandatory for this segment). The clients were told to end the eight segments by stating, "Your will is my will," meaning, "Send me what I need, even if it is not what I want." The outcomes ranged from immediate, dramatic results to subtle or no apparent results. No apparent result occurred when the technique was not being used (Rossiter-Thornton, 2000). Issues related to spirituality in psychiatric nursing are discussed in detail in Chapter 13.

Biologically Based Therapies

This domain includes natural and biologically based practices, interventions, and products; many may overlap with conventional medicine's use of dietary supplements. Examples discussed in the following sections include herbal therapies and aromatherapy. Other types of biologically based therapies include special diets (Pritikin, Ornish, vegetarian, Asian), orthomolecular medicine (unusually high-dose supplements), cell therapy, enzyme therapies, apitherapy (bee), and iridology.

HERBAL THERAPIES

Herbs, like many other CAM therapies, have been used for thousands of years. Today, 80% of the world uses herbal therapy for primary treatment. In addition, despite the lack of strong research and many ethical and legal considerations (see previous discussions), one third of American adults depend on herbs (or botanicals) to varying degrees, and insurance companies are increasingly paying for them. Rising about 18% a year, annual retail sales have increased to about $4 billion, up from $839 million in 1991 (Kotek, 1999).

An *herb* commonly refers to plant parts (including the bark, root, stem, flowers, leaves, fruit, seed, or sap) that are used as medicines. Herbal therapy also is referred to as *phytomedicine,* the practice of using plants or plant parts to achieve a therapeutic cure (Fetrow & Avila, 1999). The action of most herbs is correction of an underlying cause of the disease process, whereas synthetic drugs are often designed to alleviate the symptom or effect without addressing the underlying cause. Each herb has a complex mixture of active ingredients, often making it difficult to identify the effective agent (Kuhn, 1999). Some herbs and supplements related to mental health are listed in Table 14-2.

Use of herbals requires knowledgeable practitioners and reliable products, as there can be variation in strength and purity of herbal preparations. The USP is setting standards for purity, strength, quality, labeling, and packaging for herbal products that will be published in the *National Formulary (NF)*. Currently nine herbs and manufacturers meeting those standards can use the "NF" label: ginger, feverfew, garlic, ginkgo, Oriental ginseng, chamomile, saw palmetto, St. John's wort, and powdered valerian (Phillips, 1999). The NIH also lists information on dietary supplements and herbs at *http://www.nal.usda.gov/fnic/etext/000015.html*.

When buying herbal products, label information to look for includes the following:

- Is the product made from whole herbs or standardized extracts (matter of preference)?
- Is the plant grown organically (matter of preference)?
- Is the amount of active ingredients in each capsule similar to other products?
- Is the price consistent with other similar products; if not, why isn't it?
- Could a client be allergic to or have philosophical objections to something in this product?
- If therapeutic claims are made, is the FDA disclaimer included (a legal requirement)?
- Is the expiration date at least 3 months in the future?
- Is there a batch or lot number?
- Is there a telephone number or web site listed where one can get additional information?

Before using any herbal product, the client should consult with his or her primary healthcare provider. This is especially important for the psychiatric-mental healthcare client because many herbal and over-the-counter products interact adversely with psychiatric medications. It is also important for the client to know about the risk for allergic reactions to herbal products and how to identify allergies to herbal products. Symptoms of food allergies usually occur within 4 days (Ivker, Anderson, & Trivier, 1999).

AROMATHERAPY

Aromatherapy is the use of essential oils to treat symptoms for physiological and psychological benefits. Only 3% of the world's essential oils are used therapeutically, the other 97% are used in the perfume and cosmetic industry (Kuhn, 1999). Eighty million Americans spend approximately $70 billion per year on aromatherapy (Buckle, 1999).

It is not known if aromatherapy achieves its clinical efficacy from placebo response, the effect of touch and smell on the parasympathetic nervous system, the learned memory of the aroma, the pharmacokinetic potentiation of orthodox drugs by the essential oils, or the pharmacologically active ingredients within the essential oils that have analgesic effects. It is known that the interaction of the therapist and the client definitely influences the out-

TABLE 14-2 ▼ Selected Herbs, Minerals, and Vitamins for Mental Health Use

HERBS, MINERALS, AND VITAMINS	USES	ACTIONS AND PRECAUTIONS	DOSE
California poppy, yellow and orange	Relieves pain Acts as sedative Relieves mild anxiety	Poppy contains mild alkaloids similar to codeine and morphine. Do not use with monoamine oxidase inhibitors (MAOIs).	1 tsp/cup tea 2–3 times a day
Ginkgo biloba	Reduces senility Reduces short-term memory loss Improves peripheral circulation	Use as a circulatory aid and antioxidant. Fruit or seed should not be handled or eaten. May enhance papaverine. Possible side effects include GI distress, headache, and allergic reaction. Cautious use is recommended if taking aspirin or other blood-thinning drugs.	60 mg BID Alzheimer's—240 mg divided 2–3 times a day
Ginseng (Asian and American)	Reduces stress and fatigue Improves physical and mental function, especially with elderly clients Assists smoking cessation efforts	Use the root. Use may raise blood pressure and serum glucose levels and can increase the growth of estrogen-dependent cancer.	American—0.03% ginsenoside, 1–2 g fresh root Asian—1.5% ginseng, 1–2 g fresh root For both, 200–600 mg liquid extract daily
Guarana	Enhances cognition Reduces combat fatigue Acts as a "cerebral stimulant"	It is a food additive/dietary supplement. It contains an extremely high caffeine level: 2.6%–7%, compared to coffee beans with 1%–2% and dried tea leaves with 1%–4%.	Not recommended for use Range for use: 250–1200 mg/day
Hops	Has a sedative effect Reduces anxiety	Forms include tea, extract, or capsule. The active ingredient is in glandular hairs on its scaly, conelike fruits.	1 tsp/cup tea 2–3 times a day or 30–40 drops tincture
Kava kava	Reduces stress and anxiety Reduces insomnia	It comes from the root of the pepper tree family. It has a soothing effect on the amygdala (alarm center of brain). Do not use with tranquilizers, sedatives, or alcohol. Large doses can produce an intoxicating effect. Long-term use can lead to dry, scaly skin.	2–4 g as decoction TID for 4–12 weeks 1 tsp with 70–85 mg kava lactones

(continued)

TABLE 14-2 ▼ **Selected Herbs, Minerals, and Vitamins for Mental Health Use** (Continued)			
HERBS, MINERALS, AND VITAMINS	**USES**	**ACTIONS AND PRECAUTIONS**	**DOSE**
		Recent research has linked kava to at least 25 cases of liver toxicity, including hepatitis, cirrhosis, and liver failure; people with liver disease or liver problems or those who are taking drugs that affect the liver should talk with their health care provider before using kava (NCCAM Report, 2002)	
Passion flower	Causes mild hypnosis Reduces insomnia Reduces nervousness, restlessness, and agitation	Depresses the central nervous system (CNS) for mild sedative effect. Forms include tea, capsules, and extracts.	Infusion of 2–5 g (1 tsp) dried herb TID
Rosemary and other mints	Normalizes nerve impulses Acts as an antioxidant Relieves headache Acts as a sedative Helps improve memory and prevent dementia	Slows/inhibits action of acetylcholinesterase to acetylcholine, which stays in synapse longer. Antioxidant is carnosic acid that is concentrated in young growing leaves, peaks in the summer, lessens in older leaves, and is hardly present in old wood stems. Forms include whole essential oils for external use (see Aromatherapy section in text)	Tincture (1:5) 2–4 mL TID
St. John's wort	Treats mild-to-moderate depression, loss of interest, anorexia, fatigue, chronic fatigue immune dysfunction syndrome, and anxiety	Leaves or flowering tips can be used; hypericin is the active ingredient. May interfere with HIV drugs. Use may cause light sensitivity. Use with other drugs can be dangerous; do not take with other psychoactive medications (ie, selective serotonin reuptake inhibitors (SSRIs), tricyclics, and MAOIs). Has fewer side effects compared to antidepressants.	300–500 mg TID with meals for 4–6 weeks 0.5 mg hypericin per capsule

(continued)

TABLE 14-2 ▼ Selected Herbs, Minerals, and Vitamins for Mental Health Use (Continued)			
HERBS, MINERALS, AND VITAMINS	**USES**	**ACTIONS AND PRECAUTIONS**	**DOSE**
		May lower activity of non-sedating antihistamines, oral contraceptives, anti-epileptics, calcium channel blockers, cyclosporins, macrolides, and some antifungals.	
SAMe (S-adenosylmethionine)	Treats mild-to-moderate depression and arthritis, protects the liver, eases fibromyalgia	SAMe is a naturally occurring compound that regulates action of serotonin and dopamine. Approved as prescription drug in Italy, Germany, Spain, and Russia. Takes effect in 10 days, faster than prescription drugs. Use enteric-coated tablets with 96% pure product. Do not use for bipolar disorder. Must take 800 μg folic acid and 1000 μg vitamin B_{12} daily; the herb will not work if these vitamin levels are low.	200–800 or 1600 mg BID 1 hour before breakfast and lunch For arthritis 400–800 mg a day For fibromyalgia, 800 mg a day
Valerian	Relieves anxiety and insomnia	Forms include a tea (2–3 g dried root several times a day) or capsules. Herb is nonaddictive. Do not take with tranquilizers, sedatives, or alcohol. Possible side effects include blurred vision, excitability, and changes in heartbeat if taken in large doses or for more than 2 weeks.	300–400 mg 1–2 times a day
5-hydroxytryptophan (5-HTP)	Treats bipolar disorder in conjunction with lithium Reduces depression Relieves insomnia	This amino acid is a precursor of serotonin. Taken from *Griffonia simplicifolia* seed.	Bipolar disorder—200 mg, depression—150–300 mg, insomnia—200–600 mg

come. The Massachusetts Board of Nursing has recognized the therapeutic value of aromatherapy and has voted to accept it as part of holistic nursing care (Buckle, 1999).

Manipulative and Body-Based Methods

This category includes methods that are based on manipulation or movement of the body or both to improve health and restore function. T'ai chi, yoga, and massage are body-based methods thought to affect mental health. Other examples of body-based methods include chiropractic and osteopathic manipulation.

T'AI CHI

T'ai chi, sometimes defined as "moving meditation," is a Chinese blend of exercise and energy work with a series of choreographed, continuous slow movements performed with mental concentration and coordinated breathing. Practicing t'ai chi, the person learns to be aware of connecting with universal and earth energies, balancing energies within the body, and maintaining equilibrium with the yang and yin—opposing forces in nature (eg, active and passive, positive and negative, light and dark, male and female).

T'ai chi is a powerful centering activity and may precede meditation, prayer, or mental or physical activity. T'ai chi can help with most stress-related problems, anxiety, restlessness, problem solving, and sleep, and it can enhance socialization (because it is usually practiced within a group setting), serenity, and self-awareness (Kuhn, 1999; Fetrow & Avila, 2001). T'ai chi also can facilitate healing and rehabilitation following injury, surgery, or serious illness. After a session, 90% of clients report feeling more centered, peaceful, and happier, and their pain, stress, or illness either improved dramatically or disappeared completely (Choy, 1999). In addition, a short-term exercise program with the elderly led to significantly improved moods, increased flexibility and balance, decreased anxiety and pain, and an overall increased quality of life (Ross, Bohannon, Davis, & Gurchiel, 1999).

YOGA

Yoga dates back to 3000 BC and means "union" in Sanskrit. Yoga teaches basic principles of spiritual, mental, and physical energies to promote health and wellness. It is based on the Hindu principle of mind-body unity; a chronically restless or agitated mind will result in poor health and decreased mental clarity. Yoga was originally developed as part of a spiritual belief system focused on achieving a higher state of consciousness; in the West, yoga is practiced for its physical and psychological benefits. It is used to relieve anxiety, stress, and pain; treat addictions and migraines; enhance spatial memory; and increase auditory and visual perceptions (Kuhn, 1999; Fetrow & Avila, 2001).

Yoga uses proper breathing, movement, meditation, and postures to promote relaxation and enhance the flow of vital energy, called *prana*. There are many styles of yoga; each is a unique combination of physical postures and exercises (*asanas*), breathing techniques (*pranayamas*), relaxation, diet, and proper thinking. One style, hatha yoga, cleanses the body of toxins, clears the mind, energizes and realigns the body, releases muscle tension, and increases flexibility and strength.

MASSAGE

Massage is a systematic and scientific manipulation of the soft tissue of the body, first noted in Veda books of India in 8000 BC. P. H. Ling of Sweden (1776–1839) established the first college for massage in the United States. It became a profession in the United States in 1943, when a graduating class of the College of Swedish Massage in Chicago created the American Massage Therapy Association (AMTA).

Today there are more than 80 different kinds of massage. Benefits include decreased stress and anxiety; enhanced body–mind connection for greater mental clarity, energy, and performance; promotion of vitality, energy, and personal growth; and emotional release. Massage also has a sedative effect on the nervous system, promotes voluntary muscle relaxation, and improves self-image through reorganized posture (Kahn, 1996; Fetrow & Avila, 2001).

Energy Therapies

This domain includes therapies that focus either on energy fields that surround and penetrate the body (biofields) or those from other sources (electromagnetic fields) (Fetrow & Avila, 2001). The aim of biofield therapy is to affect the energy fields that surround and penetrate the body. Examples include healing touch, therapeutic touch, and Reiki. Bioelectromagnetic therapy involves the use of electromagnetic fields on the body. Examples include the use of magnets and electrical currents to heal nonuniting bone fractures (*Holistic Health Promotion*, 1999).

Energy therapies are based on the existence of energy fields and chakras, although energy fields have not been scientifically proven to exist. Humans, animals, and plants are made of electrons and protons that spin in a defined space, thus producing energy and forming atoms that form cells that compose organs that make up entities. According to energy field theory, these electrons give off energy or produce energy fields, chakras, or auras that may be seen, sensed, or felt by some people. When these energy fields are in disorder, the flow of essential information throughout the body is slowed, and healing is compromised. Energy from the outside, via a practitioner, can open the communication channels and facilitate tissue repair and replacement (Oschman & Oschman, 2000).

BIOFIELD THERAPIES

Healing Touch and Therapeutic Touch

Healing touch (HT) and **therapeutic touch (TT)** are two methods of energetic healing that have been derived from the ancient practice of the laying on of hands. Even though there is a spiritual aspect, there is no religious implication with either HT or TT. HT and TT incorporate the therapist's intention to heal, through either actual touch or nontouch repatterning, energy fields around the person. HT and TT are methods of consciously and intentionally directing energy through the hands of the practitioner to the client to facilitate the healing process.

Dolores Krieger, RN and PhD, and Dora Kunz, PhD, psychic and natural healer, developed the TT program in the early 1970s. TT then became a certification program of the American Nurses Association. TT is controversial; nevertheless, many hospitals, nationally and internationally, have policies that allow skilled practitioners of either modality to implement energetic treatment procedures. Healthcare consumers are requesting HT and TT before and after surgery in emergency and intensive care settings, as well as in the community (Hover-Kramer, 2002).

Janet Mentgen developed HT in 1989. The certification program is offered through the American Holistic Nurses' Association (AHNA). The communication between practitioner and client should be free and clear of attachment to any specific outcomes. The focus should be on one's intent for the greatest good of the client through centering, the healer's primary resource for such objective clarity. Personal growth and development of the practitioner is reiterated throughout HT because it enhances outcomes and profoundly changes the life of the practitioner.

HT is generally used for increased relaxation, pain relief, and an increased sense of well-being; it is even used with the dying for an easier transition. Other uses for HT are to decrease stress, resolve grief and depression, and work through codependency and child abuse issues. HT may be used in conjunction with psychotherapy; it will often facilitate deeper and more rapid healing.

Reiki

Reiki is an ancient, hands-on, Buddhist healing modality developed by the Tibetans and rediscovered by the Japanese in the 1800s; Reiki is a Japanese word meaning "universal life force." The inherent purpose of Reiki is to give the body direct access to transcendental, universal, radiant, and light energies, all at different levels on the energy spectrum. The practitioner holds his or her hands in 12 basic positions on the client's head, chest, and back (Kuhn, 1999). When "attuned" to inner processes, the practitioner can access universal energy to balance and release energy; this energy movement helps the client's body to rebalance and begin to heal. Reiki uses the four upper chakras to access this energy for strength, harmony, and balance to heal illness and reduce stress. It promotes total relaxation, which enhances the body's ability to recover from stress, injury, and disease; enhances emotional release; and reduces pain.

BIOELECTROMAGNETIC-BASED THERAPIES

Bioelectromagnetic therapy involves the use of magnetic fields in the prevention and treatment of disease and as first aid for injuries. Natural mineral magnets, lodestones, were used for thousands of years in Chinese, Egyptian, and Greek medicine for several ailments. Today, they are used for insomnia, chronic pain, broken bones, stress, and musculoskeletal disorders.

Magnetic field therapy uses two methods—static and pulsed. The static method involves placing magnets in belts, shoe inserts, and mattresses for 2 to 24 hours. Clients with pacemakers, defibrillators, or other metallic parts in their bodies should not use magnets or magnetic beds. The pulsed method involves using a machine to direct alternating electromagnetic fields (*Professional Guide to*, 2001).

THE NURSE'S ROLE

Use of complementary modalities by nurses depends on individual state licensing boards. In general, it is recommended that the nurse have the necessary credentials of the modality that is being used. Informed consent from the client is essential and will be part of the shared decision-making process. A consent form may be used, and the activity, response, and result must be documented in the medical record.

The underlying concepts in CAM concern energy—energy fields, energy centers, and changes in energy of the person. Also being an energy field, the nurse can and will affect the client regardless of whether that is the intention. Therefore, it is important and useful that there be an "energetic intention" in the interaction even if the nurse is not incorporating an energy modality into treatment. As an intentional energy source, the nurse can have greater influence with the psychiatric-mental health client. Some of the modalities are "touch free" yet tremendously powerful; the nurse may wish to incorporate such modalities into psychiatric care.

The nurse also must understand the importance and meaning of the modality for the client. What will have the greatest effects for clients is what they "believe to be true." The focus here is on the client's interpretation, expressed needs, and desired goals. Therefore, it is important for the nurse to develop an "energy-inclusive" mental healthcare plan with clients, especially if some treatment is meaningful to him or her.

▼ Reflection and Critical Thinking Questions

1. What is the most effective way to obtain information about CAM practices from the psychiatric client?
2. How would you incorporate a client's routine meditation practices into unit activity?

▼ CHAPTER SUMMARY

- CAM refers to practices that are not considered "conventional" in Western medical practice. These practices are used instead of (alternative) or in addition to (complementary) mainstream medical practices.
- CAM research focusing on psychiatric and mental

health is limited. Some research studies on St. John's wort and depression and ginkgo biloba and dementia are completed or in progress. In addition, funding for research using herbals and other indigenous therapies to treat schizophrenia and bipolar disorder has been approved.

■ The ethical and legal considerations for CAM are manifold. Many considerations are related to 1) federal regulation of herbal therapy and 2) client and primary healthcare provider collaboration on use of herbal therapies. Legal considerations include required education or training with designated actions for licensure or certification for CAM therapies.

■ The five domains of CAM are:
  ■ Alternative systems of medical practice
  ■ Mind-body interventions
  ■ Biologically based therapies
  ■ Manipulative and body-based methods
  ■ Energy therapies

■ Alternative systems of medical practice include traditional Chinese medicine, acupuncture, Ayurvedic medicine, homeopathy, and naturopathy.

■ Not all mind-body interventions are considered CAM; many mind–body interventions are used in mainstream medical practice (eg, imagery, relaxation therapy, and biofeedback). Examples of mind-body interventions that are still considered CAM include meditation, music therapy, and spiritual healing and prayer.

■ The most significant biological-based therapy is herbal therapy; aromatherapy also is used.

■ T'ai chi, yoga, and massage are body-based methods that are thought to affect mental health.

■ Energy therapies includes therapies that focus either on energy fields that surround and penetrate the body (biofields) or those from other sources (electromagnetic fields). Examples of biofield therapies include healing touch, therapeutic touch, and Reiki. Magnets (static or pulsed) are used in electromagnetic field therapy.

■ Nurses have the opportunity to obtain information from the client, relate information to the client, and facilitate the blending of CAM and traditional healing modalities. In addition, nurses can become intuitively adept at interacting and communicating with the energetic system in the body.

▼ REVIEW QUESTIONS

1. Which of the following is one of the goals of the National Center for Complementary and Alternative Medicine (NCCAM)?
   a. To promote the use of Chinese medicine
   b. To increase reimbursement for services
   c. To help people become responsible for their own healing
   d. To decrease reliance on allopathic medicine

2. Increase in the use of CAM has been attributed in part to which of the following factors?
   a. Less personal interactions between physicians and clients
   b. Safety and reliability of herbal remedies
   c. Poor coordination of traditional health care services
   d. Documented efficacy of alternative treatments

3. Which of the following conditions is the most common health problem for which CAM is used?
   a. Depression
   b. Hypertension
   c. Irritable bowel syndrome
   d. Back and neck problems

4. Drug companies do not want to research the validity of herbal remedies largely because
   a. They already have similar products.
   b. They don't have sufficient funds to research herbal medicines.
   c. Herbals cannot be patented.
   d. There isn't a big enough market for herbals.

5. Homeopathy is based on the concept that
   a. Illness can be treated with minute quantities of substances that cause the same symptoms.
   b. Spinal misalignment causes medical illness.
   c. Pessimistic thought patterns can be reversed to cure illness.
   d. Energy imbalances cause illness.

6. A 38-year-old male client is admitted to a psychiatric hospital for treatment of severe depression. A selective serotonin reuptake inhibitor is prescribed for him. The nurse is aware that the client takes large doses of vitamins, and before administering the medication, she asks the client if he has used any herbal products to treat his depression. The nurse is concerned about which of the following products?
   a. Ginseng
   b. Ginkgo biloba
   c. St. John's wort
   d. Rosemary

7. Kava kava has been linked to which of the following side effects?
   a. Pulmonary hypertension
   b. Bowel obstruction
   c. Liver failure
   d. Renal failure

8. S-adenosylmethionine (SAMe) is an herbal therapy taken for which of the following mental health problems?
   a. Depression
   b. Anxiety
   c. Phobias
   d. Short-term memory loss

9. A 45-year-old female client is being seen as an outpatient for depression. In addition to individual and group therapy, she has been taking sertraline (Zoloft). The client is upset because her mood is not improving quickly. At the next visit she complains of nausea, headache, and tremors. The nurse suspects serotonin syndrome and asks the client if she has been taking any natural remedies. Which of the following commonly used herbal therapies would put this client at risk for serotonin syndrome?
   a. Valerian
   b. Guarana
   c. 5-hydroxytryptophan
   d. Passion flower

10. Which of the following is an accurate statement about the use of CAM therapies in mental health?
   a. Their use is uncommon.
   b. They have a long history of use.
   c. They are generally as effective as pharmaceutical drugs.
   d. They have no governmental backing.

▼ REFERENCES AND SELECTED READINGS

*Achterberg, J. (1999). Imagery, ceremony and healing rituals. *Alternative Therapies in Health and Medicine, 5*(5), 76–85.

*Ameling, A. (2000). Prayer: An ancient healing practice become new again. *Holistic Nurse Practitioner, 14*(3), 40–48.

Ballentine, R. (1999). *Radical healing.* New York: Harmony Books.

Becker, N. B. (2000). NCCAM report and news briefs. *Alternative Therapies in Health and Medicine, 6*(1), 24–34.

Blumenthal, M. (1998). *The complete German Commission E monographs.* Austin, TX: American Botanical Council.

Blumenthal, M. (2000). Selected herb–drug interactions. *HerbalGram, 49,* 58–63.

Blumenthal, M., & King, P. (1996). The agony of the ecstasy. *HerbalGram, 36,* 20–24.

Brennan, B. (1988). *Hands of light: A guide to healing through the human energy field.* New York: Bantam Books.

Brinker, F. (1999). Variations in effective botanical products. *HerbalGram, 46,* 35–50.

Broadhurst, C. L., & Duke, J. A. (1999). Inside plants. *Herbs for Health, 4*(3), 26.

Bruyere, R. (1994). *Wheels of light.* New York: Simon & Schuster.

*Buckle, J. (1999). Use of aroma therapy as a complementary treatment for chronic pain. *Alternative Therapies in Health and Medicine, 5*(5), 42–51.

Chamberlain, L. (1998). *What the labels won't tell you.* Loveland, CO: Interweave Press.

*Choy, P. C. K. (1999). *T'ai chi, chi kung.* New York: The Overlook Press.

Crigliano, M. D., & Szapary, P. O. (1999). Guarana for cognitive enhancement. *Alternative Medicine Alert, 2*(6), 67–70.

Davidson, J., & Gaylord, S. (1998). Homeopathic and psychiatric perspectives on grief. *Alternative Therapies in Health and Medicine, 4*(5), 30–35.

*Dossey, L. (2000). Distant nonlocal awareness: A different kind of DNA. *Alternative Therapies in Health and Medicine, 6*(6), 102–114.

*Eisenburg, D. M., Davis, R. B., Etna, S. L., et al. (1998). Trends in alternative medicine use in the United States 1990–1997. *Journal of the American Medical Association, 280*(18), 1569–1575.

*Eliopoulos, C. (1999). *Integrating conventional and alternative therapy.* St. Louis, MO: Mosby.

*Fetrow, C. W., & Avila, J. R. (2001). *Professional's handbook of complementary & alternative medicine.* Springhouse, PA: Springhouse Corporation.

Fontaine, K. L. (2000). *Healing practices: Alternative therapies for nursing.* Upper Saddle River, NJ: Prentice Hall.

Foster, S. (1999). Go with the urge to quit: Herbal boosters for the nonsmoking life. *Herbs for Health, 4*(3), 48–51.

Fremerman, S. (1998, November/December). High anxiety. *Natural Health,* 103–111, 167–172.

*Fugh-Berman, A. (1997). *Alternative medicine: What works.* Baltimore, MD: Williams & Wilkins.

Gaynor, M. (1998). The capacity to heal. *Alternative Therapies in Health and Medicine, 4*(2), 72–78.

Gerber, R. V. (2000). *Vibrational medicine for 21st century.* New York: Eagle Brook Imprinting of HarperCollins.

*Guzzetta, C. E. (1997). Music therapy. In B. M. Dossey (Ed.), *Core curriculum for holistic nursing.* Gaithersburg, MD: Aspen Publishers, Inc.

Hagemaster, J. (2000). Use of therapeutic touch in treatment of drug addictions. *Holistic Nurse Practitioner, 14*(3), 14–20.

Hobb, C., & Schoenbart, B. (2001). Find the safest Chinese patent medicine. *Herbs for Health, 5*(6), 43–45.

Holistic health promotion and complementary therapies, Supplement #1. (1999). Gaithersburg, MD: Aspen Publishers, Inc.

*Hover-Kramer, D. (2002). *Healing touch: A resource for health care professionals* (2nd ed.). Albany: Delmar Publishing.

Husted, C., Phan, L., Hekking, A., & Niederman, K. (1999). Improving quality of life for people with chronic conditions: The example of t'ai chi and multiple sclerosis. *Alternative Therapies in Health and Medicine, 5*(5), 70–74.

*Ivker, R. S., Anderson, R. A., & Trivier, L., Jr. (1999). *The complete self-care guide to holistic medicine.* New York: Jeremy P Tarcher/Putman.

Johnston, B. A. (1999). ConsumerLab.com begins independent testing of herbal products and supplements—certification decal announced. *HerbalGram, 47,* 16.

Joy, B. W. (1979). *Joy's way: A map for the transformational journey.* Los Angeles: JP Tarcher.

*Kahn, S. (1996). *The nurse's meditative journal.* Albany: Delmar Publishers.

Kay, M. A. (1996). *Healing with plants in the American and Mexican West.* Tucson: University of Arizona Press.

Klivington, K. A. (1997). ADVANCES. *Journal of Mind–Body Health, 13*(4), 3–42.

*Kotek, K. (1999). Herbs at a glance. *Energy Times, 9*(4), 37–42.

Krieger, D. (1979). Therapeutic touch: How to use your hands to help or to heal. New York: Prentice-Hall.

Krieger, D. (1993). *Accepting your power to heal.* Santa Fe: Bear & Company.

*Kuhn, M. A. (1999). *Complementary therapies for health care providers*. Philadelphia: Lippincott Williams & Wilkins.

Kumar, A. M., Tins, F., Cruess, D. G., & Mintzer, M. J. (1999). Music therapy increases serum melatonin levels in patients with Alzheimer's disease. *Alternative Therapies in Health and Medicine, 5*(6), 49–57.

Laakmann, G., Schule, C., Baghai, T., et al. (1998). St. John's wort in mild to moderate depression. *Pharmacopsychiatry, 31*(Suppl.), 54–59.

Lad, V. (1998). *The complete book of ayurvedic home remedies*. New York: Harmony Books.

Leigh, E. (1999). Cannabis for migraine. *HerbalGram, 46,* 21.

Mayer, L., et al. (1998). Clinical efficacy of ginkgo biloba. *Phytomedicine, 5*(6), 415–424.

Murray, M. T. (1995). *The healing power of herbs* (2nd ed.). Rocklin, CA: Prima Publishing.

Muscat, M. (2000). NCCAM report. *Alternative Therapies in Health and Medicine, 5*(3), 28–32.

Myss, C. (1997). *Why people don't heal and how they can*. New York: Harmony Books.

*NCCAM report. (2002). *Alternative Therapies in Health and Medicine, 8*(2), 20–28.

Oschman, J. C. (2000). *Energy medicine: The scientific basis*. London: Churchill Livingstone.

*Oschman, J. L., & Oschman, N. H. (2000). *How healing energy works*. Philadelphia: Harcourt Publishing.

Payne, B. (1997). *Magnetic healing*. Twin Lakes, WI: Lotus Press.

*Phillips, E. (1999, July/August). Healthwatch herbal standards. *New Age Journal for Holistic Living, 28.*

Quinn, J. F., & Strelkauskas, A. F. (1993). Psychoimmunologic effects of therapeutic touch on practitioners and recently bereaved recipients: A pilot study. *Advanced Nursing Science, 15*(4), 13–26.

Quintavell, F. (1999, July/August). Bang the drum. *New Age,* 18.

Research review. Hypericin and AIDS. (1999). *HerbalGram, 47,* 29–30.

Research review. St. John's wort. (2000). *HerbalGram, 49,* 24–27.

Robinson, E., Jr., & Reinecke, M. (1998, Winter). Medicine men. *The TCU Magazine,* 6–10.

*Ross, M. C., Bohannon, A., Davis, D., & Gurchiel, L. (1999). The effects of a short-term exercise program on movement, pain and mood in the elderly: Results of a pilot study. *Journal of Holistic Nursing, 12*(2), 139–147.

*Rossiter-Thornton, J. F. (2000). Prayer in psychotherapy. Alternative Therapies in Health and Medicine, 6(1), 128, 135–137.

Roundtree, R. (2001). Potential herb–drug interactions. *Herbs for Health, 5*(6), 39–41.

Shealy, C. N. (1995). *Miracles do happen*. Rockport, MA: Element Books.

*Shealy, C. N. (1996). *The complete family guide to alternative medicine*. New York: Element Books.

St. Claire, D. (1992). *Pocket herbal reference guide*. Freedom, CA: Crossing Press.

Stevinson, C., Dixon, M., & Ernst, E. (1999). St-John's wort may bring fatigue relief. Herbs for Health, 4(3), 12.

*Strehlow, W., & Hertzka, G. (1988). *Hildegard of Bingen's medicine*. Santa Fe: Bear & Company.

*Texas State Board of Nurse Examiners. (1998, October).

The Dali Lama. (1999). The relevance of Tibetan medicine today. *Alternative Therapies in Health & Medicine, 5*(3), 67–69.

The SAMe solution. (1999, December). *Alternative Medicine Advisor, 1*(8), 1–2.

Tierra, M. (1999). Opinion standardization. *Herbs for Health, 4*(3), 6–9.

Torres-Tucker, L. (1999). The whole family. *Sharing: A Journal of Christian Healing, 67*(8), 15–17.

Tucker, A. O. (1999). Aromatherapy. *Herbs for Health, 4*(1), 46–50.

Ullman, D. (1999). *Homeopathy A–Z*. Carlsbad, CA: Hay House, Inc.

Weil, A. (1995). *Natural health, natural medicine*. Boston: Houghton Mifflin Company.

White, L. B. (2000). Herbal tricks for easing anxiety. *Herbs for Health, 5*(4), 34–39.

Starred references are cited in text.

▼ SELECTED RESOURCES

Academy for Guided Imagery
P. O. Box 2070
Mill Valley, CA 94942

Alternative and Complementary Medicine Topics
http://www.people.virginia.edu/pjb3s/Complementary_Practices.html

American Holistic Nurses Association
2733 E. Lakin Dr., Suite 2
Flagstaff, AZ 86004–2130

American Massage Therapy Association
http://www.amtamassage.org

Colorado Center for Healing Touch
12477 W. Cedar Dr., Suite 202
Lakewood, CO 80228
Phone: 303-989-7982, fax: 303-980-8683
E-mail: *ccheal@aol.com* or *HTIheal@aol.com*
http://www.healingtouch.net/us/co.shtml

Flower Essence Therapy
800-736-9222
http://flowersociety.org

Herb and Drug Interaction Data Base
4790 S.W. Watson Ave.
Beaverten, OR 97005

Integrative Body Mind Information System (IBIS)
www.IBISmedical.com
E-mail: *Interactions@IBISmedical.com*

International Academy of Classical Homeopathy
1–877-REMEDY
E-mail: *homeopath4@aol.com*

National Association of Nurse Massage Therapists
P. O. Box 1173
Abita Springs, LA 70420

National Foundation for Alternative Medicine
1155 Connecticut Avenue, NW, Suite 400
Washington, DC 20036

Nurse Healers Professional Associates
P. O. Box 444
Allison Park, PA 15101–0444

Office of Alternative Medicine
http://altmed.od.nih.gov/

Quackwatch
www.quackwatch.com

For additional information on this chapter, go to *http://connection. lww.com.*

Need more help? See Chapter 14 of the *Study Guide to Accompany Mohr: Johnson's Psychiatric-Mental Health Nursing,* 5th edition.

Continuum of Care

Community Mental Health, Support, and Rehabilitation

MARY HUGGINS, JEFFREY A. ANDERSON, & SUE ELLEN ODOM

▼ KEY TERMS

Aggregate group—A group identified as having at least one commonality among its members.

Aggregate mental health—The degree to which families and groups within a given environment contribute to, enhance, or intensify interaction among individuals along the mental health–illness continuum.

Case manager—A person who coordinates the various services that address the individual needs (eg, housing, healthcare, mental health treatment, social contacts, workups) of a mentally ill client.

Community support system—A network of caring and responsible people committed to assisting a vulnerable population to meet its needs and develop its potential without becoming unnecessarily isolated or excluded from the community.

Primary prevention—Healthcare interventions designed to prevent mental disorders or to reduce identified mental disorders and disabilities within a population.

Secondary prevention—Healthcare interventions designed to identify mental health problems early and reduce their duration and prevalence.

Systems of care—Comprehensive spectrums of mental health and other necessary services organized into coordinated networks so that providers can more appropriately address the various and changing needs of children and adolescents with serious emotional disturbances and their families.

Tertiary prevention—Healthcare interventions designed to provide rehabilitation for clients with diagnosed disorders and to minimize the residual effects for people within a community who have encountered mental health problems.

▼ LEARNING OBJECTIVES

On completion of this chapter, you should be able to accomplish the following:

■ Identify the levels of prevention of mental illness.

■ Describe potential interventions for primary, secondary, and tertiary prevention of mental health problems.

■ Define the term *community support system*.

■ Describe the philosophical context of the community support initiative.

■ Identify the essential components of a community support system.

■ Compare at least five models for the delivery of community support services.

■ Understand the development and functioning of systems of care for children who have multisystem needs and their families.

■ Explain the relationship of case management–service coordination to the effectiveness of a community support system.

■ Identify the trends that affect social policy regarding the care of persons with severe mental illnesses.

■ Describe the nurse's role in community mental healthcare using each step of the nursing process.

This chapter provides a historical and philosophical context for the promotion and protection of mental health in communities. It explains levels of prevention, which help to shape a community's health and determine the systems and programs a community needs. It describes the importance of community support systems and rehabilitation for clients to prevent recurrences or exacerbations of their psychiatric disorders. It explores the effects of the community support movement on delivery systems and projects trends that will affect the continued delivery of appropriate and effective community-based care. In addition, the chapter examines issues germane to children with mental health challenges, such as serious emotional disturbances, and recent developments in service provision for this population. Finally, the chapter addresses the nurse's role in protecting and improving a community's mental health.

COMMUNITY MENTAL HEALTH

Nursing focuses on *holistic health*, or all aspects of a person's physical, emotional, and spiritual well-being. Nurses encourage individuals, families, and communities to engage in and support various practices that will help them to avoid health problems or to prevent their recurrence. Such practices involve not only physical health but also mental health.

Each person, however, does not function as an isolated being. He or she operates within a larger society. A person interacts with other people, families, groups, and his or her community overall. Additionally, family and group systems interact, communicating with one another to produce accepted societal norms. This interaction forms a network system through which individuals, families, and groups can influence entire societies. In turn, the larger society shapes and influences the components within it. This network system forces nursing to expand its understanding of *client* to mean not only one person but also an entire community. In this way, the community becomes the client (Allen, 1997).

Nurses become used to assessing the mental health of individuals. The nurse evaluates a person's mental health by assessing how that person feels about himself or herself, how he or she feels about others, and how he or she meets everyday demands (National Mental Health Association, 1996). If the person feels good about himself or herself, interacts well with others, and functions independently, the nurse usually considers that person to be mentally healthy and designs interventions to promote or protect that state of health for as long as possible. The concept of *community mental health*, however, addresses the collective mental health of all people within a particular community. To evaluate and address a community's mental health needs, nurses must first assess internal aggregate groups. An **aggregate group** is identified as having at least one commonality among its members. Examples of aggregate groups with mental health needs might include the homeless (see Chap. 11), adolescents with mood disorders (see Chap. 24), and victims of abuse (see Chap. 17). **Aggregate mental health** can be defined as the degree to which families and groups within a given environment contribute to, enhance, or intensify the interaction among individuals along the mental health–illness continuum (Allen, 1997).

Historical Perspective

Historical, political, cultural, and economic factors have contributed to the common understanding of and circumstances surrounding community mental health. During the 1800s, people with psychiatric problems were housed in workhouses, almshouses, and jails. With no

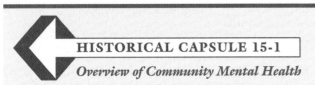

HISTORICAL CAPSULE 15-1
Overview of Community Mental Health

Approximate Date	Circumstances	Effects
1800	Housing of clients in asylums, jails, and workhouses	Separated those with mental illness from rest of population, leading to fear and stigma of mentally ill
1900	Housing of clients in state mental institutions	Overcrowding; inhumane conditions
1950	Mental Health Study Act	Research and study of mental illness
1960	Community Mental Health Centers Act	Opening of community mental health clinics
	Deinstitutionalization	Movement of mentally ill from state hospitals to community
1970	Community Support Program	Establishment of case managers
1980	Mental Health Systems Act	Legislation to address needs of mentally ill
1990	American Disabilities Act (ADA)	Legal protection of rights for mentally and physically disabled
	Healthy People 2000	Set national health goals
	National Alliance for Mentally Ill (NAMI) and National Alliance for Mental Patients (NAMP)	Established advocate groups for the mentally ill

attention given to "moral treatment," many state mental hospitals built between 1850 and 1890 rapidly became overcrowded with deplorable conditions. As the public started to become aware of these inhumane conditions, Congress eventually passed the National Mental Health Act in 1946 and established the National Institute of Mental Health (NIMH) in 1949.

NIMH provided not only research about mental illness but also training for professionals in psychiatry, psychology, social work, and nursing. NIMH also developed new services for those with mental illness. Many of the leaders of NIMH had served during World War II. They observed that environmental stress contributed to mental maladjustment and that a change to a less stressful environment decreased symptoms of psychiatric disorders. They believed that treating soldiers near the battlefield seemed to prevent prolonged debilitating effects. They later transferred their learning to the civilian sector (Worley, 1997). Ultimately, their ideas provided the foundations for early intervention and community treatment, beginning the community mental health movement.

In 1955, Congress initiated the Mental Health Study Act to examine the needs of the mentally ill. Findings led to recommendations for residential and educational programs within the community and early and intensive treatment of acute mental illness. They also suggested a need for fewer and smaller mental institutions, shifting of the care of people with mental illness to community health clinics (Grob, 1991; Isaac & Armat, 1990).

As a result of these recommendations and the continued overcrowding of clients in state mental institutions, Congress passed the Community Health Centers Act in 1963. Its provisions were for early intervention and prevention along with quality clinical mental health centers. The process of deinstitutionalization of clients from state mental institutions into the community began, saving the government many dollars (see Chaps. 1, 10, and 11). The government was supposed to make funding available for the development of community mental health clinics. Unfortunately, the needs of the mentally ill exceeded the services offered. As a result, many deinstitutionalized people became homeless, resorted to crime to survive, or both (see Chap. 11) (Worley, 1997).

In the 1970s, the first community support program (CSP) introduced the concept of the **case manager**, a person to coordinate the various functions that address the individual needs (housing, healthcare, mental health treatment, social contacts, and workups) of a mentally ill client. One case manager would be responsible for managing several mentally ill clients within a community. The intention was to reduce the need for inpatient hospitalization (Pardes, 1998).

In 1980, Congress passed the Mental Health Systems Act to address the needs of people with chronic mental illness, older adults, minorities, children, and people with psychiatric problems. The government failed to implement its provisions at the time. Subsequent policies and programs, however, incorporated several of its key concepts, among them increasing the role of individual states in developing mental health services and focusing on high-risk, high-need target populations (Pardes, 1998).

Congress passed the American Disabilities Act in 1990 to address the needs of people with mental and physical disabilities. Its major provisions mandated the mainstreaming of disabled people into everyday life, including employment, public service programs and activities, and public accommodations (Perlin, 1994). At the same time, many advocate groups for people with mental problems were developing. These included the National Alliance for the Mentally Ill (NAMI) and the National Alliance for Mental Patients (NAMP), two organizations that involve consumer and family groups (see Chaps. 1 and 10). These groups offer valuable services to the community by representing mental health issues and participating in discussions on national healthcare reform.

Legislatures currently need to address the continued needs of the mentally ill in the community setting. Some areas of concern are access to healthcare services and reimbursement mechanisms for services rendered. The power of change lies within each local community. Community health nursing can contribute to addressing these needs. Difficulties with community health services and areas for reform are discussed throughout this chapter.

Levels of Prevention

Traditionally, healthcare delivery has focused on treating ill people rather than preventing illness. With the initiation of Healthy People 2000, both society and the healthcare industry began to focus more on health promotion and health maintenance. These ideas include levels of prevention: primary, secondary, and tertiary (Table 15-1). For both individuals and communities, nurses use these different levels of prevention to identify and implement strategies to maintain and attain optimal mental health (Worley, 1997).

PRIMARY PREVENTION

The aims of **primary prevention** are to prevent mental disorders and to reduce the number of identified cases of mental disorders and disabilities within a population. Primary prevention consists of two concepts: health promotion and disease prevention. *Health promotion* aims to ensure the continued well-being of people or communities already considered healthy. Examples of health promotion measures are exercising or following a healthy diet. *Disease prevention* focuses on protecting against any potentially harmful threat. Its goal is to protect as many people as possible from any harmful consequences of a specific health threat. An example of a disease prevention strategy is to encourage immunizations for infants and children.

TABLE 15-1 ▼ Interventions According to Levels of Prevention

LEVEL OF PREVENTION	DEFINITION	EXAMPLES
Primary	Prevent problem from ever occurring	Nurse promotes self-esteem, teaches alternatives to violence, and encourages political involvement for clients.
Secondary	Early diagnosis and treatment	Nurse holds conflict management classes, teaches gun safety, conducts mental health screenings, and makes necessary referrals.
Tertiary	Continued support and rehabilitation	Nurse leads support groups, holds refresher courses on conflict management, and supports and reinforces nonviolent behavior.

Nurses design primary prevention interventions to address not only general health concerns but also to target populations known to be at high risk for mental health problems. Primary prevention includes interventions ranging from those to treat mild mental illness with limited disability to severe mental illness. Although the focus of mental health promotion is prevention, it also helps prevent relapse in those already experiencing mental distress. For example, children living in poverty or experiencing undue mental distress are included in the high-risk group. If these children do not receive appropriate, effective intervention, they are likely to continue through their adult lives with poor mental health and social outcomes. Many innovative interventions with children can improve their long-term psychological, social, and economic well-being, as discussed in Box 15-1.

Certain adults also are at high risk for mental health problems, including those experiencing adverse life situations such as unemployment, divorce, or loss of a loved one. Mental health interventions enable them to deal with the current crisis and grow from the experience. They also can prevent further deterioration and associated problems (Box 15-2).

Community mental health nurses try to incorporate health promotion by interacting with healthy people and attempting to maintain and enhance their well-being. The nurse includes family members and caregivers in developing strategies to promote mental health because caregivers who also become incapacitated are less apt to continue caring for the already mentally ill individual. Examples of mental health promotion might include promoting parent–infant bonding, developing age-appropriate social skills, developing environments that favor positive adaptation, fostering empowerment by allowing people to make

BOX 15-1 ▼ *Mental Health Promotion Interventions for Children*

- Early intervention education for preschoolers from disadvantaged communities
- Social skills training to deal with behavioral problems, improve peer relationships, enhance positive attitudes
- Cognitive skills training
- Emotional support for children experiencing death of a loved one or divorce or separation of parents
- Social support visits for parents (to target available community resources or ways to achieve educational and occupational goals)
- Training in child care for new parents
- Support groups for children with divorced parents
- Bereavement groups

BOX 15-2 ▼ *Mental Health Promotion Interventions for Adults*

- Home visits to provide social support to pregnant women from disadvantaged communities
- Cognitive-behavioral therapy
- Job-searching skills
- Problem-solving skills
- Communication techniques
- Stress management
- Respite care or some type of psychological support for long-term caregivers
- Coping skills (job loss, birth, caregiving, separation, divorce, bereavement, poverty)
- Parent–child interaction training
- Exercise programs

Adapted from Turner-Boutle, M., Sowden, A., & Gilbody, S. (1997). Mental health promotion in high-risk groups. *Nursing Times, 93*(32), 42–43.

critical decisions about their lives, and acquiring skills for coping effectively with stress (Cowen, 1994).

SECONDARY PREVENTION

Secondary prevention focuses on interventions that identify mental health problems early and reduce the duration and prevalence of mental illness. It includes early diagnosis, prompt treatment, and limitation of any disabilities. Examples of secondary prevention for the community mental health nurse include conducting screening surveys that focus on identifying mental illness in individuals within the community, referring clients for mental health treatment, and providing crisis intervention to a community that has encountered a natural or man-made disaster (see Chap. 11).

TERTIARY PREVENTION

Tertiary prevention is the final level of prevention. Its focus is rehabilitation and ways to minimize the residual effects of people within the community who have encountered mental health problems. Examples include social skills training, vocational rehabilitation, self-help groups, and sufficient residential and independent living services (Worley, 1997).

COMMUNITY SUPPORT SYSTEMS

A **community support system** is defined as a "network of caring and responsible people committed to assisting a vulnerable population to meet their needs and develop their potentials without being unnecessarily isolated or excluded from the community" (Turner, 1986). This definition encompasses a basic philosophy of care meant to address humanely the needs of adults with severe and persistent mental illnesses that seriously limit their ability to function in the primary areas of daily living.

To address issues related to deinstitutionalization and the government's inability to adequately meet the needs of people with mental illness, NIMH established the Community Support Service Branch, which was transferred to the newly formed Center for Mental Health Services in 1992. The Branch promoted community support systems throughout the country. Since its establishment, the Branch has influenced the delivery system of broad-ranged services and support needed for this population to live in the least restrictive environment possible. The Branch also recognizes the need for quality of life and focuses on moving service provision from more restrictive settings (eg, residential placements) to home and community settings (see Chap. 16).

Likewise, in response to documented poor outcomes for children with serious emotional disturbances and related mental health problems, similar changes have occurred in children's services. Substantial reform efforts intended to improve this area often are attributed to the 1984 enactment of the Child and Adolescent Service System Program (CASSP). The CASSP provides support for communities to develop mechanisms for coordinating the agencies serving children with multisystem needs and their families (Duchnowski & Kutash, 1996; Knitzer, 1996; Stroul & Friedman, 1986).

For both adults and children, much has been learned; however, much remains undone. The changing focus and locale described in the definition of community mental health is built on and refined in the definition of community support systems. Not only does an effective community support system require all the components of community mental health, it also requires elements of systems theory. In other words, this approach provides "more than a list of necessary service components . . . the range of service components must be organized into an integrated system" (Anthony & Blanch, 1989).

Components of a Community Support System

A community support system can be seen as a systems model that delivers community-based care for a specific population who traditionally required long-term hospitalization over many years. This system includes a range of supports: healthcare, mental healthcare, rehabilitation services, social networks, housing arrangements, and educational and employment opportunities. Not only does it offer these specific services, but it also offers them through several different program models (discussed later).

Typically, the community support network is coordinated by a single agency responsible for organization of the system, as well as for negotiation among the various agencies forming the network of services. This agency, then, is responsible for articulating the philosophical and operational basis for the network and promoting the active participation of all those invested: clients, family members, government officials, and healthcare providers. The community support system is not a single model: it embraces and incorporates many models to provide comprehensive services to meet the population's diverse needs. To achieve the comprehensiveness required for those with severe mental illness, the system maintains flexibility, incorporating the positive elements of several generic models while promoting a seamless system of service delivery.

Essential components of a community support system include the following:

- Identification and assertive outreach to the at-risk population to inform clients of and ensure their access to needed services
- Adequate mental healthcare, including diagnostic evaluations, management of prescribed psychotropic

medications, periodic examinations, community-based psychiatric or psychological services, and specialized counseling or treatment (eg, for substance abuse)

- Links with medical and dental services, including help in applying for medical assistance benefits
- Twenty-four hour quick-response assistance to enable both family and client to cope effectively with crises while maintaining the client's status as a functioning community member; this element requires all-day crisis services provided by trained professionals at various sites, including at home, in the criminal justice system, and on the job (see Chap. 11)
- Psychosocial and vocational services through various rehabilitative options for an indefinite duration, focusing primarily on improving the client's ability to function in normal social roles (ie, training in daily living and community living skills, social skills, interests, and leisure activities) and assisting him or her to find and use appropriate employment services
- A range of rehabilitative and supportive housing options based on choice and offering necessary support, incentives, and encouragement for the client to accept increasing responsibility for his or her own life
- Backup support, assistance, consultation, and education for families, friends, landlords, employers, and community agencies as well as referrals to family self-help or advocacy programs (eg, NAMI, Reach) to maximize the benefits of and minimize the problems associated with the client living in the community
- Recognition and involvement of concerned community members and endorsement of the natural support system, including consumer and family self-help groups, churches, community organizations, commerce, and industry in the development and implementation of community support systems
- Assistance with application for entitlements (financial, medical, housing, and other benefits) that are crucial to meeting basic human needs, including food, clothing, shelter, general medical and dental care, and personal safety
- Protection of the individual's rights, provision of information regarding basic civil rights and available resources, and access to advocacy and grievance procedures to ensure that appropriate mechanisms are in place to protect these rights
- Case management (a single person or team) responsible for helping the individual make informed choices, ensuring timely access to needed assistance, providing opportunities and encouragement for self-help, and coordinating all services to meet the individual's needs
- Provision of these components through an integrated system that responds to the individual's needs, including special needs related to his or her particular circumstances (eg, older adult, child, homelessness, parole, developmental disability, hearing impairment) (Stroul, 1987).

Guiding Principles

The overriding element of these components is respect for each person's dignity and specific needs and empowerment rather than dependency. The goal is to enable those with severe mental illnesses to remain in the community and function as independently as possible. People having such challenges are a diverse group; each person will have unique concerns, abilities, motivations, and problems. Therefore, community support systems must be based on services that provide for the following:

- Self-determination
- Individuation
- Normalization of settings as well as offerings
- Least restrictive appropriate settings
- Maximization of mutual assistance and self-help (Libermann, Kuehnel, Phipps, & Cardin, 1984)

In addition, the system must be culturally competent and accountable to its users (see Chap. 5).

Program Models

An effective community support system embraces a comprehensive spectrum of services for people with severe mental illness and their relatives. These services are not related to the specific content of a particular program model but rather are part of the program's philosophy, operating style, and leadership (Libermann et al., 1984). Several models providing access to the community support system have been identified. A community may use a model singly or in combination with other models (Stroul, 1986). The most important consideration is for the program to have the essential components of an effective community support system.

Although all program models share similarities, they differ in comprehensiveness and in the degree to which they provide or broker services. The preferred model for persons with severe mental illness embraces psychosocial rehabilitation, although the configuration of service offerings may be distinct because of factors relating to demographics or funding streams. All these models, however, embrace the principles of psychiatric rehabilitation and focus on individually tailored program plans with realistic goals based on an assessment of the individual's strengths and weaknesses.

Principles basic to psychiatric rehabilitation, and thus to all models for community support systems, are as follows (Anthony, Cohen, & Cohen, 1984):

- The primary focus is to improve the capabilities and competence of the person with mental illness. Alleviation of symptoms is secondary.
- Insight is not a primary goal. The focus is on the person's ability to function.
- The provision of services is eclectic and uses various therapeutic constructs.
- Improvement of vocational outcomes is a central focus.
- Emphasis on positive expectations and hope is essential to the process.
- A deliberate increase in dependency, as in sheltered settings, may be a first step in the process.
- The program seeks the active participation and involvement of the individual in rehabilitation, the operation of programs, and the delivery of services so that rehabilitation occurs *with,* rather than *to,* the individual.
- Development of individual skills and environmental resources is a fundamental intervention in the rehabilitation process.

The services in these program models are delivered mostly in real-life communities (in vivo), versus in hospitals, to promote the transfer of learning through modeling and immediate reinforcement. These sites include but are not limited to home, school, and work.

PSYCHOSOCIAL REHABILITATION MODEL

Also known as the clubhouse model, the psychosocial rehabilitation model evolved from Fountain House, founded by a group of clients in New York City in 1948. It is organized generally as a clubhouse with members who fully participate in the program's operation. Services usually are divided into four major areas: (1) social–recreational, (2) vocational, (3) residential, and (4) educational.

Members can participate in a variety of activities relating to the management of the program (eg, meal preparation, newsletter publication, janitorial services) as well as in decision making regarding program operation. Evaluation indicates that this model is effective in reducing hospitalizations and improving community functioning, particularly in the area of vocation and independent living for long-term members (Bond, Dincin, Setze, & Witheridge, 1984).

FAIRWEATHER LODGE MODEL

The Fairweather lodge model began in 1960. It uses the hospital as a training center for a group of clients who subsequently move into the community to live in a lodge and operate a small business. Group norms and peer support form the foundation of this model. All members of the lodge participate fully both in the lodge and the workplace, using appropriate work roles and habits. Eval-uation indicates reduced recidivism and increased community employment activities (Fairweather, 1980).

TRAINING IN COMMUNITY LIVING MODEL

Also known as the program of assertive community treatment, the training in community living model began in the 1970s in Wisconsin. It involves in vivo teaching of basic coping skills in the client's environment. This approach is directive, taking treatment to the client through role modeling and support and treating the client as a responsible citizen. The hospital is used only in extreme cases. This model emphasizes the importance of clinical management, including appropriate medications and medication monitoring. It teaches clients about symptoms, the relationship between symptoms and stress, and how to control symptoms.

Research indicates that this model is effective in helping individuals maintain stability in the community. Evidence includes increased work productivity, decreased symptomatology, decreased hospitalization, decreased unemployment, and increased satisfaction with life (Weisbrod, Test, & Stein, 1980).

CONSUMER-RUN ALTERNATIVE MODELS

These models, also known as self-help programs, are based on the idea that planning, administering, delivering, and evaluating services should be done *for* consumers *by* consumers. The program's core is voluntary participation, consumer control, and empowerment. Several such alternatives have been developed. Social, recreational, and educational services frequently are added to the core drop-in center, which also may include community and public education and advocacy at both the individual and public policy levels. Consumer alternatives also have been started in the areas of residential, crisis, and vocational services.

Several states have developed offices devoted to consumer programming and advocacy within their offices of mental health. The focus on outcomes and satisfaction with this model have provided for several grants to states to assess the effects of these programs. Initial reports indicate a highly successful overall experience, based on high attendance and high levels of reported satisfaction (Mowbry, Chamberlain, & Jenning, 1984). This additional research will provide a more comprehensive assessment including potential problem areas such as the negative effects on consumers who staff these alternatives, as well as recommendations for the provision of acceptable supports and ways to prevent negative consequences.

COMMUNITY WORKER MODELS

Community worker models rely on ordinary citizens to provide a range of community support services, generally on a part-time paid or volunteer basis. Services include friendship, emotional support, teaching of community living skills, and assistance in accessing appropriate services. The community worker complements professional mental health services by modeling appropriate behaviors and by monitoring the individual's level of functioning. In the community supportive care variation (Rhinelander model), which originated in rural Wisconsin, the county pays lay citizens to provide community support. This model emphasizes one-to-one relationships. The Compeer variation uses volunteers to provide caring, supportive relationships. It originated in Rochester, New York, as an adjunct to therapy and fills gaps when clients lack natural supports.

COMMUNITY SUPPORT PROGRAMS

Another effective model has been the community support program (CSP). The first CSP was conceived in 1977. Since then, all 50 states, the District of Columbia, and several U.S. territories have developed CSPs. Effective CSPs "have positive sanction for their activities and service function from the highest level of local and state administration" (Libermann et al., 1984). This includes visibility and continuing support from all levels of government (city, county, state, and federal) to effect services at the systems level (eg, police, housing authorities, local planning boards). This attention has helped to publicize the conditions under which the vulnerable mentally ill population must exist and to identify the needs of people with severe mental illness as a priority.

CSPs are based on values implemented at three levels: the individual, the agency, and the network. These values focus on the person: the consumer is central to the system. As such, the individual stays involved in decisions that affect the needed services. The central theme of community support is empowerment recognizing the following three tenets:

1. All people are valuable and should be afforded dignity, respect, and the opportunity to take full advantage of their human, legal, and social rights.
2. Every human being is capable of growth, development, and learning.
3. Services should be provided in a normative and socially valued way.

Key to this is a holistic understanding of each person as an individual with hope for a wide range of outcomes that includes considerable improvement and recovery for many. Severe mental illness, though devastating, is no longer a hopeless disease. Therefore, hope is essential, not only for the individual with severe mental illness, but also for the person interacting as the helper (Harding, 1994).

CHILD AND ADOLESCENT SERVICE SYSTEM PROGRAM

Outcomes for children and youth with emotional and behavioral challenges have continued to be poor. Research findings demonstrate that children with these challenges, as a group, have the poorest long-term outcomes of any group with a disability (Kutash & Duchnowski, 1997; Wagner, 1995). Friedman et al. (1996) reviewed several studies of the characteristics of children with emotional and behavioral disabilities and conclude that these children have serious problems in several domains, including social behavior, emotional and behavioral functioning, educational performance, and overall functioning. For example, these children tend to have poorer school performance and higher rates of school dropout, unemployment, and arrests than any other group with a disability (U.S. Department of Education, 1998). Research findings also demonstrate that, even after receiving years of special education services, children with emotional and behavioral challenges become adults with similar problems; they end up unemployed or incarcerated at higher rates than those found in the general population (Greenbaum et al., 1998). Researchers have found that many of these young people face unemployment, become involved in criminal activity, or both after leaving secondary school (Wagner, 1995).

In response to the multidimensional nature of emotional and behavioral challenges and the poor outcomes that children with such problems experience, reform efforts have focused on alternative ways of providing services. Beginning with the CASSP in 1984, a new philosophy of service provision for children with serious emotional disturbance evolved (Friedman, 1996). The CASSP emphasizes several important principles that have influenced the way in which services are provided (Duchnowski & Kutash, 1996):

- Services should be community based and provided in the least restrictive setting possible.
- Parents or caregivers should be partners in providing services, by both identifying needed services and designing individual service plans for their children.
- Service systems and providers should be culturally competent and provide all services within each family's unique cultural and ethnic perspectives.

Since the CASSP was enacted, additional values, including service coordination, individualization of services, local and state level leadership, and flexible funding, also have become essential aspects of comprehensive, appropriate approaches to service provision for children with serious emotional disturbances and their families.

Service systems that adopt and use these principles often are referred to as **systems of care** (Friedman, 1996). Stroul and Friedman (1986) define systems of care as comprehensive spectrums of mental health and other necessary services organized into coordinated networks so that providers can more appropriately address the various and changing needs of children and adolescents with serious emotional disturbances and their families. All systems of care use some form of service coordination, described as connecting the variety of systems, agencies, and individuals, including the family, that participate in the care of a child, and ensuring effective, ongoing communication among everyone involved so that services and interventions are consistent and directed toward common goals (Stroul, 1996). Often, a service coordinator manages this process; his or her role is to convene and guide a multiagency service coordination team. Typically, such teams are responsible for organizing and managing all the services received by the child (Friesen & Poertner, 1995). Such approaches to service provision challenge teachers, nurses, social workers, and other service providers to put aside professional biases and create partnerships both with one another and with families (Handron, Dosser, McCammon, & Powell, 1998).

The Dawn Project is an example of a system of care. Currently in its fifth year of operation, Dawn is funded jointly by county and state governments and administered through a contract with a private, nonprofit care management organization. At its core, Dawn provides a coordinated, community-based network of services for children, youth, and their families who are involved with multiple systems (Russell, Rotto, & Matthews, 1999). Part of the impetus for this project was the recognition that increasing numbers of children with serious emotional and behavioral problems were being sent away from home, including costly placements out of the county or state.

Eligibility criteria for the Dawn Project include children and youth who

- Are residents of Marion County, Indiana
- Are between 5 and 18 years of age
- Have a *DSM-IV-TR* diagnosis (*Diagnostic and Statistical Manual of Mental Disorders,* 4th edition, text revision) or special education designation
- Have functional impairments in at least two of the following domains: social, family, community, school
- Are involved in two or more child serving systems (ie, mental health, child welfare, juvenile justice, special education)
- Are at risk for or already in a residential placement

The Office of Family and Children, the Juvenile Division of the Court, or the Division of Special Education can refer children who meet these criteria to Dawn (Russell, Rotto, & Matthews, 1999). In October 1999, the Center for Mental Health Services of the Substance Abuse and Mental Health Services Administration awarded a 6-year grant to Marion County to expand the Dawn Project to include three new populations: children from Marion County who are (1) sent to the Department of Correction, (2) in state hospitals, or (3) at-risk for developing more serious emotional or behavioral problems.

Public Policy and Trends

Both CSPs and the CASSP represent system change initiatives. Such community support systems have focused on public policy issues. Certain areas of concern have become obstacles at worst, and challenges at best, to the delivery of community-based care for people with severe mental illness (Anderson, 2000):

- In the United States, approximately 20% of adults experience severe mental illness, which has a potential for debilitation similar to that of chronic heart disease. Mental and emotional disturbances affect 12% of all children, many of whom never receive needed or appropriate services.
- Approximately one third of the people who are homeless on a given night have a serious mental illness. More than half of these people also have a substance abuse problem.
- Recent estimates indicate that nearly 7% of all inmates have a serious mental illness and that 12.5% inmates require some psychiatric attention.
- Of the more than 40 million adults with mental illness requiring treatment, only 25% receive the treatment they need.
- Many of the more than 1.5 million people with HIV infection or AIDS also experience severe psychological distress.
- Culturally relevant services are not available as a matter of course for people of color or for thousands of refugees and detainees.
- Children and youth with serious emotional disturbance often have multiple needs requiring the simultaneous involvement of several child-serving agencies (eg, child services, special education, juvenile justice, mental health). Unfortunately, disparate definitions and eligibility criteria used to identify need for services have prevented agencies and providers from collaborating or even communicating about the children with whom they work, leading to a pervasive lack of coordination among service providers.

The following section discusses some of the ongoing problems faced by providers of community support services.

CHRONICITY OF SEVERE MENTAL ILLNESS

A growing body of knowledge continues to identify mental illness as a disease of the brain (see Chap. 2). Society must begin to understand that severe mental illness is a chronic, debilitating condition similar to multiple sclerosis or chronic heart disease. Such recognition counters the myth of a "quick cure." It also diminishes the belief that people with severe mental illnesses can live without supportive treatment such as medication and counseling.

Additionally, gross confusion persists about the relationships between diseases and their symptoms. Such understanding perpetuates the myth that severe mental illness precludes opportunities for rehabilitation. According to Pepper (1987), ". . . in failing to specify between chronic mental disorder and social disability, we perpetuate the myth that severe mental illness in fact, the social disability is severe mental illness is neither inevitable nor incurable characterizes patients with a chronic disability opportunity for rehabilitation

For most people, mental illness is treatable. Use of services that focus on problem-solving and coping skills in conjunction with administration of antipsychotic medications are effective ways to assist clients with the overwhelming drain of diminished coping skills resulting from severe mental illness. Healthcare providers must maintain and promote within communities a vision of recovery. They must facilitate processes that provide optimism regarding recovery while maintaining realistic expectations based on a client's specific coping abilities (Anthony, 1993; Lamb, 1994).

STALLED RESOURCES

Conflicting federal, state, and local mandates have prevented resources, including funds and staff, from making their way to the community. This can be best documented by looking at the dramatic shift of funding responsibility over the last 40 years. In the late 1960s, most costs for the mentally ill population rested with state governments (primarily in state hospitals). Recently, responsibility for the provision of community-based care has rested at the local level, with federal payments and reimbursements to support the individual. Responsibility for overall planning and policy making, however, has remained at the state level. Funding bases that were not intended to support people with mental illness have become the core for community-based treatment.

Currently, Medicaid funding, although limited in noninstitutional settings, is the major source of healthcare funding for poor people, including most people with severe mental illness. The result has been inappropriate admissions to nursing facilities and other institutions so that the client can receive appropriate care. In some states, commitment laws have become stringent to stem inappropriate admissions to state hospitals. Families of people with severe mental illness are actively trying to loosen these laws. This activity is the result of both the difficulty they have experienced in admitting their loved ones and their sense that hospitalization is necessary to appropriately address the client's needs.

POVERTY

relied solely on SSI (eg, access to healthcare) (Viccora, Perry, & Mancuso, 1993). Mental illness and stress further complicate this situation. A person who is rehospitalized or cannot work on a long-term basis loses both benefits and medical insurance.

Some legislative efforts have been developed in recognition of the person's ability to work on a sporadic or part-time basis. Efforts made in this area may be moot, however, as Congress moves toward eliminating federal programs that support housing, vocational, and basic health benefits for people with disabilities. Unless safety-net services remain intact, serious problems resulting in reinstitutionalization for thousands of people are likely.

REINSTITUTIONALIZATION

The fundamental lack of public policy and the potential dissolution of the current infrastructure have contributed to problems of "reinstitutionalization." Unlike the early institutions that housed those with mental illness in hospitals and asylums, however, the current reinstitutionalization is occurring in both hospitals and jails. As responsibility for people with severe mental illness remains in limbo, the large numbers of inadequately housed or homeless people are overwhelming local governments. These people are coming to the attention of local authorities.

EDUCATION

Another institution experiencing substantial challenges is education. Although the movement toward inclusion of children with disabilities into general education classrooms tends to require the placement in the least restrictive environment for most children with disabilities, schools have had a difficult time fully including children with more serious emotional and behavioral challenges. Lack of funding, the paucity of appropriate teacher training, and issues related to stigma all present barriers to schools' abilities to provide emotionally disturbed children with full and successful access to inclusive settings.

STIGMA

Stigma toward those with psychiatric disorders may involve employment, resulting in clients not being hired or hired for only entry-level, low-expectation positions. Stigma in housing can take the form of refusing to rent to a person with mental illness or raising the rent just above the fair market rate, thus precluding the use of a subsidy. Stigma may take the form of developing restrictive zoning regulations that regulate where the person can live. In schools, it may keep children who have been labeled with emotional disturbances out of general education classrooms and in separate, segregated settings, away from their peers without disabilities.

Stigma may take place on the street, when others avert their eyes and avoid interacting with those who have mental illnesses. Although it is clearly discriminatory to refuse jobs and housing based on a person's diagnosis, fear regarding personal safety and community welfare has allowed these practices to continue. Furthermore, the frustration of seeing a person with an "obvious illness" not being cared for has escalated the stigma and hindered acceptance of such clients into the community. When stigma becomes internalized, the individual begins to feel that they deserve an inferior status that further erodes the individual's state of hopelessness and despair. In school, for example, children with emotional disturbances may sabotage efforts at inclusion (ie, reintegration) because they have a long history of experiencing stigma in school.

At the forefront of the anti-stigma campaigns are consumer and family movements. These groups demand to be involved in the development of treatment alternatives. They provide advocacy, support, and knowledge regarding the disease—including realistic expectations—to other consumers, family members, and the general public. In many parts of the county, consumers and families are involved in anti-stigma media watches and public education and advocacy.

Consumers and family members are increasingly involved at the decision-making levels of government, helping to shape future policies and practices. In many states, legislation requires consumer–family member participation at the decision-making level, for example, the Minnesota Comprehensive Mental Health Systems Act.

REFORMS

Safety Net Services

Regulation and legislation must emphasize the establishment of community support services as essential safety nets. These services must include case management and interagency cooperation in all local areas, methods that have been shown to be effective and to increase quality of life for people involved in these programs. Historically, these services have not been eligible for Medicaid and other sources of funding. Payment for case management, day treatment, psychosocial programs, housing supports, and other community supports, as well as parity for outpatient and other healthcare coverage, is essential to any funding of community treatment alternatives.

Mainstream resources at the local and state level are equally important in the development of effective community-based alternatives to meet the needs of those being discharged from state hospital and nursing facilities (as required under the Nursing Home Reform Act of 1987) (Cook, Jonikas, & Soloman, 1992; Schaft & Randolf, 1994). The passage of the Americans With Disabilities Act and the Fair Housing Act provides for some protection of individual rights, which affords a springboard for the development of a comprehensive community support system (Bazelon Center for Mental Health Law, 1999; Kincaid, 1994; Mancuso, 1993).

Legislation

Several relatively new legal initiatives are affecting the delivery of community-based services to people with severe mental illness. *Advanced directives* allow consumers to make their intentions known regarding their choice of treatment before treatment is necessary. Clients complete these directives when they are not experiencing episodes of mental illness. The directives describe how the person prefers to be treated during a psychiatric emergency. The nurse may be requested to assist with the development of the directive.

Informed consent allows clients to make informed choices regarding their treatment plans. It is incumbent on the helping person (often, the nurse) to ensure that adequate information has been made available to the client so that he or she is informed of the choice.

Commitment and other involuntary interventions may become a reality in a situation when advanced directives and other community-based interventions break down or are not available. State laws and professional codes of ethics cover these interventions. Nurses must understand how these laws and codes pertain locally. In some cases, a less restrictive alternative can be found. The nurse can play an important role in assisting the system to identify these lesser restrictions (Weinstein & Hughes, 1998).

Due process provides protection for parents and their children with disabilities in schools. Families have the right to information and informed consent before evaluation, labeling, or placement of their child into special education and have the right to request a due process hearing if they disagree with any findings or decisions made by school personnel on their child's behalf (Hallahan & Kauffman, 2001). School nurses may be involved in these procedures and can provide valuable information about childhood mental illnesses.

Public Policy

Social and healthcare reforms require evaluation to determine their effectiveness as proposed public policy. Although interested parties have not reached total agreement on needed reforms, they have begun to view the following with some unanimity:

- A comprehensive policy for the least restrictive treatment for people with severe mental illness should range from prevention to hospitalization (noting that in *some* instances hospitalization is the least restrictive alternative) and should include accommodation for acute episodes. This policy should recognize the need for supportive housing as well as other community support services, including recreation, jobs, educational opportunities, and medical, dental, and mental health services (Bond, 1994; Carling & Ridgway, 1999; Pepper, 1987; Searight & Handal, 1987). For children, this translates into the need for, and preservation of, a continuum or cascade of available services.
- The government must direct policy and funding toward developing a comprehensive, unified, seamless network of community support services in each community. According to Pepper, ". . . state gov-

ernments, being the repositories of constitutional responsibility for the mentally ill [must] take the initiative in developing policies" (1987) that address the following areas: entitlement of citizens to intensive interventions funded by private insurance when available and by public funding when it is not; comprehensive, integrated outpatient alternatives and community support services when needed; and integrated services for persons with dual disabilities.

- The federal government needs to create active initiatives to develop federal policy regarding financial resources and regulations so that quality, community-based alternatives can become a reality (Pepper, 1987).
- Anti-stigma efforts should focus on the general population in promoting an understanding of mental illness, incorporating research that identifies the illness as a chronic disease.
- Active initiatives for healthcare reform, including parity for mental health services, must recognize that although persons with severe mental illness typically do not do well in mainstream health maintenance organizations, new systems designed to address the high-risk consumer may have potential (Mechanic & Aiken, 1987).
- For children with mental health challenges, families must be fully involved in all decisions related to the identification and service provision. All barriers (eg, meeting place and time, childcare, transportation) must be resolved, and caregivers must be made full decision-making partners in all aspects of their children's services (Anderson, 2000).

Although many other needs in the area of public policy are evident, initiatives begun by the federal CSP and CASSP must continue so that safety-net services are in place and trends resulting in untoward outcomes, such as reinstitutionalization in hospitals and jails, can be averted. Community support services have been acknowledged nationally in the role of working with existing resources to develop community alternatives (Searight & Handal, 1987). The emphasis on social integration, providing bridging for people with psychiatric disabilities to "participate in all aspects of community life" (housing, employment, school, recreation), is the basis of social integration (Reidy, 1992; Sullivan, 1994).

APPLICATION OF THE NURSING PROCESS TO COMMUNITY SETTINGS

Nurses are in a unique position to assess both individual and community supports. Furthermore, they can focus on a particular situation while retaining a holistic approach by blending the client's physical, mental, and social needs with community environmental norms.

Nurses can serve as a bridge in the gap between the medical model, hospital and rehabilitation model, and community; the psychiatrist and community caregiver; and the public and other healthcare providers (Palmer-Erbs & Anthony, 1995). Nursing education emphasizes teamwork and shared responsibility with others to an extent rarely found in other professions. Nurses understand the needs and responsibilities of 24-hour programming. When included in community teams, nurses enhance understanding of treatment alternatives, medications and side effects, and the importance of client education and teaching to reduce stress and thus alleviate episodes (Huggins, 1985). This unique background is underscored as clients in the community are treated with new antipsychotic and other drugs requiring assertive outreach and monitoring to assist the individual with compliance. Nurses understand the importance of physical movement to decrease muscle atrophy and other long-term effects resulting from lack of full range-of-motion exercise frequently associated with mental illness. Nurses also work in many schools and participate on school committees that are responsible for designing and implementing individual education programs for children and youth with emotional disturbances, in addition to other disabilities.

As services shift from the medical focus on removal of disease symptoms to the rehabilitation focus on the strengths of the individual to function in the community, the nurse brings an understating of the essential parts of the treatment process (medications, healthcare and education) to the rehabilitative process. Thus, nurses can facilitate the shift from psychiatrically disabled to psychiatrically able.

The combination of inpatient, public health, and psychiatric nursing knowledge and physical assessment skills is imperative in community-based programs. Understanding the role of stress affords the nurse the ability to provide the integrative link among community resources, housing, vocation, social relationships, and psychiatric episodes. Nurses must be able to separate the disease from the social disability (Manderscheid, 1987). Nursing education prepares nurses to educate the consumer, professional, and public regarding psychiatric disability, medication effects and side effects, effects of stress on mental disorder, and interventions to diminish harm.

Nurses traditionally have worked with natural support systems in developing care plans. In many parts of the country, nurses have initiated contact with tribal healers, curanderas, midwives, or other healers in the implementation of this plan. Integration of the nursing care process into the community support system, therefore, is a logical extension of the nurse's role.

Assessment

To assess a community's mental health issues, the nurse focuses on individuals, families, and groups within a community setting. He or she studies aggregate groups to identify problematic areas. Nurses can use many helpful public health tools to assess a particular community (Box 15-3). One important, relevant, and easily accessible tool is census data from the U.S. Bureau of Census. The Bureau gives demographic data on population (ie, age, sex), available social resources (ie, housing, transportation, community centers), available health resources (ie, hospitals, clinics), and health-related problems that might be useful for an assessment.

Vital statistics are another source for determining official records of births, deaths, marriages, divorces, and deaths within a community. The nurse uses vital statistics to compare findings among different years, thus targeting indicators of growth or shrinkage in the population.

The National Center for Health Statistics also conducts surveys and focuses on health trends using a national sample. The U.S. Department of Health and Human Services maintains data on many mental health problems such as depression, suicide, alcohol, and substance abuse. By using these data, the nurse can compare the smaller community under investigation against the larger picture.

Nurses also may find information about a community's health at local agencies, chambers of commerce, and health and hospital districts. Many agencies maintain their own records relevant to their specific population groups. For example, if a nurse is interested in a particular health issue, then he or she may want to develop a systematic data collection method to record specific findings.

In addition to all of these methods, windshield surveys are valuable ways for nurses to assess a community. To perform a windshield survey, the nurse would drive or walk through a specific community and use his or her senses to identify problem areas as well as strengths within the community. Listening, talking, and observing activities and people within the community can give the nurse a good perspective and overall picture.

An example of data collection would be the case of a school nurse concerned about violence within a middle school. The school nurse would need to collect data on the number of reported cases of abuse and violent episodes within the school. Often, schools keep such data on file as part of its record. If the school does not keep such data, then the nurse develops a method of keeping this information so that he or she can track the problem of violence. The conclusion may be that the violence within this particular school is not considered "high risk" compared with state and national averages. If the school seems to have more problems of violence than others, however, the nurse can modify current health programs or, if necessary, develop new programs to meet the needs of this school setting.

Nursing Diagnosis

When formulating a nursing diagnosis for a community, the nurse focuses on a problem identified for the aggregate group, not just an individual or family. The diagnosis focuses on a population problem identified during assessment. The assessment data support and reinforce the identified problem.

For example, during assessment, the school nurse identifies several violent activities within one particular school. The nursing diagnosis would be Violence related to the increased number of violent incidents within the middle school as evidenced by increased school fights, abuse reports, and students identified carrying weapons.

The problem focuses on the entire school population, not just on one person who is violent. Because of the increased violent episodes at school, it has become a "community" problem and as such affects all people within this particular school setting. The numbers and statistics found in the assessment data support this nursing diagnosis. It is no longer a "hunch" or "gut-feeling" on the nurse's part but has become a researchable problem.

Planning

Once the nurse establishes a diagnosis, he or she creates a plan that will help alleviate or reduce the problem. When dealing with community mental health problems, a multidisciplinary team consisting of various key individuals and agencies within the community usually is required. To continue with the example of school violence, individuals and agencies that might be beneficial for the nurse to include would be law enforcement agencies, school personnel, parents, members of the parent and teacher's association, physicians, counselors, clergy, and the students themselves. The entire school community must be involved to become active participants and agree on the plan of action.

The nurse identifies short- and long-term goals, which must be realistic and mutually agreed on by all members of the multidisciplinary team to ensure success for the community. The team refers to the short term to identify whether the problem or plan is going according to schedule. If short-term goals are not being met, then

---

BOX 15-3 ▼ *Potential Assessment Tools in a Community Assessment*

- Vital statistics
- U.S. Bureau of Census data
- National Center for Health Statistics data
- U.S. Department of Health and Human Services data
- Information from local agencies, chambers of commerce, health and hospital districts
- Windshield surveys
- Original data collection from a particular population

the plan may need to be modified so that positive goals can be achieved. An example of a short-term goal for the problem of violence within a school setting might be that by the end of a conflict management class, students will demonstrate nonviolent behavior when engaged in a confrontational situation with peers or other adults.

Long-term goals reflect the overall goal of the plan or program. What is the ultimate goal of the community for the problem identified after it has completed all interventions? An example for the problem of school violence might be that by the end of the school year, there will be a 10% reduction in reported episodes of school violence.

Implementation

Based on the previous discussed levels of prevention, the nurse can arrange methods of intervention in the same way. The focus of primary prevention is to prevent the problem in the first place. The nurse focuses on interventions that address the problem before it happens. In the case of school violence, primary prevention might include helping the faculty to set up a curriculum based on nonviolence. Strategies might include teaching students alternatives to violence and how to handle anger positively. Students need to understand the effects of adolescent violence and homicide. Teachers might use role playing and videotaping to assist students in analyzing a confrontational situation, focusing on ways to avoid fighting. The nonviolence program needs to be an entire-school effort. Classroom environments need to be conducive to nonviolence and need to include faculty and staff as well as students.

Often, people resort to violence because of individual insecurities and issues with self-esteem. The school nurse may develop programs to enhance the self-esteem of individual students as well as the entire school. The nurse may need to become involved with community leaders to develop programs geared at reducing violent exposure and improving the safety of the community. Methods may entail becoming politically active and advocating for programs and funds that support services to low-income, at-risk communities.

Secondary prevention addresses an issue after it already has been identified as a problem. During secondary prevention, identifying the problem early and assisting with treatment are pivotal. In the example of the school setting, the nurse and client (community) have identified violence as a problem within a particular school. How can the nurse assist the school to decrease violent episodes? He or she would consider the same type of conflict management program used in primary prevention. The nurse can use the same program to teach potentially violent students alternative ways of reacting to angry feelings. He or she also can focus on assisting students who already have reacted violently to learn new, nonviolent behaviors. Secondary pre-

vention also might include bringing in a law enforcement agency to provide students with an in-service program on gun safety.

The nurse also must identify "high-risk" individuals within the school setting and refer them and their families for further counseling regarding their issues with violence. Screening for a history of family or peer violence, substance abuse, depression, low self-esteem, use of weapons, and a history of central nervous injury or disease often leads to early identification. Once the nurse has identified such individuals, he or she can make appropriate referrals to mental health or other related services.

Tertiary prevention is the final, but integral, part of prevention. The nurse must continue to support and reinforce all types of interventions at the primary and secondary levels. In terms of school violence, this might include support groups for clients who have been abused or for the perpetrators. It may mean that the nurse or other teachers within the school setting need to give refresher courses on conflict management. Adults need to continuously role model nonviolent behavior for the students to learn appropriate behavior.

Evaluation

Evaluation is the final and most important part of the nursing process. The nurse returns to the original goals and determines whether they have been met. Have the interventions helped the community to meet the goals of the program. If not, why not? Evaluation should be ongoing and done periodically throughout the entire process, underscoring the importance of short- and long-term goals. In the scenario of school violence, could students count to 10 before entering into a verbal confrontation? If the answer is no, was this goal realistic for this group of students? At the end of the program, did the community find that violent episodes were reduced by 10%? If not, what could the nurse and community have done differently? Goals and evaluation of these goals give the nurse a direction in which to make a program a success.

▼ *Reflection and Critical Thinking Questions*

1. How can nurses work within the community to help ensure positive outcomes for clients with mental illness?

2. What underlying needs of clients with mental illness support the need for social and healthcare reforms?

3. How do the issues faced by adults with mental illness differ from those faced by children and adolescents with mental illness?

▼ CHAPTER SUMMARY

■ Community support is crucial to quality of life for those with severe mental illness residing in the community. The goal of community support systems is to enable those with severe mental illnesses to remain in the community while functioning at optimal levels of independence.

■ A community support system encourages participation from all people within it: clients, family members, government officials, and providers. The objective is to deliver a full range of life supportive care. Services are based on guiding principles that promote self-determination and individuation.

■ Essential components of a community support system include active outreach efforts, help in ensuring access to services, psychosocial and vocational opportunities, rehabilitative and supportive housing options, crisis intervention services, case management, and family and community education programs.

■ Reform efforts in children's social services have led to the establishment of systems of care, which create mechanisms for coordinating social services. They are designed to facilitate collaboration among parents, teachers, and other service providers so that they can gear services for students with multisystem needs toward common and agreed on goals.

■ Services must be developed with active participation from the consumer and family.

■ Consumer and family movements are very active in promoting destigmatization of mental illness, developing treatment alternatives, and helping to shape policy at all levels of government.

■ Nurses are an important link between hospital and community and bring essential knowledge and skills to a community-based treatment team or a school individual education plan team.

■ Nurses have a leadership role in the development of comprehensive systems committed to the holistic approach of intervening at both client and community levels.

▼ REVIEW QUESTIONS

1. Ned, a 60-year-old client, has come to the clinic. He mentions that he plans to retire in the next few years. He really likes his work and is unsure what he will do all day at home. The nurse encourages him to begin planning some outside activities and possibly developing hobbies that he enjoys. This is an example of
   a. Primary prevention
   b. Secondary prevention
   c. Tertiary prevention
   d. Evaluation

2. The term *community mental health* most accurately describes which of the following?
   a. A change in focus from the individual to the interaction of the individual with his or her community
   b. A place where care is delivered
   c. Services available in a community
   d. Self-help groups

3. What factors are included in an effective community support system?
   a. The needs and functioning level of people with serious mental illness
   b. A basis philosophy of care based on values and guiding principles
   c. A specific program model
   d. A and B only

4. A community support system delivers community-based care through linkages to a network of agencies. This network provides which of the following?
   a. Mental health services
   b. Rehabilitation services
   c. Social support services
   d. All of the above

5. The primary focus of a community support system is to
   a. Eliminate symptoms
   b. Focus on functioning
   c. Bring rehabilitation to the individual
   d. All of the above

6. The nurse provides all of the following services in a community support system *except*
   a. Medication monitoring
   b. Individual therapy
   c. System advocacy
   d. Mental health teaching

7. Reform efforts in the children's mental health field led to the creation of systems of care, which involve
   a. A focus on providing appropriate services in more effective, restrictive placements
   b. Full participation of parents and caregivers in all aspects of their children's services
   c. The broad involvement of experts on teams who can ensure that services are cost effective
   d. A single approach to services that can be used with all children and their families

8. Unlike clients in the 1800s and early 1900s, who often were housed in asylums and state mental institutions, reinstitutionalized clients frequently wind up housed in which of the following settings?
   a. Mental health clinics
   b. Fairweather lodges
   c. Jails
   d. Community support programs

9. The term for a person or system that coordinates the various services needed to address the individual needs (housing, healthcare, mental health treatment, social contacts, and workups) of a mentally ill client is
   a. Home care nurse
   b. Case manager
   c. Client
   d. Social worker

10. A group that has at least one commonality among its members is called a
    a. Support group
    b. Self-help group
    c. Advocate group
    d. Aggregate group

▼ REFERENCES AND SUGGESTED READINGS

*Allen, M. E. (1997). Mental health. In J. M. Swanson, & M. S. Niles (Eds.), *Community health nursing: Promoting the health of aggregates* (pp. 600–611). Philadelphia: W. B. Saunders Company.

*Anderson, J. A. (2000). The need for interagency collaboration for children with emotional and behavioral disabilities and their families. *Families in Society: The Journal of Contemporary Human Services, 81,* 484–493.

*Anthony, W. (1993). Recovery from mental illness: The guiding vision of the mental health service system in the 1990s. *Psychosocial Rehabilitation Journal, 16.*

*Anthony, W., & Blanch, A. (1989). Research on community support services: What we have learned. *Psychosocial Rehabilitation Journal, 12*(3).

*Anthony, W., Cohen, M., & Cohen, B. (1984). Psychiatric rehabilitation. In J. Talbot (Ed.), *The chronic mental patient: Five years later.* New York: Grune & Stratton.

*Anthony, W., Cohen, M., & Farkas, M. (1988). Professional pre-service training for working with long-term mentally ill. *Community Mental Health Journal, 124*(4).

*Bazelon Center for Mental Health Law. (1994). *What does "fair housing" mean to people with disabilities?* Washington: DC: The Housing Center.

*Bond, G. (1994). Applying psychiatric rehabilitation principles to employment. In R. Ancill (Ed.), *Recent findings from schizophrenia: Exploring the spectrum of psychosis.* New York: John Wiley & Sons.

*Bond, G., Dincin, J., Setze, P., & Witheridge, T. (1984). The effectiveness of psychiatric rehabilitation: A summary of research at thresholds. *Psychosocial Rehabilitation Journal, 7*(4), 6–22.

*Cannady, D. (1982). Chronics and cleaning ladies. *Psychosocial Rehabilitation Journal, 5*(1), 13–16.

*Carling, P. J., & Ridgway, P. (1998). A psychiatric rehabilitation approach to housing. In W. Anthony, & M. Farkas (Eds.), *Psychiatric rehabilitation: Program and practices.* Baltimore: Johns Hopkins University Press.

*Compeer Program. (1995). *Annual report 1984–1985.* Rochester, NY: Compeer.

*Cook, J., Jonikas, J., & Soloman, M. (1992). Models of voca-
tional rehabilitation for youth and adults with severe mental illness: Implications for America 2000 and the ADA. *American Rehabilitation, 18*(3).

*Cowen, E. (1994). The enhancement of psychological wellness: Challenges and opportunities. *American Journal of Community Psychology, 22,* 149–179.

*Duchnowski, A. J., & Kutash, K. (1996). The mental health perspective. In C. M. Nelson, R. B. Rutherford, & B. I. Wolford (Eds.), *Comprehensive and collaborative systems that work for troubled youth: A national agenda* (pp. 90–110). Richmond, KY: National Coalition for Juvenile Justice Services.

*Fairweather, G. (1980). *The prototype Lodge Society: Instituting group process principles, new directions for mental health services. The Fairweather Lodge: A twenty-five year retrospective.* San Francisco: Jossey-Bass.

*Friedman, R. M. (1996). Mental health policy for children. In B. L. Levin, & J. Petrila (Eds.), *Mental health services: A public health perspective.* New York: Oxford University Press.

*Friedman, R. M., Kutash, K., & Duchnowski, A. J. (1996). The population of concern: Defining the issues. In B. A. Stroul (Ed.), *Children's mental health: Creating systems of care in a changing society.* Baltimore: Paul H. Brookes.

*Friesen, B. J., & Poertner, J. (1995). *From case management to service coordination for children with emotional, behavioral, or mental disorders.* Baltimore: Paul H. Brookes.

*Greenbaum, P. E., Dedrick, R. F., Friedman, R. M., Kutash, K., Brown, E. C., Lardieri, S. P., et al. (1998). National Adolescent and Child Treatment Study (NACTS): Outcomes for children with serious emotional and behavioral disturbance. In M. H. Epstein, K. Kutash, & A. J. Duchnowski (Eds.), *Community-based programming for children with serious emotional disturbances and their families: Research and evaluation.* Austin, TX: Pro-Ed.

*Grob, G. N. (1991). *From asylum to community.* Princeton, NJ: Princeton University Press.

*Hallahan, D. P., & Kauffman, J. M. (2000). *Exceptional learners: Introduction to special education* (8th ed.). Boston: Allyn & Bacon.

*Harding, C. (1994). An examination of the complexities in measurement of recovery in severe psychiatric disorders. *Schizophrenia: Exploring the spectrum of psychosis.* Wiley & Sons, Ltd.

*Handron, D. S., Dosser, D. A., McCammon, S. L., & Powell, J. Y. (1998). "Wraparound," the wave of the future: Theoretical and professional practice implications for children and families with complex needs. *Journal of Family Nursing, 4,* 65–85.

*Huggins, M. (1985). A model case management system in a local CSS. *Community Support Network News, 4*(4).

*Individuals With Disabilities Education Act Amendment of 1997 (IDEA), P. L. 105–17. 20 U.S.C. § 1400 *et seq.* (1997).

*Isaac, R. J., & Armat, V. C. (1990). *Madness in the streets.* New York: The Free Press.

*Jonikas, J., & Cook, J. (1993). *Safe, secure and street smart: Empowering women with mental illness to achieve greater independence in the community.* Chicago: Thresholds National Research and Training Center.

*Kincaid, J. (1994). The ADA and Section 504: Legal mechanisms for achieving effective supported education. *Community Support Network News 10*(2).

*Knitzer, J. (1996). The role of education in systems of care. In B. A. Stroul (Ed.), *Children's mental health: Creating systems of care in a changing society*. Baltimore: Paul H. Brookes.

*Kuehnel, T., Howard, B., & Liberman, R. (1994). *Psychosocial rehabilitation competencies for mental health workers*. Los Angeles: Center for Improving Mental Health Systems. Human Interaction Research Institute.

*Kutash, K., & Duchnowski, A. J. (1997). Create comprehensive and collaborative systems. *Journal of Emotional and Behavioral Disabilities, 5*, 66–75.

*Lamb, H. (1994). A century and a half of psychosocial rehabilitation in the United States. *Hospital and Community Psychiatry, 45*(10).

*Liberman, R., Kuehnel, T., Phipps, C., & Cardin, V. (1984). *Resource book for psychiatric rehabilitation: Elements of services for the mentally ill*. Camarillo, CA: Center for Rehabilitation Research and Training in Mental Illness, UCLA School of Medicine.

*Mancuso, L. (1993). *Case studies on reasonable accommodations for workers with psychiatric disabilities*. Sacramento: Center for Mental Health Services, The California Department of Mental Health and California Department of Rehabilitation.

*Manderscheid, R. W. (1987). CSP research accomplishments. *Community Support Network News, 4*(2).

*Mechanic, D., & Aiken, L. (1987). Improving the care of patients with chronic mental illness. *New England Journal of Medicine, 317*(26), 1634–1638.

*Mowbry, C., Chamberlain, P., & Jenning, M. (1984). *Final report: Consumer run alternative services. Demonstration and evaluation projects 1982–1984*. Lansing, MI: Research and Evaluation Division, Michigan Department of Mental Health.

*National Mental Health Association. (1996). *Mental health and you*. Alexandria, VA: Author.

*Palmer-Erbs, V., & Anthony, W. (1995). Incorporating psychiatric rehabilitation principles into mental health nursing. *Journal of Psychosocial Nursing, 3*(3).

*Pardes, H. (1998). NIMH during the tenure of Director Herbert Pardes, MD (1879–1984): The President's commission on mental health and the reemergence of NIMH's scientific mission. *American Journal of Psychiatry, 155*(9), 14–19.

*Pepper, B. (1987). A public policy for the long-term mentally ill: A positive alternative to reinstitutionalization. *American Journal of Orthopsychiatry, 57*(3), 452–457.

*Perlin, M. L. (1994). Law and the delivery of mental health services in the community. *American Journal of Orthopsychiatry, 64*(2), 194–208.

*Reidy, D. (1992). Shattering illusions of difference. *Resources 4*(2), 3–6.

*Rubenstein, L., Koyanagi, C., & Manes, J. (1987). Mental health funding. *Hospital and Community Psychiatry, 38*(4), 410–412.

*Russell, L. A., Rotto, K. I., & Matthews, B. (1999). Preliminary findings from Indiana's Dawn project: A system of care for children's mental health. Expanding the research base. In J. Willis (Ed.), *Proceedings of the 11th Annual Research Conference, March 6–11, 1998*. Tampa, FL: University of South Florida, Louis de la Prate Florida Mental Health Institute, and Research and Training Center for Children's Mental Health.

*Searight, H. R., & Handal, P. J. (1987). Psychiatric deinstitutionalization: The possibilities and the reality. *Psychiatry Quarterly, 58*(3), 153–166.

*Schaftt, G., & Randolf, F. (1994). Innovative community based services for older persons with mental illness. Washington, DC: U.S. Department of Health and Human Services, Center for Mental Health Services CSP.

*Stroul, B. A. (1996). Service coordination in systems of care. In B. A. Stroul (Ed.), *Children's mental health: Creating systems of care in a changing society* (pp. 265–280). Baltimore: Paul H. Brookes.

*Stroul, B. (1987). Introduction to the special issue: The community support system concept. *Psychosocial Rehabilitation Journal, 11*(2), 5–8.

*Stroul, B. (1986). Models of community support services: Approaches to helping persons with long-term mental illness. Bethesda, MD: National Institute of Mental Health, Community Support Program.

*Stroul, B., & Friedman, R. M. (1986). *A system of care for children and youth with severe emotional disturbances* (rev. ed.). Washington, DC: Georgetown University Child Development Center, CASSP Technical Assistance Center.

*Sullivan, A. (1994). Supported education: Past, present and future. *Community Support Network News, 10*(2).

*Turner, J. (1986). *Comprehensive community support systems for severely mentally disabled adults: Definitions, components and guiding principles* (rev. ed.). Bethesda, MD: National Institute of Mental Health.

*U.S. Department of Education. (1998). *Twentieth annual report to Congress on the implementation of the Individuals With Disabilities Education Act*. Washington, DC: Author.

*U.S. Department of Health and Human Services. (1980). *Toward a national plan for the chronically mentally ill: Report to the Secretary by the Department of Health and Human Services Steering Committee on the Chronically Mentally Ill*. Washington, DC: Author.

*U.S. Department of Health and Human Services. (1991). *Caring for people with severe mental disorders: A national plan of research to improve services, National Institute of Mental Health, National Advisory Mental Health Council*. Washington, DC: Author.

*U.S. Department of Health and Human Services. (1991). *Healthy People 2000: National health promotion and disease prevention objectives*. Washington, DC: Author.

*U.S. Department of Health and Human Services. (1994). *CMHS mission* [from a bulletin of the Center for Mental Health Services]. Washington, DC: Author.

*Viccora, E., Perry, J., & Mancuso, L. (1993). *Exemplary practices in employment services for people with psychiatric disabilities*. Alexandria, VA: National Association of State Mental Health Program Directors.

*Wagner, M. M. (1995). Outcomes for youth with serious emotional disturbance in secondary school and early adulthood. *The Future of Children, 5*, 90–112.

*Weisbrod, B. A., Test, M. A., & Stein, L. I. (1980). Alternatives to mental hospital treatment: 2. Economic benefit–cost analysis. *Archives General Psychiatry, 37*, 400–408.

*Weinstein, D., & Hughes, R. (1998). *Best practices draft, IAPSRS*. Columbia, MD.

*Worley, N. (1997). Mental health nursing in the community. St. Louis: Mosby.
* *Starred references are cited in text.*

For additional information on this chapter, go to *http://connection. lww.com.*

Need more help? See Chapter 15 of the *Study Guide to Accompany Mohr: Johnson's Psychiatric-Mental Health Nursing,* 5th ed.

Behavioral Health Home Care

NINA A. KLEBANOFF

▼ KEY TERMS

Behavioral health clinical nurse specialist—A master's-prepared nurse with skills in psychiatric and mental health assessment and intervention who is eligible for or has already received certification by the American Nurses Association as a specialist in adult psychiatric and mental health nursing.

Home care—Part of a comprehensive health and mental healthcare system that aims to provide an array of health-related services to clients and families in their places of residence.

▼ LEARNING OBJECTIVES

On completion of this chapter, you should be able to accomplish the following:

- Describe the historical, philosophical, and theoretical foundations of behavioral health home care nursing practice.
- Identify the essential components of behavioral health home care nursing practice.
- Discuss appropriate candidates for behavioral health home care nursing services.
- Discuss ways that nurses modify the steps of the nursing process when caring for a client and family in their home.
- Analyze the various factors that influence trends in behavioral health home care.

▼ Clinical Example 16-1

Kristian, 34 years old, has a history of bipolar disorder, which has been treated in the past with lithium carbonate and intermittent (approximately every 2 years) hospitalizations. Recently, his spouse filed for divorce, and Kristian became suicidal. They had been married 7 years and have no children.

Kristian was hospitalized following an automobile accident in which he sustained multiple internal injuries and a broken left leg. He had stopped taking lithium before his accident; during the hospitalization, he was given phenothiazines. Shortly before discharge, he was again started on lithium carbonate. His spouse moved out of their condominium while he was in the hospital, but she agreed to assist with his care at home until he was more independent. A hospital-based social worker made the referral to a home care agency that sent a behavioral health clinical nurse specialist into the home to visit.

The nurse monitors Kristian's physical status, risk for self-harm, and adherence and response to lithium therapy. The nurse also provides supportive psychotherapy, referral to community resources, and instruction and support to him and his wife regarding his care at home. The behavioral health home care nurse arranges for physical therapy and monitoring of serum lithium levels. Kristian's spouse begins to attend support group meetings held by the local chapter of the Depressive and Manic-Depressive Association.

Behavioral health home care is a specialty service in which home healthcare nurses provide skilled nursing care on a visiting basis to clients in need of holistic care. Behavioral health home care provides the following services across the continuum of care: psychiatric and chemical dependency treatment, behavioral aspects of primary care, health teaching and wellness, and illness prevention. Because it is given in the least restrictive setting, in-home behavioral healthcare nursing focuses on the client and his or her family or caregivers. Nurses deliver services in the client's own natural setting, which enhances the therapeutic process. With a coordinated, multidisciplinary approach, behavioral health home care can reduce or prevent inpatient hospitalization. In most instances, behavioral health home care is a therapeutic and cost-effective alternative to more restrictive treatment services.

FOUNDATIONS OF BEHAVIORAL HEALTH HOME CARE

Home care, including behavioral health home care, is one part of a comprehensive health and mental healthcare system. It aims to provide an array of health-related services to clients and families in their places of residence. These residences include residential care facilities, group homes, and private homes of clients or their family members. Home healthcare is one aspect of community health nursing, *not* an alternative to institutional care (Stanhope & Lancaster, 2000). It is one of the most rapidly growing and changing fields in healthcare today, even though it is one of the oldest forms of ambulatory healthcare.

The behavioral health aspects of clients receiving home care will vary. The team providing care customizes services for each client, depending on his or her needs and problems, services available, and issues related to reimbursement. Because of the behavioral health and wellness orientation of community health nursing, a psychiatric nurse working in this setting is more aptly titled a behavioral health nurse rather than a psychiatric nurse.

History of Behavioral Health Home Care

Conceptually, home healthcare considers cultural, historical, professional, economic, political, philosophical, social, pharmacological, technological, and ecological factors. Home care has been delivered in the United States since the 1950s (Weiner, Becker, & Friedman, 1983). Approaches were patterned after the service delivered in Amsterdam (Querida, 1983). In the late 1960s and early 1970s, during the height of the community mental health movement, efforts were directed toward providing home care for the mentally ill, especially older adults. Although Medicare added "psychiatric" home care as a reimbursable service in 1979, it was not until the 1983 report of the Joint Commission of Mental Illness and Health that the process of supporting mental clients in society began, through the deinstitutionalization of mental inpatients and a focus on community care instead of hospital-based care. In 1994, the first National Psychiatric Home Care Conference was held; for the first time, the National Association for Home Care added a behavioral health forum as part of its annual meeting. Since then, nurses providing behavioral health home care have been meeting as special

interest groups during the Home Healthcare Nurses Association conventions.

Principles of Behavioral Health Home Care

Most home care agencies share the following basic principles and philosophy:

- As long as it is medically, socially, and economically possible, adults want to remain in their own homes and communities and should be permitted to do so.
- Clients who need long-term care often present many overlapping challenges and problems.
- The whole individual must be considered.
- Services must be coordinated and integrated.
- Cost-effective care requires direct payment at the level of program delivery.
- High quality long-term care should be affordable.

High-quality behavioral healthcare programs provide home visits, when necessary, on a crisis basis. They supply 24-hour telephone triage and on-site emergency response or contract for an emergency response team. They provide scheduled and immediate follow-up in the client's home after discharge from more restrictive levels of care. They also use quality improvement programs and outcome measurement systems to evaluate clinical effectiveness; clinical and financial outcomes; client, family, and caregiver levels of functioning and satisfaction; and resource use.

Additionally, the following premises guide the clinical approach of the behavioral health home care nurse and a behavioral health specialty team or service:

- Client care is maximized when integrated into a comprehensive care plan that considers the client and family and their environment, self-concept, functioning level, coping mechanisms, stressors, and sociocultural perspective.
- A client's or family's reaction to an alteration in mental health status, mental disability, or mental illness is often influenced by whether the condition is permanent, temporary, degenerative, or unknown.
- Care of a client is based on the idea of therapeutic use of self, the setting and attainment of goals for health status enhancement, and the development of the client's ability to develop personal resources within a realistic level of functioning.

Home Care Services

In addition to nursing, other suitable service components of home care, singly or in a multitude of combinations and sequences, include but are not limited to the following:

- The client will reestablish and maintain sexual activity at the level specified before the onset of depression.

Some general outcomes are expected in behavioral health home care nursing. These include maximizing the client's level of independence through health promotion, maintenance, and restoration; preventing complications in the home through health teaching, education about psychoactive medication, and sharing of information about community resources; averting or minimizing a psychiatric crisis through anticipation and planning; and delaying admission to a nursing home or other long-term care facility. Other long-term outcomes are ensuring the client's ability to maintain ties with the family network and community and maintaining a greater sense of control by helping the client to determine health, mental health, or mental illness care needs.

IMPLEMENTATION

Many factors may necessitate behavioral health nursing intervention in the home. Examples include the following:

- Potential or actual suicide attempts
- Severe depression, feelings of doom, isolation
- Refusal to leave a room or bed
- Preoccupation with somatic complaints
- Panic attacks
- Increased signs and symptoms of agitation, anxiety, and manic behaviors
- Mismanagement and exacerbation of a physical disease process
- Frequent falls secondary to an impaired state
- Increased environmental or safety hazards secondary to an impaired status or disease process
- Anorexia with weight loss of more than 10 pounds per month
- Mismanagement, noncompliance, or misunderstanding of the medication regimen
- Impaired or potential dangerous self-care and care of activities of daily living (ADLs)

The client's specific goals and outcomes lead to individual interventions in the home. The nurse uses interpersonal, intellectual, and technical skills during this phase of the nursing process. Direct interventions that behavioral health home care nurses use may include the following:

- A comprehensive in-home assessment
- Crisis intervention
- Medication administration, monitoring, and teaching about responses, indications, actions, and interactions
- Individual, couple, family, and group counseling and psychotherapy
- Verbal or written contracts with the client
- Heath guidance and referral
- Client advocacy

- Case management activities
- Mental, emotional, physical, and spiritual observation, interpretation, and evaluation
- Healthcare team coordination
- Liaison activities
- Reports to the physician about the client's response to the home environment, medication responses, medical follow-up, and new signs and symptoms relative to the client's status
- Supervision of team members (eg, home health assistant)
- Role modeling or social skills education
- Teaching
  - Diet, including special diets
  - Disease, illness, and wellness
  - Management of illness
  - Stress reduction
  - Risk factors

The behavioral health home care nurse can intervene to correct actual or potential safety hazards, such as those involving structural integrity of the residence; heating, cooling, ventilation; stairways and ramps; storage of dangerous objects and fluids; storage of medications; mats and throw rugs; gas and electrical appliances; number of residents per square footage; cooking and bathing facilities; nature of the neighborhood; and sanitation.

The nurse who works in the home care setting also intervenes in indirect ways. Indirect home care includes the nurse's actions that affect the home care situation but do not involve personal contact with the client or family. The behavioral health home care nurse may need to provide an in-service for the home care agency staff or a community group and to participate in agency orientations, team conferences, discharge planning meetings, and recertification sessions.

EVALUATION

The nurse continually evaluates the client's and family's responses to interventions to determine progress toward goal attainment and to determine the needed revision to the database, nursing diagnoses, and plan of care (ANA, 1999). He or she plans for the client's discharge from home care services early in the course of home care, ideally during the initial visit. This helps the client reach measurable, customized goals. The nurse, client, and family determine whether goals for home care have been met.

In home care, changing client needs and status necessitate a dynamic and continuous revision of, and addition to, the database and nursing care plan. Chart audits, reviews by regulatory agencies, peer reviews, and the various home health agency certification processes also evaluate the quality and effectiveness of home care services. All involved in the home care case—client, family, nurse, other home healthcare team members, physician, and others—evaluate the client's progress toward and attainment of goals. As the client and family become increasingly able to care for the client, the nurse and other home health team members decrease the intensity and frequency of their visits. Discharge from home care services includes making provisions for aftercare, if indicated, and other types of case management and coordination of community resources.

Trends in Behavioral Health Home Care Nursing

Incidence of mental illnesses, demographics, and legislative and political trends will continue to affect the future of behavioral health home care nursing practice in the United States. Preferred-provider arrangements and proprietary joint ventures to provide durable medical equipment are two examples of this changing business climate. National trends, referrer needs, and the preferences of individual communities and consumers will greatly affect the successful delivery of behavioral health home care nursing services.

As you learned in previous chapters, most people with mental illness are living in their communities. In addition, Alzheimer's disease affects 5% to 10% of the population older than 65 years and increases proportionally in people older than 85 years. Maintaining a person affected by a cognitive brain disorder in the home or facilitating a transfer to a temporary or permanent facility is often a function of the behavioral health home care nurse. Long-term service or intensive care management is needed to support this population in the home. Most home care services, however, are reimbursed on a short-term or intermittent basis. Legislation to authorize long-term home care services, including home healthcare services, has been proposed but remains to be enacted. Bills permitting directly reimbursable community nursing services, including home healthcare, are in the demonstration phase. Managed-care arrangements with capitated reimbursement are being incorporated into the home health arena.

Persistent and debilitating diseases, such as Parkinson's disease, chemical dependency, cancer, COPD, and HIV and AIDS often present with concurrent anxiety or depression. The reciprocal mind-body-spiritual relationship cannot be underscored enough.

Other needs include respite care for family members of clients who live at home to prevent hospitalization, institutionalization, caretaker burnout, client abuse, and overload. Also, women and elderly people from minority groups are especially susceptible to mental health illness problems as a result of discrimination, and they will increasingly need attention in terms of behavioral health home care. Improving coping methods and strengthening family care bonds will help to meet this burgeoning demand.

The ANA identifies societal and political forces that influence and shape the delivery of home health care nursing services. The societal forces include the following:

- The rate of living older Americans is increasing disproportionately to the total population.

- Traditionally, women have provided healthcare for youth and aging parents; more than half of all adult women now must work or choose to work outside the home and are therefore not available to care for family members.
- The traditional support system of the extended family has been almost eliminated by the increasing mobility of society and the ever-increasing rate of single-parent family units and female heads of households.
- Governmental responses to societal demands, changes, and spending trends have changed healthcare financing patterns.

Political forces identified by the ANA that influence the provision of home healthcare services include the following:

- Increased private third-party payment and government-financed healthcare programs, beginning in the 1960s, have promoted an increase in the demand for and use of healthcare services.
- Shorter hospital stays with earlier discharges of more acutely ill clients from institutions have called attention to the need for home healthcare services; these shorter hospital stays have been prompted by prospective, diagnosis-related, and managed healthcare plans (ANA, 1999).

Trends likely to affect the future of behavioral health home care nursing are moving Medicare and Medicaid participants to managed care organizations and Medicaid funding from federal to state levels. The appreciation of medical cost offsets, through behavioral health interventions, parity in behavioral healthcare insurance, the demand for clinical outcomes, and an increased desire for holistic care that is preventive and wellness oriented, will influence the acceptance and growth of behavioral health home care nursing.

▼ *Reflection and Critical Thinking Questions*

1. Briefly describe some of the components of an in-home mental wellness program.
2. Name two of the benefits of behavioral health home care nursing to clients, caregivers, family members, and physicians.
3. What steps can the behavioral health home care nurse take to ensure personal safety?
4. Discuss the placement of behavioral health home care on the continuum of mental health services.

▼ CHAPTER SUMMARY

■ Home healthcare nursing and behavioral health home care nursing are aspects of community health nursing and the community health movement.

■ Behavioral health home care nursing is *not* an alternative to institutional care; the reverse is the case.

■ The goals of behavioral health home care are to assist the client and family to gain, regain, maintain, or restore the client's optimal state of health and independence; to minimize and rehabilitate the effects of illnesses and disabilities before or after institutionalization; and to prevent institutionalization altogether when possible.

■ The nursing process is used by the behavioral health home care nurse to provide comprehensive services to clients in their places of residence.

■ Various social, legislative, and political forces make it likely that the need and demand for behavioral health home care services will continue to increase.

▼ REVIEW QUESTIONS

1. All statements are true regarding behavioral health home interventions except which of the following?
   a. Behavioral health home care is less threatening and restrictive than hospitalization.
   b. Behavioral health home care is more comfortable than hospitalization.
   c. Behavioral health home care is more expensive than inpatient hospitalization.
   d. Behavioral health home care can be part of a discharge plan.

2. Which of the following client conditions meets a criterion for homebound status?
   a. There are frequent absences from the home for shopping.
   b. The client refuses to leave home because of severe depression or paranoia.
   c. The client attends a day treatment program for socialization purposes.
   d. The client drives a car.

3. Which of the following groups are potential referral sources for behavioral health home care?
   a. Former behavioral health home care clients
   b. Members of the clergy
   c. Hospital-based psychiatric nurses
   d. All of the above

4. Which of the following services is *not* a common aspect of behavioral health home care?
   a. Psychiatric and chemical dependency treatment
   b. Behavioral aspects of primary care
   c. Cognitive-behavioral programs
   d. Health teaching and wellness

5. Which of the following is true of home care?
   a. Services are few and limited.
   b. Clients who live in residential care facilities or group homes are not eligible.
   c. Home care is an alternative to institutional care.
   d. Home care is one of the most rapidly growing and changing fields in healthcare today.

6. Home care has been delivered in the United States since
   a. The early 1900s
   b. The 1950s
   c. The 1970s
   d. The 1980s

7. Which of the following is *not* true of most behavioral health home care programs?
   a. They supply 24-hour telephone triage and on-site emergency response or contact for an emergency response team.
   b. They base services on models established by Sigmund Freud.
   c. They provide scheduled and immediate follow-up in the client's home after discharge from more restrictive levels of care.
   d. They use quality improvement programs and outcome measurement systems to evaluate clinical effectiveness; clinical and financial outcomes; client, family, and caregiver levels of functioning and satisfaction; and resource use.

8. The name for a master's-prepared nurse with psychiatric and mental health assessment and intervention skills who is eligible for or has already received ANA certification as a specialist in adult psychiatric and mental health nursing is a
   a. Behavioral health clinical nurse specialist
   b. Advance practice behavioral nurse
   c. Clinical behavioral health specialist
   d. Psychiatric clinical nurse

9. All the following are common indicators for behavioral health home care nursing *except*
   a. Mental health status changes
   b. Emotional crises
   c. Changes in the home environment
   d. Sexual dysfunction

10. When should the nurse begin to plan for the client's discharge from home care services?
    a. When the client has met 50% of the goals in the plan of care
    b. When the client asks
    c. Early in the course of home care, ideally during the initial visit
    d. When the client has made a full recovery

▼ REFERENCES AND SUGGESTED READINGS

*American Nurses Association. (1999). *The scope and standards of practice for home health care nursing.* Washington, DC: Author.

Barker, E., Robinson, D., & Brautigan, R. (1999). The effect of psychiatric home nurse follow-up on readmission rates of patients with depression. *Journal of the American Psychiatric Nurse Association, 5*(4), 116–119.

Brooker, B. (1990). A new role for the community psychiatric nurse in working with families caring for a relative with schizophrenia. *International Journal of Social Psychiatry, 36*(3), 216–224.

Burgess, A., & Lazare, A. (1990). *Psychiatric nursing in the hospital and the community.* Englewood Cliffs, NJ: Prentice-Hall.

Carson, V. B. (1995). Bay area health care psychiatric home care model. *Home Healthcare Nurse, 13*(4), 26–35.

Christoffel, K. K. (2000). Public health advocacy: Process and product. *American Journal of Public Health, 90*(5), 722–726.

Dean, C., & Gadd, E. M. (1990). Home treatment for acute psychiatric illness. *British Journal of Medicine, 301,* 1021–1023.

Duffy, J., Miller, M. P., & Parlocha, P. (1993). Psychiatric home care. *Home Healthcare Nurse, 11*(2), 22–28.

Ellenbecker, C. H., & Shea, K. (1994). Documentation in home health care practice. *Nursing Clinics of North America, 29*(3), 495–506.

Falvo, D. R. (1995). Multicultural issues in patient education and patient compliance: A special report. In *Effective patient education: A guide to increased compliance* (2nd ed.). Gaithersburg, MD: Aspen Publishers.

Frank, A., & Gunderson, J. (1990). The role of the therapeutic alliance in the treatment of schizophrenia. *Archives of General Psychiatry, 47,* 228–236.

Frisch, N. (1993). Home care nursing and the behavioral health–emotional needs of clients. *Home Healthcare Nurse, 11,* 64–65, 70.

Harris, M. D. (1993). Psychiatric evaluation and therapy. *Home Healthcare Nurse, 11,* 66–67.

Hellwig, K. (1993). Psychiatric home care nursing: Managing patients in the community setting. *Journal of Psychosocial Nursing, 31*(12), 21–24.

Holland, L. (1993). Mental health supportive home health care aides. *Caring, 12,* 44–48.

Kelley, J. H., & Lehman, L. (1993). Assessment of anxiety, depression, and suspiciousness in the home care setting. *Home Healthcare Nurse, 11,* 16–20.

Kemmerer, B. (1994). Psychiatric home health care reduces costs and improves patient satisfaction. *Psychiatry and Substance Abuse Issue Tracking, April.* Washington, DC: Health Care Advisory Board.

Kruse, E. A., & Jones, G. (1990). Development of a comprehensive suicide protocol in a home health care and social service agency. *Journal of Home Health Care Practice, 3*(2), 47–56.

Kruse, E. A., & Wood, M. (1989). Delivering mental health services in the home. *Caring, 6,* 28–34, 59.

Lehman, L., & Kelley, J. H. (1993). Nursing interventions for anxiety, depression, and suspiciousness in the home care setting. *Journal of Home Healthcare Nursing, 11,* 35–40.

Lipsman, R., Fader, D., & Harmon, J. (1992). Developing home-based mental health services for Maine's older adults. *Pride Institute of Long Term Home Health Care, 2*(1), 29–38.

*Mellon, S. K. (1994). Mental health clinical nurse specialist in home care for the 90s. *Issues in Mental Health Nursing, 15,* 229–237.

Menosky, J. (1990). Occupational therapy services for the homebound psychiatric patient. *Journal of Home Health Care Practice, 2*(3), 57–67.

Muijen, M., Marks, I., Connolly, J., et al. (1992). Home based care and standard hospital care for patients with severe mental illness: A randomized control trial. *British Journal of Medicine, 304,* 749–753.

Pigot, H. E., & Trott, L. (1993). Translating research into practice: The implementation of an in-home crisis intervention triage and treatment service in the private sector. *American Journal of Medical Quality, 8*(3), 138–144.

*Planning and program development for psychiatric home care. (1993). *Journal of Nursing Administration, 23*(11), 23–28.

*Querida, A. (1983). The shaping of community mental health care. In L. D. Breslau & M. R. Haug (Eds.), *Depression and aging causes, care, and consequences* (p. 201). New York: Springer.

Quinlan, J., & Ohlund, G. (1993). Psychiatric home care: An introduction. *Home Healthcare Nurse, 13*(4), 20–24.

Rice, R. (1993). Suicidal thoughts and ideation. *Home Healthcare Nurse, 11,* 67.

Soreff, S. M. (1994). Psychiatric home care revisited: Its scope and advantages. *Continuum, 1*(1), 71–78.

*Stanhope, M., & Lancaster, J. (2000). *Community health nursing: Process and practice for promoting health* (5th ed.). St. Louis: Mosby.

Thoaben, M., & Kozlak, J. (1990). Home health care's unique role in serving the elderly mentally ill. *Home Healthcare Nurse, 2*(3), 16–20.

Van Dongen, C. J., & Jambunathan, J. (1992). Pilot study results: The psychiatric RN case manager. *Journal of Psychosocial Nursing, 30,* 11–14.

Wagner, B. D. (1994). Innovations in the geriatric continuum of care. *Continuum, 1*(1), 51–60.

Wald, A. (1998). Psychiatric home care builds effective treatment bridges. *Nursing Spectrum, 10A*(12), 4–5.

*Weiner, L. W., Becker, A., & Friedman, T. T. (1983). Home treatment: Spearhead of community psychiatry. In L. D. Breslau & M. R. Haug (Eds.), *Depression and aging causes, care, and consequences* (pp. 201–202). New York: Springer.

* *Starred references are cited in text.*

For additional information on this chapter, go to *http://connection.lww.com.*

Need more help? See Chapter 16 of the *Study Guide to Accompany Mohr: Johnson's Psychiatric-Mental Health Nursing,* 5th edition.

the teen years, peers become a major force. Association with teens who condone antisocial or aggressive behavior becomes a strong predictor for violent behavior (Dahlberg & Potter, 2001). Sometimes, the glue of such peer groups is a dislike for school. In this case, academic failure of the group members may follow, which compounds risk. Associations with peers can take the form of gang involvement, which is associated with both gun involvement and a disproportionate amount of criminal and violent offenses (Commission for the Prevention of Youth Violence, 2000).

NEIGHBORHOOD RISK FACTORS

As mentioned in the explanation of the ecological model, a youth's macrosystem, the neighborhood and community environment, can become a risk factor for violence. Poverty and living in a poor neighborhood creates risk factors because of the various situations that are generated by poverty. As Dahlberg (1998) points out, in poor neighborhoods one finds such phenomena as high levels of transience, family disruption, firearm ownership, drug distribution networks, and high rates of school dropout, substance use, and unemployment. These dimensions of poverty become concomitant risk factors for violence.

In discussing any of the risk factors for youth violence, one must be careful not to mentally convert a risk factor into a broad generalization. Of course, not every youth growing up in poverty becomes violent. Risk is offset by protective factors. Nevertheless, poverty creates living situations that are known contributors to generating violent behavior. As the CMHS (2001) points out, living in poverty segregates people from the mainstream of society, and in doing so, isolates youth from seeing the possible opportunities to escape poverty. Further, in poor neighborhoods, unemployment is high and people are moving about looking for jobs, further disconnecting them from support systems and increasing their sense of isolation. These factors, isolation, family instability, and lack of support, all increase the risk for violence (CMHS, 2001).

PROTECTIVE FACTORS

Scientists have studied children who have overcome adversity to understand resiliency and the factors connected to a child's ability to thrive even in adverse life conditions. These *protective* factors include some characteristics with which the resilient child is born, including solid intelligence and easy disposition (Group for the Advancement of Psychiatry, 1999). A child who has a secure attachment to parents enters school with many advantages and is more likely to embark on a career of school success (Huffman, Mehlinger, & Kerivan, 2000). Children who enter school with a base of emotional security and a sense of well-being are not only ready for academic learning, they also are ready to learn critical social skills such as respecting the rights of others and the ability to give and receive support. Children with these social aptitudes function better in

school. Finally, a community can be a protective factor when it provides good schools, recreational outlets, and a system of laws and surveillance that limits youth's access to guns, alcohol, and drugs (Greenberg et al., 1999).

Public Health Approach to Youth Violence

Youth violence prevention has received tremendous attention in the last 10 years from government agencies, scientists, community activists, and health professionals. The result is scores of violence prevention programs, many of which have demonstrated short-term positive outcomes and a few demonstrating long-term efficacy (Dodge, 2001). As interventions proliferate, activists from the government and community and scientists agree that programs must be evidence based; they must address multiple risk factors over a sustained period, begin early in the child's life, and involve all parties with a stake in the outcomes (schools, parents, children, and communities) (Guerra, Attar, & Weissberg, 1997; Thornton, Craft, Dahlberg, Lynch, & Baer, 2000; Dodge, 2001).

To illustrate these principles, the Commission for the Prevention of Youth Violence (2000) cites the efforts of Galveston, Texas, where crime dropped 78% between 1994 and 1999. Galveston's accomplishment rests with its implementation of a network of programs that provided supervised recreation and a violence prevention/problem-solving curriculum in all elementary schools. Galveston also implemented secondary and tertiary prevention programs that addressed the needs of youths convicted of minor offenses and school truants, and a home-based counseling program aimed at frequent offenders. Equally noteworthy was the collaboration of the multiple agencies, law enforcement, schools, and universities in creating Galveston's programs. To facilitate understanding of the science of violence prevention, this chapter discusses one of these interventions in greater depth.

One popular violence prevention approach aims at improving youths' social problem-solving skills. These programs rest on the notion that when youths lack the strategies to deal with social situations, they are more likely to respond with aggression. Social–cognitive prevention programs aim to improve youths' conflict resolution skills by shaping how they interpret and respond to difficult social situations (Thornton et al., 2000). One such program is PATHS (Promoting Alternative Thinking Strategies) where, over a 5-year span, students are taught about their emotions, how to build positive peer relations, and how to develop problem-solving skills (Greenberg et al., 1995). Outcome data demonstrate that over the last 15 years, participants in PATHS have improved in social and emotional competencies as well as demonstrated decreases in aggressive behavior.

Nurses' Role in Youth Violence Prevention Efforts

Nurses participate in violence prevention at several levels. Nurse scientists have developed model prevention programs aimed at at-risk youth and community-based parenting programs to teach parents how to effectively deal with hard-to-manage children (Eggert, Thompson, Herting & Nicholas, 1994; Gross, Fogg, & Tucker, 1995). Nurses have been key to school-based programs that address the mental health needs of youth. They have participated in many successful home-visiting programs that provide support and education to mothers at risk (Olds et al., 1997). Nurses are in a prime position to identify children at risk by virtue of their work in primary care and health clinics. In these settings, they also can educate families about firearm safety, substance abuse problems, and violence prevention. Through these and future efforts, nurses can become meaningful participants in violence prevention.

FAMILY VIOLENCE

Intimate Partner Violence

Intimate partner violence (IPV), also called domestic violence, is not a new phenomenon but has become a major public health problem (Lent, 1997). It has reached epidemic proportions in American society and is the single major cause of injury to women in the United States, more common than rapes, mugging, and automobile accidents combined (Dutton, Mitchell, & Haywood, 1996; Grunfeld, Ritmiller, Mackay, Cowan, & Hatch, 1994; Moschella & Wilson, 1997). Approximately 2 to 4 million women are severely assaulted each year by their male partners (Bash & Jones, 1995; Holtz & Furniss, 1993; Tilden et al., 1994). IPV does occur against males; however, 94% to 98% of victims are women and children (Campbell & Humphreys, 1993). It is estimated that an intimate partner kills 42% of the women murdered each year (deVries, 1997).

IPV taxes the fabric of our society in both human and financial terms. As Poirier (1997) points out, "The monetary expense of IPV involves emergency room visits, repeated clinic visits, time lost from work because of injuries, hospitalizations, mental health counseling and the cost of maintaining domestic violence services within the community" (Poirier, 1997, p. 105). The annual estimates for injuries from family violence are $44 million in medical costs, including 21,000 hospitalizations, 99,800 days of hospitalizations, 28,700 emergency department visits, and 30,000 physician visits (Loring & Smith, 1994).

DEFINING THE SCOPE OF INTIMATE PARTNER VIOLENCE

The term *domestic violence* summons an image of an act of physical aggression between a husband and wife. However, U.S. society is home to a wide variety of relationships where persons of the same and opposite sex cohabit. In addition, there are many ways to inflict harm on another individual, physical aggression being just one method. Where should one draw the line to categorize violence between two people as an instance of IPV? Some clinicians believe the term IPV should include events such as rape, emotional abuse, stalking, or sexual harassment. Others maintain that the scope of the term should be restricted to acts meant to cause physical harm. The inconsistency in defining exactly what constitutes IPV has made study of the phenomenon difficult, especially efforts to estimate its incidence and prevalence.

Recently, clinicians and researchers have assembled a set of uniform definitions for **intimate partner violence** (Saltzman, Fanslow, McMahon, & Shelly, 1999). Intimate partners are current or former spouses or current or former nonmarital partners (dating or same-sex partners). Violent acts include both physical and sexual violence, as well as threats and psychological–emotional abuse. Physical violence includes acts used with enough force to have the potential to cause death, disability, or injury and include such actions as scratching, pushing, shoving, burning, or use of restraint on another's body. These uniform definitions are important for researchers but also for nurses charged with detecting IPV. Effective screening for IPV will occur only if healthcare professionals evaluate clients for both psychological and physical injury with an accurate perspective on the broad range of violent actions and relationships that are considered IPV.

COST TO CHILDREN

Family life is threatened and often destroyed when there is IPV in the home. Children often are the silent victims of IPV because little attention is paid to their presence at the time of an incident (Osofsky, 1995a, 1995b). Although there has been scant systematic investigation of children's exposure to IPV, a five-state study found, on the average, there were children living in the households of 75% of adult female assault victims (Fantuzzo, Borouch, Beriama, Atkins, & Marcus, 1997).

Children who live in homes where partner violence occurs are at risk for developing a range of emotional, physical, and behavioral symptoms. Research suggests that they also are at serious risk of developing a host of aggressive, antisocial, or fearful and inhibited behaviors (Christopoulos et al., 1987; Jaffe, Wolfe, & Wilson, 1990; Jaffe, Wolfe, Wilson, & Zak, 1986) and deficits in social skills (Wolfe, Jaffe, Wilson, & Zak, 1985). They are reported to have impaired concentration and difficulties in school performance and, overall, perform at a lower level than nonexposed children on a variety of measures of cognitive and motor development (Jaffe, Hurley, & Wolfe, 1990). Children who witness domestic violence demonstrate higher levels of depression and anxiety compared with children from nonviolent homes (Christopoulos et al., 1987; Holden & Ritchie, 1991). They see violence as an acceptable form of resolving interpersonal conflicts, and they are at risk for potential deviance in their future social relationships (Jaffe et al., 1990).

In addition, children from families with domestic violence are at risk for experiencing physical violence themselves. The link between marital conflict and child maltreatment has received much attention in the last 10 to 15 years. Children of battered women are at an increased risk for abuse themselves, with estimates of an overlap between spousal abuse and child abuse ranging from 30% to 60% (Hughes, Parkinson, & Vargo, 1989; O'Keefe, 1995; Suh & Abel, 1990). In sum, studies comparing children exposed to domestic violence with children from nonviolent homes indicate that this exposure

- Has an adverse impact across a range of child functioning
- Produces different adverse effects at different ages
- Increases the risk of child abuse
- Is associated with other risk factors such as poverty and parental substance abuse

Although our knowledge about the impact of IPV on children is growing, we lack information on particular types or frequencies of IPV committed against children or the impact of various degrees of exposure on children's functioning (Mohr, Lutz, Fantuzzo, & Perry, 2000).

ADDRESSING INTIMATE PARTNER VIOLENCE

Although the scientific and public interest in IVP has intensified over the last decade, a coordinated response to the problem has been slow to develop. The Surgeon General has identified family violence as a priority public health issue and has called for an organized approach to screen for, treat, and prevent further violence (U.S. Public Health Service, 1999). Yet, the inability of healthcare, judicial, and religious systems to handle the problem of IPV effectively has been well documented (Jerzierski, 1994; King et al., 1993). The healthcare community in particular has been slow to participate in the effort (Illinois Department of Public Health [IDPH], 1995). Of particular concern has been health professional's long record of poor screening and identification of IPV victims.

Problems With Detection and Screening

The literature confirms that a significant factor in the underdetection of IPV rests with the behavior of professionals (Abbott, Johnson, Koziol-McLain, & Lowenstein

1995; Campbell, Pliska, Taylor, & Sheridan, 1994; Carbonell, Chez, & Hassler, 1995; Fishwick, 1995; Reid & Glasser, 1997). Practitioners in healthcare settings often fail to identify and intervene with abused women. Healthcare providers are vigilant in assessing a client's health history, surgeries, dietary and bowel patterns, sexual activities, and current physiologic functioning but not the possibility of IPV. The underlying dynamics of health professionals' poor screening practices are complex and include both biases and knowledge deficits.

Healthcare professionals come to their practice carrying many of the societal beliefs about the occurrence of IPV—biases that create barriers to screening. For instance, healthcare workers may subscribe to the cultural belief that IPV is a personal matter between spouses and believe they have no role in this private controversy (Hoff, 1993). Healthcare professionals may believe that IPV is restricted to particular socioeconomic groups and remain naive about the prevalence of the problem, assuming it was not an issue for their client population (Fishwick, 1995).

Knowledge deficits of the healthcare professional also result in failure to identify and intervene with abused women (Tilden et al., 1994). A recent survey found that most advanced practice nurses working in women's health had received little education or training on how to identify and manage clients who they believe may have been abused by a partner. Although professionals and accrediting agencies have called for training in IVP at all levels of healthcare curricula, the response of educators has been slow (American Association of Colleges of Nursing, 1999; Short, Johnson, & Osattin, 1998). A survey of medical schools determined the instructional time devoted to family violence content was inadequate (Alpert, Tonkin, Seeherman, & Holtz, 1998).

Inadequate response to IPV by the medical system also may be a product of the traditions and structure of the medical model (Warshaw, 1995). Healthcare providers identify themselves as problem solvers but may feel frustrated and powerless when managing cases of IPV (Gremillion & Kanof, 1996; Warshaw, 1993). IPV often is a recurrent problem; the same victim is seen several times in the emergency room. It is not an issue solved easily. One cannot write an order for a woman to leave her partner; clients ultimately are responsible for leaving their mates. Thus, the IPV client may generate feelings of inadequacy and a sense of frustration, inability to act, and may create a situation that discourages the professional from future intervention efforts with IPV clients (Schorstein, 1997).

Of particular concern has been the screening behavior of emergency department (ED) staff. Research demonstrates that when abused women presented in an ED with suspicious injuries with an improbable explanation, physicians and nurses treated them impersonally and insensitively, and minimized their abuse (Campbell et al., 1994).

The ED staff did not openly confront the victim with what they believed about the source of the injuries. Instead, injuries typically were diagnosed in strictly medical terms, and the women were left to deal with the psychosocial aspects of IPV.

Several factors have been proposed to explain reluctance of ED staff to screen for IPV. In some instances, ED staff seem to be in denial about the possibility of an IVP occurrence, a denial that helps them distance themselves from the violence (Loring & Smith, 1994). Distancing enables staff to avoid feeling vulnerable and overwhelmed. Staff may see IPV as a social or legal problem rather than a healthcare issue. The client may perceive direct questions about an injury as prying or outside the scope of practice. Healthcare providers also identify with clients of similar backgrounds and as a result "domestic violence may be left off the differential diagnosis list if the patient is from the same social strata as the healthcare provider" (Gremillion & Kanof, 1996, p. 771).

Importance of Screening

Screening for domestic violence needs to be systematic and direct. The inclusion of questions that identify IPV in triage and entry point protocols significantly increases the identification of abused women. When the healthcare provider does not ask women direct questions about IPV, the incidence of discovery is approximately 5% to 7%. When the healthcare provider asks women specifically, the incidence increases to approximately 29% to 30% (IDPH, 1993; Thurston & McLeod, 1997). Screening for domestic violence also is critically important because the way in which the immediate aftermath of violence is handled is an important determinant of the survivor's psychological response (Kaufmann, 1997).

It is good healthcare policy, and, ethically, it is the duty of healthcare providers to diagnose and treat IPV (Loring & Smith, 1994; Schorstein, 1997). Several states (Colorado, Kentucky, Massachusetts, and New Jersey) have developed IPV protocols for healthcare professionals aimed at assisting IPV victims to minimize physical and psychological trauma and facilitate protection and support services. The standards for identification, treatment, and evaluation of clients with IPV are in place. The American College of Emergency Physicians (1996) policy statement on IPV emphasizes the need for evaluating clients presenting to the ED for IPV; develops multidisciplinary approaches for identification, treatment, and referral; and recognizes the special services and resources necessary for victims of IPV. The Joint Commission on Accreditation of Health Care Organizations (1997) has mandated that hospitals have objective criteria for identifying and assessing possible victims of abuse and neglect and that these standards be uniform throughout the organization. Now comes the task of implementing these standards and regulations.

NURSES' ROLE IN THE IDENTIFICATION AND TREATMENT OF INTIMATE PARTNER VIOLENCE

In the healthcare system, nurses see women in a variety of settings and often are the first point of contact for women entering primary care offices and EDs. Considering their key role, it is critical that nurses screen for IPV. In the new healthcare arena, a vital link for assessing and intervening will be the primary healthcare provider. Both physicians and nurses, through the normal course of providing care to women, are likely to encounter victims of physical, sexual, and psychological violence (Hinderliter, Pitula, & Delaney, 1998). It is imperative that nurses' index of suspicion be raised to assess for victimization and safety and to supply needed information about available community services.

Because of their unique set of skills, nurses have great potential for addressing the issue of IPV. Nursing schools train nurses to assess, and their basic curriculum includes techniques of supportive counseling. Nurses' professional value system is grounded in principles of advocacy. Nurses are natural case managers; they quickly learn how to identify and connect with community resources. An excellent body of nursing research is building concerning the difficult choices women make in leaving an abusive relationship (Campbell, Miller, Cardwell, & Belknap, 1994; Moss, Pitula, & Halstead, 1997; Ulrich, 1993). Drawing on this knowledge, nurses can increase their sensitivity to clients' dilemmas and the difficult choices they face in evaluating the strength and weaknesses of intimate relationships (King et al., 1993). A knowing, empowering response to victims could result.

As they assume their appropriate role in the effort to screen and treat victims of IPV, nurses face barriers common to all health professionals. The issue of time is a persistent problem. In numerous surveys, professionals report that time constraints pose the major barrier to IPV screening. There are, however, several ways to address this problem. A large healthcare system might have a trained IPV counselor on their staff. Advanced practice nurses in a clinical setting could be considered candidates for this role. For example, in one of the author's institutions, the maternal–child clinical nurse specialist (CNS) has special training in IPV. Her role includes on-call responsibilities as a resource to all staff and as a client advocate. This specialized CNS can also immediately direct and refer the client to shelters and to community centers for further counseling and intervention. Having access to this consultant circumvents some time barriers.

If a consultant role cannot be created, then nurses must assume the responsibility for detection and handling of IPV cases. Screening for IPV can be simple. Nurses should learn to ask two basic domestic violence questions, "Has a past or current partner ever caused you to be afraid?" and "Has a past or current partner ever physically hurt you?" (Hinderliter, Pitula, & Delaney,

RAPE AND SEXUAL ASSAULT

Rape and sexual assault are acts of violence; they are sexual behaviors that a person perpetrates forcefully on others, violating their person and shattering their sense of safety and predictability in the world. **Rape** is a crime of forced or coerced sexual penetration (oral, anal, or vaginal) of a nonconsenting person. **Sexual assault** refers to forced or coerced sexual acts performed on a nonconsenting person. **Statutory rape** refers to rape of a minor (age of minors varies from state to state). In the case of minors, consent is not an issue; the state does not consider minors capable of giving consent because of their vulnerability and dependence on adults or older peers. Therefore, sexual penetration (oral, anal, or vaginal) of a minor is a crime without consideration of consent.

Criminal statutes on rape vary from state to state, but all states define rape as a crime. Every 2 minutes, someone in the United States is sexually assaulted (U.S. Department of Justice, 2000). In the year 2000, there were 261,000 victims of rape, 92,000 completed rapes, 55,000 attempted rapes, and 114,000 sexual assaults. This statistic does not include statutory rape (rape of a minor); however, the Justice Department estimates that one of six victims is a child younger than 12 years of age.

One of every 6, or 17.7 million, American women has been the victim of an attempted or completed rape in their lifetime (National Institute of Justice & Centers for Disease Control and Prevention, 1998). About 3%, or 2.78 million, men have experienced an attempted or completed rape in their lifetime (National Institute of Justice & Centers for Disease Control and Prevention, 1998). These statistics reflect reported rapes and attempted rapes; however, most rapes and attempted rapes go unreported. Common reasons given for not reporting these crimes include the belief that rape is a private and personal matter and fear of reprisal from the perpetrator. In 1999, victims reported only 28% (less than one third) of rapes and sexual assaults to law enforcement officials (U.S. Department of Justice, 2000).

Types of Rape

RAPE BY A STRANGER

When imagining a rape, chances are that the image involves a stranger with sinister motives who suddenly attacks his unsuspecting victim. However, rape by a stranger accounts for only approximately 15% of the total rapes. A person known to the survivor (eg, acquaintance, close friend, lover, family member, or neighbor) commits most rapes. The motivations of rapists have been studied extensively by Groth (1979), who developed a classification scheme based on the most powerful motive for the rapists. The stranger rapist is more likely to use a weapon and to be more violent during the rape. The anger rapist, for example, is motivated by his overwhelming rage that explodes sporadically. These explosions usually relate to some external event (eg, an argument with a wife or girlfriend). Rape becomes the way for the anger rapist to release his pent-up anger, and sex becomes his weapon. The power rapist, conversely, is motivated by a need for power. He is thought to be compensating for feelings of insecurity and inadequacy and attempts to reassure himself of his masculinity and his control and power in the situation.

The sadistic rapist is the least common of all types; however, this type of rapist receives most of the attention by the media because of his brutal rapes, which may include murder. This type of rapist receives sexual gratification from his victim's suffering, and the rape frequently includes some type of bondage. Groth's (1979) categories of stranger rapists are not mutually exclusive. Rapists may have more than one strong motivation for raping and may have characteristics from more than one category.

DATE RAPE
AND ACQUAINTANCE RAPE

Most rapes involve people who know each other. Survivors of date rapes include women of all ages: the 50-year-old woman who accepts an offer from a coworker for assistance with installing a ceiling fan, the 20-year-old coed who becomes drunk at a party and passes out, or the 70-year-old woman who accepts a ride from a kindly looking church member. Each of these incidents may conclude without incident or, in the presence of a predatory male, may become the scene of a date or acquaintance rape.

Date or acquaintance rapes are no less traumatic or repugnant than are other types of rape; the serious physical and emotional consequences of this type of rape should not be minimized because the perpetrator and the survivor know each other. Research shows that survivors of this type of rape experience more self-blaming behaviors because they believe they should have known that the individual would rape them or they feel foolish for having trusted him. A sense of betrayal frequently is an issue for survivors of date or acquaintance rape.

The incidence of these rapes is difficult to know because victims often do not report most of them. Koss (1988) found that only 5% of women in her study who experienced date rape reported it to the police. She also found that these survivors of date rape were raped by their steady dates (35%), by men they knew but with whom they were not romantically involved (29%), by a casual date (25%), and by a husband or family member (11%). Date rape does not just happen on the first date; it may occur during any stage of a relationship.

MARITAL RAPE

The idea that rape could occur within a marital relationship was not given much consideration before 1978 and the case in Oregon of Greta and John Rideout. Greta reported that when she refused to have sex with her husband, he attacked her, beat her, and raped her. The jury, consisting of eight women and four men, ignored the medical evidence of a violent assault and found John Rideout not guilty of first-degree rape of his wife. This case highlighted the need for laws to change.

Currently, marital rape is a crime in all states; however, in 33 states, there are exemptions for prosecuting husbands for rape. These exemptions usually are related to the use of force. If the wife cannot show evidence of the use of force by her husband (eg, bodily injuries), she cannot claim she was raped by her husband. Some state supreme courts have ruled that the marital rape exemption is unconstitutional denial of equal protection for wives (Russell, 1991). Here, reasoning holds that if rape of an unmarried woman is a crime, then the same should hold true for a married woman. To intervene effectively in cases of marital rape, nurses should familiarize themselves with the laws in their state concerning rape.

Rape Trauma Syndrome

In 1974, based on their study of rape survivors, Burgess and Holmstrom described the rape trauma syndrome, a two-phase process experienced by all rape survivors. The first phase, which may go on for days or weeks, is the *acute phase of disorganization,* which appears as the survivor begins to respond to the rape. Fear, anxiety, disbelief, anger, and shock frequently are observed during this period. Physical responses include sleep disturbance, nightmares, body aches and pains related to the rape, fatigue, and loss of appetite. Physical responses vary according to the nature of the rape and the individual's perception of the incident. Ritual behaviors associated with ensuring the survivor's safety (eg, checking window and door locks repeatedly) as well as hyperalertness to potential danger (eg, scanning the environment continually for the rapist), and an increased startle response may be present.

Some survivors may openly express their feelings, whereas others may exhibit a controlled or stoic response. Both are normal responses to rape trauma, and nurses should not assume that the controlled survivor was not affected (traumatized) by the rape. One interpretation of this controlled behavior is that the survivor feels out of control and therefore is controlling the one thing she still has control over—her own behavior.

Acute phase emotional responses also may include increased irritability, difficulty concentrating, obsessive thoughts about the rape or some aspect of the rape (eg, "I keep seeing him on top of me with his hand choking me and how I couldn't breathe. . . ."). Tearfulness, anger, humiliation, shame, and guilt also are common responses during this phase. Shame and guilt frequently are related to the survivor's self-blame from reviewing and assessing her behavior associated with the rape. Family, friends, and professional helpers may inadvertently reinforce these feelings by questioning the survivor's actions or implying the survivor is to blame.

All of these symptoms may lead the survivor to feel like she is "going crazy." The world no longer makes sense to the survivor. Those of us who have not ever been traumatized live under the delusion that we are safe and that we are in control of our lives. Rape survivors have had these delusions shattered by their experience. No longer do they feel safe. They feel vulnerable and out of control of the environment and of their feelings and behaviors. One survivor described the experience this way:

> *I was afraid all the time. When I saw someone that looked like the rapist my heart would start pounding and it was all I could do to keep from running the other way. I avoided everything that reminded me of the rape but I still had these pictures in my head of him making me tell him how much I liked it. I couldn't concentrate at work and I felt tired all the time. Tired as I was, at night I couldn't sleep without medication. I was afraid to go to sleep because I often had nightmares of the rape. I felt totally out of control.*

The second phase of the rape trauma syndrome is the *long-term process of reorganization.* In this phase, the survivor works toward integration and resolution of the experience. Healthy integration and resolution involves regaining a sense of empowerment and reconnecting with others. Most survivors can benefit substantially from professional help during this phase. In therapy, the survivor has an opportunity to learn ways to feel safe again and to manage the disturbing symptoms that accompany rape trauma syndrome. Furthermore, the survivor has the opportunity to remember and work through the myriad feelings associated with the trauma. Gradually, the survivor begins to reassert control over her or his life and gains a new sense of relative safety—a new worldview.

Additional Ramifications of Rape

Rape trauma survivors also may exhibit other psychiatric disorders in response to trauma. Post-traumatic stress disorder (PTSD) is a possible diagnosis if recovery from the rape does not occur. Also, to manage symptoms (eg, anxiety, fear), the survivor may find that a glass of wine or a beer or smoking marijuana is helpful. Before long, the survivor is self-medicating her or his symptoms throughout the day. An addictive process has begun with the body developing tolerance for the alcohol or drug used by the survivor. Over time, the survivor needs more and more of the substance to get to sleep or to relax until the individual is drinking or drugging just to feel "OK" and to keep the withdrawal symptoms at bay. This survivor now has a substance abuse or dependence problem as well as PTSD.

Additionally, rape trauma survivors may develop depression, other anxiety disorders (eg, phobias, agoraphobia, or panic disorder), bipolar disorder, sexual dysfunction disorders, dissociative identity disorder, and borderline personality disorder. These disorders result from the unresolved and chronic symptoms first evident during the acute phase of disorganization of rape trauma syndrome.

Treatment for Survivors of Rape or Sexual Assault

Acute care after a rape or sexual assault generally occurs in the emergency room of a hospital. However, much of the treatment for the sexual trauma survivor takes place in outpatient settings such as rape crisis centers, victim services agencies, and the offices of mental health professionals. Treatment approaches vary and frequently are used in combination. Types of treatment interventions include psychopharmacologic and psychological.

PSYCHOPHARMACOLOGIC INTERVENTIONS

Biochemical treatment in the form of antidepressant medication (especially the selective serotonin reuptake inhibitors) and antianxiety medication is helpful in the reduction of symptoms of PTSD, depression, and anxiety. This symptom reduction frequently allows survivors to function more normally and empowers them to manage their worst symptoms. Antidepressants, notably the tricyclics, commonly are used to induce and promote sleep at bedtime. Survivors with more persistent obsessive thoughts or images of the trauma or those with psychotic symptoms may benefit from the new antipsychotic medications termed "atypicals" such as risperidone, olanzapine, and quetiapine.

PSYCHOLOGICAL INTERVENTIONS

Although biochemical intervention is useful in symptom reduction, it does not address the real issues confronting the survivor regarding how to feel safe again or what to do with her feelings of loss, anger, shame, guilt, and helplessness. It also does not address the numerous other areas of her life impacted by the sexual trauma. Trauma therapy frequently uses behavioral and cognitive approaches, individual and group treatment, as well as conjoint or family therapy as necessary.

Herman (1992) discusses the three stages of trauma treatment:

1. Safety
2. Remembrance and mourning
3. Reconnection

Safety refers to therapeutic efforts to assist the client to feel relatively safe again. This process includes teaching the survivor to manage her trauma symptoms, reestablishing her self-care and self-protection, and developing a support system. Additionally, the development of a trusting and collaborative relationship between the therapist and the client is critical to this stage of treatment.

In stage 2, called remembrance and mourning, the survivor tells her story of the trauma with as much depth and detail as she can recall. In the telling of the story, the survivor "reconstructs and transforms the traumatic memory, so that it can be integrated into the survivor's life" (Herman, 1992, p. 175). The survivor's renewed hope and energy for current concerns and life in general signals the successful conclusion of this stage. In stage 3, or reconnection, the survivor now turns her energies to creating her future. "She has mourned the old self that trauma destroyed; now she must develop a new self" (Herman, 1992, p. 196). The survivor then focuses on issues of identity and intimacy as she reengages with life and its many gifts as well as tragedies.

Adjunctive techniques that promote the goal of trauma therapy include biofeedback, relaxation training, assertiveness, hypnosis, bodywork (eg, dance, massage, yoga, self-defense training), meditation, guided imagery, journaling, grounding, and specialized groups for survivors. A new method for processing the traumatic memories of PTSD, called *eye movement desensitization and reprocessing* (Shapiro, 1995), is being used extensively for treatment of trauma survivors. This method helps to reduce the debilitating symptoms of PTSD in sexual trauma survivors. Other new methods used to treat rape survivors include trauma incident reduction (French & Harris, 1999) and emotional freedom techniques (Mountrose & Mountrose, 2000).

Rape Prevention

Rape prevention is a complex topic because it involves intervention on many different levels within the community. It includes both societal and individual interventions. *Primary prevention* of rape involves strategies that address community awareness and seek to eliminate societal values and beliefs that condone rape. For example, gender stereotypes regarding power in relationships may contribute to victimization of women (Allison & Wrightsman, 1993). Often in relationships, the male places the female in a more passive role, putting her at higher risk to be raped. These same male–female dynamics are played out in other areas of society such as the workplace and within relationships (Allison & Wrightsman, 1993). More equitable power dynamics between men and women translates into less victimization because this equity sets the scene for collaboration rather than domination of each other.

Secondary prevention includes strategies aimed at identifying situations that place the individual at greater risk of being raped or teaching individuals how to protect themselves if assaulted. Rape prevention at this level involves use of various media to educate potentially vulnerable populations. Some strategies involve hands-on interventions; for example, corporations and universities provide escort services to women who must travel at a late hour to reach their car or another part of campus. Such intervention recognizes that a woman out alone at a late hour is vulnerable to the risk of rape. These kinds of strategies not only promote the safety of women but also declare that their safety is valued. *Tertiary prevention* focuses on treatment of the survivor as soon as possible after the trauma to minimize the severity of symptoms and sequela. The content of this chapter focuses primarily on treatment of the rape trauma survivor. Many rape trauma survivors do not report their victimization and therefore do not receive treatment in a timely manner. Responsibility for early screening and identification of sexual trauma falls to all healthcare providers, whatever their focus.

Nurses' Role in the Assessment and Treatment of Survivors of Rape Trauma

Nurses' response to rape and sexual assault victims should follow the nursing process.

ASSESSMENT

Assessment begins with the nurse's first contact with the rape or sexual assault survivor; whether by telephone or in person, the nurse's attitude toward the survivor should be one of caring and support. Whatever the survivor's story, the nurse must be able to suspend his or her judgments about the rape so that he or she can render nursing care in a professional manner. Assessing blame and responsibility is not part of the nurse's professional duties. Moreover, nurses may compound the trauma of the rape if their attitude is not caring and supportive.

Not every nurse is able to work with rape trauma survivors. Even among nurses who specialize in the care of rape trauma survivors, there will be the occasional survivor with whom they cannot work effectively or therapeutically. Knowing how to recognize within yourself when your feelings are likely to interfere with your optimal care of an individual is part of your professional responsibility to the survivor. The nurse must be able to be emotionally available to the survivor so he or she can empathize (imagine what it must have been like) with the survivor's experience and at the same time view the information dispassionately. The ability to do this is directly proportional to the nurse's ability to acknowledge his or her own feelings (Clinical Example 17-1).

Instructions to the survivor who calls seeking information after a rape should stress the importance of the survivor coming to the emergency room as she is, without "cleaning herself up" in any way and especially without showering or bathing. She should bring a clean change of clothes with her to change into after the examination because she will need to leave her clothing at the hospital as evidence. If she is not wearing the clothes in which she was raped, then she should bring them with her. If possible, a supportive person should accompany the survivor to the hospital. Sometimes, survivors are reluctant to report the rape to the police. In such cases, the nurse should respect their wishes; however, they should be encouraged to seek examination and treatment for potential pregnancy, venereal diseases, AIDS, and their emotional and psychological well-being.

Once the survivor arrives at an emergency room for examination and treatment, assessment and documentation of her biopsychosocial self begins. In many communities, sexual assault nurse examiners conduct the rape examination. These registered nurses have special training in gathering evidence of the rape or sexual assault for use by the legal system in the arrest and prosecution of the perpetrator. Survivors should be encouraged to allow such evidence gathering, even if she or he is unsure about whether to report the rape to the police. The nurse can turn over the collected evidence to the police in case the survivor should decide to make a report.

▼ *Clinical Example 17-1*

One day, toward the end of a busy shift, a rape trauma survivor who was raped when she accepted a ride from a stranger comes into the emergency department. Nurse Monica is assigned to the survivor. She notices that the young woman is about her age and is attending nursing school. Monica finds herself stating to another nurse, "I can't understand why these women are so stupid. They deserve to be raped." The other nurse is surprised by Monica's comment and says so. He suggests that Monica is not in a "good place" to deal with this rape trauma survivor and that they switch clients to relieve Monica of working with the survivor. Later on, this nurse sits down and talks with Monica about her feelings. Monica discovers that she overidentified with the survivor, who reminded her of herself and her willingness to hitch rides in younger days. Had Monica not received this timely intervention from her coworker, she may have communicated some of her judgmental attitude to the survivor. This action would not have been therapeutic for the survivor.

Points for Reflection and Critical Thinking

- Discuss why nurses must be alert to their feelings about a client.
- Compare and contrast an overreaction and an underreaction to the client who has survived rape.
- Explain how Monica's feelings could have interfered with her ability to be therapeutic to, or even have harmed, the rape survivor.

The emergency room nurse plays a critical role in the care of the rape trauma survivor. He or she often is the first professional person to talk with the survivor and frequently is with the survivor at intervals throughout her stay in the emergency room. The emergency room nurse should express his or her concern for the survivor and be emotionally available to listen and support the survivor. Survivors may respond with emotion (eg, be tearful, angry, or agitated) or may appear controlled (eg, stoic, matter-of-fact, no emotion). Whatever the survivor's presentation, the nurse should express his or her concern for the survivor. The nurse's primary goal initially is to establish a trusting relationship with the survivor.

An accepting and caring attitude is critical for the survivor to begin to trust the nurse. Most survivors feel tainted by the experience, and they often feel "dirty" or somehow "bad" or guilty afterward. They are especially sensitive to rejection or blame, in part because they already may have begun to blame themselves, but also because society frequently blames victims of rape. Many fear that no one will believe them. Sometimes just being present with the survivor can be the most therapeutic thing a nurse can do to help the survivor feel safe and comfortable. Empowering the survivor also is important, and the nurse may communicate this by respecting the survivor's right to self-determination. The nurse should inform the survivor of everything that is being done or will be done for her and should respect her choices, even when the nurse personally disagrees with them.

During the initial data gathering, the nurse should ask about any previous trauma (eg, physical or sexual abuse in childhood, previous unwanted sexual incidents, previous psychiatric treatment, other traumatic events such as natural disasters, or serious car accidents or house fires). This information will be especially useful in planning for care of the survivor after discharge. Part of the nurse's assessment includes assessing for any physical trauma that requires immediate attention. Although most rape victims do not have life-threatening injuries, some do. The nurse should attend to these injuries with concern for the preservation of evidence of the crime.

TREATMENT

Planning for the treatment of the rape trauma survivor should include formulating nursing diagnoses and goals and designing interventions for the survivor's acute needs after the trauma, as well as longer term needs as she works to integrate and resolve her traumatic experience. A sample care plan for a rape trauma survivor is provided in Nursing Care Plan 17-1. Immediately after the rape, the nurse should focus on the provision of immediate medical attention and the gathering of evidence for possible use in legal proceedings. The survivor should receive a rationale for each procedure she will endure (eg, medical and legal reasons for a pelvic examination). In collaboration with the survivor, the nurse also should plan for where and with whom the survivor will leave the hospital as well as notification of significant others (eg, parents, spouse or partner, or other family members). The nurse needs to plan for the survivor to speak with a crisis counselor either while in the hospital or shortly after discharge. Client and Family Education 17-1 contains key points that the nurse should address in educating both victims and their families. To address long-term reorganization issues, the nurse needs to encourage the survivor to seek therapy or counseling services.

▼ Reflection and Critical Thinking Questions

1. When you read of a violent incident in the newspaper, do you usually feel removed from the event? Has that sense of distance changed since reading this chapter?

2. Do only particular types of people have the potential to become violent? Consider your own risk for becoming a victim or perpetrator of violence as well as protective factors.

3. Of all the types of violence in this chapter (youth, IPV, child maltreatment, elder abuse, and rape), which seems completely implausible to you? Which do you believe could never happen to you or a member of your family?

4. Assess your community, schools, and neighborhood for risk factors of youth violence.

5. Of all sections of this chapter, which topic personally touched you or generated a great deal of feeling? Why?

▼ CHAPTER SUMMARY

- Community violence is an umbrella term for numerous forms of aggression that individuals inflict on one another. It includes phenomena such as youth violence, IPV, child maltreatment, elder abuse, and rape and sexual assault.

- One way to understand community violence is to consider not just traits of the perpetrator but factors within the family, community, and culture that place individuals at risk for becoming a victim or perpetrator of violence.

- The tremendous increase in the incidence of youth violence has been explained by individual traits as well as family, school, community, and neighborhood influences.

- IPV affects the lives of 2 to 4 million women a year, yet health professionals often fail to adequately screen for IPV.

- Maltreatment affects every aspect of the child including his or her social, behavioral, emotional, intellectual, and physical development.

Nursing Care Plan 17-1

THE SEXUAL TRAUMA SURVIVOR

Alicia is a 20-year-old college student. She has been dating Jacob for 3 years, but recently they decided to see other people as well. Alicia began dating Tom, a young man whom she had met through her church. Four weeks earlier, Tom raped Alicia on their second date. She did not report the rape. Jacob has stood by Alicia and has encouraged her to seek counseling. The nurse practitioner meets with Alicia, who relates the following:

> *I had too much to drink; at first I couldn't believe it was happening. I had let him kiss me, but he just kept going. I told him to stop, but he wouldn't. He ripped my clothes off and forced me to have sex with him several times. He told me if I told anyone, they would never believe me because everyone liked him and no one liked me very much. I never should have gone out with him. Now I'm so afraid; I cry all the time. I could jump out of my skin if I hear a noise. I don't want to go to school; I can't think straight anyway. And I will not go back to church. Every night I have nightmares, or I feel him holding me down. . . . I never should have gone out with him. Even Jacob is getting sick of me; he says he doesn't know what to do and can't handle how I've changed.*

The nurse practitioner listens carefully and compassionately. She tells Alicia that she will be able to help her overcome this trauma. Together they discuss the issues that Alicia is confronting, and the nurse develops the following care plan.

Nursing Diagnosis: **Rape Trauma Syndrome** related to date rape 1 month earlier as evidenced by anxiety, distress, recurrent nightmares, flashbacks, cognitive difficulties, isolation, and fear

Goal: Alicia will feel less fear and anxiety, will not isolate herself, and will begin to integrate her trauma into her personal history and move forward. Alicia will stop blaming herself for causing the rape.

Interventions	Rationales
Use cognitive behavioral therapy (CBT) strategies to address fears. Have client talk through and gradually reexpose herself to the assault.	CBT has demonstrated effectiveness in short-term reduction of fear-related symptoms. Helping Alicia remember and visualize the rape can help to gradually reduce her anxiety and distress.
Teach client the cognitive technique of challenging automatic thoughts to help manage and defeat guilt and fear.	Alicia's story is laced with subtle self-blaming statements. Helping her recognize how automatic thoughts contribute to guilt, fear, and anxiety and helping her use more positive self-talk will empower her to stop assuming a role in causing the trauma.
Involve client in a rape survivors' support group.	Sharing her experience with others who have had similar experiences will be a source of support and compassion for Alicia, who will need a place to safely express her feelings.
Teach client anxiety reduction techniques.	They help calm the autonomic nervous system, which causes many unpleasant physical symptoms and is overly sensitive during emotional trauma.
Include supportive partner in counseling sessions, if client agrees. Help him work through his feelings of isolation, confusion, anger, powerlessness, and frustration.	Jacob's willingness to support Alicia is critical for her. Partners for rape survivors often experience distress and frustration. He can be a greater resource for her if his feelings are addressed.

Evaluation: The acute phase of rape trauma syndrome may last up to 2 or 3 months. If Alicia does not begin to show less fear and anxiety, improved sleep, less isolation, and fewer other symptoms within this time frame, more aggressive therapy, including the use of antidepressants, should be considered.

Client and Family Education 17-1

COPING WITH RAPE TRAUMA SYNDROME

Teaching Points

Family members, friends, and significant others frequently are at a loss about what to say or do to assist survivors of sexual trauma. Often, significant others exhibit strong feelings of anger and aggression toward the perpetrator. Although significant others generally have such feelings because they care for the survivor, these feelings are not helpful to the survivor who feels guilty about the rape. Nurses should allow significant others to express their feelings away from the survivor and then redirect them to discuss what the survivor needs from them now and in the future. Having some written information (a pamphlet or brochure) about rape trauma syndrome will be useful to survivors and those closest to them; written information should discuss what to expect, how to be helpful to a survivor, and what activities are beneficial to the survivor. Verbal discussion of the written information also helps because it allows survivors and their families to ask questions and relate their other concerns. Written information also is critical, however, because the participants frequently are in such a state of anxiety and concern that they do not remember what was said. Having a written guide to refer to as needed jogs the memory about what to do.

Instructions about rape trauma syndrome should include the following:

- Normal reactions to a traumatic event: cognitive, emotional, physical, and behavioral
- Negative coping strategies to avoid: use of drugs or alcohol, withdrawal
- Helpful ways to cope after the traumatic event, especially talking about the event with an experienced counselor
- Name of contact person to speak to about the rape

The information should include future medical and counseling appointments as well as guidance on symptom management (eg, exercise, relaxation, nutrition, sleep, resuming normal activities). In addition, the survivor should receive written information regarding whom to call for further information on legal issues related to the rape (eg, case number and name and number of the police investigator). Any medications needed by the survivor should be dispensed at the hospital if possible because the survivor already is overwhelmed with information and tasks related to coping with the event.

Useful Resources

www.rainn.org
RAINN (Rape Abuse and Incest National Network)
This is the National Sexual Assault Hotline (1-800-656-HOPE). It operates America's only national hotline for victims of sexual assault, offering free confidential counseling and support 24 hours a day anywhere in the country. The web site contains information about the hotline and local rape crisis centers and links to topics such as rape facts, impact of rape, and survivor stories.

www.mint.net/rrs
This site was designed for college students and contains useful facts about rape and sexual assault, safety tips, what to do if you are raped, and healing.

www.stardate.bc.ca/survivors
The Survivor's Page
This site contains writings, letters, and poetry written by survivors; survivor stories; a survivors' page newsgroup; a way to meet other survivors (electronically); and an e-mail list for partners, friends, and families of survivors.

- Older adults are increasingly victims of abuse (ie, physical, sexual, psychological, or neglect) that may occur at the hands of their caregiver.
- Rape and sexual assault are acts of violence in the form of sexual behaviors that are forcefully perpetrated on others, violating their person and shattering their sense of safety and predictability in the world.
- Rape trauma syndrome details the sequence of psychological events that rape victims may experience after an attack.
- The nursing care of the rape victim involves attending to both physical and psychological needs and requires particular sensitivity to the victim's reaction.

- To intervene with the rape victim effectively, nurses must attend to and control their own reaction to the event.

▼ REVIEW QUESTIONS

1. According to the ecologic model of violence, maternal–infant attachment behaviors are a component of which level of analysis?
   a. Macrosystem
   b. Microsystem
   c. Exosystem
   d. Ontogenic development

2. An 11-year-old male student, Michael, goes to the school nurse with a bloody nose. A fellow student had brushed against him in the hall and knocked his books out of his hands. Michael then accosted the student, shoved him, and challenged him to a fight. What type of risk factor for continued youth violence does Michael have?
   a. Peer risk factor
   b. Family risk factor
   c. Individual risk factor
   d. Neighborhood risk factor

3. The nurse at Michael's school is concerned about the number of injuries she sees that have resulted from fighting. Which of the following interventions will likely have the most effects on youth violence in her school?
   a. A social problem-solving program
   b. Family therapy for students who have been involved in fighting
   c. Referral of students involved in fighting to the school counselor
   d. Distribution of handouts about youth violence to all students

4. One of the most significant factors in the underdetection of IPV is
   a. Lack of good screening tools
   b. Knowledge deficits and biases of healthcare professionals
   c. Failure of victims to seek medical treatment
   d. Victims' lack of truthfulness about causes of injuries

5. A 5-year-old child is brought to the ED with a broken wrist. The mother states the child fell off a swing. The nurse notes multiple healing bruises on the child's back, which the mother states occurred when the child fell down the steps 5 days earlier. Based on this data, which action should the nurse take?
   a. Continue assessing the child for possible neurologic reasons for frequent falls
   b. Report the family to the child protection agency for suspected physical abuse
   c. Accept the mother's explanation and arrange for a cast to be applied to the arm
   d. Inform the physician that she suspects child abuse

6. A 78-year-old man with a history of atrial fibrillation and type 2 diabetes is brought to the ED by his 50-year-old son, who cares for him at home. On assessment, the nurse notes that the client is dehydrated, unkempt, and has a stage 3 pressure ulcer on his coccyx. He is weak but otherwise is neurologically intact. The nurse asks if the client is being well cared for at home, to which the client replies, "He does the best he can, I guess." Which of the following interpretations of the findings and the client's statement is the most likely explanation for the client's condition?
   a. The client's age and weakness
   b. Physical abuse
   c. Physical neglect
   d. The client's underlying physical condition

7. When they detect signs of elder abuse, healthcare professionals are required by law to
   a. Report the abuse to the state authorities
   b. Set up family counseling sessions
   c. Find temporary housing for the client
   d. Educate the client and family about elder abuse

8. Rape by a stranger accounts is estimated to account for what percentage of total rapes?
   a. 15%
   b. 25%
   c. 50%
   d. 70%

9. Rape trauma syndrome refers to
   a. A two-phase process including an acute disorganization phase and a long-term reorganization phase
   b. An abnormally severe psychological response to a sexual assault
   c. A four-phase process including denial, anger, bargaining, and acceptance
   d. Physical injuries incurred during the assault

10. A nurse in the ED is assessing a 42-year-old client who was brutally raped and beaten 3 hours earlier by her estranged boyfriend. The client has several facial fractures and multiple lacerations. The client states, "He has done this before." Throughout the assessment, the client does not appear upset and is cooperating matter-of-factly with the examination. The nurse attributes the client's affect to which of the following explanations?
    a. The client is handling the assault well from an emotional standpoint.
    b. The client's reaction is abnormal and suggests an underlying psychological problem.
    c. The client is concerned more about her physical injuries at this time.
    d. The client's affect is a normal reaction and may represent an effort to regain control.

▼ REFERENCES AND SUGGESTED READINGS

*Abbott, J., Johnson, R., Koziol-McLain, J., & Lowenstein, S. (1995). Domestic violence against women: Incidence and prevalence in an emergency department population. *Journal of the American Medical Association, 273,* 1763–1767.

*Aber, J. L., & Allen, J. P. (1987). Effects of maltreatment on young children's socioemotional development: An attachment theory perspective. *Developmental Psychology, 23,* 406–414.

*Alessandri, S. M. (1991). Play and social behavior in maltreated preschoolers. *Development and Psychopathology, 3,* 191–205.

*Alessandri, S. M. (1992). Mother–child interactional correlates of maltreated and non-maltreated children's play behavior. *Development and Psychopathology, 4,* 257–270.

*Allen, D. M., & Tamowski, K. J. (1989). Depressive characteristics of physically abused children. *Journal of Abnormal Child Psychology, 17,* 1–11.

*Allison, J. A., & Wrightsman, L. S. (1993). *Rape: The misunderstood crime.* Newbury Park, CA: Sage.

*Alpert, E. J., Tonkin, A. E., Seeherman, A. M., & Holtz, H. A. (1998). Family violence curricula in U.S. medical schools. *American Journal of Preventive Medicine, 14,* 273–282.

*American Association of Colleges of Nursing (AACN). (1999). Policy statement on violence as a public health problem. (On-line.) Available at: *http://www.aacn.nche.edu/publications/positions/violence.html.* Accessed November 1, 2001.

*American College of Emergency Physicians (ACEP). (1996). ACEP policy statement: Emergency medicine and domestic violence. (On-line.) Available at: *http://www.acep.org/policy/p0004163.htm.* Accessed February 1999.

*American College of Physicians. (1998). Firearm injury protection. *Annals of Internal Medicine, 128,* 236–241.

*American Psychiatric Association (APA). (2000). *Diagnostic and statistical manual of mental disorders* (4th ed., text rev.). Washington, DC: Author.

*Barahal, R. M., Waterman, J., & Martin, H. P. (1981). The social cognitive development of abused children. *Journal of Consulting and Clinical Psychology, 49,* 508–516.

*Bash, K., & Jones, F. (1995). Domestic violence in America. *North Carolina Medical Journal, 55,* 400–403.

*Bennett, K. J., Lipman, E. L., Brown, S., Racine, Y., Boyle, M. H., & Offord, D. R. (1999). Predicting conduct problems: Can high-risk children be identified in kindergarten and grade 1? *Journal of Consulting and Clinical Psychology, 67,* 470–480.

*Burgess, A. W., & Holmstrom, L. L. (1974). Rape trauma syndrome. *American Journal of Psychiatry, 131,* 981–999.

*Burgess, R. L., & Conger, R. D. (1978). Family interaction in abusive, neglectful, and normal families. *Child Development, 49,* 1163–1173.

*Campbell, J., & Humphreys, J. (1993). *Nursing care of survivors of family violence.* St. Louis: Mosby Year Book.

*Campbell, J., Miller, P., Cardwell, M., & Belknap, A. (1994). Relationship status of battered women over time. *Journal of Family Violence, 9*(2), 99–105.

*Campbell, J., Pliska, M., Taylor, W., & Sheridan, D. (1994). Battered women's experiences in the emergency department. *Journal of Emergency Nursing, 20,* 280–288.

*Campbell, S. B. (1995). Behavior problems in preschool children: A review of recent research. *Journal of Child Psychology and Psychiatry, 36,* 113–149.

*Campbell, S. B., Shaw, D. S., & Gilliom, M. (2000). Early externalizing behavior problems: Toddlers and preschoolers at risk for later maladjustment. *Development and Psychopathology, 12,* 467–488.

*Camras, L. A., & Rappaport, S. (1993). Conflict behaviors of maltreated and non-maltreated children. *Child Abuse and Neglect, 17,* 455–464.

*Carbonell, J., Chez, R., & Hassler, R. (1995). Florida physician and nurse education and practice related to domestic violence. *Women's Health Issues, 5,* 203–207.

*Carlson, V., Cicchetti, D., Barnett, D., & Braunwald, K. (1989). Disorganized/disoriented attachment relationships in maltreated infants. *Developmental Psychology, 25,* 525–531.

*Centers for Disease Control and Prevention (CDC). (1999). *National Center for Health Statistics, 47*(19). Atlanta, GA: Author.

*Centers for Disease Control and Prevention (CDC). (2000). Youth violence in the United States. (On-line.) Available at: *http://www.cdc.gov/ncipc/factsheets/yvfacts.htm.* Accessed June 2000.

*Center for Mental Health Services (CMHS). (2001). *The CMHS approach to enhancing youth resilience and preventing youth violence in schools and communities.* Washington, DC: Substance Abuse and Mental Health Services Administration.

*Christopoulos, C., Cohn, D. A., Shaw, D. S., Joyce, S., Sullivan-Hanson, J., Kraft, S. P., et al. (1987). Children of abused women. *Journal of Marriage and the Family, 49,* 611–619.

*Cicchetti, D., & Lynch, M. (1993). Toward an ecological/transactional model of community violence and child maltreatment: Consequences for child development. *Psychiatry, 56,* 96–118.

*Commission for the Prevention of Youth Violence. (2000). *Youth and violence: Medicine, nursing and public health. Connecting the dots to prevent violence.* Washington, DC: American Medical Association. (On-line.) Available at: *http://www.ama-assn.org/violence.*

*Cowen, P. S. (2001). Elder mistreatment. In M. L. Mass, K. C. Buckwalter, M. D. Hardy, T. Tripp-Reimer, M. G. Titler, & J. P. Specht (Eds.), *Nursing care of older adults: Diagnoses, outcomes, & interventions* (pp. 93–114). St. Louis: Mosby.

*Dahlberg, L. L. (1998). Youth violence in the United States: Major trends, risk factors, and prevention approaches. *American Journal of Preventive Medicine, 14,* 259–272.

*Dahlberg, L. L., & Potter, L. B. (2001). Youth violence: Developmental pathways and prevention challenges. *American Journal of Preventive Medicine, 20,* (Suppl. 1), 3–14.

*Dean, A. L., Malik, M. M., Richards, W., & Stringer, S. A. (1986). Effects of parental maltreatment on children's conceptions of interpersonal relationships. *Developmental Psychology, 22,* 617–626.

*Deblinger, E., McLeer, S. V., Atkins, M. S., Ralphe, D., et al. (1989). Post-traumatic stress in sexually abused, physically abused, and nonabused children. *Child Abuse and Neglect, 13,* 403–408.

*Denham, S. A., Workman, E., Cole, P. M., Weissbrod, C., Kendziora, K. T., & Zahn-Waxler, C. (2000). Problems from early to middle childhood: The role of parental socialization and emotional expression. *Development and Psychopathology, 12,* 23–45.

*deVries C. (1997). Domestic violence: Impacting the nation's health care delivery system. *Nursing Trends & Issues, 2*(2) 1–9.

*Dodge, K. A. (2001). The science of youth violence prevention: Progressing from developmental epidemiology to efficacy to effectiveness to public policy. *American Journal of Preventive Medicine, 20,* (Suppl. 1), 63–70.

*Dodge, K. A., & Crick, N. R. (1990). Social information-processing bases of aggressive behavior in children. *Personality and Social Psychology Bulletin, 16,* 8–22.

*Donnerstein, E., Slaby, R. G., & Eron, L. D. (1997). The mass media and youth violence. In L. D. Eron, J. H. Gentry, & P. Schlegel (Eds.), *Reason to hope: A psychosoical perspective on violence and youth* (pp. 219–250). Washington, DC: American Psychological Association.

*Downey, G. & Walker, E. (1989). Social cognition and adjustment in children at risk for psychopathology. *Developmental Psychology, 25,* 835–845.

*Dutton, M., Mitchell, B., & Haywood, Y. (1996). The emergency department as a violence prevention center. *Journal of the American Medical Women's Association, 51,* 92–95, 117.

*Egeland, B., Sroufe, L. A, & Erickson, M. (1983). The developmental consequences of different patterns of maltreatment. *Child Abuse and Neglect, 7,* 459–469.

*Eggert, L. L., Thompson, E. A., Herting, J. R., & Nicholas, L. J. (1994). Prevention research program: Reconnecting at-risk youth. *Issues in Mental Health Nursing, 15,* 107–135.

*Elder, G. H., Eccles, J. S., Ardelt, M., & Lord, S. (1995). Inner-city parents under economic pressure: Perspectives on the strategies of parenting. *Journal of Marriage and the Family, 57,* 771–784.

*Elders, J. (1994). American violence is home grown. *Focus, 22*(4), 7.

*Elliot, D. S., Hamburg, B. A., & Williams, K.R. (Eds.). (1998). *Violence in American schools: A new perspective.* Cambridge, UK: Cambridge University Press.

*Fantuzzo, J. W., Borouch, R., Beriama, A., Atkins, M., & Marcus, S. (1997). Domestic violence and children: Prevalence and risk in five major U.S. cities. *Journal of the American Academy of Child & Adolescent Psychiatry, 36,* 116–122.

*Fantuzzo, J. W., & Mohr, W. K. (1999). Prevalence and effects of child exposure to domestic violence. *The Future of Children, 9*(3), 21–32.

*Farrell, A. D., & Bruce, S. E. (1997). Impact of exposure to community violence on violent behavior and emotional distress among urban adolescents. *Journal of Clinical Child Psychology, 26,* 2–14.

*Fishwick, N. (1995). Nursing care of domestic violence victims in acute and critical care settings. *AACN Clinical Issues, 6,* 63–69.

*Ford, J. D., & Kidd, P. (1998). Early childhood trauma and disorders of extreme stress as predictors of treatment outcome with chronic posttraumatic stress disorder. *Journal of Traumatic Stress, 11,* 743–761.

*French, G. D., & Harris, C. J. (1999). *Traumatic incident reduction (TIR).* New York: CRC Press.

*Friederich, W. N., Einbender, A. J., & Luecke, W. J. (1983). Cognitive and behavioral characteristics of physically abused children. *Journal of Consulting and Clinical Psychology, 51,* 313–314.

*Fulmer, T. T. (1999). Elder mistreatment. In J. T. Stone, J. F. Wyman, & S. A. Salisbury (Eds.), *Clinical gerontological nursing: A guide to advanced practice* (2nd ed., pp. 665–678). Philadelphia: W. B. Saunders.

*Giblin, P. T., Starr, R. H., & Agronow, S. I. (1984). Affective behavior of abused and control children: Comparisons of parent–child interactions and the influence of home environment variables. *The Journal of Genetic Psychology, 144,* 69–82.

*Greenberg, M., Domitrovich, C., & Bumbarger, B. (1999). Preventing mental disorders in school-age children: A review of the effectiveness of prevention programs. Prevention Research Center for the Promotion of Human Development, Pennsylvania State University. (On-line.) Available at: http://www.psu.edu/dept/prevention. Accessed September 2001.

*Gremillion, D., & Kanof, E. (1996). Overcoming barriers to physician involvement in identifying and referring victims of domestic violence. *Annals of Emergency Medicine, 27,* 769–773.

Gross, D., Fogg, L., & Tucker, S. (1995). The efficacy of parent training for promoting positive parent–toddler relationships. *Research in Nursing and Health, 18,* 489–499.

*Groth, A. N. (1979). *Men who rape.* New York: Plenum.

*Group for the Advancement of Psychiatry, Committee on Preventive Psychiatry. (1999). Violent behavior in children and youth: Preventive intervention from a psychiatric perspective. *Journal of the American Academy of Child and Adolescent Psychiatry, 38,* 235–241.

*Grunfeld, A., Ritmiller, S., Mackay, K., Cowan, L., & Hatch, D. (1994). Detecting domestic violence against women in the emergency department: A nursing triage model. *Journal of Emergency Nursing, 20,* 271–274.

*Guerra, N. G., Attar, B., & Weissberg, R. P. (1997). Prevention of aggression and violence among inner-city youths. In D. M. Stoff, J. Breiling, & J. D. Maser (Eds.), *Handbook of antisocial violence* (pp. 375–383). New York: John Wiley.

*Guerra, N.G., Huessman, L. R., & Hanish, L. (1995). The role of normative beliefs in children's social behavior. In N. Eisenberg (Ed.), *Review of personality and social psychology: Vol. 15. Social development* (pp. 140–158). Thousand Oaks, CA: Sage.

*Halverson, K. C., Elliot, B. A., Rubin, M. S., & Chadwick, D. L. (1993). Legal considerations in cases of child abuse. *Primary Care, 20,* 407–415.

*Haskett, M. E., & Kistner, I. A. (1991). Social interactions and peer perceptions of young physically abused children. *Child Development, 62,* 979–990.

*Hinderliter, D., Pitula, C, & Delaney, K. R. (1998). Partner violence. *The American Journal for Nurse Practitioners, 2,* 32–40.

*Herman, J. L. (1992). *Trauma and recovery.* New York: Basic Books.

*Herman, J. L. (1993). Sequelae of prolonged and repeated trauma: Evidence for a complex posttraumatic syndrome (DESNOS). In J. R. T. Davidson, & E. D. Foa (Eds.), *Post-traumatic stress disorder: DSM-IV and beyond* (pp. 213–228). Washington, DC: American Psychiatric Press.

*Hoff, L. (1993). Battered women: Intervention and prevention—a psychosociocultural perspective: Part 2. *Journal of the American Academy of Nurse Practitioners, 5,* 34–39.

*Hogstel, M. O., & Curry, L. C. (1999). Elder abuse revisited. *Journal of Gerontological Nursing, 25*(7), 10–18.

*Holden, G.W., & Ritchie, K. L. (1991). Linking extreme marital discord, child rearing, and child behavior problems: Evidence from battered women. *Child Development, 62,* 311–327.

*Holtz, H., & Furniss, K. (1993). The health care provider's role in domestic violence. *Trends in Health Care, Law & Ethics, 8*(2), 47–53.

*Howes, C., & Ritchie, S. (1999). Attachment organizations in children with difficult life circumstances. *Development and Psychopathology, 11*, 251–268.

*Huffman, L. C., Mehlinger, S. E., & Kerivan, A. S. (2000). Risk factors for academic and behavioral problems at the beginning of school. In Child Mental Health Foundations and Agencies Network (Ed.), *Off to a good start: Research on the risk factors for early school problems and selected federal policies affecting children's social and emotional development and their readiness for school.* Chapel Hill, NC: University of North Carolina, FPG Child Development Center.

*Hughes, H. M., Parkinson, D., & Vargo, M. (1989). Witnessing spouse abuse and experiencing physical abuse: A "double whammy"? *Journal of Family Violence, 4*, 197–209.

*Illinois Department of Public Health (IDPH). (1993). *Domestic violence.* Springfield, IL: Author.

*Jaffe, P. G., Hurley, D. J., & Wolfe, D. A. (1990). Children's observations of violence: Critical issues in child development and intervention planning. *Canadian Journal of Psychiatry, 35*, 466–470.

*Jaffe, P. G., Wolfe, D. A., & Wilson, S. K. (1990). *Children of battered women.* Newbury Park, CA: Sage.

*Jaffe, P. G., Wolfe, D. A., Wilson, S. K., & Zak, L. (1986). Family violence and child adjustment: A comparative analysis of girls' and boys' behavioral symptoms. *American Journal of Psychiatry, 143*, 74–77.

*Jerzierski, M. (1994). Abuse of women by male partners: Basic knowledge for emergency nurses. *Journal of Emergency Nursing, 20*, 361–371.

*Joint Commission Accreditation on Hospital Organizations (JCAHO). (1997). *Comprehensive accreditation manual for hospitals* (Standard PE 1.8). Oak Brook, IL: Author.

*Kaufmann, M. (1997). Decreasing the burden of trauma for victims of violence. *Annals of Emergency Medicine, 30*, 199–203.

*Kavanagh, K. A., Youngblade, L., Reid, J. B., & Fagot, B. I. (1988). Interaction between children and abusive versus control parents. *Journal of Clinical Child Psychology, 17*, 137–142.

*King, M., Torres, S., Campbell, D., Ryan, J., Sheridan, D., Ulrich, Y., et al. (1993). Violence and abuse of women: A perinatal health care issue. *AWHONN's Clinical Issues in Perinatal & Women's Health Nursing, 4*, 163–172.

*Koss, M. P. (1988). Hidden rape: Incidence, prevalence, and descriptive characteristics of sexual aggression and victimization in a national sample of college students. In A. W. Burgess (Ed.), *Sexual assault: Vol. 2* (pp. 3–25). New York: Garland.

*Krug, E. G., Powell, K. E., & Dahlberg, L. I. (1998). Firearm-related deaths in the United States and 35 other high- and upper-middle income countries. *International Journal of Epidemiology, 27*, 214–221.

*Lent, B. (1997). Responding to our abused patients. *CMA Journal, 157*, 1539–1540.

*Loring, M., & Smith, R. (1994). Health care barriers and interventions for battered women. *Public Health Reports, 109*, 328–338.

*McFarlane, J., Greenberg, L., Weltge, A., & Watson, M. (1995). Identification of abuse in emergency departments: Effectiveness of a two-question screening tool. *Journal of Emergency Nursing, 21*(5), 391–394.

*Mercy, J. A., Rosenberg, M. L., Powell, K. E., Broome, C. V., & Roper, W. L. (1993). Public health policy for preventing violence. *Health Affairs, 12*, 7–29.

*Mitchell, J. T., & Everly, G. S. (1996). *Critical incident stress debriefing: An operations manual for the prevention of traumatic stress among emergency services and disaster workers* (2nd ed., revised). Ellicott City, MD: Chevron Publishing.

*Mohr, W.K., Lutz, M. J., Fantuzzo, J. W., & Perry, M. A. (2000). Children exposed to family violence: A review of empirical research from a developmental–ecological perspective. *Trauma, Violence, & Abuse, 1*, 264–283.

*Moschella, J., & Wilson, D. (1997). Domestic violence: Recognize abuse and do something about it. *Journal of Emergency Medicine, 22*(12), 46–50.

*Moss, V., Pitula, C., & Halstead, L. (1997). The experience of terminating an abusive relationship from an Anglo and African-American perspective: A qualitative descriptive study. *Issues of Mental Health Nursing, 18*, 433–454.

*Mountrose, P., & Mountrose, J. (2000). *Getting thru to your emotions with EFT.* Sacramento: Holistic Communications.

*Myers, W., Scott, K., Burgess, A., & Burgess, A. (1995). Psychopathology, biopsychopathology factors, crime characteristics, and classification of 25 homicidal youths. *Journal of the American Academy of Child and Adolescent Psychiatry, 34*, 1483–1489.

*National Center for Educational Statistics (1998). *U.S. Department of Education: Indicators of school crime and safety.* Washington, DC: Author.

*National Institute of Justice, & Centers for Disease Control and Prevention. (1998). *Prevalence, incidence, and consequences of violence against women survey.* Washington DC: U.S. Government Printing Office.

*National Institute of Mental Health (NIMH). (2000). Child and adolescent violence research at NIMH. (On-line.) Available at: *http://nimh.nih.gov/publicat/violenseresfact. cfm.* Accessed June 2000.

*National Research Council. (1993). *Understanding child abuse and neglect.* Washington, DC: National Academy of Sciences.

*Nix, R. L., Pinderhughes, E. E., Dodge, K. A., Bates, J. E., Pettit, G. S., & McFadyen-Ketchum, S. A. (1999). The relation between mothers' hostile attribution tendencies and children's externalizing behavior problems: The mediating role of mothers' harsh discipline practices. *Child Development, 70*, 896–909.

*NOW Legal Defense and Education Fund. (1995). *The Violence Against Women Act.* New York: Author.

*O'Keefe, M (1995). Predictors of child abuse in maritally violent families. *Journal of Interpersonal Violence, 10*(1), 3–25.

*Office of the Surgeon General (2001). Youth violence: A report of the Surgeon General. (On-line.) Available at: *http:// www.surgeongeneral.gov/library/youthviolence/youvioreport. htm.* Accessed September 2001.

*Olds, D. L., Henderson, C. R., Cole, R., Eckenrode, J., Kitzman, H., Luckey, D., et al. (1997). Long-term effects of nurse home visitation on children's criminal and antisocial behavior: Fifteen-year follow-up of a randomized trial. *Journal of the American Medical Association, 280*, 1238–1244.

*Osofsky, J. D. (1995a). Children who witness domestic violence: The invisible victims. *Social Policy Report, 9*, 1–19.

*Osofsky, J. D. (1995b). The effects of exposure to violence on young children. *American Psychologist, 50,* 782–788.

*Osofsky, J. D., Werers, S., Hann, D. M., & Fick, A. C. (1993). Chronic community violence: What is happening to our children? *Psychiatry, 56,* 36–45.

*Parnell, L. (1999). *EMDR in the treatment of adults abused as children*. New York: W.W. Norton.

*Patterson, G. R. (1982). *A social learning approach to family interaction: Vol 3. Coercive family process*. Eugene, OR: Castalia.

*Poirier L. (1997). The importance of screening for domestic violence in all women. *The Nurse Practitioner, 22*(5), 105–122.

*Prino, C. T., & Peyrot, M. (1994). The effect of child physical abuse and neglect on aggressive, withdrawn, and prosocial behavior. *Child Abuse and Neglect, 18,* 871–884.

*Quay, H. C. (1997). Inhibition and attention deficit hyperactivity disorder. *Journal of Abnormal Child Psychology, 25,* 7–13.

*Reid, J. B. (1993). Prevention of conduct disorder before and after school entry: Relating interventions to developmental findings. *Development and Psychopathology, 5,* 243–262.

*Reid, S., & Glasser, M. (1997). Primary care physicians' recognition of and attitudes toward domestic violence. *Academic Medicine, 72,* 51–53.

*Richters, J. E., & Martinez, P. (1993). The NIMH community violence project: I. Children as victims of and witnesses to violence. *Psychiatry, 56,* 7–21.

*Russell, D. E. H. (1991). Wife rape. In A. Parrot, & L. Bechhofer (Eds.), *Acquaintance rape: The hidden crime* (pp. 129–139). New York: John Wiley.

*Saltzman, L. E., Fanslow, J. L., McMahon, P. M., & Shelly, G. A. (1999). *Intimate partner violence surveillance: Uniform definitions and recommended data elements* (Version 1.0). Atlanta: Centers for Disease Control.

*Schneider-Rosen, K., & Cicchetti, D. (1991). Early self-knowledge and emotional development: Visual self-recognition and affective reactions to mirror self-images in maltreated and non-maltreated toddlers. *Developmental Psychology, 27,* 471–478.

*Schorstein, S. (1997). *Domestic violence and health care: What every professional needs to know*. Thousand Oaks, CA: Sage.

*Shapiro, F. (1995). *Eye movement desensitization and reprocessing: Basic principles, protocols, and procedures*. New York: Guilford.

*Short, L. M., Johnson, D., & Osattin, A. (1998). Recommended components of health care provider training programs on intimate partner violence. *American Journal of Preventive Medicine, 14,* 283–288.

*Suh, E. K., & Abel, EM (1990). The impact of spousal violence on the children of the abused. *Journal of Independent Social Work, 4*(4), 27–34.

*Thornton, T. N., Craft, C. A., Dahlberg, L. L., Lynch, B. S., & Baer, K. (2000). *Best practices of youth violence prevention: A sourcebook for community action*. Atlanta: Centers for Disease Control and Prevention, National Center for Injury Prevention and Control.

*Thurston, W., & McLeod, L. (1997). Teaching second-year medical students about wife battering. *Women's Health Issues, 7,* 92–97.

*Tilden, V., Schmidt, T., Limandri, B., Chiodo, G., Garland, M., & Loveless, P. (1994). Factors that influence clinicians' assessment and management of family violence. *American Journal of Public Health, 84,* 628–633.

*Ulrich, Y. (1993). What helped most in leaving spouse abuse: Implications for interventions. *AWHONNS Clinical Issues in Perinatal & Women's Health Nursing, 4,* 385–390.

*Uphold, C. R., & Graham, M. V. (1998). *Clinical guidelines in family practice*. Gainesville, FL: Barmarrae Books.

*U.S. Department of Health and Human Services, National Center on Child Abuse and Neglect (1996). *Child maltreatment, 1994: Reports from the states to the National Center on Child Abuse and Neglect*. Washington, DC: U.S. Government Printing Office.

*U.S. Department of Justice. (1998). *Violence by intimates: Analysis of data on crimes by current or former spouses, boyfriends, and girlfriends*. Washington, DC: Author.

*U.S. Department of Justice. (2000). *National crime victimization survey*. Washington, DC: U.S. Government Printing Office.

*U.S. Department of Justice. (2001). Bureau of Justice statistics: Injuries from violent crimes 1992–1998. (On-line.) Available at: *http://www.ojp.usdoj.gov/bjs/pub/press/ivc98pr.htm*. Accessed September 10, 2001.

*U.S. Public Health Service. (1999). Healthy people 2000 national health promotion and disease prevention objectives. (On-line.) Available at: *http://odphp.osophs.dhhs.giv/pubs/hp2000*. Accessed April 4, 2000.

*Vondra, J. I., Barnett, D., & Cicchetti, D. (1990). Self-concept, motivation, and competence among preschoolers from maltreating and comparison families. *Child Abuse and Neglect, 14,* 525–540.

*Warshaw, C. (1993). Domestic violence: Challenges to medical practice. *Journal of Women's Health, 2,* 73–80.

*Warshaw, C. (1995). *Establishing an appropriate response to domestic violence in your practice, institution and community: Improving the health care response to domestic violence. A resource manual for health care providers*. San Francisco: The Family Violence Prevention Fund.

*Weith, M. E. (1994). Elder abuse: A national tragedy. *FBI Law Enforcement Bulletin, 63*(2), 24–26.

*Wolfe, D. A., Jaffe, P., Wilson, S. K., & Zak, L. (1985). Children of battered women: The relation of child behavior to family violence and maternal stress. *Journal of Consulting and Clinical Psychology, 53,* 657–665.

*Wolfe, D. A., & Mosk, M. D. (1983). Behavioral comparisons of children from abusive and distressed families. *Journal of Consulting & Clinical Psychology, 51,* 702–708.

*Wolfe, D. A., Zak, L., Wilson, S. K., & Jaffe, P. (1986). Child witness to violence: Critical issues in behavioral social adjustment. *Journal of Abnormal Child Psychology, 14,* 95–104.

Starred references are cited in text.

For additional information on this chapter, go to *http://connection.lww.com*.

Need more help? See Chapter 17 of the *Study Guide to Accompany Mohr: Johnson's Psychiatric-Mental Health Nursing*, 5th ed.

UNIT IV

Nursing Care for Clients With Psychiatric Disorders

The Client With an Anxiety Disorder

JUDITH A. GREENE

▼ KEY TERMS

Acute stress disorder—An anxiety disorder in which symptoms of post-traumatic stress disorder appear within 4 weeks of exposure to the trauma and usually last less than 3 months.

Agoraphobia—A marked fear of being alone or in a public place from which escape would be difficult or help would be unavailable in the event of becoming disabled.

Anxiety—A sense of psychological distress that may or may not have a focus; it is a state of apprehension that may represent a response to environmental stress or a physical disease state.

Anxiety disorder—A group of conditions in which the affected person experiences persistent anxiety that he or she cannot dismiss and that interferes with his or her daily activities.

Compulsions—Ritualistic behaviors that a person feels compelled to perform either in accord with a specific set of rules or in a routine manner.

Generalized anxiety disorder—An anxiety disorder characterized by chronic and excessive worry and anxiety more days than not for at least 6 months and involving many aspects of the person's life; the worry and anxiety cause such discomfort that they interfere with daily life and relationships.

Obsessions—Recurrent, intrusive, and persistent ideas, thoughts, images, or impulses.

Obsessive-compulsive disorder—An anxiety disorder marked by recurrent obsessions or compulsions that are time-consuming (taking more than 1 hour per day) or cause significant impairment or distress.

Panic attack—A discrete period of intense apprehension or terror without any real associated danger, accompanied by at least 4 of 13 somatic or cognitive symptoms.

Panic disorder—An anxiety disorder marked by recurrent, unexpected panic attacks that cause the affected person to persistently worry about

recurrences or complications from the attacks or to undergo behavioral changes in response to the attacks for at least 1 month.

Phobia—A persistent, irrational fear attached to an object or situation that objectively does not pose a significant danger.

Post-traumatic stress disorder—An anxiety disorder marked by the development of characteristic symptoms after exposure to a severe or extraordinary stressor (eg, a natural disaster, an accidental or intentional human-made disaster), in which there is actual or threatened death, serious injury, or maiming to the self or others; it occurs only in response to a traumatic life experience.

Social phobia—An anxiety disorder characterized by a persistent, irrational fear of and compelling desire to avoid situations in which the person may be exposed to unfamiliar people or to the scrutiny of others; fear of behaving in a way that may prove humiliating or embarrassing.

▼ LEARNING OBJECTIVES

On completion of this chapter, you should be able to accomplish the following:

■ Define the term *anxiety*.

■ Explain what is meant by *anxiety disorder*.

■ Describe the incidence and prevalence of anxiety disorders.

■ Discuss proposed etiologies for anxiety disorders.

■ Identify symptoms of anxiety disorders.

■ Explain the different types of anxiety disorders.

■ Discuss treatments for anxiety disorders.

■ Apply the nursing process to the care of clients with anxiety disorders.

▼ Clinical Example 18-1

Ruth, 37 years old, is married with three children. She was in a fast-food restaurant when a man armed with an automatic rifle entered and began shooting. Several people were killed instantly. The man walked over to where Ruth was huddled on the floor and pointed the gun in her face but did not shoot her. The police arrived and took the man into custody.

Six months have passed since the incident. Ruth was doing "pretty well" until recently. She now describes her level of anxiety as "very high" most days and states her life doesn't seem real to her. She has dreams about the gunman pointing the gun in her face and shooting her. She wakes up from these nightmares drenched in sweat with her heart pounding. When she drives by a fast-food restaurant, something she avoids at all costs, she feels panicky and confused. Sometimes, she imagines that she hears screaming. She states she has had headaches and fatigue since the incident, and she has been irritable.

This chapter discusses anxiety disorders. As you read the chapter, consider the case of Ruth in Clinical Example 18-1. How do Ruth's history and signs and symptoms relate to this group of disorders? You will learn more about the progression of Ruth's care in Nursing Care Plan 18-1. You will also have the opportunity to apply your understanding of this client and others with anxiety disorders in the Reflection and Critical Thinking Questions at the end of this chapter.

ANXIETY

Most people are familiar with **anxiety**, which can be described as a sense of psychological distress. People may feel anxious before a job interview, when a loved one doesn't arrive home at an expected time, or when they are alone on a dark street at night. Feeling anxious, frightened, uneasy, or worried are normal responses to threatening or dangerous events.

Anxiety can be differentiated from stress. Stress is not a disorder. It is a normal part of everyday life and is not necessarily good or bad. For example, stressors that one person perceives as threatening may be easily tolerated or enjoyed by others. Therefore, the feeling of stress as a negative emotional state is substantially based on the individual's appraisal of the stressor and assessment of his or her ability to respond to it. Still, stressors are frequently cited as causes of anxiety, and when the mind interprets events as threatening, it responds.

To cope effectively with stressful, anxiety-provoking situations, the brain initiates physiological mechanisms that prepare us to combat injury and either fight or flee (the *fight or flight response*, mediated by the sympathetic nervous system). These physiological changes have widespread effects on many body systems. During a fight or flight reaction:

- Heart rate and blood pressure increase.
- Blood flows to the muscles.

- Breathing rate increases.
- Perspiration increases.
- Blood clotting ability increases.
- Saliva production decreases.
- Digestion decreases.
- Immune response decreases.
- Energy-producing stored glycogen is released.

These physiologic responses are accompanied by psychological and cognitive reactions. Anxious people have feelings of nervousness, vague discomfort, uncertainty, self-doubt, apprehension, dread, or restlessness. They may find it hard to concentrate on anything other than the threat. Their senses are heightened.

These reactions are life-saving defense mechanisms in the short term and are particularly effective against physical threats. Many people, however, feel anxious about long-term situations that they cannot influence, have feelings of anxiety with no known trigger, or worry helplessly about events taking an unlikely catastrophic turn. Others may suffer panic attacks or feel extreme fear about items or creatures that most people take in stride. In these situations, anxiety can become debilitating and chronic, with the physiological, psychological, and cognitive effects becoming chronic as well.

The Continuum of Anxiety

Anxiety can be mild, moderate, or severe, affecting cognitive, psychological, and physical function accordingly. Mild anxiety results in improved functioning; however, as anxiety increases, people become less and less able to function. Cognitive functioning becomes distorted, and bodies must endure extended periods of high physical alert.

EFFECTS ON SENSATION

Anxiety affects the ways a person perceives and processes sensory input. Mild anxiety actually heightens sensory awareness (ie, sight, hearing, taste, smell, and touch). Moderate anxiety dulls perception; however, the person can attend to greater sensory input if directed to do so. In severe anxiety, perception becomes increasingly distorted, sensory input diminishes, and processing of sensory stimuli becomes scattered and disorganized. In panic, perception becomes grossly distorted. At the level of panic, the person is incapable of differentiating between real and imaginary stimuli.

EFFECTS ON COGNITION

Anxiety greatly influences *cognition,* the ability to concentrate, learn, and solve problems. Mild and moderate levels of anxiety are still conducive to concentration, learning, and problem solving. A person of average intelligence who is mildly to moderately anxious discerns relationships between and among concepts with relative ease and can concentrate and solve problems without much difficulty.

In contrast, severe anxiety hinders cognitive function. The severely anxious person (such as a client with an anxiety disorder) has difficulty concentrating and may fail to discern even obvious relationships among concepts. The panic-stricken person suffers even greater cognitive impairment; concentration, learning, and problem solving are virtually impossible during episodes of panic.

EFFECTS ON VERBAL ABILITY

In mild anxiety, speech content and form reflect heightened sensory awareness and cognitive function. Thoughts are verbalized logically; speech rate and volume are appropriate to the context of the content and communication. The mildly anxious person typically appears alert, confident, and relatively secure.

Verbal behavior of the moderately anxious person is commonly marked by frequent changes of topic, repetitive questioning, joking, and wordiness. *Blocking,* or loss of train of thought, may also occur. Speech rate often accelerates, and speech volume often increases. The moderately anxious person may change body position frequently, use excessive hand gestures, and assume aggressive body postures toward others. Furthermore, because moderately anxious people do not perceive and process sensory input as efficiently as mildly anxious people, they tend to hesitate and procrastinate in meeting routine social and vocational expectations. Such behaviors often present an overall picture of restlessness and discontent that may provoke feelings of irritation in others toward the anxious person.

The severely anxious person displays verbal behavior that indicates highly disordered perceptual and cognitive function. He or she may verbalize emotional pain through such assertions as "I can't stand this" or "I can't think" or by vociferously demanding help and relief. Nonverbal behavior typically involves fine and gross motor tremors, grimaces, and other forms of purposeless activity, such as pacing and hand-wringing. Severely anxious people present an overall picture of extreme emotional discomfort and behavioral disorganization.

Panic-level anxiety results in even greater emotional pain and behavioral disorganization. Verbal and nonverbal behaviors suggest a psychotic-like state in which the panic-stricken person is virtually helpless and cannot negotiate simple life demands. The person may scream and run wildly or cling tenaciously to something or someone he or she accurately or inaccurately perceives as a source of safety and security. Protective and calming measures must be initiated promptly, because a prolonged panic state is incompatible with life.

Normal Versus Abnormal Anxiety

All the behaviors described previously are normal in certain situations. Even panic may be a normal response to terrifying, life-threatening situations. When does anxiety become a psychiatric disorder?

Pathological anxiety is suspected if a person feels anxious when no real threat exists, when a threat has passed long ago but continues to impair the person's functioning, or when a person substitutes adaptive coping mechanisms with maladaptive ones. Other clues that suggest that a person needs treatment include the following:

- Anxiety of greater-than-expected intensity
- Anxiety that prevents fulfillment of professional, personal, or social roles
- Anxiety accompanied by flashbacks, obsessions, or compulsions
- Anxiety that causes a curtailment of daily or social activities
- Anxiety that lasts longer than expected

Unrelieved anxiety causes physical and emotional problems, and individuals may use a variety of coping mechanisms (adaptive or maladaptive) to try to manage the anxiety. Box 18-1 lists some of these behaviors. Persistent or recurrent anxiety, however, should be evaluated to determine if the client is suffering from an anxiety disorder.

ANXIETY DISORDERS

The term **anxiety disorder** refers to a group of conditions in which the affected person experiences persistent anxiety that he or she cannot dismiss and that interferes with his or her daily activities. Persons who have anxiety disorders feel that the core of their personalities is being threatened, even when no actual danger exists.

The first surgeon general's report on mental health and mental illness confirmed widespread evidence of anxiety disorders in the United States (U.S. Public Health Service, 1999). According to this report, more than 19 million Americans suffer from an anxiety disorder each year, making anxiety disorders the most common or frequently occurring of all psychiatric syndromes. Estimates are that 13% of children and adolescents, 16.4% of adults

---

BOX 18-1 ▼ *Adaptive and Maladaptive Patterns for Coping With Anxiety*

- Withdrawal: Retreat from anxiety-provoking experiences
- Acting out: Discharge of anxiety through aggressive behavior
- Psychosomatization: Visceral or physiologic expression of anxiety
- Avoidance: Management of anxiety-laden experiences through evasive behaviors
- Problem solving: Systematic method for addressing difficult situations

aged 18 to 54 years, and 19.8% of adults aged 55 years or older have an anxiety disorder (U.S. Public Health Service, 1999).

Anxiety disorders cost the United States more than $42 billion each year. They appear to affect women more often than men. Estimates are that these disorders are often misdiagnosed and undertreated, thus compounding the problems they cause those affected by them (Greenberg et al., 1999; U.S. Public Health Service, 1999).

Currently, there are two major barriers to the care of clients with anxiety disorders. One is lack of knowledge in the general population regarding the nature of anxiety disorders, their prevalence, and their responsiveness to effective treatment. The other barrier is the social stigma that many people still attach to psychiatric illnesses and that prevent people from obtaining prompt treatment before complications arise (U.S. Public Health Service, 1999). Despite these barriers, continuity of care for individuals with anxiety disorders is essential to prevent comorbidity and complications arising from misdiagnosis and inadequate treatment (Aveline, 1997; Candilis et al., 1999; Rief, Trenkamp, Auer, & Fitcher, 2000).

Anxiety disorders include generalized anxiety disorder, phobias, panic attacks, panic disorder, obsessive-compulsive disorder (OCD), post-traumatic stress disorder (PTSD), and acute stress disorder. Each of these conditions will be discussed in more detail later in the chapter.

Etiology

According to current research, anxiety disorders have several possible causes. Any of the contributing factors alone or in combination could be determining factors in their occurrences.

NEUROBIOLOGICAL THEORIES

Hereditary predisposition plays a factor in the development of anxiety disorders. Almost 50% of all persons with panic disorder have a relative who also has it, and twin studies have shown a genetic component to OCD and panic disorder. The biological vulnerability to certain anxiety disorders varies from person to person. In the case of clients who have a family history of panic disorder, evidence suggests that their heritable neuronal state may generate a lower threshold for spontaneous emergency response episodes. This vulnerability may never be stressed, however, and a person with the same family history may not develop the disorder. Brain chemistry and developmental factors also play a role. Studies have shown that variations in the autonomic nervous system or noradrenergic system may cause some people to experience anxiety to a greater degree than others. Other studies have revealed that abnormalities in the regulation of substances such as serotonin and gamma-aminobutyric acid (GABA) may play a role in the development of anx-

iety disorders (Alsobrook & Pauls, 1994; Anagnostars & Craske, 1999; Black, 1995; Taylor & Livesley, 1995; Unnewehr, Schneider, Florin, & Margraf, 1998).

Fear and anxiety are also influenced and mediated by several interacting brain structures. The *amygdala* serves as a communications center between the parts of the brain that process sensory input and the parts that interpret this input. The amygdala can identify incoming sensory information as threatening and then instigate feelings of anxiety or fear. Also, it is theorized that emotional memories stored in the central part of the amygdala play a role in phobic disorders, while other parts of the amygdala are involved in other forms of anxiety. The amygdala also coordinates fear, memory, and emotion with heart rate, blood pressure, and other physical responses to stressful events.

Other structures thought to play a role in anxiety disorders are the *hippocampus,* which is responsible for processing threatening stimuli and plays a role in encoding this information into memories; the *locus ceruleus,* another area of the brain that will initiate a response to danger and that may be overactive in some people, making them more vulnerable to an anxiety disorder; and the *striatum,* an area of the brain involved with motor control and thought to be involved in OCD. Additional biologic factors that may contribute to the onset of anxiety disorders include physical illness (Box 18-2); exposure to substances such as cocaine, amphetamines, and caffeine (Box 18-2); and exposure to physical or psychological danger, trauma, or both (Dohrenwend, 2000; Maxmen, 1995).

PSYCHOLOGICAL THEORIES

Psychodynamic factors appear to play a role in the development of anxiety disorders. Empirical research has shown that many clients with anxiety disorder share certain features, including low self-esteem, a shy or timid nature in childhood, parents who were perceived as critical or angry, and discomfort with aggression. Long-term exposure to abuse, violence, or poverty may affect a person's susceptibility to anxiety disorders.

According to learning theory, anxiety results from conditioning, by which a person develops an anxious response by linking a dangerous or fear-inducing event (eg, a house fire) with a neutral event (eg, watching someone light a match) (see Chap. 3). In cases of general anxiety, a person may learn the anxiety response when he or she begins to liken any anxious symptoms with a full-fledged anxiety attack, causing a vicious anxiety cycle to continue.

Cognitive theorists see anxiety as a manifestation of distorted thinking and suggest that the individual's perception or attitude overestimates the danger. According to these theorists, many people with anxiety have an exaggerated need for approval and may begin to view even the most minor mistakes as catastrophes.

BOX 18-2 ▼ *Medical Disorders and Substances Associated With Anxiety*

Medical Disorders

Asthma
Cancer
Cardiac dysrhythmias
Chronic obstructive pulmonary disease
Collagen-vascular disease
Congestive heart failure
Coronary insufficiency
Cushing's syndrome
Epilepsy
Huntington's disease
Hypertension
Hyperthyroidism
Hypoglycemia
Hypothyroidism

Menopause
Multiple sclerosis
Organic brain syndrome
Pheochromocytoma
Premenstrual syndrome
Vestibular dysfunction
Wilson's disease

Substances

Anticholinergics
Caffeine
Cocaine
Hallucinogens
Steroids
Sympathomimetics

Signs and Symptoms/Diagnostic Criteria

While anxiety disorders are generally considered less serious than the personality disorders and major psychoses, they can be just as disabling. The following section focuses on the signs and symptoms of various anxiety disorders. This chapter's Information Map shows the criteria specified by the American Psychiatric Association's (APA) *Diagnostic and Statistical Manual of Mental Disorders* (4th ed., text rev.) (*DSM–IV–TR*) for the anxiety disorders discussed in this chapter.

GENERALIZED ANXIETY DISORDER

Generalized anxiety disorder (GAD) is usually characterized by chronic and excessive worry and anxiety more days than not, occurring for at least 6 months and involving many aspects of the person's life (APA, 2000). The worry and anxiety of this disorder cause such discomfort that they interfere with the client's daily life and relationships. Seldom do people suffering from this disorder experience eruptions of acute anxiety (Maxmen, 1995). Rather, they persistently exhibit signs of severe anxiety, such as motor tension, autonomic hyperactivity, and apprehensive expectation. Some clients may also exhibit chronic hypervigilance for potential threats. Displays of impatience and irritability and complaints of feeling "on edge" are common (Morrison, 1995).

Because of this tense hyperarousal, the person may be unable to concentrate, suffer chronic fatigue, and experience sleep pattern disturbances. Additionally, he or she may exhibit tenseness and distractibility in social situations. For these reasons, this disorder eventually may lead to depression (Maxmen, 1995; Morrison, 1995).

▼ *Clinical Example 18-2*

For most of her adult life, Marcia, 34 years old, has been a "worrywart." She still has nightmares about dropping out of college, even though she graduated with honors at age 22. Recently, she has become more anxious than usual, feeling that she is about to "fall off the edge of a precipice."

One year ago, Marcia was promoted to assistant buyer at a large upscale department store. "I took this position because I thought it was a great opportunity to move up the corporate ladder," she tells the nurse. She adds, "Little did I realize that I would feel so uptight, afraid of getting in over my head. My boss has no patience and wants everything done yesterday."

Marcia also complains of difficulty concentrating at work. Her primary care practitioner had prescribed diazepam (Valium) for her initially. Marcia, however, felt too drowsy while taking this medication and stopped using it. She never has had a panic attack, but she reports considerable irritation with her husband and children. Marcia also complains of insomnia. She denies depression and reports that she experiences pleasure from her ceramics class and during sex with her husband.

Marcia tried relaxation exercises and meditation but found these only added to her opportunities to dwell on job worries. Her husband encouraged her to drink a glass or two of wine before or during dinner. She found this pleasurable and that it initially relieved her job anxieties; however, Marcia soon became fearful of becoming an alcoholic.

(example continues on page 357)

⮞ Prevalence

Approximately 13% of children and adolescents, 16% of adults aged 18 to 54 years, and 20% of adults aged 55 years or older have an anxiety disorder

⮞ Risk and Contributing Factors

- Gender: women are twice as likely than are men to have an anxiety disorder
- Ethnicity: obsessive-compulsive disorder more common in whites than in Hispanics or African Americans
- Being separated or divorced
- Having experienced childhood physical or sexual abuse
- Low socioeconomic status
- Family history of similar disorders
- Substance or stimulant abuse

⮞ Summary of DSM-IV-TR Diagnostic Criteria

Acute Stress Disorder

- Client has been exposed to a traumatic event with both of the following:
  1. Experiencing, witnessing, or being confronted with an event involving actual or potential death, serious injury, or a threat to the physical integrity of self or others
  2. Response involved intense fear, helplessness, or horror
- Either during or after the event, client has at least three of the following:
  1. Numbing, detachment, no emotion
  2. Reduced awareness (e.g., "being in a daze")
  3. Derealization
  4. Depersonalization
  5. Dissociative amnesia (e.g., cannot recall an important aspect of the trauma)
- Client persistently re-experiences the trauma through recurrent images, thoughts, dreams, illusions, flashbacks, or a sense of reliving the experience. Or he or she is distressed when exposed to reminders.
- Client markedly avoids stimuli that remind him or her of the trauma.
- Client has marked symptoms of anxiety or increased arousal (e.g., difficulty sleeping, irritability, hypervigilance).
- The disturbance causes significant distress or impairs social, occupational, or other important areas of functioning or ability to pursue a necessary task.
- The disturbance lasts at least 2 days but no more than 4 weeks; it occurs within 4 weeks of the traumatic event.
- The disturbance is not the direct physiologic result of a substance or a medical condition, is not better accounted for by Brief Psychotic Disorder, and is not merely an exacerbation of a pre-existing disorder.

Generalized Anxiety Disorder

- Client has excessive anxiety and worry (apprehensive expectation) more days than not for at least 6 months about several events or activities (e.g., work, school).
- Client finds controlling the worry is difficult.
- The anxiety and worry are associated with three (or more) of the following symptoms (with at least some present more days than not for the past 6 months). **Note:** Only one item is required in children.
  1. Feeling restless, keyed up, or on edge
  2. Being easily fatigued
  3. Difficulty concentrating or mind going blank
  4. Irritability
  5. Muscle tension
  6. Sleep disturbance
- Anxiety and worry are not confined to features of an Axis I disorder.
- Anxiety, worry, or physical symptoms cause significant distress or impair social, occupational, or other important areas of functioning.
- The disturbance is not caused by a substance or a medical condition and does not occur exclusively during a mood, psychotic, or pervasive developmental disorder

Panic Disorder

- Client experiences both:
  1. Recurrent unexpected panic attacks
  2. After at least one attack, 1 month (or more) of one (or more) of the following:
     a. Concern about more attacks
     b. Worry about the implications of the attack or its consequences
     c. Significant related behavior change
- Panic attacks are not caused by substance use or a medical condition.
- Panic attacks are not better explained by another psychiatric disorder.

The two types are **without agoraphobia** and **with agoraphobia**.

Anxiety Disorders Information Map *(Continued)*

Post-Traumatic Stress Disorder

- Client has been exposed to a traumatic event with both of the following:
  1. Experiencing, witnessing, or being confronted with actual or potential death, serious injury, or threatened physical integrity of self or others
  2. Response involved intense fear, helplessness, or horror. **Note:** Children may display disorganized or agitated behavior.
- Client persistently re-experiences the trauma in one (or more) of the following ways:
  1. Recurrent and intrusive distressing recollections, including images, thoughts, or perceptions. **Note:** Young children may engage in repetitive play that uses themes or aspects of the trauma.
  2. Recurrent distressing dreams of the event. **Note:** Children may have frightening dreams without recognizable content.
  3. Acting or feeling as if the trauma were recurring (e.g., reliving the event, illusions, hallucinations, and "flashbacks," including those on awakening or when intoxicated).
  4. Intense psychological distress at exposure to cues that resemble the trauma
  5. Physical reactivity when exposed to cues that resemble the trauma
- Client persistently avoids stimuli associated with the trauma. General responsiveness is numb (not present before the trauma), as indicated by at least three of the following:
  1. Efforts to avoid thinking, feeling, or talking about the trauma
  2. Efforts to avoid activities, places, or people that remind him or her of the trauma
  3. Inability to recall an important aspect of the trauma
  4. Greatly diminished interest or participation in significant activities
  5. Feeling detached or estranged from others
  6. Restricted range of affect
  7. Sense of a short future (e.g., does not expect to have a career, normal life span)
- Symptoms of increased arousal (not present before the trauma) persist, as indicated by at least two of the following:
  1. Difficulty falling or staying asleep
  2. Irritability or anger
  3. Difficulty concentrating
  4. Hypervigilance
  5. Exaggerated startle response
- Symptoms last more than 1 month.

- The disturbance causes significant distress or impairs social, occupational, or other important areas of functioning.

Agoraphobia

- Client is anxious about places or situations from which escape might be difficult or embarrassing or in which help might be unavailable during a panic attack or panic-like symptoms. Typical fears involve being outside the home alone, in a crowd, on a bridge, or in a bus or train.
- Client avoids situations (e.g., restricts travel), endures them with marked distress, or requires a companion to participate.
- The anxiety or avoidance is not better explained by another mental disorder.

Obsessive-Compulsive Disorder

- Client has either obsessions or compulsions:
  Obsessions:
  1. Recurrent and persistent thoughts, impulses, or images that, at some time during the disturbance, are intrusive and inappropriate and cause marked distress
  2. The thoughts, impulses, or images are not simply excessive worries about real problems.
  3. Client tries to ignore, suppress, or neutralize with some other thought or action such thoughts, impulses, or images.
  4. Client recognizes that the thoughts, impulses, or images are a product of his or her own mind.
  Compulsions:
  1. Repetitive behaviors (e.g., handwashing, ordering) or mental acts (e.g., praying, counting) that the client feels driven to perform in response to an obsession, or according to rigidly applied rules
  2. The behaviors or mental acts aim to prevent or reduce distress or some dreaded situation; however, they either are not realistically connected with what they are designed to neutralize or prevent or are clearly excessive.
- Client recognizes the obsessions or compulsions are excessive or unreasonable. **Note:** This does not apply to children.
- Obsessions or compulsions cause marked distress, are time-consuming (more than 1 hour a day), or significantly interfere with occupation, education, activities, or relationships.
- If client has another mental disorder, the content of obsessions or compulsions is not restricted to it (e.g., food preoccupation with an eating disorder).

(continued)

Anxiety Disorders Information Map *(Continued)*

- The disturbance is not caused by a substance or a medical condition.

Panic Attack

Client experiences a discrete period of intense discomfort or fear, with at least four of the following symptoms developing abruptly and reaching a peak within 10 minutes:

- Palpitations, pounding heart, or accelerated heart rate
- Sweating
- Trembling or shaking
- Smothering or shortness of breath
- Feeling of choking
- Chest pain or discomfort
- Abdominal distress or nausea
- Feeling dizzy, unsteady, lightheaded, or faint
- Derealization or depersonalization
- Fear of losing control or going crazy
- Fear of dying
- Paresthesias (numbness or tingling)
- Chills or hot flushes

Specific Phobia

- Client has a marked, persistent, excessive or unreasonable fear, cued by the presence or anticipation of a specific object or situation.
- Exposure to the object almost always causes immediate anxiety, which may be a situationally bound or predisposed panic attack. **Note:** Children may cry, throw tantrums, freeze, or cling.
- Client recognizes the fear is excessive or unreasonable. **Note:** Children may not display this feature.
- Client avoids the phobic stimulus or endures it with intense distress.
- The resulting avoidance or distress interferes greatly with activities, occupation, education, or relationships, or the phobia greatly distresses the client.

- In clients younger than 18 years, the duration is at least 6 months.
- The resulting avoidance or distress is not better explained by another mental disorder.

Types include *Natural Environment* (e.g., heights, water); *Blood-Injection-Injury; Situational* (e.g., airplanes, enclosed places); and *Other* (e.g., fear of choking or contracting an illness; in children, fear of loud sounds or costumed characters).

Social Phobia

- Client markedly and persistently fears one or more social/performance situations that expose him or her to unfamiliar people or possible scrutiny. Client fears acting in a humiliating or embarrassing way or showing anxiety symptoms. **Note:** Children must also show a capacity for age-appropriate relationships with familiar people, and anxiety must occur with peers, not just with adults.
- Exposure to the feared situation almost always causes anxiety, which may take the form of a panic attack. **Note:** Children may cry, throw tantrums, freeze, or shrink from people.
- Client recognizes the fear is excessive or unreasonable. **Note:** In children, this feature may be absent.
- Client avoids feared situations or else endures them with intense anxiety or distress.
- Resulting avoidance or distress interferes significantly with occupation, education, activities, or relationships. Or client is distressed about having the phobia.
- In clients younger than age 18 years, the duration is at least 6 months.
- Resulting avoidance or distress is not caused by a substance or medical condition and is not better explained by another mental disorder.
- If client has a medical condition or another mental disorder, the fear is unrelated to it.

➡ Prevention Strategies

- Screen all clients for anxiety disorders. If a client mentions feeling especially stressed or nervous, explore the issues with him or her. Several factors, either "happy" (e.g., wedding, birth of a child) or sad (e.g., death in the family, job loss) could precipitate anxiety or an anxiety disorder or its recurrence. Discuss what is happening in the client's life.
- If a client thinks that he or she is already experiencing symptoms and fears "going crazy," reassure the client that the symptoms are real, and that treatment can help.
- Become more informed about anxiety disorders, and encourage clients to do so as well. Understanding in the form of teaching and education can help clients feel more in control.
- Refer clients to organizations that provide materials about and support for those with anxiety disorders.

(continued)

Anxiety Disorders Information Map *(Continued)*

- If the client has not yet approached a physician about signs or symptoms, encourage him or her to speak with the doctor about treatments,
- For clients taking medication to control existing anxiety disorders, stress the importance of following the medication regimen and reporting any problems to their doctor or pharmacist.
- For all clients who discuss feeling "stressed" or anxious, explore the use of relaxation techniques such as meditation.

➡ *Want to Know More?*

Anxiety Disorders Association of America
11900 Parklawn Drive
Suite 100
Rockville, MD 20852
(301) 231-9350
E-mail: AnxDis@adaa.org
http://www.adaa.org/

Association for the Advancement of Behavior Therapy
305 7th Ave.
16th Floor
New York, NY 10001-6008
(212) 647-1890
http://www.aabt.org

National Anxiety Foundation
3135 Custer Dr.
Lexington, KY 40517-4001
(606) 272-7166
http://lexington-on-line.com/naf.html

Diagnostic criteria adapted with permission from the American Psychiatric Association. (2000). *Diagnostic and statistical manual of mental disorders* (4th ed., text revision). Washington, DC: Author.

Marcia complains of a nagging uneasiness and sense of dread. She denies obsessions, compulsions, phobias, delusions, and hallucinations. She scores a 30 out of 30 on the Mini-Mental Status Examination. Her speech is clear, coherent, relevant, and spontaneous. She looks apprehensive, though she is well dressed and somewhat fidgety.

Points for Reflection and Critical Thinking

- What additional data would you consider exploring with Marcia? Explain your answer.
- In what ways can nurses help their clients separate valid concerns from things that are causing them unnecessary anxiety?

PHOBIC DISORDERS

A **phobia** is a persistent, irrational fear attached to an object or situation that objectively does not pose a significant danger (Maxmen, 1995; Morrison, 1995). The affected person experiences anticipatory anxiety followed by a compelling desire to avoid the dreaded object or situation, even though he or she usually recognizes that the fear is unreasonable or excessive in proportion to the actual threat (APA, 2000). Unlike panic attacks (discussed later in this chapter), phobias are always anticipated and never occur unexpectedly. They may be simple and specific to certain situations, events, or objects. They may also be globally incapacitating, as in the case of severe agoraphobia (discussed next). When phobias accompany panic attacks, the condition is diagnosed as a panic disorder (Morrison, 1995). The degree to which phobias are disabling depends largely on how central the phobia is in the person's life.

Agoraphobia

Agoraphobia is a marked fear of being alone or in a public place from which escape would be difficult or help would be unavailable in the event of becoming disabled. As such, it is the most severe and persistent phobic disorder. People with agoraphobia often fear such scenarios as being outside the house alone, using public or mass transportation, and being in a crowd. As a response, many people with agoraphobia avoid such situations or endure them with such agony that they rearrange their lifestyles to minimize these occurrences (eg, restrict their travel, stop leaving the house). Eventually, the limitations that agoraphobia imposes may diminish the person's enjoyment of life and lead to depression.

Social Phobia

Social phobia represents a persistent, irrational fear of and compelling desire to avoid situations in which the person may be exposed to unfamiliar people or to the scrutiny of others. Additionally, the person harbors the fear of behaving in a way that may prove humiliating or embarrassing. The person will experience marked anticipatory anxiety if confronted with such a situation and will attempt to avoid it. Examples of social phobias include fear of speaking in public, eating or taking a test in the presence of others, or using public rest rooms.

Specific Phobia

A specific phobia is a persistent, irrational fear of and compelling desire to avoid a circumstance or thing other than those specific to agoraphobia or social phobia. Common specific phobias include *acrophobia* (fear of heights), *claustrophobia* (fear of closed spaces), *blood phobia* (fear of the sight of blood or injury), and fears of birds, cats or other furry animals, house dust, microbes, snakes, or insects (APA, 2000; Morrison, 1995).

PANIC ATTACKS

Panic attacks typically are characterized by a discrete period of intense apprehension or terror without any real accompanying danger, accompanied by at least 4 of 13 somatic or cognitive symptoms (APA, 2000) (see the Anxiety Disorders Information Map). The clinical picture involves a physiologic and psychological overresponse to stressors. For example, the person experiencing a panic attack incorrectly perceives his or her circumstances to be life threatening; therefore, he or she experiences such physiologic reactions as chest pain, choking or smothering sensations, dizziness, dyspnea, fainting, hot and cold flashes, palpitations, paresthesias, sweating, and vertigo. The person may also report feelings of depersonalization or derealization, fears of dying or going crazy, or uncontrollable behaviors. Attacks typically last for several minutes, reaching a peak within 10 minutes (APA, 2000; Morrison, 1995).

During panic attacks, the person may make extreme efforts to escape from what he or she believes to be causing the panic. Consequently, his or her behavior may appear strange to others (Candilis et al., 1999). Between panic attacks, the person often remains moderately to severely anxious in anticipation of the next episode (Maxmen, 1995).

Although panic attacks are unpredictable in onset, they may occur in specific situations, such as driving an automobile. Attacks do not necessarily occur every time the person confronts the situation, however. Moreover, panic attacks may occur in other circumstances. This feature is helpful in distinguishing panic attacks from phobias (Starcevic & Bogojevic, 1997).

PANIC DISORDER

The essential features of **panic disorder** are recurrent, unexpected panic attacks that cause the affected person to persistently worry about recurrences or complications from the attacks or to undergo behavioral changes in response to the attacks for at least 1 month. Panic disorder may be with or without agoraphobia.

OBSESSIVE-COMPULSIVE DISORDER

In **obsessive-compulsive disorder** (OCD), the person experiences recurrent obsessions or compulsions that are time consuming (ie, taking more than 1 hour per day) or cause significant impairment or distress (APA, 2000). The term **obsession** used in this diagnosis refers to recurrent, intrusive, and persistent ideas, thoughts, images, or impulses. The person with OCD does not voluntarily produce obsessions but feels cognitively invaded by them, usually finding them repugnant or meaningless. Despite efforts to ignore or dismiss them, the person remains preoccupied with these obsessive ideations (Maxmen, 1995).

Compulsions are ritualistic behaviors that the person feels compelled to perform either in accord with a specific set of rules or in a routine manner. The person engages in such rituals to prevent or reduce anxiety, not to increase pleasure or satisfaction. In fact, the person can resist the compulsion for a short period, but the delay to act creates a tremendous, anxious tension that is relieved only by performing the compulsive act. Usually, the compulsion is linked with an obsession, in that the person engages in compulsive behavior to decrease the anxiety the obsession causes (APA, 2000). For example, a person who is obsessed with fear of dirt or germs may engage in repetitive, excessive hand washing or housecleaning. At the same time, the person invests the compulsive act with symbolic significance by unrealistically believing that it will magically solve problems or atone for past misdeeds. If the affected person or others intervene to stop the compulsive act, anxiety results.

At one time, there was speculation that OCD, an anxiety disorder, was closely related to obsessive-compulsive personality disorder. More recent evidence, however, suggests no real connection between the two. To illustrate, the person with obsessive-compulsive personality disorder does not experience symptoms as uncomfortable, distressful, or bothersome. Moreover, he or she does not have actual obsessions or compulsions. Clients with OCD, the anxiety disorder, experience their symptoms as alien to themselves and intrusive (Morrison, 1995).

Symptoms of OCD may be mild to severe. Whatever the degree of severity, symptoms that interfere with occupational pursuits and quality of life usually lead the affected person to seek some type of assistance. If the person does not seek treatment or treatment is unsuccessful, he or she may become so uncomfortable that he or she becomes depressed or even suicidal.

▼ *Clinical Example 18-3*

Graham, a 28-year-old registered nurse, is referred for assessment and treatment by the Employee Assistance Program at the hospital where he practices. The hospital referred Graham because he washes his hands persistently, to the point that he cannot perform clinically.

He says to the nurse therapist, "I know my hands are clean and that I'm following the necessary precautions to prevent exposure to germs, but I just feel this pressure inside me that compels me to wash my hands. I must be crazy. I can't help myself, much less anyone else." The nurse therapist notices that Graham's hands are severely chapped and appear painful. As he talks, Graham occasionally wrings his hands; during pauses in telling his story, he straightens the paperweight and files on the nurse therapist's desk.

Graham agrees to treatment with cognitive-behavioral therapy and psychoactive medications. His initial prescription is 20 mg of fluoxetine (Prozac) four times a day and 0.5 mg of lorazepam (Ativan) every 6 hours.

Points for Reflection and Critical Thinking

- What disorder does Graham seem to be exhibiting? Should the nurse therapist consider other disorders as well?
- Would you expect Graham's problems to increase or decrease following a stressful encounter with a client? Explain your response.

POST-TRAUMATIC STRESS DISORDER

Post-traumatic stress disorder (PTSD) is defined as the development of characteristic symptoms after exposure to a severe or extraordinary stressor. Unlike other psychiatric conditions, which are causally linked to a person's psychosocial and biologic makeup, PTSD occurs only in response to a traumatic life experience (APA, 2000). Traumatic events capable of causing PTSD include natural disasters and accidental or intentional human-made disasters (Box 18-3). With all these stressors, there must be actual or threatened death, serious injury, or maiming to the self or others.

PTSD is less common than many people believe. Although about 38% of the population are exposed to catastrophic stress, only about 9% of them actually develop a true post-traumatic stress reaction. Additionally, these stressors must be capable of producing intense fear, helplessness, or horror in people exposed to them. Examples of common traumatic events capable of causing PTSD include, but are not limited to, war, assault (eg, sexual assault, physical attack, robbery), kidnapping or hostage situations, torture, and severe automobile accidents (APA, 2000).

Characteristic symptoms of PTSD include the following:

- Psychic numbing and denial
- Reexperience of the traumatic event through intrusive recollections, dreams, or sudden feelings and behaviors as though the event were recurring (often referred to as *flashbacks*)
- Perceptual distortions, including illusions, intrusive images, or actual hallucinations (Andreason, 1994)
- Feelings of being pressured, confused, or disorganized when thinking about the event
- Memory impairment, especially with regard to aspects of the trauma
- Overgeneralization of other sensory inputs so that they seem related in some way to the event
- Hyperarousal and exaggerated startle reactions
- Somatic symptoms, such as fatigue, headache, and muscular pain
- Altered states of consciousness, including paranormal experiences
- Recurrent nightmares

The three cardinal features of PTSD are hyperarousal, recurrent nightmares, and flashbacks. A latency period of hours, weeks, months, or even years may separate exposure to the traumatic stressor and the onset of symptoms. Refer to Clinical Example 18-1 and Nursing Care Plan 18-1 for more information about the client with PTSD.

BOX 18-3 ▼ *Traumatic Events Capable of Producing Post-traumatic Stress Disorder*

Natural Disasters

- Earthquakes
- Floods
- Hurricanes
- Tornadoes
- Volcanic eruptions

Accidental Human-made Disasters

- Train derailments and crashes
- Auto crashes
- Work-related injuries
- Airplane crashes

Intentional Human-made Disasters

- Military combat
- Rape
- Assault
- Armed robbery
- Terrorism
- Muggings
- Stalking
- Hazing
- Abuse of all kinds (verbal, physical, sex emotional)

Nursing Care Plan 18-1

THE CLIENT WITH POST-TRAUMATIC STRESS DISORDER

The nurse at the mental health clinic, Mary, is interviewing Ruth, the client in Clinical Example 18-1. She asks Ruth about other signs and symptoms she knows are associated with PTSD. Ruth admits that she feels tremendously guilty and wonders why she wasn't killed when so many others were. She relates that she has lost interest in most things, except her children, who she now watches "like a hawk." Ruth states: "I don't let them go out in cars with friends anymore, because I'm afraid of what will happen to them." Ruth denies using any illicit drugs but says she has begun drinking wine each night to help her sleep. She says she knows something's wrong but feels powerless to help herself. She states her husband has been impatient with her to "get over it" and to be thankful she was spared.

Based on the assessment interview, Mary creates the following care plan:

Nursing Diagnosis: **Post Trauma Syndrome** related to being a victim of violent crime as evidenced by reexperiencing the trauma, psychic numbing, and hypervigilance

Goal: Ruth will recover from the intense emotional trauma and her symptoms will resolve.

Interventions	Rationales
Encourage client to discuss feelings of guilt. To help her adopt a more realistic appraisal, help her to identify evidence for and against these feelings.	Ruth's emotional response of guilt and self-blame is not unusual but is irrational and self-defeating. Asking her to rationally examine this emotional response will reveal no rational basis for this response and help her to restructure her faulty thinking pattern.
Encourage the client to talk about the event.	All forms of avoidance behaviors are common and an attempt to reduce stress. Fear levels will remain high, however, until the client confronts the fear often enough for it to dissipate. Talking about the event is a form of exposure therapy.
Encourage and assist the client to gradually expose herself to the environment in which the event occurred.	Avoiding driving by fast-food restaurants is an impractical and ineffective response to the stress. Gradual, controlled exposure will eventually desensitize Ruth to that trigger.

Evaluation: Recovery can take several months (or longer); however, effectiveness of the plan can be evaluated initially by assessing Ruth's willingness to confront rather than avoid the emotional triggers that remind her of the event. Other indicators include the following:

- ...reased feeling of self-control and power
- ...ased self-blaming
- ...d involvement in pretrauma interests

...is: Anxiety related to post-traumatic stress response as evidenced by poor ... sleep, irritability, and cognitive impairment

...will diminish, and she will experience improved mood, sleep, and

	Rationales
	Support groups are tremendous resources for people who feel alone in their disorders.
...n techniques.	Controlled breathing and relaxation techniques will decrease the sympathetic arousal that occurs when Ruth's anxiety level is high. They also will help her feel less anxious and sleep better.
...to adopt a program	Lifestyle changes will help make Ruth more resilient to stress and will prevent increasing stress.

(continued)

Nursing Care Plan 18-1 (Continued)

Evaluation: Evaluate whether Ruth practiced relaxation exercises and if she reported feeling less anxious. Other indicators include:

- Sleeping better at night
- Experiencing an increased sense of well-being

Nursing Diagnosis: Compromised Family Coping related to temporary family disorganization as evidenced by husband's comments about "getting over it"

Goal: Ruth's husband will be able to provide more emotional support to his wife.

Interventions	Rationales
Meet with the family to educate them about the disorder.	Increasing the husband's understanding of PTSD will help him to view Ruth's behavior differently and be more supportive.
Listen to the husband's concerns and accept his personal coping style without judgment.	Allowing the husband to be heard without judgment helps him to feel understood as well.
Engage the husband in the treatment plan. Teach him how to listen reflectively and ask him to encourage his wife to remain in treatment.	Partnering with family members and encouraging family decision making increases the likelihood of successful treatment.

Evaluation: Determine if the interventions have been effective by observing Ruth and her husband's interactions and by Ruth's reports of improved family coping.

ACUTE STRESS DISORDER

When symptoms of PTSD appear in a person less than 4 weeks after exposure to the trauma, a variation of PTSD called **acute stress disorder** (ASD) can be diagnosed. ASD usually lasts less than 3 months. If symptoms begin more than 6 months after the traumatic event, the condition is called delayed PTSD (APA, 2000). Without prompt, effective treatment, the client is at risk for other anxiety disorders, substance abuse, and depression (Maxmen, 1995).

Not everyone exposed to a traumatic event will develop ASD or PTSD; however, few people will be able to walk away from such trauma unscathed. Any client experiencing a traumatic event should receive at least brief psychological counseling by a healthcare provider. See Implications for Nursing Practice 18-1 for helping people cope with trauma.

Comorbidities and Dual Diagnoses

Anxiety disorders often accompany other serious psychiatric conditions. Comorbidity can impede accurate diagnosis and treatment of either condition, causing needless suffering and further psychiatric complications, including increased risk for suicidality (U.S. Public Health Service, 1999). In particular, anxiety often co-occurs with depression, substance abuse, eating disorders, personality disorders, and schizophrenia. Practitioners should suspect and actively assess clients presenting with an anxiety disorder for comorbid conditions, including other types of anxiety disorders. Some clues to look for are as follows:

- High intake of alcohol or use of prescribed or illicit mood-altering drugs
- History of barbiturate or benzodiazepine dependence
- History of frequent use of healthcare services for somatic complaints
- Negative outlook on self, others, and society
- Distorted thinking
- Obsessive or compulsive behavior
- History of an eating disorder

Implications and Prognoses

Possible complications include the development of other Axis I diagnoses (eg, major depression) with increased risk for suicidality. Chronic stress is also thought to contribute to a decline in physical health as a result of immunosuppression, increased blood pressure, and increased corticosteroid release. Even without concomitant mental or physical illness, the effects of an anxiety disorder alone can be debilitating, diminishing the client's quality of life and affecting his or her family.

Implications for Nursing Practice 18-1

Helping Clients Who Have Experienced Severe Trauma

Nurses in all specialties will encounter people who have experienced trauma. Often, more than one person is a victim of the trauma, as in catastrophic natural disasters, violent crimes, accidents, and terrorism. Nurses are in a unique position in the healthcare industry and in the community to provide initial counseling for victims of trauma. The following are general counseling points nurses can give to all clients who have been traumatized:

- Try to avoid being alone in the days immediately following the trauma. Have a relative or friend stay with you. Obtain the numbers for crises hot lines or support groups.
- Communicate your thoughts and feelings about the trauma. This can be done through talking or keeping a diary.
- Engage in some form of aerobic exercise or practice relaxation exercises to help dispel tension.
- Avoid stimulants, which will increase feelings of nervousness.
- Eat nourishing food, even if you don't want to, and try to get sufficient sleep.
- Understand that your emotions will be labile; sometimes you may feel like talking, and other times you may feel like crying. You may be irritable, angry, and jumpy. Be supportive of yourself.
- Get back into your normal routine as soon as possible, but don't overdo it. Acknowledge that you may not be up to your usual level of performance for some time.
- Continue to spend time with others, even if you feel like withdrawing.
- Expect that you may be feeling emotionally strong and then have a relapse. Anniversaries of the trauma or other reminders may trigger extreme sadness.
- Expect that you may have trouble concentrating, make more errors, or have trouble remembering things for a period after the trauma.
- If possible, reach out to others in a supportive way, such as volunteering time in the community, making a donation, or participating in Red Cross blood drives. Acts of support can alleviate some of the helplessness commonly felt after severe crisis.
- Expect trauma reactions to grow less intense and disappear within a few weeks. If you cannot carry on your life normally, or if your feelings about the trauma do not begin to subside, seek professional help.

Interdisciplinary Goals and Treatment

Treatment for anxiety disorders includes medications, psychodynamic therapies (cognitive-behavioral therapy [CBT]), or a combination of the two (Table 18-1). Goals include reduction or elimination of symptoms; resumption or enhancement of productive professional, social, and family roles; replacement of maladaptive coping strategies with adaptive ones; and improved quality of life.

PSYCHODYNAMIC THERAPIES

Psychodynamic approaches consist of individual or group therapy and involve talking with a mental health professional to learn how to manage the anxiety disorder. Individual psychoanalysis would attempt to address the childhood roots of anxiety and uncover unresolved conflicts. Other therapies may be used in combination with individual therapy.

CBT includes both cognitive and behavioral interventions. It is based on the theory that the thoughts that produce and maintain anxiety can be recognized and altered using various techniques. Cognitive interventions include problem-solving strategies, education, and help in identifying the irrational thinking that can result in anxiety. Behavioral interventions focus on changing the aberrant behaviors and abnormal responses to anxiety-provoking situations through reinforcement and exposure.

Various cognitive-behavioral methods are used to treat the different anxiety disorders. A number of CBT approaches treat both the general symptoms of anxiety and the specific disorders.

Basic Cognitive Therapy Techniques for Anxiety

The goal of basic cognitive therapy is to gain insight into the situations that provoke anxiety and then to learn new responses to those situations. It includes education and problem-solving strategies but primarily focuses on learning to identify and change the faulty thinking that can lead to emotional distress. Treatment may last 12 to 20 weeks.

Initially, the client may be asked to keep a diary of anxious feelings and any thoughts or events that accompany them. In this way, the client can begin to recognize patterns in his or her anxious responses, which will increase awareness of these anxious thoughts as they occur. The therapist or group may then challenge these deep-rooted and habitual reactions to help the client gain insight. The client will receive homework so that he or she has a concrete plan for developing new behaviors. The following week, the client will share with the group or therapist how effective the new approaches have been. As the implementation of the plan continues, the client, through self-observation and coaching, will gain insight into the faulty assumptions that trigger the anxiety and begin substituting new ways of managing stressful situations.

TABLE 18-1 ▼	Selected Cognitive-Behavioral Treatment Strategies for Clients With Anxiety Disorders	
DISORDER	**COGNITIVE-BEHAVIORAL TREATMENT**
Panic attacks	Use cognitive restructuring to reframe catastrophic thinking. Desensitize client to feared situations. Educate about the disorder. Teach breathing techniques.
Generalized anxiety disorder	Teach relaxation techniques, stress management, and biofeedback. Use cognitive interventions to reframe catastrophic thinking. Assist the client with problem solving.
Obsessive-compulsive disorder	Desensitize client to feared situations. Educate about the disorder. Teach relaxation techniques.
Acute stress disorder	Assist the client to find a support group. Engage in therapeutic dialogues with the client. Teach problem solving. Teach relaxation techniques.
Specific phobias	Desensitize client to feared situations.
Social phobia	Challenge negative beliefs. Teach realistic appraisal of social situations.
Post-traumatic stress disorder	Encourage client to attend group therapy.

Some cognitive strategies used include the following:

* *Covert rehearsal*: The client is helped to imagine himself or herself successfully confronting an anxiety-provoking situation.
* *Positive coping statements*: The client makes positive self-statements to prevent anxiety from escalating when facing emotionally difficult situations. For example, the client may face the crisis and tell himself or herself, "I can handle this. I've done it before."
* *Cognitive reframing*: The client is helped to change his or her interpretation of anxiety-provoking situations from catastrophic to realistic. For example, the client states, "I will not lose everything if I do not do well on my evaluation. If my boss has criticisms, I will work with management on a plan to address those weak points."

Systematic Desensitization and Exposure Treatment

Systematic desensitization is a classical conditioning technique by which a client learns to gradually replace a panic response with a relaxation response. It is a behavioral therapy used to treat specific phobias, social phobias, agoraphobia, and PTSD. The client progressively confronts the object of fear in very small, controlled steps while in a deeply relaxed state. In another type of systematic desensitization, the client creates a list by which he or she rates anxiety-inducing situations by degree of fear, using a scale of 0 to 10. The client begins by confronting situations that he or she rates as 1 or 2, practic-

ing relaxation techniques and gradually progressing to the higher-rated situations.

Exposure treatment is similar to desensitization in that it involves exposure to the feared object or situation, but it does not involve relaxation or a gradual approach to the source of anxiety. It does allow the client to have some control over how long he or she is exposed to the fear-causing object, if desired, and is therefore known as either *flooding* or *graduated exposure*. In flooding, the client is exposed to the anxiety-producing stimulus for as long as 1 to 2 hours; graduated exposure allows the client to control the length and frequency of exposures. Eventually, the stimulating event loses its effect.

Relaxation Techniques and Breathing Retraining

One recurrent, effective component of any cognitive-behavioral strategy for reducing anxiety is teaching the client how to reduce the physical effects of anxiety through controlled breathing techniques and relaxation exercises. For example, hyperventilation is one of the prime features of panic attacks and, in itself, results in uncomfortable physical feelings that the panic-stricken person may interpret as life threatening. People who hyperventilate may experience chest pain, dizziness, tingling of the mouth and fingers, muscle cramps, and fainting. By practicing controlled breathing techniques in the early stages of a panic attack, the client may be able to minimize the attack. Specific steps to follow for breath control are described in the Nursing Process section of this chapter.

Relaxation methods are extremely helpful in managing anxiety and stress. The *relaxation response,* a term coined by mind–body medicine pioneer Herbert Benson, M.D., is a physical state of deep rest that counters the fight or flight response (ie, it results in a feeling of peacefulness and decreased heart rate, blood pressure, and muscle tension). To gain the full benefit of the relaxation response, the client should practice relaxation techniques daily. See Client and Family Education 18-1 for tips on teaching a relaxation technique.

PHARMACOLOGIC TREATMENT

Many antianxiety medications are available, although medication is not necessarily recommended for every anxiety disorder and should not be considered the sole treatment. Each client's specific circumstances will suggest whether medication is indicated. Among those medications commonly used to treat anxiety disorders are selective serotonin reuptake inhibitors (SSRIs), benzodiazepines (BZDs), buspirone, beta-blockers, and tricyclic antidepressants (TCAs).

Selective Serotonin Reuptake Inhibitors

SSRIs have been clearly established as effective in the management of anxiety disorders and are now considered first-line treatment choices. Typical antidepressant doses of SSRIs are used to treat anxiety; however, initial doses are usually smaller to reduce the possibility of hyperstimulatory reactions. Hyperstimulatory reactions can feel very much like anxiety and may occur during the first week of treatment; lower dosages and client education about what to expect can help prevent premature discontinuation of the medication. Commonly used SSRIs

---

Client and Family Education 18-1

PROGRESSIVE RELAXATION

Teaching Points

Practicing relaxation techniques will help reduce muscle tension, anxiety, fears, and worry. Clients can and should use them when feeling anxious, but they should also use them regularly to help prevent anxiety. Teach the client and the family the following steps:

1. Sit in a comfortable chair or lie down in a quiet place away from phones or distractions.
2. Clear your mind by focusing on your breathing. Do not try to influence your breathing; just notice how the breath feels as it flows in and out. You can focus on your chest moving up and down or on the way the air feels as it moves in and out of your nose.
3. As thoughts come up, do not respond to them; rather imagine them just floating away and return to focusing on your breath. Picture a calm, peaceful place to help stop the interruption of thoughts or worries or imagine a perfectly still lake or ocean.
4. Take several controlled breaths (breathe in through the nose for 3 seconds, hold the breath for 1 second, breathe out through the mouth for 3 seconds).
5. Beginning with your hands, tense each area of your body for 8 to 10 seconds (count slowly to yourself) and then release the tension and relax for 8 to 10 seconds. Proceed up your arms to your shoulders, neck, forehead, eyes, and jaws. Then proceed to the stomach, buttocks, thighs, calves, feet, and toes.
6. After all areas have been tensed and relaxed, focus again on your breathing for a few minutes. Sit quietly for a minute or two before opening your eyes.

Additional Resources

Along with the previous points, refer clients with anxiety disorders and their family members to the following resources, as appropriate:

Anxiety Disorders Association of America
11900 Parklawn Drive, Suite 100
Rockville, MD 20852-2624
301-231-9350
www.adaa.org

Freedom from Fear
308 Seaview Avenue
Staten Island, NY 10305
718-351-1717
www.freedomfromfear.com

National Institute of Mental Health Public Inquiries
6001 Executive Boulevard
Room 8184, MSC 9663
Bethesda, MD 20892-9663
301-443-5158
www.nimh.nih.gov

Obsessive-Compulsive Foundation, Inc.
337 Notch Hill Road
North Branford, CT 06471
203-878-5669
www.ocfoundation.org

Obsessive Compulsive Information Center
Madison Institute of Medicine, Inc.
7617 Mineral Point Road, Suite 300
Madison, WI 53717
608-827-2470
www.miminc.org

include fluoxetine (Prozac), sertraline (Zoloft), paroxetine (Paxil), and fluvoxamine (Luvox).

Unlike the TCAs, SSRIs are relatively free of anticholinergic, orthostatic, and sedative effects. Common side effects include sexual dysfunction, nervousness, nausea, insomnia, and anxiety. Like the TCAs, these medications should not be given with other antidepressant medications or other serotonergic agents to avoid the risk of life-threatening serotonin syndrome. *Serotonin syndrome* is a toxic hyperserotonergic state characterized by restlessness, confusion, agitation, hyperreflexia, diaphoresis, shivering, tremors, muscle rigidity, hyperthermia, and autonomic instability. The syndrome typically develops within hours or days of the addition of a new medication or an increase in dosage. Herbal products and food supplements may contribute to the development of this syndrome. For this reason, healthcare providers must question clients carefully about what natural products they use and advise clients about over-the-counter products that influence serotonin metabolism.

Considering SSRIs may require up to 4 to 6 weeks to reach their maximum antianxiety effects, a BZD may be used in the initial phase of treatment to control anxiety.

Benzodiazepines

BZDs have long been the drugs of choice for treatment of anxiety disorders. They are highly addictive, however, and can induce severe withdrawal symptoms and intense rebound anxiety when discontinued abruptly. They potentiate the effects of alcohol and other barbiturates, are commonly abused, and have several significant side effects. The most common adverse effects are sedation, ataxia, loss of coordination, slurred speech, memory impairment, paradoxical agitation, and dizziness. They also cause psychomotor impairment; clients should not drive or operate machinery while taking them. Also, the cognitive disturbances induced by BZD therapy, especially in the early phase of treatment, can delay clients' positive engagement and response to CBT (Cates, Wells, & Thatcher, 1996). These drugs should be used with caution but are indicated for certain clients, such as those with panic disorder, those who have not responded to other medications or therapies, or those who need to reduce anxiety while waiting for other medications to show a therapeutic effect. Box 18-4 lists other guidelines for the use of BZD medications. Commonly prescribed BZDs include alprazolam (Xanax), chlordiazepoxide (Librium), diazepam (Valium), lorazepam (Ativan), clorazepate (Tranxene), and oxazepam (Serax).

Buspirone

Buspirone (BuSpar) is approved for the treatment and management of anxiety. Unlike the BZDs, buspirone lacks anticonvulsant, muscle relaxant, and hypnotic properties. It has been shown to be an effective treatment for

---

BOX 18-4 ▼ *Guidelines for Use of Benzodiazepines*

- Use the lowest dose necessary to obtain symptom relief.
- Monitor sedative effects and the client's risk for injury.
- Use for short periods.
- Use cautiously in clients with a history of substance abuse.
- Do not discontinue abruptly.

---

generalized anxiety disorder. The most common side effects include nausea, dizziness, headache, insomnia, agitation, drowsiness, and dysphoria. Buspirone does not produce tolerance and is not addictive. Unlike the BZDs, buspirone requires 1 to 2 weeks before it produces antianxiety effects, and maximal effects may not appear until 6 weeks of therapy. Often, BZDs are given during the first few weeks of treatment with buspirone to control anxiety; they are then gradually reduced and discontinued (Cates, et al., 1996).

Beta Blockers

Propranolol is considered to be less effective in treating anxiety disorders than other medications because it only affects the physical ramifications of anxiety. In clients who have prominent cardiovascular symptoms of anxiety, however, this drug may be the most effective. Like the BZDs, beta blockers should not be abruptly discontinued but should be gradually reduced to avoid rebound anxiety symptoms. Additionally, beta blockers can cause central nervous system side effects, such as depression and nightmares. Common side effects such as bradycardia and hypotension necessitate careful monitoring of the client's vital signs.

Tricyclic Antidepressants

Research has produced clinical evidence that TCAs are effective in the treatment of generalized anxiety disorder in clients without comorbid major depression. Additionally, TCAs have been shown to be highly effective in the treatment of PTSD. Commonly used TCAs include imipramine (Tofranil), clomipramine (Anafranil), amitriptyline (Elavil), desipramine (Norpramin), and nortriptyline (Pamelor). These medications are relatively easy to dose and often can be conveniently administered once daily at bedtime to take advantage of the sedative effect. Common side effects include sedation, orthostatic hypotension, and anticholinergic effects. Concurrent use of these drugs with other medications such as monoamine oxidase inhibitors (MAOIs) and SSRIs is contraindicated.

APPLICATION OF THE NURSING PROCESS TO THE CLIENT WITH AN ANXIETY DISORDER

Nurses in all healthcare settings will certainly encounter many clients experiencing anxiety, though not all will be suffering from an anxiety disorder. In either case, the goals of nursing care are to identify clients with anxiety, provide immediate interventions as indicated, and assist the client to obtain definitive treatment.

Assessment

Because anxiety and anxiety disorders are so prevalent in the general population, the nurse must carefully assess all clients for signs and symptoms of anxiety. While several formal assessment tools exist (eg, State-Trait Anxiety Inventory, the Hamilton Anxiety Rating Scale, the Beck Anxiety Inventory), the nurse may begin by simply asking the client if he or she is currently feeling anxious or worried or has recently experienced these feelings. The client's response will focus the depth of the remaining assessment. If the client answers positively, the nurse will assess him or her, through observation and interview, for the psychological, physiological, and cognitive indicators of anxiety.

The nurse should suspect an anxiety disorder when a client discusses or shows evidence of experiencing persistent anxiety to the extent that he or she cannot dismiss the feeling, it interferes with his or her daily life, or both. The nurse should remember that many physical disorders and medication reactions could result in signs and symptoms that mimic or induce anxiety. The healthcare team must rule out such problems before establishing a diagnosis of an anxiety disorder. Some of the more common signs and symptoms to assess for include the following:

Cognitive
- Fear of dying, going "crazy," or another unspecified fear
- Diminished problem-solving capability
- Preoccupation with worrisome thoughts
- Decreased ability to concentrate

Affective
- Irritable, worried, tense, or fearful affect
- Feelings of helplessness or inadequacy
- Overly excited, wary, or anguished affect

Physiological
- Palpitations, chest pain, or tachycardia
- Hyperventilation or shortness of breath
- Dizziness, headache, paraesthesia, or shakiness
- Choking sensation, dry mouth, nausea, vomiting, or diarrhea
- Muscle aches and tension, restlessness

Behavioral
- Pacing or fidgeting
- Appearance of overvigilance
- Restlessness

The nurse also asks the client about obsessive thinking patterns, worrying, compulsions and repetitive activity, specific phobias, and exposure to traumatic events. If the client answers positively to any of these questions, the nurse follows up with additional questions aimed at eliciting specific details about the behavior or response to the feared object or the trauma.

Once the nurse has determined that signs and symptoms of anxiety do exist, he or she assesses the possible underlying causes and inquires about family history, recent life events, current stress level, personal history of anxiety, medical and medication history, history of substance abuse, and other possible causes of the anxiety.

Nursing Diagnosis

Many nursing diagnoses may apply to clients with anxiety disorders depending on their specific disorder and symptomatology. Major diagnoses that can be applied to most clients with different anxiety disorders are as follows:

- **Anxiety** related to perceived threat or stress
- **Ineffective Coping** related to inadequate individual resources
- **Ineffective Breathing Pattern** related to hyperventilation related to severe anxiety

Planning

Despite the differences among clients with anxiety or panic disorders, several common goals for nursing care apply. The nurse and the client may establish the following outcomes as the goals of treatment and care:

- The client will use effective coping strategies.
- The client will report a decreased intensity of anxiety.
- The client will use breathing techniques to control anxiety and hyperventilation.

Implementation

To help the client accomplish the established goals, the nurse must first establish a supportive therapeutic relationship. This relationship is characterized by trust, empathy, respect, and calmness on the nurse's part (see Chap. 4). Displaying these behaviors consistently will lay the groundwork for a successful therapeutic relationship and enhance the effectiveness of the interventions.

ALLEVIATING ANXIETY

Successful management of an anxiety disorder involves helping the client identify thoughts and behaviors as anxiety induced and finding effective coping strategies. Some steps can be taken immediately, regardless of whether the nurse is caring for the client at home, in a clinic, or in an acute care setting.

Initiating a Therapeutic Dialogue

Simply listening and gently counseling an anxious client can be beneficial. Using therapeutic questioning techniques that draw out the client and listening reflectively can help the client feel valued, understood, and supported. The nurse avoids comments that block communication, such as statements that minimize or challenge the client's feelings (eg, "Things could be worse" or "Why do you think you'll die if you go outside?"). Likewise, false, nonchalant reassurances ("Don't worry,

you're fine") or superficial pep talks ("You can get a grip on yourself") undermine the client's trust. Clients dealing with anxiety do not feel "fine" at the moment, nor can they will themselves to "get a grip." Instead, the nurse can help the anxious client by making factual observations and offering concrete interventions ("You're hyperventilating, which is causing you to feel worse physically. Let me coach you into breathing more slowly and deeply."), by providing realistic reassurance, by listening, and by just being present with the client until uncomfortable, panicky feelings subside. Refer to Therapeutic Communication 18-1 for examples of effective and ineffective dialogues.

The nurse provides a quiet environment, displays calmness, makes clear simple statements, repeats statements calmly and quietly as often as necessary, helps the client identify events leading up to the anxiety attack, and assists the client to identify and use past successful coping techniques.

THERAPEUTIC COMMUNICATION 18-1
The Client With Generalized Anxiety Disorder

In working with Marcia, the client discussed in Clinical Example 18-2, the nurse tries to discuss the job-related anxiety she is experiencing.

Ineffective Communication

Client: What will I do if I lose my job?

Nurse: Why do you think that you will lose your job?

Client: I just feel that I might.

Nurse: Well, you seem to be worrying over nothing. I'm sure you're doing fine.

Client: I still feel like I'm going to explode under the pressure.

Nurse: Well, maybe you should look for an easier job or not work at all.

Client: (*Looks defeated and about to cry*)

Effective Communication

Client: What will I do if I lose my job?

Nurse: What has happened to make you think that you will lose your job?

Client: I just feel that I might.

Nurse: Has anything in particular happened that is worrying you?

Client: I don't know. I guess not.

Nurse: What does your boss say about your work performance?

Client: She says I do a good job as a buyer. I got a raise about 6 months ago.

Nurse: Then what is there for you to worry about?

Client: I don't know. I've always been a worrier.

Nurse: What's different now?

Client: I guess it's the promotion, more responsibility, maybe believing that I can't take the pressure.

Reflection and Critical Thinking

- Compare the approaches the nurse used in both dialogues. What techniques did the nurse in the "Effective Communication" dialogue use to improve communication with the client?
- What assumptions did the nurse in the "Ineffective Communication" dialogue make that served to shut down communication with the client?
- How would you recommend that the nurse in the second scenario proceed to continue the dialogue?
- How can nurses remember what it is like to be on the receiving end of healthcare when working with clients?

Countering Faulty Thinking

The nurse can also help the client by providing factual information that can counter the anxiety-provoking misconceptions that often underpin anxiety and panic attacks. The client can then learn to substitute an objective appraisal of the circumstances for the unrealistically threatening appraisal. The ability to restructure an anxiety-producing event as less threatening enables the client to gain control of the situation and make it more predictable. For example, the client experiencing an anxiety attack may interpret physical feelings as serious symptoms of an impending health problem (ie, heart attack or stroke). The nurse can inform the client about the very common physical feelings associated with anxiety and teach the client to objectively assess the symptoms when they occur again. The client can then say, "This is how I feel when I have an anxiety attack. This is not a heart attack. These feelings will subside soon, as they have when I have had them before."

Managing Hyperventilation

Hyperventilation is a sign of anxiety as well as a symptom that can trigger the client to panic. To decrease hyperventilation, it will be necessary to increase the carbon dioxide level in the blood. Breathing into a paper bag is effective but not always practical or acceptable to the client in certain (social, professional) situations. Also, it will not prevent a panic attack. Slow or controlled breathing exercises will treat and help prevent panic attacks by correcting habitual, faulty breathing patterns.

The nurse first helps the client identify his or her own patterns of hyperventilating. He or she can teach the client to self-monitor the respiratory rate and to begin breathing exercises if the rate is more than 12 to 16 breaths per minute (average at-rest respiratory rate is 10 to 12 breaths per minute). The nurse then demonstrates and teaches the client how to perform a slow breathing exercise. Although such exercises have variations, a common approach to use is to:

1. Hold the breath and count to 5.
2. On 5, breathe out, slowly and calmly saying the word *relax.*
3. Then breathe in for 3 seconds and out for 3 seconds, saying the word *relax* with each exhalation.
4. After 1 minute, hold the breath for 5 seconds again and then continue breathing using the 6-second cycle (3-second inhalation, 3-second exhalation).
5. Continue until hyperventilation is under control and all symptoms have subsided.

Sometimes clients report increased anxiety when they first start to use the breathing exercise. The nurse informs the client that this occasionally happens but to continue with the breathing exercises and the anxiety will eventually subside. He or she tells the client to practice the exercise four times a day and whenever he or she notices sensations of anxiety.

Suggesting Lifestyle Changes

The nurse can suggest lifestyle changes that will help reduce the amount of stress in the client's life. Lifestyle changes can reduce the severity and frequency of anxiety or panic attacks and other anxiety symptoms and may help reduce the risk of developing an anxiety disorder. Some changes to suggest include the following:

- Maintain a regular aerobic exercise program.
- Eat a well-balanced diet.
- Establish good sleep habits.
- Eliminate or minimize alcohol or recreational drug use.
- Reduce sources of stress (eg, cut back on commitments).
- Eliminate caffeine and nicotine.

TEACHING ADAPTIVE COPING STRATEGIES

Clients learn to reduce the anxiety they feel in either functional or dysfunctional ways. Functional responses lead to healthier, more productive lives. They tend to be voluntary, conscious behaviors that address and acknowledge the stressful situation and help clients to find solutions. Dysfunctional responses tend to be involuntary, inflexible, avoidance-type solutions that impair productivity. The nurse first explores with the client what techniques the client has used in the past and helps the client identify and enhance those strategies that are most beneficial. The nurse and client identify maladaptive coping strategies such as social withdrawal or alcohol use and replace them with adaptive strategies that suit the client's personal, cultural, and spiritual values. This process can be difficult, because the client may be afraid or unwilling to abandon "successful" coping strategies, as in the case of the client addicted to drugs or alcohol.

The nurse should not ask the client to give up coping mechanisms, even maladaptive ones, without offering other adaptive mechanisms. In other words, it is not appropriate to expect a client to just stop worrying, compulsively checking doors, or otherwise trying to cope with anxiety. The nurse should be prepared to suggest and teach new coping strategies and to support currently used adaptive defense mechanisms. Two possible strategies that are easy to teach are relaxation exercises and problem-solving strategies. Although easily taught and learned, the client must practice such procedures regularly for them to become habitual and to gain the full benefits.

Teaching Relaxation

Many people find relaxation techniques to be effective coping tools for managing anxiety. Regularly inducing the relaxation response reduces the general level of autonomic arousal in anxious clients. It lowers blood pressure, heart rate, metabolic rate, and oxygen demands. This physiological effect may result from effects on the production of *cortisol,* a hormone the body releases in response to stress. Cortisol is helpful during the fight or flight response, but its prolonged in chronically anxious or stressed clients can inhibit the immune system and have other deleterious effects on the body.

The relaxation response can be elicited by many methods including meditation, yoga, progressive muscle relaxation, visualization, and hypnosis. The nurse discusses with the client the method most culturally acceptable to him or her and then teaches that technique or refers the client to a professional in that field. Refer to Client and Family Education 18-1, which describes a common technique for inducing relaxation through progressive muscle relaxation.

Visualization is another technique used to manage stress and anxiety. When using visualization, the client first practices some relaxation techniques such as focused breathing or progressive muscle relaxation. The client may then be guided, by a healthcare practitioner, audiotape, or independent means, to visualize a peaceful, calming environment in which he or she works through a stressful situation. Often the client is encouraged to include a mentor, spiritual presence, or loved one in the image as a source of wisdom and guidance.

Whatever method the client chooses for relaxation and stress reduction, the nurse encourages him or her to practice it daily to receive the most benefit.

Teaching Problem-Solving Skills

Helping the client develop a method for problem solving is another intervention for teaching adaptive coping strategies. Instead of avoiding, worrying endlessly, or making a catastrophe out of anxiety-producing situations, the client can use a problem-solving technique for making decisions. The nurse can teach the client the basic steps for problem-solving:

1. Answer the question: *"What is the problem?"* Be as specific as possible. Determine a goal.
2. *List all possible solutions,* including ones you think may not work. Come up with as many as possible. Even though a solution may at first seem ridiculous, the idea may help to generate better solutions than those that are more obvious.
3. Briefly *discuss the advantages and disadvantages of each solution.* No solution will be ideal considering every good idea will have some faults and most bad ideas will also have some merit.
4. *Choose the solution or combination of solutions that will solve the problem or achieve the goal.* It may be best to choose a solution that can be quickly and easily implemented, even though it may not be the "ideal" solution. Getting started quickly and avoiding a solution that is too difficult to implement (even though it is "ideal") will make a difference in the problem.
5. *Plan how to implement the solution.* A detailed practi-cal plan of action is critical to the successful resolution of the problem.
6. *Review the results.* The effectiveness of the solution is determined during the review process. If the problem was not solved, point out to the client that difficulties are usually the result of inadequate planning, not personal failure. Identify any attempt as a partial success, consider it a learning experience, and encourage the client to try again.

Evaluation

The nurse bases evaluation of whether nursing care for a client with an anxiety disorder is effective on the client's report of his or her feelings and observed behavior changes. Reduction of cardinal symptoms associated with anxiety disorders also signifies improvement, as does the development of increased self-awareness and the ability to cope effectively with anxiety-provoking situations. Outcomes that indicate improvement include the following:

- The client identifies and uses adaptive coping strategies that are congruent with personal values.
- The client demonstrates one or more relaxation techniques.
- The client reports decreased incidence or intensity of anxiety or panic attacks.
- The client uses deep-breathing exercises to prevent and manage anxiety and panic attacks.
- The client uses problem-solving techniques to help manage difficult situations.

▼ Reflection and Critical Thinking Questions

1. Refer to Clinical Example 18-2. Marcia reports that relaxation exercises and meditation only caused her to dwell on her problems more. Analyze why you think this occurred and explain what Marcia could do differently.
2. Refer to Clinical Example 18-3. What is Graham's fear about? What function does washing his hands have in dealing with the fear? Consider the various CBTs described in the chapter and explain which one might be most effective for Graham.
3. Consider the problem-solving method outlined in the text. Compare and contrast it with the nursing process. Use it to make a decision about a current event in your life. Discuss how (or if) going through the process changed your thinking about the event.

▼ CHAPTER SUMMARY

- Anxiety is normal response to a threatening situation. Prolonged anxiety in the absence of threat, exaggerated reactions, or reactions that impair functioning are abnormal.

■ Anxiety disorders are the most common or frequently occurring of all psychiatric syndromes, affecting children, adolescents, adults, and older adults. These disorders are often misdiagnosed and undertreated, compounding the problems they cause. Anxiety disorders are more common in women than men.

■ Levels of anxiety range from mild to moderate, severe, and panic. The client may report symptoms of dread, apprehension, restlessness, and jitteriness. Physiologic signs of anxiety may include increased heart rate, blood pressure, depth and rate of respirations, and perspiration.

■ Common phobic disorders include agoraphobia, social phobia, and specific phobia.

■ A panic disorder is characterized by recurrent, unpredictable panic attacks.

■ Generalized anxiety disorder is characterized by chronic anxiety that is so uncomfortable that it interferes with daily life.

■ A person with OCD experiences recurrent obsessions (persistent thoughts, images, or impulses) and compulsions (ritualistic behaviors performed routinely).

■ Post-traumatic stress disorder is the development of certain characteristic symptoms after exposure to a severe, extraordinary, traumatic life experience.

■ Nonpharmacologic methods used to treat anxiety disorders in clients include relaxation techniques, such as deep breathing and progressive muscle relaxation; covert rehearsal; positive coping statements; cognitive reframing; systematic desensitization; and problem-solving strategies.

■ Antianxiety medications commonly used to treat antianxiety disorders are SSRIs, BZDs, buspirone, beta-blockers, and TCAs.

■ Assessment reference points for nurses include knowing the definition of anxiety and being able to recognize the signs and symptoms of different anxiety levels.

■ Important interventions nurses perform in the care of clients with anxiety disorders include assisting the client through an anxiety attack, helping clients identify sources of anxiety, reinforcing use of adaptive coping mechanisms, and teaching new coping mechanisms.

■ The nurse bases evaluation of whether nursing care for a client with an anxiety disorder is effective on the client's report of his or her feelings and observed behavior changes.

▼ R E V I E W   Q U E S T I O N S

1. Anxiety is
   a. An abnormal response to everyday stress
   b. A sense of psychological distress
   c. A physiological response to stress
   d. A normal response to everyday stress

2. Mild levels of anxiety result in
   a. A heightened sense of awareness
   b. Distorted sensory awareness
   c. Mild forgetfulness
   d. Impaired ability to concentrate

3. Generalized anxiety disorder is characterized by
   a. Excessive worry or anxiety lasting more than 6 months
   b. Flashbacks and feelings of unreality
   c. Fear of going outdoors
   d. Repetitive, ritualized behavior

4. A 30-year-old male client states he is afraid of being watched and judged by other people. He is most likely suffering from
   a. Agoraphobia
   b. Social phobia
   c. Claustrophobia
   d. Acrophobia

5. A client with panic disorder is prescribed a BZD drug. The nurse teaches the client about
   a. Serotonin syndrome
   b. Interactions with MAOIs
   c. Tardive dyskinesia
   d. Potentiation of alcohol effects

6. A client comes to the mental health clinic saying she has been "on edge" lately. She states she has been preoccupied with work, is making mistakes because she can't concentrate, and is forgetting important meetings. She says she thinks she's going "crazy." These symptoms of anxiety are
   a. Affective
   b. Physiologic
   c. Cognitive
   d. Behavioral

7. A client with generalized anxiety disorder states she is worried about her finances. She has substantial savings that are managed by a reputable financial company. She says she is afraid the company will go bankrupt and she will lose her money. Which response by the nurse is most therapeutic?
   a. "It sounds to me like you have managed your money responsibly."
   b. "Your money is insured; there is no need to worry."
   c. "Has something changed that is causing you to worry?"
   d. "Why do you think the company will go bankrupt?"

8. A 42-year-old man with a history of panic attacks complains that his attacks are becoming more frequent. He is in good health and exercises regularly. He states he occasionally drinks wine with dinner. Which of the following interventions should the nurse discuss with the client?

a. Desensitization
b. Lifestyle changes
c. Problem-solving strategies
d. Controlled breathing techniques

9. A nurse is discussing treatment options with a client who has an intense fear of snakes. The nurse correctly describes the treatment approach when she makes which of the following statements?
    a. "You will meet weekly with a psychiatrist who will discuss childhood issues with you."
    b. "You will be treated with medications; antidepressants that affect serotonin levels are the treatment of choice for phobias."
    c. "You will be gradually exposed to the object you fear until you become desensitized to it."
    d. "You will be taught a problem-solving technique that will help you manage everyday stress, which is contributing to your phobic response."

10. A 22-year-old woman who arrived in the United States 1 week earlier from a country in Central America has complained to her family that she cannot stop crying and has been having nightmares and flashbacks. A few days before she left her home country, armed men, who returned her unharmed when her family paid the ransom, had kidnapped her. The client is most likely suffering from
    a. PTSD
    b. Normal anxiety after a traumatic event
    c. Acute stress disorder
    d. Generalized anxiety disorder

▼ REFERENCES AND SUGGESTED READINGS

Albucher, R., et al. (1998). Defense mechanism changes in successfully treated patients with obsessive-compulsive disorder. *American Journal of Psychiatry, 155*(4), 558.

*Alsobrook II, J. P., & Pauls, D. L. (1994). Genetics of anxiety disorders. *Current Opinion in Psychiatry, 7,* 137–139.

*American Psychiatric Association. (2000). *Diagnostic and statistical manual of mental disorders* (4th ed., text rev.). Washington, DC: Author.

*Andreason, N. (1994). Posttraumatic stress disorder. In H. Kaplan & B. Saddock (Eds.), *Comprehensive textbook of psychiatry* (7th ed.). Baltimore: Williams & Wilkins.

Antai-Otong, D. (2000). The neurobiology of anxiety disorders: Implications for psychiatric nursing practice. *Issues in Mental Health Nursing, 21,* 71.

*Aveline, M. O. (1997). The limitation of randomized controlled trials as guides to clinical effectiveness with reference to the psychotherapeutic management of neuroses and personality disorders. *Current Opinion in Pediatrics, 7,* 387–391.

Barlow, D., Gorman, J., Shear, M., & Woods, S. (2000). Cognitive-behavioral therapy, imipramine, or their combination for panic disorder: A randomized controlled trial. *Journal of the American Medical Association, 283*(19), 2529–2536.

Beekman, A., de Beurs, E., von Balkom, A., et al. (2000). Anxiety and depression in later life: Co-occurrence and communality of risk factors. *American Journal of Psychiatry, 157,* 89–95.

*Black, B. (1995). Anxiety disorders in children and adolescents. *Current Opinion in Psychiatry, 10,* 113–115.

Blanes, T. (1995). Psychotherapy of panic disorder. *Current Opinion in Psychiatry, 8,* 161–171.

Brewin, C., Andrews, B., Rose, S., & Kirk, M. (1999). Acute stress disorder and posttraumatic stress disorder in victims of violent crime. *American Journal of Psychiatry, 156*(3), 360–366.

Bryant, R., et al. (1999). Treating acute stress disorder: An evaluation of cognitive behavior therapy and supportive counseling techniques. *American Journal of Psychiatry, 156*(11), 1780.

*Candilis, P. J., McClean, R. Y., Otto, M. W., Manfro, G. G., Worthington, J. J., Penava, S. J., Marzol, P. C., & Pollack, M. H. (1999). Quality of life in patients with panic disorder. *Journal of Nervous and Mental Diseases, 187*(7), 429–434.

Castle, D., & Groves, A. (2000). The internal and external boundaries of obsessive-compulsive disorder. *Australian and New Zealand Journal of Psychiatry, 34,* 249–255.

*Cates, M., Wells, B. G., & Thatcher, G. W. (1996). Anxiety disorders. In E. T. Herfindal & D. R. Gourley (Eds.), *Textbook of therapeutics* (6th ed.). Baltimore: Williams & Wilkins.

*Dohrenwend, B. P. (2000). Life events can trigger mental illness. *Journal of Health and Social Behavior, 41,* 1–9.

Gardos, G. (2000). Long-term treatment of panic disorder with agoraphobia in private practice. *Journal of Psychiatric Practice, 6,* 140–146.

*Greenberg, P. E., Sistsky, T., Kessler, R. C., Finkelstein, S. N., Berndt, E. R., Davidson, J. R., Ballenger, J. C., & Fyer, A. J. (1999). The economic burden of anxiety disorders in the 1990s. *Journal of Clinical Psychiatry, 60*(7), 427–435.

Griegel, L. E. (1996). Behavioral treatment of panic disorder in children and adolescents. *Current Opinion in Pediatrics, 8,* 355–360.

Hayward, C., Killen, J., & Kraemer, H. (2000). Predictors of panic attacks in adolescents. *Journal of the American Academy of Child and Adolescent Psychiatry, 39*(2), 207–214.

Lenze, E., Mulsant, B., Shear, M., et al. (2000). Comorbid anxiety disorders in depressed elderly patients. *American Journal of Psychiatry, 157*(5), 722–728.

*Maxmen, J. (1995). *Essential psychopathology and its treatment* (2nd ed., revised for *DSM-IV*). New York: W.W. Norton.

Mendlowicz, M., & Stein, M. (2000). Quality of life in individuals with anxiety disorders. *American Journal of Psychiatry, 157*(5), 669–682.

*Morrison, J. (1995). *DSM-IV made easy.* New York: Guilford Press.

Peplau, H. (1952). *Interpersonal relations in nursing.* New York: G.P. Putnam & Sons.

Peplau, H. (1963). A working definition of anxiety. In S. Burd & M. Marshall (Eds.), *Some clinical approaches to psychiatric nursing.* New York: MacMillan.

Pilowsky, D., Wu, L-T., & Anthony, J. (1999). Panic attacks and suicide attempts in mid-adolescence. *American Journal of Psychiatry, 156*(10), 1545–1549.

*Rief, W., Trenkamp, S., Auer, C., & Fichter, M. M. (2000). Cognitive behavior therapy in panic disorder and comorbid major depression. *Psychotherapy and psychosomatics, 69*(2), 70–78.

Roerig, J. (1999). Diagnosis and management of generalized anxiety disorder. *Journal of the American Pharmacological Association, 39*(6), 811–821.

Saeed, S., & Bruce, T. (1998). Panic disorder: Effective treatment options. *American Family Physician, 57*(10), 2405–2412.

Simpson, H., & Kozak, M. (2000). Cognitive-behavioral therapy for obsessive-compulsive disorder. *Journal of Psychiatric Practice, 6*, 59.

*Starcevic, V., & Bogojevic, G. (1997). Comorbidity of panic disorder with agoraphobia and specific phobia: Relationship with the subtypes of specific phobia. *Comprehensive Psychiatry, 38*(6), 315–320.

*Taylor, S., & Livesley, J. (1995). The influence of personality on the clinical course of neurosis. *Current Opinion in Psychiatry, 8*, 93–97.

*Unnewehr, S., Schneider, S., Florin, I., & Margraf, J. (1998). Psychopathology in children of patients with panic disorder or animal phobia. *Psychopathology, 31*(2), 69–84.

*U.S. Public Health Service. (1999). *Mental health: A report of the surgeon general.* Washington, DC: National Institute of Mental Health.

Yonkers, K., Zlotnick, C., Allsworth, J., et al. (1998). Is the course of panic disorder the same in women and men? *American Journal of Psychiatry, 155*(5), 596–602.

**Starred references are cited in text.*

For additional information on this chapter, go to *http://connection.lww.com.*

Need more help? See Chapter 18 of the *Study Guide to Accompany Mohr: Johnson's Psychiatric Mental-Health Nursing, 5th Edition.*

The Client With a Somatoform Disorder

CAROL J. CORNWELL

▼ KEY TERMS

Body dysmorphic disorder—A somatoform disorder in which the client is preoccupied with an imagined defect in his or her appearance (eg, a facial flaw or spot) when no abnormality or disturbance actually exists.

Conversion disorder—A somatoform disorder in which the client has at least one symptom or deficit of sensory or voluntary motor function (eg, paralysis) that cannot be explained by a neurological or general medical condition.

Culture-bound syndromes—Forms of mental illness found only in one particular culture, symbolizing that culture's unique expression of physical or mental distress.

Hypervigilance—A common symptom of somatoform disorders in which the client's heightened focus on the body and its sensations leads to chronic, prolonged misinterpretation and overreaction to physical signs.

Hypochondriasis—A somatoform disorder characterized by a client's unwarranted fear or belief that he or she has a serious disease, without significant pathology.

Hysteria—A historical term (preceding somatoform disorder) coined in the early 1900s by Sigmund Freud to describe a condition in which people could not use certain body parts despite having no physiological damage or dysfunction.

La belle indifference—In conversion disorder, a remarkable lack of affect or concern shown by a client despite a symptom that imposes significant physical disability (eg, paralysis).

Primary gain—The main benefit a person derives from the "sick role," which in the case of somatoform disorders is the blocking of psychological conflict from conscious awareness.

Psychosomatic medicine—The clinical and scientific study of the connections between the mind and body.

Secondary gain—Additional benefits that a person derives from the "sick role"; examples include being released from expected responsibilities and receiving attention from others.

Sick role—The role that all chronically ill clients assume that releases them from usual responsibilities; in somatoform disorders, clients unconsciously assume the sick role to meet their dependency needs.

Somatization disorder—A somatoform disorder characterized by many physical complaints over several years that cannot be explained by pathology or a general medical condition.

Somatoform disorders—A group of psychiatric disorders in which clients complain of extreme physiologic discomfort or disability without any identifiable pathology on testing or examination.

▼ LEARNING OBJECTIVES

On completion of this chapter, you should be able to accomplish the following:

- Define the term *somatoform disorder.*
- Differentiate somatoform disorders from organic physical disorders influenced by psychological factors.
- Discuss the epidemiology of somatoform disorders, including prevalence, gender, and age of onset.
- Describe possible psychological, neurobiological, and familial etiologies of somatoform disorders.
- Describe signs and symptoms of somatoform disorders.
- Identify the most common interdisciplinary goals and treatments for clients with somatoform disorders.
- Apply the steps of the nursing process—assessment, nursing diagnosis, planning, implementation, and evaluation—to clients who exhibit somatoform disorders.

This chapter discusses somatoform disorders. As you read it, consider the case of Rose and Andrew in Clinical Example 19-1. Think about how Rose's symptoms and history might relate to this group of disorders and how they might reflect Rose's inability to express her needs verbally. You will learn more about Rose's care and her progress in therapy in Nursing Care Plan 19-1. You also will have a chance to apply what you have learned about Rose and other clients with somatoform disorders in the

Reflection and Critical Thinking Questions at the end of this chapter.

▼ *Clinical Example 19-1*

Rose is a 62-year-old white woman. She has been married to Andrew, a 66-year-old retired schoolteacher, for 39 years. The couple has three grown children. Rose's internist of 4 years refers Rose to psychotherapy. Since becoming a client of the internist, Rose has been complaining of persistent and unrelenting pain in her head, back, arms, and joints, with occasional difficulty urinating. Just before her last visit, she had seen a kidney specialist who treated her with two courses of antibiotics, both of which have been unsuccessful in relieving her complaints of severe pain on urination. During the course of antibiotic treatment, Rose began to complain of an increasing problem with coordination and balance, often having to "hold onto the walls" as she walks through her home.

When she arrives at her therapy session, the provider asks Rose to describe her current difficulties. Rose produces a 10-page typewritten paper of her entire medical history since she was 18 years of age. She asks the provider to read it, saying, "I think it would be easier if you just read this, because it's too detailed for me to really tell you about in 1 hour." Her history includes two exploratory abdominal surgeries at 22 and 25 years of age for "extensive pain, diarrhea, and abdominal distention"; a history of irregular menses followed by a total hysterectomy at 32 years of age; and a long history of multiple, unusual symptoms that have been tested individually, usually by different physicians, and have each resulted in negative apparent physiological etiology. Regarding her history, Rose angrily states, "Those doctors don't care about me at all, and they act like my problems are 'all in my head' . . . but I can tell you right now, they're *not!*"

SOMATOFORM DISORDERS

In **somatoform disorders,** clients complain of severe symptoms that cannot be explained by any organic or physical pathology on examination. Researchers have spent years investigating and studying the ways in which thinking and the mind can profoundly affect bodily functioning without pathology (Historical Capsule 19-1). While the symptoms of somatoform disorders are truly physical, they are classified as a group of mental disorders in the American Psychiatric Association (APA) *Diagnostic and Statistical Manual of Mental Disorders,* 4th edition, text revision (*DSM-IV-TR*) (APA, 2000) because laboratory tests and physical examination reveal no demonstrable organic pathology. This chapter focuses on these disorders, in which clients present psychosocial distress through physical symptoms that have no organic basis.

HISTORICAL CAPSULE 19-1

Origins of Understanding Somatoform Disorders

In 1909, Sigmund Freud was invited by G. Stanley Hall, the first president of Clark University in Worcester, Massachusetts, to present four lectures to a gathering of psychologists. The distinguished guests included Franz Boas, the anthropologist; William James, the philosopher; Ernest Jones, who became Freud's biographer; Abraham Arden Brill, who translated Freud's works into English; and Carl Jung and Sandor Ferenczi, who had accompanied Freud from Europe (Levinson, 1994, p. 10). In these early lectures, Freud presented important clues about tracing the subtle connections between emotions and physical states, which prompted a whirlwind of intellectual and philosophical debate that continues today among those devoted to understanding and healing the mind (Levinson, 1994). Freud spoke about a common condition among his patients called **hysteria**, in which these people could not use certain parts of their bodies without any physiological evidence of damage or dysfunction. Although Freud suggested a strong sexual component to such problems, the general intrigue around psychosomatic illness began to prompt many more debates around the etiology and origins of these disorders. By the 1930s and 1940s, research about the interrelationships between the mind and body was underway in many centers, and physicians who thought in terms of "psychosomatic medicine" were treating some individuals (Levinson, 1994, p. 22).

From these early roots, the science of psychosomatic medicine has grown and flourished, and there has been continued interest in the somatic components of disease (Katon, Sullivan & Walker, 2001; MacBain, 2001). In recent years, interest in understanding the complex intricacies by which the mind influences the body and vice versa has been increasing. Psychoneuroendocrinology and psychoneuroimmunology are two areas in which research and scientific advancement continues, combining state-of-the-art concepts involving the complex interplay of psychology, emotion, the nervous system, the endocrine system, and increasingly, immune function (Ader, Felten, & Cohen, 2001).

Clients with somatoform disorders have highly elaborate self-diagnoses and symptoms that are refractory to reassurance, explanation, and standard treatments (Barsky & Borus, 1999). The anguish of clients with somatoform disorders is exaggerated by a self-fulfilling cycle in which

and meeting emotional needs is a critical prerequisite (Johns, 1999; Margo & Margo, 2000).

Expert clinicians who work with clients suffering from somatoform disorders advocate rehabilitative or chronic disease approaches to treatment that have the long-term goal of maintaining the client's optimal functioning (Becker, 1998; Epstein, Quill, & McWhinney, 1999). Clients with mild somatic symptoms that are recognized early may respond to reassurance and support. Unrecognized and untreated early symptoms progress to more debilitating disorders and unnecessarily dangerous, costly, and frustrating diagnostic procedures and treatments (Servan-Schreiber, Kolb, & Tabas, 2000).

INDIVIDUAL AND GROUP PSYCHOTHERAPIES

Individual and group psychotherapies have been advocated as the treatments of choice for clients with somatoform disorders (Campayo & Carillo, 2000; Coen, 1992, 1996; Holloway & Zerbe, 2000). Cognitive-behavioral psychotherapy can be an effective treatment with these clients (Slaughter & Sun, 1999). Coen and Sarno (1989) implemented a psychoeducational treatment program for clients with low back pain; ninety-five percent of 4000 participants with low back pain made dramatic improvements. Interventions included education, explanation of interpersonal and emotional conflicts associated with chronic pain, and avoidance of unnecessary medical procedures. Long-term recovery was achieved in 5% to 10% of these clients (Coen, 1992, 1996).

SOMATIC THERAPIES

Although psychopharmacologic agents have been of limited use in reducing symptoms of somatoform disorders alone (ie, without comorbid psychiatric diagnoses, such as anxiety or depression), the appropriate use of these medications can help in some cases. Selective serotonin reuptake inhibitors (SSRIs), given in sequential trials of one or more medications, have been found to be the drugs of choice for this group of disorders; they are cost effective and helpful (Holloway & Zerbe, 2000). Table 19-3 displays some psychopharmacologic interventions that have been studied and used in selected somatoform disorders. Alternative somatic therapies are often useful, including biofeedback, meditation, and relaxation therapies (see Chap. 14).

APPLICATION OF THE NURSING PROCESS TO THE CLIENT WITH A SOMATOFORM DISORDER

The nurse's role in caring for clients with somatoform disorders is important, regardless of the treatment setting.

Although specific somatoform disorders may respond to different interventions, nurses may work with clients who have any of these disorders using an approach with similar general outcomes and interventions designed to address basic shared components of care. The nurse intervenes to assist the client toward the overarching goal of developing and maintaining functional patterns of adaptation. Activities are directed toward:

- Developing trust and establishing a therapeutic relationship
- Demonstrating genuine concern and caring with supportive interactions
- Assisting the client to improve physical health and adapt to stress
- Enhancing the client's self-knowledge, helping him or her to examine ways to express and meet needs directly and to consider alternatives for coping other than through physical symptoms and physical illness

Ideally, one clinical care provider assumes responsibility for the client and coordinates treatment with the others. Psychiatric-mental health clinical nurse specialists are in an ideal position to work with clients with somatoform disorders over long periods and to closely coordinate care with physicians.

Assessment

Assessment is critical in the somatoform disorders because many cases are unrecognized and undiagnosed for long periods. Nurses in all settings must provide astute assessment of the client who presents with somatic symptoms. A holistic approach is especially critical when caring for clients with somatoform disorders. Viewing the client as a system greater than the sum of its parts, or subsystems, assists the nurse to assess the whole person rather than focusing only on the most obvious—the physical body. The nurse's knowledge and understanding of multidimensional causes of illness facilitates a comprehensive assessment that includes psychological, physiological, and social influences.

Analysis of assessment data focuses on a thorough examination of the possible interrelationships of all systems. During assessment, the nurse simultaneously practices therapeutic use of self and conveys understanding and genuine concern, thus developing a strong, trusting, and therapeutic relationship with the client from the start (see Chap. 4).

PSYCHOLOGICAL ASSESSMENT

Within the context of a caring, nonthreatening nurse–client relationship, the nurse obtains information about the client's behavior within interpersonal relationships (including expressing needs and feelings) and intrapersonal experiences that focus on emotional life. Because depression and anxiety

TABLE 19-3 ▼ Psychopharmacologic Treatments for Selected Somatoform Disorders		
DISORDER	**PHARMACOLOGIC TREATMENT(S)**	**REFERENCES**
Somatization disorder	In selected clinical trials, gabapentin has been found to be effective.	Garcia-Campayo & Sanz-Carrillo, 2001
	Somatization disorder symptoms improved clinically and statistically with a 14-week trial of SSRIs.	Keeley, Smith, & Miller, 2000
Hypochondriasis	Although pimozide has long been the drug of choice in treating somatic delusional disorders, risperidone has been shown to be effective in treating monosymptomatic hypochondriacal psychosis.	Elmer, George, & Peterson, 2000
	Because of the reduced incidence of cardiac and extrapyramidal abnormalities with risperidone, it should be considered first-line therapy.	
	Symptoms improved clinically and statistically with a 14-week trial of SSRIs; clients with hypochondriasis reported more side effects and treatment nonadherence than did clients with somatization disorder.	Keeley, Smith, & Miller, 2000
Body dysmorphic disorder	Clomipramine has been found to be more effective than desipramine in reducing symptoms of body dysmorphic disorder and increasing functional ability, and it is effective even in clients who are delusional.	Hollander et al., 1999
	Augmentation of SSRIs with buspirone and neuroleptics, as well as combinations of SSRIs, is promising.	Phillips, 1996
	Fluvoxamine was administered during 16 weeks with significant symptom improvement.	Phillips, Dwight, & McElroy, 1998
	SSRIs, in higher dosages than typically recommended, may be useful for body dysmorphic disorder.	Slaughter & Sun, 1999 Phillips, 1996

may be at the root of the physical symptoms, the nurse is especially sensitive to assessment strategies that include those areas. Additionally, because clients with somatoform disorders have difficulty directly expressing needs and feelings, assessment also focuses on dependent personality traits, hostility, and anger.

A comprehensive mental status examination is the foundation of the psychological assessment in psychiatric nursing. In clients with somatoform disorders, this assessment is critical to determining the coexistence of other psychiatric disorders, such as depression, anxiety, or personality disorders.

Behavior

The nurse assesses the client's general behavior, including his or her patterns of interaction during the interview. Many clients with somatoform disorders behave with an alarming, crisis-oriented presentation, focusing on their particular physical and symptomatic concerns at the time of the interview. Acknowledging the client's distress is important, while attempting to elicit information necessary for the assessment. This task can be difficult, because at the core of somatization is the client's unconscious need to focus on physical symptoms in an effort to avoid addressing emotional issues. The client's response to remaining on task will be important to assess in regard to his or her personality style and psychiatric symptomatology.

In regard to anxiety, is the client aware of excessive fear, dread, worry, apprehension, or rigid or obsessional thinking? Does the client experience physical signs and symptoms, such as restlessness, diaphoresis, palpitations, shortness of breath, or muscle tension? If the client acknowledges any of these, the nurse encourages him or her to describe specific experiences.

Because the client usually cannot meet dependency needs appropriately, the nurse focuses on how the client receives gratification, nurturance, and attention. Sensitive questions and comments that assist the client to reflect on and disclose data about self-sufficiency or perhaps possible codependency issues may be useful. Similarly the nurse uses approaches that may lead to uncovering narcissism or a tendency to be demanding within interpersonal relationships.

Mood and Affect

Mood is a key element for assessment because clients with somatoform disorders also may be experiencing comorbid depression, anxiety, or psychoses. Encouraging and caring inquiries about feelings of loneliness, helplessness, hopelessness, and self-doubt may help the client associate these feelings with communication through bodily symptoms. Repression or denial of anger may be intermingled with depression and the inability to meet dependency needs appropriately.

Assessment of anger is important. The client, for example, may "swallow" anger out of fear of rejection or abandonment. Guilt and an overriding sense of powerlessness may be present, masked by the veneer of physical symptoms. Have others commented that they perceive the client as depressed? Has the client experienced difficulty concentrating, thinking clearly, completing tasks, or enjoying usual activities, including sex and sleep?

Affect is as important as mood. Clients with somatoform disorders may have a calm affect while describing anguishing symptoms. Some clients with conversion disorders, such as a paralyzed arm or leg, may describe their situation without any affective display at all—a situation described earlier as *la belle indifference.*

Thought Process and Content

The nurse assesses thought process and content, including any psychoses (delusions or hallucinations) or thought disturbances. He or she may assess some of these areas by asking the following questions:

* What are your attitudes toward physical illness, and what do you know about the illness?
* How do you feel about being ill?
* How do you usually adapt to stress or tension?

Intellectual and Cognitive Processing

Assessing the client's level of intellectual and cognitive processing is important to evaluate his or her symptoms as well as to plan treatment approaches. The nurse may use the Mini-Mental Status Examination to establish a baseline for cognitive assessment (MiniMental LLC, 1975). In most cases, clients with somatoform disorders receive treatment from outpatient clinics and primary care practices, and intellectual and cognitive processing often is intact.

Insight and Judgment

Clients with somatoform disorders often have little to no insight into their illness. An exaggerated sense of urgency and fear about symptoms he or she is experiencing often impairs the client's judgment. What does the client perceive as his or her strengths and limitations? What events preceded or precipitated this physical illness? What relationship, if any, does the client perceive between his or her physical illness and emotions or behavior? How does the client generally meet emotional needs?

Suicidal Ideation

Reports of suicide and suicidal ideation in clients with somatoform disorders are rare. These clients may become depressed. A comprehensive mental status examination always includes questions regarding self-harm behavior and suicidal thoughts and ideations.

PHYSICAL EXAMINATION

Physical examination is an important component of the comprehensive psychiatric nursing assessment of the client with a somatoform disorder. A complete review of systems, including vital signs and laboratory work, is indicated. The nurse must elicit information about the client's current and past medical history. In particular, a complete history of help-seeking behaviors through the medical care system is essential, including any diagnostic testing, work-ups, hospitalizations, and outpatient surgeries. Through this history, the nurse may begin to put together a picture of a client who has been in and out of the healthcare system at many different points. Eliciting the client's perception about the search for medical help is important.

Vegetative Signs

Vegetative signs, such as sleep, appetite, weight gain or loss, and bowel function, are critical assessment points. This evaluation is part of the general nursing assessment and also can help to rule out comorbid psychiatric disorders, such as sleep, eating, mood, or anxiety disorders.

Energy and Psychomotor Functioning

Clients with somatoform disorders often present with complaints of low to no energy. The nurse examines the client's history of low energy and determines how it affects daily functioning. Has the client felt "slowed down" because of low energy? Does the client complain of having to rest frequently or remain in bed during the day? If so, what are the family members', employers', or friends' responses? Has the client experienced increased daily activity or spurts of energy? What tasks has this illness kept the client from performing?

SOCIAL ASSESSMENT

A comprehensive social assessment includes family functioning, social support, and cultural and ethnic ties. Everyone begins the journey of growth and development in the family system and learns patterns of behavior. Families at high risk for communicating psychological distress through physical symptoms are those in which one or both parents express needs and feelings in this way. Regardless of the setting, a thorough nursing assessment and analysis may reveal information about the family suggesting that the client is at risk for unconsciously using physical symptoms as a means of coping. The following questions may be helpful in eliciting information about family influences:

- Have any of the client's significant others or family used similar behaviors when adapting to stress?
- Did the client grow up in a family that expressed physical illnesses or symptoms frequently?
- How has the client's physical problems changed the client's or family's lifestyle?
- What interpersonal resources are available to the client?
- What roles have changed in the client's family because of the physical illness?

The nurse also assesses social support, including the client's social network and occupational and educational activities. Does the client have friends and family who participate in his or her life? Does the client have friends, family, or coworkers who are exhausted by the client's incessant worry about somatic symptoms? What is the nature and extent of the client's support systems, including individuals, groups, community organizations, and others?

Nursing Diagnosis

Nursing diagnoses for clients with somatoform disorders focus on identifying the causes of dysfunctional coping and issues related to the family and psychosocial interaction. Selected diagnoses for clients with somatoform disorders include the following:

- **Ineffective Coping** related to unresolved psychological issues as evidenced by somatization
- **Anxiety** related to perceived threat and excessive concern over physical symptoms or physical illness
- **Powerlessness** related to lifestyle of helplessness and perceived inability to effect a change in physical health as evidenced by excessive dependency
- **Chronic Low Self-Esteem** related to perceived inability to participate in daily functional activities
- **Social Isolation** related to inability to leave home and participate with others in social events
- **Interrupted Family Processes** related to client's ongoing, severe physical disability and assumption of the sick role

Planning

The nurse collaborates with the client and family to create a plan of care that includes appropriate goals and ways to meet identified goals. Possible desired outcomes are as follows:

- The client will establish a trusting relationship with the psychotherapist and his or her physician.
- The client will spend less time focusing on physical symptoms and make fewer visits to healthcare providers, the emergency department, or both.
- The client will become increasingly independent and will verbalize decreased feelings of powerlessness.
- The client will report increased feelings of relaxation and decreased anxiety.
- The client will demonstrate increased self-esteem by verbalizing positive elements of self and by reporting an increase in daily functioning.
- The client will demonstrate increased levels of participation in activities of daily living (ADLs) and more social interactions and outings away from home.
- The family will be able to manage stressors and meet the needs of its members.

Implementation

Implementation of a comprehensive, long-term treatment plan for the client with a somatoform disorder requires a multidisciplinary approach involving the physician, the psychotherapist, and other healthcare providers (Nursing Care Plan 19-1). Implementing this treatment plan often begins in the inpatient setting (if the client has been hospitalized) and continues to the outpatient setting. This section focuses on implementation of care in the outpatient setting. The primary care coordinator (ideally, a psychiatric nurse psychotherapist) and other care providers collaborate to design interventions. Coordinating care is vital to prevent the client from seeking multiple appointments with different members of the healthcare team.

ESTABLISHING A TRUSTING RELATIONSHIP

First and foremost, the care coordinator must establish a trusting relationship with the client. This includes making and keeping periodic appointments spaced at appropriate intervals—weekly at first. Appointments must be regular and planned to prevent the client from changing, canceling, or otherwise manipulating appointment times. The care coordinator, in consultation with the medical care provider, works with the client over time to communicate the terms and goals of the care plan.

A crucial component to the successful establishment of a trusting, therapeutic relationship with these clients is empathy. They need to feel as though others hear their complaints and understand what they are experiencing.

Nursing Care Plan 19-1

THE CLIENT WITH SOMATIZATION DISORDER

Rose describes her current problem to the nurse saying, "I just can't do anything from day to day. I need Andrew to help me with everything. It's been this way a long time. I'm so tired of hurting and not being able to do anything, but I know there is no help for me." Rose and Andrew's typical day revolves around assisting Rose with multiple, complicated, and time-consuming activities designed to help her feel better and to function at home. Andrew retrieves Rose's food, supplies, and anything else that she needs during the day. He reports feeling "exhausted and burned out" because of Rose's daily needs. Rose and Andrew also say that they "used to have a good social life, with our old high school friends, but that has stopped in the past year because Rose has been feeling so bad." Rose and Andrew are hopeful that therapy might help them get through this difficult time. They express an interest in meeting weekly with the therapist.

After the initial interview the nurse therapist identifies two issues to address in the beginning stages of therapy.

Nursing Diagnosis: Ineffective Coping related to unresolved psychological issues as evidenced by history of frequent bodily complaints unsupported by diagnostic testing, excessive use of medical resources, restricted lifestyle, persistent focus on physical symptoms, and inability to verbally express emotional content

Goal: The client will verbalize feelings about her life, stressors, and physical symptoms and will spend less time focusing on physical symptoms.

Interventions	Rationales
Establish a therapeutic relationship. Show empathy for the client's distress but focus on feelings rather than physical complaints.	Clients with somatization disorder often have little or no trust in the healthcare system and its providers. Therapeutic intervention is possible only when the therapist has gained the client's trust. Focusing on feelings rather than physical complaints conveys interest in Rose as a person and reduces her need to garner attention through physical complaints.
Collaborate with the primary physician to coordinate client's physical care and appropriate use of medical services.	Care coordination is an important aspect of the treatment plan. It helps ensure appropriate use of resources, medical screening, and care.
Recommend insight-oriented therapy to explore psychological motivation for somatization.	Reduced symptoms and increased functioning may result as the client gains insight into behavior patterns.
Discuss triggering factors to help client gain insight into patterns associated with increased somatization.	Recognizing triggering events will help Rose manage her behavior.
Help client gain adaptive coping strategies to replace somatization as a strategy for coping with stress. Develop techniques that do not encourage focusing on bodily sensations (eg, developing an absorbing hobby, volunteering).	Clients cannot relinquish a coping strategy, no matter how dysfunctional, until they can replace it with another.

Evaluation: Indicators that interventions have been effective are that Rose increasingly discusses emotional material, develops insight into her behaviors, demonstrates willingness to resist using medical services excessively, and manages stress through adaptive behaviors.

Nursing Diagnosis: Caregiver Role Strain (husband) related to constant care-providing tasks as evidenced by statement about feeling exhausted and burned out

Goal: Rose will become more independent in her care, thus relieving Andrew from responsibilities.

(continued)

Nursing Care Plan 19-1 (Continued)

Interventions	Rationales
Encourage client to perform one task independently each week.	As Rose gains independence in her care, she will rely less on Andrew.
Encourage Andrew to give attention to the client in ways unrelated to her physical complaints.	Doing so will minimize Rose's need to gain attention through "sick role" behavior. It also will help reestablish husband–wife roles rather than sick person–caretaker roles.
Help the husband and client identify other family members who can assist.	This support frees Andrew from the role of constant caregiver.
Encourage husband to slowly resume social activities with the client.	Social activities will help reverse the social isolation, provide an outlet for Andrew, and help Rose regain a more balanced sense of self as a friend and companion of others.

Evaluation: Indicators that interventions have been effective are reports from the couple that Rose is less reliant on Andrew to constantly provide care and that they have reassumed conjugal and social roles.

Therapeutic empathic interventions might include responses such as, "I hear that it has been a very difficult time for you. I can't imagine how it has been trying to get through all of this." Empathy serves several purposes. One is to establish a connection between the care provider and the client so that the provider conveys an understanding of the client's difficulties. The second purpose is that empathy will highlight the "feeling" or "emotional" aspect of the client's experience, which is what he or she has difficulty verbalizing. Empathic statements serve as a powerful method for establishing trust while simultaneously modeling the expression of emotional feelings to the client and encouraging him or her to engage in emotional rather than physical expressions of discomfort.

MANAGING INEFFECTIVE COPING

One primary manifestation of somatoform disorders is excessive use of healthcare services. The nurse encourages discussion about the client's frequent visits to physicians, focusing on how the client feels when scheduling and going to visits. For example, "Can you talk about Dr. Jones and how it has been for you to go to him?" The nurse avoids engaging the client in a discussion about symptoms. For example, he or she avoids statements such as, "Why did you go to see Dr. Jones?" or "What did you tell the doctor was wrong with you?"

The nurse uses the opportunity to learn about the client's perception of the physician and to assess the dynamics of the health-seeking behaviors. Clients frequently express angry, negative feelings about their healthcare providers, focusing on how providers have been unable to find a physiological cause for the client's complaints. The nurse inquires about how this feels for the client, helping him or her to express anger and frustration. Verbalization of such feelings can be powerful.

It usually takes some time before clients can begin to express feelings, and many clients with somatoform disorders have a strong tendency to revert to talking about physical problems (eg, low back pain, headaches). Gently refocusing them provides a model for moving toward expressing feelings rather than describing physical states. Over time, this modeling can help clients become more familiar with how it feels to talk about emotions instead of physical problems. The nurse provides positive reinforcement whenever the client discusses feelings or emotions (see Therapeutic Communication 19-1).

The care coordinator also can collaborate with the primary physician to facilitate periodic, appropriately timed appointments. Such planning fosters trust between the client and physician and helps establish a productive long-term relationship. At the same time, it is imperative for the care coordinator to maintain frequent contact with the primary physician. The physician should be aware of all treatment goals and ideally should participate in planning the client's care. Calling at least once every 1 to 2 months and sending copies of the client's care plan and progress notes will maintain contact and provide the physician with an overview of the therapeutic goals and interventions.

When speaking with the physician, the nurse is sure to ascertain that the doctor continues to monitor the client's physical health. Frequently, because the client somatizes so much, physicians become "immune" to their complaints and can miss critical changes in health. The nurse talks with the physician about when physical examinations and routine diagnostic tests have been scheduled. He or she conveys to the client that healthcare providers are making a team effort to protect the client's health.

THERAPEUTIC COMMUNICATION 19-1
Addressing Somatization Disorder

This therapeutic communication is between Rose from Clinical Example 19-1 and her nurse, with whom she has established a therapeutic relationship. They have been working together for 2 weeks, meeting biweekly in the psychiatric outpatient unit.

Ineffective Dialogue

Nurse: Good morning, Rose. I noticed you arrived early today and had a chance to get some coffee already. Are you ready to start? (*Tries to begin without making any references to Rose's body and focusing on the day's events*)

Rose: Yes, I got up really early today. (*Sounds and appears exhausted, and her speech lacks energy*) My back and hip pain and my dizziness bothered me all night. I could hardly sleep; I was up and down the entire night. I'm so exhausted! (*She begins to talk about her pain right away, ignoring the nurse's question about starting.*)

Nurse: Really? I'm sorry. Where was the pain centered and what was it like? (*She enters into a discussion of Rose's pain and tries to assess it. Doing so allows Rose to stay in "complaint mode" and to invest more energy into talking about her pain. Note: Rose has undergone a thorough physical examination, which revealed no arthritis, joint problems, inflammatory processes, or other medical conditions. Pain and dizziness have been long-standing complaints.*)

Rose: (*Energetically*) Well, it started at first at the bottom of my spine, then it went up my back and then down into my right hip. At the same time, I start to get real dizzy. From my hip, it goes to my legs, usually, and sometimes even my ankles. I've had trouble with that hip before, too. Last year, I ended up on bed rest when it got so sore. (*Describes her pain and in great detail*)

Nurse: But it's great that you could get up this morning. (*Realizes she has made an error and tries to refocus and give positive reinforcement about Rose's activity*)

Rose: Well, if you want to call it great, yeah. It's pathetic that "great" is a word that describes just getting out of bed. Most people do that without even thinking, so I wouldn't call it "great." This whole problem is causing me a lot of pain, and I know it is going to go around my body, joint by joint. (*Immediately rejects the nurse's attempt at positive reinforcement and proceeds to reinforce the "sick role"*)

Nurse: How do you know that? (*Attempts to encourage Rose to discuss her pain again and avert the focus to feelings*)

Rose: Because that's what it always does.

Nurse: When has it done this before?

Rose: Well, last winter, I had a really bad bout of dizziness and joint pain that circulated through all my joint—my hips, back, shoulders, knees, and then ankles. I was a mess! It was the worst thing I've ever been through! (*Continues a lively discussion of her history and the pain and comfortably avoids the work of talking about her feelings*)

Effective Dialogue

Nurse: Good morning, Rose. I noticed you arrived early today and had a chance to get some coffee already. Are you ready to start?

Rose: Yes, I got up really early today. (*Sounds and appears exhausted, and her speech lacks energy*) My back and hip pain and my dizziness bothered me all night. I could hardly sleep; I was up and down the entire night. I'm so exhausted!

Nurse: So, when you got here was the coffee made already? I know you like your coffee. (*Attempts to avoid or ignore the topic of Rose's body and refocus on a neutral subject. Even though it seems abrupt, this technique often is effective with clients who are somatizing. If the refocusing is successful, the nurse will then turn to the topic of how Rose is feeling emotionally.*)

Rose: "Yeah, it was. Your office manager is so nice. He makes the coffee as soon as he gets to work and offers me a cup when I arrive. But, I have to tell you, it was very hard to pick that coffeepot up because I was still dizzy, and my hands and fingers were so stiff." (*Quickly returns to her bodily sensations*)

Nurse: Rose, I notice that you mentioned how nice Tom is, but you very quickly began to talk about your pain again. (*Makes an observation about Rose's pattern of communication and reflects it to Rose. Doing so reinforces that Rose has difficulty staying away from the topic of her body and attempts to help Rose gain insight into her behaviors.*)

Rose: Well, yeah, I guess I did. But I thought about it because I was talking about the coffee. I can't help it. (*Defends herself and sounds irritated but acknowledges her behavior*)

Nurse: Rose, we have talked about how your focus on your body is often unconscious, so I realize that sometimes you cannot help it. You are working so hard to become better able to observe yourself and to notice it when you do this. (*Uses the effective techniques of empathy and positive reinforcement. Carefully couches this in an observation about Rose's increasing abilities of self-observation. Nurses must use caution when giving positive reinforcement; making positive comments about the client's ability to do something versus complaining about the body often pushes the client too quickly into the "well role," and the client often rejects this vehemently. If the client is not ready to acknowledge wanting to move into a "healthy" role, positively reinforcing behaviors that make the client look "healthy" will backfire.*)

Rose: Yeah, I think I am, but it is such hard work, and sometimes I feel like I'm being criticized.

(*continued*)

THERAPEUTIC COMMUNICATION 19-1 (CONTINUED)
Addressing Somatization Disorder

Effective Dialogue

Nurse: Yes, I noticed that you sounded a bit irritated with me in your response, like you needed to defend yourself. How do you feel when I raise the topic of your focusing on your body? *(Realizes that Rose is progressing with self-observation. This is difficult for clients with somatization disorder. So, she verifies Rose's stance that "she can't help it," but she also takes the opportunity to ask how Rose feels about the confrontation. This intervention is excellent, because it mirrors what the nurse would like Rose to do [talk about feelings]; she is attempting to help Rose "practice" this behavior.)*

Rose: Well, I don't know. I wasn't mad. I just felt like you were criticizing me.

Nurse: Sometimes when we get into working on the issues of your body and talking about feelings, it may seem like criticism. A very normal emotional response to criticism is anger. *(Continues to focus on one emotional or feeling aspect of the exchange. She is trying to (1) point out that anger is a normal emotion and (2) help Rose to understand that her emotions are normal responses to events. Such a technique helps Rose begin to identify emotions and to understand that they are normal.)*

Rose: I guess maybe I did feel angry. You know, when I was about 5, I remember my mom telling me that "if you don't have anything good to say about something, don't say anything at all." That used to make me feel so stupid and wrong. *(Begins to recognize her emotions and to link them with past negative experiences. This is a high-level behavior, and Rose shows excellent potential for making some changes with ongoing therapy.)*

Nurse: It sounds like that must have been very difficult for you. Picture yourself as a little girl and how it felt to hear that, when in fact, you had very normal emotions. *(Tries to provide empathy and to help Rose connect her emotions more tightly with her experience as a child)*

Reflection and Critical Thinking

- In addition to the responses of the nurse in the second dialogue, give two other examples of potentially therapeutic responses.
- How do you feel about giving positive and negative reinforcement? Can you link these behaviors to the concepts of "sick role" and "healthy role"? Give another example of how providing positive reinforcement can prematurely push a client with somatization disorder into the "healthy role."
- Carry on a conversation with another student and attempt to focus only on physical symptoms (with no references to feelings or emotions) throughout the conversation. Try to understand what it would feel like if you had somatization disorder. Ask your partner how it feels to have someone dwell on physical sensations.

Depending on how much care-seeking behavior the client displays, it may be advantageous to contract with the client not to obtain healthcare from any unknown provider without speaking with the nurse first. Often, referrals are necessary anyway for insurance purposes. If not, however, it is helpful for the client to understand that the nurse therapist is working closely with the physician to determine the best plan of care, and if the client feels the need for additional medical intervention, the therapist and physician need to be involved in this decision. A client who knows this can feel "taken care of" and reassured that the team is concerned about his or her welfare.

ADDRESSING POWERLESSNESS AND DEPENDENCY ISSUES

The care coordinator works with the client over time to address dependency needs, including establishing and maintaining a regular schedule of therapy sessions (as discussed previously). He or she does so to decrease the client's unconscious need to develop more physical symptoms to ensure that dependency needs are met. The nurse therapist and client may negotiate the length of appointments, but 30 or 40 minutes are usually best to prevent excessive dependency and increased anxiety.

During the therapy sessions, the nurse urges the client to discuss feelings rather than physical complaints. He or she can encourage this either directly, by limiting time during the session spent discussing physical complaints (eg, "Can you take the first 15 minutes to update me as to how you are feeling physically, and then we will spend the rest of the time talking about how things are going in your life at home?"), or indirectly, by guiding the discussion away from physical symptoms toward emotional feelings and reactions to events.

ENHANCING SELF-ESTEEM

Encouraging the client to complete small activities between sessions will enhance independence and self-esteem. Keeping the activities small and manageable avoids pressuring the client to divest himself or herself from the "sick role" too soon. Activities such as gathering materials for bathing or setting the table for a meal without any help from a caregiver are examples of tasks the client can perform. Taking small steps will allow the client to experience success and will minimize the anxiety that he or she may associate with being expected to abandon the sick role and become more independent.

The nurse identifies character strengths with the client or discusses the client's past history, focusing on positive events involving success and independence. He or she avoids excessive praise about the past activity (eg, statements such as "It was wonderful that you were able to do that, and it probably really helped you feel better, don't you think?"). This type of praise often increases anxiety for clients with somatoform disorders because they may perceive that the healthcare provider expects the client to quickly resume these types of independent activities. Instead, the nurse provides positive reinforcement for the client's ability to reminisce about the events (eg, "It's great that you can talk about that and describe what it was like for you."). Such responses reinforce the client's ability to talk about emotional events (instead of about physical feelings), as well as help to boost self-esteem. At the same time, they do not uproot the client from the "sick role" that is still so important.

REDUCING ANXIETY

The nurse encourages the client to engage in anxiety-reducing activities, including relaxation, meditation, and yoga. He or she frequently assesses the client's response to these therapies, because some relaxation therapies (such as progressive muscle relaxation) may cause the client to increasingly focus on bodily sensations and thus may be countertherapeutic. Quiet reading, arts and crafts, and low-impact aerobics may be alternative interventions in this case.

REESTABLISHING SOCIAL ACTIVITIES

The nurse plans for the client to participate in one social activity during the week between sessions. Such activities could be as simple as going to the grocery store or for a ride in the car with a friend. They should be activities that the client must perform outside the home for some time. The purpose is to provide an opportunity for the client to experience success at leaving the home environment and expanding his or her circle of experience. The nurse provides positive but gentle reinforcement for any activities.

REESTABLISHING FUNCTIONAL FAMILY PROCESSES

The care coordinator must assess family dynamics and functioning to determine what effects the client's illness has had on the family. The care coordinator can hold a family meeting to discover and discuss the nature of problems. This must be done carefully to avoid making the family to feel that the client's concerns are invalid.

Many times the family members of a client with a somatoform disorder have difficulty relating directly to one another. Family members may be uncomfortable verbalizing thoughts and feelings during the family meeting. Instead, they may focus on the client's symptoms or the problems that they and their loved one have experienced with the medical care system. In the family meeting, the therapist can model appropriate behaviors and discussion, with interventions such as, "Yes, I hear that her back pain has really created difficulties for the family in many ways. What has it been like for you through this time?" Such questions refocus the discussion away from physical complaints to emotional feelings about the situation.

The therapist also must work with the family to target needed supports for the client. Although dealing with a relative who has a somatoform disorder can be exhausting, family members frequently have sufficient energy to participate. If the family is willing, the therapist can schedule several sessions to provide support and to give suggestions to the family about how to help the client.

Empathizing with the client about physical discomfort is important while simultaneously encouraging the family to assist the client to become more independent. One of the most effective interventions is to provide much empathy to the client within the family setting while providing suggestions for family interventions. For example, "As we can all see, Rose is having great difficulty with her back pain, but perhaps we can help her to do some small tasks even with the pain she is feeling."

The nurse supports family members in their willingness to be involved in the client's care and to come to family meetings. In addition, he or she gives empathy about their difficult position—providing support while not being able to truly help the loved one feel better. The nurse acknowledges feelings of frustration, helplessness, and anger as normal, natural reactions to the events. This can be beneficial not only for the client to hear, but also for family members. Empathizing with their frustrations and anger can also be effective in getting these feelings "out on the table."

Another possibly helpful intervention with the family is to encourage family members to take the client out periodically, whether to dinner or to the grocery store. Doing so can assist the client to meet the goal of getting out of the home and provide an interaction around which the family can relate in a nonphysically focused manner.

Evaluation

The therapist determines whether treatment goals have been met by evaluating the client's responses to interventions. Indicators that the interventions have been effective include the following:

- The client's trust has been established within the therapeutic relationship, as reflected by keeping appointments and following the treatment plan.
- The client experiences fewer physical symptoms and visits to nonprimary healthcare providers.
- The client can discuss emotions and feelings rather than focusing on physical complaints.
- The client can make positive self-statements and manages ADLs with increasing independence.
- The client reports improvement in anxiety level.
- The client has engaged in social activities outside the home.
- The client and family can manage stressors without focusing on the client's physical status.

▼ **Reflection and Critical Thinking Questions**

1. Discuss the role that physical symptoms have played in Rose's and Andrew's life (Clinical Example 19-1). Include observations about the role of symptoms in Rose's effort to gain attention and to meet her dependency needs. Include concepts of the "sick role," somatization, and dependency needs, describing the meaning of each and how they are interrelated in Rose's case.

2. Describe major differences between somatization disorder and hypochondriasis. Discuss whether and how your treatment approach might differ between the two disorders and why your approach differs (or why not).

▼ CHAPTER SUMMARY

- Somatoform disorders are characterized by client complaints of severe physical symptoms or disabilities that are not readily explained by organic or physical pathology on testing or examination. Somatoform disorders include somatization disorder, conversion disorder, hypochondriasis, pain disorder, and body dysmorphic disorder.
- Somatoform disorders must be distinguished from psychological factors affecting medical conditions, in which an identifiable medical illness is associated with psychological factors (eg, depression, anxiety).
- Somatoform disorders are approximately 10 times more common in women than in men, with the first symptoms usually appearing in adolescence.
- Somatoform disorders result from unconscious processes in which clients use physical symptoms to express emotional needs, such as gaining attention and forcing others to meet their dependency needs.
- Clients with somatoform disorders have highly elaborate self-diagnoses and symptoms that are not responsive to reassurance, explanation, or standard treatment. Symptoms associated with somatoform disorders often unconsciously enable the client to assume the "sick role," which relieves them from social obligations and responsibilities and meets their dependency needs.
- Somatoform disorders are difficult to treat and require an interdisciplinary, chronic care approach. Clinical treatments consist of individual, group, and family psychotherapies and a selection of limited somatic therapies, most often SSRI administration.
- Using the nursing process with a client with a somatoform disorder involves assessing the client on a psychological, physiological, and social level; determining nursing diagnoses; planning care; implementing care; and evaluating the treatment plan.
- Frequent and ongoing evaluation of the treatment plan and the client's response to interventions is criti-

cal to assist the client to move toward the goals of increased health, well-being, and optimal functional status.

▼REVIEW QUESTIONS

1. When assessing the client with a somatization disorder, the nurse anticipates that the client will not
   a. Relate an exaggerated and detailed medical history
   b. Discuss feelings and express needs verbally
   c. Have a history of going to many different providers without satisfaction
   d. Unconsciously express emotions through physical symptoms

2. The major difference between somatoform disorders and factitious disorders is that
   a. In somatoform disorders, clients consciously seek to gain attention.
   b. In factitious disorders, clients are unaware that their symptoms are not real.
   c. In somatoform disorders, clients are not consciously aware that they are meeting needs through physical complaints. In factitious disorders, clients purposefully manipulate symptoms to gain attention.
   d. Factitious disorders respond much more readily to psychopharmacologic treatment than do somatization disorders.

3. Clients with conversion disorder may report severe symptoms that cause significant disruption in daily activities while maintaining a calm, unconcerned approach to the problem. This behavior has been called
   a. *La grande belle*
   b. *La belle indifférence*
   c. Manipulation
   d. Hypochondriasis

4. Nursing interventions for the client with a somatoform disorder focus first on which of the following priorities?
   a. Reducing the client's immediate symptoms
   b. Enhancing the client's ability to see connections between emotion and body
   c. Assessing the client for suicidal ideation
   d. Establishing trust in the therapeutic relationship

5. Which of the following rationales accurately explains why it is important to assess mood in clients with somatoform disorders?
   a. Clients with somatoform disorders often experience comorbid depressive illnesses that frequently are undiagnosed and untreated.
   b. Somatoform disorders often result from depression.

   c. Depressed mood is a symptom that indicates that the client is most likely suicidal.
   d. Clients with somatoform disorders often have underlying bipolar disorders.

6. The most appropriate nursing diagnosis for the client with a somatoform disorder and a long history of frequent visits to different physicians is
   a. **Hopelessness** related to chronicity of symptoms as evidenced by dependency
   b. **Ineffective Coping** related to unresolved psychological issues as evidenced by inability to express feelings verbally and difficulty establishing trust with others
   c. **Chronic Low Self-Esteem** related to chronic physical symptoms that inhibit the client's daily functioning
   d. **Caregiver Role Strain** related to excessive demands being placed on others as a result of the client's inability to perform ADLs

7. Which of the following statements accurately describes findings associated with somatoform disorders?
   a. Women experience somatoform disorders about 10 times more often than men do.
   b. Men are diagnosed with somatoform disorders about 20 times more often than women are.
   c. Somatoform disorders have not been shown to have any familial links.
   d. Somatoform disorders often begin early in childhood between 2 and 4 years of age.

8. The nurse judges the plan of care to be *ineffective* when which of the following outcomes occurs?
   a. The client experiences increased self-esteem from the increased attention shown during physician visits.
   b. The client establishes a trusting relationship with the psychotherapist and physician.
   c. The client spends less time focusing on physical symptoms.
   d. The client demonstrates increased participation in ADLs.

9. Bob, a man with somatoform disorder, has been in therapy for several weeks. When he arrives for therapy he states, "The pain in my arms and legs has been much worse this week." Which of the following responses will be most therapeutic?
   a. "Please tell me more about it."
   b. "You're focusing on your body again. Let's move on to another topic. How have you been feeling?"
   c. "Good morning Bob. Are you ready to begin now?"
   d. "I notice you look better, though."

10. Which of the following statements accurately reflects treatment for a somatoform disorder?

a. Treatment typically last 6 months to 1 year; if the client fully engages in therapy, full recovery is likely.

b. Treatment includes routinely changing therapists to prevent the client from becoming overly dependent.

c. Prognosis is generally poor; effective management is possible only when the client has established a strong, long-term relationship with a care provider or team.

d. Prognosis is generally good if the client has a strong therapeutic relationship with a care provider.

▼ REFERENCES AND SUGGESTED READINGS

*Ader, R., Felten, D. L., & Cohen, N. (Eds.). (2001). *Psychoneuroimmunology* (3rd ed.). New York: Academic Press.

*American Psychiatric Association. (2000). *Diagnostic and statistical manual of mental disorders* (4th ed., text rev.). Washington, DC: Author.

*Barsky, A. J. (1989). Somatoform disorders. In H. I. Kaplan & B. J. Sadock (Eds.), *Comprehensive textbook of psychiatry* (Vol. I, 5th ed., pp. 1009–1027). Baltimore: Williams & Wilkins.

*Barsky, A. J., & Borus, J. F. (1999). Functional somatic syndromes. *Annals of Internal Medicine, 130*(11), 910–921.

*Barsky, A. J., Peekna, H. M., & Borus, J. F. (2001). Somatic symptom reporting in women and men. *Journal of General Internal Medicine, 16*(4), 266–275.

*Barsky, A. J., Wyshak, G., & Klerman, G. L. (1986). Hypochondriasis: An evaluation of the DSM-III criteria in medical outpatients. *Archives of General Psychiatry, 43*, 493–500.

*Becker, B. E. (1998). Clinical crossroads: The rehabilitative model for somatization disorder. *Journal of the American Medical Association, 279*(9), 656.

*Bowman, E. S. (2000, May). *Treating somatization related to child abuse.* Paper presented before the American Psychiatric Association, Chicago, IL.

*Campayo, G., & Carrillo, C. (2000). Effectiveness of group psychoanalytic therapy in somatizing patients. *Actas Esp. Psiquiatr, 28*(2), 105–114.

*Clarke, D. M., & Smith, G. C. (2000). Management of somatoform disorders. *Australian Family Physician, 29*(2), 115–119.

*Coen, S. J. (1992). *The misuse of persons: Analyzing pathological dependency.* Hillsdale, NJ: Analytic Press.

*Coen, S. J. (1996). *Object relations theory and therapy.* Northvale, NJ: J. Aronson.

*Coen, S. J., & Sarno, J. E. (1989). Psychosomatic avoidance of conflict in back pain. *Journal of the American Academy of Psychoanalysts, 17*(3), 359–376.

Cunningham, S. J., Harrison, S. D., Feinman, C., & Hopper, C. (2000). Body dysmorphic disorder involving the facial region: A report of 6 cases. *Journal of Oral and Maxillofacial Surgery, 58*(10), 1180–1183.

*Elmer, K. B., George, R. M., & Peterson, K. (2000). Therapeutic update: Use of risperidone for the treatment of monosymptomatic hypochondriacal psychosis. *Journal of the American Academy of Dermatology, 43*(4), 683–686.

*Epstein, R. M., Quill, T. E., & McWhinney, I. R. (1999). Somatization reconsidered: Incorporating the patient's experience of illness. *Archives of Internal Medicine, 159*(3), 215–222.

Fava, G., Grandi, S., Rafanelli, C., et al. (2000). Explanatory therapy in hypochondriasis. *Journal of Clinical Psychiatry, 61*(4), 317–323.

*Flaskerud, J. H. (2000). Ethnicity, culture, and neuropsychiatry. *Issues in Mental Health Nursing, 21*(1), 5–29.

*Ford, C. V. (1995a). Conversion disorder and somatoform disorder not otherwise specified. In G. O. Gabbard (Ed.), *Treatments of psychiatric disorders* (2nd ed., pp. 1736–1753). Washington, DC: American Psychiatric Press.

Ford, C. V. (1995b). Introduction: Somatoform and factitious disorders. In G. O. Gabbard (Ed.), *Treatments of psychiatric disorders* (2nd ed., pp. 1714–1716). Washington, DC: American Psychiatric Press.

*Gara, M. A., & Escobar, J. I. (2001). The stability of somatization syndromes over time. *Archives of General Psychiatry, 58*(1), 94.

*Garcia-Campayo, J., & Sanz-Carrillo, C. (2001). Gabapentin for the treatment of patients with somatization disorder. *Journal of Clinical Psychiatry, 62*(6), 474.

Grant, J. E., Kim, S. W., & Crow, S. J. (2001). Prevalence and clinical features of body dysmorphic disorder in adolescent and adult psychiatric inpatients. *Journal of Clinical Psychiatry, 62*(7), 517–522.

*Green, A. R., Betancourt, J. R., & Carrillo, J. E. (2000). The relation between somatic symptoms and depression. *New England Journal of Medicine, 342*(9), 658–659.

Guereje, O., & Simon, G. E. (1999). The natural history of somatization in primary care. *Psychological Medicine, 29*(3), 669–676.

*Hodgkinson, D. J. (2001). Imagined ugliness: A symptom which can become a disorder. *Medical Journal of Australia, 174*(3), 156.

*Hollander, E., Allen, A., Kwon, J., Aronowitz, B., Schmeidler, J., & Wong, C., et al. (1999). Clomipramine vs. desipramine crossover trial in body dysmorphic disorder: Selective efficacy of serotonin reuptake inhibitor in imagined ugliness. *Archives of General Psychiatry, 56*(11), 1033–1039.

*Holloway, K. L., & Zerbe, K. J. (2000). Simplified approach to somatization disorder: When less may prove to be more. *Postgraduate Medicine, 108*(6), 89–95.

*Huber, M. (2000). Aspects of occupational disability in psychosomatic disorders. *Versicherungsmedizin, 52*(2), 66–75.

*Johns, M. (1999). Communicating effectively with a patient who has a somatization disorder. *American Family Physician, 59*(9), 2639–2640.

Katon, W., Buchwald, D., Simon, G., et al. (1991). Psychiatric illness in patients with chronic fatigue and rheumatoid arthritis. *Journal of General Internal Medicine, 6*, 277–285.

Katon, W., Egen, K., & Miller, D. (1985). Chronic pain: Lifetime psychiatric diagnoses and family history. *American Journal of Psychiatry, 142*, 1156–1160.

*Katon, W., Sullivan, M., & Walker, E. (2001). Medical symptoms without identified pathology: Relationship to psychiatric disorders, childhood and adult trauma, and personality traits. *Annals of Internal Medicine, 134*(9, Pt. 2), 917–925.

*Keeley, R., Smith, M., & Miller, J. (2000). Somatoform symptoms and treatment nonadherence in depressed family medicine outpatients. *Archives of Family Medicine, 9*(1), 46–54.

*Kent, D., Tomasson, K., & Coryell, W. (1995). Course and outcome of conversion and somatization disorders. *Psychosomatics, 36*(2), 138–144.

*Kirmayer, L. J. (2001). Cultural variations in the clinical presentation of depression and anxiety disorders: Implications for diagnosis and treatment. *Journal of Clinical Psychiatry, 62*(Suppl. 13), 22–28.

Kroenke, K., & Swindle, R. (2000). Cognitive-behavioral therapy for somatization and symptom syndromes: A critical review of controlled clinical trials. *Psychotherapy Psychosomatics, 69*(4), 205–215.

*Levinson, D. (1994). *Mind, body, and medicine: A history of the American Psychosomatic Society.* McLean, VA: American Psychosomatic Society.

*Lorenzi, P., Hardoy, M. C., & Cabras, P. L. (2000). Life crisis and the body within. *Psychopathology, 33*(6), 283–291.

*MacBain, R. N. (2001). The somatic components of disease. *Journal of the American Osteopathic Association, 101*(3), 184–190.

*Mabe, P. A., Hobson, D. P., Jones, L. R., & Jarvis, R. G. (1988). Hypochondriacal traits in medical inpatients. *General Hospital Psychiatry, 10,* 236–244.

*Margo, K. L, & Margo, G. M. (2000). Early diagnosis and empathy in managing somatization. *American Family Physician, 61*(5), 1282–1285.

Martin, R. L., & Yutzy, S. H. (1997). Somatoform disorders. In A. K. Tasman, J. Kay, & J. A. Lieberman (Eds.), *Psychiatry* (pp. 1119–1155). Philadelphia: W.B. Saunders.

McBeth, J., Macfarlane, G. J., Benjamin, S., & Silman, A. J. (2001). Features of somatization predict the onset of chronic widespread pain: Results of a large population-based study. *Arthritis and Rheumatology, 44*(4), 940–946.

*MiniMental LCC. (1975). Mini-Mental State: A practical method for grading the cognitive state of patients for the clinician. *Journal of Psychiatric Research, 12*(3), 189–198.

*Noyes, R., Roger, K., Fisher, M., Phillips, B., Suelzer, M., & Woodman, C. (1994). One-year follow-up of medical outpatients with hypochondriasis. *Psychosomatics, 35*(6), 533–545.

*Parsons, T. (1964). *Social structure and personality.* London: Collier-MacMillan.

Perkins, R. J. (1999). SSRI antidepressants are effective for treating delusional hypochondriasis [Letter]. *Medical Journal of Australia, 170*(3), 140–141.

*Phillips, K. A. (1996). Pharmacologic treatment of body dysmorphic disorder. *Psychopharmacology Bulletin, 32*(4), 597–605.

*Phillips, K. A., Dwight, M. M., & McElroy, S. L. (1998). Efficacy and safety of fluvoxamine in body dysmorphic disorder. *Journal of Clinical Psychiatry, 59*(4), 165–171.

Poikolainen, K., Aalto-Setala, T., Marttunen, M., Tuulio-Henriksson, A., & Lonnqvist, J. (2000). Predictors of somatic symptoms: A five year follow up of adolescents. *Archives of Diseases in Children, 83*(5), 388–392.

*Robbins, J. M., & Kirmayer, L. J. (1991). *Cognitive and social factors in somatization:* Research and clinical perspectives. Washington, DC: American Psychiatry.

*Servan-Schreiber, D., Kolb, N. R., & Tabas, G. (2000). Somatizing patients: Part I. Practical diagnosis. *American Family Physician, 61*(4), 1073–1078.

Sheehan, B., & Banerjee, S. (1999). Review: Somatization in the elderly. *International Journal of Geriatric Psychiatry, 14*(12), 1044–1049.

*Silverstein, B. (1999). Gender difference in the prevalence of clinical depression: The role played by depression associated with somatic symptoms. *American Journal of Psychiatry, 156*(3), 480–482.

*Singh, B. S. (1998). Managing somatoform disorders. *Medical Journal of Australia, 168*(11), 572–577.

*Slaughter, J. R., & Sun, A. M. (1999). In pursuit of perfection: A primary care physician's guide to body dysmorphic disorder. *American Family Physician, 60*(6), 1738–1742.

*Stoudemire, A. (1993). Psychological factors affecting physical condition and DSM-IV. *Psychosomatics, 34*(1), 8–11.

*Stuart, S., & Noyes, R. (1999). Attachment and interpersonal communication in somatization. *Psychosomatics, 40*(1), 34–43.

Sullivan, M., Katon, W., Dobie, R., et al. (1988). Disabling tinnitus: Association with affective disorder. *General Hospital Psychiatry, 10,* 285–291.

Walker, E. A., Roy-Byrne, P., & Katon, W. (1990). Irritable bowel syndrome and psychiatric illness. *American Journal of Psychiatry, 147,* 565–572.

*Walker, E. A., Unutzer, J., & Katon, W. J. (1998). Understanding and caring for the distressed patient with multiple medically unexplained symptoms. *Journal of the American Board of Family Practice, 11*(5), 347–356.

*Wyllie, E., Glazer, J. P., Benbadis, S., Kotagal, P., & Wolgamuth, B. (1999). Psychiatric features of children and adolescents with pseudoseizures. *Archives of Pediatric Adolescent Medicine, 153*(3), 244–248.

*Zonderman, A. B., Hegt, M. W., & Costa, P. T. (1985). Does the Illness Behavior Questionnaire measure abnormal illness behavior? *Health Psychology, 4,* 425–436.

Starred references are cited in text.

For additional information on this chapter, go to *http://connection. lww.com.*

Need more help? See Chapter 19 of the *Study Guide to Accompany Mohr: Johnson's Psychiatric-Mental Health Nursing,* 5th edition.

The Client With a Sexual or Gender Disorder

DELIA ESPARZA

▼ KEY TERMS

Arousal—Physiologic stimulation, such as touching, kissing, fondling, licking, or biting erogenous body parts, that causes changes in the genitals.

Bisexuality—An equal or almost equal attraction to or preference for members of either sex as a sexual partner.

Desire—Activation of areas in the brain that produce sexual appetite or drive.

Dyspareunia—Genital pain associated with sexual intercourse in either a man or woman.

Excitement—Psychological stimulation during the desire phase such as sexual fantasies or romantic communication.

Foreplay—Petting and fondling behaviors that cause arousal during the excitement phase.

Heterosexuality—An attraction to and preference for members of the opposite sex as sexual partners.

Homosexuality—An attraction to and preference for members of the same sex as sexual partners.

Masturbation—Self-stimulation of erogenous areas to the point of orgasm.

Orgasm—The peak of sexual pleasure. In the female, it consists of 3 to 15 strong rhythmic contractions of the orgasmic platform of the vagina. In the male, it consists of emission and ejaculation.

Paraphilias—Sexual expressions for at least 6 months that are characterized by recurrent, intense sexual urges, fantasies, or behaviors that generally involve nonhuman objects or animals, suffering or humiliation of self or partner, or children or other nonconsenting persons.

Premature ejaculation—A persistent or recurrent onset of orgasm and ejaculation with minimal sexual stim-

ulation before, on, or shortly after penetration and before the person wishes it.

Sexual dysfunction—Sexual expressions characterized by a disturbance in the processes that characterize the sexual response cycle or by pain associated with sexual intercourse.

Sexual intercourse (coitus)—Penetration of the vagina by the penis.

Sexuality—The experience of the sexual self.

Transsexual—A person who identifies with and lives as if he or she is of the opposite gender.

Transvestite—A person who cross-dresses for the purpose of sexual arousal.

Vaginismus—Recurrent or persistent involuntary spasm of the musculature of the outer third of the vagina, which interferes with sexual intercourse.

▼ LEARNING OBJECTIVES

On completion of this chapter, you should be able to accomplish the following:

- Recognize your own sexual beliefs and values to avoid imposing them on clients.
- Describe the factors that affect sexual expression.
- Discuss the phases of human sexual response.
- Understand the various methods of achieving orgasm.
- Describe normal age-related sexual changes.
- Discuss the causes of sexual dysfunction disorders.
- Describe the treatment approaches for sexual dysfunction disorders.
- Apply the nursing process to the care of a client with a sexual dysfunction.
- Discuss the types of paraphilias.

- Compare and contrast the signs and symptoms of gender identity disorders as they manifest in children and adults.

▼ Clinical Example 20-1

George is a 45-year-old married man and the father of two boys, ages 16 and 18 years. After George arrives at the office for his annual examination, the nurse reviews his chart and sees that he was diagnosed with type 1 diabetes mellitus several years ago but otherwise is healthy. Before the doctor performs the physical examination, the nurse asks George several questions related to his health. Toward the end of this interview, George looks down at the floor and quietly says, "I don't know how to say this. I guess I'm not a man anymore." The nurse responds, "Tell me more about what you're experiencing."

George explains that he and his wife have not had sex for several months because he has trouble "getting turned on." He goes on to say that he felt badly when he could not satisfy his wife and, after a few times when he "couldn't do it," he stopped making sexual advances toward her. Whenever his wife made sexual advances toward him, he "made some excuse." He asks the nurse, "Can anything be done to help me?"

George has a sexual dysfunction disorder. He is experiencing difficulty becoming aroused and maintaining an erection. Further exploration of the specifics of his problem is necessary to determine what treatment he needs. For example, his difficulty maintaining an erection could be from the effects of his diabetes. The nurse and doctor need to rule out or recognize and address the physical components of his sexual disorder. Additionally, anxiety and other emotional components may contribute to his sexual dysfunction. For example, anxiety can interfere with the arousal process, blocking the development of the penile erection.

The nurse explains to George that his difficulty could be the result of various problems and that treatment for these difficulties is available and helpful. The nurse refers George to the physician for screening and treatment of any medical problems and to a mental health professional that specializes in sex therapy (eg, clinical specialist in psychiatric-mental health nursing, psychologist, psychiatric social worker) for assistance with his sexual dysfunction.

This chapter consists of two distinct sections: normal human sexuality, and sexual and gender disorders. The three subgroups of sexual and gender disorders are sexual dysfunction, paraphilias, and gender identity disorders. Sexual dysfunction is the most common subgroup and thus receives special focus in this chapter.

As you read the chapter, consider the case of George in Clinical Example 20–1. What in George's medical history may lead the nurse to suspect a physical cause for his sexual dysfunction? Follow the progression of George's care in Nursing Care Plan 20-1 and apply your understanding of this client and others with sexual dysfunction in the Reflection and Critical Thinking Questions at the end of the chapter.

NORMAL HUMAN SEXUALITY

Sexuality, the experience of our sexual self, is so inextricably connected with our awareness of the total self that it is not limited to overtly sexual behaviors and feelings. Rather, sexuality is part of every experience we have. We cannot separate our sexuality from the rest of ourselves. When we listen to music, touch another person's skin, or feel the pleasing sensation of water spraying on our skin in the shower, our sexuality in the form of sensuality is engaged. Therefore, disorders in sexuality and gender identity are some of the most intimate concerns that human beings can have. These dysfunctions have significant consequences for self-concept, self-esteem, and overall quality of life.

Sexual Expression

Human sexual expression is diverse and tied to many intrapersonal and extrapersonal factors, including genetics, individual preferences, life experiences, culture, and health. Because values and beliefs contribute to the formation of views regarding sexual expression, the nurse must be aware of his or her own views and learn about the views of the client populations with whom he or she works. When the nurse's sexual values and expression differ from those of the client, the nurse should be alert to any tendency to apply his or her biases to the client. Instead, the professional nurse must empathize with the client's sexual concerns and difficulties. This empathy is essential for truly therapeutic interactions between the nurse and the client. If a nurse recognizes that he or she cannot be accepting and supportive of the client, then the nurse either should not work with that client or seek consultation from colleagues or supervisors on how to act professionally.

In general, sexual expression that occurs between two consenting adults, is not harmful (physically or psychologically) to either party, does not involve any form of force or coercion, and occurs in private, is thought to be within the range of acceptable sexual expression. Sexual behaviors that violate these parameters, such as pedophilia, incest, or voyeurism, are not acceptable because they violate the will of others and may fall into the category of criminal behavior (eg, incest, pedophilia).

Not everyone agrees on what types of sexual expression are harmful to the parties involved. For example, U. S. society tends to view prostitution as a criminal activity even though many believe that prostitution meets the parameters noted previously. Among the many concerns that people have about prostitution, however, is the belief that this activity is psychologically demeaning and may include physically destructive or dangerous practices by the parties involved. Overt or covert coercion or force (eg, teenage runaways forced into prostitution, prostitution to support drug addictions) frequently is part of the practice of prostitution. Interestingly, society tends to punish the seller and not the buyer of the sexual behaviors, as evidenced by the fact that prostitutes are prosecuted whereas their customers frequently experience no legal consequences (Laumann, Gagnon, Michael, & Michaels, 1994).

EFFECTS OF SEXUAL ORIENTATION ON SEXUAL EXPRESSION

Sexual orientation encompasses sexual preference, gender role, and sexual identity.

Sexual Preference

Sexual preference refers to the gender to which a person is attracted. A person may be sexually attracted to someone of the opposite sex (heterosexual preference), same sex (homosexual preference), or both sexes (bisexual preference).

A **heterosexual** is a person whose preference for sexual partners are members of the opposite sex. Most of the human population (90% or more) identifies itself as heterosexual.

For about 2% to 4% of the population, the sexual partner of choice is a member of the same sex. Preferring members of the same sex as sexual partners is called **homosexuality**. Male homosexuals sometimes are referred to as gay men, whereas female homosexuals are known as lesbians. The incidence of homosexuality varies geographically. In some major cities, for example, male homosexuals number as many as 14% of the population (Kaplan & Sadock, 1996). Nurses must be knowledgeable about health and mental health issues affecting the gay community, including coping with disenfranchisement by a predominately heterosexual population, dealing with AIDS-related loss and death, and health matters such as "safer sex" practices (Client and Family Education 20-1).

Bisexuality refers to an equal or almost equal preference for members of either sex as sexual partners. A person may identify himself or herself as bisexual, even if he or she engages in a long-term relationship with a person of the

---

Client and Family Education 20-1

SAFER SEX OPTIONS FOR PHYSICAL INTIMACY

Teaching Points

A common nursing role is educating clients in a variety of healthcare settings (community groups, clinics, hospitals) about the prevention of sexually transmitted diseases (STDs). The following is a listing of guidelines for safer sex that the nurse may wish to share with clients.

Safer Sexual Activities

- Massage
- Masturbation
- Hugging
- Hand-to-genital touching (hand job)
- Mutual masturbation
- Body rubbing
- Erotic books and movies
- Dry kissing
- All sexual activities when both partners are monogamous, trustworthy, and known by testing to be free of HIV

Possibly Safe Sexual Activities

- Wet kissing with no broken skin, cracked lips, or damaged mouth tissue
- Vaginal or rectal intercourse using latex or synthetic condom correctly
- Oral sex on a man using latex or synthetic condom
- Oral sex on a woman using a latex or synthetic barrier such as a female condom, dental dam, or modified male condom, especially if she does not have her period or a vaginal infection with discharge

- All sexual activities when both partners are in a long-term monogamous relationship and trust each other

Unsafe Sexual Activities in the Absence of HIV Testing, Trust, and Monogamy

- Any vaginal or rectal intercourse without a latex or synthetic condom
- Oral sex on a man without a latex or synthetic condom
- Oral sex on a woman without a latex or synthetic barrier such as a female condom, dental dam, or modified male condom, especially if she is having her period or has a vaginal infection with discharge
- Semen in the mouth
- Oral–anal contact
- Sharing sex toys or douching equipment
- Blood contact of any kind, including menstrual blood, or any sex that causes tissue damage or bleeding

Useful Resources

http://safersex.org
This site is an online journal of safer sex.

http://seniorliving.about.com/mbody.html
This site, geared to people older than 50 years, contains articles about safer sex.

http://www.thebody.com
This site, entitled *The Body: An AIDS and HIV Information Resource,* provides information and numerous articles on safe sex and prevention of HIV and STDs.

same or opposite sex. Some bisexuals do not feel fulfilled with a solitary (or monogamous) relationship with a member of either sex but prefer to be involved in equally intense and meaningful relationships with a man and a woman. Approximately 7% to 9% of the general population can be identified as bisexual, which includes those who refer to themselves as bisexual, although they have never had any kind of sexual experience with a person of the same sex, and those who generally prefer and are engaged in a heterosexual relationship. As with homosexuality, bisexuality is not uniformly distributed in the population. The percentage of bisexuals is likely to be highest in urban areas (Kaplan & Sadock, 1996).

The sexual behavior of homosexuals and bisexuals varies as much as the sexual behavior of heterosexuals. Sexual dysfunction, pedophilia, and promiscuity are no more prevalent among homosexuals or bisexuals than among heterosexuals. Gay men and lesbians do tend to enter into more sexual relationships than do their heterosexual counterparts, perhaps because fewer societal supports (eg, legally sanctioned marriage) exist for long-term sexual relationships among homosexuals.

Recently, community centers, organizations, and publications devoted to gay, lesbian, and bisexual activities and concerns have emerged. Gay and lesbian concerns also have become more visible in mainstream movies and television sitcoms. Community celebrities, such as politicians, actors, musicians, activists, and artists, are more open about their sexual orientation. Despite these forward strides, many people still hold values and beliefs that are discriminatory toward homosexuals. Gay men and lesbians continue to be stigmatized and persecuted by laws denying them equal rights and opportunities like those available to heterosexuals (eg, service in the military, legal recognition of marriages, antidiscrimination laws for work and housing) (Laumann et al., 1994).

Gender Role

A person's *gender role* is his or her general pattern of masculine or feminine behaviors, which are influenced strongly by cultural factors (discussed later).

Sexual Identity

Finally, *sexual identity* is whether an individual considers himself or herself to be male or female. Gender identity disorders are discussed in detail later in this chapter.

EFFECTS OF CULTURE ON SEXUAL EXPRESSION

Cultural groupings include not only racial and ethnic cultures, but also the culture of the family (each family has a unique culture); the culture of religion or spiritual philosophy; the culture of a particular geographic region; and the culture of a discipline or occupation (eg, nursing). These cultural influences are visible in a person's values, beliefs, and behaviors, including sexual expression. For example,

psychiatric nurses are bound by the American Nurses Association's Standards of Nursing Practice not to engage in sexual behavior with clients (see Chap. 1). This standard of nursing practice is an expression of the culture of nursing's values and beliefs about how nurses should conduct themselves with their clients.

Within the increasingly culturally diverse U.S. society, many variations related to sexual expression exist. Nurses should expect to encounter these variations. Furthermore, the nurse's reaction to these variations should be responsive to the client's sexual concerns. These attitudes are inherent in the nurse's efforts to treat the client with respect and dignity. For more information on culture and ethnicity in psychiatric-mental health nursing, see Chapter 5.

EFFECTS OF ILL HEALTH ON SEXUAL EXPRESSION

Illness, disability, hospitalization, and surgery are a few of the many factors that may disrupt sexual expression, sexual identity, and self-esteem. Clients manifest these disruptions in various ways, including withdrawal from the family, anger toward the hospital or clinic staff, deterioration of normal practices of hygiene and dress, and display of sexual acting-out behaviors.

In an example of a sexual acting-out behavior, the client may make sexually suggestive remarks or gestures toward nursing personnel. Nurses should respond to this inappropriate behavior in a way that clearly conveys the limits of the nurse–client relationship and communicates the intention of maintaining a professional, therapeutic, and nonsocial relationship. If the client persists, the nurse should repeat the limits of the relationship and reiterate that he or she will not tolerate the violation of these limits. The nurse should try to set limits firmly but unemotionally to reject the inappropriate behavior without rejecting the client (Implications for Nursing Practice 20-1).

Illness and hospitalization weaken most normal coping mechanisms and distance the client from significant relationships, thereby creating a need for intimacy on some level with staff members. Nursing staff should meet this need with understanding, emotional warmth, and support within the professional relationship. For example, a client may need to talk about her fear of being less feminine or less of a woman after a mastectomy or hysterectomy procedure. Similarly, a male client may seek reassurance that he is still desirable after prostate surgery or an orchidectomy. Other health problems, such as cardiac disease or diabetes, also may affect the client's sexual performance and hence his or her sexual sense of self. The nurse always should consider how a client's particular health problem is affecting or may affect the client's sexual functioning. Additionally, the nurse should be prepared to listen to and respond to these concerns.

The client who masturbates bothers many nurses. Perhaps one reason for this lack of tolerance and empathy is a mistaken belief that seriously ill people do not have

Implications for Nursing Practice 20-1

Dealing with the Sexually Inappropriate Client

Nurse Alvarez became angry when Mr. Jones patted her buttocks and commented that he "enjoyed the sight of firm and beautiful buns." She turned to find him grinning at her and saying to her "You're kind of cute when you're angry." How should Nurse Alvarez deal with this situation?

In the days after this incident, Mr. Jones no longer made any effort to touch Nurse Alvarez in any way. Nevertheless, he persistently asked her to go out on a date with him once he left the hospital and was no longer her patient. How should Nurse Alvarez deal with this situation?

On the day of Mr. Jones's discharge, Nurse Alvarez received a box of chocolates from him. Attached to the chocolates was a note saying he would call her later in the week to arrange a date. What should Nurse Alvarez do now?

One evening about 1 month after Mr. Jones's discharge, Nurse Alvarez finds him standing by her vehicle in the hospital employee parking lot. He smiles and says all he wants is a chance to talk to her. If she will just have a cup of coffee with him, he'll never bother her again if that is her wish. What should she do?

General Guidelines

There is no single right answer to the questions posed above. Each situation is different; therefore, the nurse must determine what makes the best therapeutic and professional sense in each case. Although this example shows a male client as acting in a sexually inappropriate manner toward a female nurse, the roles certainly could be reversed. Also, same-sex (male-to-male or female-to-female) inappropriate behavior occurs. The following information is meant to guide the nurse's response to the sexually inappropriate client, regardless of gender or sexual orientation:

- Be firm, clear, and consistent in setting limits on inappropriate client behavior.
- Verbalize these limits directly, calmly, and nonjudgmentally.
- Document the client's inappropriate sexual behavior from the first episode throughout the history of inappropriate occurrences.
- Also document the actions taken by the nurse and their results.
- If the client's inappropriate sexual behavior persists, seek consultation from a supervisor. Such consultation provides emotional support and the additional experience and knowledge of the supervisor. Furthermore, if the situation develops into stalking or harassment, the nurse has documentation and a witness to the harassing behavior.
- If, even though you have set firm and clear limits, the client persists in his or her sexual advances, consider removing yourself from any contact with the client.
- If client contact continues after you have taken these measures, then be aware that your safety might be in danger and take legal action (eg, restraining order, filing charges against the client for harassment or stalking) to protect yourself. Also, take precautions for your personal safety such as being escorted by security to and from your vehicle, informing neighbors to be on the lookout for a potential intruder, and making your home more secure from an intruder. These kinds of precautions also will provide witnesses to the inappropriate behavior should the matter become a legal one. Witnesses are essential in the prosecution of a stalker or harasser.

sexual needs or desires. The need for sexual release is normal, however, and does not cease because the client is ill or incapacitated. The nurse should recognize the client's need for privacy and respect it by knocking before entering a client's room or keeping the curtain drawn around the client's bed unless requested otherwise. If the nurse enters the client's room while the client is masturbating, he or she should apologize for the invasion into the client's space and provide the necessary privacy. Most important is that the nurse conveys respect and appreciation for the client's needs and individual values. Similarly, a client may need sexual activity with his or her sexual partner while hospitalized. The nurse should be sensitive to cues of these needs and respond by providing privacy.

Sexual Response

HUMAN SEXUAL RESPONSE PHASES

Masters and Johnson (1970) studied what they termed "the human sexual response cycle," which consisted of four phases: (1) excitement, (2) plateau, (3) orgasm, and (4) resolution. Kaplan's studies (1979) resulted in a reorganization of the phases of human sexual response, calling them

1. Desire
2. Excitement
3. Orgasm

The following is a brief summary of Kaplan's system and a description of resolution.

Desire

Desire involves activation of areas in the brain that produce sexual appetite or drive. This activation does not include changes in genital organs. How the activation of the brain produces sexual appetite or drive is not well understood. The individual's perception of the environment, personal preferences, and attractions to other people, as well as an absence of inhibiting influences such as pain, fear, anxiety, anger, discomfort, and mental preoccupation, contribute to the occurrence of sexual behavior. Desire, like all phases of human sexual responsiveness, is influenced by individual differences as well as by human physiologic makeup. Some individuals are more desirous of sexual activity than are others.

Excitement

Excitement begins with the psychological stimulation of the desire phase such as sexual fantasies or romantic communication. Physiologic stimulation such as touching, kissing, fondling, licking, or biting erogenous body parts causes changes in the genitals, which is termed **arousal**. These petting and fondling behaviors causing arousal during the excitement phase are called **foreplay**. The female experiences lubrication and expansion of the clitoris, whereas the male experiences penile erection and elevation of the testes. Both experience nipple erection, a generalized tensing of the muscles throughout the body, an increased heart rate, increased respirations and blood pressure, and motor restlessness. A fine rash or "sex flush" may appear over the abdomen and chest.

As the excitement phase continues, vasocongestion in the vagina results in a narrowing in the vaginal opening and the development of a swollen and tensing area called the *orgasmic platform* in the lower third of the vagina and the labia minora. The clitoris retracts from its normal position, and breasts enlarge through areolar engorgement. In males, the size of the coronal area of the glans penis increases, and the testes continue to increase in size and elevate. For males and females, the sex flush, motor restlessness, heart rate, blood pressure, and respirations continue to increase.

Orgasm

Orgasm in the female consists of 3 to 15 strong rhythmic contractions of the orgasmic platform of the vagina. These may be followed by spastic contractions. During this phase, the vagina remains enlarged and the uterus contracts irregularly. In the male, orgasm consists of emission and ejaculation and is characterized by ejaculatory contractions along the entire length of the penis with three or four expulsive contractions, then several contractions of less intensity. For both males and females, there is a generalized muscle spasm and loss of voluntary control throughout the body. Hyperventilation, blood pressure, heart rate, and sex flush reach their peak. The rectal sphincter may contract, and the urinary meatus may dilate.

Unlike the Masters and Johnson model, the Kaplan model does not include a resolution stage because Kaplan reasoned that resolution was not part of the human sexual response. The changes in the body brought about by sexual desire, excitement, and orgasm are resolved in the return to their normal state. In the female, resolution is marked by the return of the orgasmic platform to its normal size and position. The clitoris also returns to normal size and position in 5 to 30 minutes. Breasts return to normal size, and vital signs return to normal. In many women, lubrication recurs during the resolution phase, indicating an ability to reach orgasm again if stimulated. In the male, the resolution phase involves a similar return of the genitalia to their normal sizes and position; however, it also includes a *refractory period*, during which ejaculation cannot occur. The refractory period varies with the man and changes throughout the life span. During resolution, size of the penis and scrotum reduces by 50% and then returns to normal more slowly, over perhaps 2 hours. Vital signs also return to normal.

NORMAL AGE-RELATED SEXUAL CHANGES

Elderly persons experience changes in sexual abilities that they sometimes perceive as an inability to engage in sexual activity. The elderly person should be counseled regarding the normalcy of changes such as a longer refractory period after ejaculation in the man, less firmness of the male erection, a longer time required to achieve erection and reach orgasm, and occasional incidents of inability to achieve erection. Many men adapt to such changes by trying alternative sexual activities such as having their partner stimulate the penis manually or orally before attempting coitus or engaging in oral sex if erection cannot be achieved fully enough to engage in coitus. Women tend to experience a loss of lubrication and some dyspareunia with the normal physical changes of aging. Engaging in sexual activities other than coitus, trying new coital positions, or using a water-soluble lubricant may allow the elderly woman to enjoy a full sex life (Northrup, 1998; Spark, 2000).

SEXUAL AND GENDER DISORDERS

Sexual and gender disorders include sexual dysfunction, paraphilias, and gender identity disorders. Sexual dysfunction is the most prevalent of the three and the one for which nursing interventions are most common. Therefore, sexual dysfunction is the focus of the disorder section. The other two disorders are discussed in a more condensed manner.

SEXUAL DYSFUNCTION DISORDERS

Sexual dysfunction refers to sexual expression that is "characterized by a disturbance in the processes that characterize the sexual response cycle or by pain associated with sexual intercourse" (American Psychiatric Association [APA], 2000, p. 535). In other words, disruption of any of the phases of human sexual response results in a sexual dysfunction disorder. These disorders are broken into the following subgroups:

- Desire disorders
- Arousal disorders
- Orgasmic disorders
- Pain disorders

In addition, these disorders can be classified as lifelong or acquired, generalized or situational, and caused by psychological factors or combined factors.

Clinical Example 20–1 (beginning of chapter) describes a client with a sexual dysfunction disorder. Few systematic epidemiologic data are available regarding the prevalence of these disorders. Results of research that exists show wide variability. These differences are attributed to differences in assessment methods, definitions used, and characteristics of the sample populations. Much remains to be known about sexual dysfunction disorders.

Etiology

Sexual dysfunction disorders can be primary (ie, caused by various psychological and emotional conditions or a combination of psychological and medical conditions), or secondary, caused solely by a general medical condition or substance use (Table 20-1). General medical conditions that may affect sexual interest and abilities include injury, disease, or after-effects of surgery. Substance use consists of drug and alcohol abuse or use of some prescribed medications, including antihypertensives, antidepressants, and neuroleptics (see Table 20-1).

Any of these psychological or physical conditions and substances can lead to changes in sexual functioning, which may interfere in significant ways with the client's ability to perform and enjoy sexual expression. The client may require referral for tests or therapy to determine the nature of the problem because there are so many potential causes of sexual difficulties.

Signs and Symptoms/ Diagnostic Criteria

The Diagnostic Criteria for sexual dysfunction disorders are categorized according to the type of dysfunction (ie, which phase of the human sexual response cycle is affected) and the causes of the dysfunction (ie, a general medical condition or a substance [drug of abuse, medication, or toxin exposure]). Specific criteria are presented in this chapter's Sexual and Gender Disorders Information Map and in the following sections.

DESIRE DISORDERS

Hypoactive sexual desire disorder is characterized by persistently or recurrently deficient or absent sexual fantasies and desire for sexual activity. Low sexual desire may be global and may encompass all forms of sexual expression or may be situational and limited to one person or to a specific sexual activity (eg, intercourse but not masturbation). These clients do not initiate sexual activity and engage in it only reluctantly when their partner initiates it. Hypoactive sexual desire frequently is associated with problems of sexual arousal or orgasm difficulties. Also, depressive disorders are associated with low sexual desire. Some studies have found decreased levels of testosterone in men complaining of this problem. A lack of normative age- or gender-related data on frequency of sexual desire means that the therapist must exercise clinical judgment in making this diagnosis. He or she should consider factors such as age and the context of the person's life in assigning this diagnosis.

Sexual aversion disorder is characterized by persistent or recurrent extreme aversion to, and avoidance of, all (or most) genital sexual contact with a sexual partner. The aversion to genital contact may be focused on a particular aspect of sexual experience (eg, genital secretions or vaginal penetration) or may be generalized to all sexual stimuli, including kissing and touching. When confronted with a sexual situation, some individuals with severe sexual aversion disorder may experience panic attacks, extreme anxiety, feelings of terror, faintness, nausea, palpitations, dizziness, and breathing difficulties. Individuals with an aversion to sexual activity may avoid sexual situations or potential sexual partners by covert strategies (eg, going to sleep early, traveling, neglecting personal appearance, abusing drugs or alcohol, and being over-involved in work, social, or family activities).

AROUSAL DISORDERS

Female sexual arousal disorder is characterized by a persistent or recurrent inability to attain, or maintain until completion of the sexual activity, an adequate lubrication–swelling response of sexual excitement. In women, the arousal response includes vasocongestion in the pelvis, vaginal lubrication and expansion, and swelling of the external genitalia. *Male erectile dysfunction (ED)* is characterized by a persistent or recurrent inability to attain, or to maintain until completion of the sexual activity, an erection sufficient for satisfactory sexual performance. There are different patterns of ED. Some individuals

TABLE 20-1 ▼ **Psychological, Physical, and Pharmacologic Causes of Sexual Dysfunction***

CAUSES OF SEXUAL DYSFUNCTION	TYPES OF SEXUAL DYSFUNCTION
Psychological Causes	
Childhood or adult sexual abuse or trauma	Hypoactive sexual desire, sexual aversion, male and female sexual arousal disorder, male and female orgasmic disorder, vaginismus
Guilt	Female orgasmic disorder, male erectile disorder, female sexual arousal disorder, sexual aversion, vaginismus
Relationship stress, including anger or hostility toward partner and issues of control	Female orgasmic disorder, premature ejaculation, male orgasmic disorder, male erectile disorder, hypoactive sexual desire, sexual aversion, female sexual arousal disorder
Anxiety, fear, stress, including performance anxiety, fear of failure, fear of rejection, fear of pregnancy	Female orgasmic disorder, premature ejaculation, male orgasmic disorder, male erectile disorder, hypoactive sexual desire, vaginismus
Poor body image	Male erectile disorder, sexual aversion
Lack of knowledge, insufficient sexual technique	Female orgasmic disorder, male erectile disorder, dyspareunia
Cultural, religious, familial influences (past or present)	Female orgasmic disorder, male orgasmic disorder, male erectile disorder, sexual aversion
Negative attitude about sex	Male orgasmic disorder, male erectile disorder
Psychiatric illness, including anxiety (generalized) and depression	Female orgasmic disorder, male and female sexual arousal, hypoactive sexual desire
Major life changes	Hypoactive sexual desire
Physical Causes	
Infectious, inflammatory, and parasitic diseases	Female orgasmic disorder, hypoactive sexual desire, dyspareunia
Renal and urologic disorders	Male erectile disorder, dyspareunia, male and female sexual arousal disorder, hypoactive sexual desire
Local genital or pelvic pathology or trauma, congenital penile vascular or structural abnormalities	Female orgasmic disorder, male orgasmic disorder, male erectile disorder, dyspareunia, vaginismus
Endocrine disorders such as diabetes, Addison's disease, or hyperthyroidism	Female orgasmic disorder, male erectile dysfunction, hypoactive sexual desire, male and female sexual arousal disorder
Hormonal disorder	Hypoactive sexual desire, female orgasmic disorder, male erectile dysfunction, male and female sexual arousal disorder, dyspareunia
Neurologic disorders such as multiple sclerosis, Parkinson's disease, temporal lobe epilepsy, spinal cord disease, and amyotropic lateral sclerosis	Male orgasmic disorder, premature ejaculation, female orgasmic disorder, male erectile disorder, male and female sexual arousal disorder
Surgical procedures such as perineal prostatectomy, abdominal–perineal colon resection, ileostomies and colostomies (sometimes), sympathectomy (frequently interferes with ejaculation), radical cystectomy, aortoiliac surgery, retroperitoneal lymphadectomy	Female orgasmic disorder, male erectile disorder, hypoactive sexual desire
Radiation therapy	Male and female sexual arousal disorder
Aging	Female sexual arousal disorder, hypoactive sexual desire

(continued)

TABLE 20-1 ▼ Psychological, Physical, and Pharmacologic Causes of Sexual Dysfunction* (Continued)	
CAUSES OF SEXUAL DYSFUNCTION	**TYPES OF SEXUAL DYSFUNCTION**
Pharmacologic Causes	
Psychiatric Drugs Tricyclic antidepressants (eg, Tofranil, Vivactil, Elavil, Aventyl, Norpramin, Anafranil)	Male erectile disorder, hypoactive sexual desire, male and female sexual arousal disorder, male and female orgasmic disorder
Monamine oxidase inhibitors (eg, Parnate, Actomal, Nardil, Eutonyl, Marplan) Lithium Amphetamines Neuroleptics	
Major tranquilizers (eg, Prolixin, Mellaril, Serentil, Trilafon, Stelazine, Reserpine, Haldol)	
Antidepressants (eg, Prozac, Ascendin, Zoloft, Paxil)	
Antihypertensive Drugs Catapres, Aldomet, Aldactone, Apresoline, Ismelin	Male erectile disorder, male and female sexual arousal disorder
Commonly Abused Drugs Alcohol, nicotine, barbiturates, cannibus, cocaine, heroin, methadone, morphine	Female orgasmic disorder, male erectile disorder, male and female sexual arousal disorder, hypoactive sexual desire

*The nurse should be alert to the sexual consequences of every health issue with which the client may present. This is a list (not exhaustive) of psychological, physical, and pharmacologic causes of disrupted sexual performance. The list also presents the types of sexual dysfunction most often associated with the specific cause.

report the inability to obtain any erection from the outset of the sexual experience. Others complain of first experiencing an adequate erection and then losing tumescence when attempting penetration. Others report that their erection is sufficiently firm for penetration but loses tumescence before or during thrusting (APA, 2000). ED is a common problem that is increasing in incidence with the aging population. One in 10 men is thought to have ED, but few men are willing to talk about it. There are no cures for ED, but drug treatment exists and generally is well tolerated.

ORGASMIC DISORDERS

Female orgasmic disorder and *male orgasmic disorder* are characterized by a persistent or recurrent delay in, or absence of, orgasm after a normal sexual excitement phase. **Premature ejaculation** is characterized by a persistent or recurrent onset of orgasm and ejaculation with minimal sexual stimulation before, on, or shortly after penetration and before the person wishes it. Men and women exhibit a wide variability in the type or intensity of stimulation that triggers orgasm. These diagnoses should take into account the person's age, life circumstances, and the adequacy of intensity and duration of the

sexual stimulation because these disorders may be caused by psychological or medical conditions.

PAIN DISORDERS

Dyspareunia (not from a general medical condition) is characterized by genital pain that is associated with sexual intercourse in either a man or woman. Although it is most commonly experienced during coitus, it also may occur before or after intercourse. The intensity of symptoms may range from mild discomfort to sharp pain. **Vaginismus** (not resulting from a general medical condition) is characterized by the recurrent or persistent involuntary spasm of the musculature of the outer third of the vagina that interferes with sexual intercourse. The physical obstruction caused by muscle contraction usually prevents coitus. These conditions tend to be chronic unless treated (APA, 2000).

Interdisciplinary Goals and Treatments

Sexual disorders affect many areas of the client's life and frequently are intertwined with psychological disorders

Sexual and Gender Disorders Information Map

➡️ *Prevalence*

Varies according to the disorder and somewhat difficult to establish, as many clients are reluctant to share such information

- Female orgasmic disorder may be as high as 25%.
- Premature ejaculation may affect up to 40% of adult men at some point.
- Erectile dysfunction occurs in up to 20 million men in the United States.
- Hypoactive sexual desire seems to affect approximately 20% of the population.
- Gender identity disorders occur in less than 5% of the population.

➡️ *Summary of DSM-IV-TR Diagnostic Criteria*

Sexual Desire Disorders

Hypoactive Sexual Desire Disorder
- Client persistently or recurrently has deficient or no fantasies about or desires for sexual activity. Factors that affect sexuality (e.g., age, culture) help determine the appropriateness of this diagnosis.
- Client has marked distress or interpersonal difficulty because of the disturbance.
- The problem is not better explained by another condition and is not the exclusive result of a substance or general medical condition.

Sexual Aversion Disorder
- Client has persistent or recurrent extreme aversion to, and avoidance of, all (or almost all) genital sexual contact with a partner.
- Client has marked distress or interpersonal difficulty because of the disturbance.
- The problem is not better explained by another condition.

Sexual Arousal Disorders

Female Sexual Arousal Disorder
- Client persistently or recurrently cannot attain or maintain adequate lubrication and swelling response during sexual activity.
- Client has marked distress or interpersonal difficulty because of the disturbance.
- The problem is not better explained by another condition and is not exclusively caused by a substance or general medical condition.

Male Erectile Disorder
- Client persistently or recurrently cannot attain or maintain an adequate erection during sex.
- Client has marked distress or interpersonal difficulty because of the disturbance.
- The problem is not better explained by another condition and is not exclusively caused by a substance or general medical condition.

Orgasmic Disorders

Female Orgasmic Disorder
- Client persistently or recurrently has difficulty reaching (or cannot reach) orgasm. Factors the clinician must consider include age, sexual experience, and adequacy of sexual stimulation. Stimulation that triggers orgasm in women varies greatly.
- Client has marked distress or interpersonal difficulty because of the disturbance.
- The problem is not better explained by another condition and is not exclusively caused by a substance or general medical condition.

Male Orgasmic Disorder
- Client persistently or recurrently has difficulty reaching (or cannot reach) orgasm. The clinician must consider the man's age and other factors.
- Client has marked distress or interpersonal difficulty because of the disturbance.
- The problem is not better explained by another condition and is not exclusively caused by a substance or general medical condition.

Premature Ejaculation
- Client persistently or recurrently ejaculates with minimal sexual stimulation before, on, or shortly after penetration and before he desires. The clinician must consider factors that affect duration of the excitement phase, such as age and sexual experience.
- Client has marked distress or interpersonal difficulty because of the disturbance.
- The problem is not exclusively caused by a substance (e.g, withdrawal from opioids).

(continued)

Sexual and Gender Disorders Information Map *(Continued)*

Sexual Pain Disorders
Male and Female Dispareunia (Not due to general medical condition)
- Client has recurrent or persistent genital pain during sexual intercourse.
- Client has marked distress or interpersonal difficulty because of the disturbance.
- The disturbance is not caused exclusively by vaginismus or lack of lubrication. It is not better explained by another condition and is not exclusively caused by a substance.

Vaginismus (Not due to general medical condition)
- Client has recurrent or persistent involuntary spasm of the musculature of the outer third of the vagina, which interferes with sexual intercourse.
- Client has marked distress or interpersonal difficulty because of the disturbance.
- The problem is not better explained by another condition and is not exclusively caused by a substance or general medical condition.

Sexual Dysfunction Due to a General Medical Condition
- Client has clinically significant sexual dysfunction that causes marked distress or interpersonal difficulty.
- Evidence from the history, physical examination, or laboratory tests supports that the direct physiological effects of a general medical condition fully explain the sexual dysfunction.
- The disturbance is not better explained by another psychiatric disorder (e.g., depression).

Substance-Induced Sexual Dysfunction
- Client has clinically significant sexual dysfunction that causes marked distress or interpersonal difficulty.
- Evidence from the history, physical examination, or laboratory tests supports that substance use fully explains the sexual dysfunction.

Paraphilias
Exhibitionism
- For at least 6 months, client has recurrent, intense sexually arousing fantasies, urges, or behaviors that involve exposing his or her genitals to an unsuspecting stranger.
- Client has acted on these urges, or they cause marked distress or interpersonal difficulty.

Fetishism
- For at least 6 months, client has recurrent, intense sexually arousing fantasies, urges, or behaviors that involve nonliving objects (e.g., shoes).

- Client has marked distress or impaired social, occupational, or other functioning because of the fantasies, urges, or behaviors.
- The fetish object is not an article of clothing that the client uses in cross-dressing or designed specifically for tactile genital stimulation (e.g., vibrator).

Frotteurism
- For at least 6 months, client has recurrent, intense sexually arousing fantasies, urges, or behaviors involving touching and rubbing against a nonconsenting person.
- Client has acted on these sexual urges, or they cause marked distress or difficulty.

Pedophilia
- For at least 6 months, client has recurrent, intense sexually arousing fantasies, urges, or behaviors involving sexual activity with children (generally age 13 years or younger).
- Client has acted on these sexual urges, or they cause marked distress or difficulty.
- Client is at least age 16 years and at least 5 years older than the children who are the focus of the fantasies, behaviors, or urges. (The criteria would not apply to a late-adolescent client (e.g., 17 years) involved in an ongoing sexual relationship with a 12- or 13-year-old.

Sexual Masochism
- For at least 6 months, client has recurrent, intense sexually arousing fantasies, urges, or behaviors involving being made to suffer (e.g., being beaten, bound, abused).
- Client has marked distress or impaired social, occupational, or other functioning because of the fantasies, urges, or behaviors.

Sexual Sadism
- For at least 6 months, client has recurrent, intense sexually arousing fantasies, urges, or behaviors involving the psychological or physical suffering (including humiliation) of others.
- Client has acted on such urges with a nonconsenting person, or the urges cause marked distress or difficulty.

Transvestic Fetishism
- For at least 6 months, a heterosexual man has recurrent, intense sexually arousing fantasies, urges, or behaviors involving cross-dressing.
- Client has marked distress or impaired social, occupational, or other functioning because of the fantasies, urges, or behaviors.

(continued)

Sexual and Gender Disorders Information Map (Continued)

Voyeurism
- For at least 6 months, client has recurrent, intense sexually arousing fantasies, urges, or behaviors that involve watching an unsuspecting person who is naked, disrobing, or engaging in sexual activity.
- Client has acted on these sexual urges, or they cause marked distress or difficulty.

Paraphilia Not Otherwise Specified
This category includes paraphilias that do not meet the criteria for any of the specific categories. Examples include *telephone scatologia* (obscene phone calls), *necrophilia* (sexual activity with corpses), *partialism* (exclusive focus on part of body), *zoophilia* (sexual activity with animals), *coprophilia* (feces), *klismaphilia* (enemas), and *urophilia* (urine).

Gender Identity Disorder
- Client strongly and persistently identifies with the opposite sex. (The identification is beyond desiring any perceived cultural advantages of being the other sex.)
  - In a child, at least four of the following appear:
    - Repeated statements of wishing to be, or actually being, the other sex
    - In boys, preference for wearing typically female attire or cross-dressing; in girls, insistence on wearing only typically masculine clothing
    - Regular choice of roles of the opposite sex during play
    - Persistent fantasies of being the other sex
    - Desire to participate in games and hobbies typical of the other sex
    - Strong preference for playmates of the other sex

- An adolescent or adult frequently states a desire to be the other sex, often passes as the other sex, desires to live or be treated as the other sex, or is convinced that he or she has feelings and reactions typical of the other sex. Client is persistently uncomfortable with his or her sex or believes that his or her given gender role is inappropriate for him or her.
  - Male children may assert that the penis or testes are disgusting or will vanish. They may state that it would be better not to have a penis. They may reject aggressive play and toys, games, and activities commonly perceived as "male."
  - Female children may reject urinating in a sitting position. They may assert that they will grow a penis. They may reject the idea of breast growth or menstruation. They may show a marked aversion toward feminine clothing.
  - Adolescents and adults may be preoccupied with eliminating primary and secondary sex characteristics through hormones, surgery, or other means. They may believe that they were born the wrong sex.
- The disturbance does not accompany a physical intersex condition.
- Client has marked distress or impaired social, occupational, or other functioning because of the disturbance.

➡ **Want to Know More?**

American Association of Sex Educators, Counselors, and Therapists
P.O. Box 5488
Richmond, VA 23220-0488
http://www.aasect.org

Sexuality Information and Education Council of the United States (SIECUS)

130 West 42nd Street, Suite 350
New York, NY 10036-7802
Phone: 212/819-9770
Fax: 212/819-9776
www.siecus.org

With permission from the American Psychiatric Association. (2000). *Diagnostic and statistical manual of mental disorders* (4th ed., text revision). Washington, DC: Author.

and physical conditions; they also may be caused by pharmacologic agents. Professionals from many disciplines, including medicine, nursing, psychiatry, psychology, and social work, may be helpful in treating these clients. The most effective treatment for the client with a sexual disorder involves a team approach with individual team members working in conjunction to achieve the goal of optimal wellness for the client.

Some typical areas that need to be addressed in treatment of sexual disorders include the following:

- Assessment of the couple affected by the sexual disorder
- Medication management as needed to improve sexual functioning or to provide symptom management or relief
- Education regarding "normal" sexual functioning
- Training in couple communication and sexual skills
- Couple's counseling to address other issues that may exist in the couple's relationship

Treatment of specific sexual dysfunctions focuses mainly on targeting the individual and contributing causal factors (which could be psychological, physical, or pharmacologic) related to the particular disorder. For example, in treating desire disorder, the goal is to determine and treat the cause of hypoactive sexual desire disorder, which could be childhood sexual abuse, hormonal imbalances, depression, and other sexual disorders (APA, 2000). Treatment for aversion disorder focuses on managing the anxiety symptoms, using medication, behavioral desensitization, and relaxation techniques, and uncovering and working through the dynamic issue that may underlie the disorder (eg, sexual abuse or related trauma) (APA, 2000). A man with physiologic ED might be encouraged to try activities other than intercourse for sexual fulfillment. In addition, male and female clients with arousal and orgasmic disorders may be assisted to find greater sexual pleasure by trying more foreplay, experimenting with different coital positions, and improving communication about their sexual behaviors, especially what is pleasing or not pleasing to them and what behaviors facilitate their sexual satisfaction.

When the cause of the dysfunction has been determined to be drug related, these drugs should be discontinued when possible, and a drug without these side effects should be administered. If this is not possible, the nurse should explain the cause of the problem to the client and encourage the alteration of sexual activity as necessary. Such alterations could include longer periods of foreplay before attempting coitus or taking another medication (if instructed by the physician) to temporarily block the action of the drug causing the sexual problem. For example, some antidepressant medication (especially the selective serotonin reuptake inhibitors [SSRIs]) in some clients causes decreased libido, erectile dysfunction, or inorgasmia. Cyproheptadine (Periactin), taken an hour before sexual intercourse, temporarily blocks the action of the SSRI, allowing the couple to enjoy sexual intercourse (Kaplan & Sadock, 1996).

PHARMACOLOGIC THERAPY

Antianxiety medications sometimes are used with clients whose anxiety and tension interfere with their ability to engage in sexual relations. Fluoxetine (Prozac), tricyclic antidepressants, haloperidol (Haldol), lorazepam (Ativan), thioridazine (Mellaril), and the monoamine oxidase inhibitors have been used to prolong sexual activity in men with premature ejaculation.

The Food and Drug Administration (FDA) has approved one medication for treating ED: sildenafil citrate (Viagra). The drug works by blocking the action of certain enzymes involved in the erectile response, achieving smooth muscle relaxation in the corpus cavernosum area of the brain, and allowing for the inflow of blood to the penis. This treatment generally is well tolerated (Table 20-2).

A second medication, apomorphine (Uprima), is awaiting FDA approval. Uprima is taken sublingually and produces erections in men more quickly than does Viagra. Because it is a dopamine receptor antagonist, it also has a different mechanism of action than Viagra. Uprima facilitates electrical impulses from the hypothalamus in the brain down through the spinal cord. It increases nitric oxide, which occurs naturally in the body, dilating blood vessels to get more blood flowing to the penis.

SEX THERAPY

Another treatment modality for sexual dysfunction is sex therapy. Sex therapy is a particular approach to sexual counseling practiced by master-level clinicians with specialized training in this mental health specialty. Most of sex therapy currently consists of a combination of cognitive and behavioral interventions and education about sexuality. Whereas the nurse generalist may be qualified to assess the client's sexual concerns and may be prepared to educate the client regarding normal sexual function, he or she generally is not prepared to provide sex therapy.

APPLICATION OF THE NURSING PROCESS TO THE CLIENT WITH SEXUAL DYSFUNCTION

Assessment

Collecting data about the client's sexual values, practices, and concerns in a sensitive and professional way takes experience. Students and inexperienced nurses should practice conducting interviews with colleagues, friends,

TABLE 20-2 ▼ **Agents That Interact With Sildenafil**

INTERACTANTS	EFFECT AND SIGNIFICANCE	NURSING MANAGEMENT
nitrates	Sildenafil potentiates the vasodilating effect of nitric oxide from nitrates, resulting in a significant and potentially fatal decrease in BP.	Teach client that he should not use any nitrate while taking sildenafil.
amlodipine	In hypertensive clients, administration with sildenafil produces mean additionalBP reduction of 7–8 mg.	Monitor the client's BP; in most cases, this drop is not clinically significant.
beta blockers, nonspecific	Beta blockers increase the level of sildenafil's active metabolite; this is not believed to be clinically significant.	None
cimetidine	Co-administration increases the plasma concentrations of sildenafil by more than 50%.	Monitor for adverse effects; a decreased dose may be indicated; consider starting dose of 25 mg.
diuretics	Diuretics increase the level of sildenafil's active metabolite; this is not believed to be clinically significant.	None
erythromycin	A single dose of 100 mg of sildenafil administered with erythromycin at steady state (500 mg BID for 5 days) resulted in a 182% increase in sildenafil's peak concentration.	Monitor for adverse effects; a decreased dose may be indicated; consider starting dose of 25 mg.

BP, blood pressure.
From Aschenbrenner, D. S., Cleveland, L. W., & Venable, S. J. (2002). *Drug therapy in nursing.* Philadelphia: Lippincott Williams & Wilkins.

or family until they are comfortable and confident about their skills. Throughout the interview, the nurse must maintain a composed, respectful, and matter-of-fact attitude. Focused and open-ended questions about less intimate material should progress gradually to questions about more sensitive material (Table 20-3).

Framing questions in a way that normalizes a wide range of sexual behaviors or problems helps the client feel more comfortable about sharing his or her unique experience. For example, instead of asking, "Do you sometimes have difficulty achieving an erection?" the nurse could reframe the question as follows: "Men sometimes cannot have erections even when they really want to have intercourse. What is that like for you?" The nurse also is careful to use terminology that the client comprehends readily. Pictures, models, and diagrams may be helpful (see Implications for Nursing Practice 20-2).

Sexual dysfunction is not only problematic for the identified client, but also for the client's partner. The nurse may interview couples separately and together to obtain a complete picture of the difficulties. The nurse should not assume, however, that each partner will automatically be comfortable expressing his or her feelings with the other present, or that it is acceptable for the nurse to share one client's concerns, problems, or sexual history with the partner. The nurse always asks the client what he or she is comfortable with in this regard before proceeding. See Therapeutic Communication 20-1 for more information.

Information about the partnership itself includes how the partners communicate with each other about their sexual needs and preferences, how considerate each is of the other's wishes, as well as the sexual history of this partnership (eg, how soon did they become involved sexually, how satisfying has their sexual relationship been, have they experienced other sexual concerns such as infidelity or abusive sexual experiences, and what have been their best and worst times together sexually). The nurse also assesses each partner's perception of the couple's problems as a whole, such as level of satisfaction in the relationship, strengths, support system, and willingness to work on the partnership's problems.

Nursing assessments also include an understanding of the client's cultural context and sexual orientation. For example, not all clients seeking help are heterosexual couples. Assessment of homosexual or bisexual clients includes completing a modified nursing assessment (Implications for Nursing Practice 20-3). The nurse also conveys sensitivity about various lifestyle concerns (eg, homophobia, fear of hate crimes, disclosing or not disclosing a homosexual or bisexual orientation) when interviewing gay clients.

TABLE 20-3 ▼ Data Related to Sexuality to Collect From All Clients

DATA	SIGNIFICANCE OF DATA	NURSING HISTORY QUESTIONS
Age	Age identifies period in life cycle.	In what year were you born; month, day?
Sex	Each sex may react differently to life events; answers highlight gender identity problems.	Usually is evident by dress, otherwise: What sex do you consider yourself to be?
Education, occupation	Sexual practices may be related to education–socioeconomic class; change in occupation may contribute to role disturbances.	How far did you go in school? What do you do for a living? What change has there been in your ability to do your job?
Significant others	Answers indicate sources of support, stable or otherwise.	What people do you consider most helpful right now? In what way? Are they available?
Quality of relationship with significant others	Relationship may be supportive, negative, or punitive, and these affect ability to cope with sexual problems.	Are you facing any difficulty in the way you get along with these people?
Interests, hobbies	Answers indicate support systems and avocational interests that contribute to self-esteem.	What do you do with your free time? What leisure and work activities are important to you? How are these being affected now?
Spiritual/religious/philosophical beliefs	Sexual practices may be related to beliefs. Guilt may occur if religious beliefs are compromised. Client may experience conflict and anxiety if nurse suggests different practices.	With what religious denomination are you affiliated? Can you describe any spiritual or other beliefs that are helpful to you now? Do you have or want the support of a clergyperson (minister, priest, rabbi)?
Health problems, medical conditions, surgical procedures in the past and anticipated in the future; medication therapy	Some medical problems, surgical treatment, or medications result in sexual dysfunction (physiologic changes). Anxiety over outcome or change in body image may lead to functional problems.	What illness or surgery have you had in the past? Did they affect your usual way of living or work? Did they affect sexual function? Do you expect this illness/hospitalization will have effects on your usual way of living or work? In what ways? What medications do you take?
Changes in role relationships and ability to carry out the usual sexual role	Change in ability to carry out what is perceived as the usual sexual role may cause anxiety, depression, and sexual dysfunction.	What difference has there been in your functioning in the family? Describe. Can you do your usual tasks or jobs? Describe. Have there been any changes in your relationship with the way you get along with others (male, female, significant others)?
Potential changes in ability to carry out usual sexual role	Expectations of problems may cause problems (self-fulfilling prophecy).	What changes do you expect after you get home (or in the future)?
Change in perception of self as male or female because of illness or life events	Anxiety and sexual dysfunction may result from threat to gender identity.	How do you expect this illness (or life event) to affect how you see yourself as a man/woman?
Existing or potential sexual dysfunction	Answers reveal problems (sexual dysfunction).	Has there been or do you expect to have any changes in sexual functioning (sex life) because of (illness, life events)? Describe.

Note: Wording of the questions is changed depending on educational level of the client.
From Hogan, R. (1985). *Human sexuality: A nursing perspective* (2nd ed., pp. 162–163). New York: Appleton-Century-Crofts.

Implications for Nursing Practice 20-2

Discussing Sexuality With a Client

- Frequently, clients will not mention sexual concerns unless the nurse asks him or her directly and in a way that puts the client at ease. One way to help the client relax during discussions of sexuality is to connect what the nurse knows about the client's health history with potential sexual implications. For example, the nurse can ask, "Possible side effects of the blood pressure medicine you are taking are decreased libido and difficulty maintaining an erection. Have you noticed these problems? Do you have any other sexual concerns?"

- The nurse also may anticipate the client's sexual concerns. For example, the client recovering from a myocardial infarction may wonder when or if he or she can engage in sexual activity again. When the nurse provides this kind of anticipatory guidance, he or she models knowledge, interest, and willingness to address sexual concerns as part of caring for the whole client.

- Every health history interview conducted by the nurse should include questions about "unwanted sexual experiences." As many as 75% of women experience some type of unwanted sexual experience during their lifetime. Estimates in men are lower (10% to 14%); however, this figure is thought to be low because men are less likely than women to report these experiences. The nurse should not ask if the client has been "raped." Use of the term "rape" can be limiting, suggesting to clients that the nurse is interested only in past rape experiences. Also, many victims of sexual assault blame themselves for unwanted sexual experiences and therefore do not consider what happened to them as "rape." In response to a query about unwanted sexual experiences, one client responded:

"It wasn't what you would call rape or anything, but it still bothers me. Sometimes I dream about it. It was my entire fault. We had been dating for about 1 month, and I kept telling him I didn't want to have sex. One night we'd been making out, and when he tried to be more intimate, I told him I didn't want to and pushed him away. He got really mad and said I had been leading him on and what a tease I was. He grabbed me, held me down, and forced himself on me. I was so shocked, I didn't fight back like I should have. I didn't even scream. I just cried and begged him to stop. Afterwards he kept saying I had really wanted it and that I had made him do it by provoking him the way I did. I was so ashamed I never told anyone what happened. I still feel dirty and ashamed when I remember."

This client might well have answered "no" to a question about whether she had ever been raped, yet she described a traumatic rape incident that required a referral for mental health counseling to address her rape trauma issues (see Chap. 17).

- Discussion of sensitive matters, such as childhood sexual abuse, sexual dysfunction, or sexual assault, requires the nurse's time and empathy. This content will not emerge if the client feels rushed. The nurse should sit down with the client and communicate that he or she has time to listen.

- Clients frequently express intense feelings (eg, anxiety, anger, sadness, guilt) related to sexual experiences or concerns. The nurse's role includes supporting the expression of these feelings (eg, providing tissues if needed, allowing the client to express feelings uninterrupted), validating them (eg, "I'm so sorry that happened to you," "Of course you feel angry," "Many victims of rape blame themselves."), and helping the client seek further assistance if necessary (eg, "I think you could benefit from talking this over with a counselor who can help you begin to put this experience behind you. Here are the names and numbers of some local therapists and agencies that specialize in treating sexual trauma issues.")

Nursing Diagnosis

The nursing diagnoses specifically related to sexual problems are Sexual Dysfunction and Ineffective Sexuality Patterns. They apply broadly to a range of clients seeking help for a sexual dysfunction disorder. Related factors (those that are causative) and defining characteristics (the actual behaviors or problems) vary considerably and will be the significant determinants of the appropriate interventions. For example, one client's diagnosis may be Sexual Dys-

function related to diabetes-induced ED as evidenced by inability to achieve an erection. Another (male) client may be diagnosed with Sexual Dysfunction related to psychosocial abuse as evidenced by fear of sexual contact. Other diagnoses also may apply, such as Disturbed Body Image, particularly if the changed sexual pattern is related to physical illness or injury, or Situational Low Self-Esteem. As stated previously, the nurse generalist will focus on more basic issues related to the sexual problems, such as education about treatments and coping. There-

THERAPEUTIC COMMUNICATION 20-1
Respecting a Client's Wishes Regarding Sexual Issues

The nurse is working with Amy, a 30-year-old client, who mentions having sexual difficulties with her husband of 3 years.

Ineffective Dialogue	*Effective Dialogue*
Client: "I don't know what he likes. Last week, he said our sex life is no good. I don't know what I'm doing wrong." *(Appears crestfallen)*	*Client:* "I don't know what he likes. Last week, he said our sex life is no good. I don't know what I'm doing wrong." *(Appears crestfallen)*
Nurse: "Well, maybe nothing. Have you been arguing or under stress?"	*Nurse:* "Well, maybe nothing. Have you been arguing or under stress?"
Client: "No more than usual."	*Client:* "No more than usual."
Nurse: "What do you mean by usual?"	*Nurse:* "What do you mean by usual?"
Client: *(Shifts in her seat)* "Well, I *am* always on his back about the time he spends with his friends. And he works so hard. It probably is my fault."	*Client:* *(Shifts in her seat)* "Well, I *am* always on his back about the time he spends with his friends. And he works so hard. It probably is my fault."
Nurse: "It sounds like you two have problems both inside and outside the bedroom that you should address. Why don't we set up an appointment for both you and your husband to come in and discuss what's happening?"	*Nurse:* "In a relationship, both people can contribute to all sorts of problems. They also can work together to solve problems. *(Pauses)* Have you and your husband ever considered seeing a therapist together? Another possibility is that you could come here together to discuss issues."
Client: *(Looks uncomfortable)* "My husband would never feel comfortable talking about such things. I'd be embarrassed, too."	*Client:* *(Pauses, seems to think it over)* "I don't know how my husband would feel about talking about such things in front of other people. I'm afraid I'd be embarrassed in front of *him*."
Nurse: "He might surprise you! How does Tuesday the 26th at 3:00 PM sound?"	*Nurse:* "These discussions can be difficult. Talking takes courage. Why don't you think about it? Maybe you can mention it to your husband and see how he reacts and how you feel. In the meantime, you and I can talk more about specific questions you have regarding your relationship."
Client: "Well . . . OK." *(The next day, the client calls and cancels the appointment.)*	*Client:* *(Seems reassured and begins to discuss her relationship in more detail. Two weeks later, she calls to set up an appointment with her husband accompanying her.)*

Reflection and Critical Thinking

- Although the nurses in both examples proposed similar ideas, the outcomes were vastly different. Why do you think the second approach was more effective?
- What attitudes did the first nurse convey that may have contributed to the client's reluctance to pursue further discussion, with and without her husband?
- What are possible reasons why it could be damaging to prematurely involve a client's sexual partner in treatment?

fore, the diagnoses and interventions addressed here reflect that generic focus.

- **Sexual Dysfunction** or **Ineffective Sexuality Pattern** related to desire, arousal, orgasmic, or pain disorder
- **Situational Low Self-Esteem** related to sexual dysfunction or ineffective sexuality pattern

Planning

Collaborating with the client, the nurse organizes a plan of care (Nursing Care Plan 20-1). The nurse remains flexible and willing to make adaptations or changes to the plan in response to the client's needs or wishes. Again, the nurse bases specific goals on each client's particular

Implications for Nursing Practice 20-3

Sexual Assessment of Homosexual or Bisexual Clients

The following are questions the nurse can ask when taking a history from a homosexual or bisexual client:

- Do you consider yourself homosexual or bisexual? How long have you been "out" to yourself about your orientation? Do you wish to have, or have you had, any same-sex sexual experiences?
- What are your thoughts or feelings about your orientation? If you have positive feelings about being homosexual or bisexual, how do you feel you developed this outlook? If you have negative feelings about being homosexual or bisexual, how do you cope with these feelings? Do you feel you have accepted your homosexuality or bisexuality?
- Are you "out" in your life (at work or school)? Of your family and friends who know, how do they feel about your orientation?
- Whom do you consider as your support system? Do they know you are homosexual or bisexual? Do you have homosexual or bisexual friends? Has being "out" or "closeted" about your orientation caused any problems in your family, place of work, church, or social relationships? How do you deal with these problems?
- Do you have a lover or life partner? Do you and your partner have any unresolved issues that need to be addressed? How have AIDS and other sexually transmitted diseases affected your sex life and relationship? Do your family and friends know the nature of your relationship? Are they supportive?

Adapted from Smith, B. S. (1992). Nursing care challenges: Homosexual psychiatric patients. *Journal of Psychosocial Nursing, 30*(12), 15–21.

circumstances. General goals for all clients seeking sexual help include the following:

- The client will experience increased satisfaction with his or her sexuality.
- The client will express positive feelings of self-worth.

Implementation

COUNSELING THE CLIENT WITH A SEXUAL DYSFUNCTION DISORDER

The first step in helping the client with a sexual problem is establishing a therapeutic, trusting relationship. Sharing intimate, potentially embarrassing information is difficult.

The nurse's attitudes regarding sexuality powerfully influence the client's experience and response to treatment. The client must not fear criticism or rejection from the nurse. Therefore, the nurse must be aware of his or her attitudes to refrain from negative verbal and nonverbal communications that interfere with the client's sense of self or response to treatment. Unconditional acceptance of the client will facilitate a trusting and therapeutic relationship.

Providing information and helping clients gain insight are other important interventions. The nurse can discuss sexuality and its expressions with the client, providing facts as necessary and encouraging the client to ask questions and verbalize his or her fears or concerns. The nurse can use this discussion as an opportunity to discuss the effects of health issues, medical or surgical treatments, or medications on libido, self-image, and sexual function. This then can lead to a discussion of alternative or modified forms of sexual expression. Often, the client will feel satisfied with the ability to sexually please his or her partner, even if orgasm as formerly experienced becomes impossible. The nurse will be sensitive to the client's personal values and cultural norms when suggesting other forms of sexual self-expression and will discuss methods that are compatible with the client's beliefs.

Other areas in which the nurse may provide teaching and counseling include relationship counseling and communication techniques for couples. Regardless of the sexual dysfunction, improved communication skills and enhanced feelings of emotional intimacy will help the client feel more satisfied. For example, the nurse may encourage the expression of feeling by both partners, model how to elicit feedback from each other, and instruct the couple on ways of communicating in a clear and honest manner with each other. The nurse may suggest activities that will encourage the couple's development of new sexual patterns. The nurse can clarify vague information or provide new information about sexual positions or behaviors. Many sexual issues can be resolved through effective nursing intervention and may not require formal sex therapy.

The nurse also can explore deeper emotional issues or comorbid mental health problems with the client. For example, discussing a client's underlying anxiety disorder or history of childhood trauma may help the client gain insight into sexual problems. The nurse also may discuss feelings the client has directly related to the sexual problem. These feelings may include guilt, despair, anger, grief, loneliness, resentment, and depression. Any opportunity to verbalize feelings in the context of a nonjudgmental, therapeutic encounter is helpful. The nurse also can help the client overcome feelings of low self-esteem, which likely will accompany a client's diagnosis of Sexual Dysfunction or Ineffective Sexuality Patterns.

ENHANCING SELF-ESTEEM

In a society that places great value on sexuality and sexual performance, those experiencing a sexual dysfunction may feel shame, despair, and guilt over their altered abil-

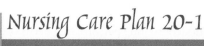

Nursing Care Plan 20-1

THE CLIENT WITH ERECTILE DYSFUNCTION

As discussed in Clinical Example 20-1, the nurse assures George that treatment for his sexual difficulties is available and helpful. The nurse then asks George how this problem has affected his relationship with his wife. George looks downcast and states that "something better change soon" because his wife is getting "fed up" and is beginning to avoid him. The nurse interviews George's wife, Betty, privately (with George's permission). Betty states that she thinks George may be having an affair and is no longer attracted to her.

Based on these interviews, the nurse creates the following care plan.

Nursing Diagnosis: Sexual Dysfunction related to physiologic changes or psychological problems as evidenced by inability to achieve an erection

Goal: The client will understand the cause of the sexual dysfunction and begin appropriate treatment for it. The couple will resume a satisfying sexual relationship and adapt to altered function (if necessary).

Interventions	Rationales
Refer client to a physician for evaluation of erectile function.	Healthcare professionals must rule out physiologic reasons for erectile dysfunction before assuming that the problem is psychological. George's history of diabetes puts him at risk for vascular and neuropathic changes that can cause erectile dysfunction.

Discuss treatment modalities with the client. Include information about
   Psychotherapy
   Drug therapy: sildenafil, testosterone, and other medications
   Vacuum devices
   Penile injection therapy
   Penile implant surgery
	Regardless of whether the erectile dysfunction has a physical cause, George may benefit from psychotherapy to help manage anxiety and improve his self-esteem. Informing George about treatments will let him know that various methods are available and effective, regardless of the cause.

Discuss alternative methods for sexual expression during treatment. Explore personal values and cultural beliefs about sexual activity and suggest methods for sexual gratification that are consistent with each client's beliefs. Encourage increased physical intimacy such as cuddling and caressing.	George and Betty still can engage in sexual activity and share physical and emotional intimacy, which will strengthen their relationship. George can help Betty achieve orgasm through other means, such as manual–genital or oral–genital stimulation.

Evaluation: George begins treatment for erectile dysfunction. George and Betty resume satisfying sexual intimacy.

Nursing Diagnosis: Compromised Family Coping related to poor communication styles as evidenced by couple's failure to communicate significant emotional information and mistaken attribution of causes for partner's behaviors

Goal: The couple's communication skills will be enhanced so that they are aware of and supportive of each other's emotional states.

Interventions	Rationales
Instruct couple on techniques of clear and honest communication. Encourage both partners to express their feelings. Help them identify their understanding of the situation. Help each client clarify what he or she needs and expects from the other. Model effective listening and how to elicit feedback from each other. Help the couple understand the medical aspects that may underlie the sexual dysfunction.	Improved communication abilities will foster greater emotional intimacy and help prevent misunderstandings and resentment.

Evaluation: George and Betty can openly and honestly express their feelings and concerns to each other and can listen and respond to each other's needs.

ities to carry out their sexual roles. Male and female stereotypes persist and may add to a client's feeling of decreased self-esteem. The partner of a client with sexual dysfunction may or may not be understanding and supportive and may increase the pressure to perform according to past abilities. Generalist nurses can help clients explore and overcome self-esteem issues. Some strategies for addressing these issues include the following:

- Listen for statements of self-worth and help the client explore his or her ideas about how sexual performance relates to self-judgments.
- Assist the client to differentiate a feeling (eg, loneliness) from a negative self-evaluation (I am unlovable).
- Help the client reexamine and reframe negative self-evaluations; teach the client to dispute negative self-evaluations.
- Encourage the client to view stereotypical measures of sexual performance as only one form of sexual expression.
- Encourage the client to include all of his or her attributes, not just sexual performance, when evaluating himself or herself.
- Encourage the client to focus on strengths and to increase activities in these areas.
- Help the client establish realistic goals and celebrate his or her successes.

Overcoming low self-esteem will have a positive effect on many aspects of the client's life, including satisfaction with his or her sexuality. People with high self-esteem are confident that they are lovable and likeable individuals, in spite of disability.

Evaluation

Ideally, evaluation should continue after the client or client couple concludes formal treatment. For example, the nurse may want to follow-up by telephone at various intervals after treatment is completed (eg, 1 month, 6 months, 1 year) to evaluate progress. Indicators that the plan of care has been effective include the following:

- Statements of improved satisfaction with sexual function, expression, and fulfillment by the clients
- Statements of positive self-regard by the client

PARAPHILIAS

According to the *Diagnostic and Statistical Manual of Mental Disorders* (4th ed., text revision), **paraphilias** are those sexual expressions characterized by "recurrent, intense sexually arousing fantasies, sexual urges or behaviors generally involving (1) nonhuman objects, (2) suffering or humiliation of oneself or one's partner, or (3) children or

other nonconsenting persons, that occur over a period of at least 6 months" (APA, 2000, p. 566). Also, to be considered paraphilias, the urges, fantasies, and behaviors must cause clinically significant distress or impair social, occupational, or other important areas of functioning.

For some clients with paraphilias, the paraphiliac behaviors are necessary for erotic arousal and sexual release (orgasm). For others, paraphiliac behaviors occur episodically (eg, during periods of stress). Although the frequency and intensity of the sexual urges, fantasies, and behaviors may vary, these disorders tend to be lifelong and chronic.

Estimates regarding the prevalence of paraphilic behavior in the general population are not available. Nevertheless, although paraphilias rarely are diagnosed in general clinical facilities, the large commercial market in paraphiliac pornography and paraphernalia suggests that many people have these disorders. The most common presenting problems in clinics that specialize in the treatment of paraphilias are pedophilia, voyeurism, and exhibitionism (see the Sexual and Gender Disorders Information Map for specific descriptions). Approximately 50% of those with paraphilias seen clinically are married. Except for sexual masochism, the female-to-male ratio of which is estimated to be 20:1, the other paraphilias are rarely diagnosed in women (APA, 2000).

Signs and Symptoms/ Diagnostic Criteria

Some clients are distressed by their paraphiliac urges, fantasies, and behaviors; others experience distress only when someone interferes with their behaviors (eg, legal consequences for child rape or molestation, voyeurism, or exhibitionism). Some clients with paraphilias may view their behaviors as an interesting part of their personal sexuality and seek to fulfill them with similarly interested partners (eg, sadomasochistic sexual practices). These individuals may be active with their partners or visit specialized prostitutes, may read books or magazines about their paraphilias, may search the Internet for information about their paraphilias, or may participate in paraphiliac subcultures. Some clients with paraphilias attend support groups that encourage responsible behavior. See the Sexual and Gender Disorders Information Map for specific diagnostic criteria and explanations of the various paraphilias.

Interdisciplinary Goals and Treatment

Frequently, involvement in treatment is not voluntary but instead is the consequence of criminal prosecution (court-ordered treatment). Sometimes, clients with paraphilias enter treatment at the insistence of their sexual partners. For example, when a husband tries to pressure his wife to assist him with his cross-dressing behavior and the wife is uncomfortable or not accepting of such behavior, she may threaten to terminate the relationship unless he gets treatment.

Treatment for paraphilic disorders often is a difficult and lifelong process. Clients who engage in paraphilic behavior, especially those whose behavior endangers the safety of others (pedophiles, violent sadists), may be treated with drugs that reduce their sexual desire, arousal, and paraphilic fantasies. Cyproterone acetate (Androcur) and medroxyprogesterone acetate (Provera) reduce testosterone levels, which results in decreased levels of deviant sexual behavior. Additionally, sertraline (Zoloft) and fluoxetine (Prozac) have been useful in reducing depressive symptoms in clients with paraphilias and decreasing some paraphilic behaviors (Bradford & Pawlak, 1993; Kafka & Prentky, 1992; Kafka, 1994).

Other treatments for paraphilias include *satiation* (a boredom technique in which sex offenders use their most erotic fantasies after orgasm in a boring, repetitive manner to extinguish their erotic quality); *signaled punishment* (a combination of aversion therapy and biofeedback of erections to deviant stimuli); and treatments aimed at the paraphiliac's deficits (eg, deficits in arousal to adult partners, deficits in assertive skills, deficits in ability to relate socially to adult partners, treatment to reduce distorted cognitions regarding their paraphilic behavior) (Kaplan & Sadock, 1996). For example, child molesters may describe themselves as victims of children's seductive behavior toward them, blaming children for their behavior. These and other personality deficits are treated using a variety of treatment modalities and approaches.

GENDER IDENTITY DISORDERS

Gender identity disorders are characterized by a strong and persistent cross-gender identification and persistent discomfort with one's assigned sex. In addition, there must be evidence of clinically significant distress or impaired social, occupational, or other important areas of functioning.

People who identify with and live as if they are of the opposite sex are called **transsexuals**. Transsexuals are not to be confused with **transvestites**, who are people who cross-dress for sexual arousal. Transvestites generally have no persistent desire for sex reassignment.

The number of transsexuals in the United States is unknown. Data from smaller countries in Europe with access to total population statistics and referrals suggest that roughly 1 per 30,000 adult men and 1 per 100,000 adult women seek sex-reassignment surgery (SRS). In child clinic samples, approximately five boys for each girl are referred with this disorder. In adult clinic samples, men outnumber women by a ratio of approximately 2 to 3:1 (APA, 2000).

Signs and Symptoms/ Diagnostic Criteria

For diagnostic criteria and manifestations of gender identity disorder, see this chapter's Sexual and Gender Disorders Information Map.

Interdisciplinary Goals and Treatment

Treatments available for clients with gender identity disorders include SRS, hormone treatment, and psychotherapy.

SEX REASSIGNMENT SURGERY

Surgical techniques for the creation of a vaginal barrel or penis are limited, expensive, and may have unpleasant side effects. At least 35% of clients complain of inadequate vaginal depth in the years after SRS, and as many as 30% regret having undergone SRS (Ettner, 1999). In male-to-female (MTF) hormone treatment in which breast enlargement is inadequate, surgical breast implants may be an option. Because of the expense and limitations of sophisticated surgeries, many clients seeking female-to-male (FTM) transformation undergo a double mastectomy with cosmetic chest resculpting and no attempt to create a penis (Ettner, 1999).

HORMONE TREATMENT

MTF hormone treatment results in less frequent erections, more rounded bodily contours, decreased testicular volume, and limited breast enlargement. FTM hormone treatment produces an increased sexual drive, amenorrhea, and hoarseness. If a client taking FTM hormone treatment begins to lift weights, a pronounced increase in muscle mass may occur. Also, some increase in the amount and coarseness of facial and body hair may occur, as may frontal balding. Nurses should discourage clients from taking hormones without a doctor's supervision and from purchasing black-market hormones and quack "feminization pills."

PSYCHOTHERAPY

Psychotherapy for adults with gender identity disorder focuses on assisting them to find a workable, comfortable sexual identity. Transsexuals often find it difficult to find partners who accept them as they are; consequently, they may experience disorders such as depression and anxiety related to their lack of an intimate connection with another. Support groups for transsexuals, as well as Internet chat rooms, newsletters, and magazines, alleviate the distress and isolation of transsexualism by providing friends, correspondence, and a safe space for them to explore their gender identities (Ettner, 1999).

▼ Reflection and Critical Thinking Questions

1. A 72-year-old man is hospitalized for total knee replacement surgery. Two days after surgery, he and his 73-year-old wife indicate they would like some privacy so that they can have sexual relations. Assuming that the client will not be harming his surgical site and that the physician has indicated no contraindication to sexual activity, examine how you would handle this situation. Evaluate the beliefs and judgments you might have.

2. Some states have laws mandating chemical castration of repeat sex offenders, particularly child molesters. Research this topic and provide arguments for and against chemical castration. Determine your own position on the subject. Consider points such as harmful side effects, whether chemical castration is cruel and unusual punishment, whether it is therapeutic treatment, and whether those undergoing chemical castration should receive a shorter sentence or parole.

3. Consider Clinical Example 20–1 and Nursing Care Plan 20-1. What are some of the issues that may have led to the breakdown in communication between George and Betty? How do male and female stereotypes contribute to their lack of communication?

▼ CHAPTER SUMMARY

- The nurse must be aware of his or her own views and learn about the views of the client populations with whom he or she works to work professionally and to avoid applying his or her own biases to clients.
- The scope of human sexual expression is diverse and influenced by many factors such as genetics, individual preferences, culture, life experiences, and health.
- In Kaplan's model, human sexual response consists of three phases: desire, excitement, and orgasm.
- Older men experience normal age-related sexual changes such as a longer refractory period after ejaculation, less firm erection, a longer time to achieve erection and reach orgasm, and an occasional inability to achieve erection. Older women normally experience loss of lubrication and some dyspareunia.
- Sexual dysfunction disorders can be primary (caused by various psychological and emotional conditions) or secondary (caused by a general medical condition or substance use). General medical conditions that may affect sexual interest and abilities include injury, disease, or consequences of surgery. Substance use consists of drug and alcohol abuse or use of some prescribed medications, including antihypertensives, antidepressants, and neuroleptics.
- Treatment of specific sexual dysfunctions focuses mainly on targeting the client and contributing causal factors (which could be psychological, physical, or pharmacologic) related to the particular disorder.
- Assessment of the client or client couple seeking help for sexual dysfunction includes assessment of the identified problem; assessment of physical health, including medication and substance use; and assessment of the couple's relationship and communication skills.
- Generalist nurses provide education and counseling for clients seeking help with sexual dysfunction.
- Nurses encourage clients seeking help for sexual dysfunction to express their feelings surrounding the problem. They should assess and address self-esteem issues.
- Paraphilias refer to those sexual expressions characterized by recurrent, intense sexually arousing fantasies, urges, or behaviors generally involving (1) nonhuman objects or animals, (2) suffering or humiliation of self or partner, or (3) children or other nonconsenting persons. They persist over at least 6 months. Several types of paraphilias include exhibitionism, fetishism, frotteurism, pedophilia, sexual masochism, sexual sadism, transvestic fetishism, and voyeurism.
- Gender identity manifests differently in children compared with adolescents and adults. Children may repeatedly state a desire to be, or insist that they are, the other sex: boys may prefer cross-dressing or simulating female attire; girls may insist on wearing only stereotypical masculine clothing; the child may exhibit a strong and persistent preference for cross-sex roles in make-believe play or may have persistent fantasies of being the other sex; or the child may have an intense desire to participate in the stereotypical games and pastimes of the other sex. In adolescents and adults, the disturbance is manifested by symptoms such as a stated desire to be the other sex, frequently passing as the other sex, desire to live or be treated as the other sex, or the conviction that they have the typical feelings and reactions of the other sex.

▼ REVIEW QUESTIONS

1. Sexuality refers to
   a. The experience of one's sexual self
   b. How often a person desires intercourse
   c. How a person defines masculine and feminine sexual roles
   d. How attractive a person feels

2. A couple who are seeking sexual counseling reveal that some of their sexual activity involves bondage (physical restraint). Which of the following comments by the nurse is most appropriate at this time?
   a. "Don't you find that demeaning?"
   b. "Do you both engage in this willingly?"
   c. "Sexual expression that is physically or emotionally harmful is not appropriate. Have you tried to refrain from this activity?"

    d. "I don't find that appealing, but I know many people do."

3. Sexual orientation refers to
    a. Heterosexuality, bisexuality, and homosexuality
    b. Sexual expression, gender role, and sexual identity
    c. Gender role, sexual identity, and cultural mores
    d. Gender role, sexual orientation, and sexual identity

4. The nurse enters the room of a 45-year-old male client recovering from orthopedic surgery. The client is alone in the room, and the nurse quickly realizes that the client is masturbating. Which response by the nurse is most appropriate?
    a. Pretend not to notice and continue with nursing activities.
    b. Gently tell the client that his behavior is not appropriate in the hospital.
    c. Apologize, leave the room, and close the door.
    d. Tell the client that you understand he needs sexual release, but ask him to do so in the evenings when fewer staff members and visitors are present.

5. A 68-year-old male client complains that his erections are less rigid than they once were and that it takes him longer to achieve an erection. Which of the following responses is best?
    a. "Erectile dysfunction is fairly common, but many treatments are available, including medications or surgery."
    b. "What you describe sounds like normal age-related changes. Is this a concern for you?"
    c. "Is this causing a problem for your partner?"
    d. "That doesn't sound like a problem; it is common in men your age."

6. Sexual dysfunction is characterized by
    a. Pain during intercourse or disturbances in the sexual response cycle
    b. Decreased desire or aversion to sexual activity
    c. Inability to achieve an orgasm
    d. Confusion over gender identification

7. A 30-year-old female client undergoing treatment for dyspareunia states she hasn't had intercourse with her husband for several months and doesn't feel like a "real woman." Which of the following actions should the nurse take?
    a. Tell the client that when intercourse becomes pleasurable instead of painful she will feel like a real woman again.
    b. Ask the client if her husband has made her feel this way.
    c. Explore the client's beliefs about her sexuality.
    d. Tell the client she shouldn't make negative self-statements or it will damage her self-esteem.

8. A couple has undergone treatment for female sexual arousal disorder. The woman states she has difficulty feeling sexually excited and has orgasms only "occasionally." Which of the following criteria is the best indicator that the treatment plan has been effective?
    a. During the last visit, the couple describes various techniques to make foreplay more exciting.
    b. Six weeks after discharge, the couple reports increased satisfaction with their sex life.
    c. Six months after discharge, the couple reports that the female partner achieves orgasm 80% of the time.
    d. During the last visit, the clients state they have tried the various techniques that the therapist suggested and have found several that are helpful.

9. Paraphilias may be characterized by sexual urges or behaviors involving
    a. Members of the same sex
    b. Members of the opposite sex
    c. Members of both sexes
    d. Nonconsenting persons

10. A 32-year-old male client is receiving counseling for issues related to his Gender Identity Disorder. He has opted not to have sex reassignment surgery and will undergo breast augmentation surgery and male-to-female hormone treatments instead. He is contemplating returning to his hometown and letting his family and friends know that he would now prefer to be thought of as a woman. Of the following nursing diagnoses, which has the highest priority?
    a. Risk for Spiritual Distress related to possible rejection by family and friends
    b. Compromised Family Coping related to family disorganization and role changes
    c. Risk for Ineffective Management of Therapeutic Regimen related to knowledge deficit about post-surgical care
    d. Disturbed Body Image related to gender identity disorder

▼ REFERENCES AND SUGGESTED READINGS

*American Psychiatric Association. (2000). *Diagnostic and statistical manual of mental disorders* (4th ed., text rev.). Washington, DC: Author.

*Bradford, J. M., & Pawlak, A. (1993). Double-blind placebo crossover study of cyproterone acetate in the treatment of the paraphilias. *Archives of Sexual Behavior, 22*(5), 383–402.

*Ettner, R. (1999). *Gender loving care: A guide to counseling gender-variant clients.* New York: W.W. Norton.

Fergusson, D., et al. (1999). Is sexual orientation related to mental health problems and suicidality in young people? *Archives of General Psychiatry, 56*(10), 876.

Gregoire, A. (1999). Assessing and managing male sexual problems. *British Medical Journal, 318*(315), 1.

Jacoby, S. (1999). Great sex: What's age got to do with it? *Modern Maturity, 42R*, 43.

*Kafka, M. P. (1994). Sertraline pharmacotherapy for paraphilias and paraphilia-related disorders: An open trial. *Annals of Clinical Psychiatry, 53*(10), 351–358.

*Kafka, M. P., & Prentky, R. (1992). Fluoxetine treatment of non-paraphilic sexual addictions and paraphilias in men. *Journal of Clinical Psychiatry, 53*(10), 351–358.

*Kaplan, H. I., & Sadock, B. J. (1996). *Concise textbook of clinical psychiatry*. Baltimore: Williams & Wilkins.

*Kaplan, H. S. (1979). *Disorders of sexual desire and other new concepts and techniques in sex therapy*. New York: Simon & Schuster.

Laumann, E., et al. (1999). Sexual dysfunction in the United States: Prevalence and predictors. *Journal of the American Medical Association, 281*, 542.

*Laumann, E. O., Gagnon, J. H., Michael, R. T., & Michaels, S. (1994). *The social organization of sexuality: Sexual practices in the United States*. Chicago: University of Chicago Press.

Lieblum, S. R. (2000). Redefining female sexual response. *Contemporary OB/GYN, 45*, 120–126.

*Masters, W. H. & Johnson, V. E. (1970). *Human sexual inadequacy*. Boston, Little Brown.

McMahon, C. G., & Touma, K. (1999). Treatment of premature ejaculation with paroxetine hydrochloride. *International Journal of Impotence Research, 11*, 241–246.

*Moran, J. R., & Corley, M. D. (1991). Sources of sexual information and sexual attitudes and behaviors of Anglo and Hispanic adolescent males. *Adolescence, 26*(104), 857–864.

Morgentaler, A. (1999). Male impotence. *Lancet, 354*, 1713–1718.

*Northrup, C. (1998). *Women's bodies, women's wisdom: Creating physical and emotional health and healing*. New York: Bantam.

*Padilla, A. M., & Baird, T. L. (1991). Mexican-American adolescent sexuality and sexual knowledge: An exploratory study. *Hispanic Journal of Behavioral Sciences, 13*(1), 95–104.

Rowland, D. L., & Burnett, A. L. (2000). Pharmacotherapy in the treatment of male sexual dysfunction. *Journal of Sex Research, 37*, 226–236.

*Smith, B. S. (1992). Nursing care challenges: Homosexual psychiatric patients. *Journal of Psychosocial Nursing, 30*(12), 15–21.

*Spark, R. F. (2000). *Sexual health for men: The complete guide*. Cambridge, MA: Perseus.

Stevens, J. (1998). When patient care gets too personal. *RN, 61*, 72.

Taylor, B. (1999). "Coming out" as a life transition: Homosexual identity formation and its implications for health care practice. *Journal of Advanced Nursing, 30*, 523.

*Ucho, L. G. (1994). Culture and violence: The interaction of Africa and America. *Sex Roles, 31*(3–4), 185–204.

**Starred references are cited in text.*

For additional information on this chapter, go to *http://connection. hww.com.*

Need more help? See Chapter 20 of the *Study Guide to Accompany Mohr: Johnson's Psychiatric-Mental Health Nursing,* 5th ed.

The Client With a Dissociative Disorder

JAN DALSHEIMER AND JANET STAGG

▼ KEY TERMS

Alter—Two or more identities or personality states.

Depersonalization disorder—A dissociative disorder characterized by a recurring or persistent feeling that one is detached from one's own thinking. Affected clients feel that they are outside their mind or body, much like an observer.

Dissociation—Altering one's usual level of self-awareness in an effort to escape an upsetting event or feeling.

Dissociative amnesia—A dissociative disorder characterized by loss of memory that is not organic and involves an inability to recall events or facts too extensive to be labeled as mere forgetfulness.

Dissociative disorders—A disruption in the usually integrated functions of consciousness, memory, identity, or perception, causing disturbance that may be sudden or gradual, transient or chronic.

Dissociative fugue—A dissociative disorder that involves sudden travel away from home coupled with an inability to remember the past and confusion about identity or the adoption of a new identity.

Dissociative identity disorder—A dissociative disorder in which the person acquires two or more identities or personality states (alters), who take control over the client's behavior.

Dissociative trance—A dissociative state in which a person's awareness of his or her immediate surroundings narrows, and he or she exhibits stereotyped behaviors such as immobilization, collapse, or loud, uncontrollable shrieking.

Possession trance—A dissociative state that involves acquiring a new identity attributed to the influence of a spirit, power, deity, or other person.

Ritual abuse—A severe form of abuse in which a child is repeatedly physically and sexually abused in ceremonies by an organized group of perpetrators.

▼ LEARNING OBJECTIVES

On completion of this chapter, you should be able to accomplish the following:

- Define dissociation.
- Describe the etiology of dissociative disorders.
- Differentiate the four types of dissociative disorders.
- Describe addictions commonly associated with dissociative disorders.
- Describe treatment modalities for dissociative disorders.
- Apply the nursing process to clients with dissociative disorders.
- Understand cultural considerations applicable to the care of clients with dissociative disorders.

▼ Clinical Example 21-1

Susan, a 20-year-old part-time college student, is admitted to a psychiatric unit for evaluation of suicidal ideation. A psychological history reveals that Susan attempted suicide 2 years ago by cutting her wrists. When Susan was a child, several male family members physically and sexually abused her for approximately 7 years. Susan first sought psychiatric treatment at 17 years of age and was diagnosed with Major Depression with Borderline Personality Disorder. Separate trials with several antidepressant medications failed to provide relief from her symptoms, which included self-destructive thoughts, feelings of hopelessness, and occasional mood swings.

During this hospitalization, Susan admits to hearing voices and having an imaginary companion who has "tried to protect her" since childhood. As her treatment progresses, she begins to exhibit different childlike behaviors and trance-like positions. Her subjective distress also increases, and she begins saying, "I just want to die," and trying to cut and burn herself. During therapy, Susan exhibits two alternate personalities, "Betty" and "Barb." Barb, the older of the two "alters," tries to protect Betty, the abused child.

This chapter discusses dissociative disorders. As you read the chapter, consider the case of Susan in Clinical Example 21-1. How do Susan's history and signs and symptoms relate to this group of disorders? You will learn more about the progression of Susan's care in Nursing Care Plan 21-1. You also will have the opportunity to apply your understanding of this client and others with dissociative disorders in the Reflection and Critical Thinking Questions at the end of this chapter.

DISSOCIATIVE DISORDERS

Despite an enormous amount of published literature on dissociative disorders, dissociation remains a poorly understood phenomenon. Because of the lack of systematic study of dissociation, little empirical information is available. The field has advanced based on anecdotal experience, poorly designed studies, and polemic arguments. Published investigations have many methodologic flaws (McHugh, 1992; North & Yutzy, 1997; Offshe & Watters, 1994; Piper, 1997). The morass of literature on dissociative phenomena includes both advocates and critics.

Currently, most psychiatrists believe that dissociation is a legitimate phenomenon. They also believe that its most dramatic manifestation, dissociative identity disorder (DID), formerly known as multiple personality disorder, is a rare condition when it occurs spontaneously but that it is easy to create iatrogenically (Gelder, Gath, Mayou, & Cowen, 1996). Student nurses reading this chapter are urged to keep an open mind and to understand that this area of psychopathology is poorly developed. More empirical study either may support or cast further question on these diagnoses in the future.

Dissociation refers to the situation of altering one's usual level of self-awareness in an effort to escape an upsetting event or feeling (Winokur & Clayton, 1994). It is a normal reaction to an emotionally overloaded situation and happens in the service of self-preservation when neither resistance nor escape is possible. This process can include actively pretending to be somewhere or someone else, experiencing amnesia, and having the ability to "cut off" pain perception from parts of the body. The cognitive outcome of dissociation is fragmentation of memory. This fragmentation can result in patchy or disorganized recall, seemingly illogical associations, and seemingly extreme affective reactions such as displaying extreme rage in reaction to relatively minor interpersonal "offenses."

All humans have the capacity to dissociate. Acts of daydreaming or amnestic episodes constitute common types of dissociation. On the Dissociative Experience Scale administered by Ross, Joshi, and Currie (1991), 29% of the general population reported that in almost one third of their conversations, they did not hear part or all of what was said. In some cultures, voluntary experiences of trance or meditation are accepted practices and should not be considered a psychiatric disorder.

Conceptually, dissociation differs from the defense mechanism of repression in several different ways. *Repression* is hypothesized to result from intrapsychic conflicts (see Chap. 3). Dissociation, on the other hand, is hypothesized to result from external trauma with amnestic barriers presumed to divide subunits of memory. Moreover, in dissociation, the information is kept out of awareness for a sharply delimited period, whereas in repression information is kept out of awareness for a variety of experiences across time (Spiegel & Maldonado, 1999). In other words, the memories that are "repressed" in dissociation are specific to events. They are not the result of "forgetting" as a way to avoid anxiety associated with intrapsychic conflicts that may have nothing to do with specific events.

When is dissociation a problem? Because mild states usually do not cause a person much difficulty in daily functioning, dissociation can be conceptualized on a continuum (Figure 21-1) or as a typology. In the continuum model, pathologic dissociation occurs when a person experiences more frequent or "deeper" states of dissociation. Everyday functioning deteriorates as a person moves from left to right along the continuum. In the typology model, pathologic dissociation represents a different kind of dissociative experience altogether. Each model seems to account for some of what is seen clinically (Putnam, 1997).

Dissociation leading to impaired functioning requires treatment. The degree of disruption of the self and the intensity and types of interventions vary in the dissociative disorders. People may not remember their identity and travel far away from home (dissociative fugue), they may lose their memory (dissociative amnesia), they may assume two or more identities or personalities (DID), or they may feel that they are not in touch with their body (depersonalization disorder).

Epidemiology

Fifty years ago, DID was thought to be so rare that it was considered nonexistent. During the 1980s and 1990s, however, the number of reported cases increased precipi-

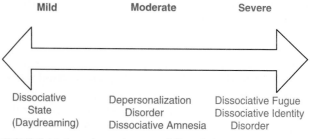

FIGURE 21-1   A continuum of dissociation.

tously and exponentially. Some experts assert that this increase is related to heightened public and therapist awareness of these conditions. Others say that publicity concerning these disorders provokes related behaviors and diagnoses of these disorders in suggestible individuals (Gelder et al., 1996). Regardless, no adequate studies have been performed to estimate the prevalence of dissociative disorders in the general population (North & Yutzy, 1997).

Cultural Considerations

Cultural considerations regarding dissociative disorders include the acknowledgment that trance states are seen in some cultures, including Indonesia, Malaysia, the Arctic, India, and Latin America. Indeed, dissociative phenomena have occurred around the world. They seem to be more prevalent in the less heavily industrialized, developing countries (Spiegel & Maldonado, 1999).

Trance states are seen or induced as part of a system of spiritual beliefs. In **dissociative trance,** a person's awareness of his or her immediate surroundings narrows. The person also may exhibit stereotyped behaviors such as immobilization, collapse, or loud shrieking beyond his or her control. **Possession trance** in these cultures involves acquiring a new identity that is attributed to the influence of a spirit, power, deity, or other person. For diagnostic purposes, an individual must be experiencing dysfunction and stress, and the behaviors noted must not be a normal part of a broadly accepted collective cultural or religious practice (American Psychiatric Association [APA], 2000).

Research shows that DID can be misdiagnosed in the Latino population because "ataque de nervios" is accepted as a diagnosis for this group, yet it has symptoms similar to DID. Amnesia is a predominant symptom of "ataque" and often is a culturally acceptable reaction to stress within the Latino community. The condition has a lifetime prevalence of 12% in Puerto Rico (Lewis-Fernandez, 1993).

Etiology

The etiology of dissociative disorders is not known. Results of the few genetic studies examining dissociative disorders have been inconclusive (Gelder et al., 1996). One study finds that most parents of adolescents with the disorder have high rates of dissociative problems themselves.

BIOLOGIC FACTORS

Various substances or medical conditions can induce dissociative symptoms. For example, a seizure disorder or prolonged use of alcohol may cause amnesia. Clients experiencing such symptoms, then, must undergo a thorough medical evaluation before a definitive diagnosis of dissociative disorder is made.

People with dissociative disorders appear to be particularly susceptible to hypnotism when tested for this capacity. They also seem to be highly suggestible and have low sedation thresholds (APA, 2000; Winokur & Clayton, 1994). The ability to dissociate is believed to be partly related to having the biologic capacity to do so when subjected to repeated stress (Fink, 1991). Physiologic studies suggest that dissociative reactions may be precipitated by excessive cortical arousal, which triggers reactive inhibition of signals in sensorimotor pathways by way of negative feedback relationships between the cerebral cortex and the brainstem reticular formation (Winokur & Clayton, 1994).

PSYCHOLOGICAL AND SOCIAL FACTORS

Dissociative disorders are believed to be a way for individuals to defend themselves against painful or distressing circumstances (Maxmen & Ward, 1995). Some scholars (Kluft, 1995; Putnam, 1997) contend that abused people are especially likely to dissociate to defend against feeling the pain of remembering what has been done (or is being done) to them (Box 21-1). After reviewing the literature on this subject, however, Pope, Hudson, Bodkin, and Oliva (1998), as well as Merckelbach and Muris (2001), con-

---

BOX 21-1 ▼ *Dissociative Disorders and Ritual Abuse*

Ritual abuse has been defined as a severe form of abuse in which a child is repeatedly physically and sexually abused in ceremonies by an organized group of perpetrators. Such groups may be pseudoreligious (as in satanic cults), or they may not associate themselves with a religious belief. Ritual abuse frequently is violent and may involve threats of death or the witnessing of death of other victims, both human and animal (Fraser, 1990).

During the mid-1970s, widespread allegations of satanic ritual abuse (SRA) began to surface, and the publication of a book entitled *Michelle Remembers* (1980) triggered a public panic. Although presented as fact, the book later proved to be a hoax. Because of widespread concerns, a study of SRA allegations was sponsored by the National Center on Child Abuse and Neglect. Researchers investigated more than 12,000 accusations and surveyed more than 11,000 psychiatric, social service, and law enforcement personnel. They found no evidence for a single case of satanic cult abuse (Goodman, Quin, Bottoms, & Shaver, 1994). Substantiating these findings, a study published in 1992 by Kenneth Lanning of the Federal Bureau of Investigation concluded that there is no solid evidence of a single case of SRA.

clude that not a single study provides methodologically sound evidence that dissociative amnesia is more prevalent in victims of abuse than in the general population.

ROLE OF FAMILY DYNAMICS

Although the empirical literature does not support the popular contention that dissociative phenomena are more common in individuals who have been abused as children, some clients with dissociative disorders have a background of family dysfunction. Some scholars believe that family dynamics such as those present in abusive families may result in dissociative behaviors. Chapter 17 provides a discussion of dysfunctional family systems and child abuse and the psychological consequences.

Signs and Symptoms/ Diagnostic Criteria

The *Diagnostic and Statistical Manual of Mental Disorders*, 4th edition, text revision (*DSM-IV-TR*) defines **dissociative disorders** as "a disruption in the usually integrated functions of consciousness, memory, identity, or perception." The disturbance may be "sudden or gradual, transient or chronic" (APA, 2000, p. 519). This definition includes four disorders:

1. **Depersonalization disorder** is characterized by a recurring or persistent feeling that one is detached from one's own thinking. Affected clients feel that they are outside their mind or body, much like an observer.
2. **Dissociative amnesia** is characterized by loss of memory that is not organic and involves an inability to recall events or facts too extensive to be labeled as mere forgetfulness.
3. **Dissociative fugue** involves sudden travel away from home coupled with an inability to remember the past and confusion about identity or the adoption of a new identity.
4. **Dissociative identity disorder**, in which the person acquires two or more identities or personality states (**alters**) who take control over his or her behavior. As with amnesia, DID involves an inability to recall important personal information that is too extensive to be labeled as forgetfulness (Historical Capsule 21-1).

The *DSM-IV-TR* also includes a fifth category, *dissociative disorder not otherwise specified* (NOS). The disorders in this category have a dissociative symptom as a primary feature but do not meet the criteria for any of the four dissociative disorders. Examples of disorders in this category include brainwashing, loss of consciousness not attributable to a medical condition, and trance disorder. In this definition, trance disorder is not a normal part of a broadly accepted collective cultural or religious practice.

Comorbidities and Dual Diagnoses

Experts on dissociative disorders have found a link between addictive behaviors, particularly eating disorders, and dissociative disorders (Barber, 1991; Levin, Kahan, Lamm, & Spauster, 1993). Some clients with eating disorders report trance-like experiences during episodes of binge eating or purging. Some feel "unreal" when binge eating (Barber, 1991).

Clients with DID who have an additional diagnosis of eating disorder may develop the eating dysfunction as a coping mechanism to handle abuse. They may find that binge eating acts as a form of self-medication, a way of comforting oneself and escaping frightening feelings. Some clients with anorexia were told that they are not worthy to eat and adopt starvation as a punishing technique (Barber, 1991).

When a client with an eating disorder presents for treatment, it is wise to assess for symptoms of a dissociative disorder. Presence of atypical eating behaviors, such as the onset of anorexia and bulimia later in life, combined with a history of multiple symptoms and previous treatment failures, could signal dissociative disorder. In this case, the dissociative disorder should be the focus of primary treatment with the eating disorder considered secondary (Levin et al., 1993).

Clients who develop dissociative patterns of behavior often meet the criteria for other diagnoses, such as alcohol or drug abuse and anxiety disorders (Gelder et al., 1996). Severe depression is present in 70% to 100% of these individuals, and approximately 75% report "high periods." Panic attacks are common: at least 90% of these clients present psychotic symptoms. Of clients with DID, 69% to 84% are diagnosed with concomitant personality disorders, including antisocial personality disorder (Gelder et al., 1996) and borderline personality disorder (North & Yutzy, 1997).

Interdisciplinary Goals and Treatment

The treatment goal for the client with DID is to learn how to control the symptoms and distress. How to accomplish this is the subject of a controversy that has as its basis a philosophical split among mental healthcare providers. One group of therapists believes that DID is a unique diagnosis, requiring involved exploration of alters and recovered memories and other distinct treatment modalities. The other group believes that the dramatic symptoms of DID—multiple alters and recovered memories—are induced by well-meaning but misguided therapists and that other diagnoses can explain the basic symptomatology of these clients, such as somatoform or personality disorder. This second group further believes that therapists must take care to avoid insinuating the presence of

Dissociative Disorders Information Map

⇨ Prevalence

Rates vary and remain controversial

⇨ Risk and Contributing Factors

- Gender: women are far more likely than men to experience Dissociative Identity Disorder or Depersonalization Disorder
- Having experienced childhood physical or sexual abuse
- Low self-esteem
- Family history of similar disorders
- Substance or stimulant abuse
- Problems with Self-Concept

⇨ Summary of DSM-IV-TR Diagnostic Criteria

Dissociative Fugue

- Client suddenly and unexpectedly travels away from home or customary workplace and cannot recall his or her past.
- Client is confused about identity or assumes a new identity (partial or complete).
- The disturbance does not occur exclusively during Dissociative Identity Disorder and is not caused by a substance or medical condition.
- Symptoms cause significant distress or impair social, occupational, or other important areas of functioning.

Dissociative Amnesia

- Client cannot recall important, usually traumatic or stressful, personal information. This predominant problem is too extensive to simply label as forgetfulness.
- The disturbance does not occur exclusively during Dissociative Identity Disorder, Dissociative Fugue, Posttraumatic Stress Disorder, Acute Stress Disorder, or Somatization Disorder. It is not caused by a substance or neurologic or other medical condition.
- Symptoms cause significant distress or impair social, occupational, or other important areas of functioning.

Depersonalization Disorder

- Client persistently or recurrently feels detached from (an outside observer of) his or her thoughts or body (e.g., client feels like he or she is in a dream).
- During depersonalization, reality testing remains intact.
- Depersonalization causes significant distress or impairs social, occupational, or other important areas of functioning.
- Depersonalization does not occur exclusively during another mental disorder and is not caused by a substance (e.g., medication) or medical condition (e.g., temporal lobe epilepsy).

Dissociative Identity Disorder

- Client has two or more distinct identities or personalities. Each has its own consistent pattern of perceiving, relating to, and thinking about environment and self.
- At least two identities or personalities recurrently control the client's behavior.
- Client cannot recall important personal information. Lack of recall is too extensive to explain as ordinary forgetfulness.
- The disturbance is not caused by a substance or medical condition. **Note:** In children, symptoms cannot be attributed to "imaginary friends" or other fantasy play.

⇨ Want to Know More?

The International Society for the Study of Dissociation
60 Revere Drive, Suite 500
Northbrook, IL 60062
Telephone: 847-480-0899
Fax: 847-480-9282
www.issd.com

New York Society for the Study of Multiple Personality
    and Dissociation
Columbia University Teachers College
525 West 120th Street
New York, NY 10027

Sidran Foundation
200 E. Joppa Road, Suite 207
Towson, MD 21286
Phone: 410-825-8888
Fax: 410-337-0747
www.sidran.org

alters or a history of abuse in suggestible clients. Naturally, these diametrically opposed conceptual models yield very different treatment approaches. Because the nurse may encounter clients under either treatment approach, both are presented here.

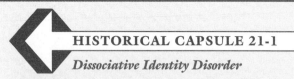

HISTORICAL CAPSULE 21-1

Dissociative Identity Disorder

Dissociative identity disorder is not an aberration peculiar to 20th century North America. Ancient history shows that all cultures have recognized fragmentation of the self. Colin Ross, an eminent researcher and therapist in the field of dissociative disorders, believes that the client with DID suffers from an Osiris complex, named after Osiris in Egyptian myth. According to this myth, Osiris was killed by his brother, Set, who then cut Osiris into many pieces and scattered them over a wide area. Isis, Osiris' wife, gathered up the fragments, embalmed them, and resurrected Osiris as king of the land of the dead. Isis and Osiris had a son, Horus, who defeated Set in battle and became king of the earth. This myth portrays fragmentation, death, healing, and resurrection of the self in a new form. This is the cycle through which the successfully treated client with DID must pass (Ross, 1997).

In the late 19th century and until about 1910, case studies of DID and fugues were recorded. In 1890, the psychologist William James discussed multiple personality in a theoretical chapter on the consciousness of self. Little new work was done on DID, however, from 1910 to 1980.

Clinical interest in DID resurged in the 1970s, partly because of the women's movement, which helped to bring child abuse and incest out of the closet. In 1980, DID was given official diagnostic status in *DSM-III*. Writings about DID began to proliferate, leading to research and treatment refinement. The 1990s saw the development of the International Society for the Study of Dissociation (ISSD), an organization that boasted approximately 2,600 members in late 1995.

Currently, the dissociative disorders are widely researched and have increasing political organization. The most likely development in the first decade of the 21st century will be an increase in the scientific foundation of the disorders and international study of the field (Ross, 1997).

TREATMENT APPROACH

Proponents of DID as a distinct diagnosis with a unique treatment approach assert that treatment must involve fusion of all "alters" into a single personality. Although no studies document the validity of their techniques, they claim that the process of integration of "alters" involves unlearning an overreliance on dissociation and acquiring a new set of adaptive coping strategies (Ross, 1997). Thus, treatment involves breaking down amnestic barriers and integrating altered conscious states. Proponents recommend prolonged treatment with intensive psychotherapy.

Although the practice is controversial and has been condemned by the False Memory Syndrome Foundation, proponents of DID support clients in recalling early memories to produce "abreactions"; that is, feelings associated with the traumatic events (Stafford, 1993). Talking with a therapist in a safe environment may help the client remember earlier, painful times, or hypnosis may be useful in bringing about such memories (Box 21-2). Working through the original feelings with a trusting per-

BOX 21-2 ▼ *Repressed Memories: Are They Real?*

University of Washington researcher and experimental psychologist Elizabeth Loftus asserts that no scientific evidence supports the belief that people can suddenly remember long-forgotten memories. Loftus does not dispute that many people are abused as children or that they may try to avoid the memories as adults. She contends, though, that no evidence supports that people can completely repress memories and then remember them later in life in complete detail. Loftus and other scientists are concerned that if a client cannot remember abuse, some therapists will "suggest" it until the person does "remember." Loftus believes that memories become distorted and cannot be recalled in their original form (1993).

Colin Ross, MD, a leading researcher and writer on DID, states that working with severely abused clients and listening to their stories is like watching hours of atrocity films. Is every detail that a client describes true? Ross, who estimates that approximately 5% of clients on adult psychiatric inpatient units have DID (Ross, Anderson, Fleisher, & Norton, 1991), believes that skepticism is warranted when hearing terrifying stories of abuse, particularly satanic ritual abuse. Other therapists treating DID also might agree that every detail of what a client recounts does not have to be believed. What becomes most important, however, is attending to the client's pain and suffering.

son in a safe environment is thought to help clients reintegrate their self. Proponents of DID say that the therapist may find it necessary to work with all the alters as different persons in therapy for them to accept each other. They also suggest that because integration of the personalities may not be possible, the therapist should help the client to acquire new coping skills to deal with maladaptive behaviors.

Because they assert that DID is an extremely severe disorder, proponents of the diagnosis posit that only psychotherapists who are trained in working with these clients should provide individual therapy. Others disagree, saying that the treatment of dissociation requires no such special background and that it might in fact be counterproductive (North & Yutzy, 1997). Proponents of the DID diagnosis admit that their clients often severely deteriorate during treatment and that as psychotherapy progresses, clients may become more dissociative, anxious, or depressed. Some experts report that clients can develop hundreds or even thousands of "alters" (Kluft, 1984; Putnam, 1989; Ross, 1989).

In the last decade, cases of severe deterioration of such clients resulted in hospitalizations, costing enormous amounts of money. Critics assert that such deterioration and dissociation result from therapists encouraging the display of "alters" and treating them as if they were real (Offshe & Watters, 1994; Piper, 1997). Criticism of these practices by professional organizations and senior mental health professionals, as well as huge lawsuits filed against therapists who used some of the more questionable "therapeutic practices," have resulted in the decline of specialized DID hospital units and the promulgation of years of individual psychotherapy (Acocella, 1999).

Currently, most of the mainstream psychiatric literature recommends treating clients with presumed DID using therapeutic approaches similar to those used in the treatment of somatoform and borderline personality disorders (North & Yutzy, 1997). Indeed, the entire trend in psychological treatment in the last 20 years has been away from "insight"-oriented and long-term therapies toward psychopharmacologic and short-term cognitive behavior therapies that help clients to address their current problems (Acocella, 1999).

INDIVIDUAL THERAPY

The onset of dissociative amnesia and dissociative fugue often is acute, and supporting the client in talking about recent events may prompt rapid recovery of memory. If talking alone is not effective, hypnosis may help prompt the client to reveal events and feelings and ultimately assist in restoring the person's memory. Many experts, however, deny that hypnosis is an effective memory-retrieval tool, and little empirical evidence substantiates its use as such. Indeed, a mountain of evidence suggests that hypnosis is not an effective method of recovering memory and that it

increases suggestibility (Offshe & Watters, 1994). An interview using amobarbital sodium (Amytal Sodium, "truth serum") also may be an effective approach if conducted soon after the onset of the amnesia. Some psychiatric experts, however, assert that such techniques should be avoided because they typically yield increasing numbers of new personalities (North & Yutzy, 1997). Supporting the client with depersonalization disorder to talk about antecedent events surrounding the client's feelings of anxiety and then planning behavioral techniques to cope with stressful situations are effective treatment strategies.

GROUP THERAPY

Although group therapy may be helpful for people with a dissociative process that is less severe than DID, the value of group therapy must be carefully assessed for clients with DID. Group work may be too intense and threatening for these clients, and the type of group should be evaluated carefully. Generally, a highly structured group with a clear focus and time frame seems to be most useful.

As clients with dissociative disorder progress in their recovery, a 12-step group may be a helpful adjunct to individual therapy when their work includes recovery from addictions. Because 12-step programs promote belief in a higher power, however, this concept must not overwhelm or threaten the client.

PHARMACOTHERAPY

Psychotropic medication is not a primary treatment for dissociative disorders (Barach, 1994). Antianxiety medications such as lorazepam, however, may be helpful for short-term management of severe anxiety. Antidepressant medication also may be indicated, but clients should be evaluated on an individual basis for necessity and category of drug. With clients who have DID, it is common for the different alters to report conflicting responses and side effects to the same medication. Also, for clients with DID who hear voices, antipsychotic medications generally are ineffective. Although clients with DID display high levels of anxiety and depression, no medication has been documented to be of specific value for treating the dissociative phenomenon itself (Markowitz, 1996).

ART THERAPY

Art therapy is a helpful adjunct when well timed and led by a trained professional who has knowledge of dissociative disorders. Art therapy encourages clients to tell their stories in a nonthreatening way; it is a safe alternative to acting out feelings destructively and a means to erode denial gently. Art often may present the whole picture of a client long before the client's consciousness can grasp what has happened in the past. For clients with DID, art also can be a useful tool for promoting integration of alters. The different personalities can participate in a common activity and contribute toward a collective whole (Frye & Gannon, 1993).

MILIEU MANAGEMENT

Clients with dissociative disorders may be hospitalized in psychiatric inpatient units when their symptoms interfere grossly with daily functioning, when they are out of touch with reality, or when they are a danger to self or others. All disciplines that work with clients with dissociative disorders are responsible for effective milieu management, but no other discipline is involved as much as nursing. Staff nurses set the tone of the unit and see that guidelines are upheld (see Nursing Care Plan 21-1). Some of these guidelines include the following:

- Expect clients with dissociative disorders to show involvement in the unit and exhibit appropriate behavior. This expectation conveys a sense of self-responsibility and ultimately empowerment as the client learns coping skills.
- Convey that clients must verbalize, not act on, impulses related to violent and self-injurious behavior. This includes contracting with the client for safety (Stafford, 1993). As with all clients, physical restraints should be used only as a last resort because of the trauma they impose.

Other issues of concern include understanding that clients with DID may not easily accept new staff members or new peers (Stafford, 1993). People new to the milieu should allow the client physical and psychological space to allow her or him to determine closeness. Also, staff should use touch judiciously with DID clients and always ask if a gesture of touch is acceptable to the client. Because the client may have an exaggerated startle response, nurses must never touch the person from behind, where the client cannot see movement. The best guideline is not to touch the client unless there is sound therapeutic rationale for doing so and the client's permission has been obtained.

FAMILY EDUCATION

Dissociative disorders are difficult illnesses to explain and teach to family members. Clients frequently are misdiagnosed for years and treated for illnesses such as schizophrenia or bipolar disorder with psychotic features. Education of the client is expedited when the client becomes aware of the gaps in time and memory. Family education begins at the time of diagnosis. Simple explanation of the disorder, including its diagnostic criteria, is the best way to teach families about the illness. The most important feature that families need to learn is that the gaps in time and memory are critical safety issues for the client. For example, the client may get into the car and start driving without any idea of destination or reason for driving, ending up in a strange place with people he or she does not know. Family members need to be aware of this possibility and be prepared to activate an emergency search plan to locate the client and bring him or her home quickly and safely.

APPLICATION OF THE NURSING PROCESS TO THE CLIENT WITH A DISSOCIATIVE DISORDER

Assessment in Adults

Assessment of DID is imprecise. Adherents of the concept have claimed that scores of behaviors should signal the possible presence of guest personalities. Among these are changing hairstyles between sessions, changing posture, covering the mouth, rolling the eyes upward or blinking, having a headache, scratching an itch, or wearing a particular color of clothing or jewelry (Lowenstein, 1991; Ross, 1989; Putnam, 1998). More mainstream assessment of the client's behavior requires attention to multiple details, as evinced by asking the following questions:

- Does the client exhibit inconsistencies in physical behaviors such as switching right or left handedness, voice changes, or marked differences in clothing and hairstyles on different occasions?
- Has the client ever found himself or herself at a place, unable to remember how he or she got there? This behavior indicates a "blackout," which, in the absence of other dissociative disorder symptoms, could indicate alcohol abuse.
- Has the client written notes or created artwork of which he or she has no memory?
- Is there evidence of substance abuse or an eating disorder?

Assessment of the client's thoughts and perceptions provides essential information about past and present experiences. The following questions are helpful to assess thought and perception:

- What is the client's earliest childhood memory? If the client reveals having an abusive childhood, the nurse should ascertain the type of abuse, how long the abuse occurred, and the number of people involved.
- Did the client ever have an imaginary childhood friend? If so, what was the nature of the relationship? Does the client still have conversations with this friend?
- Does the client have gaps in memory? Are there periods that he or she cannot remember?
- Is the client sometimes accused of lying but does not think that he or she has lied?

- Does the client sometimes feel as if he or she is standing outside of himself or herself, as if watching another person?
- Does the client exhibit rapid changes in mood and thought process during one interview?
- Does the client express psychophysiological complaints such as severe headache, chest pain, or a fluctuation in pain threshold?

Assessment in Children

Diagnosing dissociative disorders in children may be more difficult than in adolescents and adults because the symptoms may be subtler and dissociation may present in various forms. The child with a dissociative disorder may not recall information that most children would readily remember, such as the name of a teacher or best friend or important events. Pathologic lying tends to be universal as the child tries to cover up not knowing certain information. Trance-like states may result in the child being labeled as having attention problems in school. Difficulty concentrating is common, as are auditory hallucinations that present as critical voices. Some experts assert that the voice may sound like the abuser's voice. Behavioral problems may include aggression coupled with anger, self-injurious behaviors, and sexual acting out. Sleep disturbance and intermittent depression are common (Putnam, 1991).

Several assessment instruments are available to measure symptoms of pathology in children. Some depend on feedback from the parent or other caregiver, and some involve direct feedback from the child. No behavior or symptom rating, however, can be used to assess for dissociative pathology on an ongoing basis. The instruments, although helpful, have their limitations (Pinegar, 1995).

Examples of two standardized instruments most frequently used to measure the severity of emotional distress in children are the Child Behavior Checklist and the Louisville Behavior Checklist. Because the parents complete these instruments, information of a child's unusual behavior to which a caregiver may be sensitive could be revealed. An obvious disadvantage is that if the parent completing the instrument is the perpetrator, responses may be distorted. Another test, used by nurse–researchers, is the Traumatic Events Drawing Series, which evaluates stress responses of children to sexual abuse. Completed by the child, it is thought to be highly effective for examining the effects of sexual abuse. The Child Abuse and Trauma Questionnaire has five scales that measure physical abuse or punishment, psychological abuse, sexual abuse, neglect, and negative home atmosphere. It is completed by the child and considered to have good reliability. A drawback, however, is that there is latitude for a wide variety of interpretations of answers. For example, what might be considered abuse in one family or culture may not be considered abuse in another setting (Pinegar, 1995).

Nursing Diagnosis

Possible nursing diagnoses for a client with a dissociative disorder include the following:

- **Disturbed Personal Identity** related to childhood trauma
- **Risk for Self-Mutilation** related to feelings of stress and use of maladaptive coping mechanisms
- **Anxiety** related to fragmented identity and nonintegrated self
- **Ineffective Coping** related to perception of inability to control stressors and traumatic events
- **Ineffective Role Performance** related to amnestic episodes

Planning

Throughout the process of the client's recovery, the treatment team must maintain a sense of collaboration and congruency to provide a milieu of safety and consistency. As much as possible, the team should include the client in the planning to foster the development of empowerment and self-responsibility. Nursing Care Plan 21-1 presents the care of Susan from Clinical Example 21-1.

Goals for the client with DID include the following:

- The client will have decreased episodes of dissociation, depersonalization, use of alters, or fugue.
- The client will be able to recall recent and past events.
- The client will demonstrate adaptive coping strategies and gain emotional control.
- The client will refrain from acts of self-harm.
- The client will resume social, work, and family roles and function.
- The client will have increased feelings of security.

Implementation

The nurse's role in managing the care of the client with a dissociative disorder is to support and reinforce the gains made in therapy sessions. The nurse accomplishes this by providing emotional support, grounding, and a sense of security. Specific techniques include the following:

- Educate the client about the recovery process. Clients may have idealistic fantasies that the treatment team can give them a "quick fix." Clients need to know that part of the treatment of DID may involve uncovering painful feelings and memories to begin recovery.
- Provide a safe, nonjudgmental environment to encourage the client to diminish defensive responses. A simple, structured environment is most helpful.

Nursing Care Plan 21-1

DISSOCIATIVE IDENTITY DISORDER

Susan, whose history is presented in Clinical Example 21-1, is diagnosed with DID. Her mental health care team initiates a program designed to limit the use of "alters," increase her feelings of safety, and improve her ability to manage strong emotions. Susan relates that she feels threatened and unsafe; the anxiety these feelings engender is relieved when she cuts or burns herself.

   Susan's therapy goals include resolving her identity disturbance; working out the issues, conflicts, and pain resulting from her childhood abuse; and developing adaptive coping strategies. One important immediate goal is to diminish self-harm/self-mutilation behaviors.

Nursing Diagnosis: Risk for Self-Mutilation related to intense feelings of anxiety and history of physical abuse

Goal: Susan will remain physically safe and will replace maladaptive coping mechanisms with adaptive ones.

Interventions	Rationales
Negotiate a "no self-harm" contract, both verbally and in writing, and identify situations that trigger self-harm impulses.	Agreeing to the "no self-harm" contract increases Susan's safety and helps Susan gain control over her behavior. Identifying triggers also will help Susan gain control by helping her recognize risky situations so that she can act before becoming overwhelmed by her emotions.
Work with Susan to develop steps that she can take when the urge to harm herself occurs. Suggest activities such as deep breathing, seeking out a staff member to talk to, drawing pictures of what's bothering her, writing in a journal, or engaging in sports to overcome the urge. Recognize that Susan can use any activity that appeals to her and is not harmful to replace self-injurious behavior.	Replacing maladaptive coping mechanisms with positive actions teaches Susan that there are alternatives to self-harm.
Help the client to identify at least one "safe" person per shift that she can go to for support and problem solving during a self-harm crisis.	Identifying one "safe" person promotes Susan's sense of security and safety and places responsibility on Susan for seeking out this person during a crisis period.
Refer the client to a support group for people who self-harm as a way to handle intense emotions.	Support from others will help Susan learn new coping techniques and alleviate the isolation and shame she may feel about engaging in this behavior.

Evaluation: Susan complies with the contract and begins to use other strategies when urges to inflict self-harm occur. She still feels strong urges to harm herself when she is angry but does not always act on them. She reports feeling an increased ability to manage her emotions.

Nursing Diagnosis: Disturbed Personal Identity related to childhood trauma and abuse

Goal: Susan's feelings of depersonalization and dissociation will diminish.

Interventions	Rationales
Orient client to the "here and now" using physical grounding techniques. Such techniques include lighting areas if dark; asking the client to keep her eyes open, stand up, or hold the hands of staff member; having the client maintain eye contact or walk around and look at present surroundings; suggesting the client chew on ice chips.	Orientation measures can break the dissociative state by focusing Susan on physical reality. Experiencing stimuli through the senses connects Susan to the "here and now."

(continued)

Nursing Care Plan 21-1 (Continued)

Interventions	Rationales
Orient the client to the "here and now" using verbal grounding techniques. Such techniques include stating the place, day, time, and date; calling her by her legal name, not an "alter" name; identifying yourself and validating the client's adult status by having her look at her size in relation to yours.	Verbal grounding techniques will remind Susan that she is in the present, is safe, and is an adult.
Encourage the client to assume more responsibility for her behavior. Discuss fears and perceptions about assuming responsibility for behavior. Encourage independence but be available for help and assistance when needed. Facilitate family support and provide positive feedback for behavior changes.	Assuming responsibility for her behavior will help Susan gain control over her emotional state and diminish her reliance on dissociation and other maladaptive coping mechanisms.
Support client's therapy program by encouraging the expression of feelings; helping the client identify strengths and positive attributes; demonstrating empathy, warmth, and a nonjudgmental attitude; and avoiding unconsciously reinforcing maladaptive behaviors.	An integrated, supportive, and stable milieu will help Susan make progress in her own efforts to gain ego integrity and stability.

Evaluation: Susan uses "alters" less and begins taking more personal responsibility for her behaviors.

- Monitor the client's pace in uncovering memories. Moving too fast may be seen behaviorally in attempts at self-mutilation, symptoms of psychosis, and increased incidences of dissociation
- Assist the client in learning "grounding" techniques (see Nursing Care Plan 21-1). These concrete techniques bring the client into the present and remind him or her that he or she is a safe adult.
- Help the client to identify times when strong emotions begin to be overwhelming. Journaling antecedent events and developing a concrete plan for managing emotions are helpful strategies.
- Assist the client in planning for discharge from the hospital. A measure that the client can use is compiling a list of people who can be contacted for support as needed. These people may include family members, friends, members of 12-step groups, and people staffing "hotlines." Lists should be posted where the client can see them, reminding him or her of options and lending a sense of control. Identifying safe places and comforting activities when feeling stressed will help the client continue to gain a feeling of self-responsibility and control (Benham, 1995). See Therapeutic Communication 21-1 and Implications for Nursing Practice 21-1.

The client may practice new coping skills while in the hospital. These include calling a friend to talk about feelings of anxiety, focusing on topics that decrease anxiety; using reassuring self-talk; engaging in moderate exercise; and focusing on a favorite activity such as painting, reading, singing, or watching a relaxing video (Benham, 1995).

Evaluation

Just as illness is a matter of degree, so too is recovery. Generally, a client recovering from a dissociative disorder slowly will begin to trust people worth trusting. He or she will have appropriate personal boundaries and begin to trust feelings. The client will begin to try new activities with less fear and will be able to use new coping strategies to deal with anxiety. The client will sleep better at night and will have times of contentment during the day.

▼ Reflection and Critical Thinking Questions

Now that you have completed this chapter, consider Clinical Example 21-1 and the related nursing care presented in Nursing Care Plan 21-1. Answer the following questions.

1. Hearing stories of physical and sexual abuse is stressful. What feelings did Susan's situation evoke in you?
2. What feelings do you have regarding those who abuse children? Is child abuse a societal or individual issue?
3. What purposes did the symptoms of depersonalization serve for Susan?

THERAPEUTIC COMMUNICATION 21-1
The Client With a Dissociative Disorder

Jennifer, 24 years old, is experiencing an episode in which she does not know where she is or what is going on around her. The nurse is attempting to calm her down and orient her.

Ineffective Communication	Effective Communication

Ineffective Communication

Jennifer: (*Crying and pacing*) Help me, help me!

Nurse: (*Looks frustrated*) Tell me what's wrong. How can I help?

Jennifer: I'm afraid. I don't know what to do. Who are you?

Nurse: I'm the nurse. It's time for you to take your medications. (*Gives orders without providing an explanation*)

Jennifer: Why do I need medication? I'm afraid you're trying to hurt me!

Nurse: You'll feel better if you cooperate. Please just take the medicine. (*Dismisses the client's feelings*)

Jennifer: (*Begins to sob uncontrollably*)

Effective Communication

Jennifer: (*Crying and pacing*) Help me, help me!

Nurse: (*Remaining calm*) Tell me what's wrong. How can I help?

Jennifer: I'm afraid. I don't know what to do. Who are you?

Nurse: I'm the nurse. My name is Mary. I will be giving your medications today and helping you if you have a crisis or feel unsafe. (*Provides enough specific directions to orient to the "here and now"*)

Jennifer: What do I do now?

Nurse: A very important part of therapy is attending group. You should go to your groups according to your program schedule. (*Reinforces the schedule of the unit to convey structure and safety and to promote therapeutic involvement*)

Jennifer: What if I don't remember what to do or where I am?

Nurse: I am here to help you know what to do next and to remind you where you are even if I have to tell you over and over again. Just ask me until your thoughts are clear enough for you to remember.

Reflection and Critical Thinking

- What assumptions did the first nurse make that led the interaction between her and Jennifer to go so poorly?
- Why is it important to orient the client with a dissociative disorder to the here and now?
- How can reinforcing a schedule and explaining the purpose of interventions help to ease dissociative symptoms?

4. Before your work in psychiatric nursing, what did you believe about DID (formerly called multiple personality disorder)? Were Susan's symptoms similar to, or different from, those that you would have expected to see with this disorder?

▼ CHAPTER SUMMARY

- Dissociative disorders are thought by some scholars to be caused by trauma. The individual attempts to deal with this trauma by escaping into the mind. Behaviors of the person, however, are dysfunctional.
- Types of dissociative disorders include depersonaliza-

tion disorder, dissociative amnesia, dissociative fugue, and dissociative identity disorder (DID, formerly called multiple personality disorder). The most severe of the dissociative disorders is DID.

- The nurse should examine cultural considerations when diagnosing a dissociative disorder. He or she also should explore group and religious norms and the person's degree of functioning.
- Treatment modalities for dissociative disorders may include individual and group therapy, art therapy, and milieu management.
- The nursing assessment for DID should include detailed questions about the client's family history and the client's present level of functioning. The nurse must consider the total client picture because many

The Client With a Personality Disorder

JUDITH GREENE

▼ KEY TERMS

Personality—The totality of a person's unique biopsychosocial characteristics that consistently influences his or her inner experience and behavior across the life span.

Personality disorder—A collection of

personality traits that have become fixed and rigid to the point that they impair the affected client's functioning and cause distress; this disorder also can be considered a lifelong pattern of behavior that affects many

areas of the client's life, causes problems, and is not produced by another disorder or illness.

Splitting—The perception of people and life experience in terms of "all good" or "all bad" categories.

▼ LEARNING OBJECTIVES

On completion of this chapter, you should be able to accomplish the following:

- Define *personality disorder*.
- Discuss the various etiological theories of the development of personality disorders.
- Explain the prognosis of personality disorders.
- Identify the types of personality disorders and their differentiating characteristics.
- Describe the treatment options available for clients with personality disorders.
- Apply the nursing process to the care of a person with a personality disorder.

▼ Clinical Example 22-1

Margaret is a 22-year-old woman whose parents bring her to therapy. They have become concerned that Margaret has no friends or social life whatsoever and has become increasingly isolated. The nurse performing the interview notes that Margaret has a flat affect and seems cold and detached. She states she has no interest in forming friendships and would prefer to be alone. When asked about social relationships, Margaret states she has never had a boyfriend and can't understand why this is of interest to anyone. Margaret does not have a job and spends most of her time in her room, sewing needlepoint pillows.

When the nurse asks the client what she hopes to get from therapy, Margaret states she is afraid of people and

possibly could see a benefit to therapy if she was less afraid of others.

This chapter discusses personality disorders. As you read it, consider the case of Margaret in Clinical Example 22-1. How do her history and signs and symptoms relate to this group of disorders? You will learn more about the progression of Margaret's care in Nursing Care Plan 22-1. You also will have the opportunity to apply your understanding of this client and others with personality disorders in the Reflection and Critical Thinking Questions at the end of this chapter.

PERSONALITY DISORDERS

Personality may be defined as the totality of a person's unique biopsychosocial characteristics that consistently influences his or her inner experience and behavior across the life span. Personality is as essential to self-identity as is physical appearance. It may even be considered the psychological equivalent of physical appearance, as neither changes easily nor quickly (Greene, 1997).

Several theorists have explained the processes determining formation of human personality. Freudian, Ericksonian, and Sullivanian theories of personality development generally emphasize the importance of nurturance, while biogenetic hypotheses and theories emphasize the importance of gene transmission in the formation of personality. Social learning and cognitive behavioral theorists assert that personality characteristics are acquired through various cognitive processes interacting with the environment (Johnson, 1994). When personality development goes awry for whatever reason, clinical conditions currently referred to as personality disorders can occur.

Personality disorder can be defined as a collection of personality traits that have become fixed and rigid to the point that the person experiences inner distress and behavioral dysfunction. A personality disorder also can be considered a lifelong pattern of behavior that affects many areas of the person's life, causes problems, and is not produced by another disorder or illness (American Psychiatric Association [APA], 2000; Morrison, 1995). Another definition of personality disorder is "an enduring pattern of inner experience and behavior that deviates markedly from the expectations of the individual's culture" (APA, 2000).

Personality disorders are considered serious psychiatric conditions because of their associated symptoms. Their seriousness is underscored by the fact that they increase the risk of developing comorbid psychiatric disorders such as major depression, anxiety disorder, and substance abuse (APA, 2000; Marinangeli et al., 2000; Rettew, 2000; U.S. Public Health Service, 1999). Information is limited about the incidence and prevalence of personality disorders because people with them often do not seek help from professionals. In addition, because diagnostic criteria for personality disorders have changed frequently, their actual incidence and prevalence remains unverifiable (Maxmen, 1995; Ballas, 2001). Because personality disorders often occur with other major psychiatric disorders, however, estimates are that at least 10% to 25% of adults have some form of personality disorder (Centers for Disease Control and Prevention [CDC], 1998).

Etiology

Little information is available or verifiable about what actually causes personality disorders despite several theories regarding personality development. In fact, some support the position that what the *DSM-IV-TR (Diagnostic and Statistical Manual of Mental Disorders,* 4th edition, text revision) refers to as "personality disorders" actually represent variants of normal personality structure rather than disease processes (Widiger & Costa, 1994). Contrary to this position, others claim that psychosocial factors such as abuse, neglect, trauma, inadequate parenting, or a combination of these factors produce personality disorders (Carter, Peter, Mulder, & Luty, 2001; Caspi, 2000; Parker et al., 1999; Reich & Zanarini, 2001). Still others assert that nature, not nurture, is responsible for producing personality disorders. For example, support is growing for the

position that personality disorders in both children and adults have a substantial genetic component (Coolidge, Thede, & Jang, 2001). Finally, there are those who think that the truth probably lies somewhere in the middle and support the idea that a combination of psychosocial and biological factors are responsible for the formation of personality itself and personality disorders (Hamer, Greenberg, Sabol, & Murphy, 1999; Ballas, 2001).

Signs and Symptoms and Diagnostic Criteria

The *DSM-IV-TR,* which involves a multiaxial assessment, lists personality disorders on Axis II. Axis II is used to report personality disorders to ensure that healthcare providers will not overlook their treatment if overshadowed by the more pronounced symptoms of Axis I disorders (APA, 2000).

According to the *DSM-IV-TR,* personality disorders manifest symptomatologically in two or more of the following areas:

- Cognition—ways of perceiving and assigning meaning to self, others, and events
- Affectivity—the range, intensity, and appropriateness of emotionality
- Interpersonal behavior
- Impulse control (APA, 2000)

Additionally, the behavior of clients with personality disorders is enduring and inflexible and pervades a wide range of personal and social contexts. Furthermore, it can be traced to the affected person's adolescence or early adulthood. According to the *DSM-IV-TR,* for a personality disorder to exist, the enduring personality pattern cannot be better explained by another psychiatric disorder, substance abuse, intoxication, or a medical condition such as head trauma (APA, 2000).

The *DSM-IV-TR* groups 10 specific personality disorders into three clusters according to descriptive similarities (APA, 2000). *Cluster A,* which includes paranoid, schizoid, and schizotypal personality disorders, represents people whose behavior is odd or eccentric. *Cluster B* includes antisocial, borderline, histrionic, and narcissistic personality disorders; people with these disorders often appear dramatic, emotional, or erratic. *Cluster C,* including avoidant, dependent, and obsessive-compulsive personality disorders, represents people with anxious or fearful behavior.

CLUSTER A PERSONALITY DISORDERS

Clients with Cluster A personality disorders manifest signs and symptoms associated with the more adaptive end of the schizophrenic spectrum (Maxmen, 1995). In addition to appearing odd or eccentric, those affected

➡️ *Prevalence*

Varies according to disorder—common range is 11% to 23%

General Personality Disorder

- Client shows an enduring pattern of inner experience and behavior that deviates markedly from cultural expectations. This pattern is manifested in two (or more) of the following areas:
  - Cognition
  - Affectivity
  - Interpersonal functioning
  - Impulse control
- The enduring pattern is inflexible and pervasive across a broad range of personal and social situations.
- The enduring pattern leads to clinically significant distress or impairs social, work, or other important areas of functioning.
- The pattern is stable and long lasting, and its onset can be traced back at least to early adulthood.
- The enduring pattern is not better accounted for as a manifestation or consequence of another mental disorder.
- It is not from the direct physiological effects of a substance or general medial condition (e.g., head trauma).

Schizotypal Personality Disorder

- Client shows a pervasive pattern of social and interpersonal deficits marked by acute discomfort with, and reduced capacity for, close relationships as well as by cognitive or perceptual distortions and eccentricities of behavior. These findings begin by early adulthood in various contexts, as indicated by five (or more) of the following:
  - Ideas of reference (excluding delusions of reference)
  - Odd beliefs or magical thinking that influences behavior and is inconsistent with subcultural norms (e.g., superstitiousness, belief in clairvoyance; in children and adolescents, bizarre fantasies or preoccupations)
  - Odd thinking and speech
  - Unusual perceptual experiences, including bodily illusions
  - Suspiciousness or paranoid ideation
  - Inappropriate or constricted affect
  - Odd, eccentric, or peculiar behavior or appearance
  - Few close friends or confidants other than first-degree relatives
  - Excessive social anxiety that does not diminish with familiarity and is usually associated with paranoid fears rather than negative self-judgments

Paranoid Personality Disorder

- By early adulthood, client shows pervasive distrust and suspiciousness of others, interpreting their motives as malevolent, in several contexts, as indicated by at least four of the following:
  - Suspicion, without sufficient basis, that others are exploiting, harming, or deceiving him or her
  - Preoccupation with unjustified doubts about the loyalty or trustworthiness of friends or associates
  - Reluctance to confide in others because of unwarranted fear that they will maliciously use the information against him or her
  - Reading of hidden demeaning or threatening meanings into benign remarks or events
  - Persistent grudges
  - Perceived attacks on character or reputation that are not apparent to others and angry reactions or counterattacks
  - Recurrent suspicions, without justification, about fidelity of spouse or partner
- The disorder does not occur exclusively during schizophrenia, a mood disorder with psychotic features, or another psychotic disorder. It is not the result of direct physiological effects from a general medical condition.

Schizoid Personality Disorder

- Client is pervasively detached from social relationships and has a restricted range of emotional expression in interpersonal settings. These findings begin by early adulthood and are seen in various contexts, as indicated by four (or more) of the following:
  - No desire for or enjoyment of close relationships (including family)
  - Consistent selection of solitary activities
  - Little, if any, interest in sexual experiences with others
  - Pleasure in few, if any, activities
  - No close friends or confidants other than first-degree relatives
  - Indifference to praise or criticism
  - Emotional coldness, detachment, or flattened affectivity
- The condition does not occur exclusively during schizophrenia, a mood disorder with psychotic features, another psychotic disorder, or a pervasive developmental disorder. It is not from the direct physiological effects of a general medical condition.

(continued)

- The condition does not occur exclusively during schizophrenia, a mood disorder with psychotic features, another psychotic disorder, or a pervasive developmental disorder.

Antisocial Personality Disorder
- Since 15 years of age, client shows a pervasive pattern of disregard for and violation of the rights of others, as indicated by three (or more) of the following:
  - Failure to conform to social norms with respect to lawful behaviors, as indicated by repeatedly performing acts that are grounds for arrest
  - Deceitfulness, as indicated by repeated lying, use of aliases, or conning others for personal profit or pleasure
  - Impulsivity or failure to plan ahead
  - Irritability and aggressiveness, as indicated by repeated physical fights or assaults
  - Reckless disregard for safety of self or others
  - Consistent irresponsibility, as indicated by repeated failure to sustain consistent work behavior or honor financial obligations
  - Lack of remorse, as indicated by being indifferent to or rationalizing having hurt, mistreated, or stolen from others
- Client is at least 18 years of age.
- Client showed evidence of conduct disorder before 15 years of age.
- Antisocial behavior does not occur exclusively during schizophrenia or a manic episode.

Borderline Personality Disorder
By early adulthood, client shows a pervasive pattern of instability in interpersonal relationships, self-image, and affect and marked impulsivity in several contexts, as indicated by five (or more) of the following:
- Frantic efforts to avoid real or imagined abandonment
- Unstable and intense interpersonal relationships characterized by alternating extremes of idealization and devaluation
- Identity disturbance (markedly and persistently unstable self-image or sense of self)
- Impulsivity in at least two potentially self-damaging areas (e.g., spending, sex, substance abuse)
- Recurrent suicidal behavior, gestures, or threats, or self-mutilation
- Affective instability from a marked reactivity of mood (intense episodic dysphoria, irritability, or anxiety usually lasting a few hours and only rarely more than a few days)
- Chronic feelings of emptiness

Histrionic Personality Disorder
By early adulthood, client shows a pervasive pattern of excessive emotionality and attention seeking in several contexts, as indicated by five (or more) of the following:
- Discomfort in situations in which he or she is not the center of attention
- Inappropriate sexually seductive or provocative behavior toward others
- Rapidly shifting and shallow expression of emotions
- Use of physical appearance to draw attention to self
- Style of speech that is excessively impressionistic and lacking in detail
- Self-dramatization, theatricality, and exaggerated expression of emotion
- Suggestibility (easily influenced by others or circumstances)
- Overvaluation of relationships (considers them more intimate than they are)

Narcissistic Personality Disorder
By early adulthood, client shows a pervasive pattern of grandiosity (in fantasy or behavior), need for admiration, and lack of empathy in several contexts, as indicated by five (or more) of the following:
- A grandiose sense of self-importance
- Preoccupation with fantasies of unlimited success, power, brilliance, beauty, or ideal love
- Belief that he or she is "special" and can be understood by, or should associate with, only other special or high-status people or places
- Desire for excessive admiration
- A sense of entitlement (unreasonable expectations of favorable treatment or automatic compliance with his or her expectations)
- Interpersonal exploitation (takes advantage of others to achieve his or her own ends)
- Lack of empathy
- Arrogant, haughty behaviors or attitudes

Avoidant Personality Disorder
By early adulthood, client shows a pervasive pattern of social inhibition, feelings of inadequacy, and hypersensitivity to negative evaluation in several contexts, as indicated by four (or more) of the following:
- Avoidance of occupational activities that involve significant interpersonal contact, because of fears of criticism, disapproval, or rejection
- Unwillingness to get involved with people unless certain of being liked
- Restraint within intimate relationships because of the fear of being shamed or ridiculed
- Preoccupation with being criticized or rejected in social situations

(continued)

Personality Disorders Information Map *(Continued)*

- Inappropriate, intense anger or difficulty controlling anger (e.g., frequent displays of temper, recurrent fights)
- Transient, stress-related paranoid ideation or severe dissociative symptoms

Obsessive-Compulsive Personality Disorder

By early adulthood, client has a pervasive pattern of preoccupation with orderliness, perfectionism, and mental and interpersonal control, at the expense of flexibility, openness, and efficiency, in several contexts, as indicated by four (or more) of the following:

- Preoccupation with details, rules, lists, order, organization, or schedules to the extent that the major point of the activity is lost
- Perfectionism that interferes with task completion (e.g., cannot complete a project because his or her own overly strict standards are not met)
- Excessive devotion to work and productivity to the exclusion of leisure activities and friendships (not accounted for by obvious economic necessity)
- Overconscientiousness, scrupulousity, and inflexibility about matters of morality, ethics, or values (not accounted for by cultural or religious identification)
- Inability to discard worn-out or worthless objects even when they have no sentimental value
- Reluctance to delegate tasks or to work with others unless they submit to exactly his or her way of doing things
- A miserly spending style toward both self and others (viewing money as something to hoard for future catastrophes)
- Rigidity and stubbornness

- Inhibition in new interpersonal situations because of feelings of inadequacy
- View of self as socially inept, personally unappealing, or inferior to others
- Unusual reluctance to take personal risks or to engage in any new activities because they may prove embarrassing

Dependent Personality Disorder

By early adulthood, client has a pervasive and excessive need to be taken care of that leads to submissive and clinging behavior and fears of separation in several contexts, as indicated by five (or more) of the following:

- Difficulty making everyday decisions without excessive advice and reassurance from others
- Need for others to assume responsibility for most major areas of his or her life
- Difficulty expressing disagreement with others because of fear of loss of support or approval (Does not include realistic fears of retribution)
- Difficulty initiating projects or doing things on his or her own (because of a lack of self-confidence in judgment or abilities rather than a lack of motivation or energy)
- Going to excessive lengths to obtain nurturance and support from others, to the point of volunteering to do things that are unpleasant
- Discomfort or helplessness when alone because of exaggerated fears of being unable to care for himself or herself
- Urgent seeking of another relationship as a source of care and support when a close relationship ends
- Unrealistic preoccupation with fears of being left to take care of himself or herself

➡ Want to Know More?

Avoidant Personality Group Homepage
http://www.geocities.com/HotSprings/3764/

Borderline Personality Disorder Research Foundation
The Rockefeller University
1230 York Ave., Box 36
New York, NY 10021
Phone: 212-327-7344
http://www.borderlineresearch.org/

Borderline Personality Disorder Sanctuary
http://www.mhsanctuary.com/borderline/

Cognitive Therapy for Personality Disorders
http://www.mhsource.com/pt/p960241.html

With permission from American Psychiatric Association. (2000). Diagnostic and Statistical Manual of Mental Disorders (4th ed., text revision). Washington, DC: Author.

with these disorders often seem cold, withdrawn, suspicious, and irrational.

Paranoid Personality Disorder

People with *paranoid personality disorder* are suspicious and quick to take offense and usually cannot acknowledge their own negative feelings toward others. However, they often project these negative feelings onto others. They have few friends and may project hidden meaning into innocent remarks. They may be litigious and guarded, and they may bear grudges for imagined insults or slights. Marital or sexual difficulties are common and often involve issues related to fidelity. People with paranoid personality disorder are quick to react with anger and counterattack in response to imagined character or reputation attacks. Despite their tendency to interpret the actions of others as deliberately threatening or demeaning, these people do not lose contact with reality (APA, 2000; Maxmen, 1995).

Schizoid Personality Disorder

Clients with *schizoid personality disorder* show an indifference to social relationships, a flattened affectivity, and a cold, unsociable, seclusive demeanor. They take pleasure in few, if any, activities. People with this disorder usually never marry, have little interest in exploring their sexuality, and frequently live as adult children with their parents or other first-degree relatives. Because they are lifelong loners, they often succeed at solitary jobs others would find intolerable (APA, 2000; Frey, 1999; Maxmen, 1995; Ballas, 2001).

Schizotypal Personality Disorder

People with *schizotypal personality disorder* display an enduring and pervasive pattern of social and interpersonal deficits marked by extreme discomfort with and intolerance for close relationships. They also have disturbed thought patterns and manifest odd behavior, speech, and appearance. They may be suspicious and display ideas of reference without delusions of reference. Additionally, they may be superstitious and believe that they are capable of unusual forms of communication such as telepathy and clairvoyance. Schizotypal clients have a constricted or otherwise inappropriate affect and lack friends or confidantes other than first-degree relatives. They experience great social anxiety that does not diminish with familiarity and that seems to be associated with paranoid fearfulness rather than issues of low self-esteem (APA, 2000; Frey, 1999; Ballas, 2001; Morrison, 1995).

CLUSTER B PERSONALITY DISORDERS

Clients with Cluster B disorders display dramatic, emotional, and attention-seeking behaviors. They also can display labile and shallow moods. They tend to become involved in all kinds of intense interpersonal conflicts during their lifetimes.

Antisocial Personality Disorder

Antisocial personality disorder also refers to *psychopathic personality* and *sociopathic personality*. Those with this disorder display aggressive, irresponsible behavior that often leads to conflicts with society and subsequent involvement in the criminal justice system. People with this disorder commonly display behaviors such as fighting, lying, stealing, abusing children and spouses, abusing substances, and participating in confidence schemes. These people, while often superficially charming, lack genuine warmth (APA, 2000; Herpertz and Henning, 1997; Maxmen, 1995).

While the diagnosis of antisocial personality disorder is limited to clients older than 18 years of age, the person also must have had a history of conduct disorder before 17 years of age (APA, 2000). Antisocial personality disorder has been difficult to diagnose and treat (Frey, 1999). A recent study, however, may have shed some light on diagnosing clients with this disorder. This study found that people with antisocial personality disorder have less gray matter in the prefrontal cortex, the area of the brain that acts to control and regulate behavior (Raine, 2000). Further research in this area may help to resolve an ongoing debate concerning whether this disorder represents a true psychiatric disorder or a legal problem (Kaylor, 1999).

Borderline Personality Disorder

By early adulthood, clients with *borderline personality disorder* evidence instability in mood, impulse control, and interpersonal relationships. Their overall behavior is unpredictable and erratic. They tend to view people, circumstances, and their overall life experience in terms of extremes—either all good or all bad. This tendency is referred to as **splitting** (APA, 2000; Koerner and Linehan, 1996).

Clients with borderline personality disorder view themselves as victims and assume little responsibility for themselves or their problems. They become intensely and inappropriately angry if they believe others are ignoring them. They may impulsively try to harm or mutilate themselves. These actions are usually manifestations of extreme anger, cries for help, or efforts to numb themselves to emotional discomfort (Maxmen, 1995). There also may be marked and persistent identity disturbance regarding self-image, sexual orientation, long-term goals, and career choices (APA, 2000; Koenigsberg, 1995). Additionally, they display extreme affective instability and emotional reactivity in the form of intense dysphoria, irritability, anxiety, or all of these. These episodes usually last just a few hours and rarely more than just 1 day (APA, 2000; Greene, 1997).

Histrionic Personality Disorder

Clients with *histrionic personality disorder* have a long-standing pattern of excessive emotionality and attention-seeking behaviors. In fact, clients with this disorder strive to be at center stage by focusing exclusively on their own desires and interests during conversations with others. They also often dress provocatively and express themselves in dramatic and highly emotional ways to gain attention. Despite their theatricality, their speech style is superficial and lacking in detail.

Because of feelings of insecurity, people with this disorder often engage in seductive behaviors to gain approval. Their extreme dependence on the favor of others may result in their moods appearing shallow or excessively reactive to their surroundings. Additionally, they can be naïve, gullible, and easily influenced, while simultaneously given to temper tantrums as a result of low tolerance for frustration. Hence, people with this disorder often appear inconsistent and unpredictable. They usually blame failure or disappointment on others and tend to suppress or repress affect-laden material without acquiring any insight about their own inner experience and behavior (APA, 2000; Frey, 1999; Greene, 1997; Maxmen, 1995; Ballas, 2001).

Narcissistic Personality Disorder

Clients with *narcissistic personality disorder* have a lifelong pattern of self-centeredness, self-absorption, inability to empathize with others, grandiosity, and extreme desire for the admiration of others. They feel that they are unusually special and often exaggerate their accomplishments to appear more important than they actually are. Despite their grandiose ideas, these clients have fragile self-esteems and are overly sensitive to what others think or say about them. As sensitive as they are to the opinions of others, they are particularly insensitive to the needs or feelings of others and lack empathy. In fact, they often feel entitled to special treatment from others; when it is denied, these clients can become demanding, angry, and offended (APA, 2000; Frey, 1999; Greene, 1997; Ballas, 2001). Additionally, narcissists can be haughty, arrogant, and capable of taking advantage of others to achieve their own ends. They also are often intensely envious of others and believe others are envious of them (APA, 2000).

The diagnosis of narcissistic personality disorder is applied to adults only. All children and adolescents are naturally narcissistic to a degree. Hence, these characteristics in a child or adolescent do not necessarily portend the existence of this disorder in adulthood (Maxmen, 1995).

CLUSTER C PERSONALITY DISORDERS

Clients with Cluster C personality disorders are often anxious, tense, and overcontrolled. These disorders may occur with Axis I anxiety disorders and require effort to distinguish between the two axes (Maxmen, 1995; Morrison, 1995; Rettew, 2000).

Avoidant Personality Disorder

People with *avoidant personality disorder* have a pattern of social discomfort, timidity, and fear of negative evaluation beginning in early adulthood. They are preoccupied with what they perceive as their own shortcomings and will risk forming relationships with others only if they believe acceptance is guaranteed (APA, 2000; Morrison, 1995). While most clients with avoidant personality also may be diagnosed with social phobia, most clients with social phobia do not qualify for the diagnosis of avoidant personality disorder (Morrison, 1995). That is, avoidant personality disorder pervades all social situations, while social phobia is confined to specific situations (eg, speaking or eating in public).

People with this disorder often view themselves as unattractive and inferior to others and are often socially inept. Consequently, they usually avoid occupations that have social demands. They are reluctant to take risks or try new activities for fear of being embarrassed, shamed, or ridiculed (APA, 2000).

Dependent Personality Disorder

Clients with *dependent personality disorder* have a pervasive and excessive need to be taken care of, leading to submissive and clinging behavior and fears of separation (APA, 2000). Additionally, they need the approval of others to such an extent that they have tremendous difficulty making independent decisions or starting projects. In effect, they do not trust their own ability to make decisions and often believe that others have better ideas or judgment than they do. People with dependent personality disorder fear abandonment, feel helpless when alone, and are miserable when relationships end. Consequently, they urgently seek another relationship to provide them with care and support if a relationship ends. They may go to great lengths, even suffering abuse, to stay in a relationship. Because they feel an intense need to be taken care of, people with this disorder become extremely anxious if placed in a position of authority. As a result of their intense need for reassurance, they often have occupational difficulties (Maxmen, 1995; Ballas, 2001; Morrison, 1995).

Obsessive-Compulsive Personality Disorder

Perfectionism, rigidity, controlling behavior, and extreme orderliness characterize people with *obsessive-compulsive personality disorder* (APA, 2000). These lifelong traits exist at the expense of efficiency, flexibility, and candor (Maxmen, 1995). Their rigid perfectionism often results in indecisiveness, preoccupation with detail, and an insistence that others do things their way. Thus, they may have difficulty being effective in their occupational and social roles. Additionally, people with obsessive-compulsive personality disorder may have difficulty expressing affection and may appear depressed. In fact, they are at risk to develop clinical depression (Maxmen, 1995).

Resisting authority and insisting that they and they alone are right are common behavioral patterns in people with obsessive-compulsive personality disorder. Hoarding worthless objects, displaying stinginess, working excessively, showing stubbornness, and moralizing also occur to a high degree in people with this disorder (Greene,

1997). Unlike Axis I obsessive-compulsive disorder (see Chap. 18), clients with obsessive-compulsive personality disorder do not have actual obsessions or compulsions (Maxmen, 1995). Instead, these clients are involved in an inner struggle to gain self-control through the control of others and the environment.

Comorbidities and Dual Diagnoses

Persons with personality disorders are at risk for Axis I disorders such as major depression with or without psychotic features, anxiety disorders, and suicide crises. It appears that clients with all types of personality disorders may be at risk for substance abuse and dependence (Ballas, 2001). While clients with obsessive-compulsive and dependent personality disorders are believed to be at risk for depression, it is important to note that persons with narcissistic personality disorder can become depressed to the point of suicide crisis if their grandiosity is threatened (Greene, 1997; Maxmen, 1995).

Implications and Prognosis

Because little information is available about the actual prevalence and incidence of personality disorders, determining an accurate prognosis is difficult (Ghodse, 1995; Maxmen, 1995). Based on reported clinical observations, however, the following outcomes are believed to occur:

- Worsening of symptoms over time
- Improvement of symptoms over time
- Treatment dropout preventing further follow-up
- Treatment refusal causing an unknown variable in the study of this disorder (Morrison, 1995)

At one time the prognosis for all personality disorders was grim because these conditions were considered untreatable. Recent findings, however, suggest the opposite (Barber & Ellman, 1996; Koenigsberg, 1995; Perry, Banon, & Ianni, 1999; Strand & Benjamin, 1997). As clinicians become more optimistic about and skillful in treating these disorders, hopefully more complete and reliable information will become available regarding their prognoses.

Interdisciplinary Goals and Treatment

Clients with personality disorders are typically resistant to seeking psychiatric treatment. They seek help when they become acutely uncomfortable with themselves, when they develop an Axis I disorder, or when they are forced to seek treatment (eg, clients with antisocial personality disorder primarily).

While people with borderline personality disorder are believed to be the most frequent recipients of psychiatric care in both inpatient and outpatient settings, the other disorders are also represented in various treatment settings (Morrison, 1995; National Institute of Mental Health [NIMH], 2001). For example, clients with paranoid and schizoid personality disorders may find themselves pressured by their families to seek treatment because of their odd behavior (Ballas, 2001). Clients with schizotypal personality disorder may develop psychotic symptoms, requiring either inpatient or outpatient services. Many clients with antisocial, histrionic, dependent, and borderline personality disorders also require treatment for substance abuse (Ghodse, 1995).

Clients with personality disorders also present themselves regularly to healthcare settings for other reasons. For example, these clients often present to trauma or medical surgical services as a result of the untoward effects of substance abuse or impulse control difficulties, which have caused physical injury or other problems requiring treatment (U.S. Public Health Service, 1999).

Whatever the reason for seeking or being forced to seek treatment, clients with personality disorders, once considered untreatable, are now deemed treatable. Individual and family therapies using cognitive strategies have been found to be particularly helpful (Koenigsberg, 1995; Perry, Banon, & Ianni, 1999).

Goals of treatment vary because personality disorders manifest in different ways. Long-term restructuring of personality would require years of psychotherapy, which is prohibitively costly and may be unsuccessful. So treatment is often short term. Also, as stated previously, many clients with personality disorders do not seek treatment unless compelled to do so by a personal crisis, and they may terminate treatment quickly. Therefore, treatment frequently focuses on immediate problem solving, enhancement of coping skills, and improvement of social relationship skills. Increased tolerance of anxiety without resorting to maladaptive coping mechanisms would be a positive outcome. Other goals include increased self-awareness and amelioration of the more destructive personality traits. Refer to Table 22-1 for goals of treatment for specific disorders.

Pharmacologic agents such as antidepressants, lithium carbonate, or antipsychotic medication are sometimes used for certain clients; however, no single medication has been shown to have long-term benefits. Alcohol or drug abuse problems must be treated for therapy to progress. Brief hospitalization may be necessary during stressful periods or if suicide or other self-destructive behaviors are present.

INDIVIDUAL PSYCHOTHERAPY

Clients with personality disorders are likely to benefit from individual psychotherapy (Greene, 1997; Maxmen, 1995; Ballas, 2001). The client must be motivated to benefit from individual therapy, which may be insight oriented, supportive in nature, or oriented in cognitive-behavioral tech-

TABLE 22-1 ▼ Goals of Treatment for Specific Personality Disorders

PERSONALITY DISORDER	GOALS
Cluster A	
Paranoid	Solve immediate crisis or problem.
Schizoid	Solve immediate crisis or problem.
Schizotypal	Complete social skills training.
Cluster B	
Antisocial	Improve social relationships. Enhance insight into antisocial feelings and behaviors. If client is incarcerated, develop goals for life when released from custody.
Borderline	Prevent suicide. Function independently, maintain emotional balance, and engage in cognitive restructuring.
Histrionic	Prevent suicide. Gain insight into unrealistic expectations and fears.
Narcissistic	Develop a healthier sense of individuality. Recognize others as separate people. Improve coping mechanisms.
Cluster C	
Avoidant	Enhance social functioning. Solve immediate crisis or problem.
Dependent	Complete assertiveness training. Engage in cognitive restructuring.
Obsessive-compulsive	Experience specific symptom relief.

niques. Because of the complexities associated with clients who have personality disorders (and usually have comorbid issues), a combination of these approaches may be indicated, depending on the client's motivation, progress, and presenting symptoms. Through participation in individual therapy, affected clients gradually may develop insight into their problems and learn to acquire or generate emotional support and stability in more appropriate ways. Additionally, cognitive-behavioral therapy using rational-emotive techniques, behavioral contracting, thought stopping, positive coping statements, and covert rehearsal also may help clients with personality disorders make needed behavioral changes during the course of individual therapy (Frey, 1999; Greene, 1997; Ballas, 2001).

GROUP THERAPY

Group therapy that provides psychoeducational experiences and teaches assertiveness skills, positive coping skills, relaxation techniques, and nonchemical coping (ie, no alcohol, street drug, or prescription drug abuse) can benefit most clients with personality disorders, with perhaps the exception of paranoid personality disorder. Addition-

ally, group therapy can be useful to assist clients with borderline, avoidant, and dependent personality disorders to eventually recognize how their personality disorders interfere with their relating in social contexts (Frey, 1999). Group therapy also reduces social isolation, which affects many people who have personality disorders (Greene, 1997; Ballas, 2001).

FAMILY EDUCATION AND THERAPY

Clients with borderline, dependent, histrionic, and avoidant personality disorders may benefit from family treatment approaches (Greene, 1997; Maxmen, 1995). Family members and significant others can be involved in treatment with the written consent of clients. Given the nature of some of the personality disorders, affected clients may not consent to family involvement. In such cases, the use of a family systems theoretical framework during the course of individual therapy may be beneficial to decrease overinvolvement and fusion (Greene, 1997). When clients and their families or significant others agree to engage in family therapy sessions, progress in reducing overinvolvement, acting out, and inappropriate dependence is possible.

▼ Clinical Example 22-2

"I'm here to see you because my wife has threatened to divorce me if I don't do something" said John, 28 years old. His wife, Gloria, who accompanied him, made the appointment 2 weeks ago. John obviously resented this. As the session progressed, Gloria described what she experienced as selfishness and miserliness from John. She complained that John insists on exact schedules for meals and sleep and refuses to allow her to shop for groceries or other articles unless she agrees to do exactly as he instructs. She added that he refuses to allow her to throw away worthless objects such as sacks, old clothes, wrapping paper, or boxes and insists on keeping them stored in various places throughout their home. She also complained about a lack of affection from her husband.

John stated that Gloria is wasteful, scatterbrained, and disorganized, and he must keep close check over their finances because otherwise ". . . we'd go broke." He also complained that she is too emotional and sentimental.

John stopped coming to therapy after two sessions, claiming, "it ought to be obvious by now to any competent therapist that it is my wife, not me, who needs help." Gloria continued in individual therapy to address her decisional conflicts related to whether she would remain married to John. After about 6 months of therapeutic work, she decided to divorce John.

Initially, John behaved as though nothing had changed and stubbornly refused to accept any responsibility for failure of the marriage. He became more emotionally reactive when Gloria sought her share of their property and financial holdings. In addition to the stress of the divorce and property settlement, John was summoned into his boss' office to discuss his increasing difficulty in delegating work effectively. Employees under his supervision had also complained that he reserved all overtime work for himself, thereby increasing his paycheck at their expense. His boss stated clearly that he must make some changes in his relationships with his coworkers and employees, and in his overall work patterns.

John experienced the demand for change in both his personal and occupational lives to be overwhelming. As a result he became extremely depressed and sought psychiatric treatment. Previously, he had had periods of depression from which he recovered in a few days. He had never experienced, however, the depth of depression he felt on the day he presented for help. In fact, John was entertaining suicidal ideas and feeling hopeless and helpless about taking control of his life.

John received the following diagnoses:

- Axis I: Major depression, single episode, severe 296.23
- Axis II: Obsessive-compulsive personality disorder, severe 301.4
- Axis III: Deferred
- Axis IV: Separation with impending divorce and job stress
- Axis V: GAF = 40 to 50 present; past 70

John received individual psychotherapy using cognitive-behavioral techniques combined with 100 mg of sertraline (Zoloft) daily to treat his diagnosis of major depression. He was treated on an outpatient basis and readily contracted to refrain from self-harm. With the assistance of cognitive reframing, John could place the loss of his spouse and current job difficulties into perspective with what had been a fairly successful life. Because John had experienced significant and timely relief from what he had experienced as intense emotional pain, he decided to continue individual therapy even after he no longer required antidepressant therapy. He had gained self-awareness and insight and wanted to ensure as much as possible that he not repeat or fall back into his previous behavioral patterns. While John did not like change, he decided that change driven from within himself during therapy was much more to his liking than change driven from external sources.

From Barber and Ellman, 1996; Koenigsberg, 1995; Maxmen, 1995; Perry, Banon, and Ianni, 1999.

APPLICATION OF THE NURSING PROCESS TO A CLIENT WITH A PERSONALITY DISORDER

Assessment

Clients with personality disorders seldom seek psychiatric assistance unless they develop comorbid conditions (Maxmen, 1995; Ballas, 2001; Morrison, 1995). Therefore, assessing clients for personality disorders who present with symptoms of depression and other mood disturbances, anxiety, psychosis, substance abuse, or suicide crisis is important. The co-occurrence of personality disorders can complicate the treatment and course of Axis I diagnoses and other psychiatric syndromes (Ghodse, 1995; Maxmen, 1995; Shea, 1996; Wonderlich, Petersen, & Mitchell, 1997).

Whatever the reason for presenting to the healthcare system, clients with personality disorders can cause considerable difficulties for those who attempt to care for them. Consequently, others label them as complainers, drug seekers, grumps, or manipulators. In fact, they often trigger negative countertransference from their providers, or the displacement of negative feelings onto the client. To ensure that the nurse remains calm and objective while assessing the client with a personality disorder, self-monitoring is essential (Nehls, 2000). Monitoring oneself in terms of expressing concern and setting boundaries also has been reported to increase the effectiveness of therapeutic relationships with clients with personality disorders. By practicing self-monitoring, nurses found that they were more effective in relationships with clients who have personality disorders and, as a result, were more helpful over time (Nehls, 2000).

Nursing Diagnosis

Because of the high rate of comorbidity, nursing diagnoses pertaining to other applicable psychiatric disorders, such as affective disorders, anxiety disorders, substance abuse, and even schizophrenia, need to be addressed to ensure optimal care. The following list contains some nursing diagnoses that reflect behavioral targets of intervention in clients with personality disorders:

- **Noncompliance** related to personality disorder
- **Ineffective Coping** related to entrenched maladaptive personality traits
- **Risk for Suicide** secondary to psychiatric illness

Planning

Planning and implementing treatment plans for clients with personality disorders require a collaborative treatment team approach (Perry, Banon, & Ianni, 1999). As stated previously, those with personality disorders may resist treatment or accept it for only short periods. Nurses will need to consider this factor when developing a treatment plan and setting goals with the client and family.

Major goals for the care of clients with personality disorders include the following:

- The client will participate in therapy.
- The client will exhibit improved coping skills and tolerance of anxiety.
- The client will experience physical safety.

Implementation

While standard care plans address the treatment of clients with personality disorders, the nurse must individualize care plans to ensure the inclusion of comorbid issues. Ideally, the treatment plan synthesizes goals and approaches of all applicable psychiatric diagnoses. See Nursing Care Plan 22-1.

PROMOTING PARTICIPATION IN TREATMENT

The nurse helps clients develop trust in themselves, others, and the environment. He or she uses a straightforward, matter-of-fact approach while avoiding an overly warm approach. The nurse demonstrates punctuality, respect, and genuineness to the client. It is a good idea for the nurse to avoid interpreting the client's behavior; clients with personality disorders may experience interpretations as intru-

sive and controlling (Koenigsberg, 1995). The nurse uses open-ended questions to assist clients to focus on their own behavior and its consequences. It is also important for the nurse to be consistent and congruent with clients who have personality disorders; failure to do so may provoke increased manipulative and acting-out behaviors.

The nurse encourages clients to follow through with treatment for their disorder and for comorbid issues. He or she also must encourage adherence to medication regimens for comorbid diagnoses. The nurse, however, also should monitor the client closely for prescription drug abuse because clients with personality disorders are at risk for substance abuse and dependence (Ghodse, 1995; Ballas, 2001).

ENLISTING THE FAMILY IN THE TREATMENT PLAN

Family members of clients with personality disorders have endured heartache, worry, concern, and possibly abuse because of their loved one's mental illness. It is vitally important to include family members in the treatment plan, engage their help, acknowledge their experiences and efforts in coping with and caring for the client, provide support, and improve possible treatment outcomes for the client. See Client and Family Education Box 22-1 for specific teaching and intervention points.

IMPROVING COPING SKILLS

The nurse encourages clients to assume responsibility for their thoughts, feelings, and behaviors without blaming, shaming, or punishing them. A good approach is to present the idea that behavioral change is within the realm of possibility rather than to demand behavioral change (Maxmen, 1995). The nurse asks questions that assist clients to think through actual or intended behaviors. Doing so can help clients predict the consequences of their behaviors. One thing to keep in mind regarding client behavior is that the nurse should avoid requesting or recommending the use of psychotropics to control manipulative, acting-out behaviors because they are a function of personality, not brain chemistry (Maxmen, 1995).

In addition to implementing techniques that will improve coping skills, the nurse can suggest that clients learn how to manage stress better. Deep-breathing exercises, regular aerobic exercise, and progressive muscle relaxation are tools that the client can use to help dampen the negative effects of stress and possibly limit the need to use maladaptive coping strategies.

REDUCING INAPPROPRIATE BEHAVIORS

As stated previously, the client with a personality disorder may display negative behaviors that can interfere with therapy, just as they interfere with the client's interpersonal relationships. It may be necessary to tolerate a cer-

Nursing Care Plan 22-1

THE CLIENT WITH SCHIZOID PERSONALITY DISORDER

Margaret states that she would like to have a job but has been too uncomfortable around others to consider it. Because Margaret has identified her fear of others as a problem and decreasing that fear as a desired outcome of care, the nurse develops a care plan focusing on this problem. The nurse also understands that pressing Margaret into an ambitious plan for recovery will frighten her and likely lead to early termination of treatment. Helping Margaret overcome her fear of others will take substantial skill, care, and effort by both the nurse and Margaret.

Nursing Diagnosis: **Fear** related to personality disorder as evidenced by the statement, "I am afraid of other people"

Goal: Client's fear of others will diminish, and she will be able to better tolerate social situations.

Interventions	Rationales
Establish a therapeutic relationship. Proceed slowly and focus more on the technical aspects of treatment. Do not confront the client on her need for distance within the therapeutic relationship. Be consistent and stable.	This approach will help Margaret to feel the nurse's concern but will not press her beyond comfortable limits. Margaret's fear of others includes a fear of the nurse. The nurse can model safety and security in social relationships first within the context of the therapeutic relationship.
Explore client's fears about others and use cognitive restructuring techniques to address irrational thought patterns. Encourage client to examine the unrealistic nature of her fears and fantasies.	Thinking patterns predict behavior, and cognitive restructuring can replace faulty thinking patterns that lead to negative behavior patterns. Many clients with schizoid personality disorder have fears of unbearable dependency and fantasies about friendships. Examining these fears and fantasies is the first step toward being able to abandon them.
Encourage client to form one social relationship. Provide social skills training, as necessary. Consider group therapy as a forum for beginning social interaction.	Margaret may be able to experiment with social relationships within the safety of a group therapy setting. The therapist will need to protect Margaret from confrontation or criticism by other clients about her inability to participate or share in the group.
As therapy progresses, encourage client to find a job that will allow some social interaction but not so much that it will overwhelm the client.	Margaret may not be able to manage jobs that involve even a moderate degree of social interaction. She recognizes, however, that her fears are preventing her from working, and her desire to work can become an important motivating force to continue therapy.

Evaluation: It is probable that progress will be slow as Margaret first overcomes her fears enough to share her thoughts and feelings within the context of a therapeutic relationship. Working through her thought patterns and fears of social interaction may take many months, if not longer. Indicators that the interventions have been effective include the following:

• Continued participation in treatment
• Willingness to share meaningful personal information with the nurse therapist
• Greater participation in social relationships

tain amount of acting-out behavior, as the client may be testing if he or she can trust the therapeutic relationship. At times, however, the nurse will have to confront clients about their behaviors and set appropriate limits to move therapy forward.

CONFRONTING THE CLIENT

The nurse intervenes, using confrontation with clients who attempt to use manipulation or display other inappropriate behaviors. Doing so may assist the client to

a. Cluster A
b. Cluster B
c. Cluster C
d. Cluster D

5. Odd, eccentric, cold, withdrawn, and irrational describe the symptoms associated with which cluster of personality disorders?
   a. Cluster A
   b. Cluster B
   c. Cluster C
   d. Cluster D

6. Cluster B includes which of the following personality disorders?
   a. Dependent and obsessive-compulsive personality disorders
   b. Histrionic and narcissistic personality disorders
   c. Schizoid and schizotypal personality disorders
   d. Depersonalization disorder and dissociative identity disorder

7. Clients who display behaviors such as fighting, lying, and stealing and who were diagnosed with a conduct disorder before 17 years of age may have which of the following personality disorders?
   a. Borderline personality disorder
   b. Antisocial personality disorder
   c. Narcissistic personality disorder
   d. Histrionic personality disorder

8. Obsessive-compulsive personality disorder is characterized by
   a. Ritualistic, repetitive behavior such as hand washing
   b. Rigid, controlling, perfectionistic behaviors
   c. Fear of negative evaluation by others
   d. An intense need for reassurance

9. The nurse is interviewing a client diagnosed with schizoid personality disorder. She notes that the client has a flat affect and is not communicative. The nurse accurately attributes this behavior to which of the following causes?
   a. The comorbid major depression associated with schizoid personality disorder
   b. The hostility associated with schizoid personalities
   c. The severely limited social interest associated with schizoid personality disorder
   d. The paranoid delusions associated with schizoid personality disorder

10. A client with narcissistic personality disorder is terminating treatment soon. The nurse considers the plan of care effective when the client exhibits which of the following outcomes?
    a. The client can see others as individuals.
    b. The client can make social contacts.
    c. The client no longer expresses suicidal thoughts.
    d. The client agrees to participate in assertiveness training.

▼ REFERENCES AND SUGGESTED READINGS

*American Psychiatric Association. (2000). *Diagnostic and statistical manual of mental disorders* (4th ed., text rev.). Washington, DC: Author.

Andrews, J. A., Foster, S. L., Capaldi, D., & Hop, H. (2000). Adolescent and family predictors of physical aggression, communication, and satisfaction in young adult couples: A prospective analysis. *Journal of Consulting Clinical Psychology, 68*(2), 195–208.

*Ballas, C. (2001). Personality disorders. In *MEDLINEplus Medical Encyclopedia*. U.S. National Library of Medicine. [Online.] Available: *http://www.nlm.nih.gov/medlineplus/ency/article/000939.htm.*

*Barber, J. P., & Ellman, J. (1996). Advances in short-term dynamic psychotherapy. *Current Opinion in Psychiatry,* 188–192.

Bateman, A., & Fonagy, P. (1999). Effectiveness of partial hospitalization in the treatment of borderline personality disorder: A randomized controlled trial. *American Journal of Psychiatry, 156*(10), 1563–1569.

Boone, M. L., McNeil, D. W., Masia, C. L., Turk, C. L., Carter, L. E., & Ries, B. J., et al. (1999). Multi-modal comparisons of social phobia subtypes and avoidant personality disorder. *Journal of Anxiety Disorders, 13*(3), 271–292.

*Carter, J. J., Peter, R., Mulder, R. T., & Luty, S. E. (2001). The contribution of temperament, childhood neglect, and abuse to the development of personality dysfunction: A comparison of three models. *Journal of Personality Disorders, 15*(2), 123–135.

*Caspi, A. (2000). A study to investigate the effects of early childhood traits on the development of adult personality. *Journal of Personality and Social Psychology, 78,* 158–172.

*Centers for Disease Control and Prevention. (1998). Self-reported frequent mental distress among adults—United States 1993–1996. *Morbidity and Mortality Weekly Report, 47*(16), 326–331.

*Centers for Disease Control and Prevention. (1998). Self-reported frequent mental distress among adults—United States 1993–1996. *Morbidity and Mortality Weekly Report, 47*(16), 326–331.

*Coolidge, F. L., Thede, L. L., & Jang, K. L. (2001). Heritability of personality disorders in childhood: A preliminary investigation. *Journal of Personality Disorders, 15*(1), 33–40.

Farmer, C. M., O'Donnell, B. F., Niznikiewicz, M. A., Voglmaier, M. M., McCarley, R. W., & Shenton, M. E. (2000). Visual perception and working memory in schizotypal personality disorder. *American Journal of Psychiatry, 157*(5), 781–788.

*Frey, R. (1999). Personality disorders. In *Gale Encyclopedia of Medicine*. Gale Research in Association with The Gale Group and Looksmart. [On-line.] Available: *www.FindArticles.com.*

*Ghodse, H. (1995). Substance misuse and personality disorders. *Current Opinion in Psychiatry, 8,* 177–179.

*Hamer, D. H., Greenberg, B. D., Sabol, S. Z., & Murphy, D.

L. (1999). Role of serotonin transporter gene in temperament and character. *Journal of Personality Disorders, 13*(4), 312–328.

*Herpertz, S., & Henning, S. (1997). Psychopathy and antisocial syndromes. *Current Opinion in Psychiatry, 10,* 436–440.

*Johnson, S. (1994). *Character styles.* New York: W.W. Norton & Co.

*Kaylor, L. (1999). Antisocial personality disorder: Diagnostic, ethical, and treatment issues. *Issues in Mental Health Nursing, 20*(3), 247–258.

Klein, M. H. (1996). Current issues in neuroses and personality disorders. *Current Opinion in Psychiatry, 9,* 109–111.

*Koenigsberg, H. W. (1995). Psychotherapy of patients with borderline personality disorder. *Current Opinion in Psychiatry, 8,* 157–160.

*Koerner, K., & Linehan, M. M. (1996). Cognitive and interpersonal factors in borderline personality disorder. *Current Opinion in Psychiatry, 9,* 133–136.

Leichsenring, F. (1999). Splitting: An empirical study. *Bulletin Menninger Clinic, 63*(4), 520–537.

*Marinangeli, M. G., Butti, B., Scinto, A., Di Cicco, L., Petruzzi, C., & Daneluzzo, E., et al. (2000). Patterns of comorbidity among DSM-III-R personality disorders. *Psychopathology, 33*(2), 69–74.

*Maxmen, J. (1995). *Essential psychopathology and its treatment* (2nd ed., revised for *DSM-IV*). New York: W.W. Norton & Co.

*Morrison, J. (1995). *DSM-IV made easy: The clinician's guide to diagnosis.* New York: Guildford Press.

*National Institute of Mental Health. (2001, January). *Borderline personality disorder* (NIH Publication No. 01-4928).

*Nehls, N. (2000). Being a case manager for persons with borderline personality disorder: Perspectives of community mental health center clinicians. *Archives of Psychiatric Nursing, 14*(1), 12–18.

Nehls, N. (1999). Borderline personality disorder: The voice of patients. *Residential Nursing and Health, 22*(4), 285–293.

*Parker, G., Roy, K., Wilhelm, K., Mitchell, P., Austin, M., & Hadzi-Pavlovic, D. (1999). An exploration of links between early parenting experiences and personality disorder type and disordered personality functioning. *Journal of Personality Disorders, 13*(4), 361–374.

*Perry, J. C., Banon, E., & Ianni, F. (1999). Effectiveness of psychotherapy for personality disorders. *American Journal of Psychiatry, 156*(9), 1312–1321.

*Raine, A. (2000). Brain differences in antisocial personality disorder. *Archives of General Psychiatry, 57,* 119–129.

*Reich, D. B., & Zanarini, M. C. (2001). Developmental aspects of borderline personality disorder. *Harvard Review of Psychiatry, 9,* 294–301.

*Rettew, D. C. (2000). Avoidant personality disorder, generalized social phobia, and shyness: Putting the personality back into personality disorders. *Harvard Review of Psychiatry, 8,* 283–297.

*Shea, M. T. (1996). The role of personality in recurrent and chronic depression. *Current Opinion in Psychiatry, 9,* 117–120.

*Strand, J., & Benjamin, L. S. (1997). Resistance to change in individuals with personality disorder. *Current Opinion in Psychiatry, 10,* 132–135.

*U.S. Public Health Service. (1999). *Mental health: A report of the Surgeon General.* Washington, DC: National Institute of Mental Health.

Washington Associated Press. (2000, January 10). *Mental illness drives bodybuilders. Reporting on the addition of the diagnosis of muscle dysmorphia or body dysmorphic disorder, also referred to as bigorexia, to the next revision of the American Psychiatric Association's Diagnostic and Statistical Manual.*

*Widiger, T. A., & Costa, P. T., Jr. (1994). Personality and personality disorders. Personality and psychopathology [Special issue]. *Journal of Abnormal Psychology, 78*–91.

Wilkinson-Ryan, T., & Westen, D. (2000). Identity disturbance in borderline personality disorder: An empirical investigation. *American Journal of Psychiatry, 157*(4), 528–541.

*Wonderlich, S., Petersen, C., & Mitchell, J. (1997). Body image, psychiatric comorbidity, and psychological factors in the eating disorders. *Current Opinion in Psychiatry, 10,* 141–146.

Starred references are cited in text.

For additional information on this chapter, go to *http://connection.lww.com.*

Need more help? See Chapter 22 of the *Study Guide to Accompany Mohr: Johnson's Psychiatric-Mental Health Nursing,* 5th edition.

The Client With an Eating Disorder

SUSAN D. DECKER

▼ KEY TERMS

Amenorrhea—Absence of or abnormal cessation of menstruation.

Anorexia nervosa—A life-threatening eating disorder characterized by disturbed body image, emaciation, and intense fear of becoming obese.

Binge eating—Uncontrollable consumption of large amounts of food.

Binge eating disorder—An eating disorder characterized by recurrent episodes of binge eating with accompanying marked distress and impaired control over such behavior.

Bulimia nervosa—An eating disorder characterized by binge eating followed by purging.

Emotional reasoning—A cognitive distortion by which a person relies on his or her subjective emotions to determine reality.

Purging—Attempting to eliminate the body of excess calories; examples of purging methods include self-induced vomiting, use of laxatives, and excessive exercise.

▼ LEARNING OBJECTIVES

On completion of this chapter, you should be able to accomplish the following:

■ Describe the incidence of eating disorders and the populations most commonly affected by them.

■ Discuss possible etiologies of eating disorders.

■ Distinguish between anorexia nervosa and bulimia nervosa.

■ Describe the DSM-IV-TR diagnostic criteria for anorexia nervosa and bulimia nervosa.

■ Describe interdisciplinary goals and treatment of clients with eating disorders.

■ Apply the nursing process to the care of clients with eating disorders.

▼ Clinical Example 23-1

Jody, a 20-year-old cross-country runner, is in her junior year of college. At 5'8" and 117 lb, she is proud that her body fat is only 14%. She would like it to be even lower. The fastest runner on the team is very thin, and Jody runs extra miles every day to try to lose weight.

Jody's roommate, Mary, is worried about Jody because Jody weighs herself several times a day, eats very little, has stopped having menstrual periods, and is becoming irritable and withdrawn. After hearing Jody vomiting in the bathroom on several occasions,

Mary decides to confront Jody with her concerns. She tells Jody what she has observed and explains that she is concerned and wants to help. After responding with initial defensiveness, Jody admits that she is terrified that she will gain weight. She adds that she is experiencing low energy and leg pains.

After talking with Mary, Jody agrees to meet with Kate, the family nurse practitioner at the campus health center. Kate encourages Jody to discuss what is happening and listens carefully and objectively. Although she is honest and forthcoming about the behaviors that caused Mary such concern, Jody says that she doesn't really think she has a problem. Kate replies, "I hear what you're saying and I hope you are right, that this is not a problem. I am still very worried about what I have seen and heard. Just to be sure, I'd like to do a physical examination today and have you come back tomorrow so we can talk some more." Jody bursts into tears but agrees to Kate's plan.

This chapter discusses eating disorders. As you read the chapter, consider the case of Jody in Clinical Example 23-1. How does Jody's history and signs and symptoms relate to this group of disorders? How can Kate effectively address Jody's needs? You will learn more about the progression of Jody's care in Nursing Care Plan 23-1. You also will have the opportunity to apply your understanding of this client and others with eating disorders in the Reflection and Critical Thinking exercise at the end of this chapter.

EATING DISORDERS

Eating disorders affect more than 8 million people in the United States, with 86% of affected individuals developing the disorder before 21 years of age (Carter, Stewart, Dunn, & Fairburn, 1997). Two of the most prevalent eating disorders are anorexia nervosa and bulimia nervosa. **Anorexia nervosa** is a life-threatening condition characterized by disturbed body image, emaciation, and intense fear of becoming obese. **Bulimia nervosa** is a disorder characterized by uncontrollable consumption of large amounts of food (**binge eating**), followed by attempts to eliminate the body of the excess calories (**purging**).

Both anorexia and bulimia traditionally have been most commonly diagnosed in white, affluent, well-educated adolescent girls and young women. Incidences of both disorders, however, appear to be increasing among girls and women of color and in diverse socioeconomic groups (Rogers, Resnick, Mitchell, & Blum, 1997; Weiss, 1995; Williamson, 1998). The literature suggests that between 0.5% and 2% of young women meet the criteria for anorexia or bulimia (Marcus & Levine, 1998). Accurately determining the incidence of bulimia is particularly difficult because most affected clients carry out their binging and purging secretly, and the weights of these clients may be relatively normal.

Anorexia and bulimia are relatively uncommon in boys and men. Popular emphasis on fitness and the stringent requirements for weight in certain sports (eg, wrestling), however, have made males increasingly vulnerable (Olivardia et al., 1995).

Although commonly thought of as disorders of youth, manifestations of eating disorders do not necessarily disappear after young adulthood (Lyons, 1998; Perkins, Fritz, Barber, & Turner, 1997). A survey by the National Association of Anorexia Nervosa and Related Disorders indicates that among 1400 respondents with anorexia and bulimia, 5% were older than 60 years, 1.8% were older than 50 years, 2.7% were aged 40 to 49 years, and 20.5% were aged 30 to 39 years. The remaining respondents, 70%, were younger than 30 years (Brozan, 1983). The age of onset tends to be older for clients with bulimia than for clients with anorexia.

Many more individuals engage in less severe forms of disordered eating. Although this chapter focuses specifically on anorexia and bulimia, nurses should be aware of these other conditions. **Binge eating disorder** (BED), a new diagnostic category proposed for inclusion in the *Diagnostic and Statistical Manual of Mental Disorders,*

4th edition, text revision (*DSM-IV-TR*), affects approximately 2% of adults, with as many as 40% of these individuals being men (Marcus & Levine, 1998). This disorder is characterized by recurrent episodes of binge eating, with accompanying subjective and behavioral indicators of marked distress and impaired control over such eating (American Psychiatric Association [APA], 2000). Obesity, a state of excessive weight, is a condition with significant physical and psychologic overtones and ramifications. Many researchers view obesity as the result of compulsive eating behavior. It certainly is associated with morbidity and is not a healthy state (Research in Psychiatric-Mental Health Nursing 23-1).

Etiology

> At age 13, I was totally immersed in self-starvation. Weighing less than 60 pounds . . . all the time I kept running into people who hadn't seen me in awhile. They all looked shocked, they all said the same thing: "You're so thin! You don't look like yourself any more!" I thrived on their reactions. It's so reassuring to hear that I don't look like my supposed "self" anymore.
> —Annie Ciseaux, 1980

Why would a teenage girl determinedly starve herself when others view her as grotesquely thin? Why can't her parents make her eat? Why does a young woman ingest enormous amounts of food and furtively vomit?

Multiple theories have been proposed to explain the development of eating disorders. Eating disorders can be best understood in terms of a multifactorial etiology. Most experts agree that anorexia and bulimia develop from a complex interaction of individual, family, and sociocultural factors (Figure 23-1). A vulnerable personality, sociocultural emphasis on slimness, family functioning style, major life changes or stressors, dieting, genetic factors, and the onset of puberty all may contribute to the development of eating disorders. Exploring the different etiologic theories is the best way to gain an understanding of eating disorders.

BIOLOGIC THEORIES

Because of the complex nature of eating and the mechanisms behind it, researchers have had to address the effects of dieting on neurobiology and neuroendocrine systems as well as identify biologic abnormalities in clients with eating disorders. Because eating behavior can effect change in neurobiology and vice versa, teasing out cause from effect has been particularly problematic. Whether the biologic abnormalities seen in clients with eating disorders contribute to the disorders or are secondary to the dysregulation in the eating behavior remains unclear. It is clear, however, that several neurochemical disturbances are associated with both anorexia and bulimia.

Research in Psychiatric–Mental Health Nursing 23-1
THE PHENOMENON OF COMPULSIVE OVEREATING IN A SELECTED GROUP OF PROFESSIONAL WOMEN

Purpose: To explore the meaning of compulsive overeating, or binge eating, in the lives of adult professional women

Background: The reasons why many people eat without being hungry are complex. The may include lack of love, physical and emotional abuse, unexpressed rage, grief, anxiety and low self-esteem. Binge eating also has been associated with higher rates of certain psychiatric disorders, including depression, panic disorder, obsessive–compulsive disorder, and personality disorders.

Method and Sample: The population for this study consisted of six adult professional women who ranged in age from 25 to 55 years. The small sample size is consistent with qualitative research methodology. With the consent of the participants, the researcher conducted and audiotaped open-ended interviews with them.

Findings: Data analysis reveals seven themes that characterized the lived experience of the participants:

- Childhood perceptions of being overweight were interspersed with periods of thinness.
- Food choices during binging most frequently were chocolate, candy, doughnuts, cake, and foods high in fat and salt.
- Binge eating frequently was done secretly.

- All participants perceived a loss of control over their eating patterns.
- Reasons for overeating included stress, anxiety, loneliness, boredom, isolation, celebrations, and the desire to reward oneself.
- Emotional consequences of overeating were guilt, shame, denial, rationalization, and blaming.
- All participants engaged in compensatory behaviors such as exercising, dieting, participating in self-help groups, getting help from family members, or turning to religion or faith.

Application to Nursing Practice: The researcher asked participants what would be helpful prevention or intervention strategies. The most frequent suggestion was for education to begin in childhood and continue through adulthood. Nurses can direct primary prevention efforts at aggregates as early as elementary school and continue through the college years. Nurses must have good assessment skills, incorporating questions related to eating behaviors into initial interviews with clients in all settings. A thorough understanding of compulsive overeating and binge eating should result in increased empathy, caring, and acceptance by the nurse.

Lyons M.A. (1998). The phenomenon of compulsive overeating in a select group of professional women. *Journal of Advanced Nursing, 27,* 1158–1164.

Research strongly suggests that eating disorders may originate in part from hypothalamic, hormonal, neurotransmitter, or biochemical disturbances. Both the noradrenergic and serotonergic systems are involved in regulating eating behavior, with norepinephrine activating feeding in general and serotonin inhibiting it. Abnormalities in both the noradrenergic and serotonergic systems have been identified in anorexia as well as in bulimia. The binge eating behavior observed in bulimia is consistent with dysregulation in either or both of these systems (Kaye & Weltzin, 1991). Some research also suggests that dopamine may play a role in anorexia. Decreased levels of homovanillic acid, which is a major metabolite of dopamine, have been found in the cerebral spinal fluid of clients with the disorder. Also, reduced peptides (specifically, cholecystokinin), which contribute to normal regulation of eating, may play a role in the lack of satiety demonstrated by clients with bulimia during periods of binge eating. Currently, however, study findings are suggestive more than conclusive. Researchers must conduct more studies before they can make definitive statements about the biologic foundations for eating disorders.

Evidence for the role of genetics in the development of eating disorders has been considered for more than 100 years (Strober, 1991, 1995). Studies of twins and the sisters and daughters of people with eating disorders suggest a biologic or genetic link. Lilenfeld, Strober, and Kaye (1997) report that approximately 50% of the variance in the development of anorexia and bulimia can be attributed to genetic influences. Evidence from clinical samples of clients suggests that a family history of depression or substance abuse may be a strong risk factor for bulimia. The exact role of genetics in the development of eating disorders, however, still is a matter of speculation.

Studies from the National Institute of Mental Health suggest that anorexia, bulimia, and obsessive-compulsive disorder are associated with excessive levels of the brain hormone vasopressin. Studies with laboratory animals show that vasopressin, which is released in response to physical and emotional stress, prolongs behaviors learned under conditioned circumstances. In the same way that animals injected with vasopressin retain learned associations longer, vasopressin may enhance the conditioned obsessive-compulsive cycle of vigorous dieting, exercise,

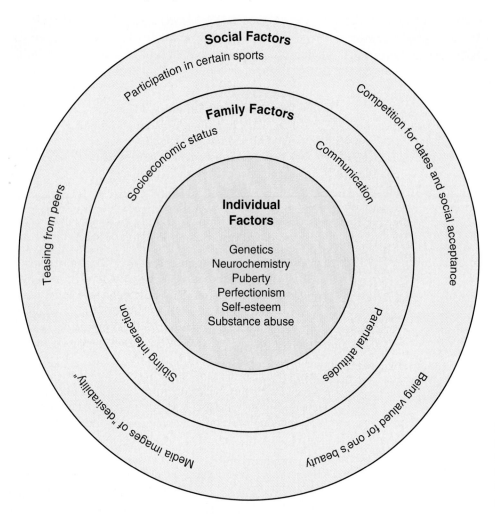

FIGURE 23-1 The etiology of eating disorders is multifactorial, with individual, family, and social factors combining to contribute to their development.

binging, and purging in people with eating disorders (Freund, Graham, Lesky, & Moskowitz, 1993).

BEHAVIORAL THEORIES

Supporters of behavioral theory argue that the client with an eating disorder initially may engage in dieting and gain approval for weight loss. As weight loss continues to a dangerous level, however, this approval turns to concern. The client continues to receive attention centered on the issue of weight. Thus, the attention may reinforce maladaptive eating behaviors.

SOCIOCULTURAL THEORIES

Few studies examine the prevalence of eating disorders among various cultures. Anorexia nervosa, however, appears to be less prevalent in countries with an inadequate food supply. This finding may support a sociocultural theory of eating disorders. Western cultural contexts are thought to determine the differential risk in the development of eating disorders in direct and indirect ways. Some social scientists argue that the socialization of girls to evaluate themselves against certain "idealized"

standards of appearance lays the groundwork for a negative body image. When they cannot meet this ideal and begin to diet compulsively, the stage may be set for them to develop an eating disorder. Studies showing that weight concern is endemic among adolescent girls tend to support this argument. Concerns about being "fat" have been found in children as young as 7 or 8 years of age in Western cultures (Hsu, 1990).

Physical attractiveness of a certain kind is highly valued, and girls are subjected to images of this kind of attractiveness from a very early age. Certain notions of what it means to be "feminine" and "beautiful" shape their social conduct. Girls learn very early that being "pretty" is what draws attention and praise from others.

FAMILY-BASED THEORIES

Families of daughters with eating disorders have been portrayed in very negative ways in the past. The old "family systems model" projected an image of such families as being overly concerned with external appearances and overly involved with one another (being enmeshed; having poor personal boundaries; being overprotective, rigid, and unable to accept changes that accompany puberty; avoiding conflict; and displaying perfectionistic tendencies). Despite the widespread acceptance of some of these notions that resulted from observational studies by Minuchin et al. (1975), reliable empirical literature to support these patterns of behavior are scant and have methodologic shortcomings. Family advocates suggest that certain overprotective patterns, rather than helping to cause eating disorders, may be displaying normative behavior for parents with a child who has a chronic and potentially life-threatening illness.

Whereas establishing causality may be impossible, studies provide some evidence to support that disturbed patterns of interaction exist in families of girls with anorexia. In such situations, from the viewpoint of family structure, the appropriate hierarchy of "parent in charge of child" is reversed in the area of food and eating. The child–adolescent is eating or not eating as she desires, and parents have very little influence over eating behaviors. Feeling extremely helpless, parents often make extraordinary efforts to appease the child in hope of getting the child to eat.

Signs and Symptoms/ Diagnostic Criteria

Before the diagnosis of a primary eating disorder is made, other psychiatric diagnoses, such as depression or schizophrenia, and a physiologic basis for anorexia must be ruled out. The *DSM-IV-TR* criteria for anorexia and bulimia clearly delineate the clinical features of these disorders (see Eating Disorders Information Map). Eating disorders that do not meet full criteria for anorexia or bulimia are classified as eating disorders not otherwise specified (NOS). BED without compensatory behavior currently is included under the NOS category.

ANOREXIA NERVOSA

Although anorexia was described as early as the 17th century, healthcare professionals and the general public have become increasingly aware of eating disorders in recent years. Anorexia is characterized by a voluntary refusal to eat and typically a weight less than 85% of what is considered normal for height and age. Clients with anorexia have a distorted body image and, to the bewilderment of others, view their emaciated bodies as fat. Some clients consider their whole bodies as too fat, whereas others fixate on one or more particular parts (eg, stomach, legs). Although clients with anorexia eat very little themselves, they may be obsessed with food and spend time cooking for others, saving recipes, or talking about foods. They often obsessively pursue vigorous physical activity to burn "excess calories."

In addition to psychological symptoms, the client suffers from multiple physiologic consequences of starvation. Physiologic changes resulting from extreme weight loss may include **amenorrhea** (the absence of or abnormal cessation of menstruation), lanugo hair, hypotension, bradycardia, hypothermia, constipation, polyuria, and electrolyte imbalances. Common laboratory abnormalities include increased serum cholesterol levels; increased serum carotene levels; decreased serum zinc and copper levels; increased blood urea nitrogen, cortisol, and growth hormone levels; anemia; leukopenia; and normal serum albumin. Low serum calcium levels may cause leg cramps.

Families of clients with anorexia typically describe them as model children: compliant, obedient perfectionists who want to please parents and teachers. They generally are high achievers in academic and athletic endeavors. Symptoms commonly begin after life changes, such as starting high school, moving to a new city or school, or going away to camp. Although families of clients with anorexia may not appear to have major interpersonal difficulties, unresolved and denied conflicts often exist among family members. Sisters of clients with anorexia also are at risk for developing an eating disorder.

BULIMIA NERVOSA

Bulimia is characterized by episodic, uncontrolled, rapid ingestion of large quantities of food. This disorder may occur alone or in conjunction with the food-restricting behavior of anorexia. Clients with bulimia nervosa compensate for excessive food intake by self-induced vomiting, obsessive exercise, and use of laxatives and diuretics. They may consume an incredible number of calories (an average of 3415 calories per binge episode) in a short period, induce vomiting, and perhaps repeat this behavior several times a day.

Clients with bulimia may develop dental caries as a result of frequent contact of tooth enamel with food and acidic gastric fluids. Other physiologic complications may include electrocardiographic changes, parotid gland enlargement, esophagitis, gastric dilation, menstrual irregularity, and electrolyte imbalances.

The typical client with bulimia is a young, college-educated woman who achieves highly at work or school. Despite her achievements, she tends to be passive, dependent, and unassertive. Her family may be disorganized, noncohesive, in conflict, and characterized by confusing sex role expectations for women (Clinical Example 23-2).

Comorbidities and Dual Diagnoses

Numerous studies show an association between depression and eating disorders, but determining whether mood disorders lead to eating disorders or vice versa is difficult. Antidepressant and antianxiety medications have been used effectively to treat bulimia (Marcus & Levine, 1998). Many clients with anorexia also exhibit

Eating Disorders Information Map

➡️ *Prevalence*

Approximately 0.5 to 2%

➡️ *Risk and Contributing Factors*

- Age: typical onset adolescence to early adulthood; rare after age 40 years
- Gender: more than 90% of cases occur in women
- Culture: far more prevalent in industrialized societies
- Ethnicity: in the United States, more common in whites and Hispanics than in blacks or Asians
- Genetics: increased risk among first-degree biologic relatives
- Low self-esteem
- Feelings of ineffectiveness and lack of control
- Dieting

Anorexia Nervosa

- Client refuses to maintain weight at or above normal for age and height. Weight loss or failure to gain expected weight during a growth period causes body weight to be below 85% of expected.
- Although underweight, client intensely fears gaining weight or becoming fat.
- Client experiences a disturbance of body weight or shape. These factors unduly influence self-evaluation, or client denies how serious the current low body weight is.
- A female client who has already begun menstruating experiences *amenorrhea,* at least three consecutive absent menstrual cycles. She still meets this criterion if periods resume only after hormone administration.

In the *restricting type*, client has not regularly engaged in binge eating or purging during this episode. In the *binge eating and purging type*, client has regularly engaged in binge eating or purging during this episode.

Bulimia Nervosa

- Client engages in recurrent binge eating, characterized by both of the following:
  1. Eating in a discrete period (e.g., within 2 hours) an amount of food that is definitely more than most people would eat during a similar period under similar circumstances
  2. A sense of no control (e.g., feeling that he or she cannot stop eating) during the episode
- Client engages in recurrent inappropriate behavior to compensate for weight gain. Examples include misuse of laxatives, diuretics, enemas, or other medications; self-induced vomiting; excessive exercise; or fasting.
- Binge eating and inappropriate compensatory behaviors persist at least twice a week for 3 months.
- Body shape and weight unduly influence self-evaluation.
- The disturbance is not exclusive to episodes of AN.

In the **purging type**, client has regularly engaged in self-induced vomiting or misuse of laxatives, diuretics, or enemas during the current episode. In the **nonpurging type**, client has used other inappropriate compensatory behaviors (e.g., fasting) but has not regularly engaged in purging behaviors during the current episode.

➡️ *Prevention Strategies*

- Screen all clients, and especially young girls and women, for signs and symptoms of eating disorders.
- When working with preteen and teenage clients, be sure to include discussions of menses, puberty, and weight gain during this life stage; peer pressure; and media influences. Emphasize that a person's worth is not connected to how many pounds he or she weighs.
- When working with clients who are dieting or mention concern with their weight, ask them to discuss their feelings, relationships, and current stressors.

(continued)

Eating Disorders Information Map (Continued)

- Help families explore eating behaviors, rituals, and practices.
- Emphasize to families that teasing about weight can be damaging.
- Avoid mentioning a client's appearance related to weight, even if the client looks good. The client can misperceive such comments, which may contribute to preoccupation with body image.

➡ *Want to Know More?*

American Anorexia/Bulimia Association, Inc.
165 W. 46th St., Suite 1108
New York, NY 10036
(212) 575-6200
http://www.aabainc.org

Center for the Study of Anorexia and Bulimia
8550 Arlington Blvd., Suite 300
Fairfax, VA 22031
(800) 944-9662
http://www.4woman.gov/nwhic/references/
   mdreferrals/csab.htm

Eating Disorders Awareness and Prevention
603 Stewart St., Suite 803
Seattle, WA 98101
http://www.edap.org

National Association for Anorexia and Associated
   Disorders
P. O. Box 7
Highland Park, IL 60035
(847) 831-3438
http://www.anad.org/

National Eating Disorders Organization
6655 South Yale Ave.
Tulsa, OK 74136
(918) 481-4044
http://www.nmisp.org

Diagnostic criteria adapted with permission from the American Psychiatric Association. (2000). *Diagnostic and statistical manual of mental disorders* (4th ed., text revision). Washington, DC: Author.

▼ *Clinical Example 23-2*

Fifteen-year-old Julie, a sophomore in high school, is 5′8″ tall and weighs 115 lb. A teacher refers Julie to the school nurse after hearing Julie vomit in the school bathroom on several occasions. In talking with Julie, the nurse initially observes that her teeth are in very poor condition. When the nurse asks about the vomiting, Julie looks embarrassed but confides that she is worried about gaining weight and vomits when she eats too much. When the nurse asks how long she's been vomiting, Julie reports that she went on a diet to lose weight during the summer before her freshman year in high school. Several other girls whom she admired were on diets, and Julie, although not overweight, gradually ate less and less. Between July and December, her weight dropped from 114 to 87 lb. Julie states that her parents didn't worry at first but eventually became upset about her weight loss. She recalls that they tried to bribe her with food and fought with each other about her refusal to eat. That whole period now seems somewhat unreal to her.

Right before Christmas in her freshman year, Julie's mother took her to the family physician. The doctor told Julie she would have to be admitted to the hospital if she didn't eat. No other intervention occurred at this time. Julie was a "straight A" student; the idea of being hospitalized and missing school frightened her. She agreed to start eating and did so that day. She rapidly regained the lost weight by eating everything she wanted. She can't remember exactly when the thought occurred to her that she could eat as much as she wanted without gaining weight if she could vomit. She soon learned that if she drank a lot of water after eating she could easily induce vomiting. With this discovery, she began eating larger amounts of food. So that her family wouldn't be suspicious that food was disappearing so quickly, she began buying, and then stealing, candy and cookies from the grocery store and hiding them in her room. She still is engaging in this behavior. Julie states that her parents do not suspect that she is doing this. She says that her parents were happy when she started eating, and they've never discussed her weight loss again.

Julie tells the school nurse that she sometimes wonders if she is crazy and that she is ashamed of her teeth. She wonders if vomiting has anything to do with dental decay, even though she brushes her teeth immediately after vomiting. The nurse provides Julie with some basic information about anorexia nervosa and bulimia. Julie is relieved to hear that others have the same problems. The nurse explains that there is an association between frequent eating, vomiting, and dental caries but that Julie should not blame herself. She didn't get anorexia and bulimia on purpose and couldn't have prevented it.

With Julie's permission, the nurse calls her parents in for a conference. The nurse explains what Julie is going through and that she needs assistance to cope more effectively. Without blaming the family, the nurse explains that it would help Julie if all family members would meet with a counselor experienced in eating disorders. Julie's parents initially react by denying that Julie has a problem. They say that she does well in school and eats well. They add that everyone in their family has poor teeth. After hearing in more detail, however, about Julie's vomiting and stealing of food, they agree to attend a family session.

Points for Reflection and Critical Thinking

1. What biologic, social, family, and other factors may have contributed to Julie's development of an eating disorder?
2. Was the intervention by the family physician appropriate? If not, how would you have modified this approach? How does your response relate to the importance of client teaching?
3. What are the goals of family therapy? Based on the information provided, what factors may hinder the family's progress? What factors may assist their progress?

bulimic behavior. Some researchers propose that eating disorders are basically a form of depressive mood disorder. For example, many clients with bulimia share a family history of mood disorders. These clients also typically have difficulty with direct expression of feelings, are prone to impulsive behavior, and may have problems with alcohol and other substance abuse.

Implications and Prognosis

Many clients with anorexia or bulimia never seek or receive treatment. Some recover spontaneously, whereas others have long-term problems. Herzog, Nussbaum, and Marmor (1996) report that of clients treated for anorexia, 50% have a good outcome, 30% have an intermediate outcome, and 20% have a poor outcome. Death from starvation, infection, or suicide may occur in up to 21% of cases.

Interdisciplinary Goals and Treatment

The treatment of clients with eating disorders is a complex and frequently long process. Client improvement often is gradual and characterized by two steps forward and one back. Clients may resist treatment.

In many settings, the nurse, physician, psychotherapist, social worker, dietitian, and occupational therapist work together to formulate the treatment plan. Communication and consistency among members of the multidisciplinary team are critical. The primary nurse often coordinates client care among team members.

Treatment of eating disorders most commonly occurs in community-based settings. In the current climate of healthcare reform, managed care and short-term treatments predominate (Davis, 1998). Treatment of eating disorders increasingly occurs in school, community mental health centers, clinics, private offices, day treatment centers, and groups.

Clients with anorexia nervosa are hospitalized more frequently than are those with bulimia. The primary reasons for hospitalizing clients with anorexia are low weight, depressed mood, low serum potassium level, lack of response to outpatient treatment, and family discouragement and demoralization. Reasons for inpatient treatment of bulimia include the client's desire for treatment, low weight, dangerously low potassium levels, or a diagnosis of maladaptive personality patterns such as an impulse disorder or borderline personality disorder (see Chap. 22).

BEHAVIORAL THERAPY

Behavioral therapy programs generally begin in an inpatient setting. Although programs vary, the client typically starts with no privileges. He or she gains privileges in response to appropriate eating behaviors. A criticism sometimes aimed at behavior modification techniques is that the provider manipulates and controls client behavior without dealing with underlying issues (Clare & Cuthbertson, 1998). Several research studies conclude that behavior modification is useful to restore lost weight and generally is more successful when used in conjunction with cognitive and family therapies.

COGNITIVE THERAPY

Cognitive therapy focuses on how a person thinks about something and how that thinking affects subsequent feelings and actions. A discussion of particular cognitive therapy approaches that the nurse can use when working with clients is discussed in the Implementation section.

COGNITIVE-BEHAVIORAL THERAPY

A combination of behavioral and cognitive strategies exists as cognitive-behavioral therapy (CBT) (Leitenberg, 1994; Wilson, 1995). Fairburn (1993) developed this manual-based treatment for promoting healthy eating behaviors, decreasing binge eating and purging, modifying irrational attitudes and thoughts, and preventing relapse. CBT has shown itself particularly effective with clients with bulimia and BED. A self-help version of the CBT manual may be an effective, low-cost intervention modality. CBT also can be implemented as a group psychoeducational strategy.

INTERPERSONAL THERAPY

Interpersonal therapy (IPT) (Wilson, 1995) is short term, noninterpretive, and highly focused on a limited number of interpersonal changes agreed on by the client and therapist. The therapist does not address healthy eating behaviors or concern about shape or weight based on the belief that improved interpersonal functioning will improve self-esteem and defuse the importance of body weight and shape in self-evaluation.

SOLUTION-FOCUSED BRIEF THERAPY

In response to increasing pressures to treat clients as cost-effectively as possible, solution-focused brief therapy (SFBT) reflects a paradigm shift away from pathology to one in which the clinician views the client as basically healthy, inherently resourceful, and able to solve his or her own problems. The clinician's role is to learn the client's unique view of the problem and what needs to be different as a result of treatment. Although the SFBT approach originated from economic pressures, it has many virtues. Rather than looking for causes and taking deep excursions into the past, SFBT empowers clients to recognize and acknowledge their own abilities and resourcefulness (McFarland, 1995).

The two key techniques of SFBT are "asking the miracle question" and "searching for exceptions." In the first, the therapist works with the client to explore "How would your life be different if your eating disorder were miraculously gone?" In the second, they examine "What are the times like when you are managing your eating behavior more successfully?"

FAMILY THERAPY

Family therapy may occur in conjunction with inpatient treatment or entirely on an outpatient basis. Family therapy is particularly important when the client is to return to the home after treatment.

Family therapy focuses on fostering open, healthy interaction patterns among members. One innovative program uses family meal therapy as the primary technique in a multicomponent approach to changing eating behaviors (Forisha, Grothaus, & Luscombe, 1990). Family therapy is challenging because clients and families may deny the presence of an eating disorder. Even when they admit that a problem exists, they may minimize the extent of the client's illness. Families also may typically insist that there is no conflict and that they get along very well. To complicate matters, the client may not be thinking clearly and may be unable to reason effectively enough to participate meaningfully in a program of therapy.

Behavior family systems therapy (BFST) is an approach that blends behavior modification, cognitive therapy, and family therapy. It relies on empirically tested behavioral and cognitive techniques (Robin, Bedway, Siegel, Moye, & Gilroy, 1997; Robin et al., 1999). BFST for anorexia nervosa begins *after* the client is medically stable. It consists of four phases:

1. Assessment: The multidisciplinary team, consisting of dietitian, physician, psychologist, nurse, and other professionals, comes together to coordinate care with the client and family. Team members engage the family in treatment and check the client's weight weekly. They conduct history, behavioral analyses, and social and functional analyses.
2. **Control rationale:** The therapist encourages parents to "take charge" of the client's eating and deals with their reactions to control rationale. The therapist also coaches parents to develop an appropriate behavioral weight program.
3. **Weight gain:** The therapist begins to refine the weight-gain program and introduces nonfood-related issues. He or she begins cognitive therapy interventions (eg, cognitive restructuring). Family psychotherapy and psychoeducation take place.
4. **Weight maintenance:** Control over food gradually returns to the client. Team members teach healthy ways of maintaining weight. Family interactions become more the focus of treatment. The therapist fosters client individuation.

Specific family therapy approaches for nurses to use are included in the Implementation section.

GROUP THERAPY

Clients with eating disorders also may benefit from group therapy. Groups may have specific therapeutic goals, such as fostering self-esteem or gaining insight into feelings and behavior. They also may be organized as primarily supportive or self-help groups. Members gain self-acceptance by sharing concerns with others and receiving constructive support and feedback from peers (Owen & Fullerton, 1995).

PHARMACOLOGIC INTERVENTIONS

Medications are useful for some clients with eating disorders (Marcus & Levine, 1998). Although pharmacologic intervention generally is not a primary intervention in anorexia, antidepressants or antianxiety drugs may benefit clients with depressive, anxiety, or obsessive-compulsive symptoms. Antidepressant medications also appear to have therapeutic benefits in many clients with bulimia. Antidepressant medications may include tricyclic antidepressants (TCAs), monoamine oxidase inhibitors, and selective serotonin reuptake inhibitors, specifically fluoxetine and sertraline. Clients who display obsessive-compulsive traits particularly may benefit from treatment with clomipramine (Anafranil) or fluoxetine (Prozac). Lithium, the TCAs, and anticonvulsants also have been reported to be useful in treating bulimia in adults. They are not, however, recommended for treating children with bulimia.

APPLICATION OF THE NURSING PROCESS TO CLIENTS WITH EATING DISORDERS

Eating disorders are a great challenge for nursing because of their accompanying complex physical and psychosocial problems. Sensitivity to the needs of clients with eating disorders helps the nurse intervene constructively with those who resist help and persist in self-destructive behaviors. Forming an alliance with the client is crucial. A supportive but firm approach by the nurse is helpful in engaging the client in the therapeutic relationship. See Therapeutic Communication 23-1.

Assessment

Because clients with eating disorders may be secretive and unwilling to portray themselves as having problems, the nurse must be skilled in eliciting feelings and thoughts. The client with an eating disorder may exhibit disturbances in many areas. Assessment, therefore, can be complex. Knowledge of the diagnostic criteria and etiology of eating disorders and use of an organizational framework can guide the nurse in asking relevant assessment questions. An organizational assessment framework based on functional health patterns is presented in Table 23-1.

HISTORY AND PHYSICAL EXAMINATION

The client with an eating disorder requires a careful, thorough physical assessment. The behaviors associated with eating disorders involve manipulation or deprivation of foods and fluids. These behaviors can result in severely disturbed, even life-threatening metabolic processes.

Because so many physical problems are the result of disturbances in nutrition, the nurse must first evaluate the client's nutritional status. The nurse begins by obtaining an accurate weight, history of previous high and low weights, and chronology of recent weight fluctuations. The nurse questions how fast weight loss or gain occurred and if any associated circumstances surrounded the event such as medical illness, psychiatric illness, situational crisis, or major life changes. Because the client may be reluctant to reveal details about dieting or binge–purge behaviors, the nurse may ask the client to describe food and fluid intake for a typical day.

Physical examination may reveal numerous symptoms related to disturbances in nutrition and metabolism. Possible findings include dehydration, hypokalemia, cardiac dysrhythmia, hypotension, bradycardia, dry skin, brittle hair and nails, lanugo, frequent infections, dental caries, inflammation of the throat and esophagus, swollen parotid glands (from purging), amenorrhea, and hypothermia.

Elimination disturbances are very common in clients with eating disorders. The nurse asks about related problems that the client may be experiencing. Constipation may result from restricted food intake, self-induced vomiting, and slowed gastrointestinal motility. Excessive laxative use causes diarrhea and loss of protein, fluid, and potassium in stools. Long-term laxative use may lead to eventual reliance on laxatives for bowel elimination. Polyuria may be present in the client with severe weight loss.

Hormonal imbalances result from excessive weight loss. Reproductive hormones regress to prepubertal levels. Clients experience amenorrhea, breast atrophy, lanugo, and loss of axillary and pubic hair. Infertility accompanies amenorrhea, but this typically resolves once the client regains weight and menses resume.

Another concern for the nurse to address during the physical examination is the client's patterns of activity and rest. Assessment questions include what kind of exercise the client engages in, if he or she is involved in organized sports at school, whether he or she has difficulty sleeping, and if he or she often is tired or has a lot of energy. Often, these patterns are markedly disordered, with some clients engaging in compulsive activity at all times to burn calories. Some exercise compulsively, are restless, and frequently experience insomnia. Early morning awakening is common. A lowered pulse rate often occurs in response to excessive exercise and starvation.

In addition to a physical examination and interview, the nurse may pursue laboratory and cardiac testing for the client with an eating disorder to assess for electrolyte abnormalities and cardiac dysfunction. Some clients with bulimia may require an endoscopy to detect esophageal abnormalities incurred by frequent vomiting.

PSYCHOSOCIAL ASSESSMENT

Clients with eating disorders typically lack awareness of the connection between their eating behaviors and underlying feelings, needs, and conflicts. These clients tend to exhibit intellectualization and all-or-none reasoning. They are more comfortable with abstract concepts than with recognizing and expressing feelings. These clients also tend to have perfectionistic personalities and to give up if something is not exactly right. They may overgeneralize and believe that all life's problems will be solved if they lose enough weight. The cognitive distortion, emotional reasoning, is characteristic (Table 23-2). **Emotional reasoning** means relying on one's emotions to determine reality. An example of emotional reasoning in a client with an eating disorder is "I know I'm fat because I feel fat."

THERAPEUTIC COMMUNICATION 23-1
Moving with Resistance

Elise, a 16-year-old with bulimia nervosa, has come to the school mental health clinic at the insistence of her sister, who is concerned about Elise's purging. Elise presents with a sense of agitation, and during the interview she seems quite distracted. She asks for a glass of water. She stands, moves about, and generally appears unsettled and anxious. When asked if she wants to sit, she replies, "I prefer to stand."

Ineffective Dialogue

Nurse: "Tell me why you are here"

Elise: (*Walks toward door*) "You know, I need a break. I'm going to sit out in the waiting room. If you want to talk to me there, that's fine."

Nurse: (*Looks at watch and shakes her head*) "I don't think that's appropriate. Let's get started. We only have 40 minutes."

Elise: (*Hand on doorknob*) "Frankly, I don't think I need help, and this was a big mistake. I'm not nuts."

Nurse: (*Sighs and sits behind her desk*) "Elise, you must want to be helped for something. You're here, aren't you?"

Elise: (*Getting defensive*) "Well that wasn't my idea. My sister and boyfriend forced me. I am just fine."

Nurse: (*Notices Elise's behavior is defensive*) "You're very defensive. There must be something behind all that defensiveness."

Elise: "Fine, then you have a good time trying to root around for what it is." (*Slams door on her way out*)

Effective Dialogue

Nurse: "What are some of the things that concern you?"

Elise: (*Walks toward door*) "You know, I need a break. I'm going to sit out in the waiting room. If you want to talk to me there, that's fine."

Nurse: "Before we step out, why don't we talk frankly for a minute. I guess that both you and I realize that this situation is stressful for you. It's hard to share important and personal information with a stranger." (*Remains patient with Elise, sensing that she is trying to express something other than her words*)

Elise: "I don't know, I guess you're going to get inside my head. Isn't that what psychotherapy does, shrink heads?"

Nurse: "I guess that depends on what you mean. What were you expecting today?"

Elise: (*Says with some exasperation but less tension*) "I don't know. I guess I was expecting to lie down on some couch. I also thought that coming here meant that I was some kind of a nut."

Nurse: "First of all, there are no couches. We'll talk for about 40 minutes and only about those things that *you* think are important." (*Trying to restore some sense of control to Elise*) "You don't have to talk about anything that is too painful. That's your decision. We'll move at your pace. Is that OK with you?"

Elise: "Yeah, I guess that will be fine."

Nurse: "By the way, you said that you were afraid that you were 'some kind of a nut.' Are you worried that you'll be seen as unstable or 'nuts,' as you say?" (*Redirecting Elise to what might be bothering her*)

Elise: "Yes, the thought had crossed by mind."

Nurse: "What exactly are you worried about?"

Elise: "My sister thinks I'm crazy. So does my boyfriend. They're convinced of it, and I'm beginning to wonder myself."

Reflection and Critical Thinking

- What types of communication did Elise exhibit in both scenarios? Assess the reason for Elise's fear of losing control. Why might she be anxious about this interview?
- What nonverbal cues did Elise and the nurse give in both scenarios?
- What methods of communication did the nurse use in the second scenario that ultimately were more effective than those used in the first?

TABLE 23-1 ▼ Functional Health Patterns Assessment Guide

PATTERN	QUESTIONS
Health perception–health management	• How has your general health been? • Do you feel that you need treatment for a health issue? • Have others been concerned about your health or your weight? • Do you use laxatives or diuretics to control weight?
Nutritional–metabolic	• Have you ever fasted to lose weight? • Have you ever tried to vomit after eating?
Elimination	• Do you have to use laxatives to have a bowel movement? • Do you have diarrhea often?
Activity–exercise	• Do you feel weak or dizzy or have muscle cramping? • Do you ever have palpitations? • Do you follow a strict exercise regimen? • Do you panic if you cannot exercise as much as you'd like?
Sleep–rest	• Do you have difficulty sleeping?
Cognitive–perceptual	• Would you describe yourself as a perfectionist? • Do you repeat things until you get them right? • Have you ever not been able to get something out of your mind? • Do you find yourself repeatedly thinking about the same things? • How do you feel if you lose control, such as getting very angry or eating too much? • What do you do when you feel you are losing control? • Have you ever had times when you have eaten uncontrollably? What did you feel, and what did you do?
Self-perception–self-concept	• What do you like the best about your body? • What do you like the least about your body? • If you could change how you look, how would you be different? • What do you like the best about yourself? • What do you like the least about yourself? • How would you describe yourself to others? • How would others (family, friends) describe you? • What are your strengths? • What are your weaknesses?
Role–relationships	• How is your relationship with your parents? • How would you describe your family? • Do you have many friends? • Do you have a best friend? • What do you like to do with your friends? • What is school like? • Do you study a lot? • In what activities are you involved at school? • Do you feel pressure to do well in school? If so, from whom?
Sexuality–reproductive	• Have your periods become irregular or stopped completely? (for female clients) • How do you feel about the body changes that occur at adolescence (eg, in females, breast development, menstruation, broadening of hips)? • Is dating something that you enjoy? • Have you had any sexual experiences? • How do you feel about your sexual experiences (or lack of them)?
Coping–stress tolerance	• How do you make decisions about everyday things? • How do you spend your free time? (For example, do you usually ask someone for advice or think things out for yourself?) • Is your life right now pretty much the way you want it? If not, what would you change? What can you do to make these changes? • What do you do to feel better when you are sad or upset?

(continued)

TABLE 23-1 ▼ **Functional Health Patterns Assessment Guide** (Continued)	
PATTERN	**QUESTIONS**
	• Have you ever felt like hurting yourself when you are down? • Have you ever thought about committing suicide? • Have you ever used alcohol or drugs to feel better? • Have you ever stolen anything (eg, food or money)? If so, how do you feel about that? • Do you get along with your parents? What happens when you argue with them? What do you argue about? What happens when you talk to them about a problem or concern? • How do you get along with your siblings? Can you talk to them about your feelings and problems? • Do your friends help you if you have a problem?
Value-belief	• What is important to you? • What do you care about? • What is the meaning of life for you?

Clients with eating disorders experience considerable anxiety about becoming obese. Emaciated clients with anorexia have distorted body images, seeing themselves as too fat even when others view them as alarmingly thin (Figure 23-2). They generally have low self-esteem even though they achieve well at school, sports, and work. Their expectations often are unrealistically rigid and high. They look to others for approval and perceive a lack of control over themselves and situations. They do not have the sense that their actions will significantly effect a desired outcome.

Clients with eating disorders frequently become isolated from family and friends. They often exhibit immature interaction patterns and remain inappropriately dependent and childlike in their relationship with their parents. They may stop dating and gradually abandon good friends. As the disorder persists, deficits in social skills increase. They often remain good students and spend much time alone studying. Isolation also may result from preoccupation with weight, food, and exercise.

Eating disorders are maladaptive attempts to meet life's demands, roles, and stresses. The client may have difficulty in the following areas:

• Asking for help and nurturance
• Making decisions
• Meeting role expectations of adolescence
• Expressing emotions
• Exerting control (perceived powerlessness)

Because the client with an eating disorder may have little self-knowledge or self-awareness, he or she may have poorly defined values and beliefs. In addition, eating disorders occur most often when the client is struggling to establish his or her own identity and formulate a philosophy about the meaning of existence.

The nurse needs to ask questions designed to uncover these various psychosocial characteristics and needs to explore in depth any area that is of concern (see Table 23-1).

Nursing Diagnosis

Because of the multisystem nature of eating disorders, data analysis may suggest several nursing diagnoses. Clients who are medically unstable should have nursing diagnoses specific to their medical problems (eg, Deficient Fluid Volume, Decreased Cardiac Output).

Most nursing diagnoses for clients with eating disorders center on psychosocial problems. They may include the following:

• **Imbalanced Nutrition: Less than Body Requirements** related to refusal to ingest or retain ingested food, physical exertion in excess of caloric intake
• **Disturbed Thought Processes** related to all-or-none thinking, intellectualization, obsessions, overgeneralization, and malnutrition
• **Disturbed Body Image** related to unresolved psychosocial conflicts
• **Chronic Low Self-Esteem** related to unrealistic expectations from self or others, lack of positive feedback, striving to please others to gain acceptance
• **Powerlessness** related to belief that one's actions will not result in desired outcomes
• **Ineffective Coping** related to unmet developmental tasks (trust, autonomy), dysfunctional family system
• **Interrupted Family Processes** related to ineffective communication patterns, denial of problems

TABLE 23-2 ▼ **Manifestations of Cognitive Distortions in Clients With Eating Disorders**

DISTORTION	EXPLANATIONS	EXAMPLE
Catastrophizing/magnification	Giving an event or its consequences more merit than is realistic	"These jeans feel tight today. I know everyone can tell that I've gained 3 lb."
Dichotomous thinking	Reasoning by extremes; seeing everything as "black or white"	"If I'm not thin, I must be fat." "I've already eaten two slices of pizza and wrecked my diet. I might as well eat the whole thing."
Emotional reasoning	Relying on emotions to determine reality	"I know I'm fat because I feel fat."
Overgeneralization	Basing beliefs on one or a few, not necessarily related, considerations	"I don't have a boyfriend. It must be because I'm fat." "Liz is so thin and has the perfect life. I should lose weight so my life can be better."
Personalization	Overinterpreting an event as having personal significance	"Dad made a face when I grabbed a piece of candy from the jar. He must think I'm overweight."
Selective abstraction	Focusing on only some information while choosing to ignore other information	"I've lost 10 lb, but I still can't fit into a size 8. I'm a failure."

and conflicts, unresolved issues of control, inability to manage conflict

Planning

Planning involves collaborating with the client and usually the family to formulate an appropriate treatment approach and to set goals. Short-term goals focus on decreasing anxiety, stopping weight loss, restoring the individual to an acceptable weight, and normalizing eating behaviors. Appropriate goals include the following:

- The client will have adequate dietary intake to meet body requirements and maintain weight that is appropriate to age and height.
- The client will verbalize diminished fears and exhibit decreased anxiety regarding weight gain and loss of control.
- The client will not engage in binge eating or purging activities.
- The client will maintain an appropriate activity level.

Long-term goals focus on helping the client and, if possible, the family to resolve the psychological issues that precipitated the eating disorder and to develop more constructive coping mechanisms. These goals may include the following:

- The client will exhibit a realistic thinking process and body perception.

- The client will verbalize adequate self-esteem.
- The client will perceive control over actions.
- The client will recognize maladaptive coping behaviors and demonstrate adaptive coping behaviors.
- The client will recognize and verbalize emotions and needs.
- Family will demonstrate constructive communication patterns.
- Family will manage conflict constructively.

In Clinical Example 23-1 at the beginning of this chapter, you read about Jody, who has anorexia nervosa. Nursing Care Plan 23-1 shows the care that Kate, the nurse practitioner, designs for Jody.

Implementation

The nurse is challenged to establish a relationship of open communication and trust (Woolsey, 1998). Because many clients with eating disorders never seek treatment, nurses commonly encounter the more severely ill clients in the hospital setting. Clients with eating disorders may be admitted to general psychiatric units or to units or facilities specializing in the treatment of eating disorders. Families frequently are frustrated, angry, and scared after months of trying to get the client to eat. Temporarily removing the client from the home may relieve the family's distress and set the stage for behavior changes in the client and her family (Implications for Nursing Practice 23-1).

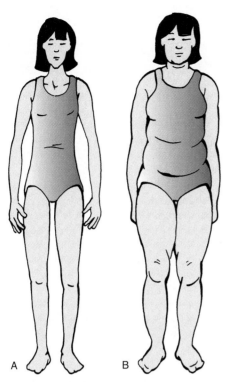

FIGURE 23-2 An example of distorted body image in anorexia. Part A depicts how the client with anorexia actually looks to the world. Part B depicts how the client with anorexia sees herself.

RESTORING NUTRITIONAL BALANCE

Restoring nutritional balance is a priority for clients with severe eating disorders. Most experts in this area believe that conducting meaningful psychotherapy with these clients is impossible until they are nutritionally stable. Clients who are clearly malnourished should be under the care of an internist until they are medically stable and no longer pose a risk of developing a severe medical complication related to starvation. Medical management requires a holistic approach that considers more than the client's "psychological needs." For example, because an increased workload by an already compromised cardiac reserve can lead to congestive heart failure, refeeding the very low weight client with anorexia means that nurses must carefully monitor cardiac function. Another important intervention is to carefully monitor electrolyte levels when refeeding clients with anorexia. They are at risk of developing a "refeeding syndrome" in which hypokalemia can occur.

Refeeding also involves establishing a contract that spells out the expected behaviors, rewards, privileges, and consequences of noncompliance. Such a contract may be useful in eliminating power struggles with the client. Contracts typically address how much weight the client will gain and in what time frame. Typically, the priority is to achieve a healthy weight at which menses resumes and bone demineralization does not occur.

The first goal is for the client *to stop losing weight.* Engaging the client is important, as is giving her an opportunity to eat on her own. In inpatient settings, if more supervision is needed, restricting the client's access to bathrooms for 2 hours after meals may be necessary to prevent the client from engaging in self-induced vomiting.

When the client is medically stable, the treatment team may confer with the family to discuss transition to home. Clients also should be integral parts of determining their treatment and care. If clients believe that they have contributed to the planning of rewards and privileges, they will perceive more control over their environment and bodies and more likely will adhere to the treatment regimen.

All health team members must consistently carry out the terms of the contract. Even though clients may rebel against contract terms, it reassures them to know that consistent limits are being maintained and that they can trust the staff to help maintain control.

Hospitalized clients with anorexia frequently express frustration with limitations placed on them regarding exercise. Examining the type of exercise may help in setting sound guidelines for exercise protocols. Rigorous aerobic exercise generally is contraindicated when weight gain is a goal. Allowing the client to engage in moderate resistance training (eg, weight lifting), however, would increase the lean body mass as the client gains weight and minimize the gain in "fat weight," which is a great fear of the client. Developing a contract that allows the client to participate in exercise of this nature would acknowledge the benefits of exercise in a healthy lifestyle, enable the client to feel more in control, and help the client to develop a more positive body image while gaining weight (Michielli, Dunbar, & Kalinski, 1994).

The nurse communicates caring to the client through a kind, firm, matter-of-fact approach. For example, when a client is upset that her activities are being restricted, the nurse responds, "When you gain 5 pounds, you will earn privileges to participate in more activities. This is your choice." The nurse avoids offering punitive responses, arguing about limits, bribing, cajoling, and being excessively vigilant and overprotective. Through his or her interactions, the nurse conveys to the client, "You are a worthwhile person, and I care about you; I have expectations of you, and you are capable of meeting these expectations."

ENCOURAGING REALISTIC THINKING PROCESSES

People with eating disorders tend to have perfectionistic personalities and to think in all-or-none terms (see Table 23-2). This kind of thinking helps to explain the characteristic extreme fear of becoming obese. For example, a client who eats two cookies might conclude, "I couldn't control myself; I might as well give up and eat the whole

Nursing Care Plan 23-1

THE CLIENT WITH ANOREXIA NERVOSA

Jody, the client in Clinical Example 23-1, begins to receive care for anorexia nervosa. Kate, the nurse practitioner, performs a physical examination on Jody. She finds Jody to be somewhat cachectic looking, with very dry skin and limp, dull hair. Her heart rate is 50 beats per minute, and her blood pressure is 88/50 mm Hg. Jody tells Kate that she has not had a period in several months.

Kate orders blood studies and an electrocardiogram. Results show decreased hemoglobin and potassium levels, other electrolyte abnormalities, and sinus bradycardia.

On the following day, Kate continues her discussion with Jody and asks about family dynamics. Jody reveals that her mother is very controlling. She also relates that conflicts within the family never are handled in a straightforward way.

Based on the assessment data, Kate devises the following care plan:

Nursing Diagnosis: Impaired Nutrition: Less than Body Requirements related to reduced food intake and increased exercise to bring about weight loss

Goals: Jody will gain 1.5 lb per week until she reaches her ideal weight of 135 lb.

Jody's vital signs, hemoglobin count, and electrolyte levels will return to normal.

Interventions	Rationales
Develop a behavior modification contract for gradual weight gain. The plan should include the following: • Ingesting 1800 to 2000 calories per day • Limiting exercise to 30 minutes per day • Establishing a system of rewards for compliance with contract (or restrictions for noncompliance)	A well-defined behavioral modification program will provide consistency, decrease power struggles, and enhance compliance.
Meet with a dietitian to determine a diet plan that includes nutritious foods that the client likes.	Including Jody in meal planning will enhance her sense of control.
Monitor the client's vital signs, food and fluid intake and output, and weight. Weigh the client daily at the same time and under the same conditions.	Hypotension and bradycardia may occur as a result of starvation. Monitoring intake, output, and weight is necessary to ensure Jody's health.
Arrange for a family member or friend to supervise meals and remain with the client up to 1 hour after eating.	Direct observation will diminish Jody's opportunities to avoid eating, hoard or hide foot, or vomit.
Discuss with the client the need to avoid exercising excessively. Discuss how healthy exercise is an important component of physical and mental fitness, but that the client needs to stop relying on exercise for weight reduction.	Clients with eating disorders may engage in excessive exercise to burn calories. By focusing on physical fitness, Jody may begin to associate exercise with health-promotion goals instead of weight loss.
Provide a liquid diet through nasogastric or nasoduodenal tube if necessary to maintain an adequate oral intake.	A liquid diet will provide adequate nutrition and fluid if Jody is unwilling to eat and drink.
Use a supportive, firm, nonjudgmental, and matter-of-fact approach in regulating eating behavior.	The client with an eating disorder will not view a matter-of-fact approach as punishment. Such an approach also helps to alleviate feelings of guilt. Through this approach, Jody can experience feelings of acceptance.

Evaluation: Jody must gain 18 lb to reach her goal weight of 135 lb. She should reach this goal in 12 weeks. Evaluation includes determining if Jody has met her goal of a weekly weight gain of 1.5 lb. Other indicators of effective interventions are normal hemoglobin and electrolyte values.

Nursing Diagnosis: Chronic Low Self-Esteem related to perfectionism, dependence on the appraisals and approval of others, disturbed body image, and inadequate social skills

(continued)

Nursing Care Plan 23-1 (Continued)

Goal: Jody will gain a realistic appraisal of her body image, exhibit age-appropriate autonomy, and interact comfortably with peers.

Interventions	Rationales
Use cognitive restructuring techniques:	Client can confront irrational beliefs and substitute them with more realistic ones.
For disturbed body image: Assist client to review her own and others' bodies realistically.	External, objective feedback will help Jody attain a healthier, more realistic body image.
For low self-esteem: Help client acknowledge relationship between overly high self-expectations and feelings of inadequacy.	Realistic expectations of self will increase Jody's sense of self-esteem.
Help client identify her strengths and resources.	Realistic positive reinforcement and feedback will enhance Jody's self-esteem.
Encourage client to make decisions and choices for self.	Opportunities to practice independent functioning will help Jody develop improved self-confidence and self-esteem.
For inadequate social skills: Enhance client's communication and socialization skills by promoting information, role-playing, and participation in group activities with peers.	Enhanced social skills will improve Jody's peer relationships and contribute to improving her self-esteem.

Evaluation: The nurse and client can measure Jody's progress in developing a greater sense of self-esteem and a realistic body image by evaluating the changes in her self-comments, descriptions of herself, verbalizations of self-acceptance, and willingness to focus on positive attributes. Observing and discussing her social interaction with peers can help to measure her progress in age-appropriate social skills.

Nursing Diagnosis: Dysfunctional Family Processes related to denial of problems and conflicts, unresolved control issues, and dysfunctional communication patterns

Goals: Jody and her family will manage conflict constructively and communicate directly with one another.

The family will encourage autonomy of all its members.

Interventions	Rationales
Encourage family members to identify and express conflicts openly.	Communicating assertively fosters individuality and personal efficacy among family members.
Encourage family members to speak for themselves by making "I," rather than "we," statements.	Family members need to learn to distinguish and be responsible for their own feelings, words, and actions.
Explore ways for each member to increase autonomy.	Children have more power to make decisions and accept responsibility for own behavior.
Role-model direct, constructive communication patterns for family members.	Role-modeling of open communication provides an example and gives family members permission to express their thoughts and feelings openly.

Evaluation: The family's struggle to overcome its dysfunctional patterns will be an ongoing process. The nurse and family can measure improvement in this area by observing and discussing family interaction and willingness to encourage age-appropriate autonomy and open communication among members.

Implications for Nursing Practice 23-1

Preventing Eating Disorders

When working with clients and populations who may be at risk for eating disorders, nurses should remember to discuss the "3 Cs":

- **Communication**—How to recognize and express feelings
- **Conflict Resolution**—How to express needs when they are not being met
- **Coping**—What to do when the client cannot directly solve a problem

bag of cookies." The client has rigidly defined appropriate behaviors for herself in terms of "walking on a tightrope," with the need for constant vigilance to keep from falling off. The client needs to learn balance and moderation in thinking and behavior.

The nurse can reassure the client that life is more like walking in a big meadow and that she can safely move in many directions. The nurse encourages the client to try out new behaviors, explaining that although doing so may be frightening, the client gradually will learn to be more confident about her behavioral choices in all areas, including eating. See Client and Family Eduation 23-1.

IMPROVING BODY IMAGE

The disturbed body image of the client with an eating disorder is related to disordered thinking such as overgeneralization (believing that all problems will be solved when sufficient weight is lost), powerlessness, and self-esteem issues. Social factors also affect the client's body image issues. The nurse can help the client recognize the influence of maladaptive thoughts by asking the client to keep a diary in which he or she records situations and events that cause concern about physical appearance and weight. In discussing these situations, the nurse and client can begin to identify anxiety-provoking events and develop strategies for managing such situations without resorting to self-damaging behaviors. Such strategies include avoiding anxiety-provoking situations or persons, or, if that is not possible, learning to desensitize oneself to certain situations. For example, clients might practice a form of progressive relaxation if they become agitated when they are at the mall, faced with images of extremely thin mannequins. Or they might try the cognitive technique of "disputation" if they have distorted thoughts about their bodies (see Chap. 3).

BUILDING SELF-ESTEEM

Low self-esteem in clients with eating disorders is associated with overly high self-expectations, need for approval

Client and Family Education 23-1

EATING DISORDERS

Teaching Points

The nurse counsels and educates the client with an eating disorder and his or her family members by offering the following suggestions:

- Provide unconditional love.
- Focus on the person rather than on the eating disorder.
- Give the client the power to make decisions and facilitate changes in matters other than eating.
- Demonstrate united support for one another and the plan for the client's treatment.
- Prepare for hospitalization if the client becomes medically unstable or for rehospitalization if he or she experiences a relapse.

Useful Resources

Families may find the following resources useful:

Books

Brisman, J., Siegel, M., & Weinshel, M. (1997). *Surviving an eating disorder: Strategies for family and friends.*
Buckroyd, J. (1996). *Anorexia and bulimia: Your questions answered.*
Holbrook, T. (2000). *Making weight: Men's conflicts with food, weight, shape, and appearance.*
Natenshon, A.H. (1999). *When your child has an eating disorder.*
Sargent, J.T. (1999). *The long road back: A survivor's guide to anorexia.*
Treasure, J. (1997). *Anorexia nervosa: A survival guide for families, friends, and sufferers.*

Web Sites/Organizations

www.aabainc.org/join/index.html
American Anorexia/Bulimia Association (AABA), Inc.
This site gives information about the AABA, a nonprofit organization dedicated to the prevention and treatment of eating disorders through research, education, and advocacy. The AABA serves as a national authority on eating disorders and related concerns and promotes attitudes that enhance healthy body image.

www.edreferral.com
Eating Disorder Referral and Information Center
This site provides information and treatment resources for various eating disorders.

www.bulimia.com
Eating Disorders Resources
This site specializes in publications and education about eating disorders.

and acceptance from others, and possible deficiencies in social skills. The nurse helps the client see the association between overly high self-expectations and feelings of ineffectiveness and helps the client identify her positive attributes and achieve self-approval. Along with undergoing individual therapy, the client may improve her social skills by participating in group psychotherapy with clients who have similar needs. Successful participation with peers in activities such as recreational or occupational therapy also can enhance self-esteem.

EXPLORING FEELINGS OF POWERLESSNESS

The client's perception of control and autonomy increases as she learns to express her emotions and needs more directly, think in a less rigid fashion, and establish more realistic self-expectations. The nurse encourages the client to assume responsibility for choices and decisions. For the client to take risks and grow, she must trust that the nurse cares about her well-being and will maintain appropriate limits. The nurse assures the client that she will learn to trust in her ability to exert appropriate behavioral controls and act autonomously.

ENCOURAGING EFFECTIVE COPING

When working with clients with eating disorders, the nurse encourages the client to discuss feelings. Clients need to learn that strong feelings, especially those of a "negative" nature, are acceptable and that one can experience and express strong feelings without losing control. Because the client may fear that strong feelings will lead to loss of control, the nurse repeatedly helps to distinguish between feelings and behaviors. The nurse teaches the client that it is normal to have strong feelings that may provoke anxiety and communicates that the client can express those feelings toward another person without being hurtful. As an adjunct therapy, assertiveness training also may help to increase the client's ability to express feelings directly and constructively.

RESTORING FAMILY PROCESSES

When working with clients who have eating disorders, some family therapists recommend focusing on the four dysfunctional interaction patterns identified by Minuchin et al. (1974, 1975): enmeshment, overprotectiveness, rigidity, and lack of conflict resolution. Nurses can work with clients in these four areas in several ways.

Enmeshment and Overprotectiveness

When working with families, the nurse helps all members to make "I" statements instead of "we" statements; for example, "I feel sad" and "I am so angry!" as opposed to "We are all so upset!" The nurse encourages members to speak for themselves and not for each other.

Parents in enmeshed families frequently try to protect their children by speaking for them, as in "She feels happy most of the time." Members are not accustomed to identifying and expressing their own feelings and need frequent prompting from the nurse: "You look upset; what are you feeling right now?" Because enmeshed families typically have weak or inappropriate boundaries between generations, the nurse may ask siblings to sit together as a unit distinct from the parents. Such seating arrangements reinforce appropriate boundaries and help to disrupt dysfunctional alliances that may exist between a parent and child.

Conflict Avoidance and Rigidity

Families of clients with eating disorders tend to brush conflicts under the carpet. It may be an unspoken family rule that feeling sad or upset and having problems are unacceptable. The nurse helps family members to bring existing conflicts to shared awareness. If members try to avoid or deny conflict, the nurse refocuses them on the conflictual issue. The nurse helps members to express their conflict constructively—without shouting, threatening, accusing, or demanding—so that other family members can listen and respond.

Because the client with anorexia may be accustomed to diverting parental conflict onto herself, the nurse keeps the parents talking to each other and instructs them not to involve the adolescent. For example, "Jane is not part of this conflict. This is between you and your wife. Keep talking to her, and don't involve Jane in it." Family members may have difficulty listening to each other's concerns and requests. The nurse models appropriate communication skills and helps members to repattern their communications with one another.

Evaluation

Evaluation of care for the client with eating disorders involves determining if the goals identified in the planning stage were met or if the client and family have made progress toward meeting the goals.

The nurse evaluates the client's physical and psychosocial responses to interventions. Desired physical outcomes include weight gain, normal laboratory values and vital signs, and return of secondary sexual characteristics and menstruation. Desired psychosocial outcomes include a realistic perception of body image, direct expression of feelings, improved self-esteem, a sense of control over self and environment, and constructive family process.

As a client recovers, she may feel guilty about and ashamed of her behavior while ill. Such feelings can persist long after the client attains normal weight. The nurse reassures the client that she could not have prevented herself from becoming ill and that her behavior while ill was an ineffective attempt to cope with stressors. The nurse stresses that the client now has increased coping skills and will not need to resort to the immature responses that she used previously.

The nurse also evaluates the family's interaction patterns. Desired outcomes are that family members communicate directly with each other and deal openly with conflicts and that parents relinquish previous patterns of overcontrol and overprotectiveness to allow the client an appropriate degree of autonomy.

Even if the client and family appear to have met these goals, most clients require follow-up treatment to reinforce behavioral changes and prevent a return of disordered eating. Follow-up should span at least 4 years because of the high rate of relapse.

▼ Reflection and Critical Thinking Questions

Now that you have completed this chapter, consider Clinical Example 23-1 and the related nursing care presented in Nursing Care Plan 23-1. Answer the following questions.

1. Was Kate's initial intervention therapeutic? Can nursing interventions be therapeutic even if the client reacts emotionally to them?

2. One of Kate's concerns will be whether Jody's continuation in sports will jeopardize her health. What factors should Kate consider when discussing sports with Jody? If Jody cannot participate in sports, is she at risk for depression?

3. What role, if any, can Jody's roommate, Mary, play in a treatment plan for Jody?

4. What efforts can schools and their athletic programs make toward preventing eating disorders and identifying them in students? What obstacles may stand in the way of schools taking such measures?

▼ CHAPTER SUMMARY

- Anorexia nervosa and bulimia nervosa primarily affect adolescent and young women.
- Anorexia nervosa and bulimia nervosa share many etiologic factors and may be viewed as existing along a single spectrum of eating disorders.
- Although multiple theories exist, most experts agree that eating disorders develop from a complex interaction of individual, family, and sociocultural factors.
- Clients with eating disorders exhibit disturbances in many or all of the functional health patterns.
- Treatment of clients with eating disorders occurs in community-based and inpatient settings and is a complex and often lengthy process.
- In the current climate of healthcare reform, short-term therapies such as CBT, IPT, and SFBT are being used increasingly.

- Desired client outcomes include normalization of weight and eating patterns, improved self-esteem, and development of realistic thought processes, adaptive coping mechanisms, and constructive family processes.
- Most clients require follow-up treatment to reinforce behavioral changes and prevent a return of disordered eating.

▼ REVIEW QUESTIONS

1. A 21-year-old female client is 5′4″ and weighs 145 lb. She states that two or three times per week she consumes "too much" food and induces vomiting after she becomes sick. She reports that she has done this for several years. The nurse suspects the client may have
   a. Anorexia nervosa
   b. Binge eating disorder
   c. Bulimia nervosa
   d. Eating disorder NOS

2. A 17-year-old client admits to recent use of diuretics and laxatives to lose weight quickly. She is 5′ tall, weighs 90 lb, and has lost 15 lb in 3 weeks. The nurse is most concerned about which of the following possible physiologic consequences of the client's behavior?
   a. Dehydration
   b. Low sodium level
   c. Low potassium level
   d. Anemia

3. The weight maintenance phase of Behavior Family Systems Therapy (BFST) consists of which of the following activities?
   a. The family is engaged in treatment, and the client's weight is checked weekly.
   b. The therapist encourages the parents to take charge of the client's eating and coaches parents to develop an appropriate behavioral weight program.
   c. The therapist streamlines the weight-gain program and introduces nonfood-related issues.
   d. The therapist fosters client individuation and encourages the client to gradually reassume control over food.

4. The nurse at a community mental health center has been coordinating the care of a client with anorexia nervosa. The 5′3″, 16-year-old adolescent has maintained her weight at 110 lb for 6 months. This week, the client appears tired. Her weight has dropped to 104 lb. Her laboratory test results reveal a potassium level of 2.3 mEq and a hemoglobin level of 12 mg/dL. The client states that she has been depressed, restricting foods, and using laxatives. The nurse determines that which of the following management actions is most appropriate?

a. Calling the social worker involved in the client's care to arrange home visits

b. Calling the physician to discuss the need for anti-depressants and potassium supplements

c. Calling the physician to discuss the need for inpatient care

d. Developing a contract with the client that outlines consequences for food restriction and laxative use

5. A client with an eating disorder has been involved in follow-up care for 4 years after her hospitalization for anorexia nervosa. The nurse considers which of the following indicators to be most important when evaluating the effectiveness of the plan of care?

a. The client has maintained her target weight for the last 3 years.

b. The client reports that she has learned to accept her body.

c. The client interacts with her peers.

d. The client has moved into her own apartment.

6. Sixteen-year-old Paula Smith, after returning to school last fall, was referred to the school nurse by several teachers. Paula had had a noticeable weight loss over summer vacation, and faculty members were concerned that she was either ill or anorexic. Betty, the school nurse, arranges a health conference with Paula and contacts Paula's parents. Paula's parents are most likely to describe Paula as

a. Hostile

b. Anxious

c. Manipulative

d. Well-behaved

7. Paula's primary nurse uses a "client contract" approach with her. This technique serves the important function of

a. Providing the client with a feeling of responsibility and control over her behavior

b. Providing the therapist with a strategy for client compliance

c. Allowing the client a tool to negotiate behavior

d. Establishing an effective assessment tool

8. Paula states that she feels fat and ugly. What would be the nurse's most therapeutic response to her statement?

a. "I don't think you are fat and ugly."

b. "Can you help me to understand what you mean by that?"

c. "You are a good 30 lb underweight for your height."

d. "What parts of your body do you like the least?"

9. The nurse asks Paula a question. Paula's mother answers for her. How should the nurse respond?

a. "Thank you for your view, Mrs. Smith. Paula, I'd like to hear what you have to say."

b. "Paula, do you usually let your mother speak for you?"

c. "Paula, do you agree with your mother's answer?"

d. "Paula, does it make you angry when your mother answers for you?"

10. During a family meeting, Paula's parents begin to open up about their conflicts regarding past decisions about child rearing. Paula adds to the discussion, giving her view of events. Paula's mother comments, "We are all so upset by this!" What statement by the nurse is most therapeutic?

a. "Yes, Mrs. Smith, it's understandable that you might feel upset. This isn't easy for any of you. Paula, can you tell your mom and dad a little more about what you said?"

b. "Mrs. Smith, why do you feel that everyone is upset?"

c. "Mr. and Mrs. Smith, parents sometimes do not listen to their children. Please pay attention to Paula's comments."

d. "Mrs. Smith, tell me about your feelings. Then we will hear from Mr. Smith and Paula."

▼ REFERENCES AND SUGGESTED READINGS

Agras, W. S., Walsh, B. T., Fairburn, C. G., Wilson, G. T., & Kraemer, H. C. (2000). A multicenter comparison of cognitive-behavioral therapy and interpersonal psychotherapy for bulimia nervosa. *Archives of General Psychiatry, 57*(5), 459–466.

*American Psychiatric Association. (2000). *Diagnostic and statistical manual of mental disorders* (4th ed., text rev.). Washington, DC: Author.

Ammerman, S., Shih, G., & Ammerman, I. (1996). Unique considerations for treating eating disorders in adolescents and preventive intervention. *Topics in Clinical Nutrition, 12*(1), 79–85.

Anstine, D., & Grinenko, D. (2000). Rapid screening for disordered eating in college-aged females in the primary care setting. *Journal of Adolescent Health, 26*(5), 338–342.

*Brozan, N. (1983, July 18). Anorexia: Not just a disease of the young. *The New York Times*.

Bulik, C. M., Sullivan, P., Wade, T., & Kendler, K. (2000). Twin studies of eating disorders: a review. *International Journal of Eating Disorders, 27*, 1–20.

*Carter, J., Stewart, D. A., Dunn, V., & Fairburn, C. (1997). Primary prevention of eating disorders: Might it do more harm than good? *International Journal of Eating Disorders, 22*, 167–172.

Chally, P. (1998). An eating disorders prevention program. *Journal of Child and Adolescent Psychiatric Nursing, 11*(2), 51–63.

*Ciseaux, A. (1980). Anorexia nervosa: A view from the mirror. *American Journal of Nursing, 80*(8), 1468–1470.

*Clare, L., & Cuthbertson, G. (1998). Ethical issues in the treatment of women with eating disorders. *Mental Health Nursing, 18*(1), 15–17.

*Davis, W. (1998). Eating disorders and case management. *The Case Manager, 9*(1), 35–39.

Eisler, L., Dare, C., Russell, G., Szmukler, G., et al. (1997). Family and individual therapy in anorexia nervosa. *Archives of General Psychiatry, 54*, 1025–1030.

Fairburn, C. G., et al. (1999). A cognitive behavioural theory of anorexia nervosa. *Behavioral Research Therapy, 37*, 1.

*Fairburn, C. G., Jones, R., Peveler, R. C., Hope, R. A., & O'Conner, M. (1993). Psychotherapy and bulimia nervosa: Longer term effects of interpersonal psychotherapy, behavior therapy and cognitive–behavior therapy. *Archives of General Psychiatry, 50*, 419–428.

*Forisha, B., Grothaus, K., & Luscombe, R. (1990). Dinner conversation: Meal therapy to differentiate eating behavior from family process. *Journal of Psychosocial Nursing and Mental Health Services, 28*(11), 12–16.

French, S., et al. (1997). Ethnic differences in psychosocial and health behavior correlates of dieting, purging and binge eating in a population-based sample of adolescent females. *International Journal of Eating Disorders, 22*, 315–322.

*Freund, K., Graham, S., Lesky, L., & Moskowitz, M. (1993). Detection of bulimia in a primary care setting. *Journal of General Internal Medicine, 8*, 236.

Gardner, R. M., Friedman, B. N., & Jackson, N. A. (1999). Body size estimations, body dissatisfaction, and ideal size preferences in children six through thirteen. *Journal of Youth and Adolescence, 28*(5), 603–618.

*Herzog, D., Nussbaum, K., & Marmor, A. (1996). Comorbidity and outcome in eating disorders. *Psychiatric Clinics of North America, 19*, 843.

*Hsu, L. K. G. (1990). *Eating disorders.* New York: Guilford Press.

Katzman, D., Zipursky, R., Lambe, E., & Mikulis, D. (1997). A longitudinal magnetic resonance imaging study of brain changes in adolescents with anorexia nervosa. *Archives of Pediatric and Adolescent Medicine, 151*, 793–797.

*Leitenberg, H. (1994). Comparison of cognitive–behavior therapy and desipramine of bulimia nervosa. *Behavioral Research Therapy, 32*(1), 37–45.

*Lilenfeld, L., Strober, M., & Kaye, W. H. (1997). Genetics and family studies of anorexia nervosa and bulimia nervosa. *International Practice and Research, 3*, 177–197.

*Lyons, M. A. (1998). The phenomenon of compulsive overeating in a selected group of professional women. *Journal of Advanced Nursing, 27*, 1158–1164.

*Marcus, M., & Levine, M. (1998). Eating disorder treatment: An update. *Current Opinion in Psychiatry, 11*, 159–163.

*McFarland, B. (1995). *Brief therapy and eating disorders.* San Francisco: Jossey-Bass.

*Michielli, D., Dunbar, C., & Kalinski, M. (1994). Is exercise indicated for the patient diagnosed as anorectic? *Journal of Psychosocial Nursing, 32*(8), 33–35.

*Minuchin, S. (1974). *Families and family therapy.* Cambridge, MA: Howard University Press.

*Minuchin, S., Baker, L., Rosman, B., Liebman, R., Milman, L., & Todd, T. (1975). A conceptual model of psychosomatic illness in children: Family organization and family therapy. *Archives of General Psychiatry, 32*, 1031–1038.

Neumark-Sztainer, D. (1996). School-based programs for pre-venting eating disturbances. *Journal of School Health, 66*(2), 64–71.

*Olivardia, R., Pope, H., et al. (1995). Eating disorders in college men. *American Journal of Psychiatry, 152*, 1279.

*Owen, S., & Fullerton, M. (1995). A discussion group in a behaviorally oriented inpatient eating disorder program. *Journal of Psychosocial Nursing, 33*(11), 35–40.

*Perkins, A., Fritz, J., Barber, C., & Turner, J. (1997). The prevalence and correlates of eating disorder tendencies in older women. *Journal of Women and Aging, 9*(3), 67–84.

Putukian, M. (1998). The female athlete triad. *Clinics in Sports Medicine, 17*(4), 675–696.

*Robin, A. I., Bedway, M., Siegel, P. T., Moye, A. W., & Gilroy, M. (1997). Therapy for adolescent anorexia nervosa: Addressing cognitions, feelings, and the family's role. In E. D. Hibbs & P. S. Jensen (Eds.), *Psychosocial treatments for child and adolescent disorders: Empirically based strategies for clinical practice* (pp. 239–259). Washington, DC: American Psychological Association Press.

*Robin, A. I., Siegel, P. T., Moye, A. W., Gilroy, M., Dennis, A. B., & Sikand, A. (1999). A controlled comparison of family versus individual therapy for adolescents with anorexia nervosa. *Journal of the Academy of Child and Adolescent Psychiatry, 38*(12), 1482–1489.

*Rogers, L., Resnick, M., Mitchell, J., & Blum, R. (1997). The relationship between socioeconomic status and eating-disordered behaviors in a community sample of adolescent girls. *International Journal of Eating Disorders, 22*, 15–23.

Stice, E., Akutagawa, D., Gaggar, A., & Agras, W. S. (2000). Negative effect moderates the relation between dieting and binge eating. *International Journal of Eating Disorders, 27*(2), 218–219.

Strober, M., et al. (2000). Controlled family study of anorexia nervosa and bulimia nervosa: Evidence of shared liability and transmission of partial syndromes. *American Journal of Psychiatry, 152*, 1630.

*Strober, M. (1995). Family genetic perspectives on anorexia nervosa and bulimia nervosa. In K. Brownell & C. G. Fairburn (Eds.), *Eating disorders and obesity: A comprehensive handbook* (pp. 212–218). New York: Guilford Press.

*Strober, M. (1991). Family genetic studies of eating disorders. *Journal of Clinical Psychiatry, 52*, (Suppl), 9–12.

Turner, J., Batik, M., & Palmer, L. J. (2000). Detection and importance of laxative abuse in adolescents with anorexia nervosa. *Journal of the American Academy of Child and Adolescent Psychiatry, 39*(3), 378–385.

Wade, T., et al. (2000). Anorexia nervosa and major depression: Shared genetic and environmental risk factors. *American Journal of Psychiatry, 157*(3), 469.

Walsh, B. T., Wilson, G. T., Loeb, K. L., Devlin, M., et al. (1997). Medication and psychotherapy in the treatment of bulimia nervosa. *American Journal of Psychiatry, 154*, 523–531.

Watkins, P., Cartiglia, M., & Champion, J. (1998). Are Type A tendencies in women associated with eating disorder pathology? *Journal of Gender, Culture and Health, 3*(2), 101–109.

*Weiss, M. (1995). Eating disorders and disordered eating in different cultures. *The Psychiatric Clinics of North America, 18*(3), 537–553.

*Williamson, L. (1998). Eating disorders and the cultural forces behind the drive for thinness: Are African American women really protected? *Social Work in Health Care, 28*(1), 61–73.

*Wilson, G. T. (1995). Psychological treatment of binge eating and bulimia nervosa. *Journal of Mental Health, 4,* 451–457.

Wiser, S., & Telch, C. F. (1999). Dialectic behavior therapy for binge eating disorder. *Journal of Clinical Psychology, 55*(6), 755–768.

*Woolsey, M. (1998). When food becomes a cry for help. *Journal of the American Dietetic Association, 98*(4), 395–398.

Zipfel, S., Lowe, B., Reas, D. L., Deter, H., & Herzog, W. (2000). Long-term prognosis in anorexia nervosa: Lessons from a 21-year follow-up study. *Lancet, 355,* 721–722.

Starred references are cited in text.

For additional information on this chapter, go to *http://connection. lww.com.*

Need more help? See Chapter 23 of the *Study Guide to Accompany Mohr: Johnson's Psychiatric-Mental Health Nursing,* 5th ed.

The Client With a Mood Disorder

CAROL J. CORNWELL

▼ KEY TERMS

Affect—The outward expression of emotion; it is of shorter duration, more variable, and more reactive than the underlying *mood*, which is more pervasive and stable.

Cyclothymia—A disorder resembling bipolar disorder, with less severe symptoms, characterized by repeated periods of nonpsychotic depression and hypomania for at least 2 years (1 year for children and adolescents).

Dysthymia—A milder form of depressive illness in which symptoms are less severe than those of depressive disorder but may be chronic.

Electroconvulsive therapy (ECT)—A therapy that involves the application of a small dose of electricity to one or both sides of the brain to induce a seizure.

Hypomania—A subcategory of mania, slightly less severe and without the

psychotic features or severely impaired functioning that would require hospitalization.

Manic episodes — Periods of an abnormally and persistently elevated, expansive, or irritable mood.

Mood—A pervasive, sustained emotional coloring of one's experience.

Phototherapy—Use of artificial light therapy to prevent and treat depression with a seasonal pattern.

▼ LEARNING OBJECTIVES

On completion of this chapter, you should be able to accomplish the following:

- Describe examples of mood disorders.
- Discuss the incidence and prevalence of major mood disorders in the United States.
- Analyze differences between theories of the etiology of mood disorders.
- List the symptoms of depressive and bipolar disorders using criteria from the American Psychiatric Association's *Diagnostic and Statistical Manual of Mental Disorders,* 4th edition, text revision.
- Discuss interdisciplinary treatment modalities for clients with mood disorders.
- Apply the nursing process to the care of clients with mood disorders.

▼ Clinical Example 24-1

Jill, 35, and her husband Shane, 37, have been married for 12 years and have three children, ages 10, 7, and 4. They arrive at the psychiatric-mental health nurse practitioner's office after getting a referral from Jill's primary care physician. During the past month, Shane has

noticed that Jill has difficulty staying asleep through the night, awakening at around 3 AM each morning. She has stopped attending the children's sports and school activities, which were a source of great pleasure and pride for her, and she has been sleeping for up to 3 to 4 hours during the day, which is uncharacteristic of the usually energetic Jill. Shane has been becoming more concerned about Jill because she has been neglecting her day-to-day hygiene and has not been participating in any child-care activities, household activities, or arts and crafts, in which she had previously taken delight. Her work as a part-time reporter for the local paper also has been suffering because she has been unable to focus on writing and is too exhausted to interview people. Jill begins to cry during the interview, stating, "I didn't want to come today. Now you know that I'm a terrible mother, and I haven't even been doing my job as a wife and partner, either." Despite Shane's encouragement and attempts to dissuade Jill from these thoughts, she is adamant that she has become "a terrible person, and I'm really no good to anyone anymore. I just wish I were not here to bother everyone."

This chapter discusses mood disorders, specifically major depressive disorder, dysthymic disorder, and bipolar disorder. As you read the chapter, consider the case of Jill in

Clinical Example 24-1 and Danielle in Clinical Example 24-2 below. How do these clients' histories and signs and symptoms relate to this group of disorders? You will learn more about the progression of Jill's and Danielle's care in Nursing Care Plans 24-1 and 24-2. You will also have the opportunity to apply your understanding of these clients and others with mood disorders in the Reflection and Critical Thinking Questions at the end of this chapter.

▼ *Clinical Example 24-2*

Danielle is a 45-year-old mother of two who has just been admitted to the acute inpatient psychiatric unit. According to Roger, her husband of 10 years, Danielle has "been depressed off and on since she was 25 but has never been diagnosed with a psychiatric disorder." During the past 6 months, Roger has noticed that she has been staying up more and more during the night. Danielle is a wedding videographer, and Roger reports that she has been taking her video camera out during the night and taping scenes all over the city. She has also become very irritable, snapping at their two children, ages 3 and 9, for small infractions, which is uncharacteristic of Danielle. According to Roger, Danielle is typically a loving, caring, nurturing mother and enjoys her children a great deal, often attending their soccer games at school and never missing an open house. The previous night, Danielle was found by the local police, driving 80 miles per hour down the main street of the city while taking video shots. She was stopped and became belligerent to the officer, shouting obscenities. The officer reported that Danielle claimed she was the "president's personal video assistant, and I have to finish this job before I meet him this morning!" The officer then brought her to the local emergency room, where she was admitted involuntarily to psychiatry.

MOOD DISORDERS

Mood is defined as a pervasive, sustained emotional coloring of one's experience. Extreme changes in mood can signal a mood disorder. These disorders have been described for more than 40 centuries, with ancient sufferers such as Nebuchadnezzar, Saul, and Herod. Hippocrates (460–377 BC) hypothesized that black bile (melancholia), a toxic product of digestion, caused depression. This belief may have been the first "biological" causal theory of mood disorders. Many famous people have experienced the pain of mood disorders, including Fyodor Dostoyevsky, Edgar Allan Poe, Nathaniel Hawthorne, Abraham Lincoln, Winston Churchill, and more recently, Mike Wallace, Kitty Dukakis, Joan Rivers, and first ladies Betty Ford and Barbara Bush. Mood disorders know no socioeconomic or racial boundaries.

Mood disorders, which include major depressive disorder, dysthymic disorder, and bipolar disorder, are associated with disturbances in psychological, physiological, and social functioning. They are characterized by many symptoms, of which mood is only one. Other symptoms include vegetative signs (eg, problems with sleep, appetite, weight, libido), cognitive features (eg, distorted attention, memory, thinking), impulse control problems (eg, suicide, homicide), behavioral features (eg, withdrawal, pleasure, fatigability), and somatic features (eg, headache, stomachache, muscle tension) (Stahl, 1996).

Because mood is an unseen entity, mood disorders often go undetected. The average client with bipolar disorder has seen four physicians before his or her disorder is correctly diagnosed (Bowden, 2001). If untreated, clients may suffer for months or even years with an illness that is highly treatable. The economic costs to society and personal costs are enormous. In the United States alone, the estimated monetary costs for mood disorders exceeded $44 billion in 1990. The personal costs are reflected by higher mortality and impairment in multiple areas of functioning. The World Health Organization (WHO) estimates that depressive disorders are the leading cause of disability in the United States and other economies worldwide (Murray & Lopez, 1996).

Epidemiology

About 18.8 million American adults, or about 9.5% of the U.S. population 18 years of age or older, have a depressive disorder in a given year (National Institute of Mental Health [NIMH], 2001). Nearly twice as many women (6.5%) as men (3.3%) suffer from major depressive disorder every year, with the average age of onset being the mid-20s. Dysthymic disorder affects about 5.4% of the U.S. population (NIMH, 2001). About 40% of adults who meet criteria for dysthymia also meet criteria for major depressive disorder or bipolar disorder during a given year. Bipolar disorder affects about 1.2% of Americans, with men and women being equally as likely to develop this disorder. The average age for a first manic episode is the early 20s (NIMH, 2001).

Clients at highest risk for recurrent depressive disorders include those whose first depression was before age 25, those who have had more than 16 weeks of depression in their lifetimes, and those who have had a recurrence of depression within 2 months of discontinuing an antidepressant (Bowden, 2001).

Mood disorders in children and teenagers are a significant problem in America. Studies have reported that up to 2.5% of children and up to 8.3% of adolescents in the United States suffer from mood disorders (Birmaher, Ryan, & Williamson, et al., 1996). One longitudinal prospective study found that early-onset depression often continues into adulthood, which indicates that mood disorders in youth may also predict more severe illness in adult life (Weissman, Wolk, Goldstein, et al., 1999). See

Chapter 29 for an in-depth discussion of mood disorders in children and adolescents.

Mood disorders in older adults also are a significant problem. About 6% of Americans 65 years of age or older (or about 2 million of the 34 million adults in this age group in 1998) have a diagnosable depressive illness (major depressive disorder, bipolar disorder, or dysthymic disorder) (Narrow, 1998) in a given year (see Chap. 30).

Suicide is a frequent companion to mood disorders and has been identified recently as an emergent national public health priority. In 1998, suicide was the eighth leading cause of death for all Americans and the third leading cause of death for people between the ages of 15 and 24 years (McIntosh, 2001; Murphy, 2000). Older Americans are disproportionately likely to commit suicide. Although people 65 years of age or older make up about 13% of the U.S. population, this age group accounted for 19% of all suicide deaths in 1997 (Hoyert, Kochanek, & Murphy, 1999). The highest rate is for white men ages 85 years and older; in 1997 there were 64.9 deaths per 100,000 persons in this group, about 6 times the national U.S. rate of 10.6 per 100,000 (Hoyert et al., 1999). Suicide is a complex behavior, and most people who commit suicide successfully have an underlying mental or substance abuse disorder or both (Blumenthal & Kupfer, 1990; Centers for Disease Control and Prevention [CDC], 2001; Harris & Barraclough, 1997) (Implications for Nursing Practice 24-1).

Etiology

Increasingly sophisticated scientific technologies make it possible to target the causes of mood disorders more clearly and concisely. Although a definitive cause has not been discovered, research in recent years has focused primarily on neurobiology and the neurosciences. Scientists agree that a combination of or interaction among several factors, such as genes, the environment, individual life history and development, and neurobiologic makeup, cause mood disorders. Hyman (2000) speaks about the necessity for continued and vigorous research on finding vulnerability genes for the depressive disorders. Regarding research initiatives, NIMH representatives have indicated, "We want to understand how mood states are represented in the brain, how genes and environmental factors during development affect the regulation to mood—and its representation in the brain. We also want to understand how salient stimuli affect mood at both brain and experimental levels in health and disease" (Hyman, 2000, p. 437).

GENETIC FACTORS

In general, extensive research continues in the area of behavioral genetics, or how genes influence human behavior, as related to the etiology of depressive and bipolar disorders. Many studies have contributed to the growing body of knowledge regarding genetic factors in

Implications for Nursing Practice 24-1

Suicide Survivors: Helping Those Left Behind

The suicide of a friend or loved one deeply and painfully affects approximately 200,000 people a year. These people, referred to as suicide survivors or suicide grievers, experience the sudden, often violent loss of a loved one. The loss of a loved one by suicide is not the same as the loss of a loved one to a physical health problem or even an accidental death. Suicide is stigmatized in our society, and the survivors do not experience the same outpouring of support as others who suffer a loss. In fact, suicide survivors don't "get over" the loss but instead are forever changed by it. They suffer a range of difficult emotions and may, themselves, develop depression, suicidality or, if they witnessed the suicide or found the body, post-traumatic stress disorder (PTSD).

As a nurse, you can offer support and guidance to the survivors to help them come to terms with this agonizing loss by discussing the emotions that suicide survivors report to help the family member(s) or friend(s) feel less alone. Explain that the emotions usually do subside with time, but there is no set time frame for the process. Let them know that these painful feelings may recur, particularly during a special holiday or on the anniversary of the suicide. Some of the emotional responses suicide survivors may experience include:

- Feelings of unreality, shock, disbelief, and emotional numbness
- Grief, sadness, and despair
- Confusion over not knowing why the loved one chose suicide
- Anger toward the mental health practitioner, another family member, or a friend for failing to prevent the suicide
- Self-anger and guilt for failing to prevent the suicide
- Feelings of anger toward and betrayal by the loved one who committed suicide
- Social stigmatization and isolation

In addition to helping the family member or friend work through the feelings of loss, grief, and anger, suggest that the suicide survivor seek professional mental health counseling for a time after the suicide. Suicide survivors have a real risk for developing depression or PTSD, which can be prevented or appropriately treated with counseling or psychotherapy. Also, help the family member find a support group for suicide survivors and encourage him or her to talk openly with other family members and friends of the deceased. Stress the importance of not withdrawing from others, but of maintaining social support systems.

major depressive disorders (Klein, Schwartz, Rose et al, 2000). Three decades of family studies reveal that the range in age-adjusted risk of depression for first-degree relatives of a depressed individual is from 5% to 25% (Moldin, Reich, & Rice, 1991; Tsuang & Faraone, 1990). The results of three adoption studies on unipolar depression are consistent with twin data that provide evidence for a genetic component in the etiology of unipolar depression (Cadoret, 1978; Mendlewicz & Rainer, 1977; Wender, Kety, Rosenthal, Schulsinger, Ortmann, & Lunde, 1986).

Regarding bipolar disorder, the mode of inheritance is complex. It most likely involves a combination of multiple interacting genes. The number of loci, the recurrence risk ratio that each locus confers, and the degree of interlocus interaction are unknown, but it seems there is not a single, major locus that accounts for how bipolar disorder aggregates within certain families (Tsuang & Faraone, 1990). Data from more than 40 family and twin studies consistently show that the risk to relatives of those with bipolar disorder is greater than the risk to relatives of those without (Goodwin & Jamison, 1990; Tsuang & Faraone, 1990; Weissman, et al., 1984; Winokur, Tsuang, & Crowe, 1982). No genetic region has yet been identified as the location of bipolar susceptibility. Most current evidence points to a susceptibility loci on chromosomal regions 18p, 18q, and 21q, but these findings are not confirmed (De Bruyn, Souery, Mendelbaum, Mendlewicz, & Van Broeckhoven, 1996; Detera-Wadleigh et al., 1997). Ongoing studies into the genetic etiology of the mood disorders will provide knowledge that may help identify susceptible individuals and thus promote primary prevention efforts.

PHYSIOLOGIC FACTORS

Among the theories about the etiology of the mood disorders, physiologic factors have taken precedence. With the explosion of research and knowledge in the area of molecular biology in the past decade, scientists are coming closer than ever to unraveling the mysteries of the biophysiological mechanisms underlying mood disorders.

Several brain areas are involved in mood disorders (Figure 24-1) (Nemeroff, 1998), most of which are located in the limbic system. Reduced neurologic activity in the areas of the brain that are regulated by the neurotransmitters norepinephrine (NE) and serotonin contribute to mood disorders. NE-producing cells project from the locus ceruleus to other parts of the brain.

Biogenic Amines

Originally, the biogenic amine hypothesis held that depression resulted from a deficiency in the biogenic amines, which are neurotransmitters synthesized by enzymes in the nerve terminal. This idea was first hypothesized when clients who were being treated for hypertension with the biogenic amine-depleting agent reserpine became depressed. Conversely, some clients who were taking iproniazid, a biogenic-enhancing agent used to treat tuberculosis, were experiencing euphoria. The monoamines that

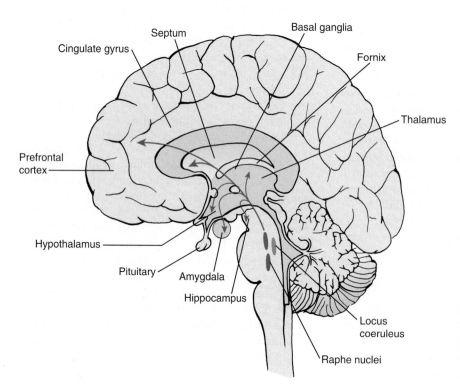

FIGURE 24-1 Brain regions involved in mood disorders. Except for the pituitary gland, all regions are broadly considered part of the limbic system, and all normally receive signals from neurons that secrete serotonin (5-HT), norepinephrine (NE), or both. Reduced activity in the circuits that use 5-HT and NE apparently contribute to depression. The arrows indicate some 5-HT pathways. (Adapted from Nemeroff, C. B. [1998]. The neurobiology of depression. *Scientific American, 278* [6], 42–49.)

have been implicated in the mood disorders are the cate-cholamines, NE and dopamine (DA), and the indolamine called serotonin (5-HT). The monoamine hypothesis of depression holds that the biological basis for depression is a deficiency in NE, 5-HT, or both (Leonard, 1997, 2000; Racagni & Brunello, 1999).

Norepinephrine. The noradrenergic neuron uses NE as its major neurotransmitter (Figure 24-2A). The major hypothesis about monoamines and depression has been that the absolute concentrations of NE, 5-HT, or both are deficient in depression. Evidence also supports, however, that metabolism may be altered with altered numbers, affinities, or both of the 5-HT and NE receptors and uptake sites. More recently, focus has been on the possibility that second messenger systems are involved, as well as the notion of "cross-talk" between the NE and 5-HT systems, which are related to mood disorders (Leonard, 2000).

Dopamine. The neurotransmitter DA is synthesized by two of the three enzymes that also synthesize NE; how-ever, DA neurons do not have dopamine beta hydroxylase (DBH) and thus cannot break down DA into NE (Figure 24-2B) (Stahl, 1996). This leaves DA to be stored and released from the dopaminergic neuron. There are many DA receptor subtypes. The most extensively studied is the DA2 receptor. It is stimulated by dopaminergic agonists such as those used in treating Parkinson's disease, and it is blocked by DA antagonist neuroleptics for the treatment of schizophrenia.

Serotonin. Serotonin, or 5-HT, is the neurotransmit-ter within the serotonergic neuron (Figure 24-3). Plasma transports the amino acid tryptophan into the brain, which uses tryptophan as the precursor to 5-HT in the seroton-ergic neuron. Two enzymes then convert tryptophan into 5-HT—tryptophan hydroxylase and aromatic amino acid decarboxylase. As with NE and DA, monoamine oxidase (MAO) destroys 5-HT, converting it into an inactive metabolite. The amount of 5-HT in the synapse and types of receptors affect the cell's response to 5-HT; 5-HT receptors come in at least 13 "flavors" (Nemeroff, 1998).

Psychoneuroendocrine and Immune Relationships

The hypothalamic-pituitary-adrenal (HPA) axis is classically considered the stress axis and has complex feed-forward and feedback mechanisms that interact with multiple body systems (Figure 24-4) (Nemeroff, 1998). The hypothalamus, pituitary gland, adrenal gland (HPA axis), and endocrine system are closely connected. The hypothalamus, interacting with the central nervous sys-tem (CNS), acts on the pituitary through corticotropin-releasing hormone (CRH), which then stimulates the adrenal medulla, through adrenocorticotropic hormone (ACTH), to secrete catecholamines and cortisol. Both

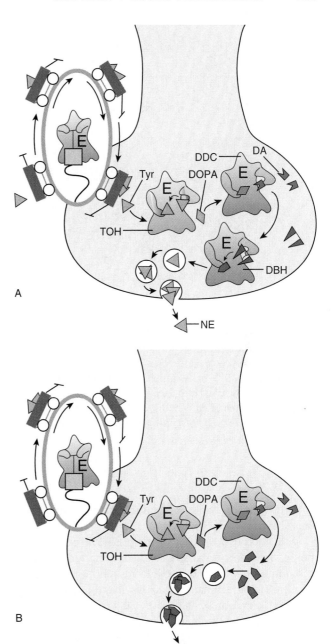

FIGURE 24-2   (**A**) Production of norepinephrine (NE) starts with transport of its amino acid precursor, tyrosine (Tyr), into the nervous system through an active transport pump. This pump is separate from the active transport pump for NE itself. Once Tyr is pumped inside the neuron, three enzymes act upon it in sequence: (1) tyrosine hydroxylase (TOH), which converts Tyr into DOPA; (2) DOPA decar-boxylase (DDC), which converts DOPA into dopamine (DA); and (3) dopamine beta hydroxylase (DBH), which converts DA into NE. (**B**) DA is produced in dopaminergic neurons from its precursor Tyr, which is transported into the neuron by an active transport pump. Two of the same enzymes that synthesize NE convert DA: TOH, which produces DOPA, and DDC, which produces DA. (Adapted from Stahl, S.M. [1996]. *Essential psychopharmacology: Neuroscientific basis and practical applications.* Cambridge: Cambridge University Press.)

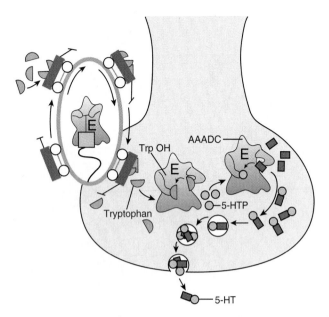

FIGURE 24-3 Serotonin (5-HT) is produced from enzymes after its amino acid precursor tryptophan is transported into the 5-HT neuron. Tryptophan is then converted into 5-hydroxy-tryptophan (5-HTP) by tryptophan hydroxylase (Trp OH). 5-HTP is then converted into 5-HT by decarboxylase (AAADC). (Adapted from Stahl, S.M. [1996]. *Essential psychopharmacology: Neuroscientific basis and practical applications.* Cambridge: Cambridge University Press.)

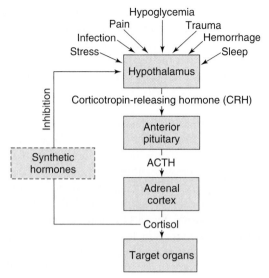

FIGURE 24-4 The hypothalamic-pituitary-adrenal (HPA) axis actively responds to stress. Mounting evidence suggests that chronic overactivity of the axis, particularly of CRH, contributes to depression.

are known to modulate the endocrine and immune systems (Nemeroff, 1998).

Sustained hyperactivity of the HPA axis occurs in response to uncontrollable stressors. This results in the hypersecretion of adrenal glucocorticoids and corticotropin-releasing factor (Leonard, 2000). In major depression, the protracted elevation of glucocorticoid levels causes a desensitization of the central glucocorticoid receptors and probably also those receptors located on macrophages, an important component of the immune response (Leonard, 2001). In fact, many aspects of cellular immunity are activated during depressive illness, even though other immunologic markers are suppressed. Cells of the immune system produce bioactive neuroendocrine hormones and have receptors for many of these hormones. The immune system may be thought of as a sensory organ for external stimuli such as bacteria, viruses, and tumors, whereas the CNS detects classic sensory stimuli.

The classic and recent works of Ader and colleagues have provided ample evidence of linkages between the autonomic nervous system and the immune system in response to various natural and experimental conditions involving the stress response (Ader, 2000a, 2000b; Ader, Cohen, & Felten, 1990; Glaser et al., 1999; Larson, Ader, & Moynihan, 2001). There is evidence that the hyper-

secretion of cortisol and proinflammatory cytokines that are secreted by activated macrophages of the immune system result in the malfunctioning of noradrenergic and serotonergic neurotransmission in the brain (Leonard, 2001). Increasingly, studies are finding that, in addition to providing communication between immune cells, the cytokines also signal the brain to produce neurochemical, neuroendocrine, neuroimmune, and behavioral changes (Kronfol & Remick, 2000). This emerging field of study on cytokines provides rich information about the physiologic milieu within which the psychological, neurologic, endocrine, and immune systems may interact in the etiology of mood disorders.

PSYCHOLOGICAL FACTORS

Before the discovery of psychotropic medications in the early 1950s and the associated growth in biochemical and neurological understanding of the brain and its function, psychological theories prevailed regarding the etiology of most mental illnesses, including the mood disorders. In other words, many practitioners and researchers believed that psychosocial factors were important in "causing" depressive disorders. In recent years, with the advent of more specific and refined medications for the mood disorders, it is now clear that the etiology of these disorders has a strong biological component and that, in fact, most depressive disorders are primarily "caused by" neurochemical imbalances and physiological disturbances in brain chemistry. Many clinicians believe that the mood disorders result from a complex interplay between biological and psychological factors, which are usually impossible to separate. Biological factors, however, have emerged as the most salient of the etiological factors in these and in many other psychiatric disorders.

Even though much literature on current treatments for all mood disorders focuses on psychopharmacological interventions, psychosocial factors do play a profound role in how the individual *responds* to these illnesses. Psychological and social issues significantly influence how clients and their families cope with chronic illnesses, such as the mood disorders, after they develop. Historically, psychosocial theories were discussed in regard to their role in "causing" depressive illness; however, in the following sections, they are discussed in regard to their implications for ongoing treatment. Thus psychodynamic, cognitive, and feminist theories are not seen as "causes" of depressive illness; rather they are seen as frameworks from which to plan effective psychosocial interventions. Hyman (2000) states that more potent psychosocial interventions are needed in the realm of treatment adherence; for example, during a manic episode, the client with bipolar disorder sees no need to take his or her medications because he or she feels so good. It is critical that providers establish therapeutic relationships to provide consistent, client-specific therapies during disease recurrences. Therefore, it is essential to understand some of the traditional and historical theoretical foundations that underlie nonpharmacologic treatments for mood disorders.

Psychodynamic Factors

Many therapists and counselors whose clinical training is in psychodynamic therapy continue to extensively use psychodynamic theories of depression to guide psychotherapy (Bowden, 2001). The preponderance of research regarding the efficacy of psychodynamic and psychoanalytic therapy in depression reports that these therapies are most effective if combined with psychotropic medications (Keller, McCullough, Klein et al., 2000). Briefly, psychodynamic theories postulate that clients who are depressed have unexpressed and unconscious anger as a reaction to being helpless or dependent on others. In these situations, clients cannot express their emotions because of their dependency on the object of their anger, so they turn their anger inward. Psychodynamic theorists would state that this anger begins during the child's development, when basic, early, developmental needs are not met. The child then begins to see the world as a hostile, unpredictable place in which the child blames himself or herself and feels angry and inferior. Freud said that depression results, as well as a fragile sense of self-esteem and competence (Freud, 1957). Psychoanalytic theorists posit a link between mood disorders that occur later in life and unmet dependency needs in childhood. Many therapists who work with clients with mood disorders use the psychoanalytic model to assess their clients (eg, in regard to their feelings of helplessness, dependency needs, and anger) and then use the basic tenets of the theory to design interventions that enhance the client's function and self-perception in those areas.

Learned Helplessness

Although learned helplessness as an etiological, or causal factor, in affective disorders has received less attention since the advent of molecular biology and the explosion of knowledge in the neurophysiology of depression, it continues to be used in many areas as a context from which to understand depression and its symptoms and from which to develop therapeutic treatments. A review of the literature in which learned helplessness is cited within the abstract or article reveals that more than 180 articles (many clinical and some research articles) have been published since 1997. Since the learned helplessness paradigm continues to receive attention in the literature and in practice, it may help the reader to understand its basic theoretical concepts.

Seligman first proposed the theory of learned helplessness as an antecedent to depression (Seligman, Friedman, & Katz, 1974). The original theoretical model proposed that people who are susceptible to mood disorders have encountered a lifetime of experiences that have taught them that they are ineffective and have no influence on the factors that cause their suffering. Behaviors that define learned helplessness, such as passivity, negative expectations, and feelings of helplessness, hopelessness, and powerlessness, are symptoms of major depression.

Several studies in recent years have used a "learned helplessness paradigm" as a context for supporting research and intervention efforts with clients suffering from depression and other disorders that have depressive components (Andersen, 1999; Ellgring, 1999; Greer, 2000). Learned helplessness has even been used as a paradigm to explore neurobiological effects of certain neurotropic factors in the brain (Altar, 1999).

It may be helpful to view the learned helplessness paradigm as more relevant to the client's experience following the emergence of mood disorders instead of as a precipitator, or "causal" agent. In any case, the theory of learned helplessness continues to emerge in the literature as a commonly used framework for psychotherapeutic interventions.

Cognitive Factors

Cognitive theory states that clients experience depression because of errors in thinking and unrealistic attitudes about themselves and the world. The cognitive view holds that cognitive (thinking) errors precede mood changes. These errors involve faulty thinking about oneself, having a negative view about one's ability to achieve goals, and being unable to experience pleasure. Self-depreciation and unrealistic expectations cause recurrent dissatisfaction, which leads to depression. For more information about cognitive theory, see the Interdisciplinary Goals and Treatment section later in this chapter and Chapters 3 and 8.

Feminist Factors

Beeber (1996), an advanced practice psychiatric-mental health nurse who has done extensive research and practice in the area of mood disorders in women, discusses them within the context of contemporary American society. Stating that the larger social environment affects the incidence and prevalence of mood disorders in women, Beeber points out that contemporary women often struggle with the discrepancy between their personal goals and aspirations and the reality of cultural definitions and boundaries surrounding gender issues. Box 24-1 presents a powerful excerpt from Beeber's work, in which she discusses depression in women as "an expression of biological, interpersonal, and social processes that coalesce to create a vulnerability for women" (Beeber, 1996, p. 236).

Signs and Symptoms / Diagnostic Criteria

The mood disorders can be categorized in various ways, depending on the number of symptoms, their severity, and persistence. If depression is seen as existing on a continuum

from health to illness and as sometimes serving a useful function (Figure 24-5), the reaction of grief and the process of mourning would be placed at the healthy end of the continuum. Major depression, dysthymia, and bipolar disorders have been argued to be distinct, biologically different disorders. They can be grouped by their severity and distance from euthymic state (Figure 24-5). This chapter will review the *Diagnostic and Statistical Manual of Mental Disorders,* 4th edition, text revision (*DSM-IV-TR)* spectrum of mood disorders, including major depressive disorder, dysthymia, the bipolar disorders (bipolar I and bipolar II), and cyclothymic disorder (American Psychiatric Association [APA], 2000). For detailed descriptions of *DSM-IV-TR* criteria, see this chapter's information map.

MAJOR DEPRESSIVE DISORDER

Depression that seems to occur without any relationship to external events is sometimes called *endogenous depression.* This is in contrast to *reactive* or *exogenous depression,* the cause of which is evident from the client's history. The differing terms used to label depression are the result of the efforts of mental health caregivers to provide accu-

---

BOX 24-1 ▼ *Depression and Women*

The prevalence of depression in women and the insidious nature of this disorder present a clear and present danger to the personal development of women. Except in its most severe forms, depression masquerades as fatigue, laziness, confusion, lack of organization, and a variety of qualities that are maligned in the contemporary American quest for productivity and efficiency. As these qualities resonate with deeply held attitudes that women are not capable of achieving excellence, the appearance of these behaviors is not viewed with alarm, but rather a perception that the expected has materialized. Qualities associated with depression—such as social withdrawal, blunted reactivity to situations, and diminished ability to act efficaciously—invite those around the depressed woman to back away, ignore the problems, and overlook the gradual decline. These attitudes confirm the depressed woman's perception that her contribution was never intrinsically worth much at all. Consequently, the young woman who is failing a course, the mother who cannot energetically nurture her young children, the career woman whose productivity is faltering, and the older woman who isolates herself after her husband dies are all treated with a shrug, or worse, a moralistic "get yourself moving" approach. The losses are immeasurable because in many ways, traditional forms of women's work do not lend themselves to traditional measure of worth. Although there is a reason to be concerned about the potential lethality of depression by virtue of its rela-

tionship with suicide, death in more subtle ways must also be of concern to those who care for women.

Another danger that depression presents to women is the progressive nature of the disorder. Far from being a quiescent phenomenon, depression produces unrelenting symptoms that, over time, destroy meaningful human connections to work and love. Depression ideally requires aggressive, sustained interventions within a context of a deep, professional commitment to another person. The episodic, short-term nature of the American mental health care system does not allow for this type of relationship, creating a treatment response that is primarily symptom focused; it aims to restore previous functioning rather than to seek a better-than-previous functional outcome. Treatment systems are restricted, and the options that are offered to a client often reflect an institution's philosophy rather than the treatment options that are best for the person in question.

Within this context, depression as a health problem for women emerges as a challenge for psychiatric nursing that requires a commitment to holism, humanism, and care in the context of the professional relationship.

From Beeber, L. S. (1996). Depression in women. In A. B. McBride & J. K. Austin, *Psychiatric-mental health nursing: Integrating the behavioral and biological sciences.* Philadelphia: W.B. Saunders.

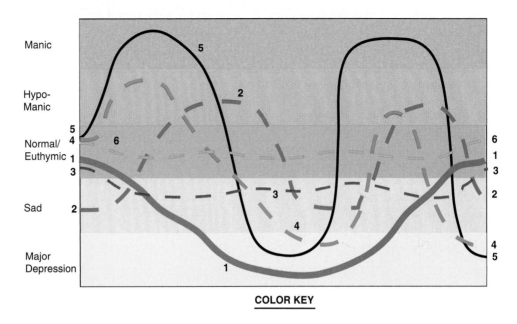

COLOR KEY

FIGURE 24-5   Mood disorder patterns.

1 = Blue = Major Depressive Episodes
3 = Magenta = Dysthymic Disorder
5 = Black = BiPolar I Disorder

2 = Purple = Cyclothymic Disorder
4 = Green = BiPolar II Disorder
6 = Yellow = Normal/Euthymic

rate descriptions of the depressive process. Accurate classification and descriptions of depression aid in diagnosis, guide treatment, and facilitate professional communication and research efforts.

According to the *DSM-IV-TR* (APA, 2000), a client diagnosed with major depressive disorder must have either a depressed mood or a loss of interest or inability to derive pleasure from previously enjoyable activities. Other symptoms include recurrent thoughts of suicide, decreased or increased appetite, inability to concentrate, difficulty making decisions, feelings of worthlessness and self-blame, decreased energy, motor disturbances (agitation or severe slowness), disturbed sleep (insomnia or excessive sleeping), substance abuse, and social withdrawal. Also, the client with depression often disregards grooming, cleanliness, and personal appearance. Stooped posture and dejected facial expression are nonverbal messages of depression. These clients may present disheveled, downcast, without eye contact, and tearful. Conversely, they may be agitated but usually do not exhibit bizarre or unusual behaviors. Many clients with depression remain in their rooms, beds, or chairs. They resist attempts by others to engage them in the environment. They tend to exhibit withdrawn behavior within a very circumscribed environment (such as a bed or room).

For diagnostic purposes, symptoms must be present most of the day nearly every day for at least 2 weeks, and they must cause significant distress or impair functioning. Major depressive disorder is further classified according to severity, longitudinal course of recurrent episodes, and

descriptions of the most recent episode. A special case of depression, postpartum depression, is discussed briefly in Box 24-2.

Typically, major depressive episodes last several weeks to several months and are followed by periods of relatively normal mood and behavior. The average major depressive episode lasts about 4 months; however, it can last for 12 months or more without remitting.

DYSTHYMIC DISORDER

The word *dysthymia* comes from the Greek prefix *dys,* meaning difficult or bad, and *thymos,* meaning mind. The *DSM-IV-TR* considers **dysthymia** a milder form of depressive illness in which the symptoms, such as poor appetite, overeating, difficulty falling asleep, excessive sleep, low energy, fatigue, low self-esteem, poor concentration, or difficulty making decisions, are less severe than in depressive disorder but are chronic. Diagnostic criteria for dysthymic disorder include depressed or irritable mood most of the day, occurring more days than not for at least 2 years (1 year in children and adolescents). During this time, the client has had no more than 2 months in which symptoms are not present and has not experienced a manic or depressive episode.

The chronic nature of dysthymia is a cause for concern, because it often presents as a lifelong struggle against depression, which can assume various forms and cause significant distress. In an attempt to escape negative self-esteem, feelings of self-depreciation, emptiness, low energy

Prevalence

- Lifetime risk for depression is approximately 7 to 12% for men and 20 to 30% for women.
- Prevalence of bipolar disorders is 0.5 to 2%.

Risk and Contributing Factors

Depression
- Gender: higher in women than in men
- Prior episode of depression
- Family history
- Stressful life event
- Current substance use
- Medical illness
- Few social supports

Bipolar Disorders
- Gender: higher in women than in men
- Family history
- Age: symptoms are more likely to develop in people younger than 50 years

Summary of DSM-IV-TR Diagnostic Criteria

Major Depressive Disorder

- Over 2 weeks, client has experienced a change from previous functioning with depressed mood or decreased interest or pleasure and at least four of the following:
  - Significant weight loss without dieting or weight gain or markedly decreased or increased appetite
  - Hypersomnia or insomnia
  - Psychomotor agitation or slowness
  - Fatigue or energy loss
  - Feelings of worthlessness or guilt
  - Difficulty concentrating or indecisiveness
  - Recurrent thoughts of death, either with or without suicide ideation
- Symptoms cause significant distress or impair social, occupational, or other functioning.
- Symptoms are not caused by a substance or a general medical condition.

Dysthymic Disorder

- For at least 2 years, client has depressed mood, based on either subjective report or observation from others.
- During depression, client displays at least two of the following:
  - Poor appetite or overeating
  - Hypersomnia or insomnia
  - Fatigue or energy loss
  - Feelings of hopelessness
  - Difficulty concentrating or indecisiveness
- During the disturbance, client has never been without the above symptoms for more than 2 months.
- Client has not had major depressive disorder.
- Client has never had a manic, mixed, or hypomanic episode and does not meet criteria for cyclothymic disorder.
- Symptoms are not caused by a substance or a general medical condition.
- Symptoms cause significant distress or impair social, occupational, or other functioning.

Bipolar I Disorder

- Client has one or more manic or mixed episodes and one or more major depressive episodes.
- Episodes are not better explained by other psychiatric disorders.
- Episodes are not the direct result of a substance or other medical condition.

Manic Episode

- Mood is abnormally and persistently elevated and expansive or irritable for at least 1 week.
- Client participates excessively in pleasurable activities with a high potential for painful results.
- Need for sleep is decreased.
- Client has inflated self-esteem or grandiosity.
- Goal-oriented activity or agitation is increased.
- Client is easily distracted, talks excessively, or has racing thoughts.
- Functioning in several areas is markedly impaired.

Major Depressive Episode

- Client has a depressed mood most of the day.
- Interest in nearly all activities is markedly decreased.
- Client shows significant weight loss without dieting, weight gain, or decreased/increased appetite.
- Client experiences hypersomnia or insomnia.
- Psychomotor agitation or slowness is present.
- Client experiences fatigue or energy loss.
- Client has feelings of worthlessness or guilt.
- Client has difficulty concentrating or is indecisive.
- Thoughts of death are recurrent, either with or without suicide ideation.

Mixed Episode

- Client meets criteria for both manic and major depressive episodes nearly every day for 1 week or longer.
- Client requires hospitalization to prevent harm to self or others.
- Client displays psychotic features.

(continued)

Mood Disorders Information Map *(Continued)*

Cyclothymic Disorder

- For at least 2 years, client has had numerous periods with hypomanic symptoms and numerous periods of depressive symptoms, but has not met criteria for major depressive disorder.
- Client has not been without symptoms for more than 2 months at a time.
- Client has had no manic, mixed, or major depressive episodes during the 2-year period.
- Symptoms are not the direct result of a substance or other medical condition.
- Symptoms significantly impair functioning or cause significant distress.

Hypomanic Episode

- Client has a persistently elevated, expansive, or irritable mood for at least 4 days. This mood is clearly different from client's usual mood.
- Client meets symptoms for a manic episode.

- Client's function has unequivocally changed, which others have observed.
- Condition is not severe enough to markedly impair social, occupational, or other functioning or require hospitalization.

Bipolar II Disorder

- Client has a history of one or more major depressive episodes or has major depression now.
- Client has a history of one or more hypomanic episodes or has hypomania now.
- Client has never had a manic or mixed episode.
- Symptoms cause significant distress or impair social, occupational, or other functioning.

➡ Prevention Strategies

- Screen all clients for mood disorders, especially if they have risk factors for these conditions.
- If a client thinks that he or she is already experiencing symptoms, reassure the client that the symptoms are real, and that treatment can help.
- Refer clients to organizations that provide materials about and support for those with mood disorders (see below).
- If the client has not yet approached a physician about signs or symptoms, encourage him or her to do so.
- For clients taking medication to control existing mood disorders, stress the importance of following the medication regimen and reporting any problems to their doctor or pharmacist.

➡ Want to Know More?

Mental Health Infosearch
http://www.mhsource.com
Mental Health Net
http://www.cmhc.com/

National Depressive and Manic Depressive Association
730 North Franklin, Suite 501
Chicago, IL 60610
(800) 82-NDMDA
(312) 642-0049
http://ndmda.org/

National Foundation for Depressive Illness
P.O. Box 2257
New York, NY 10116
(212) 370-7190
http://www.depression.org

National Institute of Mental Health (NIMH)
Information Resources and Inquiries Branch
Office of Scientific Information, Room 15C
5600 Fishers Lane
Rockville, MD 20857
(301) 443-4513
http://nimh.nih.gov/

National Mental Health Association
1021 Prince Street
Alexandria, VA 22314-2971
(800) 969-NMHA
http://aoa.dhhs.gov/aoa/dir/181.html

Society for Light Treatment and Biological Rhythms
(updated 2001)
P. O. Box 591687, 174 Cook St.
San Francisco, CA 94159-1687
(415) 751-2758 (FAX)
http://www.sltbr.org

With permission from the American Psychiatric Association. (2000). *Diagnostic and statistical manual of mental disorders* (4th ed., text revision). Washington, DC: Author.

A special case of depressive illness, postpartum depression, has also been a focus for research and study recently. In July 2001, postpartum depression was brought into national attention when, in Houston, Texas, a young mother of five murdered her children during an episode of postpartum psychosis (for story, see this web site: *http://slate.msn.com/default.aspx?id=*11419.) The young woman had been in treatment for psychosis, but she had discontinued her antipsychotic medication 2 weeks prior to the murders. During the postpartum period, women who have preexisting mood disorders or are currently in treatment for mood disorders are at higher risk for developing postpartum depression.

The story about the young Houston mother generated interest and increased public awareness around the issue of postpartum psychosis. Although up to 70% of women report having negative mood symptoms during pregnancy, the prevalence of pregnant women who actually meet criteria for major depression is between 10% and 16%, with only one to two per 1,000 women progressing to postpartum psychosis (Misri, Kostaras, Fox, et al., 2000). The genetics of postpartum psychosis are an emerging area of research (Coyle, Jones, Robertson, et al., 2000).

and fatigue, pessimism about the future, and hopelessness with suicidal ideations, the client may engage in certain activities to generate excitement. He or she may focus heavily on work, spend money, engage in sexual behavior, or become preoccupied with religious and mystic involvement in the struggle against depression. The client with dysthymia may turn to substance abuse or food to dull or escape psychic pain. Many times, the client with dysthymia has become accustomed to the chronic, negative, oppressive effect of the disorder and, therefore, does not readily recognize symptoms as being abnormal. Nurses practicing in acute care settings, physician offices, and the community play a critical role in primary prevention by identifying these clients.

BIPOLAR DISORDERS

The bipolar disorders include bipolar I disorder, bipolar II disorder, and cyclothymic disorder (see Figure 24-5). These disorders are characterized by mood swings, ranging from intense euphoria (mania) to profound depression.

Many nursing professionals work specifically with clients who have mood disorders, especially bipolar disorders. Research studies in nursing often focus on the client's and family's response to living with such a chronic illness. Cutler (2001) describes a study that explored client perceptions of their ability to care for themselves and whether these perceptions were related to management of symptoms after discharge from an acute care hospitalization (Research in Psychiatric-Mental Health Nursing 24-1). The study reflects the high caliber of research that psychiatric-mental health nurses conduct today and the ways this research significantly contributes to nursing practice.

Bipolar I Disorder

Bipolar I disorder is characterized by one or more manic episodes, usually alternating with major depressive episodes. **Manic episodes** are periods of an abnormally and persistently elevated, expansive, or irritable mood. During a manic episode, the client will typically exhibit three or more of the following symptoms:

- Extreme mood swings, irritability, sudden attacks of misplaced rage
- Sleep disturbances, awakening earlier each day, inability to stay in bed
- Decreased work output, distraction, restlessness
- Spending sprees
- Sexual promiscuousness
- Exaggerated self-esteem, delusions of grandeur
- Elation
- Excessive activity
- Flight of ideas
- Excessive and illogical rhyming, punning, and word associations; pressured speech

Clients with mania often dress flamboyantly and in an exaggerated manner. They may present in bizarre clothing, jewelry, or makeup, with hyperactive and excessively intrusive behaviors. For example, women may tend to wear heavier makeup than normal. Clients with mania will usually choose bright colors. Initially, other people may view clients with mania as sociable or fun to be around, but eventually others disengage because of the client's hyperactive and intrusive behaviors. Clients with mania also tend to laugh and talk excessively, usually inappropriately. Because of feelings of euphoria, grandiosity, and power, they attempt to control the environment by invading others' personal space and stretching environmental boundaries (eg, trying to go into the nurses' station or report room). At the same time, they have little to no insight that their behaviors are inappropriate.

Manic episodes usually begin suddenly and last from a few days to a few months. While in a manic phase, as described in Clinical Example 24–2, the client does not often realize that he or she is behaving strangely and resists treatment. It is common for the person to have abrupt mood changes, with rapid shifts from euphoria to anger or depression. The client may have a hypomanic episode or a relatively mild manic phase occurring with severe depression.

▶ *Research in Psychiatric-Mental Health Nursing 24-1*
SELF-CARE AGENCY AND SYMPTOM MANAGEMENT IN CLIENTS TREATED FOR MOOD DISORDER

Purpose: To assess client perception of self-care ability and to explore whether self-care ability could predict posthospitalization symptom management

Background: Many clients with mood disorders have multiple illness episodes during their lives, and 75% of clients treated for depression relapse within 2 years. Symptom management of clients with mood disorders, such as depression and bipolar illness, influences their quality of life and relapse. Many research studies have focused on the importance of self-care ability, including medication adherence and symptom management, in keeping the client stable after an acute illness episode. However, no studies have focused on predicting outcomes such as symptom management after an acute hospitalization. This study attempted to fill that gap in the literature.

Method and Sample: This report includes data from a larger study, which was a descriptive, correlational study with predictive components. In this article, the researchers examined the relationship between the predictor variable—self-care agency—and the dependent variable—symptom management. A purposive sample of 45 subjects was studied. Subjects were interviewed twice—once while in the hospital just before discharge and then again 2 months after discharge. Tools included the Perception of Self-Care Agency Questionnaire (PSCAQ) and a symptom management checklist developed by the researcher.

Findings: Stepwise multiple regression analyses of self-care agency with symptom management resulted in self-care agency explaining 37% of the variance in symptoms management at 2 months' posthospitalization. Two months after discharge, subjects reported an average of only three current symptoms out of a possible 12. Thirteen subjects said they had no symptoms. Symptoms reported most frequently were difficulty sleeping (44%), sadness most of the time (33%), extreme anxiety (33%), racing thoughts (29%), and thoughts of suicide (24%). After hospital stabilization, clients with bipolar illness reported needing ongoing nursing support to cope with their long-term relapse potential. Clients' perceptions of high self-care agency after discharge may be helpful in maintaining stability when symptoms of the illness recur, and this prevents a sense of being overwhelmed by a return of symptoms.

Application to Nursing Practice: This study has implications for nursing care of clients with mood disorders. The researchers used Orem's theory, which focuses on the identification of the client's deficits in the area of self-care and the nurse's role in helping clients to restore their self-care abilities. Nurses need to assist clients in estimating their self-care abilities and areas of self-care, such as symptom management, to promote autonomy and ongoing follow-up of treatment and to reduce recidivism in clients with mood disorders. This can begin in the hospital, as nurses observe the client's level of self-management of hygiene, dressing, grooming, and nutrition; ability to organize self-care activities; distortions of thought about caring for self; the ability to ask for help; and the ability to relate to others with minimal conflict and maximal clarity. In addition, nurses need to design client education programs in order to prevent relapse. Such a program could be designed around the three general strategies used by study clients for symptom management: seeking help from others, activities by oneself, and cognitive techniques. Nurses also need to participate in interdisciplinary outreach programs through community mental health centers to strengthen the client's social support and to follow up on problematic symptoms identified at the time of discharge.

Cutler, C. G. (2001). Self-care agency and symptom management in patients treated for mood disorder. *Archives of Psychiatric Nursing, 15*(1), 24–31.

Hypomania is a subcategory of mania and is slightly less severe. It does not have the psychotic features or severely impaired functioning that would require hospitalization, such as those that occur in manic states. Bipolar I disorders are coded based on the clinical picture during the most recent episode.

Bipolar II Disorder

Bipolar II disorder is characterized by having had a major depressive episode (either current or past) and at least one hypomanic episode. Most hypomanic episodes in bipolar II disorder occur immediately before or after a major depressive episode. Bipolar II disorder differs from bipolar I in that the client has never had a manic or mixed episode. Bipolar II clients may have had an episode in which they experienced a persistently elevated, expansive, or irritable mood (hypomania) for at least 4 days, and it is a mood that is clearly different from their usual mood. With Bipolar II, however, the client does not experience hypomanic symptoms severe enough to cause marked social or occupational dysfunction or to require hospitalization.

Bipolar II disorder is sometimes difficult to diagnose, particularly if the client presents for the first time with a depressive episode. The nurse must carefully gather the history to determine whether the client has experienced a past hypomanic episode. Commonly, a diagnosis of bipolar II is made after one nurse practitioner or physician has treated a client for some time and become familiar with that client's presentation and symptom history.

Cyclothymic Disorder

Cyclothymia is a disorder resembling bipolar disorder, with less severe symptoms. Cyclothymic disorder almost presents as a "subclinical" bipolar I disorder. Clients with cyclothymic disorder experience repeated periods of nonpsychotic depression and hypomania for at least 2 years (1 year for children and adolescents). The opposing manifestations of depression and hypomania are seen in the following pairs of symptoms: feelings of inadequacy (during depressed periods) and inflated self-esteem (during manic periods), social withdrawal and uninhibited social interaction, sleeping too much and too little, and diminished and increased productivity at work. Cyclothymic disorder is diagnosed only if a major depressive or manic episode has never been present.

Implications and Prognosis

The implications of unrecognized, undiagnosed, and untreated mood disorders are astounding, and costs are high, both economically to society and personally to individuals and families. In the United States alone, the estimated monetary costs for depression exceeded $44 billion in 1990 (Agency for Healthcare Policy and Research [AHCPR], 1999). The personal costs are reflected by higher mortality rates and impaired multiple areas of functioning. The WHO estimates that major depression is the fourth most important cause worldwide of loss in disability-adjusted life years, and that it will rise to second place by the year 2020 (AHCPR, 1999).

Although many mood disorders go unrecognized and untreated, the prognosis for clients who receive treatment is good. In fact, mood disorders are among the most treatable mental illnesses. With psychotherapy, pharmacotherapy, and somatic treatments, most clients who suffer from mood disorders can return to normal functioning.

Interdisciplinary Goals and Treatment

Because of the significant challenges in caring for clients who are living with depressive disorders, it is most effective to employ an interdisciplinary approach to long-term management. Many nurses work in acute care settings, step-down programs, day treatment programs, and community-based programs to provide the complex care these clients need. These programs always have an interdisciplinary approach and often include various professionals, such as physicians, social workers, case managers, and activities therapists. In addition, many nurse practitioners are working in outpatient clinics, seeing clients with mood disorders in psychotherapy and following these clients independently, while maintaining contacts with physician consultants and other professionals when necessary.

Current research is ongoing into the etiology and treatment of bipolar disorders. Recently, the NIMH launched the Systematic Treatment Enhancement Program for Bipolar Disorder (STEP-BD), the largest study of bipolar disorders ever undertaken (Box 24-3). The study is an interdisciplinary effort that incorporates nursing interventions as well as several other multidisciplinary modalities to study and treat this devastating illness. Treatment modalities for the client with a mood disorder include psychotherapy, pharmacotherapy, and somatic therapy.

PSYCHOTHERAPY

Psychotherapy, including family therapy, continues to be used extensively for treatment of depression, most often as an adjunct to pharmacologic treatment (Bowden, 2001). Most research studies report that the combination of psychotherapy and medications is more effective than either approach is alone in treating depressive disorders (Keller et al., 2000). Psychosocial treatments for bipolar disorder include psychoeducation, group therapy, cognitive-behavioral therapy (CBT), couples therapy, family therapy, and interpersonal psychotherapy (Swartz & Frank, 2001). This array of psychosocial treatments can assist the clients' adherence to medications, ability to cope with environmental stress triggers, and social–occupational functioning.

Family and marital psychoeducational interventions and individual interpersonal therapies have received the most empirical support in experimental trials (Craighead & Miklowitz, 2000). Although research is limited, converging reports suggest that of the psychosocial approaches commonly used, CBT, family therapy, and interpersonal therapy are most useful in bipolar depression (Swartz & Frank, 2001). In a recent review of 32 peer-reviewed reports involving 1052 clients, important gains were often seen of increased clinical stability and reduced hospitalization, as well as other functional and psychosocial benefits, as measured by objective tests (Huxley, Parikh, & Baldessarini, 2000).

COGNITIVE-BEHAVIORAL THERAPY

CBT is one of the most researched psychosocial interventions in psychiatry, and many studies have found CBT to be significantly effective in the treatment of depressive disorders (Lejuez, Hopko, & Hopko, 2001; Segal, Whitney, Lam, & CANMAT Depression Work Group, 2001).

BOX 24-3 ▼ Systematic Treatment Enhancement Program for Bipolar Disorder Launched at the National Institute of Mental Health

The Systematic Treatment Enhancement Program for Bipolar Disorder (STEP-BD) is the largest treatment study ever conducted for bipolar disorder, also known as manic-depressive illness. It is a long-term outpatient project that aims to find out which treatments, or combinations of treatments, are most effective for treating episodes of depression and mania and for preventing recurrent episodes. The coordinating center will establish a network of up to 20 treatment centers in which clients will be treated by specially trained psychiatrists and clinical specialists. These practitioners will use common assessment procedures and implement therapeutic interventions as called for by treatment guidelines that integrate pharmacological interventions and several psychosocial interventions. During a 5-year period, 5000 people with bipolar disorder will be enrolled in the study to ensure a broad sample inclusive of all bipolar subtypes, ethnic groups, and treatment settings. The coordinating center will analyze data from these centers to determine the impact of a wide variety of treatments on disease-specific outcomes, quality of life or functional outcomes, and economic outcomes. Additional data will be collected that focus on adherence to guidelines, as well as the influence of treatment setting and of regional and ethnic factors on treatment outcomes.

The proposed studies were designed to address key questions in areas considered to be of major clinical importance. Given the limitations of time and budget, the objectives are designated as primary and ancillary. The four primary objectives of STEP-BD are 1) implement common clinical practice procedures across a network of clinicians treating large numbers of bipolar clients in diverse treatment settings, 2) determine the most effective strategies for treatment of the depressed phase of bipolar illness, 3) determine which maintenance strategies most effectively prevent recurrence of affective episodes, and 4) provide a systematic means for translation of novel treatments and new findings into clinical practice.

The ancillary objectives of STEP-BD are 5) determine the benefit of specific interventions for bipolar clients with comorbid psychoactive substance abuse or dependence, 6) determine the prognostic significance of common comorbid conditions, 7) determine the benefit of specific interventions for rapid cycling, 8) determine the benefit of specific treatment strategies for acute mania, 9) determine the best treatment for bipolar women who are or want to become pregnant, and 10) Determine the validity of proposed subtypes of bipolar illness.

Hyman, in discussing the STEP-BD program at the NIMH, states that it is one of a new generation of clinical trials that has few exclusion criteria and longer-term treatment and follow-up periods. The study will assess functional outcomes as well as symptom reduction, and it will be implemented at diverse clinical sites, which will allow generalizability to much of the American population.

STEP-BD is being conducted at 17 research centers around the United States. For more information about STEP-BD, call toll free: 1-866-398-7425 or visit the STEP-BD web site *http://www.stepbd.org*.

Cognitive therapies may take place in individual or group contexts. The goal is to assist the client to identify and correct distorted, negative, and catastrophic thinking, thereby relieving depressive symptoms. Evidence has shown that using cognitive therapy can reduce subsequent relapse after the period of initial drug treatment has been completed (Teasdale, Segal, & Williams, 1995). The goal of behavioral therapies is to modify maladaptive behaviors through homework assignments, structured schedules, and various other techniques.

Aaron Beck developed the first model of cognitive therapy, a time-limited, structured intervention based on the idea that an individual's moods and emotions are a result of his or her thoughts and ideas (Beck, 1972; Beck, Rush, Shaw, & Emery, 1979). Believing that changing one's thoughts and ideas could influence affect and mood, Beck formulated a treatment model in which the therapist takes an active, directive position to help the client uncover and revise distorted thinking and to help the client use reality-based judgments to formulate experience (Wright & Thase, 1992). Beck noticed that clients with depression tend to have a certain combination of similar negative attitudes, which he labeled the "cognitive triad" of depression (Figure 24-6). This triad of thought patterns includes negative views of the self, the world, and the future. He also found that clients with depression tend to generalize by drawing global conclusions from a single, isolated life event, and then they ignore incoming data that could provide evidence to the contrary. He developed therapeutic interventions that focus on working actively with the client to change faulty thought patterns, and he found that these interventions were highly successful in depressed individuals.

CBT treatment specifically designed to systematically increase exposure of the client with depression to positive activities has been found to improve affect and cognition

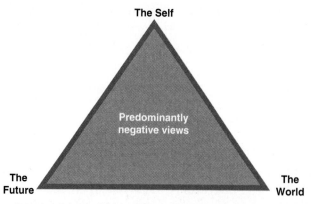

FIGURE 24-6 Beck's cognitive triad of depression. In this model, the client with depression sees the future marked by continuing trouble, full of hardship, deprivation, and frustration. He or she sees the world as negative, demanding, hostile, and full of obstacles. He or she sees the self as deficient and inadequate and attributes unpleasant experiences to personal defects.

significantly (Lejuez, Hopko, & Hopko, 2001). One study found that the combination of CBT and the antidepressant nefazodone resulted in higher rates of remission compared to clients who received either treatment alone (Keller et al., 2000). Another study of 102 subjects meeting criteria for major depressive disorder examined the efficacy of desipramine alone, CBT alone, and a combination of the two. Although all treatments resulted in significant improvement, the combination was superior in reducing depressive symptoms, particularly in those clients who were more severely depressed (Thompson et al., 2001). Chapter 8 provides additional information about CBT techniques.

PHARMACOLOGIC THERAPY

Psychopharmacologic treatments for mood disorders are grouped traditionally into two major categories: antidepressants and mood stabilizers (see Chap. 12).

Antidepressants

Antidepressants are the first-line drugs of choice for mood disorders (with the exception of mania or hypomania), including the depressive phase of bipolar disorders. With few exceptions, antidepressants have proven highly effective for all clients who suffer from depressive disorders. If one antidepressant is not effective, others are tried to determine which is optimal for a given client.

In general, all the antidepressants exert their effects at the level of the neuron, altering 5-HT and NE as well as several other neurochemicals. Their effects include changing the receptor itself, altering the metabolism and breakdown of the neurochemical, or blocking the reuptake of the neurochemical at the presynaptic receptor. These effects occur soon after a client takes the medication, but the clinical effects of reducing depressive symptoms usually take between 2 to 6 weeks, depending on the medication used.

Because each client is unique, the treatment team must arrive at the medication of choice through trial and error. The ultimate effect of reducing depressive symptoms is almost identical for all classes of antidepressants. For example, the Veterans Health Administration (VHA) clinical practice guidelines for major depressive disorder (Bobo et al., 2001; Snow, Lascher, & Mottur-Pilson, 2000) state that either tricyclic antidepressants (TCAs) or selective serotonin reuptake inhibitors (SSRIs) are equally efficacious. Therefore, the antidepressant is often chosen based on its side-effect profile and on the client's unique needs and symptom constellation (Snow et al., 2000). If the client has used an effective medication in the past, then providers should strongly consider that medication for subsequent depressive episodes. Before assuming treatment failure with any antidepressant, the client should remain on the drug long enough to ensure that an appropriate dose titration and target dose range have been achieved; the client should continue taking any given antidepressant for a minimum of 4 to 6 weeks (Snow et al., 2000).

Often, antidepressant therapy is a long-term process, requiring patience from client and clinician. This is often challenging when a client has a depressive disorder. It is sometimes necessary to try several types and dosages of antidepressants before arriving at the optimal one. Encouragement and supportive nursing interventions are especially important during the phase of medication initiation with clients who are experiencing severe depression (see Application of the Nursing Process to the Client With a Mood Disorder later in this chapter).

Some deterrents to maintaining antidepressant therapy include the length of time for clinical symptoms to subside and some side effects. In addition, some medications (most often the TCAs) are highly lethal and have a narrow therapeutic window. Providers must consider the risk of overdose when prescribing these drugs to clients who are suicidal. Prescriptions for a limited amount of medication may be necessary for acutely suicidal, at-risk clients. In most cases, the TCAs are not considered for clients who are acutely suicidal because of these factors.

When instituting antidepressant therapy, it is important to carefully document the baseline target symptoms, including their severity and frequency, and the effects of these symptoms on the client's functional status (Burger et al., 1998). Antidepressant regimens should continue at the same dose for at least 4 months after the initial alleviation of symptoms; this decreases the possibility of short-term relapse. If at 6 weeks the client does not show improvement with appropriate dosage titration, another antidepressant should be tried (Bobo et al., 2001).

Antidepressants can precipitate manic episodes in clients with bipolar disorder (Box 24-4). They also can activate latent psychosis in some susceptible clients. Therefore, close symptom monitoring is critical in these clients. Abrupt discontinuation of antidepressants also may cause severe rebound symptoms and a rapid return of the origi-

Use of antidepressants without a mood stabilizer should be avoided in bipolar disorder (Sachs, Koslow, & Ghaemi, 2000). If a client can be treated with lithium alone, obviously the risk for antidepressant-induced mania is avoided. If lithium is not sufficient, however, a combination of lithium and an antidepressant appears to reduce the risks for affective switch and for the induction of a long-term, rapid-cycling course.

In general, antidepressant treatments for unipolar depression are efficacious for bipolar depression as well. Antidepressants must be chosen carefully, however, in clients who experience rapid shifts from mania to depression, because some of them may trigger rapid mood switches to a manic state. Of the antidepressants, bupropion and the SSRIs carry less risk for inducing hypomania, mania, and rapid cycling compared with TCAs (Compton & Nemeroff, 2000). Tapering antidepressant medication after periods of sustained remission in clients with bipolar disorder is beneficial in limiting the risk for affective switch and acceleration of the cycle rate.

nal depression. Thus, discontinuation should proceed with a very slow taper, guided by the elimination half-life of the parent compound and its metabolites and close symptom monitoring (Bobo et al., 2001).

According to the *VHA/DOD Clinical Practice Guideline for the Management of Major Depressive Disorder in Adults* (Bobo et al., 2001), generally clients should receive antidepressant medications for the following indications:

- Moderate or severe symptoms of depression
- Significant impairment in social or occupational functioning as a result of depression
- Suicidal ideation

Strong indications for antidepressants include past history of a positive response to such medications, negative response to psychotherapeutic interventions, recurrent depressive episodes, family history of depression, and client preference for drug therapy (Bobo et al., 2001). Antidepressants may be divided into several categories, each of which is reviewed in the following sections:

- Serotonin reuptake inhibitors (SRIs)
- Novel (atypical) antidepressants
- Cyclic antidepressants
- Monoamine oxidase inhibitors (MAOIs)

Chapter 12, Psychopharmacology, describes the mechanisms of action and full side-effect profiles for each anti-

depressant group. The discussions that follow provide individual, class-specific side effects and special issues for each class.

Serotonin Reuptake Inhibitors. The SRIs are available in different formulations, each with different target neurotransmitters:

- SSRIs: fluoxetine (Prozac), sertraline (Zoloft), paroxetine (Paxil), fluvoxamine (Luvox), and citalopram (Celexa)
- Serotonin antagonist and reuptake inhibitor (SARI): nefazodone (Serzone)
- Serotonin norepinephrine reuptake inhibitor (SNRI): venlafaxine (Effexor)

The SSRIs were the "first-generation" serotonergic agents; later generations include the SARIs (which act as both serotonin antagonists and reuptake blockers) and the SNRIs (which block the reuptake of both 5-HT and NE).

In general, the mechanism of action of the SSRIs is to block reuptake of 5-HT into the neuron by blocking the 5-HT reuptake pump (Figure 24-7), thereby increasing the level of 5-HT available in the synapse.

The SSRIs are typically considered first-line drugs of choice for depressive disorders, unless elements of the client's history or medical conditions warrant use of an alternative. For example, with certain gastrointestinal disorders, such as chronic diarrhea or peptic ulcer disease, the TCAs are a better first choice than the SSRIs. Another example is a client presenting with psychotic depression

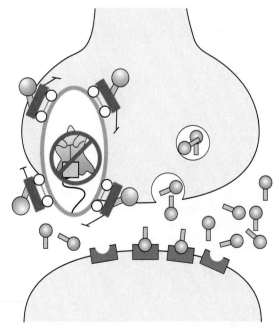

FIGURE 24-7   The SSRIs block the 5-HT reuptake pump on the presynaptic neuron. (Adapted from Stahl, S. M. [1996]. *Essential psychopharmacology: Neuroscientific basis and practical applications.* Cambridge: Cambridge University Press.)

who may begin ECT as a first-line treatment of choice, rather than beginning with oral medication.

SSRIs are considered first-line choices because of their decreased incidence of side effects. Their most common side effects affect the gastrointestinal system (nausea, vomiting, diarrhea) and CNS (headache, nervousness, anxiety, light-headedness) (Karch, 2002). Loss of libido is also reported relatively frequently. The SSRIs have very few to no anticholinergic or cardiotoxic side effects, unlike other antidepressants.

One possibly lethal reaction to SSRIs is serotonin syndrome. It typically occurs following the use of serotomimetic agents (SSRIs, TCAs, tryptophan, dextromethorphan, or meperidine) alone or combined with MAOIs. Serotonin syndrome also has been observed in clients who take St. John's wort, a popular herbal medication that increases 5-HT levels, in combination with another serotomimetic agent. The administration of certain combinations of these drugs results in hyperactivity of 5-HT in the CNS, which causes serotonin syndrome (Nisijima et al., 2000).

In particular, if the client is switching from an SSRI (eg, fluoxetine [Prozac]) to an MAOI, providers should allow a "washout" period of at least 5 weeks (half-life of fluoxetine) before beginning the MAOI. Conversely, if the client is switching from an MAOI to fluoxetine, the provider should allow a washout period of at least 2 weeks (half-life of MAOI). If switching to and from other SSRIs, the washout period should be at least the half-life of the alternative drug. Symptoms of and treatment for serotonin syndrome are listed in Box 24-5.

Novel (Atypical) Antidepressants. Generally, the novel antidepressants, including trazodone, mirtazapine, bupropion, maprotiline, and amoxapine, are considered safer medications than the cyclic antidepressants or MAOIs. They are considered second-line choices for antidepressant therapy.

Trazodone (Desyrel) is considered a novel antidepressant, although it is actually an SSRI. Side effects of trazodone are similar to SSRIs, but this drug has a few more cardiovascular side effects than typical SSRIs. Side effects include agitation, drowsiness, dizziness, fatigue, gastrointestinal irritation, nausea, vomiting, dry mouth, decreased libido, diarrhea, hypertension or hypotension, tachycardia, shortness of breath, syncope, and palpitations (Karch, 2002). Unlike the typical SSRIs, trazodone should be considered with caution for clients with recent myocardial infarction (MI) or history of cardiovascular disease. Suicidal or potentially suicidal clients should have limited access to trazodone.

Mirtazapine (Remeron) is a newer tetracyclic drug that appears to act similarly to TCAs, which inhibit the presynaptic reuptake of NE and 5-HT. Major adverse effects include headache, dizziness, drowsiness, weakness, blurred vision, nausea, vomiting, dry mouth, and changes in libido. Mirtazapine has a similar side effect as the novel antipsychotic Clozaril, in that it may cause

---

BOX 24-5 ▼ *Symptoms of and Treatment for Serotonin Syndrome*

Symptoms

Confusion

Disorientation

Mania

Restlessness or agitation

Myoclonus

Rigidity

Hyperreflexia

Diaphoresis

Shivering

Tremors

Diarrhea

Nausea

Ataxia

Headache

Autonomic instability

Coma

Low-grade fever

Flushing

Rhabdomyolysis (rarely)

Death (rarely)

Treatment

1. Immediately discontinue all serotonergic drugs.
2. Give anticonvulsants for seizures if needed.
3. Serotonin antagonist drugs (eg, cyproheptadine and propranolol) may help. Strong 5-HT2A antagonists, such as risperidone, have been shown to counteract lethality in a mouse model of serotonin syndrome (Nisijima et al., 2000).
4. Other drugs may also be used to counteract specific symptoms. Some examples include clonazepam for myoclonus, lorazepam for restlessness and agitation, chlorpromazine for hyperthermia, and diazepam for muscle rigidity.

agranulocytosis and neutropenia; blood work should be monitored with this drug. Symptoms such as fever, sore throat, or other signs of infection during therapy should be followed up immediately.

Bupropion (Wellbutrin, Zyban) is an unusual antidepressant in that its mechanism of action is unknown. It differs from other antidepressants, although it is known to weakly block the reuptake of 5-HT and NE, and it also slightly inhibits the reuptake of DA (Karch, 2002, p. 206). Adverse side effects include agitation, insomnia, headaches including migraines, tremors, seizures, dry mouth, constipation, dizziness, tachycardia, and weight loss.

Maprotiline (Ludiomil) and amoxapine (Asendin) are thought to act similarly to the TCAs by blocking reuptake of NE and 5-HT. These two novel antidepressants share a similar side-effect profile, including sedation and anticholinergic (atropine-like) effects, confusion and disturbed concentration, dry mouth, constipation, nausea, and orthostatic hypotension.

Cyclic Antidepressants. This category includes the TCA tertiary amines (amitriptyline, clomipramine, doxepin, imipramine, and trimipramine); TCA secondary amines (amoxapine—described above, desipramine, nortriptyline, and protriptyline); and tetracyclics (maprotiline, also categorized as a novel antidepressant and described previously). Before the introduction of the SSRIs and novel antidepressants, TCAs were considered the first-line drugs of choice for depression. The newer medications have fewer side effects, however, and do not have the cardiotoxic effects or narrow therapeutic window of TCAs. In most cases, TCAs are now used only when SSRIs and novel antidepressants have been ineffective in relieving depressive symptoms or when there has been documented prior success of TCAs relieving depressive symptoms in a client.

Briefly, TCAs work by blocking the reuptake of NE and DA in much the same way as the SRIs except that they work on the noradrenergic neuron (Figure 24-8) by blocking the reuptake pumps there.

The cyclic antidepressants, as a rule, should not be used in clients at risk for suicide. The therapeutic window is narrow, making use of TCAs dangerous. Bobo and colleagues (2001) report that an analysis of coroner data suggests that TCAs are associated with elevated death rates in overdoses compared with SSRIs.

TCAs also must be used cautiously in clients who are hypersensitive to any of the tricyclic drugs, who may be taking MAOIs, who have had a recent MI, or who are lactating. In addition, they should be evaluated thoroughly and considered carefully in clients who have preexisting cardiovascular disorders (eg, severe coronary artery disease, progressive heart failure, angina pectoris, paroxysmal tachycardia, symptomatic or unstable ischemic heart disease), closed-angle glaucoma, symptomatic benign prostatic hypertrophy, troublesome constipation,

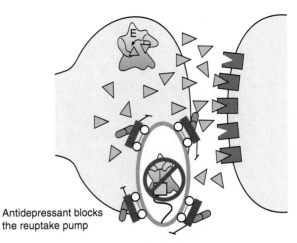

Antidepressant blocks the reuptake pump

FIGURE 24-8   The TCAs block reuptake of DA and NE into the presynaptic neuron. (Adapted from Stahl, S. M. [1996]. *Essential psychopharmacology: Neuroscientific basis and practical applications.* Cambridge: Cambridge University Press.)

seizure disorders, impaired hepatic or renal function, or manic-depressive disorders (TCAs may precipitate mania) (Karch, 2002, p. 121).

Monoamine Oxidase Inhibitors (MAOIs). The MAOIs, including phenelzine (Nardil) and tranylcypromine (Parnate), are used infrequently since the development of the SSRIs. They may be used to treat atypical depression or depression in a client who does not respond to other classes of antidepressants. The MAOIs work quite differently than the SSRIs or the novel or cyclic antidepressants. Instead of blocking reuptake of neurotransmitters, they block the activity of MAO, an enzyme that breaks down the catecholamines (NE in particular) within the neuron itself (Figure 24-9).

The MAOIs increase levels of tyramine (by inhibiting the breakdown of catecholamines, such as NE). Therefore, if the client overdoses, takes other medications that interact with MAOIs, or eats foods that contain tyramine, NE will accumulate, leading to hypertensive crisis, a critical condition requiring immediate medical intervention (Box 24-6). Other less severe adverse effects of the MAOIs include dizziness, vertigo, headache, constipation, nausea, dry mouth, and weight changes (Karch, 2002).

Mood Stabilizers

Mood stabilizers, including lithium and the anticonvulsants discussed next, are the first-line drugs of choice for clients with bipolar disorders. Drugs in this class bring the depressive and manic mood cycles within a more normal range. Generally, however, they all have been shown more effective for mania than for depression within the bipolar spectrum (Bowden, 2001). Therefore, clients with significant depressive symptoms during this phase of the bipolar spectrum or whose depressive symptoms do not respond well to mood stabilizers alone also often need antidepres-

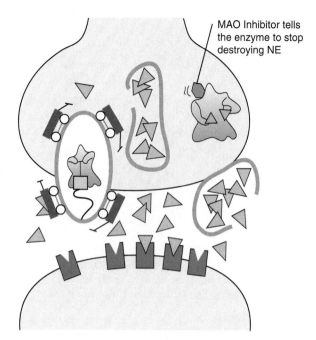

MAO Inhibitor tells
the enzyme to stop
destroying NE

FIGURE 24-9   The MAOIs block the destruction of NE
within the presynaptic neuron, thus increasing NE's release into
the synapse. (Adapted from Stahl, S. M. [1996]. *Essential psychopharmacology: Neuroscientific basis and practical applications*. Cambridge: Cambridge University Press.)

sant therapy. Use of combinations of mood stabilizers is
common but requires extensive knowledge of potential
pharmacokinetic interactions. In addition, close monitoring and frequent follow-up are critical elements of caring
for clients taking these medications.

Lithium. Lithium is the only drug whose prophylactic activity in bipolar disorder has been proven unequivocally. It remains the first-line drug of choice in the long-term treatment of stabilizing mood in the bipolar disorders
(Bowden, 2001; Bowden, Calabrese, McElroy et al., 2000;
Maj, 2000). Recent evidence, however, points to the notion that lithium therapy (even when supplemented by antidepressants and antipsychotics) is not adequate for most
clients with bipolar disorder, particularly those who experience rapid cycling (Post et al., 2000).

Historically, lithium's mechanism of action in stabilizing mood has been largely unknown. Recent studies are
revealing that lithium's actions may result from its effects
on lithium-specific enzymes, including inositol monophosphatase and the protein kinase glycogen synthase kinase 3.
Lithium-specific enzymes are widely expressed, need to
have metal ions for catalysis, and are generally inhibited by
lithium. The challenge is to determine which target, if any,
is responsible for a given response to lithium within the cell
(Phiel & Klein, 2001).

The importance of monitoring lithium levels in the
blood cannot be overemphasized. Lithium toxicity has a
fairly narrow therapeutic window; related adverse effects

BOX 24-6 ▼ *Hypertensive Crisis Alert*

Symptoms of hypertensive crisis include:

- Occipital headache, which may radiate frontally
- Palpitations
- Neck stiffness or soreness
- Nausea
- Vomiting
- Sweating
- Dilated pupils
- Photophobia
- Tachycardia or bradycardia
- Chest pain
- Orthostatic hypotension, sometimes with
  falling
- Disturbed cardiac rate and rhythm

(From Karch, A. M. (2002). *2002 Lippincott's nursing
drug guide* (pp. 942–943). Philadelphia: Lippincott
Williams & Wilkins.)

---

are shown in Table 24-1. At the start of therapy, lithium
levels must be checked twice each week in samples drawn
immediately before a dose and 8 to 12 hours after the prior
dose (Karch, 2002, p. 694). For maintenance therapy, the
lithium serum level should be between 0.6 to 1.2 mEq/L;
serum levels should be monitored every 2 months when
stabilized (Karch, 2002). Side effects of lithium that may
occur unrelated to serum levels include headache, hyperkalemia, tachycardia-bradycardia syndrome, dermatologic
effects such as pruritus and rashes, hypercalcemia, weight
gain, and swollen or painful joints.

Anticonvulsant Medications. Some of the anticonvulsant medications (carbamazepine and divalproex) are
used either as adjuncts to or replacements for lithium in
stabilizing mood in bipolar disorders. They also are used in
clients who do not respond to lithium or experience intolerable side effects during use. Divalproex (Depakote) is
being used, instead of lithium, with increasing frequency as
an alternative first-line treatment in bipolar disorders. In
recent studies of divalproex and lithium, compared to
placebos, both drugs delayed mania recurrence. Divalproex stabilized the client's condition for twice as long as
lithium and was better tolerated than lithium (Bowden et
al., 2000; Calabrese et al., 1999).

The mechanism of action of the anticonvulsant medications continues to be investigated; hypotheses involve
their ability to modulate metabolism and other aspects of
the gamma-aminobutyric acid (GABA) system (Stahl,
1996). Common but not physiologically severe side effects include sedation, dizziness, drowsiness, unsteadiness, nausea and vomiting, tremors, and gastrointestinal
problems (Karch, 2002, p. 226). Less common but more

TABLE 24-1 ▼ Lithium Toxicity and Associated Serum Levels*

LITHIUM SERUM LEVEL	SYMPTOMS OF TOXICITY
< 1.5 mEq/L	CNS: lethargy, slurred speech, muscle weakness, fine hand tremors GI: nausea, vomiting, diarrhea, thirst GU: polyuria
1.5–2.0 mEq/L (mild-to-moderate toxicity)	CNS: coarse hand tremors, mental confusion, hyperirritability of muscles, drowsiness, incoordination GI: persistent GI upset, gastritis, salivary gland swelling, abdominal pain, excessive salivation, flatulence, indigestion CV: ECG changes (QT interval changes)
2.0–2.5 mEq/L (moderate-to-severe toxicity)	CNS: ataxia, giddiness, fasciculations, tinnitus, blurred vision, clonic movements, seizures, stupor, coma CV: serious ECG changes (arrhythmias), severe hypotension Respiratory: fatalities secondary to pulmonary complications GU: large output of dilute urine
> 2.5 mEq/L (life-threatening toxicity)	Complex involvement of multiple organ systems and death

*Toxic lithium levels are close to therapeutic levels (a small therapeutic window). Therapeutic levels in acute mania: 1 to 1.5 mEq/L. Therapeutic levels in maintenance: 0.6 to 1.2 mEq/L.
CNS = central nervous system; CV = cardiovascular; ECG = electrocardiogram; GI = gastrointestinal;
GU = genitourinary
Reproduced with permission, from Karch, A.M. (2002). *2002 Lippincott's nursing drug guide*. Philadelphia:
Lippincott Williams & Wilkins.

physiologically significant are the side effects of increased body weight and metabolism and dose-related hepatic and hematologic effects. Rare but more severe toxicities include skin, bone marrow, life-threatening pancreatitis, and hepatic toxicity as a result of hypersensitivity (Swann, 2001). The most important interventions for the management of side effects of anticonvulsant drugs are detecting them early, discontinuing the medication, and aggressively treating the toxicity.

Medications for Refractory Mania

Several newer medications from various classes to treat bipolar mood cycles are currently being studied. The medications mentioned here are being used for mania that is refractory to any other first-line or second-line drug therapies, and so they are typically tried after first-line drugs, such as lithium and divalproex, have failed.

Anticonvulsants. Lamotrigine (Lamictal), an anticonvulsant, has been found to be superior to placebos in preventing recurrences of depression in long-term treatment of clients with bipolar disorders, including rapid cyclers (Calabrese et al., 1999, 2000; Gitlin, 2001). Lamotrigine also has been found particularly effective for the depressive component of bipolar disorder (Bowden, 2001). A potentially life-threatening side effect of lamotrigine is Stevens-Johnson syndrome and toxic epidermal necrosis with multiorgan failure (Karch, 2002, p. 664). Dizziness, ataxia, nausea, and rashes are other, less lethal, side effects. Clients on lamotrigine require careful monitoring for any

dermatologic conditions or rashes, particularly during the introduction and titration phases of drug treatment. Topiramate (Topamax), another newer anticonvulsant used in bipolar disorder, has been associated with weight loss and is currently still under research for refractory mania.

Atypical (Novel) Antipsychotics. Novel antipsychotics are effective in treating acute mania; however, with the exception of clozapine, their efficacy as true mood stabilizers continues to be largely unknown. A recent report found that antipsychotics with the most rapid onset in acute mania are haloperidol, risperidone, and olanzapine. Chlorpromazine and thiothixenes had the slowest rate of onset, 2 weeks or more (Tohen, Jacobs, & Feldman, 2000).

Novel antipsychotic agents have become a mainstay in the maintenance adjunctive treatment of bipolar disorders, because they are more effective and safer alternatives (fewer motor side effects, such as tardive dyskinesia and the more lethal neuroleptic malignant syndrome [Schweitzer, 2001]) than many of the typical antipsychotic agents. Studies are currently ongoing with clozapine, risperidone, olanzapine, and quetiapine. Although long-term studies of these agents are lacking, preliminary reports suggest that they serve an important role as adjunctive treatments (Ghaemi, 2000). Differences in efficacy have not been established through rigorous experimental studies; however, differences in the side effect of weight gain have been found. For example, olanzapine causes significant weight gain, to the same extent as clozapine and greater than that observed with risperidone (Schweitzer, 2001).

Olanzapine increasingly is considered a first-line drug of choice for treatment of bipolar disorder, particularly from an efficacy and adverse side effect point of view; however, more studies are needed to justify the costs associated with olanzapine compared to typical antipsychotics (Lund & Perry, 2000). Given the state of current research on this drug, however, it is not yet indicated as a monotherapy for bipolar disorder.

Other Medications. Gabapentin (Neurontin), an antiepileptic agent, has yet to be proven efficacious by a controlled study. Its mechanism of action is unknown but is thought to be related to its ability to inhibit polysynaptic responses and block pretetanic potentiation (Karch, 2002, p. 547). Its few adverse side effects include dizziness, insomnia, somnolence, ataxia, gastrointestinal upset, and fatigue. Other novel treatments for bipolar disorder currently under investigation include high-dose thyroid hormones, calcium channel blockers (including nimodipine), and omega-3 fatty acids (Gitlin, 2001; Levy & Janicak, 2000).

SOMATIC NONPHARMACOLOGIC INTERVENTIONS

The traditional first-line nonpharmacologic therapy *for mood disorders* is ECT. Phototherapy is used commonly for depression with a seasonal pattern. In addition, at least three new somatic, nonpharmacologic interventions are under investigation for treating clients with bipolar disorders: sleep deprivation (SD), transcranial magnetic stimulation (TMS), and vagal nerve stimulation (VNS).

Electroconvulsive Therapy

First used in 1938, **electroconvulsive therapy (ECT)** involves the application of a small dose of electricity to one or both sides of the brain to induce a seizure. Exactly how ECT works remains unclear, but the seizure most likely modifies the chemical milieu, or environment, of the neurotransmitters believed to contribute to depression.

Although ECT has received negative attention and stigmatization from movies, it is a safe intervention with relatively few long-term side effects. The nurse should keep in mind that ECT may elicit strong feelings of fear and anxiety in clients and families. The client may envision electrocution or death or may anticipate permanent intellectual changes. The physician and nurse must carefully explain what the treatment is like and prepare the client and family for aftereffects.

The nurse prepares the client for ECT in a manner similar to preparation for surgery. He or she ensures that the client has no food or drinks the morning of the treatment, voids just before the procedure, removes dentures, and wears a hospital gown or loose clothing. The client must give informed consent and sign the appropriate forms. A compete physical examination is required, including a

spinal x-ray. The nurse monitors vital signs before and after treatment. ECT is usually administered in a room designated for this purpose. The nurse places the client on a stretcher or firm bed and inserts a rubber mouthpiece in the mouth to maintain an airway. Usually the client receives a short-acting anesthetic and a muscle relaxant just before the electric shock is administered.

Electrodes are applied unilaterally or bilaterally to the client's temples, and the shock is administered. The client experiences a typical grand mal seizure with tonic and clonic phases. The nurse and others in attendance should not attempt to restrain the client but should guide the extremities to prevent injury during the seizure activity.

When the seizure ends, oxygen may be given as a safety measure because apnea may occur physiologically in any general convulsive seizure. Airways and oxygenation equipment should be readily available in the treatment area. Once the client is transferred to the recovery area, consciousness quickly returns. The nurse positions the client on the side while the client awakens to prevent aspiration of oral secretions. The nurse monitors vital signs during the recovery period. It is normal for the client to be confused temporarily. The nurse must observe the client carefully to ensure his or her safety and must reorient him or her to the surroundings.

The client may or may not be hospitalized for ECT treatments. The number of treatments given depends on the client's response to treatment. Nursing observations during this time are important in the decision making regarding future treatments.

A frequent aftereffect of ECT is memory impairment, ranging from a mild tendency to forget details to severe confusion. This may persist for weeks or months after treatment but does usually resolve significantly. The nurse prepares the client and family for this confusion and assures them that it is expected and that full return of memory will occur eventually.

Phototherapy

Phototherapy for depression has been proven most effective for clients who have mild to moderate symptoms of mood disorders associated with a seasonal pattern. This treatment consists of using artificial light therapy for one or two 30-minute to 3-hour daily sessions. The seasonal pattern of depression is thought to be related to lack of light and decreased melatonin production. Recent evidence, however, has shown that disturbances in brain serotonin systems also play a role in the pathogenesis of seasonal affective disorder and that phototherapy may compensate for the underlying serotonin deficit. The catecholaminergic systems may be involved in the mechanism of action of phototherapy (Neumeister, Praschak-Rieder, Willeit, et al.,1999).

Nurses can promote health in clients by teaching them about the relationship of light to mood and the benefits of daily sunshine. They also can advocate for better lighting in the workplace.

Sleep Deprivation

SD has been studied for several other medical disorders, and it is under investigation for use in the depressive phase of bipolar disorder. SD has been found to have a strong and rapid effect on depressed mood in more than 60% of all diagnostic subgroups of affective disorders (Wirz-Justice & Van den Hoofdakker, 1999). In more than 36 studies published in the last 3 decades, SD has been found to produce marked, acute antidepressant effects in most clients with depression (Szuba et al., 1994; Wirz-Justice & Van den Hoofdakker, 1999). SD is thought to exert its effects by suppressing cholinergic activity, which is thought to be excessive, relative to the transmission of monoamine, in both depression and Parkinson's disease (Demet, Chicz-Demet, Fallon, & Sokolski, 1999). Other reports discuss the effects of SD being linked to changes in disturbed circadian- and sleep–wake-dependent phase relationships and concomitant increases of slow-wave sleep pressure, as well as counteraction of the hyperarousal state in depression through SD sleepiness (Wirz-Justice & Van den Hoofdakker, 1999).

Transcranial Magnetic Stimulation

Although TMS is often used for seizure disorders, recently it has received attention for its therapeutic effects in depressive disorders. Several studies have shown TMS to improve depression (George, Nahas, Zozel et al., 1999; George, Nahas, Molloy et al., 2000a). One study found an antimanic effect of right prefrontal TMS (Nahas et al., 1999). Imaging studies in clients with depression have pointed to dysfunctional limbic and prefrontal cortex activity. It is hypothesized that TMS works by stimulating the brain in the dorsolateral prefrontal cortex, which then changes brain activity both locally and in paralimbic areas through transsynaptic connections. Little is known, however, about the role of various stimulation parameters such as the intensity or frequency of stimulation, and more research is needed in this area (Nahas et al., 1999). TMS has been under recent investigation as an alternative to ECT, which presents a higher risk to clients (Szuba, O'Reardon, & Evans, 2000).

TMS is a noninvasive procedure that affects the brain by stimulating the cerebral cortex and inducing electrical currents in neurons (Nahas et al., 1999). The powerful magnetic field generated by TMS acts as a vector that passes through the scalp and the skull and then converts into an electrical energy in the brain. TMS has been compared to ECT in regard to its mechanism of action and therapeutic effects (Krystal et al., 2000). It differs, however, in that it does not induce a seizure, does not require anesthesia, and does not cause cognitive side effects (George et al., 1999).

Vagus Nerve Stimulation

Vagus nerve stimulation (VNS) was first used in clients with epilepsy who were resistant to traditional treatments. It is built on a long history of research involving the relationship of autonomic signals to limbic and cortical function, and it is one of the newest methods to physically alter brain function (George et al., 2000b). Since the late 1980s, VNS has been studied in clients with treatment-resistant depression as well. Because 80% of the fibers in the vagus nerve are afferent, it was hypothesized that the episodic stimulation of this nerve using an implanted electrode would change blood flow in the medial temporal cortex and hippocampus. Studies done so far indicate that the improvement from VNS is maintained for up to 1 year after the 12-week treatment (Prater, 2001).

APPLICATION OF THE NURSING PROCESS TO THE CLIENT WITH A MOOD DISORDER

Nurses in psychiatric-mental healthcare frequently encounter clients with depression or mania. In many cases, depression coexists with other psychiatric disorders and, therefore, may be a consideration for many additional clients with different primary diagnoses.

Assessment

Nursing assessment of depressive and manic behaviors involves systematic, thorough consideration of the client's safety, psychological functioning or mental status (including affect, thought processes, and intellectual processes), physiological and psychomotor activity, and behavioral and social activity.

SAFETY ASSESSMENT

Safety is a nursing priority for clients suffering from either depression or bipolar disorder, although the focus of interventions may differ slightly depending on the disorder. Suicide is a primary concern for clients with depression. The client with agitated depression may threaten to harm others and requires a thorough violence assessment (see Chap. 26). The client with mania is at greater risk for accidents because of the hyperactive state, loss of inhibition, and lack of judgment, although, of course, the nurse must also assess for suicide. In addition, clients with mania may be angry, hostile, and irritable, causing them to lash out at others unexpectedly. Therefore, the nurse would perform both suicide and violence assessments for clients with mania.

Suicide Risk Assessment

Nurses assess all clients with depression for suicide risk. Suicide assessment is a critical component that psychiatric-mental health nurses must learn, practice, and refine. The novice psychiatric-mental health nurse asks for assistance when learning how to do a suicide assessment and seeks and obtains additional training and mentoring regarding the nuances and details of assessing the acutely suicidal client.

Factors that increase the risk for suicide include expression of current thoughts or plans about committing suicide, active mental illness (such as severe depression, psychosis, bipolar disorder), substance abuse disorder, past history of suicidal attempts or behaviors, formulation of a plan, availability of means for completing the suicide, disruption of important personal relationships, or failure at personal endeavors (Bobo et al., 2001). It is a myth that forthright questioning about suicidal thoughts or plans will increase the risk for suicide; direct, nonjudgmental questioning is most effective. In fact, clients often report feeling relieved that someone has asked them in detail about their suicidal thoughts. Box 24-7 provides assessment questions to guide the nurse when completing a comprehensive suicide assessment.

Violence Assessment

Violence may indicate that the client perceives a threat or cannot get his or her needs met through nonviolent means. Specific factors contributing to violent behavior include psychiatric or medical disorders and environmental, situational, or social factors (Bobo et al., 2001). The nurse considers the following as warning signs for violence: ideas about or intent to harm others, a history of violent behavior, severe agitation or hostility, and active psychosis.

MENTAL STATUS EXAMINATION

The mental status examination (MSE) is the comprehensive and thorough assessment of the client's mental state

---

BOX 24-7 ▼ *Suicide Assessment*

Questions to Ask for a Comprehensive Suicide Assessment

- Ask the client directly if he or she has thoughts of suicide:
  - "Have you had thoughts about death or about killing yourself?"
  - "Are the thoughts pervasive or do they come and go (intermittent)?"
  - "Do these thoughts stay with you for awhile, or do they tend to come and go?"
  - "Have you heard voices telling you to hurt or kill yourself?"
  - "Do thoughts tend to have some connection to certain situations?"
  - "Has anything happened lately that has prompted you to think about suicide more?"
  - "Are there situations or ideas that always seem to be present when you are thinking about suicide?"
- Ask the client if he or she has a plan; ask for details about how extensive the plan is and identify means or method and lethality:
  - "Do you have a plan for how you would kill yourself?"
  - "Are there means available (eg, pills, a gun and bullets, or poison)?"
  - "Have you actually rehearsed or practiced how you would kill yourself?"
  - "How strong is your intent to do this?"
- Can the client resist the impulse to commit suicide?
  - "Are you an impulsive person?"
  - "Can you resist the impulse to do this?"

- "What would keep you from committing suicide?"
- "Tell me about your hopes for the future."
- Has the client ever had ideas about or attempted suicide?
  - "Have you ever thought about hurting or killing yourself?"
  - "Have you tried to hurt or kill yourself in the past? When?"
- Has anyone in the client's immediate or extended family or a significant other ever committed suicide?
  - "What was that person's relationship to you?"
  - "What were the circumstances of his or her death?"
  - "What was your experience of this event?"

Questions to Ask if Assessing a Recent Suicide Attempt

- What were the means; how did you try to commit suicide?
- Where was the attempt made?
- Did anyone know about the attempt beforehand or during the attempt?
- Who found you?
- How many attempts have you made in the past?
- Did you have a plan that you had thought out and prepared, or was the attempt done more on an impulsive feeling?
- Did you have any physical harm or impairment from the attempt?
- How did you get treated, and what was required?

Adapted from Bobo et al., 2001. *VHA/DOD clinical practice guideline for the management of major depressive disorder in adults.* Washington, DC: Department of Veterans Affairs.

during each assessment. Mental status changes over time, sometimes rapidly. The frequency of performing the MSE will depend on the client's behavior, symptoms, medications, specific needs for ongoing monitoring (eg, the client who is on suicide precautions), and other environmental factors.

Appearance and General Behavior

The first assessment component of the MSE is appearance, which includes age, grooming, clothing, posture, hygiene, and stature. If the client is depressed, he or she may be poorly groomed and disheveled, with a dejected facial expression. Clients with mania may appear flamboyant with an exaggerated manner and dress.

In describing general overall behavior, nurses must avoid value judgments and give examples to support their descriptions. They cannot forget to include the motor activity that the client demonstrates during the MSE.

Mood and Affect

Because mood disorders manifest themselves mainly as disturbances in mood and affect, the client's emotional tone may be the most observable deviation from healthy behavior. The nurse can assess a client's mood by examining the content of his or her verbal communication, tone of voice, facial expression, posture, and gestures. The assessment is direct, based on verbalization by the client, and indirect, through observation of the client's behavior.

Affect refers to the facial expressions the client exhibits during the interview. In depression and mania, affect may or may not be congruent to mood (ie, it may or may not match the observed mood). In depression, affect is usually more constricted but is most often appropriate to content. In mania, affect is typically very happy, with laughter, giggling, or exaggerated displays of joy. Many times in the client with mania, affect has a wide range and great flexibility and is inappropriate to the context.

Thought Process and Content

Thought content refers to the ideas, vocabulary, and actual subject matter about which the client speaks. For example, thought content is reflected in comments about family, job, or a recent stressful situation. Thought process refers to the way in which thinking occurs and is expressed by the client. The degree of logic and clarity of thought determine whether the client's thought processes are coherent. The nurse can assess thought process and content by formal questioning, with the use of structured and sometimes written questionnaires (such as the Mini-Mental Status Examination) or by informal discussion.

Clients with depression may exhibit confusion, difficulty concentrating, and thought blocking. Thought content often revolves around issues of loss and abandonment, worthlessness, guilt, and hopelessness. In the client with mania, thought processes are disturbed, with flight of ideas, ideas of reference, loose association, and often tangential and bizarre ideas. Thought content may revolve around issues of superiority, competition, and self-aggrandizement.

Perceptual Disturbances

Perception refers to awareness of events through the senses: tactile, olfactory, auditory, visual, and gustatory. Perceptions are subjective and internal. The nurse can elicit the client's perceptual experiences by verbal exploration and sometimes by observation of the client's behaviors. Perceptual disturbances (eg, delusions and hallucinations) often cause intense anxiety for clients.

Clients with depression often present with perceptual disturbances, such as hallucinations or delusions, particularly those of the persecutory type, especially if the depressive illness has psychotic features. Clients with bipolar disorders often have hallucinations and delusions because they have great difficulty screening out environmental stimuli.

Judgment and Insight

Judgment and decision-making capabilities are an important part of the MSE in the client with a mood disorder, because of the implications for the safety of the client and others. Depression can cause disturbed judgment, possibly related to anergia and withdrawal. On the other hand, clients with bipolar disorder may outwardly display impulsive, aggressive, and often dangerous behaviors that reflect disturbances in their ability to assess for danger and harm.

Insight is the client's ability to look inward, evaluate his or her own behavior, and have some ideas about what might be causing difficulty. Insight is often limited in clients who have major depression, because they cannot step back from themselves to assess the situation objectively. Clients in the manic phase of illness often have limited to no insight into their illness; they often cannot acknowledge that their behaviors are creating difficulty for themselves or others.

PHYSIOLOGICAL STABILITY ASSESSMENT

A primary nursing concern for the client with a mood disorder is physiological integrity and function. Often these clients avoid eating, have difficulty sleeping, and suffer from other physiological consequences of their inability to engage in self-care behaviors. Vegetative signs, energy, and psychomotor functioning may be considered physiological areas for assessment and intervention.

In clients with depression, vegetative signs include problems with appetite, sleep, nutrition, elimination, libido, and sexuality. Depression may decrease or increase appetite. The nurse fully assesses for recent weight gain or loss, appetite changes, nutritional intake, and bowel habits. Mania causes hyperactivity, resulting in the inability to sit still for the time needed to eat a full meal. Clients with mania often neglect their nutritional needs and fluid needs as a result of inattention.

Markedly disturbed sleep patterns are common in clients with mood disorders. Early morning awakening is common in clients with depression, and sleep disturbances contribute to fatigue and exhaustion. In mania, sleep patterns are disturbed as well, most often with lack of sleep for days at a time or disturbed sleep–wake cycles. These clients may have patterns of brief napping and then activity for extended periods.

Libido is usually lowered during depressive episodes. Conversely, many clients with mania report feelings of hypersexuality and hyperarousal. They may become promiscuous, increasing their exposure to HIV and other sexually transmitted diseases (STDs) and injurious situations.

FAMILY ISSUES ASSESSMENT

The family may be worried about or angry with the client and may not understand the disease. Families of a client with mania may become burned out, angry, and frustrated from trying to manage the manic behaviors at home. Finally, adherence to the medication regimen is the single most important factor in preventing relapse; however, many clients cease taking their medications when they feel well. Therefore, assessing the family's and client's knowledge about the disease and its treatment is essential, as is including them in care planning (Client and Family Education 24-1).

Nursing Diagnosis

Common diagnoses for clients with mood disorders are as follows:

- **Risk for Suicide** related to impaired judgment and distorted thinking (client with depressive or bipolar disorder) or impulsivity (client with bipolar disorder)
- **Risk for Violence** toward others related to impulsivity and impaired judgment (client with bipolar disorder) or agitation and low tolerance level (client with agitated depression)
- **Ineffective Health Maintenance** related to lack of attention, lack of concern for self, and low self-esteem (client with depressive disorder) or low attention threshold, hyperactivity, and lack of attention to self-care needs (client with bipolar disorder)
- **Impaired Social Interaction** related to distorted thinking, feelings of low self-esteem, disorientation, or restlessness
- **Disturbed Thought Processes** related to biochemical imbalances or psychological stress
- **Ineffective Therapeutic Regimen Management** related to lack of knowledge about medications and lack of incentive to maintain medication regimen upon discharge

Planning

Goals for clients with mood disorders include the following:

- The client will remain safe throughout the hospitalization, without harming self or others.
- The client will demonstrate self-control in milieu activities and interactions with others, including maintaining appropriate boundaries and refraining from aggressive or risky behaviors.
- The client will have adequate food and fluid intake, will maintain balanced rest, sleep, and activity, and will maintain personal care.
- The client will engage in appropriate social behavior.
- The client will demonstrate logical, reality-based thought processes.
- The client will consistently maintain the medication regimen, including taking medications as ordered and following up with his or her care provider for appropriate postdischarge visits and laboratory work.

Nursing Care Plans 24-1 and 24-2 discuss care for a client with depression and with bipolar disorder, respectively.

Implementation

PROTECTING THE CLIENT FROM SUICIDE

Interventions to prevent suicide are similar for clients with depression or bipolar disorder. The first step is to assess the client's level of risk for suicide. If the client is at risk, the nurse immediately places him or her on suicide precautions with frequent or continuous one-to-one observation and reassessment. In addition, the nurse locates the client's room central to the nursing station. He or she restricts the client to unit-based activities and removes dangerous objects (eg, glass, ties, belts, razors) from the environment. If the client needs to use these objects, the nurse monitors such use at all times. Considering the bathroom is the most common area for successful suicide completion in inpatient psychiatric settings, the nurse monitors the client carefully and locks the bathroom for safety, if needed.

Building a therapeutic relationship increases the likelihood that the client will convey suicidal thoughts to the nurse. The nurse establishes trust through brief, frequent contacts; empathy; and a nonjudgmental attitude that conveys caring and respect. He or she encourages the client to verbalize feelings and discuss current stressors. In particular, the nurse asks the client to talk about suicidal feelings when they surface. Then the nurse and client explore the sadness, anger, or other feelings that may have precipitated the suicidal thoughts. Because suicidal clients are often ambivalent about dying, the nurse encourages the client to verbalize why he or she would want

HELPING YOUR LOVED ONE WITH BIPOLAR DISORDER

Teaching Points

The family members of the person with bipolar disorder can experience a wide range of emotions about their loved one, including frustration, anger, and helplessness. The nurse can provide education and support to family members so that they are better able to cope with their own feelings and help their loved one. Begin by educating the family about bipolar disorder and its treatment. Other points to incorporate include recommending that family members:

- Learn the warning signs of mania and depression. Suggest that they plan with their loved one, while he or she is well, what to do when they notice these symptoms. For example, the family may want to make arrangements for withholding credit cards and banking privileges.
- Support their family member in adhering to the treatment plan, taking medications as ordered, and seeing his or her mental health practitioner on a regular basis.
- Offer to attend therapy sessions, if appropriate.
- Help the client refrain from using alcohol and drugs.
- Avoid interpreting their loved one's mood changes as rejection or an indication of their own inability to help. Remind them that this is the disease.
- Learn the warning signs of suicide. Tell them to take any threats or comments the person makes seriously and to seek help immediately from the person's mental health provider.
- Tell their loved one that his or her presence is deeply meaningful and important and that his or her suicide would be a tremendous loss.
- Share caretaking responsibilities with another family member or friend when the need is acute to prevent feelings of burnout.
- Understand that there is a difference between a good day and hypomania and between a bad day and depression. Let them know that their loved one can have good days and bad days that are not part of the illness.
- Take advantage of the help available from support groups.

Resources of Interest for Professionals and Families

For more information about mood disorders:

National Institute of Mental Health (NIMH)
Office of Communications and Public Liaison
Information Resources and Inquiries Branch
6001 Executive Blvd., Rm. 8184, MSC 9663
Bethesda, MD 20892-9663
Phone: (301) 443–4513; Fax: (301) 443–4279
Fax-back System, Mental Health FAX4U: (301) 443–5158

E-mail: *nimhinfo@nih.gov*; web site: *http://www.nimh.nih.gov*

Child & Adolescent Bipolar Foundation
1187 Willmette Avenue, PMB #331
Willmette, IL 60091
Phone: (847) 256–8525
Web site: *http://www.bpkids.org*

Depression and Related Affective Disorders Association (DRADA)
Johns Hopkins Hospital, Meyer 3–181
600 North Wolfe Street
Baltimore, MD 21287-7381
Phone: (410) 955–4647 or (202) 955–5800
E-mail: *drada@jhmi.edu*; web site: *http://www.med.jhu.edu/drada*

National Alliance for the Mentally Ill (NAMI)
Colonial Place Three
2107 Wilson Blvd., 3rd Floor
Arlington, VA 22201
Toll free: 1–800-950-NAMI (6264)
Phone: (703) 524–7600; fax: (703) 524–9094
Web site: *http://www.nami.org*

National Depressive and Manic-Depressive Association (NDMDA)
730 North Franklin Street, Suite 501
Chicago, IL 60610
Toll free: 1–800-826–3632
Phone: (312) 642–0049; fax: (312) 642–7243
Web site: *http://www.ndmda.org*

National Foundation for Depressive Illness, Inc. (NAFDI)
P.O. Box 2257
New York, NY 10116
Toll free: 1–800-239–1265
Web site: *http://www.depression.org*

National Mental Health Association (NMHA)
1021 Prince Street
Alexandria, VA 22314-2971
Toll free: 1–800-969-NMHA (6642)
Phone: (703) 684–7722; fax: (703) 684–5968
E-mail: *infoctr@nmha.org*; web site: *http://www.nmha.org*

Resources for Suicide Information and Prevention

NIMH
Office of Communications and Public Liaison
Public Inquiries: (301) 443–4513
Web site: *http://www.nimh.nih.gov*
American Association of Suicidology
Phone: (202) 237–2280
Web site: *http://www.suicidology.org*
American Foundation for Suicide Prevention
Phone: (212) 363–3500
Web site: *http://www.afsp.org*
Suicide Prevention Advocacy Network USA, Inc.
Phone: (770) 998–8819
Web site: *http://www.spanusa.org*

Nursing Care Plan 24-1

THE CLIENT WITH DEPRESSION

The therapist listens to Jill and Shane (from Clinical Example 24-1) and then discusses her concern over Jill's condition. She performs a comprehensive mental status examination and evaluation, including a suicide assessment. Jill states that she does not have a plan for committing suicide; she just wishes that she "weren't here." The therapist determines that Jill is a low to moderate risk for suicide, places her on an antidepressant, and arranges for the couple to come in weekly for follow-up.

The nurse therapist formulates the following plan of care for Jill:

Nursing Diagnosis: Risk for Suicide related to depression and feelings of self-blame and worthlessness as evidenced by the comment, "I'm really no good to anyone anymore. I just wish I were not here to bother everyone."

Goal: Jill will not harm herself.

Interventions	Rationales
Perform a suicide assessment and determine client's level of risk.	Assessing Jill's risk for suicide is critical in validating concerns that she may be suicidal and in determining the level of care needed to prevent suicide.
Repeat assessment frequently over the next 2 months.	Repeating the suicide assessment is important as suicidality increases when energy levels improve before the client's mood does.
Develop a contract with the client in which the client agrees to not harm herself and to immediately contact the therapist if she has suicidal thoughts.	Establishing a plan for Jill to implement if she has more intense suicidal thoughts will help prevent self-injury or death.

Evaluation: The effectiveness of the plan to prevent self-harm through frequent assessment and a contract is determined by Jill adhering to the contract and not harming herself.

Nursing Diagnosis: Disturbed Sleep Pattern related to depression as evidenced by nighttime inability to sleep and daytime lethargy

Goal: Jill will reestablish a natural pattern of sleep.

Interventions	Rationales
Encourage the client to establish normal sleep–wake routines by refraining from napping during the day.	Daytime sleeping will interfere with Jill's ability to sleep at night.
Suggest establishing nighttime routines that induce sleep, such as taking a hot bath or reading a book.	Avoiding stimulating activities and replacing them with calming ones will help Jill prepare for a more restful sleep.
Instruct client about medications and the sleep–wake schedule.	Antidepressants do help with restoring normal sleep patterns, but the client may also want to consider a hypnotic agent. If suicide risk is suspected, plans will need to be made for the safe administration of medications in the home environment.

Evaluation: Jill reports improved sleep patterns and feeling more well rested.

Nursing Diagnosis: Situational Low Self-Esteem related to depression as evidenced by the comment, "I'm a terrible mother, and I haven't even been doing my job as a wife and partner, either."

Goal: Jill will be able to see her self-worth.

(continued)

Nursing Care Plan 24-1 (continued)

Interventions	Rationales
Use cognitive-behavioral strategies to help client see how chronic thinking patterns influence mood and self-judgments.	Restructuring faulty thinking patterns can help turn depressive, pessimistic thinking patterns into self-affirming, optimistic ones.
Encourage client to recall past experiences in which she felt a sense of accomplishment and pride. Help the client identify areas of personal strength that contributed to the past events.	Helping Jill recall positive past experiences will contribute to her feelings of self-worth.
Help the client plan activities with her children and husband that she can accomplish each day that will help her regain confidence in her role performance as wife and mother. Make sure the plans are not overly ambitious so the client experiences successes each day.	Focusing on manageable activities will help Jill experience a sense of accomplishment, which contributes to higher feelings of self-esteem.
Explore the client's value system with her to help her see or develop congruity between her sense of self and that which she values.	Exploring underlying values and Jill's sense of connection with her beliefs will identify other target areas for therapy as her depression resolves.

Evaluation: Jill's improved feelings of self-worth, expressions of satisfaction with her role performance, and sense of connectedness to her value system are the best indicators that the plan of care has been effective.

Nursing Care Plan 24-2

THE CLIENT WITH BIPOLAR DISORDER IN THE MANIC PHASE

The charge nurse on the psychiatric unit, Janet Bell, RN, observes Danielle (from Clinical Example 24-2) in the milieu before the admission assessment. She notes that Danielle is walking rapidly up and down the hallway, poking her head into other client rooms and asking what they are doing. Danielle is dressed in a hot-pink outfit, with thick layers of makeup on her eyes and lips that match her dress. Danielle tries to engage other clients in an elaborate card game. When no one will play, she flings the cards at another client, cursing. Janet approaches Danielle from the front and gently asks if she can talk with her. They go to a quiet room where Janet conducts the admission assessment.

Throughout the interview, Danielle exhibits pressured speech and jumps quickly from one topic to the next. Danielle dismisses her husband's concerns and states she's been doing "great, better than ever!" Janet tries to engage Danielle in a discussion of treatment goals, but Danielle's comments about what she expects from treatment are extravagant and unrealistic—she expects to win an Oscar for the video she will produce. No matter what the topic, Danielle jokes briefly about it and returns to her plans for fame and fortune. Based on her observations and the interview, Janet develops a plan of care.

Nursing Diagnosis: Risk for Other Directed Violence related to psychiatric illness as evidenced by poor impulse control when angry

Goal: Danielle will manage her anger appropriately and will not harm or threaten others.

Interventions	Rationales
Perform a violence assessment and determine client's level of risk.	Assessing the client's risk for violence will help the staff establish guidelines and interventions.
Discuss anger management with client and determine what behaviors are appropriate when angry.	Providing limits and outlets for Danielle's anger will give her a concrete framework for managing angry impulses.

(continued)

Nursing Care Plan 24-2 (Continued)

Interventions	Rationales
Role model appropriate anger management and give the client feedback on her behavior.	Role modeling and feedback reinforce constructive coping.
Limit the client's environment and remove dangerous objects. Use sedative medication as needed and physical restraint or seclusion as a last resort.	Preventing violence by limiting Danielle's interaction with others is the best approach if her anger and outbursts escalate. Medication can be used effectively; however, seclusion and restraint should be used only if all other methods have failed.

Evaluation: Anger management strategies for Danielle can be considered effective if the following outcomes are met:

- Danielle refrains from harming others.
- Angry outbursts diminish.
- Danielle uses strategies for coping with anger and frustration.

Nursing Diagnosis: Disturbed Thought Processes related to psychiatric illness as evidenced by unrealistic, grandiose comments; pressured speech; flight of ideas; and incongruent affect

Goals: Danielle will exhibit reality-based thinking, appropriate thought content, and appropriate social activity.

Interventions	Rationales
Use a calm, forthright approach with the client and provide clear directions for the client.	Providing structure and expectations communicates that staff members are effectively managing the milieu, which should diminish power struggles and increase feelings of security for Danielle who is bordering on being out of control.
Establish firm expectations for behavior and communicate these limits clearly to the client. Have all staff members enforce limits consistently.	Consistently implementing limits will help prevent Danielle from trying to manipulate staff members and will help her to gain control of her own behavior.
Avoid getting into power struggles or trying to dissuade the client from her grandiose, delusional ideas.	Power struggles and arguments with staff members will increase Danielle's manic behavior.
Accept acting-out behavior neutrally; do not respond with irritation or anger. Avoid feeding into client's jokiness and maintain a professional demeanor.	Not participating in Danielle's manic perceptions and thwarting her conscious or unconscious attempts to upset staff will help prevent escalation of the manic behavior.
Redirect client into productive or more appropriate activities.	Manic clients are highly distractable; staff members can use this factor to their advantage by redirecting Danielle's energy when needed.

Evaluation: It may take 1 to 2 weeks for Danielle's medication to begin effectively stabilizing her mood, which will correct the delusional grandiose thinking. During this time, the effectiveness of the interventions can be evaluated by noting if Danielle maintains an affect consistent with her mood and maintains limits set by staff members.

Nursing Diagnosis: Risk for Deficient Fluid Volume and Imbalanced Nutrition: Less than Body Requirements related to excessive physical activity and inattention to physical needs

Goal: Danielle will ingest adequate fluids and nutrients.

(continued)

ENCOURAGING TREATMENT AND MEDICATION ADHERENCE

Interventions to assist clients with mood disorders to manage their medication regimens are similar regardless of the specific disorder. The nurse begins by providing clients with information about the medication and needed aftercare, such as frequency of laboratory testing, needed follow-up care, and discharge planning. For example, the client taking lithium must learn that blood levels must be checked twice a week initially and every 2 months after stable therapeutic levels have been reached. Likewise, clients prescribed Clozaril must understand the importance of monitoring for agranulocytosis. If possible, the nurse helps the client obtain a notebook or cards on which to record information about the medications, including mechanisms of action, dosages, side effects, and ongoing monitoring needs. He or she helps the client review the information until the client is familiar with each medication and its actions.

To help link the importance of taking the medication with relapse prevention, the nurse lists the target symptoms of the medications and identifies symptoms of imminent relapse. He or she problem-solves with the client about early management of symptoms so severity does not increase. Next, the nurse explores what the client perceives as barriers to obtaining medications, participating in follow-up with the psychiatric care provider, and having necessary laboratory tests done. The nurse works with the client to overcome real or perceived barriers.

The nurse addresses the issue of nonadherence matter-of-factly and discusses the client's view and factors that may affect his or her ability or willingness to adhere to the therapeutic regimen. It is often during periods of remission that clients become less vigilant and more apt to reduce their adherence to medication management and follow-up psychiatric care. The nurse works with the client and family regarding the importance of adhering to the treatment regimen, especially during periods in which symptoms are under control. He or she reinforces the link between symptom control and medication adherence. The nurse educates the family about medication management, adherence, target symptoms, and symptoms of recurrence.

As Hyman (2000) states, "One obvious area in which more potent psychosocial interventions are needed is the realm of treatment adherence. This is a particularly difficult problem in bipolar disorder because of the fact that during manic episodes people often feel well or even better than well and see no need to take medicine; however, many relapses are related to termination of medical treatments during periods of relative stability or early relapse" (p. 439).

Evaluation

Improvement in symptoms is gradual but noticeable as medication and psychodynamic interventions take effect.

Specific indicators that interventions are effective include the following:

- The client reports fewer or no suicidal thoughts.
- The client refrains from harming himself or herself or acting aggressively toward others.
- The client maintains physiologic health, including ingesting adequate calories and fluids, maintaining a balance between rest and activity, and independently managing self-care.
- The client participates appropriately in milieu activities and social interactions.
- The client expresses a positive sense of self-worth without delusions of grandeur.
- The client demonstrates logical thought processes.
- The client reports reduced anxiety and agitation.
- The client adheres to the therapeutic regimen and discusses the importance of doing so after discharge.

▼ Reflection and Critical Thinking Questions

1. Now that you have completed this chapter, consider Clinical Example 24-1 and the related nursing care presented in Nursing Care Plan (NCP) 24-1. Answer the following questions.

- List the symptoms that Jill has that lead you to think about major depressive disorder.
- What other information would you want to get from Jill and Shane?
- List at least three nursing diagnoses from the North American Nursing Diagnosis Association (NANDA), other than those discussed in NCP 24-1, that would be appropriate for Jill at this time.
- What are the immediate priorities in planning care for Jill?
- Discuss the longitudinal course of Jill's symptoms and talk about ways you might work with her over time to assist her in maintaining optimal functioning during times of relapse.

2. In Clinical Example 24–2, Danielle evidences clinical features of bipolar I disorder. Consider the nursing care presented in NCP 24-2 and answer the following questions.

- List the symptoms that Danielle has which lead you to think about bipolar disorder.
- What other information would you want to get from Danielle and Roger?
- What thoughts do you have about the severity, longitudinal course, and chronicity of Danielle's symptoms?
- List at least three NANDA nursing diagnoses, other than those discussed in NCP 24-2, that would be appropriate for Danielle at this time.
- What are the immediate priorities in planning care for Danielle?

▼ CHAPTER SUMMARY

■ Mood disorders include major depressive disorder, dysthymic disorder, and bipolar disorder.

■ Mood disorders are a significant problem in America, and suicide, which is closely associated with mood disorders, is an emergent national public health priority.

■ The etiology of mood disorders is complex and involves multiple interactions among genetic factors, physiologic factors, and psychological factors.

■ Signs and symptoms and diagnostic criteria for the mood disorders are categorized by diagnosis and are highly specific.

■ Mood disorders are often unrecognized and go untreated; however, when clients receive appropriate treatment, the mood disorders are highly treatable with good outcomes. There are multiple treatment modalities for clients with mood disorders, including individual, group, and family psychotherapies; pharmacotherapy; and somatic therapies.

■ Psychiatric-mental health nurses must use the nursing process to assess, plan, implement, and evaluate care for individuals who have mood disorders. Nursing assessment is the first step of the nursing process and involves systematic, thorough consideration of the client's *safety,* psychological functioning or mental status, physiological and psychomotor activity, and social and behavioral functioning. From data gathered during the assessment process, the nurse identifies the client's potential or actual problems in functioning, formulates nursing diagnoses, and specifies client behavior outcomes that guide the planning of interventions. Following interventions, the nurse evaluates the effectiveness of the interventions in contributing to desired outcomes, makes changes and improvements, and continues with the assessment process.

▼ REVIEW QUESTIONS

1. Georgie, a 32-year-old woman, has a history of bipolar disorder but stopped taking her lithium 2 months ago. Her family found her in a bar, claiming to be a millionaire, dressed provocatively, and buying everyone drinks. She is admitted to the psychiatric unit and has received two 300-mg doses of lithium carbonate. On the unit, she is somewhat irritable and has been running up and down the hallway, asking male clients if they will lie down with her. She also has been entering other clients' rooms dressed only in her underwear. The nurse notes that her behaviors reflect
   a. Poor judgment
   b. Euthymia
   c. Increased attention span
   d. Poor planning and insight

2. The first priority for nursing interventions with Georgie upon her admission to the unit would be
   a. Monitoring for lithium toxicity and hypertensive crisis
   b. Close monitoring of her behavior and taking appropriate actions to ensure she does not injure other clients and maintains behavioral control
   c. Taking Georgie out of the milieu, medicating her for agitation, and putting her on 1:1 supervision
   d. Teaching Georgie that her behavior negatively affects other clients and staff

3. You would expect to see Georgie's lithium levels become therapeutic in about
   a. 24 hours
   b. 48 hours
   c. 1 to 2 weeks
   d. 3 to 4 weeks

4. After Georgie has been taking lithium for 2 weeks, she complains of vomiting, having diarrhea, and slurring her words. Which of the following represents the most appropriate nursing action?
   a. Tell Georgie that these are symptoms of mild toxicity that will go away as she becomes reaccustomed to the lithium.
   b. Immediately call the physician to inform her of Georgie's symptoms and hold her next lithium dose.
   c. Check to see that her last lithium level was safely between 1 and 2 mEq/L.
   d. Tell her to lie down, immediately drawing a blood glucose and giving her orange juice.

5. Therapeutic lithium levels range between
   a. 2.0 to 7.9 mEq/L
   b. 0.01 to 0.05 mEq/L
   c. 1.0 to 1.5 mEq/L
   d. 2.5 to 3.0 mEq/L

6. A 35-year-old client with depression lost his job and most of his investments because of his own unethical business practices. He states his family would be better off without him because of the shame he has brought to them. How should the nurse respond to this statement?
   a. "Tell me more about the shame you feel."
   b. "Are you thinking of killing yourself?"
   c. "Has your wife told you she wants a divorce?"
   d. "You appear depressed."

7. Dysthymia refers to
   a. A less severe form of depressive disorder
   b. A less severe form of bipolar I disorder
   c. Normal sad moods that most people feel from time to time
   d. A mood disorder related to dysfunction of the thymus gland

8. A 30-year-old physically fit female client with a history of depression returns to the mental health clinic for follow-up care. She takes 100 mg of sertraline daily. In addition, she states she tries to stay mentally and physically well by taking yoga classes, walking regularly, and taking vitamins and St. John's wort. She also relates that she is a lacto-ovo-vegetarian and gets most of her protein from cheese. Given this data, what should the nurse tell the client?
   a. "You should avoid cheese as it can, in conjunction with your medication, precipitate hypertensive crises."
   b. "You're doing a great job taking care of yourself. You've made several healthy lifestyle choices."
   c. "You should stop taking the St. John's wort as it can, in conjunction with your medication, precipitate serotonin syndrome."
   d. "You're doing a great job with your lifestyle choices. I suggest you do more intensive aerobic exercise, as aerobic exercise has been shown to stabilize mood."

9. A 25-year-old male client has been in inpatient treatment for severe depression for 3 weeks. He will be discharged soon, and the nurse is evaluating the effectiveness of the plan of care. Which outcome is the most appropriate indicator that the client's depression is resolving sufficiently for safe discharge?
   a. The client has resumed caring for his physical appearance and always appears clean and well groomed.
   b. The client denies wanting to commit suicide.
   c. The client expresses a willingness to begin tapering his medication.
   d. The client will sit in the public areas and will speak when addressed.

10. Which of the following variables has the most impact on relapse prevention for clients with depressive or bipolar disorders?
   a. Strong social support
   b. High socioeconomic status
   c. Stress-management skills
   d. Medication adherence

▼ REFERENCES AND SUGGESTED READINGS

*Ader, R. (2000a). Classical conditioning in the treatment of psoriasis. *Cutis, 66*(5), 370–372.

*Ader, R. (2000b). On the development of psychoneuroimmunology. *European Journal of Pharmacology, 405*(1–3), 167–176.

*Ader, R., Cohen, N., & Felten, D. (1995). Psychoneuroimmunology: Interactions between the nervous system and the immune system. *Lancet, 345*(8942), 99–103.

*Agency for Healthcare Policy and Research. (1999, March). Treatment of depression—newer pharmacotherapies (summary). *Evidence Report/Technology Assessment, 7.* (On-line.) Available at: *http://www.ahrq.gov/clinic/deprsumm.htm.*

*Altar, C. A. (1999). Neurotrophins and depression. *Trends in Pharmacological Science, 20*(2), 59–61.

*American Psychiatric Association. (2000). *Diagnostic and statistical manual of mental disorders* (4th ed., text rev.). Washington, DC: Author.

*Andersen, S. (1999). Patient perspective and self-help. *Neurology, 52*(7, Suppl. 3), S26–S28.

*Beck, A. T. (1972). *Depression: Causes and treatment.* Philadelphia: University of Pennsylvania Press.

*Beck, A. T., & Rush, A. J. (1989). Cognitive therapy. In H. I. Kaplan & B. J. Sadock (Eds.), *Comprehensive textbook of psychiatry* (Vol. 2, 5th ed., pp. 1542–1543). Baltimore: Williams & Wilkins.

*Beck, A. T., Rush, A. J., Shaw, B. F., & Emery, G. (1979). *Cognitive therapy of depression.* New York: Guilford.

*Beeber, L. S. (1996). Depression in women. In A. B. McBride & J. K. Austin (Eds.), *Psychiatric-mental health nursing: Integrating the behavioral and biological sciences* (pp. 235–268). Philadelphia: W.B. Saunders.

*Birmaher, B., Ryan, N. D., Williamson, D. E., et al. (1996). Childhood and adolescent depression: A review of the past 10 years. Part I. *Journal of the American Academy of Child and Adolescent Psychiatry, 35*(11, Pt. 1), 1427–1439.

Blumenthal, S. J. (1988). Suicide: A guide to risk factors, assessment, and treatment of suicidal patients. *Medical Clinics of North America, 72,* 937–971.

*Blumenthal, S. J., & Kupfer, D. J. (Eds.). (1990). *Suicide over the life cycle.* Washington, DC: American Psychiatric Press.

*Bobo, W. V., et al. (2001). *VHA/DOD clinical practice guideline for the management of major depressive disorder in adults* (Rev. ed.). Washington, DC: Department of Veterans Affairs.

Bodner, R. A., Lynch, T., Lewis, L., & Kahn, D. (1995). Serotonin syndrome. *Neurology, 45*(2), 219–223.

*Bowden, C. L. (2001, May). *Recurrent depression.* Presentation at 5th annual meeting of the American Psychiatric Association, Atlanta, GA.

*Bowden, C. L., Calabrese, J. R., McElroy, L., et al. (2000). A randomized, placebo-controlled 12-month trial of divalproex and lithium in treatment of outpatients with bipolar I disorder. *Archives of General Psychiatry, 57,* 481–489.

Brunello, N., Akiskal, H., Boyer, P., Gessa, G. L., Howland, R. H., Langer, S. M., et al. (1999). Dysthymia: Clinical picture, extent of overlap with chronic fatigue syndrome, neuropharmacological considerations, and new therapeutic vistas. *Journal of Affective Disorders, 52*(1–3), 275–290.

*Burger, S. G., et al. (1998). *Pharmacotherapy companion to the depression clinical practice guideline* (p. 26). Columbia, MD: American Medical Director's Association.

*Cadoret, R. (1978). Evidence for genetic inheritance of primary affective disorder in adoptees. *American Journal of Psychiatry, 133,* 463–466.

*Calabrese, J. R., Bowden, C. L., McElroy, S. L., et al. (1999). Spectrum of activity of lamotrigine in treatment of refractory bipolar disorder. *American Journal of Psychiatry, 156,* 1019–1023.

*Calabrese, J. R., Suppes, T., Bowden, C. L., Sachs, G. S.,

Swann, A. C., McElroy, S. L., et al. (2000). A double-blind, placebo-controlled, prophylaxis study of lamotrigine in rapid cycling bipolar disorder. Lamictal 614 Study Group. *Journal of Clinical Psychiatry, 61*(11), 841–850.

*Center for Mental Health Services. (2001). *National strategy for suicide prevention: Goals and objectives for action* (Publication Inventory Number SMA01–3517). (On-line.) Available at: *http://www.mentalhealth.org/publications/allpubs/SMA01–3517/default.asp.*

*Centers for Disease Control and Prevention. (2001). Ten leading causes of death for the United States. (On-line.) Available at: *http://webapp.cdc.gov/sasweb/ncipc/leadcaus10.html.*

*Compton, M. T., & Nemeroff, C. B. (2000). The treatment of bipolar depression. *Journal of Clinical Psychiatry, 61*(Suppl. 9), 57–67.

*Coyle, N., Jones, I., Robertson, E., et al. (2000). Variation at the serotonin transporter gene influences susceptibility to bipolar affective puerperal psychosis. *Lancet, 356*(9240), 1490–1491.

*Craighead, W. E., & Miklowitz, D. J. (2000). Psychosocial interventions for bipolar disorder. *Journal of Clinical Psychiatry, 61*(Suppl. 13), 58–64.

*Cutler, C. (2001). Self-care agency and symptom management in patients treated for mood disorder. *Archives of Psychiatric Nursing, 15*(1), 24–31.

*De Bruyn, A., Souery, D., Mendelbaum, K., Mendlewicz, J., & Van Broeckhoven, C. (1996). Linkage analysis of families with bipolar illness and chromosome 18 markers. *Biological Psychiatry, 39*, 679–688.

*Demet, E. M., Chicz-Demet, A., Fallon, J. H., & Sokolski, K. N. (1999). Sleep deprivation therapy in depressive illness and Parkinson's disease. *Progress in Neuropsychopharmacology and Biologic Psychiatry, 23*(5), 753–784.

Depression Guideline Panel. (1993). Depression in primary care: Volume 1. Detection and diagnosis (AHCPR Publication No. 93–0550). *Clinical Practice Guideline, 5.* Rockville, MD: Agency for Health Care Policy and Research.

Detera-Wadleigh, S., Badner, J. A., Goldin, L. R., Berrettini, W., Sanders, A. R., Rollins, D. Y., et al. (1996). Affected-sib-pair analyses reveal support of prior evidence for a susceptibility locus for bipolar disorder, on 21q. *American Journal of Human Genetics, 58*, 1279–1285.

*Detera-Wadleigh, S. D., Badner, J. A., Yoshikawa, T., Sanders, A. R., Goldin, L. R., Turner, G., et al. (1997). Initial genome scan of the NIMH Genetics Initiative bipolar I pedigrees: Chromosomes 4, 7, 9, 18, 19, 20, and 21q. *American Journal of Medical Genetics, 74*, 254–262.

Eggert, L. L., & Herting, J. R. (1991). Preventing teenage drug abuse: Exploratory effects of network social support. *Youth & Society, 22*, 482–524.

Eggert, L. L., Seyl, C., & Nicholas, L. J. (1990). Effects of a school-based prevention program for potential high school dropouts and drug abusers. *International Journal of Addictions, 24*, 773–801.

Eggert, L. L., Thompson, E. A., Herting, J. R., & Nicholas, L. J. (1994). Prevention research program: Reconnecting at-risk youth. *Issues in Mental Health Nursing, 15*, 107–135.

Eggert, L. L., Thompson, E. A., Herting, J. R., & Nicholas, L. J. (1995). Reducing suicide potential among high-risk youth: Tests of a school-based prevention program. *Suicide & Life-Threatening Behavior, 25*(2), 276–296.

*Ellgring, J. H. (1999). Depression, psychosis, and dementia: Impact on the family. *Neurology, 52*(7, Suppl. 3), S17–S20.

Eriksson, E. (2000). Antidepressant drugs: Does it matter if they inhibit the reuptake of noradrenaline or serotonin? *Acta Psychiatric Scandinavia Supplement, 402*, 12–17.

*Freud, S. (1957). Mourning and melancholia. In *Standard edition of the works of Sigmund Freud* (Vol. 14). London: Hogarth.

Geller, B., & Luby, J. (1997). Child and adolescent bipolar disorder: A review of the past 10 years. *Journal of the American Academy of Child and Adolescent Psychiatry, 36*(9), 1168–1176.

*George, M. S., Nahas, Z., Kozel, F. A., Goldman, J., Molloy, M., & Oliver, N. (1999). Improvement of depression following transcranial magnetic stimulation. *Current Psychiatry Reports, 1*(2), 114–124.

*George, M. S., Nahas, Z., Molloy, M., et al. (2000a). A controlled trial of daily left prefrontal cortex TMS for treating depression. *Biological Psychiatry, 48*, 962–970.

*George, M. S., Sackeim, H. A., Marangell, L. P., Husain, M. M., Nahas, Z., Lisanby, S. H., et al., (2000b). Vagus nerve stimulation. A potential therapy for resistant depression? *Psychiatric Clinics of North America, 23*(4), 757–783.

Gershon, E. S., Hamovit, J. H., Guroff, J. J., Dibble, E., Leckman, J. F., Sceery, W., et al. (1982). A family study of schizoaffective, bipolar I, bipolar II, unipolar, and normal control probands. *Archives of General Psychiatry, 39*, 1157–1167.

*Ghaemi, S. N. (2000). New treatments for bipolar disorder: The role of atypical neuroleptic agents. *Journal of Clinical Psychiatry, 61*(Suppl. 14), 33–42.

*Gitlin, M. J. (2001). Treatment-resistant bipolar disorder. *Bulletin Menninger Clinics, 65*(1), 6–40.

*Glaser, R., et al. (1999). The differential impact of training stress and final examination stress on herpesvirus latency at the United States Military Academy at West Point. *Brain, Behavior, and Immunity, 13*(3), 240–251.

*Goodwin, F. K., & Jamison, K. R. (1990). *Manic-depressive illness.* New York: Oxford University Press.

*Greer, S. (2000). Fighting spirit in patients with cancer. *Lancet, 355*(9206), 847–848.

*Harris, E. C., & Barraclough, B. B. (1997). Suicide as an outcome for mental disorders. *British Journal of Psychiatry, 170*, 205–229.

Henney, J. E. (2000). Risk of drug interactions with St. John's wort. From the Food and Drug Administration. *Journal of the American Medical Association, 283*(13), 1679.

Horwath, E., Johnson, J., Klerman, G. L., et al. (1992). Depressive symptoms as relative and attributable risk factors for first-onset major depression. *Archives of General Psychiatry, 49*(10), 817–823.

*Hoyert, D. L., Kochanek, K. D., & Murphy, S. L. (1999). Deaths: Final data for 1997 (DHHS Publication No. 99–1120). *National Vital Statistics Reports, 47*(19). Hyattsville, MD: National Center for Health Statistics.(On-line.) Available at: *http://www.cdc.gov/nchs/data/nvs47_19.pdf.*

*Huxley, N. A., Parikh, S. V., & Baldessarini, R. J. (2000). Effectiveness of psychosocial treatments in bipolar disorder: State of the evidence. *Harvard Review of Psychiatry, 8*(3), 126–140.

*Hyman, S. E. (1999). Introduction to the complex genetics of mental disorders. *Biological Psychiatry, 45*(5), 518–521.

Hyman, S. E. (2000). Goals for research on bipolar disorder: The view from NIMH. *Biological Psychiatry, 48,* 436–441.

Hyman, S. E., & Rudorfer, M. V. (2000). Depressive and bipolar mood disorders. In D. C. Dale & D. D. Federman (Eds.), *Scientific America; Medicine* (Vol. 3, Sect. 13, Subsect. II, p. 1). New York: Healtheon/WebMD Corp.

*Karch, A. M. (2002). *2002 Lippincott's nursing drug guide.* Philadelphia: Lippincott Williams & Wilkins.

*Keller, M. B., McCullough, J. P., Klein, D. N., et al. (2000). A comparison of nefazodone, the cognitive behavioral-analysis system of psychotherapy, and their combination for the treatment of chronic depression. *New England Journal of Medicine, 342,* 1462–1470.

Killgore, W. D. (2000). Academic and research interest in several approaches to psychotherapy: A computerized search of literature in the past 16 years. *Psychology Report, 87*(3, Pt.1), 717–720.

Klein, D. N., Schwartz, J. E., Rose, S., et al. (2000). Five-year course and outcome of dysthymic disorder: A prospective, naturalistic follow-up study. *American Journal of Psychiatry, 157*(6), 931–939.

*Kronfol, Z., & Remick, D. G. (2000). Cytokines and the brain: Implications for clinical psychiatry. *American Journal of Psychiatry, 157*(5), 683–694.

*Krystal, A. D., West, M., Prado, R., Greenside, H., Zoldi, S., & Weiner, R. D. (2000). EEG effects of ECT: Implications for TMS. *Depression and Anxiety, 12*(3), 157–165.

*Larson, M. R., Ader, R., & Moynihan, J. A. (2001). Heart rate, neuroendocrine, and immunological reactivity in response to an acute laboratory stressor. *Psychosomatic Medicine, 63*(3), 493–501.

Lebowitz, B. D., Pearson, J. L., Schneider, L. S., et al. (1997). Diagnosis and treatment of depression in late life. Consensus statement update. *Journal of the American Medical Association, 278*(14), 1186–1190.

*Lejuez, C. W., Hopko, D. R., & Hopko, S. D. (2001). A brief behavioral activation treatment for depression: Treatment manual. *Behavior Modification, 25*(2), 255–286.

*Leonard, B. E. (1997). The role of noradrenaline in depression. *Journal of Psychopharmacology, 11*(4 Suppl.), S39–S47.

*Leonard, B. E. (2000). Evidence for a biochemical lesion in depression. *Journal of Clinical Psychiatry, 61*(Suppl. 6), 12–27.

*Leonard, B. E. (2001). The immune system, depression and the action of antidepressants. *Progress in Neuropsychopharmacologic and Biologic Psychiatry, 25*(4), 767–804.

*Levy, N. A., & Janicak, P. G. (2000). Calcium channel antagonists for the treatment of bipolar disorder. *Bipolar Disorder, 2*(2), 108–119.

Llewellyn, A., Stowe, Z. N., Strader, J. R., Jr. (1998). The use of lithium and management of women with bipolar disorder during pregnancy and lactation. *Journal of Clinical Psychiatry, 59*(Suppl. 6), 57–64; discussion on p. 65.

*Lund, B. C., & Perry, P. J. (2000). Olanzapine: An atypical antipsychotic for schizophrenia. *Expert Opinion in Pharmacotherapy, 1*(2), 305–323.

*Maj, M. (2000). The impact of lithium prophylaxis on the course of bipolar disorder: A review of the research evidence. *Bipolar Disorder, 2*(2), 93–101.

Mann, J. J., Huang, Y., Underwood, M. D., Kassir, S. A., Oppenheim, S., Kelly, T. M., et al. (2000). A serotonin transporter gene promotes polymorphism (5-HTLPR) and prefrontal cortical binding in major depression and suicide. *Archives of General Psychiatry, 57,* 729–738.

*McIntosh, J. L. (2001). *1998 official final statistics: USA suicide.* Prepared for the American Association of Suicidology. [On-line.] Available: www.suicidology.org.

*Mendlewicz, J., & Rainer, J. D. (1977). Adoption study supporting genetic transmission in manic-depressive illness. *Nature, 268,* 326–329.

*Misri, S., Kostaras, X., Fox, D., et al. (2000). The use of selective serotonin reuptake inhibitors during pregnancy and lactation: Current knowledge. *Canadian Journal of Psychiatry, 45*(3), 285–287.

*Moldin, S. O., Reich, T., & Rice, J. P. (1991). Current perspectives on the genetics of unipolar depression. *Behavior Genetics, 21,* 211–242.

Mueser, K. T., Goodman, L. B., Trumbetta, S. L., Rosenberg, S. D., Osher, F. C., Vidaver, R., et al. (1998). Trauma and posttraumatic stress disorder in severe mental illness. *Journal of Consulting and Clinical Psychology, 66*(3), 493–499.

*Murphy, S. L. (2000). Deaths: Final data for 1998. (DHHS Publication No. [PHS] 2000–1120; data to be published in the 1998 annual volume of *Vital Statistics of the United States*). *National Vital Statistics Report, 48*(11), 86.

*Murray, C. J. L., & Lopez, A. D. (Eds.). (1996). *Summary: The global burden of disease: A comprehensive assessment of mortality and disability from diseases, injuries, and risk factors in 1990 and projected to 2020.* Cambridge, MA: Published by the Harvard School of Public Health on behalf of the WHO and the World Bank, Harvard University Press. (On-line.) Available at: *http://www.who.int/msa/mnh/ems/dalys/intro.html.*

*Nahas, Z., Molloy, M. A., Hughes, P. L., Oliver, N. C., Arana, G. W., Risch, S. C., et al. (1999). Repetitive transcranial magnetic stimulation: Perspectives for application in the treatment of bipolar and unipolar disorders. *Bipolar Disorders, 1*(2), 73–80.

*Narrow, W. E. (n.d.). One-year prevalence of depressive disorders among adults 18 and over in the U.S.: NIMH ECA prospective data. Population estimates based on U.S. Census-estimated residential population age 18 and over on July 1, 1998. Unpublished manuscript.

*National Institute of Mental Health. (2001). *The numbers count: Mental disorders in America.* (NIMH Publication No. 01–4584). Rockville, MD: Author.

National Institute of Mental Health Genetics Workgroup. (1998). *Genetics and mental disorders.* (NIH Publication No. 98–4268). Rockville, MD: Author.

*Nemeroff, C. B. (1998). The neurobiology of depression. *Scientific American, 278,* 6.

*Neumeister, A., Praschak-Rieder, N., Willeit, M., Stastny, J., & Kasper, S. (1999). Monoamine depletion in non-pharmacological treatments for depression. *Adv. Exp. Med. Biol. 467,* 29–33.

Nierenberg, A. A., Burt, T., Matthews, J., & Weiss, A. P. (1999). Mania associated with St. John's wort. *Biological Psychiatry, 46*(12), 1707–1708.

*Nisijima, et al. (2000). Risperidone counteracts lethality in an animal model of the serotonin syndrome. *Psychopharmacology, 150*(1), 9–14.

Pearson, J. L., Conwell, Y., & Lyness, J. M. (1997). Late-life suicide and depression in the primary care setting. In L. S. Schneider (Ed.), *Developments in geriatric psychiatry. New directions for mental health services* (No. 76, pp. 13–38). San Francisco: Jossey-Bass.

*Phiel, C. J., & Klein, P. S. (2001). Molecular targets of lithium action. *Annual Review of Pharmacology and Toxicology, 41,* 789–813.

*Post, R. M., Frye, M. A., Denicoff, K. D., Leverich, G. S., Dunn, R. T., Osuch, E. A., et al. (2000). Emerging trends in the treatment of rapid cycling bipolar disorders: A selected review. *Bipolar Disorder, 2*(4), 305–315.

*Prater, J. F. (2001). Recurrent depression with vagus nerve stimulation. *American Journal of Psychiatry, 158,* 816–817.

*Racagni, G., & Brunello, N. (1999). Physiology to functionality: The brain and neurotransmitter activity. *International Clinical Psychopharmacology, 14*(Suppl. 1), S3–S7.

Regier, D. A., Narrow, W. E., Rae, D. S., et al. (1993). The de facto mental and addictive disorder service system. Epidemiologic Catchment Area prospective 1-year prevalence rates of disorders and services. *Archives of General Psychiatry, 50*(2), 85–94.

Rothschild, A. J., Bates, K. S., Boehringer, K. L., & Syed, A. (1999). Olanzapine response in psychotic depression. *Journal of Clinical Psychiatry, 60*(2), 116–118.

*Sachs, G. S., Koslow, C. L., & Ghaemi, S. N. (2000). The treatment of bipolar depression. *Bipolar disorder, 2*(3, Pt. 2), 256–260.

Sachs, G. S., Printz, D. J., Kahn, D. A., Carpenter, D., & Docherty, J. P. (2000, April). The expert consensus guideline series: Medication treatment of bipolar disorder. *Postgraduate Medicine,* Spec No., 1–104.

Sachs, G. S., & Thase, M. E. (2000). Bipolar disorder therapeutics: Maintenance treatment. *Biological Psychiatry, 48*(6), 573–581.

*Schweitzer, I. (2001). Does risperidone have a place in the treatment of nonschizophrenia patients? *International Clinical Psychopharmacology, 16*(1), 1–19.

*Segal, Z. V., Whitney, D. K., Lam, R. W., & CANMAT Depression Work Group. (2001). Clinical guidelines for the treatment of depressive disorders. III. Psychotherapy. *Canadian Journal of Psychiatry, 46*(Suppl. 1), 29S–37S.

Seligman, M. P., Friedman, R. J., & Katz, M. M. (Eds.). (1974). *Depression and learned helplessness in the psychology of depression: Contemporary theory and research.* New York: John Wiley & Sons.

*Snow, V., Lascher, S., & Mottur-Pilson, C. (2000). Pharmacologic treatment of acute major depression and dysthymia. *Annals of Internal Medicine, 132*(9), 738–742.

Soares, J. C., & Mann, J. J. (1997a). The anatomy of mood disorders—review of structural neuroimaging studies. *Biological Psychiatry, 41*(1), 86–106.

Soares, J. C., & Mann, J. J. (1997b). The functional neuroanatomy of mood disorders. *Journal of Psychiatric Research, 31*(4), 393–432.

Spitz, R. A. (1946). Anaclitic depression. In P. Greenacre (Ed.), *Psychoanalytic study of the child* (Vol. 2). New York: International Universities Press.

*Stahl, S. M. (1996). *Essential psychopharmacology: Neuroscientific basis and practical applications.* Cambridge, MA: Cambridge University Press.

Stoll, A. L., Severus, W. E., Freeman, M. P., Rueter, S., Zboyan,

H. A., Diamond, E., et al. (1999). Omega 3 fatty acids in bipolar disorder: A preliminary double-blind, placebo-controlled trial. *Archives of General Psychiatry, 56*(5), 407–412.

Strakowski, S. M., & DelBello, M. P. (2000). The co-occurrence of bipolar and substance use disorders. *Clinical Psychology Review, 20*(2), 191–206.

Strakowski, S. M., Sax, K. W., McElroy, S. L., Keck, P. E., Jr., Hawkins, J. M., & West, S. A. (1998). Course of psychiatric and substance abuse syndromes co-occurring with bipolar disorder after a first psychiatric hospitalization. *Journal of Clinical Psychiatry, 59*(9), 465–471.

Suppes, T., Webb, A., Paul, B., Carmody, T., Kraemer, H., & Rush, A. J. (1999). Clinical outcome in a randomized 1-year trial of clozapine versus treatment as usual for patients with treatment-resistant illness and a history of mania. *American Journal of Psychiatry, 156*(8), 1164–1169.

Svensson, T. H. (2000). Brain noradrenaline and the mechanisms of action of antidepressant drugs. *Acta Psychiatric Scandinavia Supplement, 402,* 18–27.

*Swann, A. C. (2001). Major system toxicities and side effects of anticonvulsants. *Journal of Clinical Psychiatry, 62*(Suppl.14), 16–21.

*Swartz, H. A., & Frank, E. (2001). Psychotherapy for bipolar depression: A phase-specific treatment strategy? *Bipolar Disorders, 3*(1), 11–22.

*Szuba, M. P., Baxter, L. R., Jr., Altshuler, L. L., Allen, E. M., Guze, B. H., Schwartz, J. M., et al. (1994). Lithium sustains the acute antidepressant effects of sleep deprivation: Preliminary findings from a controlled study. *Psychiatry Research, 51*(3), 283–295.

*Szuba, M. P., O'Reardon, J. P., & Evans, D. L. (2000). Physiological effects of electroconvulsive therapy and transcranial magnetic stimulation in major depression. *Depression and Anxiety, 12*(3), 170–177.

*Teasdale, J. D., Segal, Z., & Williams, J. M. (1995). How does cognitive therapy prevent depressive relapse and why should attentional control (mindfulness) training help? *Behavioral Research and Therapy, 33*(1), 25–39.

Thase, M. E., & Sachs, G. S. (2000). Bipolar depression: Pharmacotherapy and related therapeutic strategies. *Biological Psychiatry, 48*(6), 558–572.

Thompson, L. W., Coon, D. W., Gallagher-Thompson, D., Sommer, B. R., & Koin, D. (2001). Comparison of desipramine and cognitive/behavioral therapy in the treatment of elderly outpatients with mild-to-moderate depression. *American Journal of Geriatric Psychiatry, 9*(3), 225–240.

*Tohen, M., Jacobs, T. G., & Feldman, P. D. (2000). Onset of action of antipsychotics in the treatment of mania. *Bipolar Disorder, 2*(3, Pt. 2), 261–268.

Tohen, M., Sanger, T. M., McElroy, S. L., Tollefson, G. D., Chengappa, K. N., Daniel, D. G., et al. (1999). Olanzapine versus placebo in the treatment of acute mania. Olanzapine HGEH Study Group. *American Journal of Psychiatry, 156* (5), 702–709.

*Tsuang, M. T., & Faraone, S. V. (1990). *The genetics of mood disorders.* Baltimore: Johns Hopkins University Press.

U.S. Department of Health and Human Services. (1999). *Mental health: A report of the Surgeon General.* Rockville, MD: U.S. Department of Health and Human Services, Substance Abuse and Mental Health Services Administration,

Center for Mental Health Services, National Institutes of Health, National Institute of Mental Health.

U.S. Public Health Service. (1999). *The Surgeon General's call to action to prevent suicide.* Washington, DC: Author.

Vainionpaa, L. K., Rattya, J., Knip, M., Tapanainen, J. S., Pakarinen, A. J., Lanning, P., et al. (1999). Valproate-induced hyperandrogenism during pubertal maturation in girls with epilepsy. *Annals of Neurology, 45*(4), 444–450.

*Weissman, M. M., Gershon, E. S., Kidd, K. K., Prusoff, B. A., Leckman, J. F., Dibble, E., et al. (1984). Psychiatric disorders in the relatives of probands with affective disorders. *Archives of General Psychiatry, 41,* 13–21.

*Weissman, M. M., Wolk, S., Goldstein, R. B., et al. (1999). Depressed adolescents grown up. *Journal of the American Medical Association, 281,* 1701–1713.

Wender, P. H., Kety, S. S., Rosenthal, D., Schulsinger, F., Ortmann, J., & Lunde, I. (1986). Psychiatric disorders in the biological and adoptive families of adopted individuals with affective disorders. *Archives of General Psychiatry, 43,* 923–929.

*Winokur, G., Tsuang, M. T., & Crowe, R. R. (1982). The Iowa 500: Affective disorder in relatives of manic and depressive patients. *American Journal of Psychiatry, 139,* 209–212.

*Wirz-Justice, A., & Van den Hoofdakker, R. H. (1999). Sleep deprivation in depression: What do we know, where do we go? *Biological Psychiatry, 46,* 445–453.

*Wright, J. H., & Thase, M. E. (1992). Cognitive and biological therapies: A synthesis. *Psychiatric Annals, 22,* 451–458.

Starred references are cited in text.

For additional information on this chapter, go to *http://connection. lww.com.*

Need more help? See Chapter 24 of the *Study Guide to Accompany Mohr: Johnson's Psychiatric-Mental Health Nursing,* 5th edition.

The Client With a Thought Disorder

BARBARA SCHOEN JOHNSON; GERALDINE S. PEARSON

▼ KEY TERMS

Affect—An observable behavior that expresses feeling or emotional tone; it refers to more fluctuating changes in emotional "weather."

Affective flattening or blunting—A reduced intensity of emotional expression and response.

Alogia—A poverty of thinking that is inferred from observing the client's language and speech.

Anhedonia—The loss of capacity to experience pleasure subjectively.

Apathy—The seeming absence of caring about self or others.

Avolition—The inability to start, persist in, and carry through any goal-directed activity to its logical conclusion.

Delusions—Fixed, false beliefs about external reality that reasoning cannot correct; these include but are not limited to the following types: *grandiose* (beliefs involving inflated self-worth, power, or knowledge), *persecutory* (beliefs that one is being attacked, harassed, cheated, or conspired against), and *somatic* (beliefs that give false attributions to the appearance or functioning of one's body).

Dual diagnosis—Diagnosis of a serious mental illness in addition to a sub-stance abuse disorder or an addiction to a substance.

Extrapyramidal side effects—The most common and distressing side effects associated with traditional antipsychotic medications; they include *akathisia* (severe restlessness), *dystonia* (muscle spasms or contractions), chronic motor problems such as tardive dyskinesia, and the pseudoparkinsonian symptoms of rigidity, masklike faces, and stiff gait.

Hallucinations—A sensory perception with a compelling sense of reality; types include *auditory* (involving the perception of sound); *gustatory* (involving the perception of taste); *olfactory* (involving the perception of odor); *tactile* (involving the perception of being touched or of something under the skin); *visual* (involving sight, such as seeing images, people, flashes of light); and *somatic* (involving the perception of a physical experience localized within the body).

Mood—A sustained emotional "climate."

Schizophrenia—A heterogeneous disorder of the brain with features including thought disturbances and preoccupa-tion with frightening inner experiences (eg, delusions and hallucinations), affect disturbances (eg, flat or inappro-priate affect), and behavioral or social disturbances (eg, unpredictable, bizarre behavior or social isolation).

Tardive dyskinesia—An extrapyramidal symptom characterized by abnormal, involuntary, and irregular choreoa-thetoid (writhing) movements, pre-dominantly in the head and facial region.

Thought disorders—Serious and often persistent mental illnesses character-ized by disturbances in reality orien-tation, thinking, and social involve-ment.

Vulnerability model (stress-vulnerability model)—Psychosocial theory that states that schizophrenia is characterized by vulnerability rather than continuous symptoms.

Water intoxication—A problem that sometimes accompanies schizophre-nia, in which a client drinks excessive water, thereby developing polyuria and hyponatremia; when severe enough, this condition can result in seizures, coma, cerebral edema, and even death.

▼ LEARNING OBJECTIVES

On completion of this chapter, you should be able to accom-plish the following:

- Define schizophrenia.
- Compare other thought disorders with schizophre-nia.
- Discuss the proposed etiologies of schizophrenia.
- Identify signs and symptoms of schizophrenia.
- Describe the subtypes of schizophrenia.
- Compare the benefits versus risks of antipsychotic med-ications.
- Explain the continuum of care for people with schizo-phrenia.
- Apply the nursing process to the care of a person with schizophrenia.
- Identify self-care for nurses working with clients with schizophrenia.

▽ *Clinical Example 25-1*

"I just came here to help people," says James, a 20-year-old single man, when he is admitted to the hospital for the third time. His parents bring James to the acute treatment center because of his increasingly bizarre behavior, decreased sleep, and isolation during the 3 days before admission. They noticed that he was pacing around the house, eating and sleeping very little, talking to himself, making strange statements, and displaying unusual mannerisms. His parents also said that James seemed to "have no expression on his face" for the 2 weeks before his behavior became unusual.

Carol, the nurse on duty in the admitting room at the hospital, notes that James was treated with Prolixin and Cogentin when he was admitted to the hospital 2 months ago. The medications stabilized his psychotic symptoms, and James was discharged with instructions to receive follow-up care at his local community mental health center. James's mother states that James stopped taking his medication several weeks ago because "he said the government was trying to control his mind. We can't force him to take his medication because he gets very agitated."

When James was 14 years old, he suffered head trauma from a skateboarding accident and resultant loss of consciousness. Little family history of mental illness is known, although his father and brother both abuse alcohol. James has smoked marijuana and abused alcohol for at least the past 2 years.

James admits to Carol that he hears voices that "tell me to do things," although he would not say what things he was told to do. He tells Carol that the voices scare him. He looks over his shoulder as if hearing voices and is distracted easily by noises in and outside the interview room. Carol knows from experience that James is experiencing auditory hallucinations. He makes clicking noises in quick succession before answering questions. In addition, his answers are often "hidden" in language that does not seem to make sense. He states he has "special powers" and can break glass and blocks of ice with his fist and communicate with others through the radio.

Carol explains to James that she would like him to stay in the hospital so that she, James, and his doctor can determine how best to help James control the voices that scare him. James does not make eye contact but nods his head.

This chapter discusses **thought disorders**—serious and often persistent mental illnesses characterized by disturbances in reality orientation, thinking, and social involvement. Schizophrenia is the most prevalent of the thought disorders and will be the main focus of discussion in this chapter. Other psychotic disturbances related closely to schizophrenia will be discussed briefly.

In Clinical Example 25-1, what is it about James's thinking, behavior, and affect that give evidence of a thought disorder? You will learn about the progression of James's care in Nursing Care Plan 25-1. You also will have the opportunity to apply your understanding of this client and others with thought disorders in the Reflection and Critical Thinking Questions section at the end of this chapter.

SCHIZOPHRENIA AND OTHER THOUGHT DISORDERS

Schizophrenia, a common and serious neurobiologic illness that affects 1 in 100 people worldwide and about 2.5 million Americans, is discussed in this section. Other psychotic disturbances closely related to schizophrenia include schizophreniform disorder, schizoaffective disorder, delusional disorder, brief psychotic disorder, shared psychotic disorder, and psychotic disorder not otherwise specified. These are described in Box 25-1. They are also discussed in more detail in the Thought Disorders Information Map.

Schizophrenia is most likely not a single disease of the brain but a heterogeneous disorder (ie, a group of several distinct disorders of the brain) with some common features, including thought disturbances and preoccupation with frightening inner experiences (eg, delusions and hallucinations), affect disturbances (eg, flat or inappropriate affect), and behavioral or social disturbances (eg, unpredictable, bizarre behavior or social isolation) (Kaplan & Sadock, 1996). These disturbances seem to be related to a disorder of brain circuitry. Increasing evidence for its etiologies points to abnormalities that arise early in life, probably before birth, which disrupt the brain's normal development.

The word *schizophrenia* originally referred to a "splitting off" of one's thoughts from one's emotions. Thus, the word has become confused in the public's mind with "split personality" or "multiple personality." Nurses must be careful not to confuse schizophrenia with dissociative disorders such as dissociative identity disorder, in which a client actually displays more than one personality (see Chap. 21).

Schizophrenia is a treatable disorder or group of disorders. If untreated, it can devastate the lives of affected persons and severely disrupt their families and their relationships with their families. Persons with schizophrenia may be totally withdrawn from the external environment. They may regress to such an extent that they fail to perform personal hygiene and activities of daily living, participate in interpersonal relationships, and even notice physical illness or pain. These symptoms often result in marked social and occupational dysfunction.

The onset of symptoms usually occurs during the late teenage years to the early 20s. Schizophrenia, however, has been diagnosed in children as young as 5 years and in per-

BOX 25-1 ▼ *Other Thought Disorders: Psychotic Disorders*

Schizophreniform disorder—Symptoms are the same as schizophrenia but of shorter duration, specifically, symptoms that last at least 1 month but less than 6 months.

Schizoaffective disorder—During an uninterrupted period of illness, there is either a mood episode at the same time as active symptoms of schizophrenia, preceded or followed by 2 weeks of delusions or hallucinations without mood symptoms.

Delusional disorder—The person has nonbizarre delusions of 1 month's duration, and functioning is not impaired outside of the delusion. Types include jealous, persecutory, somatic, grandiose, and erotomanic.

Brief psychotic disorder—For more than 1 day but less than 1 month, the person has delusions, hallucinations, disorganized speech, and grossly disorganized or catatonic behavior but no negative symptoms. Client then returns to premorbid level of functioning. This may occur in the postpartum period.

Shared psychotic disorder (formerly called folie à deux)—Two people in a close relationship (eg, twins, mother and child) hold similar delusions.

Psychotic disorder not otherwise specified (NOS)—The person has persistent nonbizarre delusions with periods of overlapping mood episodes or auditory hallucinations.

From American Psychiatric Association. (2000). *Diagnostic and statistical manual of mental disorders* (4th ed., text rev.). Washington, DC: Author.

---

sons in their 40s (Box 25-2). Schizophrenia is found in all cultures, races, and social classes. In industrialized nations, however, a disproportionate number of persons with schizophrenia are in the low socioeconomic groups. A possible explanation for this fact may be that the illness interferes with productivity and moves affected clients into a lower socioeconomic group. In addition, the stresses that those who live in poverty experience may trigger the vulnerability of some persons to schizophrenia.

The remarkable thing about schizophrenia, given its severity and prevalence, is how little attention it receives (Torrey, 1995). Its cost in the United States is estimated to be $15 to $25 billion annually, including costs of inpatient and outpatient care, federal and state assistance, and lost wages (Kaplan & Sadock, 1996). Schizophrenia is the most expensive of all chronic illnesses, because it strikes just at the age when the person should become a contributing wage earner. Although research in the 1990s began to identify the biologic aspects of schizophrenia, a definitive cause remains unknown. Inadequate treatment ("too little too late") and lack of preventive efforts are the norm.

The Stigma of Schizophrenia

"Schizophrenics are the lepers of the 20th century," says Dr. Fuller Torrey, an expert in serious and persistent mental illnesses and an outspoken advocate for clients and families (Torrey, 1995). Stigma has long been and continues to be a problem for people with mental illness and their families (Historical Capsule 25-1). Although it seems that, with the dawn of the 21st century, mental illness should be treated "like any other disease," this is not the case (see Chap. 1).

Because it is a mental illness with severe symptoms that are difficult to conceal from relatives and friends, schizophrenia, in particular, is likely to result in stigmatization of clients and families. Those with schizophrenia suffer the effects of the illness itself, often inadequate clinical care and rehabilitation, as well as the stigma of shame and family burden. A recent study showed that many family members do not tell others about their relative's psychiatric hospitalization. In addition, families with higher education are more likely to perceive that others are avoiding them (Phelan, Bromet, & Link, 1998).

Etiology

Schizophrenia is thought to have multiple etiologies. Although various etiologic theories have been posed in the past, the advent of more sophisticated neurobiologic testing such as magnetic resonance imaging (MRI) has shown that people with schizophrenia have specific alterations in their brains that make them different from those without schizophrenia. Such alterations include neurochemical imbalances, irregular patterns of certain brain cells, and information coordination difficulties.

Despite the strong evidence that schizophrenia is a biologically based brain disorder, researchers also suspect that psychosocial (ie, ecological) factors influence a person's vulnerability to this disorder. Many researchers hypothesize that psychological stress may trigger the activation (or expression) of a "schizophrenia gene" (although no such gene has been found), which makes a person vulnerable to the disorder (see Chapters 1 and 3 for discussion of environmental–genetic interactions). Because schizophrenia is most likely a group of disorders

Thought Disorders Information Map

⇨ *Prevalence*
Schizophrenia occurs in approximately 1% of the population. Rates of other thought disorders vary from 0.5 to 15%.

⇨ *Summary of DSM-IV-TR Diagnostic Criteria*

Schizophrenia
- Client has two or more of the following *characteristic symptoms* for a significant portion of 1 month (or less if successfully treated):
  - A. Delusions
  - B. Hallucinations
  - C. Disorganized speech (e.g., frequent derailment or incoherence)
  - D. Grossly disorganized or catatonic behavior
  - E. Negative symptoms (i.e., affective flattening, alogia, or avolition)
- Client has significant social/occupational dysfunction since the disturbance began, which is markedly below the client's level before onset. When onset is in childhood or adolescence, client fails to achieve expected interpersonal, academic, or occupational achievement.
- Signs of the disturbance are continuous for at least 6 months. The period must include at least 1 month of symptoms (or less if successfully treated). During any prodromal or residual periods, signs of the disturbance may be only negative symptoms or two or more symptoms listed in the first criterion in an attenuated form (e.g., unusual perceptual experiences).
- Schizoaffective disorder and mood disorder with psychotic features have been ruled out because either (1) no mood episodes have accompanied the active-phase symptoms; or (2) total duration of accompanying mood episodes has been brief relative to the active and residual periods.

Substance/general medical condition exclusion: The disturbance is not caused by a substance or general medical condition.

Relationship to a Pervasive Development Disorder. If client has a history of a Pervasive Development Disorder, the additional diagnosis of Schizophrenia is made only if prominent delusions or hallucinations are also present for at least 1 month (or less if successfully treated).

Schizophrenia Subtypes
Paranoid Type
- Client is preoccupied with one or more delusions or auditory hallucinations.

- Client shows none of the following: disorganized speech, disorganized or catatonic behavior, flat or inappropriate affect.

Disorganized Type
- All of the following are prominent:
  - Disorganized speech
  - Disorganized behavior
  - Flat or inappropriate affect
- Client does not meet criteria for catatonic type.

Catatonic Type
Client has schizophrenia in which at least two of the following dominate:
- Motor immobility as evidenced by catalepsy (including waxy flexibility) or stupor
- Excessive motor activity with no apparent purpose and uninfluenced by external stimuli
- Extreme negativism (resistance to all instructions or maintenance of a rigid posture against attempts to be moved) or mutism
- Peculiarities of voluntary movement such as posturing (voluntary assumption of inappropriate or bizarre postures), stereotyped movements, prominent mannerisms, or prominent grimacing
- Echolalia or echopraxia

Undifferentiated Type
Client has schizophrenia with the characteristic symptoms, but he or she does not meet the criteria for paranoid, disorganized, or catatonic type.

Residual Type
- Client does not have prominent delusions, hallucinations, disorganized speech, and grossly disorganized or catatonic behavior.
- Continuing evidence of the disturbance appears, as indicated by negative symptoms or two or more characteristic symptoms in an attenuated form.

Schizophreniform Disorder
Client meets the same criteria as for schizophrenia; however, the episode (including prodromal, active, and residual phases) lasts at least 1 month but no longer than 6 months.

(continued)

Thought Disorders Information Map (Continued)

Brief Psychotic Disorder

- Client has one (or more) of the following symptoms:
  - Delusions
  - Hallucinations
  - Disorganized speech
  - Grossly disorganized or catatonic behavior
- Duration is at least 1 day but less than 1 month, with eventual full return to normal functioning.
- The disturbance is not better explained by a Mood Disorder With Psychotic Features, Schizoaffective Disorder, or Schizophrenia. It is not caused by a substance or general medical condition.

Schizoaffective Disorder

- Client has an uninterrupted period of illness with a major depressive episode, a manic episode, or a mixed episode along with the characteristic symptoms of schizophrenia.
- During the same period, client has had delusions or hallucinations for at least 2 weeks without prominent mood symptoms.
- Symptoms of a mood episode last for a substantial portion of the total illness.
- The disturbance is not caused by a substance or general medical condition.

Delusional Disorder

- Client has nonbizarre delusions (i.e., involving real-life situations) for at least 1 month.
- Client has never had the characteristic symptoms of schizophrenia.
- Apart from the effects of the delusions, the disturbance does not markedly impair functioning, and client's behavior is not obviously strange.
- Any mood episodes that have accompanied the delusions have been brief compared with the delusional periods.
- The disturbance is not caused by a substance or general medical condition.

Shared Psychotic Disorder

- A client develops a delusion in the context of a close relationship with another person(s), who has an already-established delusion.
- The delusion is similar to that of the person who already has the established delusion.
- The disturbance is not better accounted for by another thought or mood disorder. It is not caused by a substance or general medical condition.

➡ Prevention Strategies

To prevent relapses of schizophrenia in clients, encourage clients and their families as follows:

- Follow the medication regimen accurately.
- Participate regularly in any other form of treatment.
- Know the early warning signs of relapse, and notify the physician immediately if such signs develop.
- Discuss any troubling side effects of medications with health care personnel, and be aware that changes to such medications can help.
- Avoid the use of drugs and alcohol.
- Practice stress reduction techniques.
- Maintain physical health by following a healthy diet, exercising, and sleeping regularly.
- Participate in support groups, which can provide assistance in many areas and provide outlets for shared discussion, learning, and experience.

➡ Want to Know More?

National Alliance for the Mentally Ill
200 N. Glebe Rd., Suite 1015
Arlington, VA 22203-3754
1(800) 950-NAMI

National Mental Health Consumers' Self-Help
  Clearinghouse
Newsletter, *The Key*
311 S. Juniper St., Suite 1000
Philadelphia, PA 19107
1 (800) 553-4539

Schizophrenics Anonymous
15920 West Twelve Mile
Southfield, MI 48076
(313) 477-1983
http://www.schizophrenia.com

The Schizophrenia Society of Canada
75 The Donway West, Suite 814
Don Mills, Ontario
M3C 2E9 416-445-8204
www.schizophrenia.ca/

With permission from the American Psychiatric Association (2000). *Diagnostic and statistical manual of mental disorders* (4th ed., text revision). Washington, DC: Author.

BOX 25-2 ▼ *Schizophrenia Across the Life Span*

Most people with schizophrenia experience their first symptoms during their late teens and early 20s. Rarely, however, schizophrenia begins in childhood and has been reported in children as young as 5 years old. Childhood schizophrenia is an identifiable entity that shares some of the anatomical abnormalities common in the adult manifestation of the disorder. These abnormalities are identified through magnetic resonance imaging (MRI) and include deviations in total cerebral volume, thalamic area, and ventricle size (O'Leary et al., 1996).

While childhood schizophrenia was previously thought to be a form of autism or pervasive developmental disorder (see Chap. 29), it is now viewed as a clinical phenomenon that occurs earlier and is more dramatic and devastating than adult-onset schizophrenia. Jacobsen and Rapoport (1998) report that childhood psychosis is 5 times as rare as adult-onset schizophrenia but probably has the same etiology as adult schizophrenia; that is, genetic mutations and faulty development of the brain in utero.

Childhood schizophrenia has a devastating effect on child development. The onset tends to be insidious compared to the episodic nature of the adult disorder. The brain abnormalities appear to be more severe in children; similarly, children tend to deteriorate in their functioning after a psychotic break. The child with schizophrenia is much less likely to master the normal developmental tasks of early childhood and latency. Their social relationships with family and peers, functioning in school, and mastery of some separation and independence from parents are poor. These children require early, intensive psychiatric services to help them cope with their difficulties. There has been some reported success in treating children with schizophrenia with atypical antipsychotic medication such as clozapine (Clozaril) or olanzapine (Zyprexa). In addition, they require intensive community and educational services to help them function within their school and community.

Most clients first experience the symptoms of schizophrenia during their late teens and 20s. Their life is disrupted just at the point of embarking on higher education and career goals and entering into their productive years. This disruption affects every part of their lives—interpersonal, family, occupational, social, and financial. Stabilization through medication and community supports may take considerable time and effort.

Schizophrenia can begin later in life with an onset after age 45 years. Late-onset schizophrenia is more common in women and is more likely to be marked by paranoid delusions and hallucinations. It is less likely to include negative and disorganized symptoms (APA, 2000). Although the course of late-onset schizophrenia tends to be persistent, these clients respond well to antipsychotic medications in lower doses.

Adapted from American Psychiatric Association. (2000). *Diagnostic and statistical manual of mental disorders* (4th ed., text rev.). Washington, DC: Author. Jacobsen, L. K., & Rapoport, J. (1998). Research update: Childhood-onset schizophrenia: Implications of clinical and neurobiological research. *Journal of Child Psychology and Psychiatry, 39,* 101–113. O'Leary, D. S., Andreasen, N. C., Hurtig, R. R., Kesler, M. L., Rogers, M., Arndt, S., et al. (1996). Auditory attentional deficits in patients with schizophrenia: A positron emission tomography study. *Archives of General Psychiatry, 53*(7), 633–641.

with heterogeneous causes, this chapter presents both biologic and psychosocial theories.

BIOLOGIC THEORIES

Current data about schizophrenia reveal a complex picture of brain dysfunction that includes neuroanatomic, neuropathologic, and metabolic disturbances and various neuropsychological deficits. These findings support the belief that schizophrenia is not one disorder but a group or collection of disorders involving brain function. Ongoing research and improved assessment techniques are helping scientists test their theories of biologic etiology more directly.

Genetic Influences

Many studies strongly suggest that genetics plays a part in the development of schizophrenia. A higher incidence of the disorder occurs in the relatives of people with schizophrenia than in the general population. First-degree relatives (ie, parents, siblings, and children) of a person with schizophrenia have a greater risk of developing the illness than second-degree relatives (eg, grandparents, grandchildren, aunts, uncles, and half-siblings). Children with one parent who has schizophrenia are 13% more likely to develop schizophrenia than those who don't have a parent with schizophrenia; when both parents have schizophrenia, the child has a 46% risk of developing the illness.

Twin studies have long illustrated the genetic link in schizophrenia. Studies of monozygotic (identical) twins have found that if one twin becomes schizophrenic, the likelihood that the other twin will become schizophrenic is greater than 50%, which is significantly higher than it would be for fraternal (or nonidentical) twins. Also, the incidence of schizophrenia in children adopted as infants by parents without schizophrenia, but whose biological mothers had schizophrenia, equals the rate in children

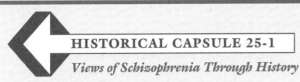

HISTORICAL CAPSULE 25-1
Views of Schizophrenia Through History

Emil Kraepelin (1856–1926)

- Named the syndrome *dementia praecox,* a condition occurring precociously or early in life, followed by a gradual but continuous downhill course leading to intellectual deterioration
- Proposed that etiology was related to endogenous factors such as organic pathology or an error in metabolism, not to societal influences
- Identified the symptoms of hallucinations, delusions, disorders of thought and speech, poor insight and judgment, flat affect, and reduced attention to the outside world

Eugen Bleuler (1857–1930)

- Swiss psychiatrist who renamed the syndrome *schizophrenia* to indicate "splitting" of various mental functions
- Divided symptoms into two major categories:

  1. Fundamental symptoms (also known as the "four As")
     - Associative disturbance: thought disorder
     - Affective disorder: flat or blunted affect or affect inappropriate or incongruous to the thought or situation
     - Autism: detachment from external reality and withdrawal into fantasies
     - Ambivalence: simultaneous existence of opposing feelings, thoughts, and desires

  2. Accessory symptoms, or symptoms frequently present but not specific to schizophrenia, including hallucinations, delusions, and catatonic posturing

Sigmund Freud (1855–1939)

- Emphasized importance of psychological factors in etiology of schizophrenia
- Believed hallucinatory psychoses originated from frightening and unbearable ideas

Adolf Meyer (1866–1950)

- Supported the view of psychological factors contributing to development of schizophrenia
- Proposed a longitudinal study of clients with schizophrenia to determine etiologies

Carl Jung (1875–1961)

- Viewed the client with schizophrenia as an "introvert" directing energy into self
- Proposed that an emotional disorder could cause a metabolic disturbance and, eventually, physical brain damage
- Proposed that symptoms of schizophrenia were "reproductions of the archetypes deposited in our collective unconscious"

Harry Stack Sullivan (1892–1949)

- American psychoanalyst who proposed that impaired interpersonal relations, rather than intrapsychic forces, were significant in the development of schizophrenia
- Believed that children who became adults with schizophrenia had impaired interpersonal relations with their parents and other significant people
- Interacted with clients as a participant rather than an observer in psychotherapy of those with schizophrenia, which became his major life work

Fuller Torrey and Current Research Into Brain Diseases

- Demonstrated that schizophrenia is a biologic disorder marked by various anatomic and physiologic differences of the brain
- Showed probable biological bases of schizophrenia include genetic, viral, immunologic, and neurochemical etiologies

From Arieti, S. (1974). *Interpretation of schizophrenia* (2nd ed.). New York: Basic Books. Cancro, R. (1983). Individual psychotherapy in the treatment of chronic schizophrenic patients. *American Journal of Psychotherapy, 37*(October), 493–501.

---

raised by their biological mothers who had schizophrenia. Similarly, the incidence of schizophrenia in children who were given up for adoption by mothers who did not have schizophrenia equals the rate of schizophrenia seen in the general population (about 1%).

The exact mode of inheritance of schizophrenia has not been identified; opinion about its cause is divided between *monogenic* (one gene) factors and *polygenic* (many genes) factors. One hypothesis proposes the existence of a single susceptibility gene, whereas another theory states that schizophrenia is a genetically heterogeneous group of disorders. This latter possibility, the polygenic hypothesis, proposes that schizophrenia results from the interaction of many genes, and none of them acting individually would be strong enough to produce schizophrenia.

Associations between specific chromosomal sites and schizophrenia have led to the possibility of chromosomal markers for schizophrenia. The most commonly reported markers include the long arms of chromosomes 5, 11, and 18; the short arm of chromosome 19; and the X chromosome (Kaplan & Sadock, 1996).

Schizophrenia also may occur through the interaction of genetic susceptibility with environmental stress or significant environmental risk factors. While recent studies have failed to locate a major gene for susceptibility to schizophrenia, genetic influences increase the risk of schizophrenia but not of other psychotic disorders. Further research may clarify the genetic basis of schizophrenia.

Most investigators agree that schizophrenia is best conceptualized as a "multiple-hit" illness, similar to cancer. In other words, a person may carry a genetic predisposition for schizophrenia; however, this vulnerability is not "released" unless other factors also intervene (see Chap. 2). Although most such factors are considered environmental in the sense that they are not encoded in DNA and thus could potentially produce mutations or influence gene expression, most are also biological rather than psychological and include factors such as birth injuries and nutrition. Current studies of the neurobiology of schizophrenia examine a multiplicity of factors, including genetics, anatomy (primarily through structural neuroimaging), functional circuitry (through functional neuroimaging), neuropathology, electrophysiol-ogy, neurochemistry, neuropharmacology, and neurodevelopment (Andreasen, 1999b).

Neurochemical and Neuroanatomic Changes

The most recent research into the etiology of schizophrenia has focused on brain imaging and the neurochemical and neuropathologic changes that occur in the brains of clients with the disorder. These changes involve the brain's structure, metabolism, blood flow, electrical activity, and neurochemistry.

Imaging studies of schizophrenia have shown neurodevelopmental defects in brain circuitry and abnormal brain metabolism. Positron emission tomography (PET), which produces slice images of radioisotope density, has indicated relative metabolic underactivity of the frontal lobes of clients with schizophrenia (Figure 25-1). These PET scans have shown decreased activity in the basal ganglia, which can be reversed with antipsychotic medications (also known as neuroleptic medications).

The symptoms of schizophrenia are related to deficits or dysregulation in one or more neurotransmitter systems. Disturbances with the neurotransmitters dopamine, serotonin, norepinephrine, acetylcholine, cholecystokinin, glutamate, and gamma-aminobutyric acid (GABA) have been commonly linked to schizophrenia (Buchsbaum & Hazlett,

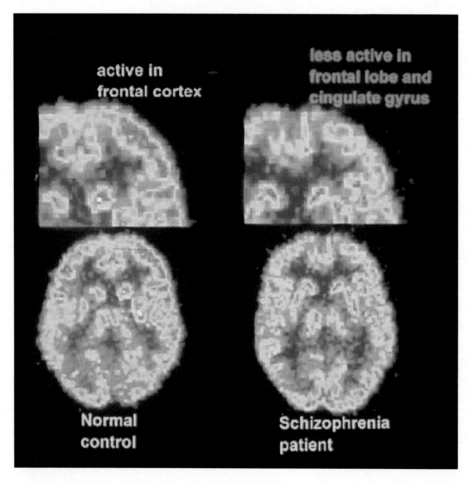

FIGURE 25-1   Positron emission tomography scanning showing metabolic differences in a control subject (*left*) and a client with untreated schizophrenia (*right*).

1998; Kaplan & Sadock, 1996). Although it is thought to oversimplify this complex disease, the dopamine hypothesis of schizophrenia proposes that an overactivity of dopamine results in the illness. Also an insufficiency of norepinephrine at certain central synapses of the brain, an imbalance between dopamine and norepinephrine, or both could be among the biological factors present in schizophrenia. These biochemical differences in the nervous system of the person with schizophrenia cause them to process sensory information abnormally, resulting in disturbances of attention, inadequate social interaction, isolation, and hypersensitivity.

Several lines of evidence support the speculation that schizophrenia is a neurodevelopmental disorder that results from brain injury early in life. For example, clients with schizophrenia are more likely than control subjects without schizophrenia to have a history of birth injury and perinatal complications, which could result in a subtle brain injury and thereby set the stage for the development of schizophrenia. The viral theory of schizophrenia, another neurodevelopmental hypothesis, proposes that exposure to a virus in utero may be a factor in the development of schizophrenia (Andreasen, 1999a). This idea has gained considerable attention in recent years because of the high incidence of schizophrenia following prenatal exposure to influenza during epidemics (Buchsbaum & Hazlett, 1998; Kaplan & Sadock, 1996).

Neuroanatomical imaging and study may link schizophrenia to certain patterns of hemispheric brain dysfunction. These studies have suggested left hemisphere overactivation and consequent temporal abnormalities and delays in processing sensory information. Hallucinations have been correlated with accelerated glucose metabolism in the left temporal lobe. PET scans show a relative decrease in metabolic activity in the frontal lobes with a low metabolic rate in the basal ganglia, both of which increase when antipsychotic medications are administered.

Other pathologic findings in schizophrenia include dysfunctions of eye movements, impaired modulation of stimulus input that allows too much information to reach higher brain centers, laterality differences in which the left hemisphere may be less efficient than the right, impaired selective attention, and directed attention in the form of vigilance.

Neuroanatomical differences also have been identified in clients with schizophrenia, including several structural brain abnormalities. Cerebral ventricular enlargement is the most consistently replicated finding, but sulcal enlargement and cerebellar atrophy are also reported. These abnormalities appear to be present from the earliest stages of the illness and may be related to the symptoms of impaired motivation, socialization, and complex problem solving. Ventricular enlargement is associated with poor premorbid functioning, negative symptoms, poor response to treatment, and cognitive impairment.

Neuroanatomical studies also indicate a slightly decreased volume of the putamen, substantia nigra, and various portions of the limbic system, especially the temporal lobe and hippocampus. The limbic system, because of its role in the control of emotions, and the basal ganglia, because of their involvement in movement and movement disorders, have long been implicated in the development of schizophrenia. Postmortem studies on clients with schizophrenia have found a decreased size of the area of the brain that makes up the limbic system. In some studies, the basal ganglia are reduced in volume (Kaplan & Sadock, 1996).

Reduced numbers of neurons have been reported in several cortical areas. Frontal lobe abnormalities may account for some of the cognitive, attention-related, and affective symptoms of schizophrenia. The decrease in frontal lobe size, however, has been less consistently replicated than studies documenting ventricular enlargement, with negative studies appearing equally to positive studies. Much more research must be conducted before it can be definitively said that frontal lobe size is a factor in schizophrenia.

PSYCHOSOCIAL THEORIES

While biologic theories are currently believed to explain the etiology of schizophrenia, psychosocial theories also have been proposed and have been influential to the development of the understanding of schizophrenia.

According to the **vulnerability model** (sometimes called the **stress-vulnerability model**), schizophrenia is characterized by vulnerability rather than continuous symptoms. Under the stress of biologic and psychosocial factors, a person may be predisposed to "break down;" hence the archaic expression "nervous breakdown." There is no actual empirical evidence to support this model, and professional consensus is that a complex interplay of environmental and biologic factors is responsible for the expression of the disease.

The risk factors (stressors) identified in the vulnerability model may include poverty, major life stressors (eg, leaving home for college), substance abuse, and other environmental or interpersonal stressors. Moderators or buffers to these risk factors or stressors can be such things as perceived social support, intact family, higher education, and stability of community (O'Connor, 1994).

A recent study supporting the influence of risk factors in the development of schizophrenia found that initial or early episodes of the disease are more likely to be associated with recent life events than are later episodes of the illness. Life events refer to situations or events that significantly change personal circumstances. Examples include pregnancy, marriage, divorce, or death of a loved one (Castine, Meador-Woodruff, & Dalack, 1998).

Past views held that interpersonal influences, particularly disordered communication and interaction, contribute to the development of schizophrenia. While most researchers and clinicians acknowledge the influence of a supportive family and healthy patterns of communication in mental health, there is no evidence, nor has there ever been any evidence, that family communication patterns cause schizophrenia. Theories of family communication and interaction have been discarded as a cause of this brain-based disorder. A spokesperson for the National Alliance for the Mentally Ill (NAMI) says that major mental illness is a family problem only in the sense that the illness of one member affects all family members. Family systems theory, which places the etiology of schizophrenia on family communication patterns, is "irrelevant, stigmatizing, and misleading," according to NAMI (Conn, 1990).

Signs and Symptoms and Diagnostic Criteria

At one time the syndrome of schizophrenia was conceptualized as being of two types: Type I, in which positive symptoms prevailed, and Type II, in which negative symptoms prevailed. Recent studies, however, have proposed more complex delineations of psychopathology than that offered by the positive and negative dichotomy. Indeed, the symptoms and signs of schizophrenia are so diverse that they cover the entire range of human thought, emotion, and behavior. Students should approach this section knowing that it is not prudent to make simple distinctions or generalizations about schizophrenia. There is much to be learned, and what may be "true" today may be found invalid tomorrow.

According to the American Psychiatric Association (APA) *Diagnostic and Statistical Manual of Mental Disorders*, 4th edition, text revision (*DSM-IV-TR*), schizophrenia is a disturbance that lasts at least 6 months and includes at least 1 month of two or more active-phase symptoms such as bizarre delusions, hallucinations (eg, a running commentary of two voices conversing with each other), disorganized speech, grossly disorganized or catatonic behavior, and negative behavior. These symptoms interfere markedly with social or occupational functioning (APA, 2000). The duration of the illness must last 6 months, including prodromal or residual symptoms, with an active phase of 1 month of symptoms. In the *DSM-IV* and *DSM-IV-TR* (APA, 1994, 2000), schizophrenia is defined by characteristic positive or negative symptoms. A list of common symptoms of schizophrenia, divided into positive and negative categories, appears in Box 25-3.

Perhaps it is most accurate to say that people with schizophrenia manifest alterations in their cognitive functioning. Cognition entails the entire gamut of skills necessary for people to process information correctly. Through cognition, people learn about the world and their place in it. Cognition includes such important functions as memory, attention, and judgment. Persons with schizophrenia

may have difficulties with many areas of their cognitive functioning (Box 25-4).

Researchers have found three dimensions of psychopathology in schizophrenia:

1. The disorganization dimension
2. The psychotic dimension
3. The negative dimension (Andreasen, 2000)

For purposes of discussion, the positive and negative symptoms of schizophrenia are discussed under these three major areas.

THE DISORGANIZATION DIMENSION

The *disorganization dimension* of schizophrenia involves one kind of thought disturbance—formal thought disorder. Formal thought disorder affects the relationship and associations among the words a person uses to express thought (ie, the verbal form that the thought takes). It is important to keep in mind, however, that clients with mania or depression manifest thought disorder frequently and may have similar difficulties with their cognition and cognitive processes as people with schizophrenia (see Chap. 24). None of the disorders of thought are thought to be disorder specific (Andreasen, 1999a). That said, many persons with schizophrenia have disturbances in their conceptual thinking that make their ideas difficult to follow. These disturbances are manifested by disorganized speech, disorganized or bizarre behavior, and incongruous affect.

Disorganized Speech

Because thinking and speech are related intimately, disorganized thought is manifested by disorganized, bizarre speech. Disorganized speech as a manifestation of formal thought disorder has historically been considered one of the primary characteristics of schizophrenia (Andreasen & Black, 2000). Researchers believe that clients with schizophrenia cannot process complex thoughts or express coherent sentences as a result of malfunctioning in their information-processing abilities (Andreasen, 1999b). Their information processing may be blocked, accelerated, or delayed because of alterations in brain structure and functioning.

The lack of a logical relationship between thoughts and ideas may be manifested by speech that is vague, diffuse, unfocused (loose associations), or incoherent (eg, emitting words that are totally unrelated—"word salad") or by a client's inability to get to the point of a conversation (tangentiality). An example of loose associations from a client with schizophrenia follows.

"Let's see, there was one I would have liked if it wasn't for the instructor, well I go along with his, he was always wanted me to do the worse in the class, it seemed like, and I'd always get the bad, the grade, in my grading, and he tried to make other people like they were good enough to be in Hollywood or something, you

BOX 25-3 ▼ Positive and Negative Symptoms of Schizophrenia

Positive Symptoms	Negative Symptoms
Positive formal thought disorder	*Alogia*
• Derailment • Tangentiality • Incoherence • Illogicality • Circumstantiality • Pressure of speech • Distractible speech • Clanging	• Poverty of speech • Poverty of content of speech • Blocking • Increased response latency
Bizarre behavior	*Affective flattening or blunting*
• Clothing, appearance • Social, sexual behavior • Aggressive, agitated behavior • Repetitive, stereotyped behavior	• Unchanging facial expression • Decreased spontaneous movements • Paucity of expressive gestures • Poor eye contact • Affective nonresponsiveness • Lack of vocal inflections
Delusions	*Avolition*
• Persecutory • Jealous • Guilt, sin based • Grandiose • Religious • Somatic • Delusions of reference • Delusions of being controlled • Delusions of mind reading • Thought broadcasting • Thought insertion • Thought withdrawal	• Impaired grooming and hygiene • Lack of persistence at work or school • Physical anergia
	Anhedonia
	• Few recreational interests or activities • Little sexual interest or activity • Impaired intimacy or closeness • Few relationships with friends or peers
Hallucinations	*Attentional Impairment*
• Auditory • Voices commenting • Voices conversing • Somatic-tactile hallucinations • Olfactory • Visual	• Social inattentiveness • Inattentiveness during testing

Adapted from Andreasen, 1985

---

know. I'd be the last one down the ladder. That, that's the way they wanted the grading to be in the first place according to whose, theirs, they, they have all different reasons that I, I think that they use that they want one, won't come out."

—Andreasen, 1985, p. 61

Other types of thought disorder include *perseveration* (repeating oneself), distractibility, *clanging* (sound associations replace conceptual connections), *neologisms* (made-up words whose meaning is only known to the person), echolalia, and thought blocking. Some illustra-

tions of bizarre and disorganized speech associated with formal thought disorder are illustrated in Box 25-5.

Persons with schizophrenia also may use words in peculiar ways (Horwath & Cournos, 1999). An example is the following response by a woman who was asked why she was in the hospital. She replied, "Being unhealthy. In my head I feel like I'm a bleed." Clients may experience thought blocking, which is a sudden derailment of a train of thought with a complete interruption in the flow of ideas. Thought blocking is a disconcerting experience that may leave clients feeling embarrassed or confused.

BOX 25-4 ▼ *Disordered Cognitive Functioning in Schizophrenia*

Thought Content

Delusions

- Grandiose
- Nihilistic
- Paranoid
- Religious
- Somatic

Hallucinations

Formal Thought Disorder

Loose associations

Tangentiality

Incoherence, word salad, neologisms

Illogic

Poverty of speech

Attention

Difficulty in attending

Poor concentration

Distractibility

Difficulty in using selective attention

Memory

Impaired ability to retrieve or use stored memory

Impairment of short- and long-term memory

Decision Making and Judgment

Indecisiveness

Difficulty initiating tasks

Impaired judgment

Illogical thinking

Lack of insight

Lack of planning and problem-solving skills

Impaired abstract thinking

Difficulty initiating tasks

Disorganized Behavior

Another aspect of the disorganization dimension is disorganized motor or social behaviors. Persons with schizophrenia may have profound psychomotor retardation or excitement, and they may exhibit bizarre posture. Catatonic schizophrenia, in particular, is marked by episodes of bizarre

BOX 25-5 ▼ *Illustrations of Bizarre and Disorganized Speech*

Loose Associations

Nurse: What brought you to the hospital?

Client: I was home when a drum began beating. I flew too low.

Clanging

Nurse: Are you ready to take your stomach medicine?

Client: Peptobismuth, petrobismuth, peptibismark, (for Pepto-Bismol); I'm gonna fly, cry, lie, buy, die.

Neologisms

Nurse: What are you holding?

Client: It's a fumebook. You know, a special temple to protect you.

Word Salad

Nurse: What would you like, Lucy?

Client: The thing that goes, the nails who made me barf.

behavior in which clients assume and maintain strange postures. In a catatonic stupor, clients may be unresponsive to questions or other stimuli, mute, and immobile, yet they may be fully conscious. Some clients may have a peculiar rigidity. They may allow their limbs to be moved, but then they may hold them for hours in the position in which they are placed. This is called *waxy flexibility*. In catatonic excitement clients may show uncontrolled and aimless motor activity. They may engage in repetitive stereotypic movements with no apparent purpose, such as rocking back and forth for hours. Clients also may manifest normal mannerisms out of context, such as grimacing for no reason.

In addition, social behavior often deteriorates. Clients may withdraw from others and isolate themselves. They may become unkempt and wear the same clothing for weeks at a time. Their surroundings may become cluttered and unfit for habitation. For example, they may refuse to bathe or clean up after themselves or their animals. Clients also may become pack rats, hoarding papers and other nonessentials. In addition, persons with schizophrenia may exhibit socially inappropriate behaviors, such as defecating or masturbating in public.

Incongruous Affect

The final component of the disorganization dimension is incongruity or inappropriateness of affect (Andreasen & Black, 2000). The word **affect** in psychiatric terminology refers to an observable behavior that expresses feeling or emotional tone. In contrast to **mood**, which is a more sustained emotional "climate," affect refers to more fluctuating changes in emotional "weather" (APA, 2000). Clients with incongruent affect express themselves in a way that is not congruent to the situation or content of thought. They may smile or giggle for no apparent reason, or they may laugh uproariously while describing truly frightening experiences.

THE PSYCHOTIC DIMENSION

The psychotic dimension involves two classic "psychotic" symptoms that reflect a client's confusion about the loss of boundaries between self and the external world: delusions and hallucinations. Delusions and hallucinations are very real to clients with schizophrenia; clients who have these problems are not simply "imagining things." Delusions and hallucinations are physiologic events for clients, and important imaging studies have dramatically illustrated brain activity during hallucinatory activity.

Delusions

Delusions involve disturbances in thought content rather than perception. They are firmly held false beliefs that reasoning cannot correct and for which there is no support in reality. The delusions may have different content and may be persecutory, grandiose, somatic, nihilistic, religious, or referential. Clients with paranoid schizophrenia generally have persecutory delusions; they might believe that neighbors, friends, or family are planning to harm them or are tormenting or ridiculing them; that others are spying on them; or that people or important organizations are taking control of their bodies or minds. Clients also could have grandiose delusions in which they believe that they are persons of great wealth, talent, influence, power, or beauty. A client with grandiose delusions may belief himself or herself to be a different famous or historically significant individual, such as Jesus Christ, Madonna, or George Washington. Clients with schizophrenia also may have somatic delusions that concern their bodies. For example, they might believe that they are incredibly ugly and that certain aspects of their appearance (eg, their noses) disgust others. Persons having nihilistic delusions may believe that they are dead or dying or even that they no longer exist. Persons with religious delusions may believe that they have a special relationship with God or some other deity. In addition, they may think that they are the greatest sinner that ever lived or that they have a special mission from God. In referential delusions, the person believes that other people's words, newspaper articles, television shows, or song lyrics are directed specifically at him or her.

Delusional beliefs also are accompanied by thought broadcasting, thought insertion, and thought withdrawal. In *thought broadcasting,* clients believe that others can perceive their thoughts (as though they are being broadcast out loud). Clients exhibiting *thought insertion* are convinced that their thoughts are not their own but rather the thoughts of another that have become implanted in their heads. In *thought withdrawal,* clients believe that their thoughts are somehow being removed from their heads.

The content and frequency of the delusions vary according to one's culture. For example, in the United States clients may worry about the Federal Bureau of Investigation (FBI) or Central Intelligence Agency (CIA), whereas in other cultures they may worry more about demonic possession or possession by evil spirits (Andreasen & Black, 2000).

Hallucinations

Hallucinations are another manifestation of thought disorder. **Hallucinations** are sensory perceptions with a compelling sense of reality. During auditory hallucinations, the most common form of hallucinations, the person may hear the voice of God or a close relative, two or more voices that keep up a running commentary about his or her behavior, or a voice that commands the person to commit a certain act. Usually the voices are obscene and condemn, accuse, or insult the person. They may call the client names and make other nasty remarks. A client may hear voices with opposing views about the same subject, such as one voice commanding the client to kill, with another voice warning the client not to kill. Auditory hallucinations also may involve the sounds of bells, whistles, whispers, rustlings, and other noises, but most often, they are of voices talking.

Visual hallucinations (eg, monsters or frightening scenes) are less common than auditory hallucinations in clients with schizophrenia. They are likely to be threatening experiences and are often accompanied by delusional ideas and other sensory perceptions. For example, a client with religious delusions may hear and see the Buddha beckoning to him or her. Persons with schizophrenia also may have tactile (touch), olfactory (smell), and gustatory (taste) hallucinations, but these are fairly uncommon.

THE NEGATIVE DIMENSION

The *DSM-IV-TR* (APA, 2000) lists three negative symptoms as characteristic of schizophrenia: alogia, affective blunting, and avolition. Other negative symptoms common in schizophrenia include anhedonia and attentional impairment. Negative symptoms account for the substantial degree of morbidity and impairment associated with schizophrenia. They are the most intractable and difficult to treat, and they reflect a deficiency of mental functioning that is normally present.

Alogia is a poverty of thinking that is inferred from observing the client's language and speech (APA, 2000). People with alogia may have great difficulty producing fluent responses to questions and instead may manifest brief and very concrete replies (Andreasen & Black, 2000). Spontaneous speech also may be reduced. Speech content may be empty and impoverished (poverty of speech). Sometimes the words themselves may be adequate or even plentiful, but they convey little information because they are too abstract, repetitive, or stereotypic (poverty of content).

Negative affect disturbances include flat or blunted affect. **Affective flattening** or **blunting** is a reduced intensity of emotional expression and response. The difference between flat and blunted affect is in degree. A person with flat affect has no or nearly no emotional expression. He or she may not react at all to circumstances that usually evoke strong emotions in others. A person with blunted affect, on the other hand, has a significantly reduced intensity in emotional expression. He or she may react to circumstances—but only slightly.

Persons with affective flattening or blunting fail to change their facial expressions in response to a given circumstance. Their movements lack spontaneity, their expressive gestures are slow and infrequent, their voice lacks inflection, and their speech is considerably slow. They may appear wooden and robot-like; a loss of sense of self may accompany affective flattening. For example, a client may report that he or she has no feelings whatsoever and feels "dead" inside.

Complicating the picture of the reduced intensity in emotional response is that significant depressive symptoms occur in up to 60% of people with schizophrenia (Andreasen, 1999a). Depression often is difficult to recognize and diagnose, however, because the symptoms of major depression and schizophrenia often overlap.

Avolition is the inability to start, persist in, and carry through any goal-directed activity to its logical conclusion (APA, 2000). In its most severe manifestation avolition severely impairs social and occupational functioning. Clients seem to have lost their will or drive. They cannot sustain work or engage in self-care activities. Some clients may actually initiate a project and then disappear, abandoning it for weeks or even months. They may wander aimlessly or fail to show up to their jobs, if they have them. Others often accuse them of laziness. Avolition, however, is not laziness but a loss of basic drives and capacity to formulate and pursue goals.

Anhedonia is the loss of the capacity to experience pleasure subjectively. Clients may describe themselves as feeling empty and no longer able to enjoy activities, such as hobbies, family, and friends, which once gave them pleasure. This symptom is particularly tragic because clients are very much aware that they have lost the capacity for pleasure. A recent study suggests that anhedonia may result from abnormalities in the complex functional interactions between the mesolimbic and frontal brain regions (Crespo-Facorro et al., 2001).

Clients also manifest impairment of attention. This can be seen in their inability to concentrate. This attentional impairment may result from having to attend to multiple stimuli. For example, they may be listening to their inner voices and thus be unable to attend to the external world of social interactions.

OTHER SYMPTOMS

Lack of insight is a common symptom of schizophrenia. People with this illness may not believe that they are ill or that their behavior is odd or abnormal in any way. Lack of insight is one of the most difficult aspects of schizophrenia to treat (Andreasen & Black, 2000). It may remain even if the other symptoms, such as delusions and hallucinations, are successfully brought under control.

SUBTYPES OF SCHIZOPHRENIA

Schizophrenia can be divided into five subtypes, largely based on the particular set of signs and symptoms a client exhibits:

- *Paranoid*—The client is preoccupied with delusions of persecution or grandeur (organized around a coherent theme), ideas of reference, or frequent auditory hallucinations. He or she may appear tense, suspicious, guarded, reserved, hostile, or aggressive.
- *Disorganized*—The client demonstrates markedly regressed, disorganized, silly, inappropriate, and uninhibited behavior; disorganized speech; flat or inappropriate affect; poor reality contact; poor grooming and social skills; a prominent thought disorder; and possibly grimacing, strange mannerisms, or other odd behaviors.
- *Catatonic*—The client demonstrates motoric immobility or stupor, rigidity, excessive motor activity, extreme negativism, stupor, and peculiarities of movement, such as posturing, echolalia and echopraxia, mutism, and waxy flexibility.
- *Undifferentiated*—The client's behavior and speech clearly indicate schizophrenic psychosis but fail to meet the criteria of paranoid, disorganized, or catatonic types.
- *Residual*—The client with schizophrenia does not have active, positive symptoms, such as hallucinations and delusions, but continues to demonstrate negative symptoms, such as withdrawal from others or flat affect (APA, 2000).

WATER INTOXICATION IN SCHIZOPHRENIA

A few clients with chronic schizophrenia drink excessive amounts of water, thereby developing a state of **water intoxication**, characterized by polyuria and hyponatremia. When this condition becomes severe enough it can result in seizures, coma, cerebral edema, and even death. The reasons for drinking excessive amounts of water are unknown, but possibilities include a response to delusional belief, changes in the secretion of antidiuretic hormone, or abnormalities in the hypothalamic region, which regulates thirst and fluid intake (Gelder, Lopez-Ibor, & Andreasen, 2000).

Preventing water intoxication can be a challenge. Treatment includes restricting water intake, although clients can be very creative at finding water. Some have been known to drink from toilets in the absence of any other water source. Treatment of severe water intoxication involves the administration of furosemide (Lasix) and intravenous (IV) normal saline. IV hyperosmolar saline may be given cautiously in an emergency. Treatment is necessarily slow because too rapid replacement of saline may result in permanent brain damage (Kokko, 2000).

Comorbidities and Dual Diagnoses

An estimated 50% to 75% of persons with severe mental illness, such as schizophrenia, also have substance abuse problems. When people with serious illness have a substance abuse disorder or are addicted to a substance, they are referred to as having a **dual diagnosis**. Alcohol is the most abused substance, followed in frequency by cannabis and cocaine use. More than 75% of clients with schizophrenia smoke cigarettes. The combination of substance abuse and schizophrenia is associated with increased symptoms, more frequent relapses, more treatment noncompliance, homelessness, and violent behavior (Tiihonen, Isohanni, Rantakallio, Lehtonen, & Moring, 1998).

Whereas others often take substances for the pleasurable "high," those with severe mental illness usually take drugs as a way to cope with the symptoms of their disorders (eg, hallucinations). This is called "self-medication." Treatment programs often fail to address the dual needs of the addicted person with schizophrenia; effective treatment addresses both disorders in an integrated manner. See Chapter 27 for a discussion of substance abuse and treatment.

In addition to substance abuse, clients with schizophrenia often are also diagnosed with anxiety disorders, specifically obsessive-compulsive disorder (OCD) and panic disorder. See Chapter 18 for a discussion of these disorders.

Implications and Prognosis

Clients with schizophrenia are at high risk for suicide. About 10% to 15% of those with schizophrenia commit suicide; 50% attempt suicide at least once. Risk factors for suicide in this population include depressive symptoms, young age at the disorder's onset, and a high level of premorbid functioning (Kaplan & Sadock, 1996).

Clients with schizophrenia also have a higher mortality rate from accidents and medical illnesses. Identifying medical illness is extremely difficult when the client is psychotic or otherwise cannot clearly communicate the medical symptoms he or she is experiencing.

Unfortunately for clients and families, the prognosis for persons with schizophrenia has been described only in pessimistic terms. Approximately 20% to 30% of clients with schizophrenia, however, are able to lead somewhat normal lives. Another 20% to 30% continue to have moderate symptoms, while the illness significantly impairs 40% to 60% (Kaplan & Sadock, 1996). Recent studies have shown no chronic deterioration of cognitive functions as previously thought (Rund, 1998). The development of hope is essential for clients' recovery from schizophrenia and for their families.

Although there have been cases in which the person has only one episode (during adolescence) and never has another, the course of schizophrenia is typically one of exacerbations and remissions. The course of relapses and periods of higher functioning can be foreshadowed by the pattern of symptoms in the first 5 years of the illness. Each psychotic episode leaves the client with a lower level of functioning. Specifiers to describe the course of schizophrenia may be added after the first year of symptoms. These course specifiers include "episodic with or without interepisode residual symptoms," "continuous," or "a single episode in full or partial remission" (APA, 2000).

The repeated admission of clients with schizophrenia to psychiatric hospitals is referred to as the "revolving door syndrome." The two most predictive factors of repeated or "revolving door" admissions are substance abuse and failure to follow medication regimens.

Interdisciplinary Goals and Treatment

Both pharmacologic and psychosocial interventions are necessary to safeguard the client and promote his or her recovery. A recent study demonstrated that the combination of medication and psychosocial treatment that targets social cognitive deficits reduces relapse rates in persons with schizophrenia by as much as 50% (Hogarty & Ulrich, 1998). In addition, continuity of care, including discharge planning and ongoing care within the community, are essential interventions for clients with schizophrenia.

Overall goals of treatment for a person with schizophrenia include the following:

- Safety in all settings
- Stabilization on antipsychotic medication
- Client and family education about schizophrenia and its treatment
- Physical care of client
- Psychosocial support of client and family

The scope and breadth of needs of the person with schizophrenia are too great for any one professional to meet. An interdisciplinary team works together to provide the comprehensive care necessary to achieve these goals. Professionals from psychiatry, nursing, psychology, and social work supply therapeutic services to clients with schizophrenia.

Case management and rehabilitation services are also essential to recovery. The most effective treatment model to help persons with schizophrenia and their families requires coordination of multidisciplinary care by a case manager. The case manager's role is to ensure that the client receives effective services, to help various care providers communicate with one another about the client's care, to function as a liaison to family members, and to work directly with the client to assess needs and arrange services. Clinical pathways, a tool often used by case managers, help the team monitor the client's progress over time (Table 25-1).

TABLE 25-1 ▼ Clinical Pathway: Schizophrenic disorder (295.1x, catatonic 295.2x, delusional 297.10, brief reactive psychosis 298.80)

Patient Name: _____ **Case Manager:** _____ **Physician:** _____ **Medical Record #** _____
Admit date: _____ **Expected LOS:** _____ **UR days certified:** _____ **Discharge date:** _____
Actual LOS: _____

DAY/DATE:	0–8 HOURS	8–24 HOURS	DAY 2	DAY 3	DAY 4	DAY 5
ASSESSMENTS & EVALUATIONS	Nursing Assessment Nutritional screening, wt Admit note, Precautions	H & P, Social HX, RT/TA; Dr. Initial TX Plan/ Admit Note Prec. Eval. AIMS Scale	Precaution Evaluation Document sleep patterns Observe/ document nonverbal behavior	Psych Eval done Social Hx done Precaution Evaluation	Assess readiness for discharge	Assess for goals achieved
PROCEDURES	Lab ordered-Admit profile UA, UDS, UCG, EKG, Other:	Lab done: UA, UDS, UCG, EKG Other:	Lab results checked Abnormals called to Dr.	Physician progress note r/t abnormal lab values		
CONSULTS	IT ordered Y/N FT ordered Y/N GT ordered Y/N	GT started Psych Testing Order Y/N	Schedule MTP meeting	IT started, FT started Psych Testing Done Home Contract		Psych Testing results
TREATMENT PLANNING	N1: _____ Axis III _____		RT/TA started School started	Master TX Plan Update/ Revise, RT/ TA		
INTERVENTIONS	Assess S/H or Aggr. monitor anxiety stimulus	Monitor sleep pattern, orient X 4	Encourage group interaction	Give honest and consistent feedback	Encourage oral hygiene, adeq. fluid intake 2000 ml	Assess client support network, output resources
MEDICATIONS	Meds ordered, Inf. Con.	Assess for EPS	Drug interaction ✓'d, Dr. signs Inf. Con. ✓ for EPS	Meds evaluated/ readjusted Assess for EPS	Observe/ document response to Rx, ✓ for EPS	Discharge instructions for medication self-admin
LEVEL	Level ordered		Re-evaluate	Re-evaluate	Re-evaluate consider PHP	Re-evaluate
TEACHING	Patient Rights Orient to Unit	Orient to Program	Goals setting, relaxation techniques	Meds reinforced; Altered perceptions as symptom	Coping skills for unusual perceptions	Teach family S/S of Rx non-compliance

(continued)

TABLE 25-1 ▼ Clinical Pathway: Schizophrenic disorder (295.1x, catatonic 295.2x, delusional 297.10, brief reactive psychosis 298.80) (Continued)

DAY/DATE:	0–8 HOURS	8–24 HOURS	DAY 2	DAY 3	DAY 4	DAY 5
NUTRITION/ DIET	Type: _____	Chart daily intake	Chart daily intake	Chart daily intake	Chart daily intake	Chart daily intake
CARE CONTINUUM	Initial D/C Plans	Placement Search Outcome survey		Discharge Plan updated/ rev		After care plan written Outcome survey
PATIENT OUTCOMES	Controls violent impulses	ADLS w/assist, oriented × 3	Tolerates peer interaction	Improves insight	Uses adaptive coping skills	Goal directed inter- actions

Strategic Clinical Systems, Inc., 3715 Mission Ct., Granbury, TX 76049 (817) 326-4239. PsychPaths, © Copyright 1994. All Rights Reserved. Darla Belt, RN & Vickie Pflueger, RNC—Authors.
(EKG = electrocardiogram; FT = family therapy; GT = group therapy; H & P = history and physical; IT = individual therapy; MTP = master treatment plan; RT/TA = recreational therapy/therapeutic activities; S/H = suicide/homicide precautions; S/S = signs and symptoms; Signs Inf Con = signs informed consent; TX = treatment; UA = urinalysis; UDS = urine drug screen; UCG = urine test for pregnancy; ✓ for EPS = check for extrapyramidal symptoms.)

An optimal model of interdisciplinary treatment for those with schizophrenia includes the following:

- Assessment of current functioning
- Medication management
- Client and family education
- Skills training
- Family counseling
- Vocational training and rehabilitation
- Housing assistance
- Crisis intervention and brief inpatient services
- Continuity of care providers
- Network of ongoing social support

PHARMACOLOGIC INTERVENTIONS

Because failure to take prescribed medications is the primary reason most people with schizophrenia relapse, adherence to a medication schedule is critical to successful treatment and relapse prevention.

Antipsychotic (sometimes called neuroleptic) medications are needed to treat the symptoms of schizophrenia during both the acute and long-term phases of the illness. They do not, however, cure schizophrenia. Early intervention with medication decreases some of the associated long-term comorbid, or coexisting, conditions. Medication treatment also makes the client more amenable to other social, cognitive, and rehabilitative therapies.

Two types of antipsychotics are used to treat schizophrenia: traditional and atypical (Table 25-2). Traditional antipsychotics have been in use since 1952 and are successful in treating schizophrenia that is manifested by mostly positive symptoms. Their associated side effects (especially extrapyramidal side effects [EPSs]), however, are numerous and distressing, and they often cause the client to become noncompliant (Table 25-3). Atypical antipsychotics were developed in response to recent neurobiologic-based research findings in schizophrenia. These atypical antipsychotics, which are effective against both positive and negative symptoms, are less likely to induce EPSs (including tardive dyskinesia) and, thus, promote adherence (Kasper, 1998). Elderly clients are particularly sensitive to EPSs, and, therefore, respond better to atypical antipsychotics (see Chap. 12).

Antipsychotic medications are usually taken orally in liquid or tablet form, but intramuscular (IM) injections also can be given for immediate action. In addition, Haldol and Prolixin can be given in depot injections that continue to release the medication over 2 to 4 weeks.

Traditional (Conventional) Antipsychotics

Traditional antipsychotics treat the positive symptoms of schizophrenia such as hallucinations and delusions. A comprehensive discussion of the mechanisms of action and side effects of some of the most traditional antipsychotic medications is provided in Chapter 12. Traditional antipsychotics include the following:

- Chlorpromazine (Thorazine)
- Fluphenazine (Prolixin)
- Haloperidol (Haldol)
- Trifluoperazine (Stelazine)
- Thioridazine (Mellaril)
- Thiothixene (Navane)
- Perphenazine (Trilafon)

TABLE 25-2 ▼ Traditional and Atypical Antipsychotic Medications

MEDICATIONS	USUAL ADULT DAILY DOSAGE
Traditional (Conventional) Antipsychotic Medications	
High potency	
haloperidol (Haldol)	2–20 mg/day
fluphenazine (Prolixin)	2–20 mg/day
Medium potency	
thiothixene (Navane)	5–30 mg/day
trifluoperazine (Stelazine)	5–30 mg/day
perphenazine (Trilafon)	8–64 mg/day
molindone (Moban)	50–225 mg/day
loxapine (Loxitane)	25–100 mg/day
Low potency	
chlorpromazine (Thorazine)	200–800 mg/day
thioridazine (Mellaril)	150–600 mg/day
Long-acting depot antipsychotic medications	
depot haloperidol	50–200 mg as a monthly injection
depot fluphenazine	6.25–50 mg as injection every 2–3 weeks
Atypical (Novel) Antipsychotic Medications	
risperidone (Risperdal)	2–8 mg/day
clozapine (Clozaril)	150–600 mg/day
olanzapine (Zyprexa)	5–20 mg/day
quetiapine (Seroquel)	150–750 mg/day
ziprasidone (Geodon)	40–160 mg/day

The most common and distressing side effects associated with traditional antipsychotic medications are acute **extrapyramidal side effects (EPSs)**. These side effects may make clients feel worse than then they did before taking medication, contributing to nonadherence. EPSs include *akathisia* (severe restlessness), *dystonia* (muscle spasms or contractions), chronic motor problems such as tardive dyskinesia, and the pseudoparkinsonian symptoms of rigidity, masklike faces, and stiff gait (Barnes & McPhillips, 1998). EPSs are generally treated by reducing the dose of the medication, trying a different medication, or adding a medication that reduces or eliminates side effects. Some medications that reduce or eliminate EPSs are as follows (Box 25-6):

TABLE 25-3 ▼ Side Effect Profiles of Antipsychotic Medications

MEDICATION	SEDATION	AUTONOMIC	ANTICHOLINERGIC	EPSs
Traditional Antipsychotics				
High potency	+	+	+	+ + + +
Medium potency	+	+	+	+ + +
Low potency	+ + +	+ + +	+ + +	+ +
Atypical Antipsychotics				
risperidone (Risperdal)	+	+ +	−	+(low doses) + + + (high doses)
clozapine (Clozaril)	+ + + +	+ + + +	+ +	+
olanzapine (Zyprexa)	+	+ +	+	−
quetiapine (Seroquel)	+ + +	+ +	+	+

The greater the number of +, the more the characteristic is present; − indicates absence.

BOX 25-6 ▼ *Medications Used for Side Effects of Antipsychotics*

Anticholinergics—Used to treat parkinsonism and dystonia; may reduce akathisia
  benztropine (Cogentin) 1–6 mg
  trihexyphenidyl (Artane) 5–15 mg
Dopamine agonist—Used for its antiparkinsonian effect, without anticholinergic problems; may be less effective than anticholinergics
  amantadine (Symmetrel) 100–400 mg
β *blocker* (only central-acting not peripheral β blockers) — Used to treat akathisia; contraindicated in clients with diabetes and asthma
  propranolol (Inderal) 30–100 mg
Benzodiazepines—Should not be used for clients with substance abuse; use with caution with clozapine because of the risk of respiratory depression and arrest

  clonazepam (Klonopin) 1.5–4 mg
  lorazepam (Ativan) 2–8 mg
Antihistamine—Used in IM form for rapid relief of acute dystonia; used to treat akathisia when sedation is needed
  diphenhydramine (Benadryl) 25–150 mg

Adapted from Frances, A., Docherty, J. P., & Kahn, D. A., (Eds.). (1996). The Expert Consensus Guideline Series: Treatment of Schizophrenia. *The Journal of Clinical Psychiatry, 57* (Suppl. 12B). (On-line.) Available at: *www.psychguides.com.*
Weiden, P. J. (1997). Quetiapine ('Seroquel'): A new "atypical" antipsychotic. *Journal of Practical Psychiatry and Behavioral Health,* 368–374.

* Dopamine releasers, such as amantadine (Symmetrel)
* Anticholinergic drugs, such as trihexyphenidyl (Artane), benztropine (Cogentin), biperiden (Akineton), procyclidine (Kemadrin), and ethopropazine (Parsidol)
* Antihistamines almost exclusively limited to diphenhydramine (Benadryl)

Tardive dyskinesia (TD) is a type of EPS characterized by abnormal, involuntary, irregular, choreoathetoid (writhing) movements, which may include lip smacking, neck twisting, facial grimacing, and tongue and chewing movements. TD can occur after several months to years of treatment with traditional antipsychotics; about one third of those treated develop TD. Treatment usually involves discontinuing or decreasing the medication. Assessment by means of the Abnormal Involuntary Movement Scale (AIMS) will promote early detection of TD.

Other side effects associated with traditional antipsychotics include orthostatic hypotension; anticholinergic effects of dry mouth, blurred vision, constipation, and urinary retention; endocrine effects of amenorrhea, breast enlargement, galactorrhea, and male erectile dysfunction; photosensitivity of the skin; tachycardia; sedation; weight gain; and agranulocytosis (Kaplan & Sadock, 1996). A life-threatening complication associated with traditional antipsychotic medications is neuroleptic malignant syndrome (NMS). This is marked by elevated temperature, severe EPSs (eg, rigidity and dystonia), autonomic dysfunction (eg, hypertension, tachycardia, diaphoresis), and an elevated creatine phosphokinase (CPK) level. NMS requires immediate medical attention, transfer to an intensive care unit, and administration of bromocriptine and dantrolene (Kaplan & Sadock, 1996).

Atypical (Novel) Antipsychotics

Atypical antipsychotics relieve both the positive and negative symptoms (eg, apathy, avolition, social withdrawal) of schizophrenia, and are less likely to cause distressing EPSs typically seen with the traditional antipsychotic medications. Atypical antipsychotic medications are discussed in depth in Chapter 12. They include the following:

* Clozapine (Clozaril)
* Risperidone (Risperdal)
* Olanzapine (Zyprexa)
* Quetiapine (Seroquel)
* Ziprasidone (Geodon)

Since its release in the United States in 1989, clozapine (Clozaril) has been effective in treating refractory schizophrenia (ie, schizophrenia that does not respond to ordinary treatment). People with refractory schizophrenia make up about 30% of the total population of those with schizophrenia and are particularly prone to assaults and suicide. Clozapine use has resulted in decreased negative symptoms, increased impulse control, reduced violence to self and others, and improved quality of life. Although it is not associated with EPSs, including TD, it has the potentially fatal side effect of agranulocytosis (1% to 2% incidence); adverse reactions including lowered seizure threshold, hypotension, sedation, and elevated liver enzymes; and unpleasant side effects, such as weight gain (Sousa, 1999). Because agranulocytosis can be a life-threatening condition, nurses must provide extensive education to clients taking clozapine and their families, monitor weekly hematologic counts, and report and document any drop in white blood cell counts. Generally, clozapine is not used as a first-line agent because of the danger posed by some of the more severe side effects.

Risperidone (Risperdal), an atypical antipsychotic approved for first-line treatment of psychotic disorders, is effective in treating both positive and negative symptoms with reduced EPSs and dyskinetic side effects. The most commonly reported side effects are drowsiness, orthostatic hypotension, light-headedness, anxiety, dizziness, nausea, akathisia, constipation, and weight gain.

Another atypical antipsychotic approved for first-line use, olanzapine (Zyprexa) has demonstrated even lower EPSs than risperidone. Side effects are somnolence, nausea, light-headedness, dizziness, constipation, substantial weight gain, and headache (Jibson & Tandon, 1998). Quetiapine (Seroquel) is a relatively new atypical antipsychotic, and incidences of EPSs and akathisia have been rarely reported. It also seems to be well tolerated in elderly clients with psychoses (McManus, Arvanitis, & Kowalcyk, 1999). Side effects include drowsiness, dizziness, postural hypotension, agitation, dry mouth, and weight gain (Jibson & Tandon, 1998).

In mid-2000, the Food and Drug Administration (FDA) approved the release of the newest atypical antipsychotic ziprasidone (Geodon), which is effective in treating negative, positive, and depressive symptoms of schizophrenia. Although side effects include somnolence, orthostatic hypotension, headache, nausea, constipation, dysphagia, and potential dysrhythmias, it is considered weight neutral (does not make users gain weight). Another antipsychotic medication in development and close to FDA release for the treatment of schizophrenia is iloperidone.

PSYCHOSOCIAL INTERVENTIONS

While pharmacotherapy is the staple of treatment for schizophrenia, it alone is not sufficient. Clients require additional types of therapy to address the psychosocial ramifications of the illness. Psychosocial care assists clients and families in coping with stress and solving problems; educates them about the illness, its treatment, and self-care; enhances medication compliance; and provides rehabilitative support to help clients master skills of independent living.

Milieu Management

Milieu management refers to providing an environment rich with therapeutic possibility. The inpatient client with a thought disorder will likely have impaired judgment and reality testing. Also, safety needs will be paramount. Healthcare staff members assume responsibility for the client's well-being and physical care when he or she cannot meet those basic needs. Symptom management and family education are ongoing in the milieu. Recreational and activities therapies can be used to increase the client's social and recreational skills.

Individual and Group Therapy

For the client with a thought disorder, individual and group therapies that offer support, education, and behav-ioral and cognitive skills training (see the following section) are recommended to improve functioning and address specific problems, such as medication noncompliance or social isolation (see Chaps. 8 and 9). Conversely, individual and group therapies that focus on gaining insight into unconscious material are not recommended for most clients with schizophrenia because it is thought that therapies that result in regression and transference can be harmful to the client with a thought disorder (Lehman, Steinwachs, & the Co-Investigators of the PORT Project, 1998). Rather, the focus of individual therapy should be on building a therapeutic relationship, helping the client stay oriented to reality, and helping the client improve coping skills. This relationship can help the client experience guidance, support, and reinforcement for his or her health promotion efforts and successes.

Group therapy sessions can focus on social skills, concentrating on appropriate interpersonal interaction. The therapist will role-play with the client, modeling and identifying suitable social actions and responses. Various scenarios are acted out repeatedly on key social behaviors, during which the client receives feedback and support. Treatment also addresses practical matters such as personal care, living skills, and money management.

Cognitive-behavioral Therapy

Cognitive-behavioral therapy aims to improve remotivation, resocialization, and reality testing by means of goal setting and increasing coping and problem-solving skills, self-esteem, and the client's sense of control. Distorted thoughts are replaced with more rational and logical thoughts that have better outcomes for the client. The change in attitude, values, and thinking results in changed behavior (Blair & Ramones, 1997). In a recent study, cognitive-behavioral therapy was shown to reduce the number and severity of positive symptoms in clients with chronic schizophrenia, compared to those who received supportive counseling (Tarrier et al., 1998). Clients also reported learning rational self-talk and other cognitive skills from their family and friends. Social skills training helped the client improve relationships with others.

Vocational Rehabilitation

Another aspect of psychosocial therapy involves employment training. Some clients with schizophrenia can be gainfully employed and should be offered vocational rehabilitation, particularly if they:

- Identify employment as a goal
- Have a history of successful employment
- Have a history of few psychiatric hospitalizations
- Have good work skills

Vocational rehabilitation involves speedy placement in a real job, coupled with assistance and coaching from a therapist or job coach. The client is supported as he or she transitions back to work and is encouraged to become involved in vocational educational services and counseling as the best model for successful employment (Lehman, Steinwachs, & the Co-Investigators of the PORT Project, 1998).

CONTINUUM OF CARE

The person with schizophrenia requires a seamless system of comprehensive care. Continuity of care must occur as the client moves to and from various settings. Continuum of care issues include medication and symptom monitoring, follow-up care, use of appropriate resources and services, and ongoing training and assistance with the skills needed for independent living.

Discharge Planning

During an acute psychotic episode, the client's care in the inpatient setting should include collaborative treatment planning with the family members or friends who will be involved in his or her care in the community. Introduction to community resources, appointments to accessible community agencies, and information about phone help lines and how to contact care providers should be part of the discharge teaching. Connecting clients and family members to NAMI support groups can provide an invaluable learning experience for them as well as an enormous source of emotional and social support. When clients are outpatients, client and family needs are usually met through community mental health centers.

Care in the Community

The continuum of care within the community must provide for the extensive needs of the client with schizophrenia. Transportation, nutrition, social activities, substance abuse education, medication monitoring, psychoeducation, and access to decent, safe, and affordable housing are services that extend beyond traditional care boundaries but are essential in the rehabilitation of the client. Employment is associated with better quality of life for clients with schizophrenia; employers should be prepared to give direct and constructive feedback to the client. The person is neither helpless nor frail and should not be regarded as such.

Unfortunately, deinstitutionalization from state hospitals has led to reinstitutionalization of many clients with long-term psychiatric problems in jails, nursing homes, and shelters, and it has placed many clients on the streets. The problems of those with schizophrenia, including substance abuse and medical illness, are complex (see Research in Psychiatric-Mental Health Nursing 25-1). Elderly clients require both physical and psychological assessment and management, medication monitoring, housing, rehabilitation, and community support. Rehabilitation clubhouses can decrease recidivism, or repeated hospitalization, through supportive, vocational, and educational services (Delaney, 1998).

The Community Mental Health Center Act of 1963 brought about the construction of local community men-

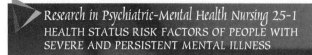

Research in Psychiatric-Mental Health Nursing 25-1
HEALTH STATUS RISK FACTORS OF PEOPLE WITH SEVERE AND PERSISTENT MENTAL ILLNESS

Purpose: To address the assessment of physical health needs in persons with severe and persistent mental illness in community residential programs.

Background: Fifty percent of people with mental illness are estimated to have a known, comorbid medical disorder; another 35% are estimated to suffer from undiagnosed and untreated medical disorders. The three major lifestyle habits that increase the risk of life-threatening physical illness are physical inactivity, smoking, and poor nutrition.

Method and Sample: The researchers conducted surveys and interviews of 154 consumers of mental health services (85% of whom had schizophrenia) and 16 residential managers to assess physical health needs, current use of available health services, and willingness to participate in health promotion programs to improve lifestyle habits.

Findings: Compared with the general population, the persons with severe and persistent mental illness spent more time sleeping and engaged in fewer activities requiring any degree of physical exertion. Forty-one percent of the consumers voiced some complaint about their physical health. Several risk factors that affect physical health surfaced, including smoking (75%), lack of exercise (60%), overweight or underweight (42%), poor diet and nutrition (40%), medication intake (22%), alcohol consumption (22%), and drug abuse (15%). Consumers indicated their willingness to participate in health promotion programs.

Application to Nursing Practice: Nurses need to conduct health education programs, built on an illness prevention and health promotion model, specifically for consumers with severe and persistent mental illness. Nurses and other mental health staff should understand the benefits of health promotion activities in this population. Teaching techniques for this population will have to consider specific learning problems such as shorter attention span, limited grasp of complexity, short-term memory deficits, poorer fund of general knowledge, and limited ability to adapt to new situations and information.

Farnam, C. R., Zipple, A. M., Tyrrell, W., & Chittinanda, P. (1999). Health status risk factors of people with severe and persistent mental illness. *Journal of Psychosocial Nursing, 37*(6), 16–21.

tal health centers where clients could receive services in their own communities. Community-based care for those with schizophrenia includes assertive community treatment

(ACT), intensive case management (ICM), ongoing medication management, and housing, rehabilitation, social, and vocational supports (see Chap. 16). More effective than traditional approaches, ACT teams and ICM were developed to meet the client's multiple and complex healthcare needs (Mueser, Bond, Drake, & Resnick, 1998).

Assertive Community Treatment. ACT is a program of individualized, consistent, comprehensive, and continuous services to clients with schizophrenia and other severe and persistent mental illnesses. ACT services are provided by a team, not an individual mental health worker, and delivered where people live, work, and play. These services include helping clients with symptom management, medication monitoring, housing, vocational needs, parenting skills, nonpsychiatric medical care, and daily responsibilities and problems. ACT is designed for those clients "in greatest need" because of frequent relapse, repeated hospitalization, dual diagnosis, homelessness, incarceration, or resistance or avoidance of involvement in usual mental health services. The cost of ACT programs is about $8,000 to $12,000 a year per client, considerably less than the average cost of hospitalization in a state facility (more than $100,000/year), residential treatment ($50,000/year), or incarceration ($18,000/year) (Edgar, 1998–1999). ACT services reduce the most devastating outcomes of severe psychiatric illnesses, such as incarceration, repeated hospitalizations, and homelessness.

Intensive Case Management. ICM is another model of community care. It involves assessment, referral, coordination, and integration of a cohesive program of services tailored to the needs of the individual client. In addition, the case managers in ICM serve as advocates for the client (Mueser, Bond, Drake, & Resnick, 1998). A more useful model includes a case manager who is also a clinician with skills in helping to strengthen family coping.

APPLICATION OF THE NURSING PROCESS TO THE CLIENT WITH A THOUGHT DISORDER

Assessment

Assessment of the client with a thought disorder may occur in various care settings, from the outpatient clinic, to the home, to the inpatient psychiatric unit. The nurse may be assessing the client with a known history of schizophrenia or a client unknown to the mental healthcare system. Although formal assessment tools for schizophrenia exist, many nurses will assess clients without such tools, relying instead on interviews and observation of the client.

Assessment begins with an interview and focuses on establishing what signs and symptoms the client is exhibiting, how impaired the thought processes are, whether the client is at risk for self-injury or violence directed at others, and what support systems the client has. The nurse may wish to interview the client with a family member or friend to obtain all information regarding the family history, previous episodes of psychotic symptoms, onset of symptoms, and thoughts of suicide or violent behavior.

ASSESSING MOOD AND COGNITIVE STATE

The nurse assesses the client's mood, affect, and behavior, including the range of emotional expressiveness, motivation, and interpersonal skills, while keeping in mind the client's cultural background. The nurse is alert for signs and symptoms such as:

- Absence of expression of feelings
- Language content that is difficult to follow
- Pronounced paucity of speech and thoughts
- Preoccupation with odd ideas
- Ideas of reference (ie, believing that mundane objects have special meanings)
- Expressions of feelings of unreality
- Evidence of hallucinations such as comments that the way things appear, sound, or smell is different

Additionally, the nurse asks the client if he or she has had difficulty concentrating or performing intellectual activities at a previous level. The client's ability to concentrate is a factor necessary for effective participation in rehabilitation. In a recent study, persons with schizophrenia identified the ability to concentrate as a major turning point in their recovery (Baier & Murray, 1999).

Other signs and symptoms to assess include sleep disturbances, somatic complaints, and social withdrawal. The nurse also inquires about recent stressors, which can precipitate a psychotic episode in the client with a thought disorder, and signs and symptoms of impending relapse. These warning signs include disrupted sleep cycle, significant mood changes (mostly depression), decreased appetite, and somatic complaints such as headache, malaise, and constipation. Relapse leads to client withdrawal, resistance, and preoccupation with psychotic symptoms.

ASSESSING POTENTIAL FOR VIOLENCE

Some clients with schizophrenia can become violent, either directing injury at themselves or at others. The nurse assesses the client for his or her potential for violence by inquiring about the following:

- A history of violent or suicidal behavior
- Extreme social isolation
- Feelings of persecution or being "controlled" by others

- Auditory hallucinations that tell the client to commit violent acts
- Concomitant substance abuse
- Medication noncompliance
- Feelings of anger, suspiciousness, or hostility

The nurse makes other members of the team aware of the client's potential for violence, because protecting the client and others from serious harm is a priority.

ASSESSING SOCIAL SUPPORT

Availability and responsiveness of a social support network and the client's role in the family and community are important factors in nursing assessment. The presence of caring, supportive family and friends influences the client's recovery process; its absence contributes to feelings of hopelessness. Assessing the availability of significant others helps the nurse in planning educational and other aspects of treatment.

ASSESSING KNOWLEDGE

The nurse assesses the client's and family's knowledge of schizophrenia, its treatment, and the potential for relapse. Adherence to medication and other therapeutic schedules is bolstered when clients and families understand the biological basis of the illness, signs of recovery and relapse, and their roles in treatment. Not only do the client and family benefit from knowledge about the disease process, but they also benefit from knowledge about treatment modalities, goals of care, and types of services available in their community. The nurse assesses if the client and family are receiving all the services for which they are eligible.

Nursing Diagnosis

Nursing diagnoses that guide the nursing care of the client with schizophrenia include the following:

- **Disturbed Thought Processes** related to biochemical imbalances, as evidenced by hypervigilance, distractibility, poor concentration, disordered thought sequencing, inappropriate responses, and thinking not based in reality
- **Disturbed Sensory Perception (auditory or visual)** related to biochemical imbalances, as evidenced by auditory or visual hallucinations
- **Risk for Other-Directed or Self-Directed Violence** related to delusional thoughts, hallucinatory commands, history of childhood abuse, or panic, as evidenced by overt aggressive acts, threatening stances, pacing, or suicidal ideation or plan
- **Social Isolation** related to alterations in mental status and an inability to engage in satisfying personal relationships, as evidenced by sad, flat affect; absence

of supportive significant others; withdrawal; uncommunicativeness; and inability to meet expectations of others
- **Noncompliance** with medication regimen related to health beliefs and lack of motivation, as evidenced by failure to adhere to medication schedule
- **Ineffective Coping** related to disturbed thought processes as evidenced by inability to meet basic needs
- **Interrupted Family Processes** related to shift in health status of a family member and situational crisis, as evidenced by changes in the family's goals, plans, and activities and changes in family patterns and rituals
- **Risk for Ineffective Family Management of Therapeutic Regimen** related to knowledge deficit and complexity of client's healthcare needs

Planning

Preparing the treatment plan is a collaborative effort between the entire mental health team and the client and family. No single treatment helps every client; rather, a plan must be tailored to each client's strengths, needs, and limitations. Although standardized nursing care plans exist for specific diagnoses, they must be individualized for each person (Nursing Care Plan 25-1). Major goals for the care of a client with schizophrenia are as follows:

- The client will experience improved thought processes and fewer psychotic symptoms.
- The client will not engage in violent behavior.
- The client will acquire improved social skills and engage in satisfying social interaction.
- The client and family will gain knowledge about the disease process and treatment.

Implementation

Implementing a plan of care for the client with schizophrenia involves careful attention to the therapeutic relationship. Nurses who work with clients with schizophrenia must be straightforward, hopeful, and accepting and should view the client with unconditional regard and dignity. They must work within the confines of the client's ability and willingness to participate in treatment. Furthermore, nurses should demonstrate acceptance of the client and his or her behavior without judgment. Although the behavior may disgust or anger the nurse, it is a symptom of the illness and not purposefully directed at the mental health staff. Failure to establish a therapeutic relationship based on trust and unconditional regard will make successful intervention difficult at best.

Nursing Care Plan 25-1

THE CLIENT WITH A THOUGHT DISORDER

As discussed in Clinical Example 25–1, James agrees to stay in the hospital to receive treatment. He is admitted to a locked psychiatric unit. Carol is concerned about James's fears surrounding the auditory hallucinations, particularly considering he is afraid to reveal the content. Carol suspects that the voices may be telling James to hurt himself or others. Client safety—his and others—is a priority. Other issues that Carol and the treatment team would like to address in the early stages of treatment include restarting James's medications, building the therapeutic relationship, and helping him manage his delusional thoughts and hallucinations.

Nursing Diagnosis: Risk for Self-Directed or Other-Directed Violence related to psychotic symptomatology as evidenced by auditory hallucinations that tell him "to do things"

Goal: James will not harm himself or anyone else.

Interventions	Rationales
Assess client's behavior from the standpoint of potential for violence. Ask client directly if the voices tell him to harm himself or others. Be alert for signs of self-harm and keep client in a protected environment under frequent observation until delusions and hallucinations subside.	Preventing other-directed violence is possible if healthcare providers heed warning signs such as intimidating behaviors and verbal threats. Warning signs of self-directed violence may be less overt; protecting, observing, and asking James about them may be the only tools available to staff.
Provide reassurance, comfort, and the opportunity to discuss delusional thoughts.	Caring interventions help build a therapeutic relationship and may increase the likelihood that James will reveal the content of his auditory hallucinations.
Determine a plan of action with other team members if violence appears imminent. Discuss plan with client; ask client to tell staff when or if he feels he may harm himself or others.	Having a plan in place will help the staff more effectively manage a violent situation. Engaging James in the plan may help him gain control over his thought processes, increase the likelihood that he will comply with the plan, and help build a therapeutic relationship.

Evaluation: A positive outcome would be that James feels trusting enough to reveal the content of his hallucinations and informs the staff if and when he feels he may act on violent impulses or hallucinatory "commands."

Nursing Diagnosis: Noncompliance related to disturbed thought processes as evidenced by refusal to take medication

Goal: Client will take his medications.

Interventions	Rationales
Discuss use of depot injections to manage short-term medication compliance.	James's refusal to take his medication at home suggests that compliance will remain an issue. Depot injections ensure that therapeutic levels of neuroleptic medication can be maintained for 2 weeks at a time.
Initiate medication compliance therapy. Help the client achieve insight into the benefit of taking medication by helping him review the history of his illness, symptoms, and medication side effects and encouraging him to consider the benefits versus the drawbacks of drug treatment. Encourage medication compliance and provide information about neuroleptic medication.	Medication compliance therapy, which involves medication education, support, and insight into the disorder, has been shown to increase long-term medication compliance.

(continued)

Nursing Care Plan 25-1 (Continued)

Evaluation: Medication compliance will likely be an ongoing issue for James, as it is for many clients with schizophrenia. The nurse can evaluate the effectiveness of medication compliance therapy indirectly by observing a change in James's attitude about taking medications, by observing James take oral medications as prescribed while in inpatient care, by James's ongoing participation in outpatient follow-up care, and by James's and his family's reports.

Nursing Diagnosis: Disturbed Thought Processes related to possible neurochemical dysregulation and effects of head trauma as evidenced by nonreality based thinking

Goal: James's thinking will become more reality-based, and his delusions will subside.

Interventions	Rationales
Focus on client's underlying feelings, not the content, about the delusion (eg, "You seem troubled by these thoughts," not "Why would the government want to control your thoughts?"). Do not reinforce or argue about the delusion. Rather, express doubt about the content matter-of-factly. ("People don't have 'special powers.'")	Focusing on nondelusional content (such as feelings) and discouraging an animated discussion of the delusional content (which would only end up reinforcing the delusion) will help the client see that his thoughts are not real.
Encourage client to validate his delusional ideas with the staff (reality testing) and to discuss any delusional beliefs before acting on them.	Asking the client to bring delusional content to the caregivers' attention provides opportunities for reinforcing reality-based thinking and may prevent bizarre or possibly violent behavior generated by the delusional beliefs.
Administer neuroleptic medication as ordered and as needed.	Antipsychotic medication is the most powerful tool in the treatment of schizophrenia. Even if James receives depot injections, he may require additional medication if psychotic symptoms escalate.

Evaluation: James's thinking will become more reality based as he responds to the medication and the staff interventions. Evaluation includes noting that James begins to recognize when delusional beliefs are occurring, asks for validation from the staff, reports a decreased frequency of delusions, and displays more logical, appropriate thought processes.

Nursing Diagnosis Disturbed Sensory Perception related to biochemical imbalances as evidenced by auditory hallucinations

Goal: James will not respond to hallucinatory commands, and hallucinations will subside.

Interventions	Rationales
Keep client in a safe, protected, restricted environment. Avoid excessive activity and stimulation.	Close observation of the client with active hallucinations in a secure environment is essential to maintain the safety of the client and others. Excessive sensory stimulation could overwhelm and agitate James.
Encourage client to tell staff when he is hallucinating and to reveal the content of the hallucinations. Monitor hallucinations for harmful content.	James may act on the hallucinations. Staff should be aware of the content, especially if it is potentially harmful.
Focus on feelings about, rather than details of, the hallucination (eg, "You seem to be afraid," not "Why would the voices tell you to hurt yourself?").	Focusing on James's feelings, which are real, minimizes emphasis on the hallucination.

(continued)

Nursing Care Plan 25-1 (Continued)

Interventions	Rationales
Do not argue with the client about whether the hallucinations are real; state, if asked, that you do not perceive the visual, auditory, tactile, or olfactory stimuli that the client perceives.	Arguing with the client or expressing disbelief in the hallucinations does not affect the client's belief in the reality of the hallucination and can disrupt trust and the therapeutic relationship. Expressing that you do not see, hear, or otherwise experience the hallucinatory stimuli indirectly encourages James to question the reality of the experience.

Evaluation: Judgment about the effectiveness of the interventions will be based on whether James feels comfortable expressing the content of the hallucinations to the staff, does not act on any hallucinatory commands, begins to question the reality of the hallucinations, and reports a decrease in, and eventually the total cessation of, hallucinations.

INTERVENING IN DISTURBED THOUGHT PROCESSES AND SENSORY PERCEPTIONS

The focus of care for the client with acute psychosis in the early stages of treatment will be on improving his or her reality testing. Although pharmacotherapy plays the major role in diminishing psychotic symptoms, nonpharmacologic interventions help as well.

Reinforcing Reality

The nurse clarifies and validates reality for the client with schizophrenia by involving him or her in present-oriented conversations and activities, describing real events, and clarifying the reality of a situation. Nurses apply this principle to a client's delusions. For example, in response to the client's assertion that his or her body has turned to concrete, the nurse might reply, "I am looking at you, and your body looks like it is still made of flesh." It is important, however, not to engage in arguments about delusional content because arguments and lengthy discussions may further strengthen the delusions. No one can argue away perceptions of depersonalization, hallucinations, or delusions. The delusion is real to the client. Rather, the nurse should state the facts in a simple, concise, and nonthreatening way. He or she should gently introduce doubt about the delusion (eg, "No, Mr. L., I don't understand why the FBI would be interested in following you").

Reality-based activities, such as looking at pictures in a magazine or taking a walk, are therapeutic because they allow the client to interact in a satisfying interpersonal relationship and diminish the time that he or she is in poor reality contact. Many times the client cannot interact, but staying with him or her provides a vital link with the real world. Nurses should not permit clients to isolate themselves because doing so only increases withdrawal and poor reality orientation.

Understanding Language Content

The client's illogical, symbolic, and disorganized speech will often hold a message that he or she cannot express clearly. The nurse listens for themes and reflects back to the client the meaning that the nurse has deciphered. The nurse does not dismiss the client's verbal and nonverbal behaviors as meaningless or nonsense. In effect, the nurse tries to decode the communication that the client offers and validates its meaning.

Much of the communication that the client presents will be confusing to the nurse. The nurse must clarify, not assume to understand, vague, ambiguous statements. He or she should never pretend to understand or agree with a client's illogical or delusional thinking. Rather, he or she asks for clarification. At all times, nurses are role models for healthy, clear communication.

Intervening in Hallucinations

The person who hallucinates is preoccupied and frightened by what he or she hears or sees. The hallucination is real to the client, and the nurse cannot argue away, dismiss, or ignore it. Although the hallucination is a real perception to the client, nurses make it clear that they do not hear the voices or see the visual hallucination that the client experiences.

Nurses do, however, communicate concern that the client is bothered, upset, or frightened by the hallucination. For example, it is therapeutic to say, "No, I don't hear that voice saying bad things about you, but I imagine it is frightening for you to hear it. I would like to help you feel less frightened."

The nurse does not leave the person who is hallucinating alone; the nurse's presence is a reassuring force that may calm the client. Drawing him into activities and conversation that are reality based may distract him or her from the hallucination as well as reinforce reality. Some people with schizophrenia have found that elevated anxiety precedes their hallucinations, and therefore, have developed skills to deal with anxiety. Other important interventions for managing hallucinations include using the following:

- Dismissal intervention (ie, telling the voices to go away)
- Various coping strategies (eg, jogging, telephoning, playing games, seeking out others, employing relaxation techniques)
- Competing stimuli (eg, listening to music or another's or one's own voice to overcome auditory hallucinations and visual stimuli to overcome visual hallucinations; the nurse might say, "Listen to my voice, don't listen to that other voice. You know me. I'm Barbara. I'm here with you now. Listen to me.")

MANAGING VIOLENT BEHAVIOR

The first step in managing violent behavior is intervening before violence occurs. The nurse is alert to inappropriate and possibly previolent behaviors such as irritability, intimidating behavior, refusal to cooperate with unit routines, motor restlessness, intense staring, loud speech, or overt threats. The nurse at this point should not overwhelm the client with too much talk or closeness. Touch should be avoided except in the most judicious use, as it will likely be perceived as threatening and harmful.

It is usually appropriate to initiate urgent intervention when these behaviors are present. The client will likely require chemical restraint, with oral medication being the most acceptable route to the client. An IM injection and seclusion would be the next step if oral medication fails or will not be taken by the client. Physical restraint is the least acceptable intervention but may be unavoidable in some instances.

LESSENING SOCIAL ISOLATION

Despite the fact that the severe psychotic symptoms of schizophrenia can subside with pharmacologic treatment, many clients with schizophrenia still have severely restricted social lives. Their impaired communication, lack of motivation, inattention to self-care, and difficulty establishing and maintaining relationships with others leave them socially isolated. The psychosocial approaches described earlier can help clients improve social functioning and enjoy a better quality of life. It should be noted, however, that these interventions are not usually implemented until psychotic symptoms are under control. Nurses can lay the groundwork for these interventions by establishing a therapeutic relationship and then implement these interventions as clients' thought processes improve.

Developing Trust

The person with schizophrenia is likely to be anxious and fearful around others. Through therapeutic communication and trustworthy nonverbal behavior, the nurse builds a trusting relationship with the client. This is accomplished through acceptance, a nonjudgmental attitude, and genuineness. A genuine desire to help is perceived accurately by the client, just as fear and repulsion are accurately perceived; nonverbal behavior is usually trustworthier than words.

Because of his or her illness, the client with schizophrenia has likely had unsatisfying or unsuccessful interpersonal relations and is unwilling or unable to take risks in encounters with another person. Establishing rapport with the client becomes a gradual process built on consistent and pleasant interactions. As rewarding experiences occur, the client may be able to interact with greater numbers of people. The ultimate message here is that others can care for him or her, not just take care of him or her.

Initiating Interaction

The nurse needs to initiate interaction with the client because his or her behavior is often one of withdrawal and isolation. The nurse's approach should be nonthreatening and calm—one that gives the client plenty of space. For example, the nurse should sit near the client but not so near that he or she might perceive that his or her personal space is being violated. This approach communicates that the nurse is willing to respond to cues and progress at the client's pace.

Modeling Affect

Persons with schizophrenia often display flat, blunted, or inappropriate affects. Nurses model appropriate affect in their communication with clients and others through facial expressions and body language that match the tone or content of the message. For example, a nurse has a sad facial expression and somber movements when discussing a sad event. The nurse should not reinforce inappropriate or bizarre behavior by smiling, laughing, nodding, or becoming angry with the client.

PROMOTING ADHERENCE TO MEDICATION REGIMENS

A person with schizophrenia may fail to take his or her medication, as prescribed, for a number of reasons. The client may be disturbed by the medication's side effects, may believe he or she doesn't need the medication, may believe he or she doesn't have an illness, or may believe that the medication is poison. Eighty percent of persons with schizophrenia who stop taking their medication have a relapse within a year, compared with 30% who continue their medication and relapse. The most common causes of relapse and rehospitalization for "revolving-door" inpatients are medication nonadherence and medication nonresponse (ie, having little relief of symptoms from the medication).

Nurses are responsible for assessing and encouraging medication adherence (Therapeutic Communication 25-1). Accepting the diagnosis of schizophrenia is not a nec-

THERAPEUTIC COMMUNICATION 25-1
Language Problems in Schizophrenia

Frank Oliver is a 41-year-old man with schizophrenia, disorganized type, continuous. Although he has had five prior psychiatric hospitalizations, Frank has been managing fairly successfully in the community through medication monitoring and ACT interventions. Two weeks ago, however, he experienced an acute psychotic episode and was hospitalized.

While administering 10 mg of Haldol, 1 mg of Cogentin, and 500 mg of Depakote to Frank, the nurse, Jenna Ivey, reviews his knowledge and beliefs about his medications.

Ineffective Dialogue

Jenna: "Frank, you haven't done very well with taking your medications. Do you know what you're supposed to be taking?"

Frank: "Depakote every day, Cogentin 300 mg every day, and a pink pill with a description on it. Total containment."

Jenna: "What do you mean by 'total containment'? And those amounts aren't right. At bedtime you take 10 mg of Haldol, 1 mg of Cogentin, and 500 mg of Depakote."

Frank: "Right. A precocious repercussion."

Jenna: "Frank, that doesn't make sense."

Frank: "Make sense."

Jenna: "OK, let's try again. Do you know why you take these medications?"

Frank: "Doctors and policemen. You said to."

Jenna: "I'm not a policeman, Frank. Why do you think that?"

Frank: "Locked up. Upstairs. In, out."

Jenna: "Do you mean because you're in a locked unit you feel like you're in jail? You're here for your own good, Frank."

Frank: "Not the light."

Jenna: "I give up! We'll talk about this later, maybe tomorrow when you're feeling better."

Frank: "Okay."

Effective Dialogue

Jenna: "Here are your medicines, Frank. What are the names and amounts of these medicines that you take every day?"

Frank: "Depakote every day, Cogentin 300 mg every day, and a pink pill with a description on it. Total containment."

Jenna: "You named two of your three medicines correctly, Frank, but you didn't quite have the amounts right. Let's go over that again. At bedtime you take 10 mg of Haldol, 1 mg of Cogentin, and 500 mg of Depakote."

Frank: "Relate it to the immediate facility and permanency."

Jenna: "Frank, I'd like to ask you a few questions about your medicines."

Frank: "Okay."

Jenna: "How do these medicines help you?"

Frank: "They help me overcome the fact that I'm not working right now. Makes me feel all right when I see good people."

Jenna: "You feel all right when you see good people?"

Frank: "Yes, I do."

Jenna: "What are the symptoms of your illness that these medicines help you with?"

Frank: "Clean, work, happy, have no conflict or complaint. Romans and Galatians, Proverbs. Sometimes my eye automatically closes. Sometimes it pops right out of my head. Automation."

Jenna: "Are you having a problem with your eye, Frank?"

Frank: "No, I don't think it's fair for me to say right now."

Jenna: "You don't want to answer that now?"

Frank: "No."

Jenna: "Frank, it's important for us to know if you are having any side effects or problems from your medicines so we can help you. And you need to know what to do if you have any side effects from your medicines."

Frank: "I would smoke, don't drink beer, and try not to be relentless."

(continued)

THERAPEUTIC COMMUNICATION 25-1 (CONTINUED)
Language Problems in Schizophrenia

Jenna: "I think it would be good if we sat down together, Frank, and talked more about your medicines. Would you be willing to do that after I finish giving medicines to the others?"

Frank: "Okay."

Reflection and Critical Thinking

- In both dialogues, what therapeutic techniques did Jenna use to communicate with Frank? Identify any blocks or barriers to therapeutic communication.
- What statements did Jenna make in the first scenario that were less effective than the statements in the second scenario? Describe the effects of her statements.
- How does the conclusion of the conversation in the second scenario differ from the one in the first scenario?
- Describe Frank's communication style and themes. What do you think he was trying to say?
- What methods of communication did Jenna use in the second scenario that ultimately were more effective than those she used in the first?

essary condition for medication adherence. Some people will take their medication and realize that they are vulnerable to relapse, even though they are not convinced they have schizophrenia (Baier & Murray, 1999). Providing education to the client and family and promoting increased client autonomy and involvement usually results in increased adherence to medication regimens. To do this, nurses must know the medication's action, use, dosage, route of administration, desired effects, side effects, toxic effects, contraindications, and nursing implications (see Tables 25-2 and 25-3). Clients and families also must know this information, as well as how to intervene if an adverse reaction occurs.

PROMOTING IMPROVED INDIVIDUAL COPING SKILLS

Stress management techniques such as breathing and relaxation exercises, imagery, nutritional improvement, and aerobic exercise are useful stress management measures to help clients with schizophrenia. Nurses teach clients to discover and practice the stress-relieving activities that work for them.

Learning their own signs of impending relapse is critical for the clients and families so they can contact their care provider and adjust medication or implement other necessary interventions. Factors that promote recovery are adhering to medication, self-monitoring symptoms, understanding the illness and its treatment, having adequate housing, working at a vocation or job, receiving support of significant others, participating in community rehabilitation, and developing spirituality.

STRENGTHENING FAMILY PROCESSES

The challenges and problems faced by the family with a schizophrenic member are immense. The schizophrenic client's failure to care for personal needs, difficulty managing money, social withdrawal, strange personal habits, suicide threats, and interference with family schedules are such that fear for the safety of the ill member and other family members are realistic concerns. The family's resources often deteriorate so much that the members' well-being and family stability are threatened. Chronic sorrow may develop in response to unending caregiver responsibilities.

Teaching and encouraging the use of independent living skills promote independent functioning for the client. As the client progresses in his or her ability to accept more responsibility, he or she is given greater responsibility. Clients and families should be taught to care for their physical needs and to renew themselves through pleasurable activities, hobbies, and other interests.

Family members must be taught that schizophrenia is a "no fault" brain disease, and there is no reason for blame. Family-to-family education, now available in 40 states, has proved to be an effective means of both education and support. Nurses promote measures that increase the family's social network and reduce stigma.

Barriers to recovery are not just clinical symptoms of schizophrenia and stigma. Another barrier can be hopelessness, including the hopeless attitudes of nurses and other mental healthcare providers. Hope is offered to clients and families through therapeutic relationships, successful experiences, family-to-family and client-to-client education, and symptom management skills.

PROVIDING CLIENT AND FAMILY EDUCATION

Family members need education about schizophrenia and its treatment, access to help in crises, participation in decision making, information about resources, and respite care. The optimal approach to working with families is to recognize their contribution towards restoring health to the client.

Nurses provide education (sometimes called psychoeducation) about the nature of schizophrenia, symptom management, necessity of medication adherence, signs of relapse, collaboration in treatment planning, and lifestyle accommodation. Education may also become treatment by seeking to develop insight and address therapeutic issues. For example, education can empower clients by increasing their sense of control and mastery over their lives and teaching coping and problem-solving skills (Blair & Ramones, 1997). Families of consumers have come together to educate families of newly diagnosed persons and each other in an effective nationwide program sponsored by NAMI.

Teaching Symptom Management

People with schizophrenia need to learn to monitor their symptoms and recognize when the symptoms are worsening so they can seek appropriate help. Clients can learn how to deal with current behaviors and to detect early signs of relapse, which may be mood changes, changes in sleeping or eating, or preoccupations. Significant others can also perform this monitoring function.

Persons with schizophrenia often lack insight into their illness in variable degrees. They may deny that they have the illness, that the medication has any effect on their unusual thoughts or behavior, or that certain triggers (eg, lack of sleep, stress) lead to relapses. However, if the client acknowledges that he or she has schizophrenia and understands the illness and its treatment, he or she will be able to participate in his or her care and recovery.

In a recent study, clients with schizophrenia reported that insight was being able to recognize and control distortions in their perceptions and thoughts, and they attributed their insight to taking medications. Other means of insight development were rational self-talk, labeling of unusual experiences as symptoms, and information and feedback provided by family members (Baier & Murray, 1999).

Evaluation

Evaluation of the effectiveness of treatment on client symptoms should be based on whether clients reach higher levels of functioning. Achieving this goal requires availability and accessibility of appropriate community supports. Nursing interventions must be reassessed continuously to determine whether therapeutic outcomes

have been reached. The evaluation process constantly examines changes in client thinking, affect, and behavior, which leads to redesigning therapeutic plans in collaboration with the client and family. Some outcomes that indicate improvement include:

- Decreased frequency of hallucinations and delusions
- Ability to recognize that hallucinations or delusional thoughts are occurring
- More logical and reality-based thought processes
- Improved ability to concentrate
- Improved ability to interact with others
- Appropriate affect and mood

▼ *Reflection and Critical Thinking Questions*

Now that you have completed this chapter, consider Clinical Example 25-1 and the related nursing care presented in Nursing Care Plan 25-1. Answer the following questions.

1. What are the signs and symptoms that support the diagnosis of paranoid schizophrenia in James?
2. If you just met James for the first time, what feelings would you most likely experience?
3. What factors would contribute to his achieving a more independent and satisfactory lifestyle?
4. Identify three interventions, in order of priority, for James. Provide rationales for your choices.

▼ CHAPTER SUMMARY

- Schizophrenia, the most common and severe psychotic disorder, affects 1% of the population. Its onset occurs during late adolescence and early adulthood.
- Other psychotic disorders include schizophreniform disorder, schizoaffective disorder, delusional disorder, brief psychotic disorder, shared psychotic disorder, and psychosis not otherwise specified.
- Schizophrenia is most likely not a single disease of the brain but a heterogeneous disorder (ie, a group of several distinct disorders of the brain) with some common features, including thought disturbances and preoccupation with frightening inner experiences (eg, delusions and hallucinations), affect disturbances (eg, flat or inappropriate affect), and behavioral or social disturbances (eg, unpredictable, bizarre behavior or social isolation).
- The major theories of etiology are biologic, including genetic, neurochemical, and neuropathologic; viral; immunologic; and structural abnormalities.
- People with schizophrenia manifest alterations in their cognitive functioning (ie, memory, attention and judgment). Researchers have found that there are three dimensions of psychopathology in schizophrenia: the

disorganization dimension, the psychotic dimension, and the negative dimension; positive (hallucinations or delusions) and negative (alogia or attentional impairment) symptoms of schizophrenia fall into these three dimensions.

■ There are five subtypes of schizophrenia, including paranoid, disorganized, catatonic, undifferentiated, and residual.

■ Antipsychotic medications are the primary treatment for a client with schizophrenia. There are two types of antipsychotics: traditional or atypical. Traditional antipsychotics primarily treat the positive symptoms of schizophrenia and are associated with numerous and distressing EPSs. The atypical antipsychotics treat both the positive and negative symptoms of schizophrenia and typically cause fewer side effects.

■ Continuity of care for the schizophrenic client is essential. It involves discharge planning and aggressive care within the community setting.

■ Nursing intervention for the client with schizophrenia focuses on safety, acceptance, medication education and adherence, intervention in hallucinations and delusions, social skills, self-care, and education.

▼ REVIEW QUESTIONS

1. Schizophrenia is a
   a. Disorder of neuroanatomy
   b. Group of disorders involving a disorder of neurotransmitters
   c. Collection of disorders involving brain function
   d. Disorder of brain metabolism

2. Schizophrenia is primarily marked by
   a. Inattention and anger
   b. Violent and impulsive behavior
   c. Thought disturbance such as delusions
   d. Affective disturbance such as dysphoria

3. Which of the following statements most accurately describes treatment of schizophrenia?
   a. Cognitive behavioral therapies decrease affective disturbance.
   b. Atypical neuroleptics treat the positive and negative symptoms.
   c. Antipsychotic medication cures schizophrenia.
   d. Psychoanalytical, insight-oriented therapy diminishes hallucinations and delusions.

4. Prevention of relapse occurs by
   a. Taking additional medication on days when the client is "feeling bad"
   b. Taking stress management classes
   c. Blocking hallucinations during daily activities
   d. Reporting changes in sleeping, eating, and mood

5. The three primary negative symptoms of schizophrenia include

   a. Alogia, hallucinations, and delusions
   b. Alogia, affective blunting, and avolition
   c. Affective blunting, delusions, and avolition
   d. Hallucinations, delusions, and avolition

6. A client in a locked unit has been staring at a staff member, pacing and muttering under his breath. The nurse astutely interprets this behavior to mean that the client
   a. Wants to speak with the staff member, but his thinking is too disorganized to accomplish this.
   b. Is having auditory hallucinating.
   c. Feels threatened by the staff member and may become violent.
   d. Is having visual hallucinations.

7. An 18-year-old male client who has just begun taking Haldol comes to the nurse complaining of severe muscle spasms. The nurse assesses the client and notes that his heart rate is 104, his blood pressure is 160/90, and his temperature is 101°F. Based on this data, which of the following actions should the nurse make?
   a. Check the chart for an "as-needed" order for Artane or Cogentin or other medication for EPSs because the client is experiencing EPSs. Record the client's symptoms and the intervention in the chart.
   b. Immediately call the physician and report the findings.
   c. Ask the client if he has been exposed to flu or cold viruses and administer acetaminophen for his elevated temperature.
   d. Schedule an exam for later in the week with the physician, who will evaluate the client's cardiovascular status.

8. A 27-year-old female client is being seen in individual therapy for ongoing treatment of schizophrenia. The therapist focuses on which of the following issues during therapy sessions?
   a. The client's history of childhood trauma
   b. Personal care and money management
   c. Socialization and medication compliance
   d. Coping skills and the therapeutic relationship

9. A 22-year-old male client with a history of schizophrenia is being treated on an open inpatient unit. He had stopped taking his medication at home and had became increasingly psychotic, proclaiming that he was God and stating that he had special powers. He has been improving since restarting his medication, and the team expects that he will be discharged within a few days. This is his third hospitalization in 1 year. He also has a history of alcohol and drug abuse. He had once had his own apartment and a job at a local department store, but lately he has been homeless and unemployed. Based on this data,

what plans will the treatment team most likely make for his ongoing outpatient care?
  a. Refer the client to the mental health clinic.
  b. Arrange for ICM.
  c. Arrange for ACT.
  d. Continue to see the client in outpatient individual therapy.

10. A client being admitted to the psychiatric unit tells the nurse that the FBI is after her and that agents have been watching her for some time. Her husband brought her in for treatment because she had refused to leave her home or speak with anyone other than him. Which of the following nursing diagnoses best reflects this client problem?
  a. Disturbed Sensory Perception
  b. Disturbed Thought Processes
  c. Impaired Social Interaction
  d. Acute Confusion

11. A client with schizophrenia has been in outpatient care through the mental health clinic. Which of the following observations best suggests that the plan of care has been effective?
  a. The client has been compliant with taking her medications and attending therapy sessions.
  b. The client reports that she no longer has hallucinations.
  c. The client has resumed employment and has been attending social functions at the community center.
  d. The client no longer believes that she has special powers.

▼ REFERENCES AND SUGGESTED READINGS

*American Psychiatric Association. (2000). *Diagnostic and statistical manual of mental disorders* (4th ed., text rev). Washington, DC: Author.

*Andreasen, N. C. (1985). *The broken brain: The biologic revolution in psychiatry.* New York: Harper & Row.

*Andreasen, N. C. (1999a). A unitary model of schizophrenia. *Archives of General Psychiatry, 56,* 781–787.

*Andreasen, N. C. (1999b). Understanding the causes of schizophrenia. *New England Journal of Medicine, 340,* 645–647.

*Andreasen, N. C. (2000). Schizophrenia: The fundamental question. *Brain Research Review, 31*(2–3), 106–112.

*Andreasen, N. C., & Black, D. W. (2000). *Introductory textbook of psychiatry.* Washington, DC: American Psychiatric Association.

*Arieti, S. (1974). *Interpretation of schizophrenia* (2nd ed.). New York: Basic Books.

:*Baier, M., & Murray, R. L. (1999). A descriptive study of insight into illness reported by persons with schizophrenia. *Journal of Psychosocial Nursing, 37*(1), 14–21.

*Barnes, T. R., & McPhillips, M. A. (1998). Novel antipsychotics, extrapyramidal side effects and tardive dyskinesia.

International Clinical Psychopharmacology, 13(Suppl. 3), S49–S57.

*Blair, D. T., & Ramones, V. A. (1997). Education as psychiatric intervention: The cognitive-behavioral context. *Journal of Psychosocial Nursing, 35*(11), 29–36.

Blanchard, J. J., Brown, S. A., Horton, W. P., & Sherwood, A. R. (2000). Substance use disorders in schizophrenia: Review, integration, and a proposed model. *Clinical Psychological Review, 220*(2), 207–234.

*Buchsbaum, M. S., & Hazlett, E. A. (1998). Positron emission tomography studies of abnormal glucose metabolism in schizophrenia. *Schizophrenia Bulletin, 23*(3), 343–364.

*Cancro, R. (1983). Individual psychotherapy in the treatment of chronic schizophrenic patients. *American Journal of Psychotherapy, 37*(October), 493–501.

*Castine, M. R., Meador-Woodruff, J. H., & Dalack, G. W. (1998). The role of life events in onset and recurrent episodes of schizophrenia and schizoaffective disorder. *Journal of Psychiatric Research, 32,* 283–288.

*Conn, V. S. (1990). Commentary: The case against family systems theory. *Journal of Child and Adolescent Psychiatric and Mental Health Nursing, 3*(1), 29–33.

*Crespo-Facorro, B., Paradiso, S., Andreasen, N. C., O'Leary, D. S., Watkins, G. L., Ponto, L. L. B., et al. (2001). Neural mechanisms of anhedonia in schizophrenia: A PET study of response to unpleasant and pleasant odors. *Journal of the American Medical Association, 286*(4), 427–435.

DeHert, M., McKenzie, K., & Peuskens, J. (2001). Risk factors for suicide in young people suffering from schizophrenia: A long-term follow-up study. *Schizophrenia Research, 47*(2–3), 127–134.

*Delaney, C. (1998). Reducing recidivism: Medication versus psychosocial rehabilitation. *Journal of Psychosocial Nursing, 36*(11), 28–34.

*Edgar, E. (1998–1999). PACT across America: An advocacy strategy. *NAMI Advocate, 20*(3), 19.

*Frances, A., Docherty, J. P., & Kahn, D.A., (Eds.). (1996). The Expert Consensus Guideline Series: Treatment of schizophrenia. *The Journal of Clinical Psychiatry, 57*(Suppl. 12B). (On-line.) Available at: *www.psychguides.com*.

*Gelder, M., Lopez-Ibor, J. J., & Andreasen, N. C. (2000). *New Oxford textbook of psychiatry* (3rd ed.). Oxford: Oxford University Press.

Hagen, B. R., & Mitchell, D. (2001). Might within the madness: Solution-focused therapy and thought-disordered clients. *Archives in Psychiatric Nursing, 15*(2), 86–93.

Hirayasu, Y. (2000, May). *Management of schizophrenia with comorbid conditions.* Paper presented at the American Psychiatric Association 153rd Annual Meeting, Chicago, IL.

*Hogarty, G. E., & Ulrich, R. F. (1998). The limitations of antipsychotic medication on schizophrenia relapse and adjustment and the contributions of psychosocial treatment. *Journal of Psychiatric Research, 32*(3–4), 243–250.

*Horwath, E., & Cournos, F. (1999). Schizophrenia and other psychotic disorders. In J. L. Cutler & R. Marcus (Eds.), *Psychiatry.* Philadelphia: W.B. Saunders.

*Jacobsen, L. K., & Rapoport, J. (1998). Research update: Childhood-onset schizophrenia: Implications of clinical and neurobiological research. *Journal of Child Psychology and Psychiatry, 39,* 101–113.

*Jibson, M. D., & Tandon, R. (1998). New atypical antipsychotic medications. *Journal of Psychiatric Research, 32,* 215–228.

*Kaplan, H. I., & Sadock, B. J. (1996). *Concise textbook of clinical psychiatry.* Baltimore: Williams & Wilkins.

*Kasper, S. (1998). How much do novel antipsychotics benefit the patients? *International Clinical Psychopharmacology, 13*(Suppl. 3), S71–S77.

*Kokko, J. (2000). Fluids and electrolytes. In L. Goldman & J. C. Bennet (Eds.), *Cecil textbook of medicine* (21st ed., pp. 540–558). Philadelphia: W.B. Saunders.

*Lehman, A. F., Steinwachs, D. M., & the Co-Investigators of the PORT Project. (1998). *The Schizophrenia Patient Outcomes Research Team (PORT) treatment recommendations.* Rockville, MD: Agency for Healthcare Research and Quality. (On-line.) Available at: *http://www.ahrq.gov/clinic/schzrec.htm.*

*McManus, D. Q., Arvanitis, L. A., & Kowalcyk, B. B. (1999). Quetiapine, a novel antipsychotic: Experience in elderly patients with psychotic disorders. *Journal of Clinical Psychiatry, 60*(5), 292–298.

Mercier-Guidez, E., & Loas, G. (2000). Polydipsia and water intoxication in 353 psychiatric inpatients: An epidemiological and psychopathological study. *European Psychiatry, 15*(5), 306–311.

*Mueser, K. T., Bond, G. R., Drake, R. E., & Resnick, S. G. (1998). Models of community care for severe mental illness: A review of research on case management. *Schizophrenia Bulletin, 24*(1), 37–74.

Newcomer, J., Craft, S., Fucetola, R., et al. (1999). Glucose-induced increase in memory performance in patients with schizophrenia. *Schizophrenia Bulletin, 25*(2), 321–335.

North American Nursing Diagnosis Association. (1999). *NANDA nursing diagnoses:* Definitions and classification, 1999–2000. Philadelphia: Author.

*O'Connor, F. W. (1994). A vulnerability-stress framework for evaluating clinical interventions in schizophrenia. *Image: Journal of Nursing Scholarship, 26*(3), 231–237.

*O'Leary, D. S., Andreasen, N. C., Hurtig, R. R., Kesler, M.
L., Rogers, M., Arndt, S., et al. (1996). Auditory attentional deficits in patients with schizophrenia: A positron emission tomography study. *Archives of General Psychiatry, 53*(7), 633–641.

*Phelan, J. C., Bromet, E. J., & Link, B. G. (1998). Psychiatric illness and family stigma. *Schizophrenia Bulletin, 24*(1), 115–126.

*Rund, B. R. (1998). A review of longitudinal studies of cognitive functions in schizophrenia patients. *Schizophrenia Bulletin, 24*(3), 425–435.

*Sousa, S. (1999). Refractory schizophrenia: What works pharmacologically? *Journal of Psychosocial Nursing, 37*(2), 19–23.

Soyka, Z. (2000). Substance misuse, psychiatric disorder, and violent and disturbed behavior. *British Journal of Psychiatry, 176,* 345–350.

*Tarrier, N., Yusupoff, L., Kinney, C., McCarthy, E., Gledhill, A., & Haddock, G., et al. (1998). Randomised controlled trial of intensive cognitive behaviour therapy for patients with chronic schizophrenia. *British Medical Journal, 317* (7154), 303–307.

*Tiihonen, J., Isohanni, M., Rantakallio, P., Lehtonen, J., & Moring, J. (1998). Schizophrenia, alcohol abuse, and violent behavior: A 26-year followup study of an unselected birth cohort. *Schizophrenia Bulletin, 24*(3), 437–441.

*Torrey, E. F. (1995). *Surviving schizophrenia: A family manual* (3rd ed.). New York: HarperCollins.

Weiden, P. J. (1997). Quetiapine ('Seroquel'): A new "atypical" antipsychotic. *Journal of Practical Psychiatry and Behavioral Health,* 368–374.

Wuerker, A. K. (2000). The family and schizophrenia. *Issues in Mental Health Nursing, 21*(1), 127–141.

* *Starred references are cited in text.*

For additional information on this chapter, go to *http://connection. lww.com.*

Need more help? See Chapter 25 of the *Study Guide to Accompany Mohr: Johnson's Psychiatric-Mental Health Nursing,* 5th edition.

The Client Who Displays Angry, Aggressive, or Violent Behavior

BONNIE LOUISE RICKELMAN

▼ KEY TERMS

Aggression—Harsh physical or verbal responses that indicate rage and a potential for destructiveness.

Anger—An emotional response to perceived frustration of desires or needs.

Hostility-related variables—Emotions, attitudes, and behaviors that occur regularly and predictably in people prone to aggression and violence.

Impulsivity—A symptom of an underlying disorder or a pervasive personality trait that causes a person to perform actions with little or no regard for the consequences.

Restraint—The use of a physical or mechanical device to involuntarily restrict the free movement of all or a portion of a person's body to control his or her physical activity.

Seclusion—The placement of a client alone in a hazard-free room that often is locked and in which others can maintain direct observation of him or her.

Temperament—Constitutional or biologically based personality dispositions that are partly inherited, evident early in life, and somewhat stable across situations and over time.

▼ LEARNING OBJECTIVES

On completion of this chapter, you should be able to accomplish the following:

- Define the broad range of responses that constitute aggressive behavior, including pertinent variables related to violence.
- Discuss significant sociodemographic, inpatient, outpatient, and other ecologic factors related to people who are mentally ill and prone to violence.
- Discuss the psychological, neurobiologic, and social–environmental determinants of aggression in terms of pertinent theory and research findings.
- Discuss relevant legal issues regarding the treatment of aggressive and violent clients.
- Apply nursing care guidelines to assess, diagnose, establish client goals, intervene, and evaluate outcomes for clients with aggressive and violent behavior.

▼ Clinical Example 26-1

"I'm here because she says I drink too much," says Peter, looking scornfully at his wife, Debra. Peter is being admitted to an inpatient drug and alcohol treatment program. He is sarcastic and noncommunicative during the admission interview, ridiculing Debra's comments and belittling her.

Debra relates that Peter drinks half a bottle of vodka and several beers daily and takes amphetamines occasionally. Peter has been injured in several fights at bars and has slapped or pushed Debra on several occasions. He has grown increasingly controlling of her and will not let her have the car keys or any money. Although Peter blames his wife for his current circumstances, the employee assistance program manager at Peter's company referred him to treatment when he failed a random urine-screening test for drugs. Peter's continued employment is contingent on his recovery from alcohol and drug abuse. He has not had a drink for 72 hours and shows no signs of alcohol withdrawal syndrome.

Peter is admitted to an open unit and oriented to the facility and the milieu activities. He complains about the "rinky dink" recreation area and laughs openly at other clients. Another male client yells at him from across the room, "What's your [expletive] problem?" Before Peter can answer, the nurse asks him if he would like to play basketball. He agrees, and the psychiatric technician takes Peter outside to play. The other clients resume their game of pool.

After 30 minutes, Peter returns and appears calmer. The nurse asks if she might speak with him to discuss his hospitalization and develop a plan of care.

This chapter discusses angry, aggressive, and violent behavior in terms of adults who have been diagnosed with psychiatric disorders and are receiving care in a mental health facility. It defines terms relevant to a conceptual understanding of aggression and presents current perspectives regarding psychobiologic, social, and environmental determinants of aggressive behaviors. The chapter emphasizes the essential components of the nursing process, namely assessment, diagnosis, planning, implementation, and evaluation, when addressing aggressive and violent behaviors. In addition, it provides pertinent clinical examples and nursing care plan guidelines. For information on the escalating problem of violence in the community, youth violence, and care of clients who are victims of violent acts, see Chapter 17.

As you read this chapter, consider the case of Peter in Clinical Example 26-1. How do his history and signs and symptoms relate to this group of disorders? How can nurses effectively address his needs? You will learn more about the progression of Peter's care in Nursing Care Plan 26-1. You also will have the opportunity to apply your understanding of Peter and others who display angry, aggressive, and violent behaviors in the Reflection and Critical Thinking Questions at the end of this chapter.

AGGRESSIVE BEHAVIOR, HOSTILITY-RELATED VARIABLES, AND VIOLENCE

Aggressive behavior generally is considered to include anger and physical or verbal aggression. **Anger** is an emotional response to perceived frustration of desires or needs. It can be positive when a person directs it toward actual injustices or if it motivates a person to organize and institute constructive and beneficial changes. Anger loses any constructive effect when it turns inward, flails ineffectively at others with little or no cause, bullies others having less strength or power, harms or hurts the self or others physically or emotionally, or is out of control. The ways that a person deals with anger tend to persist over time. **Aggression** is harsh physical or verbal responses that indicate rage and a potential for destructiveness. *Violence* is used for behaviors and responses that are destructive.

Hostility-related variables are emotions, attitudes, and behaviors that occur regularly and predictably in people prone to anger and aggression. Negative emotionality, including irritability, resentment, and impulsivity, have been linked with aggressive behaviors and the potential to develop certain medical conditions such as essential hypertension, cardiovascular hyperactivity, and atherosclerotic heart disease (Scarpa & Raine, 1997; Siegman, 1993). **Impulsivity**, viewed as a symptom of an underlying disorder or a pervasive personality trait, includes actions performed with little or no regard for the consequences (Gallop, McCay, & Esplen, 1992). Characteristics of impulsivity include unpredictable behavior, threats toward others, irresponsible acts, low tolerance for frustration, poor problem-solving skills, disturbed interpersonal relationships, restlessness, and general disregard for social rules and customs.

Three criteria generally characterize impulse-control disorders:

1. The inability to control the impulse to behave in a way that is viewed as harmful to oneself or others
2. A sense of increasing tension (increased feelings of pressure, discomfort, or energy) before acting on the impulse, which the person may or may not consciously resist
3. A sense of excitement, gratification, and tension-release during the act; clients with impulse-control disorders typically experience some degree of regret or remorse after the act, although such feelings usually are transient because of a tendency to rationalize the behavior

Violent acts are the primary focus for legal assessment of dangerousness in all clinical and forensic settings. Dangerousness includes actions with a high risk of harming or injuring self or others. The intent to harm another person is an important criterion when evaluating and differentiating situations of accidental harm or injury as opposed to situations in which harm is done deliberately to other people or property (Berman & Coccaro, 1998).

Profiles of Aggressive and Violent Behaviors in Persons With Psychiatric Diagnoses

Incidents of aggressive behavior, including physical violence, occur in all clinical diagnostic categories and are not exclusively manifested by clients with a diagnosed psychiatric disorder (Harris & Rice, 1997). Findings from research studies of sociodemographic factors, psychiatric inpatients, psychiatric outpatients, and families with seriously mentally ill members, however, have rekindled the long-standing debate about the relationship between serious mental illness and incidence of violence.

SOCIODEMOGRAPHIC FACTORS

Common socioeconomic status (SES) factors used to study aggression and violence include employment status, education, income, age, and gender. In a study of 162 mentally ill criminal defendants, unemployment was found to be a significant correlate of violence (Menzies & Webster, 1995). Other SES correlates of violence include low educational attainment and decreased residential stability (Hastings & Hamberger, 1997).

Deinstitutionalization has resulted in thousands of people being displaced from the sheltered inpatient settings of state hospitals to situations of homelessness. Approximately one third of the estimated 600,000 homeless people are single adults who have severe mental illness such as schizophrenia or bipolar disorder (Task Force on Homelessness and Severe Mental Illness, 1992). Unsupervised, these individuals may become involved in antisocial acts and violence. The lack of adequate nutrition; higher incidence of drug, alcohol, and physical abuse; and increased severity of disease may also contribute to the spectrum of aggressive responses in homeless people with mental illness. See Chapter 11 for discussions of forensic nursing, crisis management, and homelessness.

Studies on violence and age generally support the idea that violence rates peak in the late teens and early 20s (Hastings & Hamberger, 1997). A study of violence in emergency departments found that young clients (mean age younger than 28 years) were nearly twice as violent (57% versus 30%) as older clients (Berman & Coccaro, 1998). Chapter 17 discusses the growing problem of youth violence.

In terms of gender, most research findings indicate that men have a greater tendency to behave violently than do women. In women with a serious psychiatric diagnosis, however, the rate of violence is similar to that of men (Hastings & Hamberger, 1997).

INPATIENT FACTORS

A series of studies exploring aggression and violence found that, in contrast to nonviolent inpatients who primarily had a characteristic interaction style of accommodation, violent inpatients primarily had an exploitative, coercive interaction style (ie, using others for self-gain) (Morrison, 1992, 1994). These studies identify a coercive, interaction style as a primary precursor to the use of aggression and violence by people with mental illness.

Additional research reveals the importance of staff members' interaction styles with clients as related to violent incidents on psychiatric units (Lancee, Gallop, McCay, & Toner, 1995). Interpersonal precursor events that have been linked with escalating client violence include occasions when clients are angered or frustrated by the behavior of other clients, such as disputes over cigarettes or food, or by staff behavior who, in the process of caring for the client, may intrude on or frustrate the client. Examples of such staff behavior include preventing the client from leaving the ward, engaging in disputes over medication, generally enforcing rules or denying requests, physically restraining the client, taking something from the client, ignoring the client, or requesting the client to do or refrain from doing something (Whittington, 1994).

OUTPATIENT FACTORS

Most studies since the 1960s indicate that people who have been hospitalized primarily in public psychiatric facilities tend to have postdischarge arrest rates one to three times higher than those of the general population (Asnis, Kaplan, Hundofean, & Saeed, 1997). Higher levels of arrests for violent behavior have been found in people diagnosed with antisocial personality disorder, paranoid schizophrenia, and substance abuse and a history of noncompliance with medications (Mulvey, 1994; Tardiff, Marzuk, Lem, & Portera, 1997). Study findings reveal that about 25% to 30% of male and female clients with a psychiatric disorder and history of violent behavior exhibit violent behavior again within 1 year of discharge and tend to attack the same persons (McNiel & Binder, 1994; Tardiff et al., 1997).

The use of time during outpatient clinic visits to help clients understand their medications, the importance of compliance, and the consequences of noncompliance cannot be overemphasized. Proper referral and involvement of family and significant others are crucial in deterring recidivism.

FAMILY FACTORS

The National Alliance for the Mentally Ill (NAMI) has conducted extensive surveys of families in which a family member had been diagnosed with a serious mental illness such as schizophrenia, bipolar disorder, or major depression. In one survey of 1401 families, findings indicate that 10.6% of seriously mentally ill individuals had physically harmed another person, whereas 12.2% had threatened harm (Steinwachs, Kasper, & Skinner, 1992). In addition, gender differences were found among those who threatened harm (24.9% of men versus 12.5% of women), but no substantial gender difference was found among those who harmed another person (11.9% of men, 9.5% of women). Another study found that among clients who had physically attacked someone within the previous 2 weeks of admission to a psychiatric hospital, family members had been the object of their attacks 56% of the time (Straznickas, McNeil, & Binder, 1993). In addition, it was found that people who were more likely to threaten and commit violent acts had a diagnosis of schizophrenia and were financially dependent on family members (Estroff, Zimmer, Lachicotte, & Benoit, 1994). Most of the targets of such violence were mothers living with an adult offspring with schizophrenia. Such findings highlight the need for careful family assessment and preventive intervention and referral (see Chap. 10).

Determinants of Aggression

Aggressive and violent behaviors have multiple determinants, including neurobiologic, psychological, and social–environmental factors. Key factors linked with a lack of impulse control and violent behavior include various medical and neurobiologic conditions, including imbalances in neurotransmitter systems, temperament, cognitive appraisal, and dual diagnoses such as mental illness and substance abuse (Mulvey, 1994).

NEUROBIOLOGIC FACTORS

Brain neuroimaging studies indicate that aggressive behavior is associated with deficits or damage to portions of the brain located in the limbic structures and frontal and temporal lobes. Limbic tumors often result in personality changes, with irritability as a predominant symptom. Such tumors may destroy inhibitory mechanisms for aggression. Rabies and encephalitis, as well as brain injury that damages portions of the limbic system or the frontal lobe, are associated with loss of impulse control. Theorists believe that connections between the amygdaloid complex and the hypothalamus and between the hippocampal cortex and frontal lobes modulate the control and expression of aggressive behavior (Garza-Trevino, 1994). Compulsive aggressive behavior has been reported in clients with lesions in the hypothalamic, or bifrontal, anterior cingulate, and temporal areas of the brain (Paradis, Horn, Lazar, & Schwartz, 1994). Also, as many as 70% of clients with brain injuries secondary to blunt head trauma exhibit irritability and aggression (Kavoussi, Armstead, & Coccaro, 1997).

When the complex functions of the frontal lobe are examined, it becomes apparent what serious disorders may occur when these functions are disrupted. Self-disciplinary functions, including the abilities to resist distraction, inhibit inappropriate behavior, and exert social control, are located in the frontal lobe, as is the ability to judge or weigh the merits of behavior. The orbitofrontal syndrome (damage to specific areas of the frontal lobe) is associated with impulsive outbursts of rage and violent behavior, disinhibition, hyperactivity, distractibility, and mood lability (Kavoussi et al., 1997). Debate continues as to whether intermittent, explosive reactions may result from undetected temporal lobe epilepsy (TLE). Some experts believe that people with TLE are easily provoked to violence by feelings of injustice in the periods between seizures (interictal periods). The interictal behavioral syndrome theory views such violence as a result of changes in the sensitivity of the limbic system and brain stem because of repeated, uncontrolled electrical discharges, a phenomenon known as *kindling* (*The Harvard Mental Health Letter*, 1991).

The term *low serotonin syndrome* specifies conditions characterized by episodes of mood changes, impulsive behavior, or both. Among the monoamine neurotransmitters (ie, serotonin, dopamine [DA], and norepinephrine [NE]), serotonin has been studied most extensively for its modulation of aggressive and impulsive behavior. Several studies have found a low concentration of 5-hydroxy-indoleacetic acid (5-HIAA), a metabolite of serotonin, in the cerebrospinal fluid (CSF) of subjects with a history of violence toward others and violent suicide attempts compared with those with no such history (Berman & Coccaro, 1998; Kavoussi et al., 1997). Results of CSF studies of DA in humans generally are similar to those of serotonin and reveal that the level of the DA metabolite, homovanillic acid, is inversely correlated with aggressive behavior (Berman & Coccaro, 1998).

Regarding NE and aggressive behavior, some studies have found lower CSF levels of the NE metabolite, 3-methoxy-4-hydroxyphenylglycol (MHPG), in violent offenders compared with healthy volunteers (Kavoussi et al., 1997). When both 5-HIAA and MHPG levels from CSF were examined, however, CSF 5-HIAA was found to be a better predictor of aggression in humans.

Other researchers who studied healthy subjects have found a link between increased monoamine oxidase (MAO) activity in the brain and increased total scores on the Buss and Durkee Aggression Questionnaire (Buss & Durkee, 1992) and increased scores on the negativism and verbal aggression scales (Castrogiovanni, Capone, Maremmani, & Marazziti, 1994). Such findings indicate that MAO activity may be linked to the behavioral expression of aggression: MAO metabolizes serotonin and thus contributes to decreased serotonin levels in the brain.

PSYCHOLOGICAL FACTORS

Temperament Theory

Researchers have shown an increasing interest in **temperament**, defined as constitutional or biologically based personality dispositions that are partly inherited, evident early in life, and somewhat stable across situations and over time (Allen, 1994). Temperament is thought to remain consistent throughout the life span, and although most studies focus on infants and children, some researchers have found that adults at risk for adjustment problems had experienced difficult temperaments as preschoolers. The temperament style that is most relevant to potential aggressive behavior is that of negative emotionality.

Negative emotionality, commonly known as a "difficult" temperament, is manifested by irregularity in biologic functions; behavioral inhibition, including shyness and the tendency to become fearful in new or novel situations and to withdraw from them; slow adaptability; and an intense and negative mood. For example, on the first day of preschool, the behaviorally inhibited child stands silently alone, whereas the behaviorally uninhibited child freely explores the environment and interacts with others. Notice that research studies have found that a predisposition to negative emotionality increases the likelihood of impulsive antisocial or aggressive behavior (Scarpa & Raine, 1997). Although negative emotionality may be difficult to change, nurses can encourage people with this trait to become more positive thinkers and to gain confidence and more positive emotional experiences.

Cognitive Theory

A cognitive model explains how one's attributions, appraisals, expectancies, and self-talk mediate between stimuli and aggressive reactions. Appraisals of events are highly individualistic. Certain ways of interpreting situations and events produce an aggressive disposition and expectations that result in negative self-fulfilling prophecies. The role of attributions in anger arousal has been proposed as follows (Reeder, 1991):

1. A person perceives events as aversive based on his or her expectations of the event and how he or she interprets the event's meaning.
2. When a person expects a certain outcome and receives a different one, he or she appraises the extent to which the unwanted outcome is provocative (eg, frustrating, threatening), which influences the level of anger arousal and the resulting behavior.
3. When a person appraises an impending event as aversive and anger inducing, he or she is likely to react with anger when the event occurs.

The kind of self-talk used by a person also influences expectations and appraisals (Stuart, Wright, Thase, & Beck, 1997). Such self-talk has been called automatic thought or private speech. For example, suppose two people are served the wrong order in a restaurant. Person A may think, "These things always happen to me," or "Waiters are dumb," and may react angrily by cursing and shouting at the waiter. On the other hand, person B may think, "Mistakes sometimes happen. It's no big deal," and may react calmly by stating the error to the waiter and asking for it to be corrected. Person A likely perceived the mistake as aversive or catastrophic whereas person B did not. Although the situation is the same, the self-talk is different, and the perceptions and emotional outcomes are different.

SOCIAL–ENVIRONMENTAL FACTORS

Social learning theory often is applied to explain aggressive behavior that a person learns from exposure to aggressive models or as the result of random positive reinforcement of direct experience (Maiuro, 1993). Exposure to aggressive models may occur in the family; in a subculture such as gangs; or through media such as television, movies, and video games. Wiegman and van Schie (1998) investigated the link between the amount of time seventh and eighth grade children in Enschede, The Netherlands, spent playing aggression-oriented video games and the resultant aggressive and prosocial behavior. Findings indicate that children, especially boys, who prefer aggressive video games are more aggressive and show less prosocial behavior than those with a low preference for these games. Some researchers and theorists believe that television, video, and movie violence portrays coercive behavior as resulting in obtaining material rewards, social recognition, or successful retaliation against enemies. In essence, the media glorifies violence and teaches people how to aggress. Subcultures, such as gangs, may promote violent crime as a means of achieving recognition and status. Aggressive sports and war also may lead to imitation of aggressive behavior.

Legal Issues

Four primary legal issues regarding violent behavior include involuntary commitment to mental hospitals, protection of potential victims of a client's aggression, maintenance of clients' rights, and preservation of the rights of staff. In general, involuntary commitment is allowed only for clients who are diagnosed as mentally ill and who clearly are dangerous to themselves or others in terms of inflicting serious physical injury. States vary in the interpretation of anticipated harm. Rigorous interpretation criteria may include anticipated harm as "imminent," "a clear and present danger," or an overt act of violence within the last month (*The Harvard Mental Health Letter*, 1991). Less rigorous interpretations may permit involuntary commitment of clients on the basis of threats or the expressed and reasonable fears of potential victims.

About half of the states are implementing the requirement for the least-restrictive treatment alternative by permitting commitment to outpatient treatment settings rather than to a hospital when possible for individuals who meet the traditional commitment criteria of dangerousness to self or others. Another relatively recent least-restrictive option that has been adopted only by a few states is preventive commitment (Slobogin, 1994). Unlike outpatient commitment, preventive commitment allows commitment to outpatient treatment and, in some states, to inpatient treatment as well for individuals who do not yet meet the usual commitment criteria but will do so soon if intervention is not forthcoming. The statute governing preventive commitment is called a predicted deterioration standard (Slobogin, 1994).

Another least-restrictive treatment option is conditional release, currently available in about 40 states (Slobogin, 1994). Conditional release requires continued supervision of a person after discharge from a hospital. The hospital or a court in criminal cases informs the client of the release conditions (eg, attending group therapy or reporting to a clinic for medication supervision). If the client violates the conditions of release, immediate rehospitalization may result or, in some cases, may follow a court hearing. Conditional release tests the individual's ability to function in the community (supposedly under supervision) and frees up hospital beds.

As a result of the Tarasoff decision (*Tarasoff v. Regents of the University of California*, 1976), it is mandatory to report any clear threats made by psychiatric clients to harm specific people. Psychiatrists, psychotherapists and other mental health care providers must warn authorities (specified by law) and potential victims of possible dangerous actions of their clients, even if the clients protest (Mason, 1998; McNiel, Binder, & Fulton, 1998).

Regarding the rights of clients within hospitals and clinics, voluntary clients may refuse any treatment, although they may be asked to leave. In most states, involuntary clients have a right to refuse antipsychotic drugs unless they are found incompetent. In any case, medications can be administered legally by qualified personnel in an emergency (ie, client is dangerous to self or others).

A new area of law pertaining to psychiatric care is the Psychiatric Advance Directive. This directive specifies to a doctor, institution, or judge what types of confinement and treatment a client does or does not want or appoints a friend or family member as an "agent" to make mental healthcare decisions for the client if he or she is incapable of doing so. For specific information regarding the Psychiatric Advance Directive, clients and their families should contact the protection and advocacy system in their state because state laws and requirements vary.

Interdisciplinary Goals and Treatment

With clients who are aggressive and violent (or potentially so), major types of treatment strategies include verbal interventions, limit setting, cognitive-behavioral therapy, group and family therapy, pharmacologic (medications), and, if other interventions fail, physical seclusion and restraint. These interventions may be used separately or in combination according to protocols in given treatment settings. Overall goals of treatment as they specifically relate to aggression and violence among psychiatric clients are that the client does not threaten or harm anyone and that the client gains insight into and skill at managing aggressive impulses.

VERBAL INTERVENTIONS

People want to be listened to and understood. Verbal intervention is emphasized when interacting with aggressive clients at all levels of escalation. It generally is most useful, however, with clients exhibiting milder levels of aggression. Verbal intervention can prevent an escalation of aggressive behavior.

The Prevention and Management of Aggressive Behavior program developed by the Human Resources Division of the Texas Department of Mental Health and Mental Retardation emphasizes three phases of verbal intervention in preventing the escalation of aggressive behavior: making contact, discovering the source of distress, and assisting the person with alternative behaviors and problem solving. These verbal intervention strategies are discussed in more detail in the Nursing Process section.

LIMIT SETTING

Limit setting is a process through which someone in authority (often, the nurse) reminds clients of the boundaries of acceptable behavior and sets limits as warranted (DeLaune, 1991). It is helpful to assess the client's need and desire for control and then to set limits that he or she will not perceive as punitive. Usually, clients find it reassuring to know that they will not be allowed to be destructive to themselves, others, or property. Knowing established limits gives the client a framework within which to function more freely and adequately, maintain self-esteem, learn new behaviors, and gain new self-awareness. Guidelines for communicating with poten-

tially aggressive clients whose behavior requires limit setting can be found in the Nursing Process section.

COGNITIVE INTERVENTIONS

Cognitive therapy is a brief, directive, collaborative form of psychotherapy that is useful in assisting clients to confront their dysfunctional and irrational thinking, test the reality of their thinking and behavior, and learn to use more positive and assertive responses in interactions with others. Types of cognitive interventions include guided discovery and anger management.

Guided Discovery

The "guided discovery" technique is one form of cognitive retraining that has been successful with clients who have depression or anger-control problems (Reeder, 1991; Rickelman & Houfek, 1995). In this approach, specific learning experiences are designed to teach clients how to recognize the connection between their thoughts, feelings, and behaviors; identify their automatic negative thinking and replace it with more positive thinking; and identify dysfunctional expectations and appraisals, substituting more reality-based interpretations.

Anger Management

Another key cognitive-behavioral treatment program for assaultive clients is anger-management training. In this program, clients learn ways to identify and monitor their own anger cues, behavioral and physiologic signals related to anger arousal, signs of impending loss of control, and how to rechannel aggressive responses in the early stages of arousal. Clients also learn to differentiate acceptable emotional responses (anger, frustration, fear) from inappropriate and destructive behavioral responses (verbal abuse, physical assault) (Tardiff, 1999).

Assaultive clients tend to experience anger responses as automatic, reflexive, deeply ingrained reactions because they have used them so often in previous confrontative episodes. Less anger is aroused if a client can define a situation as a problem that calls for a solution rather than as a threat that calls for an attack. The further a person has progressed into a provocation sequence, the less likely the person is to initiate anger control. Defining a situation as a problem and seeking a solution is not an easy skill to master. If a client can experience some success in using cognitive problem-solving methods rather than emotional reactionary responses, however, he or she may begin to take pride in new ways of coping with anger. In problem-solving skills training, clients learn to be aware of others' points of view and to anticipate and understand the consequences of their own emotional and behavioral responses.

BEHAVIOR THERAPY: TOKEN ECONOMY

A key expectation in mental health treatment settings is that clients will act or behave in socially appropriate ways.

Discharge planning for clients who have been violent may involve intensive case management and strong links with community centers that provide mental health services, treatment for substance abuse, social and welfare services, and probation and other criminal justice services.

2. Organization of pertinent observational data and interaction incidents into useful client assessment data: For example, for the potentially violent client, such data might include any behavioral patterns typical of the client escalating into violence and any particular interventions that were successful in helping the client regain self-control.

3. Collecting outcome data: In the ever-changing healthcare system, nurses must document client outcomes related to nursing interventions, including which of the client's symptoms improved and to what extent. Close monitoring of medication effects and client compliance with the treatment plan is essential.

APPLICATION OF THE NURSING PROCESS TO THE CLIENT DISPLAYING ANGRY, AGGRESSIVE, OR VIOLENT BEHAVIOR

Assessment

Watching for behavioral cues and listening carefully for the tone in the client's communication enables the nurse to prevent angry and hostile feelings from escalating into dangerous actions. Clients may reveal these behavioral clues through comments, actions, or mood. Alternatively, the client's history may alert the nurse to the potential for violence. The nurse may see signs of escalating aggressiveness in the following features of the client:

- *Thinking and perception:* Is the client making aggressive statements? What is his or her view of the world and others? Does the client suffer from delusions or hallucinations that could be potentially harmful to self or others? (For example, a wife becomes convinced that her husband is trying to kill her and the "voices" she hears in her head tell her to kill him).

- *Motor activity and body language:* Does the client exhibit increased psychomotor agitation (fidgeting, pacing) along with a tense posture, clenched fists, or a tightened jaw?

- *Mood or affect:* Has the client's affect or verbalization increased in intensity, or has there been a noticeable change in the usual manner in which a client expresses wants and needs? (For example, the client speaks using an angry tone of voice and gets louder as he states that he wants the staff to let him out of

the hospital.) During initial interviews, or when the nurse suspects a possibility of suicidal or homicidal behavior, the nurse should ask, "Do you feel like hurting yourself or anyone else?" Experts agree that asking this question does not suggest ideas of violence to the client but rather promotes alternative problem solving in place of acting-out behavior.

- *Physical state:* Does the client have conditions such as seizures, delirium, or brain lesions that may influence sudden violent behavior with no warning?

- *Context:* Does the client have a history of violent behavior? Some studies indicate that the best predictor of violence is a history of violence (McNiel & Binder, 1994). A history of violent outbursts against self or others may include repeated criminal behavior or suicide attempts and the use of alcohol, other addictive drugs, or hallucinogenic drugs that diminish the client's control over behavior (Littrell, 1998). (See Box 26-1.)

Nursing Diagnosis

The nursing diagnoses primarily relevant to potentially aggressive and violent clients are Risk for Other-Directed Violence related to psychopathology, poor impulse control, or history of violence and Ineffective Coping related to psychopathology or disturbance in pattern of threat appraisal. See Nursing Care Plan 26-1 for further discussion.

Planning

Goals for the potentially violent client include the following:

- The client will refrain from acting on violent impulses.
- The client will report feelings of loss of control and ask for help from staff.
- The client will discuss feelings of anxiety, anger, frustration, and aggression and describe positive ways to prevent escalation.
- The client will state awareness of cognitive appraisals of precipitating events, ways to reframe thoughts and behavioral responses more constructively, and awareness of personal competencies in problem solving and coping.
- The client will use assertive communication skills and maintain self-control of aggressive and violent inclinations.

Implementation

The nurse and other mental healthcare professionals must carefully weigh the principles of safety and least-restrictive

BOX 26-1 ▼ *Risk Factor Profiles for Violent Behavior*

Demographic
- Young age
- Male gender
- Lack of employment
- Limited education

History
- Violence to self or others
- Antisocial behavior
- Arrests for criminal acts
- Violence within family of origin (eg, physical abuse, sexual abuse)
- Aggressive childhood behavior, including cruelty to animals

Psychiatric Diagnosis
- Antisocial personality disorder
- Substance abuse
- Psychoses (especially paranoid schizophrenia and violence-prone delusions or hallucinations)
- Schizoaffective disorder
- Impulsive aggression

Medical
- Traumatic brain injuries
- Other central nervous system dysfunctions

Social–Environmental
- Association with antisocial peers
- Low residential stability
- Living with and financially dependent on family members(s)
- Living within a violent milieu
- Access to lethal weapons

Cognitive
- Negative perceptions and appraisals of impending events as aversive and anger-inducing

Behavioral
- Poor impulse control
- Escalating anger or agitation
- Coercive, exploitative interaction style
- Antisocial and criminal acts
- Statement of intent to harm self or others

environment while caring for aggressive and violent clients. Staff members must maintain attitudes of caring and concern and use a nonauthoritarian approach while setting appropriate limits. Even a floridly psychotic client whose tension increases before violence may respond positively to nonprovocative, nonjudgmental interpersonal contact. Nurses planning the care of the client with angry, aggressive, or violent behavior must address immediate needs such as preventing the behavior from escalating and ensuring the safety of other clients and staff.

MAINTAINING THE SAFETY OF CLIENTS AND STAFF

When interacting with angry and potentially aggressive clients, staff should be concerned for the safety of themselves, the client, and others. Some general guidelines for safety awareness include the following (Cembrowicz & Ritter, 1994; Zook, 1996):

- Take a position just outside the client's personal space (slightly out of arm's reach).
- If possible, stand on the client's nondominant side (usually the side on which he or she wears a wristwatch).
- Keep an open posture with your hands in sight.
- Keep the client in visual range.
- Make sure the door of a room is readily accessible.
- Avoid letting the client get between you and the door.

- Retreat from the situation and summon help if the client's aggression escalates to violence.
- Avoid being alone with a violent client.

DEFUSING ANGER AND AGGRESSION THROUGH VERBAL INTERVENTIONS

Simply speaking in a therapeutic manner with an angry client can help defuse anger and foster insight. Conversely, engaging in a power struggle by subtly or overtly trying to establish authority over the angry client can result in an escalation of aggression. When managing a potentially aggressive client, implement the following steps:

1. *Make contact:* Appear calm and in control. Speak in a normal, nonprovocative, and nonjudgmental tone of voice. Be alert to verbal and nonverbal behaviors that indicate how the client may be feeling. Based on observations, ask what the client is feeling. State your observations of what you see the client doing behaviorally and how you think he or she might be feeling. Check your understanding with the client.

2. *Discover the source of distress:* Attempt to discover the client's concern and respond with empathy, interest, and willingness to help. Encourage the client to describe and clarify his or her experience to increase the client's awareness of problematic feelings and what triggers them. Use open-ended questions such as who, what, when, where, and how rather than closed-ended, yes-or-no questions. Open-ended questions elicit more

Nursing Care Plan 26-1

THE AGGRESSIVE, POTENTIALLY VIOLENT CLIENT

Peter from Clinical Example 26-1 meets with the nurse. She asks him about his relationship with his wife and his history of fighting. He states that Debra's and other people's shortcomings easily frustrate him and that fighting in bars is just a way to let off steam. "I guess it is kind of stupid, though," he adds. He also says that he knows it isn't right to hit his wife and that he thinks she might leave him if he continues. He says he just can't control his anger. "I watched my dad do the same things, and my mom took us and left."

Peter also admits that he has gotten into trouble at work several times for "mouthing off" and blames the fact that he has not been promoted to supervisor on this. The nurse says, "I hear you saying that your anger is causing you trouble in many areas of your life and that you would like to be able to control your anger better." "Yes," says Peter, "That's correct."

The nurse develops a plan of care for Peter's aggressive behavior and poor anger management skills. Ongoing treatment for and recovery from substance abuse are integral to the success of the following plan of care; please refer to Chapter 27 for nursing care of clients with substance abuse problems.

Nursing Diagnosis: **Ineffective Coping** related to poor role models for coping behaviors as evidenced by substance abuse and hurtful and self-defeating behaviors

Goal: The client will learn to be assertive, not aggressive, and will learn adaptive coping techniques.

Interventions	Rationales
Suggest that the client keep an anger journal in which he records the situations that provoked anger and all the attendant thoughts and feelings.	Keeping a journal will help Peter gain insight about anger-triggering events and any self-talk that promotes outbursts.
Help client to replace anger-stimulating self-talk with more suitable self-talk. Teach thought-stopping techniques.	Self-talk is powerful and self-fulfilling. Cognitive restructuring leads to behavior changes.
Role-model respect for the feelings of others; explore with the client the concept of dignity and the rights of others.	Aggressive behavior is characterized by lack of respect for others. Peter must learn to value the dignity of others and how to show respect.
Teach the use of "I" statements and taking responsibility for one's own feelings.	Doing so helps client avoid "I'm right, you're wrong" arguments and encourages a calmer discussion.
Help client identify acceptable coping strategies when tension is high. Possibilities include aerobic activity, relaxation techniques, discussion with staff or trusted friends, cognitive restructuring, and other techniques that are acceptable to the client or that he has successfully used before.	An alternative coping strategy must be in place before Peter can abandon his former strategy of dominance and aggressiveness.

Evaluation: Peter gains insight into his behaviors, develops assertive rather than aggressive interpersonal behaviors, and successfully uses a coping technique that does not threaten, harm, or intimidate others.

Nursing Diagnosis: **Risk for Other-Directed Violence** related to poor impulse control and ineffective coping skills as evidenced by history of spousal abuse and fighting

Goal: The client will maintain self-control, thereby avoiding harm to self or others.

Interventions	Rationales
Remove potentially dangerous objects (ie, sharp objects, belts, glass items, drugs).	External control of the environment prevents impulsive actions when a client lacks internal controls.

(continued)

Nursing Care Plan 26-1 (Continued)

Interventions	Rationales
Convey an attitude of caring and concern toward client.	A caring attitude will promote feelings of trust and self-worth in Peter.
Approach the client in calm, nonthreatening manner and speak in a soft, even tone of voice.	A calm attitude and demeanor models positive behavior and precludes power struggles.
Discuss behavioral expectations and consequences.	Such discussion teaches Peter about behaviors that are socially acceptable.
Offer opportunity for client to express concerns and to talk about events, thoughts, and feelings (especially anger) that may have triggered current reaction.	This expression allows Peter to confront unresolved issues and gain self-awareness about own behavior.
Obtain a behavioral contract from client that he will not behave in an aggressive or threatening manner to others.	The contract will encourage Peter to assume self-control.

Evaluation: Peter does not become aggressive or violent to others.

meaningful descriptions. Yes-or-no questions are useful when specific information is requested, such as "Are you feeling angry?" A series of yes-or-no questions, however, may seem like an interrogation. Avoid using "why" questions because they may seem accusatory rather than empathetic and may put the client on the defensive. When the client responds, listen and paraphrase the client's feelings and the source or reasons given for feelings. Ask if your understanding is correct.

3. *Focus on the client's competency and alternative problem solving:* Often, we are aware of only the deficit side of various disturbing behaviors and the affect of an angry person rather than the person's competency to prevent anger escalation by maintaining control and rebuilding constructive functioning (Simms, 1995). If possible, talk with the client about his or her ideas regarding a plan of action that would help deal with the situation. Doing so affirms the client's competence and provides information for further problem solving. Discussing the following is useful:
   - What does the client want?
   - What has the client tried in the past to get what he or she wants?
   - How well did it work?

Recognizing what has been tried and how well it worked can help the client avoid repeating ineffective behavior, make more adaptive choices, and avoid limit-setting situations. See Implications for Nursing Practice 26-1 for additional, situation-specific interventions to prevent escalation of client aggression.

SETTING LIMITS TO PREVENT VIOLENT BEHAVIOR

Setting firm but fair limits helps clients to establish appropriate boundaries and can increase feelings of security.

Before setting a limit, the nurse describes the client's unacceptable behavior; communicates expected behavior; and offers acceptable alternatives such as walking with the nurse, talking about feelings and thoughts, or participating in recreational therapy. Clients usually can "save face" when they are given a choice of more constructive alternatives than their intended aggressive behavior.

The nurse states the limit in a matter-of-fact manner, not as advice, bribery, or punishment. The limit tells the client specifically what he or she is to do or not to do in the situation. Also, the nurse helps the client understand the reason for the limit and the consequences if he or she tests the limit or continues inappropriate behavior. Explaining the consequences is of therapeutic value because it gives the client a sense of responsibility for the outcomes or results of his or her behavior.

The nurse enforces the limit, which must be reasonable and one that the nurse can realistically and uniformly enforce. Applying limits uniformly means that all clients are expected to adhere to certain standards of behavior. Injustices tend to incite anger in most people in any setting. When a client tests a limit, he or she usually experiences some anxiety, and having staff respond predictably to ensure the safety and protection of the client and others provides security and confidence.

TEACHING ANGER MANAGEMENT AND COPING SKILLS

Anger, which can lead to aggression and violence, results from many variables including personality, temperament, impulsivity, low frustration tolerance, and poor coping skills and cognitive patterns. Different events trigger different people to anger. Clients can learn to control anger by recognizing what triggers their anger, how behaviors contribute to a volatile situation, and how self-talk can either help or hinder adaptive coping.

Implications for Nursing Practice 26-1

Situation-Specific Interventions to Prevent Escalation of Client Aggression

- When the client asks questions in a demanding way, such as "Why isn't my doctor here?" or "Why can't you give me my medication now?," avoid becoming defensive or authoritarian. Address the client's concern in a factual, respectful, and supportive manner (Zook, 1996). Studies by nurse researchers indicate that anger in hospitalized clients tends to escalate when they are confronted with an authoritative, superior attitude on the part of nurses and other healthcare staff (Lancee, Gallop, McCay, & Toner, 1995; Morrison, 1994).

- When the client makes refusals, such as "I'm not going to take that medicine," or "I'm not going to group," remain calm and avoid a power struggle with the client. Useful responses include a supportive acknowledgement of the client's concern and asking the client to explain the reasons behind the refusal (Zook, 1996). After hearing the client's story, explain the consequences of the refusal and help the client toward solutions or alternatives.

- When the client directs verbal anger at you, allow the client to "vent," then express understanding. For example, "I can see that you are disappointed" (or whatever feeling the client is expressing). Work with the client toward constructive solutions.

- When the client uses intimidation like "I'm going to sue everyone who works on this unit," avoid trying to justify the situation or defend your actions. Show empathy for the client's feelings. For example, "I know you're frustrated at having to wait for your treatment." Receiving the nurse's understanding may help calm the client.

- When the client's behavior continues to escalate toward violence, assess the need for limit-setting.

The nurse may want to suggest that the client keep a journal to obtain insight into patterns of behavior. Clients can write about their angry feelings and consciously try to identify precursors to feeling out of control or enraged. Often, the client is able to identify situations that trigger anger and are thereby empowered to implement other strategies that will modulate angry responses before acting on them.

One such strategy is cognitive restructuring. Changing the automatic self-talk that feeds into anger is an effective method for anger management. Assist the client to begin to recognize the self-talk that encourages anger. For example, the client may say to himself, "This person is trying to make me look bad. I want to hurt this guy." The client can be taught to recognize this thought and replace it with a more acceptable thought such as, "This isn't my problem, it's his. Relax."

Another effective method for controlling aggression is to teach the angry and aggressive client assertiveness skills. Although typically associated with dependent and passive clients, assertiveness training also benefits aggressive clients by teaching them appropriate tools for meeting their needs without infringing on the rights of others. Assertive statements follow a pattern:

1. "When. . . . " (Concretely describe the other individual's behavior.)
2. "The effects are. . . . " (Objectively describe the effect of the other individual's actions.)
3. "I feel. . . . " (Honestly describe feelings.)
4. "I prefer. . . . " (Respectfully suggests desired outcome or behavior.)

A correlate to assertiveness training is teaching better communication and problem-solving skills. Empathic communication can help the chronically angry client improve his or her social and familial relationships. The client can be taught about making "I" statements ("I feel hurt by your remarks") instead of "you" statements ("You hurt my feelings") to avoid making judgments by relating feelings rather than opinions and to develop better listening skills. The client should learn to ask for feedback to enhance his or her ability to communicate. The client's family or loved ones should be included in this process.

Finally, the client should be instructed in relaxation techniques and deep-breathing exercises, which dampen the sympathetic response and stimulate a parasympathetic response. Regularly practicing relaxation exercises helps decrease the overall response to stressful situations; using techniques in a specific situation also is helpful.

Evaluation

When evaluating the care of the client who has displayed angry, aggressive, or violent behavior, consider the following indicators of success:

- Did implementation of the plan of care prevent an escalation of aggressive behavior, although emotions may have been intense?
- Was everyone's safety maintained?
- Did healthcare personnel follow the institution's written guidelines and strategies for dealing with aggressive behavior?
- Did the client (and nursing staff) learn any new problem-solving techniques or resources for handling aggressive behaviors in the future?
- Was the client's dignity respected?

Expected outcomes for the client include the ability to report feelings of loss of control and ask for help from appropriate staff. The client discusses antecedents to feelings of anxiety, anger, frustration, and aggression and describes positive ways to prevent escalation. He or she verbalizes awareness of cognitive appraisals of precipitating events, ways to reframe thoughts and behavioral responses more constructively, and awareness of personal competencies in problem solving and coping. The client uses assertive communication skills and can maintain self-control of aggressive and violent inclinations as evidenced by a calm demeanor and no aggressive and violent behavior. He or she is optimistic about using more constructive cognitive skills and changing methods of coping with anger in future frustrating situations.

Before discharge, the client and family members or significant others verbalize knowledge of available community support services, such as ongoing anger-management groups, and their intent to use phone numbers of a crisis hotline or other resources if needed.

▼ *Reflection and Critical Thinking Questions*

1. Consider Peter in Clinical Example 26-1. What factors put Peter at high risk for violent behavior? Is he currently dangerous?

2. Is limit setting appropriate for all clients who are potentially violent?

3. With staff shortages and decreased length of hospital stay, what increased client safety concerns occur in hospitals?

4. What kinds of community support resources need to be in place to accommodate commitment to outpatient treatment settings and preventive commitment?

▼ CHAPTER SUMMARY

- Although the range of aggressive behaviors, including violence, occurs in all clinical diagnostic categories, certain subgroups of psychiatric diagnoses have been linked with violent behavior, such as antisocial personality disorder, paranoid schizophrenia, schizoaffective disorder, and substance abuse.

- Antecedent events that have been linked with client violence on inpatient units include a coercive interaction style, arguments with other clients, and arguments with staff whose behavior in the process of caring for the client is interpreted by the client as intrusive and frustrating or indifferent.

- Theories and research-based findings regarding the biologic determinants of aggressive and violent behavior point to factors such as neurobiologic deficits, neurotransmitter dysregulation, or injuries in the limbic system or frontal or temporal lobes of the brain.

- When developing a nursing care plan for the client who is at high risk for aggressive and violent behavior, the nurse gathers information such as a history of aggressive or violent behavior and substance abuse; factors associated with increasing anxiety levels, agitation, and inclinations toward violence; cognitive appraisals of life events and aggressive responses; inability to generate alternative problem solving; and inability to communicate angry feelings.

- When planning therapeutic interventions, the nurse and client choose desired client outcomes based on the client's needs and ability to maintain self-control of aggressive and violent inclinations.

- Three major types of intervention strategies include verbal, pharmacotherapeutics, and physical (seclusion and restraint), which may be used separately or in combination as indicated by client needs and treatment setting protocols with adherence to the principles of safety and least-restrictive environment.

- Prevention of violent behavior through de-escalating angry feelings and supporting the client who attempts to control violent inclinations in socially acceptable ways are preferable to applying seclusion and restraint.

- Therapeutic strategies with reported success in helping clients toward greater self-awareness and positive management of anger include cognitive therapy, behavior therapy, anger management groups, and other group and families.

- Discharge planning should incorporate education for the client and family or significant others based on an assessment of learning needs regarding the risks and characteristics of violent behavior, de-escalation strategies, and community support resources. In addition, pertinent nursing care plan information regarding the client should be communicated to appropriate referral agencies to ensure continuity of care, effective monitoring, and support.

- Evaluation requires a close examination of client and nursing efforts to determine whether client goals and behavior outcomes were met and to decide what additional therapeutic interventions might be more effective in reinforcing clients' efforts in exerting internal control of aggressive and violent inclinations.

▼ REVIEW QUESTIONS

1. According to recent research studies, which of the following risk factors is the best predictor of violent behavior?
   a. Argumentative personality style
   b. A history of violent behavior
   c. Decreased brain serotonin
   d. Negative thinking

2. Which of the following statements regarding the cognitive theory of anger arousal is false?

a. Negative perceptions and appraisals of self, other people, and the world influence a person's anger arousal.

b. Individuals who interpret certain situations and events as aversive and provocative tend to react with anger when the event occurs.

c. Individuals' appraisals of events are unrelated to their expectations about the events.

d. The kind of self-talk that individuals use influences their expectations and appraisals of events that happen to them.

3. Which of the following events on a psychiatric unit are most likely to precipitate an episode of aggressive or violent behavior in a violence-prone client (Mr. A.)?

a. A psychiatric technician asks Mr. A. if he would like to have some juice during snack time.

b. The nurse notices Mr. A. frowning, cursing, and pacing up and down the hall, and she asks him if he is feeling upset about something.

c. The nurse reminds Mr. A. that it is time to take his medication, which he has been doing willingly.

d. Another client on the unit picked up Mr. A's pack of cigarettes and said that they were his.

4. Which of the following statements about the emergency use of seclusion and restraint is false?

a. It is not necessary to explain to the client who is displaying violent behavior that restraint and seclusion may be used.

b. Specific written guidelines and a manual for the use of intervention procedures should be available in mental health institutions.

c. Justification for the emergency use of seclusion and restraint is legally based on professional clinical judgment and professional standards of care.

d. A professional nurse can act as the leader to direct the actions of a team of staff in implementing emergency seclusion and restraint procedures for a client whose behavior is violent and out of control.

5. Which of the following medications is most commonly used to treat aggressive behavior associated with acute psychoses?

a. Diazepam
b. Haloperidol
c. Lithium
d. Fluoxetine

6. Which type of intervention is most appropriately used by the nurse when interacting with aggressive clients at early levels of anger escalation?

a. Administration of sedating medication
b. Seclusion
c. Restraint

d. Talking with the client to discover the source of distress and alternatives to violent behavior

7. Which of the following statements best reflects the legal implications of the Tarasoff decision (*Tarasoff v. Regents of the University of California*, 1976)?

a. Clients' threats to harm a potential victim are not reportable to police as long as the clients are under the care of a psychiatrist.

b. It is mandatory that mental healthcare providers warn appropriate police authorities and potential victims of possible dangerous actions threatened by clients.

c. The Tarasoff decision has resulted in a "duty to warn" potential victims of clients' threats only in the state of California.

d. Seclusion and restraint interventions are automatically required for clients who are potentially violent.

8. All the following statements reflect outcome goals of anger-management training for violence-prone clients *except:*

a. Gaining awareness of one's own thoughts, feelings, and behaviors that are related to anger arousal

b. Rechanneling aggressive responses in the later stages of anger arousal

c. Reappraising certain arousal situations as a problem that calls for a solution rather than as a threat that calls for an attack

d. Gaining awareness of others' points of view and the consequences of one's own emotional and behavioral responses

9. Which of the following statements is false regarding the legalities of treating violent clients within hospitals and clinics?

a. Although involuntary clients may refuse antipsychotic medication, the nurse may administer such medication as prescribed if the client is dangerous to self or others.

b. Involuntary commitment criteria and interpretation vary among the states.

c. If violent clients, hospitalized or not, make clear threats to harm specific people, the mental healthcare provider who hears such a threat cannot be held responsible if potential victims are not warned and are harmed.

d. Specific advocacy groups favor less strict commitment standards.

10. Which of the following conditions has been consistently linked with medication noncompliance among discharged, previously violent clients?

a. Substance abuse
b. Broodiness
c. Feelings of resentment
d. Coercive interaction style

▼ REFERENCES AND SUGGESTED READINGS

*Allen, J. G. (1994). Temperament: The biological shaper of personality. *The Menninger Letter, 2*(10), 4–5.

*Allen, L. A. (1999). Treating agitation without drugs. *American Journal of Nursing, 99*(4), 36–42.

*Altimari, D., & Weiss, E. (1998). Reform urged in use of restraints. Deadly restraints: A Hartford Courant investigative report. [On-line]. Available: *http://www.courant.com/news/special/restraint/reform1.stm.*

*American Psychiatric Association. (2000). *Diagnostic and statistical manual of mental disorders* (4th ed., text rev.). Washington, DC: Author.

American Psychiatric Nurses Association (2000). Position statement on the use of seclusion and restraint (pp. 1–15). [On-line]. Available: *http://www.apna.org.*

*Asnis, G. M., Kaplan, M. L., Hundofean, G., & Saeed, W. (1997). Violence and homicidal behaviors in psychiatric disorders. *Psychiatric Clinics of North America, 21*(2), 405–424.

*Bazelon, D. L. (1998). Bazelon Center for Mental Health Law. [On-line]. Available: *http://www.bazelon@nicon.com.*

*Berman, M. E., & Coccaro, E. F. (1998). Neurobiologic correlates of violence: Relevance to criminal responsibility. *Behavioral Sciences and the Law, 16,* 303–318.

*Buss, A. H., & Durkee, A. (1992). The aggression questionnaire. *Journal of Personality and Social Psychology, 63*(3), 452–459.

*Castrogiovanni, P., Capone, M. R., Maremmani, I., & Marazziti, D. (1994). Platelet serotonergic markers and aggressive behavior in healthy subjects. *Neuropsychobiology, 29*(3), 105–107.

*Cembrowicz, S., & Ritter, S. (1994). Attacks on doctors and nurses. In J. Shepherd (Ed.), *Violence in health care: A practical guide to coping with violence and caring for victims* (pp. 13–41). New York: Oxford University Press.

*Corrigan, P. W., Yudofsky, S. C., & Sliver, J. M. (1993). Pharmacological and behavioral treatment for aggressive psychiatric inpatients. *Hospital and Community Psychiatry, 44*(2), 125–133.

*Delaney, K., Ulsafer-Van Lanen, J., Pitula, C. R., & Johnson, M. E. (1995). Seven days and counting: How inpatient nurses might adjust their practice brief hospitalization. *Journal of Psychosocial Nursing, 33*(8), 36–40.

*DeLaune, S. C. (1991). Effective limit setting: How to avoid being manipulated. *Nursing Clinics of North America, 26*(3), 757–764.

*Estroff, S. E., Zimmer, C., Lachicotte, W., & Benoit, J. (1994). The influence of social networks and social support on violence by persons with serious mental illness. *Hospital and Community Psychiatry, 45*(7), 669–678.

*Fava, M. (1997). Psychopharmacologic treatment of pathologic aggression. *The Psychiatric Clinics of North America, 20*(2), 427–451.

*Ferguson, L. E. (1993). Steps to developing a critical pathway. *Nursing Administration Quarterly, 17*(3), 58–62.

Frederickson, B., Maynard, K., Helms, M., Haney, T., Siegler, I., & Barefoot, J. (2000). Hostility predicts magnitude and duration of blood pressure responses to anger. *Journal of Behavioral Medicine, 23*(3), 229–243.

*Gallop, R., McCay, E., & Esplen, M. J. (1992). The conceptualization of impulsivity for psychiatric nursing practice. *Archives of Psychiatric Nursing, 6*(6), 366–373.

*Gallop, R, McCay, E., Guha, M. & Khan, P (1999). The experience of hospitalization and restraint of women who have a history of childhood sexual abuse. *Health Care for Women International, 2*(4), 401–416.

*Garza-Trevino, E. S. (1994). Neurobiological factors in aggressive behaviors. *Hospital and Community Psychiatry, 45*(7), 690–699.

*Geracioti, T. D. (1994). Valproic acid treatment of episodic explosiveness related to brain injury. *Journal of Clinical Psychiatry, 55*(9).

*Glazer, W. M., & Dickson, R. A. (1998). Clozapine reduces violence and persistent aggression in schizophrenia. *Journal of Clinical Psychiatry, 59*(Suppl. 3), 8–14.

*Goldsmith, H. F., Manderscheid, R. W., Henderson, M. J., & Sacks, A. J. (1993). Projections of inpatient admissions to specialty mental health organizations: 1990 to 2010. *Hospital and Community Psychiatry, 44*(5), 478–483.

*Haas, S., Vincent, K., Holt, J., & Lippmann, S. (1997). Divalproex: A possible treatment alternative for demented, elderly aggressive patients. *Annals of Clinical Psychiatry, 9*(3), 145–147.

*Harris, G., & Rice, M. E. (1997). Risk appraisal & management of violent behavior. *Psychiatric Services, 48*(9), 1168–1176.

*Hastings, J. E., & Hamberger, K. (1997). Sociodemographic predictors of violence. *The Psychiatric Clinics of North America, 20*(2), 323–33.

*Health Care Financing Administration (1999). Medicare and Medicaid programs; Hospital conditions of participation: Patients' rights; Interim final rule. [On-line.] Available: www.access.gpo.gov.

*Human Resources Development. (1991). *Prevention and management of aggressive behavior: Lesson plan on communication* (pp. 2–15). Austin, TX: The Texas Department of Mental Health and Mental Retardation.

*Kant, R., Smith-Seemiller, L., & Zeiler, D. (1998). Treatment of aggression and irritability after head injury. *Brain Injury, 12*(8), 661–666.

*Kavoussi, R., Armstead, P., & Coccaro, E. (1997). The neurobiology of aggression. *The Psychiatric Clinics of North America, 20*(2), 395–403.

Kavoussi, R. J., Liu, J., & Coccaro, E. F. (1994). An open trial of sertraline in personality disordered patients with impulsive aggression. *Journal of Clinical Psychiatry, 55*(4), 137–141.

*Lancee, W. J., Gallop, R., McCay, E., & Toner, B. (1995). The relationship between nurses' limit-setting styles and anger in psychiatric patients. *Psychiatric Services, 46*(6), 609–613.

*Lidz, C. W., Mulvey, E. P., & Gardner, W. P. (1993). The accuracy of predictions of violence to others. *Journal of the American Medical Association, 269,* 1007–1011.

*Littrell, K. (1998). Current understanding of violence and aggression: Assessment and treatment. *Journal of Psychosocial Nursing, 36*(12), 18–24.

*Maiuro, R. D. (1993). Intermittent explosive disorder. In D. L. Dunner (Ed.), *Current psychiatric therapy* (pp. 482–489). Philadelphia: W. B. Saunders.

*Martinez, R. J., Grimm, M., & Adamson, M. (1999). From the other side of the door: Patient views of seclusion. *Journal of Psychosocial Nursing, 37*(3), 13–22.

*Mason, T. (1998). Tarasoff liability: Its impact for working with patients who threaten others. *International Journal of Nursing Studies, 35,* 109–114.

*Megan, K., & Blint, D. (1998). Why they die: Little training, few standards, poor staffing put lives at risk. Deadly restraints: A Hartford Courant investigative report. [Online]. Available: *http://www.courant.com/news/special/restraint/day2.stm.*

*Menzies, R., & Webster, C. D. (1995). Construction and validation of risk assessments in a six-year follow-up of forensic patients: A tridimensional analysis. *Journal of Consulting & Clinical Psychology, 63,* 766–778.

*McNiel, D. E., & Binder, R. I. (1994). The relationship between acute psychiatric symptoms, diagnosis and short-term risk of violence. *Hospital and Community Psychiatry, 45*(2), 133–137.

*McNiel, D. E., Binder, R. L., & Fulton, F. M. (1998). Management of threats of violence under California's Duty-to-Protect statute. *American Journal of Psychiatry, 155*(8), 1097–1101.

*Mohr, W. K., Mahon, M. M., & Noone, M. J. (1998). A restraint on restraints: The need to reconsider the use of restrictive interventions. *Archives of Psychiatric Nursing, 12*(2), 95–106.

*Morrison, E. F. (1992). A coercive interactional style as an antecedent to aggression in psychiatric patients. *Research in Nursing Health, 15,* 421–431.

*Morrison, E. F. (1994). The evolution of a concept: Aggression and violence in psychiatric settings. *Archives of Psychiatric Nursing, 7*(4), 245–253.

*Mulvey, E. P. (1994). Assessing the evidence of a link between mental illness and violence. *Hospital & Community Psychiatry, 45,* 663–668.

*Norris, M. & Kennedy, C. (1992). The view from within: How patients perceive the seclusion process. *Journal of Psychosocial Nursing and Mental Health Services, 23*(3), 555–563.

*North American Nursing Diagnosis Association. (1998). NANDA nursing diagnoses: Definitions and classification 1997–1998. Philadelphia: Author.

*Paradis, C. M., Horn, L., Lazar, R. M., & Schwartz, D. W. (1994). Brain dysfunction and violent behavior in a man with a congenital subarachnoid cyst. *Hospital & Community Psychiatry, 45*(7), 714–718.

*Pilowsky, L. S., Ring, H., Shine, P. J., et al. (1992). Rapid tranquilization: A survey of emergency prescribing in a general psychiatric hospital. *British Journal of Psychiatry, 160,* 831–835.

*Reeder, D. M. (1991). Cognitive therapy of anger management: Theoretical and practical considerations. *Archives of Psychiatric Nursing, 5*(3), 147–150.

*Rickelman, B. L., & Houfek, J. (1995). Toward an interactional model of suicidal behaviors: Cognitive rigidity, attributional style, stress, hopelessness, and depression. *Archives of Psychiatric Nursing, 9*(3), 158–168.

*Scarpa, A., & Raine, A. (1997). Psychophysiology of anger and violent behavior. *Psychiatric Clinics of North America, 20*(2), 375–394.

Siegman, A., Townsend, S., Civelek, A., & Blumenthal, R. (2000). Antagonistic behavior, dominance, hostility, and coronary heart disease. *Psychosomatic Medicine, 62*(2), 248–257.

*Siegman, A. W. (1993). Cardiovascular consequences of expressing, experiencing, and repressing anger. *Journal of Behavioral Medicine, 16*(6), 539–569.

*Simms, C. (1995). How to unmask the angry patient. *American Journal of Nursing, April,* 7–40.

*Slobogin, C. (1994). Involuntary community treatment of people who are violent and mentally ill: A legal analysis. *Hospital and Community Psychiatry, 45*(7), 685–689.

*Spivak, B., Mester, R., Wittenberg, N., Maman, Z., & Weizman, A. (1997). Reduction of aggressiveness and impulsiveness during clozapine treatment in chronic neuroleptic-resistant schizophrenic patients. *Clinical Neuropharmacology, 20*(5), 442–446.

*Stanislav, S. W., Fabre, T., Crismon, M. L., & Childs, A. (1994). Buspirone's efficacy in organic-induced aggression. *Journal of Clinical Psychopharmacology, 14*(2), 126–130.

*Steinwachs, D. M., Kasper, J. D., & Skinner, E. A. (1992). Family perspectives on meeting the needs for care of severely mentally ill relatives: A national survey. Arlington, VA: National Alliance for the Mentally Ill.

*Straznickas, K. A., McNeil, D. E., & Binder, R. L. (1993). Violence toward family caregivers by mentally ill relatives. *Hospital and Community Psychiatry, 44,* 385–387.

*Stuart, S., Wright, J. H., Thase, M. E., & Beck, A. T. (1997). Cognitive therapy with inpatients. *General Hospital Psychiatry, 19*(1), 42–50.

*Tardiff, K. (1999). Violence. In R. E. Hales, S. C. Yudofsky, & J. A. Talbot (Eds.), *Textbook of psychiatry* (3rd ed., pp. 1405–1428). Washington, DC: The American Psychiatric Press.

*Tardiff, K., Marzuk, P. M., Lem, A. C., & Portera, L. (1997). A prospective study of violence by psychiatric patients after hospital discharge. *Psychiatric Services, 48*(5), 678–681.

*Tariot, P. N., Erb, R., Podagorski, C. A., Cox, C., Patel, S., Jakimovich, L., et al. (1998). Efficacy and tolerability of carbamazepine for agitation and aggression in dementia. *American Journal of Psychiatry, 155*(1), 54–61.

*Task Force on Homelessness and Severe Mental Illness. (1992). *Outcasts on Main Street: Report of the Task Force on Homelessness and Severe Mental Illness.* Rockville, MD: National Institute of Mental Health.

The Harvard Mental Health Letter. (1991). Violence and violent patients: Part 1. *7*(12), 1–4.

*Whittington, R. (1994). Violence in psychiatric hospitals. In T. Wykes (Ed.), *Violence and health care professionals* (pp. 23–43). New York: Chapman & Hall.

*Wiegman, O., & van Schie, E. G. (1998). Video game playing and its relations with aggressive and prosocial behavior. *British Journal of Social Psychology, 37*(Pt. 3), 367–378.

*Zook, R. (1996). Take action before anger builds. *RN, 54*(4), 46–50.

**Starred references are cited in text.*

For additional information on this chapter, go to *http://connection.lww.com.*

Need more help? See Chapter 26 of the *Study Guide to Accompany Mohr: Johnson's Psychiatric-Mental Health Nursing,* 5th ed.

CHAPTER 27

The Client Who Abuses Drugs and Alcohol

CAROL J. CORNWELL

▼ KEY TERMS

Alcohol (ethanol)—A legal chemical substance (drug) that commonly leads to abuse and dependency.

Blackout—A phenomenon in which a person functions normally while drinking but later has no memory of what occurred during that period, with no accompanying loss of consciousness.

Blood alcohol level (BAL)—Milligrams of alcohol per milliliter of blood.

Club drugs—A group of synthetic drugs commonly used in nightclubs and as recreational drugs.

Delirium tremens (DTs)—Most serious form of withdrawal from alcohol; occurs after cessation or reduction in prolonged heavy drinking; can be a medical emergency and needs immediate treatment.

Dual diagnosis—A diagnosis of a coexisting substance abuse or dependency disorder and a major psychiatric disorder; the disorders are unrelated and meet the *DSM-IV-TR* diagnostic criteria for each specific disorder.

Fetal alcohol syndrome—A syndrome characterized by a group of congenital birth defects caused by the mother's drinking while pregnant.

Proof—Concentration of ethyl alcohol in a beverage.

Substance abuse—Use of alcohol or other drugs repeatedly to the extent that functional problems occur; it does not include compulsive use or addiction.

Substance dependency—Continued use of alcohol or other drugs despite negative consequences, such as significant functional problems in daily living.

Tolerance—A phenomenon that occurs after heavy drug or alcohol use in which the user needs more of the drug to achieve the same effect.

Wernicke-Korsakoff syndrome—Alcoholic amnesia related to thiamine deficiency.

▼ LEARNING OBJECTIVES

On completion of this chapter, you should be able to accomplish the following:

- Define substance abuse and dependency.
- Explain current diagnostic categorization of various types of substance abuse and dependency disorders.
- Discuss the common etiological concepts related to substance abuse and dependency.
- Discuss the incidence and significance of substance abuse and dependency.
- Discuss the importance of recognizing dual diagnoses and co-morbidity in clients with substance abuse and dependency, and the implications for prognosis.
- Describe the effects of substance abuse disorders on physiology, behavior, society, and the family.
- Discuss interdisciplinary treatment interventions for the client with a substance abuse disorder.
- Apply the components of the nursing process to the client who abuses or is dependent on substances.

▼ Clinical Example 27-1

Eric is a 38-year-old, white, married man who lives with his wife of 2 years and his 1-year-old daughter. He was admitted to an alcohol rehabilitation program 2 days ago after being arrested for disorderly conduct in a local bar. He had been at the bar—a popular hangout where he stops daily on his way home from work—since 5:00 PM Friday evening. At 7:30 PM, he began an argument with another customer that progressed quickly into a fistfight. The bar owner called the police, and both men were arrested. This is Eric's second arrest for disorderly conduct, and the judge ordered inpatient detoxification and treatment for alcoholism.

This is Eric's fourth admission for alcohol abuse in the last 7 years. He works at a local machine shop where his alcohol abuse has threatened his position. During his last admission to the rehabilitation program 6 months ago, his employer made his continued employment contingent on participating in a long-term, outpatient alcohol treatment program. He had been in this program for 3 months until dropping out 1 week before his current arrest.

Eric has experienced a continuing decline in function over the last 10 years, including increased tolerance and withdrawal symptoms from alcohol. Recently, Eric began to have gastric distress that required an abdominal workup. The workup revealed mild cirrhosis of the liver and esophageal varices.

His wife has considered a legal separation until he can become sober; however, she has been unable to make the move out of their home. She assumes all responsibility for their daughter because Eric often is at the local bar and does not participate in activities to maintain their home or family life.

This chapter discusses clients who abuse substances that affect the central nervous system (CNS). It examines systems of substance classification, various concepts related to the etiology and dynamics of substance abuse and dependency, physical and behavioral changes that occur in people who abuse and become dependent on substances, and interdisciplinary treatment interventions. Furthermore, the chapter focuses on application of the nursing process to care of the client with a substance abuse disorder.

All drugs of abuse and dependency share certain factors. In addition, factors are specific to each drug. This chapter addresses the similarities of substance abuse and dependency and the factors that are particular to each drug classification, such as alcohol. The discussion emphasizes the commonalities underlying these disorders with the idea that the problem of abuse and dependency and the manifestations or functional disturbances resulting from the problem may differ. For example, the manifestations of dependency on alcohol differ from those of dependency on cocaine, but the core problem remains the same: the abuse of, or the dependency on, a substance.

As you read this chapter, consider Eric's symptoms (from Clinical Example 27-1) and the degree to which his alcohol dependency has affected all areas of his life. You will learn more about the progression of Eric's care in Nursing Care Plan 27-1. You also will have the opportunity to apply what you will learn about substance abuse and dependency in the Reflection and Critical Thinking Questions at the end of this chapter.

SUBSTANCE ABUSE AND DEPENDENCY

Substance Use Disorders, as defined by the *Diagnostic and Statistical Manual of Mental Disorders,* 4th edition, text revision (American Psychiatric Association [APA], 2001),

is an umbrella term that includes substance abuse and substance dependency. **Substance abuse** occurs when a person uses alcohol or other drugs repeatedly to the extent that functional problems manifest; however, it does not include compulsive use or addiction. A person diagnosed with substance abuse does not experience the withdrawal syndromes that occur with substance dependency. Conversely, **substance dependency** is diagnosed when the person continues using alcohol or other drugs despite negative consequences such as significant functional problems in daily living. A person with substance dependency is likely to experience tolerance as the use of the substance escalates and withdrawal when the drug of abuse is stopped.

Historical Context

People have used and abused drugs, including wine, narcotics, and marijuana, for thousands of years (Columbia University, 2000). During the 19th century, physicians extracted and prescribed substances such as morphine, laudanum, and cocaine without any regulation for a wide variety of conditions. Traveling salesmen placed these substances in patented medicines and sold them in drugstores or by mail. Morphine was used freely during the Civil War and was provided along with hypodermic needles to soldiers in kits. After the war, opium dens flourished in the United States; by the early 1900s, an estimated 250,000 opium addicts were in the United States.

U.S. drug laws mirror the changing perceptions of substance abuse. The first national drug law was the Pure Food and Drug Act of 1906, requiring labeling of patent medicines that contained certain drugs. In 1919, an amendment, subsequently repealed in 1933, was added to the constitution prohibiting the use of alcohol. By 1970, more than 55 federal drug laws and many state laws included punitive measures for illicit drug use. The Center for Substance Abuse Treatment (CSAT) of the Substance Abuse and Mental Health Services Administration (SAMHSA), U.S. Department of Health and Human Services (DHHS), was created in October 1992 with a congressional mandate to expand the availability of effective treatment and recovery services for alcohol and drug problems. These agencies continue to provide myriad programs and services in the area of substance abuse and mental health.

Epidemiology

With the advent of the Internet and rapid information technology, the latest national statistics on substance abuse and dependency in America are best found on the Internet site of SAMHSA (2001). Findings from the most recent National Household Survey are highlighted in Box 27-1. For the first time, the survey provides state-by-state estimates of illicit drug, alcohol, and cigarette

BOX 27-1 ▼ Highlights From the National Household Survey

- Illicit drug use among people aged 12 to 17 years began to decline in 1997 and continued to do so through 1999; during the same time period, illicit drug use among the overall population, aged 12 and older, remained constant.
- According to the trend data in the report, in 1999, an estimated 9% of youths aged 12 to 17 reported current illicit drug use, meaning they used an illicit drug at least once during the 30 days before to the time of the survey interview.
- There is a significant, consistent downward trend over the last 3 years in illicit drug use, from 11.4 % (1997), to 9.9% (1998), to 9.0% (1999).
- Current drug use varies substantially among states, ranging from a low of 4.7 % to a high of 10.7% for the overall population, and from 8.0 % to 18.3 % for youths aged 12 to 17 years.

From Substance Abuse and Mental Health Services Administration (SAMHSA), Office of Applied Studies. (2001, October 12). *National Household Survey on Drug Abuse (NHSDA): National household survey.* [On line.] Available: http://www.samhsa.gov/statistics/statistics. html.

use according to age group, as well as information about the brands of cigarettes that Americans smoke. These new, expanded data on demographic and geographic populations are a valuable tool for states and community-based organizations to better tailor their programs to their communities (see Web Sites of Interest at end of chapter for SAMHSA data).

Several new substances have emerged on the scene in recent years. **"Club drugs"** are a group of drugs used in nightclubs and by groups of people as recreational drugs. These drugs are primarily synthetic and have gained a false reputation that they are less addictive than mainstream drugs such as heroin. The Drug Abuse Warning Network (DAWN) report for 2000 indicates that the use of club drugs steadily rose from 1994 to 1998 (Figure 27-1) (DEA, 2000).

The 1999 National Household Survey on Drug Abuse explores the incidence and prevalence of heavy alcohol and drug use in the United States. More than 13% of young adults between 18 and 25 years of age were heavy alcohol users in 1999 (Figure 27-2). This figure represents approximately 4 million young adult heavy drinkers. Among young adults, men (20%) drank heavily more than women (7%). Whites had the highest rate of heavy alcohol use (16%) of any racial or ethnic group, followed by American Indians/Alaska Natives and Hispanics (both at 10%) and blacks and Asians (both at 6%).

Young adults, both men and women, who are full-time undergraduates in college tend to drink heavily compared with those who are not full-time undergraduates enrolled in college (18% and 12%, respectively) (Figure 27-3). Full-time undergraduate men drink more heavily (about 1 in 4) than do women (about 1 in 10).

Heavy alcohol use is associated with alcohol dependence, which is characterized by increased tolerance, withdrawal symptoms when alcohol is not used, unsuccessful efforts to cut down on alcohol use, and interference with everyday life (APA, 2000). The survey found that the rate of alcohol dependence for persons between 18 and 25 years of age was higher than for persons between 12 and 17 years of age or 26 years of age or older. Both heavy drinking and alcohol dependence peaked at 21 years of age (Figure 27-4).

Alcohol often has been referred to as a "gateway" drug that eventually opens the door to illicit drug use. The

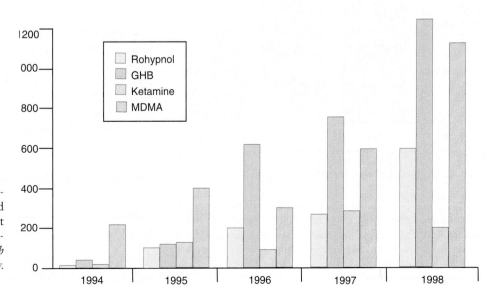

FIGURE 27-1 Estimated emergency room mentions for selected club drugs. Drug Enforcement Administration: Intelligence Division. [2000]. *An overview of club drugs.* [On-line.] Available: www. usdoj.gov/dea.

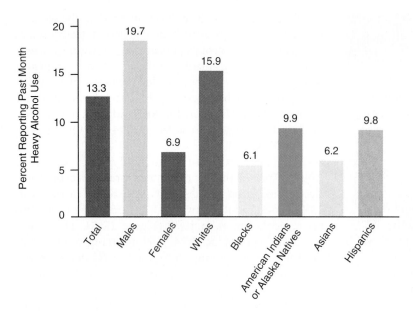

FIGURE 27-2 Percentages reporting past month heavy alcohol use among young adults aged 18 to 25 by demographic characteristics: 1999. (From Substance Abuse and Mental Health Services Administration [SAMHSA], Office of Applied Studies [1999]. *National Household Survey on Drug Abuse [NHSDA],* October 12, 2001. Used with permission.)

NHSDA survey also looked at the rate of illicit drug use past month and its association with heavy drinking. Among young adults between 18 and 25 years of age, the rate of past month illicit drug use was higher with increasing levels of past month alcohol use (Figure 27-5). Among heavy drinkers, 44% had used illicit drugs in the past month compared with 26% of "binge" drinkers, 11% of nonbinge drinkers, and 5% of nondrinkers. This connection between heavy drinking and illicit drug use is found for marijuana and for illicit drugs other than marijuana.

In addition to the National Household Surveys, the DAWN (2000) of SAMHSA publishes a periodic *Emergency Department Data Report* compiling and analyzing data regarding drug-related emergency department visits in the continental United States. In 2000, there were an estimated 601,776 drug-related emergency department visits in the continental United States with 1,100,539 mentions of a particular drug (on average, 1.8 drugs per visit). Among these drug-related emergency department visits, dependence (217,224, or 36% of visits) and suicide (193,061, or 32 %) were the most frequently cited motives for taking the substances. Overdose (264,240, or 44%) was the most common reason given for contacting the emergency department.

Between 1999 and 2000, emergency department visits involving clients seeking detoxification increased by 24% (from 72,960 to 90,625), and visits involving overdose increased by 14% (from 232,283 to 264,240). Also in the report was that emergency department visits involving the club drug MDMA (3,4-methylenedioxymethamphetamine, or Ecstasy) increased by 58%, from 2850 visits in 1999 to 4511 in 2000 in the continental United States. The number of heroin- or morphine-related visits increased by 15%, from 84,409 to 97,287.

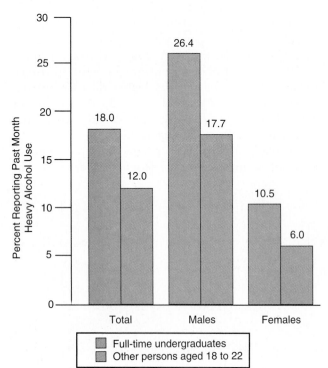

FIGURE 27-3 Percentages reporting past month heavy alcohol use persons aged 18 to 22, by college enrollment status and gender: 1999. (From Substance Abuse and Mental Health Services Administration [SAMHSA] Office of Applied Studies [1999]. *National Household Survey on Drug Abuse [NHSDA],* October 12, 2001. Used with permission.)

Prenatal Alcohol and Drug Abuse

Drug and alcohol use and smoking are significant risk factors for poor perinatal outcomes in the United States and therefore have been the focus of attention. The SAMHSA report, *Alcohol and Tobacco Use Among Pregnant Women,* indicates that in 1999, an estimated 17% of pregnant

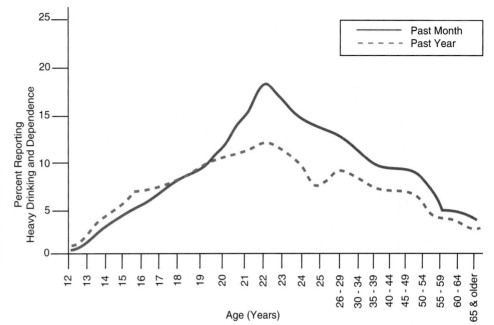

FIGURE 27-4 Percentages reporting past month heavy drinking and past year alcohol dependence among persons aged 12 or older, by age: 1999. (From Substance Abuse and Mental Health Services Administration [SAMHSA], Office of Applied Studies [1999]. *National Household Survey on Drug Abuse [NHSDA]*, October 12, 2001. Used with permission.)

women smoked cigarettes in the past month, compared with 31% of nonpregnant women. Younger pregnant women were more likely than their older counterparts to smoke cigarettes and binge drink. The 1999 data indicate that reductions in tobacco and alcohol use in women during pregnancy are not permanent. Rates of smoking and drinking in the year after giving birth were similar to those among all nonpregnant women.

The harmful effects of tobacco and alcohol on the human embryo and fetus are well documented (Centers for Disease Control and Prevention, 2001; National Institute on Alcohol Abuse and Alcoholism, 2000). **Fetal alcohol syndrome** (FAS) is a serious syndrome characterized by a group of congenital birth defects caused by chronic drinking while pregnant (Box 27-2). Cocaine also has adverse effects on the fetus and neonate when used during pregnancy. Box 27-3 depicts some of the perinatal outcomes that are caused by cocaine use during pregnancy. More treatment and intervention programs for alcohol and substance abuse are needed that target pregnant women.

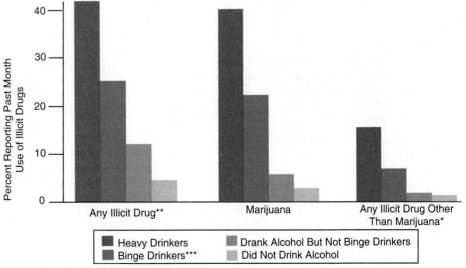

FIGURE 27-5 Percentages reporting past month use of illicit drugs among persons aged 18 to 25, by level of past month alcohol use: 1999. (From Substance Abuse and Mental Health Services Administration [SAMHSA], Office of Applied Studies [1999]. *National Household Survey on Drug Abuse [NHSDA]*, October 12, 2001. Used with permission.)

*"Any illicit drug other than marijuana" indicates use at least once of any of these listed drugs, regardless of marijuana/hashish use; marijuana/hashish users who also had used any of the other listed drugs were included.
***"Any illicit drug" indicates use at least once of marijuana/hashish, cocaine (including crack), heroin, hallucinogens (including LSD and PCP), inhalants, or any prescription-type psychotherapeutic used nonmedically.
***Binge drinkers reported that they drank five or more drinks on the same occasion on at least 1 day in the past 30 days.

BOX 27-2 ▼ Fetal Alcohol Syndrome

Alcohol is a teratogenic drug; that is, when taken during pregnancy, it crosses the placenta and can cause adverse effects in the fetus. Many alcohol-related birth defects have been associated with alcohol use during pregnancy. The most clearly defined effect on the fetus is a specific pattern of neonatal defects called fetal alcohol syndrome (FAS). FAS is the leading known preventable cause of mental retardation (Stratton et al., 1996). Behavioral and neurologic problems associated with prenatal alcohol exposure often lead to decreased academic performance as well as legal and employment difficulties in adolescence and adulthood (Thomas et al., 1998). There has been a recent impetus to increase public awareness of the risks involved in drinking while pregnant; however, increasing numbers of women continue to do so (Ebrahim et al., 1999).

FAS is defined by four criteria: maternal drinking during pregnancy, a characteristic pattern of facial abnormalities,

growth retardation, and brain damage, which often is manifested by intellectual difficulties or behavioral problems (Stratton et al., 1996). It is manifested by a group of congenital birth defects including the following:

- Prenatal and postnatal growth deficiency
- A particular pattern of facial malformations, including a small head circumference, flattened midface, sunken nasal bridge, and a flattened and elongated philtrum (the groove between the nose and upper lip)
- Central nervous system dysfunction
- Varying degrees of major organ system malfunction

When signs of brain damage appear after fetal alcohol exposure in the absence of other indications of FAS, the condition is termed *alcohol-related neurodevelopmental disorder* (Stratton et al., 1996).

BOX 27-3 ▼ Perinatal Outcomes Affected by Cocaine Use During Pregnancy

Use of cocaine in pregnant women has increased rapidly in the last decade. The following depicts the devastating consequences that may occur in cocaine-affected pregnancies.

Maternal Complications

- Spontaneous abortion
- Higher incidence of abruptio placenta with increased stillbirth
- Increased cocaine-induced uterine contractibility
- Tachycardia, dysrhythmias, angina
- Increased rate of prematurity
- Seizures
- Cerebral vascular accidents
- Hypertension
- Anorexia resulting in weight loss
- Respiratory lung damage if cocaine is smoked
- HIV infection if intravenous route is used

Effects on the Fetus

- Cerebral artery injury and infarction
- Acute hypertension
- Low birth weight
- Intrauterine growth retardation
- Decreased head circumference
- Decreased length
- Skull defects
- Increased cardiac anomalies
- HIV infection if intravenous route is used

Effects on the Newborn

- Increased rate of sudden infant death syndrome

- Abnormalities on the Brazelton Neonatal Behavioral Assessment Scale
- Poor suck-and-swallow pattern
- Fine motor tremors of hands, arms, legs
- Unusual response to stimuli
- Vomiting, poor feeding
- Weak pull-to-sit development
- Irritability, difficulty sleeping
- Intolerance to cuddling
- Difficult to comfort
- Seizures in babies whose mothers use cocaine while breast-feeding

Mother-Infant Bonding

- Infants exposed to cocaine may be unable to bond with their mothers.
- To form attachment, the newborn and mother bond through an interactive process.
- The infant responds to the mother's eye contact, speaking, cuddling, talking and grasping.
- Mothers who are addicted to cocaine may be unable to respond to the infant, because of the effects of the drug, and, therefore, the infant cannot attach.
- If the mother is able to be responsive to the infant, but the infant fails to respond back to behavioral cues from the mother, this may produce feelings of frustration, anger, and inadequacy in the mother.
- This, in turn, may create a pattern of the mother's negative response to the infant and put the infant in danger of physical and emotional abuse.

Cultural Considerations

Substance abuse and dependency are found in all cultures and ethnic groups. There are sociocultural variations, however, in substance abuse patterns, the drug preferred, and several aspects of treatment, prevention, and rehabilitation. For example, a low incidence of alcoholism but a high incidence of opiate dependency is reported in the Asian culture and population (APA, 1994; U.S. Congress, 1994). Researchers attribute the low incidence of alcoholism to a possible genetic intolerance to alcohol, manifested by unpleasant physical symptoms when even small amounts of alcohol are ingested (Goodwin, 1979; U.S. Congress, 1994). There also is a low incidence of alcohol dependency in the American Jewish population but a high incidence in the Native American and Irish populations and relatively high incidence in Scandinavian and German populations. The reasons for these phenomena are related to cultural drinking habits and accepted use of alcohol (U.S. Congress, 1994). Since the 1950s, research related to cultural aspects of alcohol abuse and dependency has increased. The importance of ethnic factors and cultural diversity and their effect on substance abuse and dependency are being emphasized. Knowledge acquired through study and research has special application in drug prevention and treatment programs.

Etiology

Recently, mechanisms of drug abuse and addiction have been studied intensively. Emerging multidimensional models strongly relate these disorders to neurophysiologic processes and are replacing unidimensional, purely psychologically based models. Research and exploration in this area reveals new information daily.

Therefore, the etiology of substance abuse and dependency is complex and difficult to determine. Age, sex, culture, and social setting are factors that affect drug use, as well as the availability of drugs, cost, peer pressure, and the drug-oriented American culture, which extols the use of alcohol and prescription drugs for relief of tension and pain. Each person responds to a specific drug according to the dosage, frequency, route of administration, and biologic, behavioral, social, and psychological factors. Determining the etiology of substance-related disorders includes consideration of all of these areas. The following discussions reviews psychosocial, behavioral, and biologic factors in substance abuse and dependency and is followed by a brief presentation of theoretical concepts regarding the etiology of substance abuse.

PSYCHOSOCIAL AND BEHAVIORAL FACTORS

Psychosocial and behavioral factors that contribute to or occur in tandem with substance abuse disorders have been studied extensively. Affective disorders, such as depression and post-traumatic stress disorder, are correlated with higher incidences of alcohol and substance abuse (Handelsman et al., 2000; Ouimette, Kimerling, Shaw, & Mood, 2000; Weaver, Turner, & O'Dell, 2000). Symptoms that are associated with affective disorders, including alexithymia, hostility, anxiety, and social withdrawal, also are linked to substance abuse (Handelsman et al., 2000; Ouimette et al., 2000; Rebelo, 1999). Variations in problem-solving techniques and coping styles are associated with substance abuse disorders, with cognitive and problem-solving styles being more effective in reducing symptoms (Rebelo, 1999; Weaver et al., 2000; Winter, 2001). The stress response and perceived stress also have been an area of study. Higher perceived stress is associated with a greater severity of substance abuse, and chronic drug use has been hypothesized to change (perhaps permanently) the stress response and coping styles of an individual (Rebelo, 1999; Sinha, 2001; Weaver et al., 2000).

Although psychosocial and behavioral factors often were considered "the cause" of substance abuse disorders, recently they have been viewed as operating within the context of "vulnerability" factors in susceptible individuals. In addition, they often are studied after the occurrence of drug or alcohol abuse and are shown to play important roles in abuse, addiction, and in the process of recovery.

BIOLOGIC FACTORS

Recently, biologic theories have flourished regarding the neurophysiologic mechanism of substance abuse and addiction. Although the question revolves around the familiar "nature or nurture" argument (in the case of alcoholism, Goodwin, 1976, 1979), molecular biology, genetics, and neurophysiology are increasingly elucidating answers.

Strong familial genetic links are being found in all of the substance abuse disorders. Regarding alcohol, children of alcoholics are at significantly higher risk for developing alcoholism and drug dependency than are children of nonalcoholic parents (Jaffe, 2000; Prescott & Kendler, 1999). Other studies show similar links between substance use disorders (such as heroin use) and genetic ties within family systems (Pickens et al., 2001)

In addition to familial genetics, molecular genetics and neurophysiologic contributions are areas of research in drug abuse vulnerability. Recent findings include the identification of brain regions that are linked to vulnerability to nicotine or alcohol abuse (Uhl, Liu, Walther, Hess, & Naiman, 2001); self-exposure to drugs that alters molecular, cellular, and neurophysiologic "set points" in the brain (Kreek, 2001); genes that display altered expression after the administration of drugs of abuse (Kuhar, Joyce & Dominguez, 2001); and over-expression of certain dopaminergic genes in specific brain regions (Thanos et al., 2001). Increasingly, the physiologic mechanisms of drug abuse and addiction are being elucidated. Understanding the physiologic features and genetics of drug abuse and addiction is critical to treatment and to the education of clients and their families.

THEORETICAL CONCEPTS

Several theories have been studied and reported to explain the nature and cause of substance abuse and dependency. Two of the most popular treatment philosophies include cognitive theories about behavioral change and implicit theories used by 12-step programs such as Alcoholics Anonymous (AA) and Narcotics Anonymous (NA) (Bell, Montoya, & Richard, 1998). Cognitive theorists see behavior change as a series of rational choices. In these models, the individuals' perception of the personal consequences of their behavior is a critical element of behavior change and, by definition, of choosing certain behaviors (ie, drug abuse).

Recent behavioral change theories view "perceived outcomes or consequences of behavior as weighted by their subjective importance to an actor, independent of that actor's perception of their severity or of the actor's susceptibility" (Bell et al., 1998, p. 2). This notion may be helpful in explaining the initiation and cessation of chronic drug use. Learning about how people assign weights to outcomes could be important in understanding what motivates drug users to initiate the self-change process leading to treatment.

The implicit theory used in 12-step programs such as AA and NA focuses more on the emotional components of behavior change rather than on the cognitive components. Elements of the 12-step theory are popular among those who have gone through that treatment modality as well as among substance abuse paraprofessionals (ie, substance abuse counselors). Because some of the descriptions of the 12-step theory are viewed as imprecise and "mystical," they tend to be less popular among academically trained social scientists and health professionals (Bell et al., 1998). Twelve-step theory defines hitting bottom as an emotional and cognitive experience that impels the individual toward changing behavior. According to 12-step theory, one cannot change one's behavior until the emotional and cognitive components of one's attitude toward drug use have been transformed. Research studies support the description of hitting bottom as central to the behavior change process (Bell et al., 1998).

Another popular theory among healthcare professionals is that of learning theory, involving a conditioned response mechanism. The drug use initially may produce pleasant physical responses, desired social consequences, increased feelings of self-confidence, or relief from tension or anxiety. The conditioned response always is positive in the beginning; however, even after severe negative consequences occur, the repetitive or learned behavior continues, although the initial reasons for the behavior are no longer in operation.

In summary, psychological and behavioral theories about substance abuse and the factors that perpetuate it have revealed important information about individual coping style and life stress. However, psychological theories do not explain the phenomenon of how individuals become addicted to substances, how the addictive process is perpetuated, or the difficulty experienced by individuals when attempting to stop using abuse substances.

Comorbidities and Dual Diagnoses

The terms *comorbidity* and *dual diagnosis* describe a client with coexisting substance abuse or dependency and a major psychiatric disorder; the disorders are unrelated and meet the *DSM-IV-TR* criteria. The following are examples of clients who meet the specific dual diagnosis criteria:

- The client who has a major psychiatric disorder and uses psychoactive substances to cope with the symptoms or treatment of the disorder (eg, a client with schizophrenia who uses alcohol or other drugs for relief from side effects of medications): If this client did not meet the criteria for substance dependency, then treatment for the psychiatric illness would relieve both problems, and treatment and rehabilitation would focus primarily on the major psychiatric disorder.
- The client who has psychoactive drug dependency and presents with psychiatric symptoms as a result of intoxication, withdrawal, or other effects of the psychoactive substance being used (eg, a client who has a psychotic episode produced by the use of cocaine): Treatment and rehabilitation would focus on substance dependency to alleviate the symptoms.
- The client with a dual diagnosis of two basically unrelated psychiatric disorders that may interact to exacerbate each other (eg, a client with bipolar disorder and alcohol dependence): Treatment and rehabilitation need to address both the bipolar disorder and the substance dependency.

Reports estimate that dual diagnoses in chronically mentally ill clients range from 30% to 40% of the outpatient and 60% to 80% of the inpatient population (Drake, Tegue, & Waeren, 1990). Traditional methods of treatment for major psychiatric disorders and substance dependency (ie, substance dependency programs) have not been successful in treating clients with dual diagnoses. Ongoing research on the identification, treatment, and rehabilitation of clients with dual diagnoses is needed.

Implications and Prognosis

Substance-related disorders are a significant healthcare problem in America and globally. The use of alcohol and other drugs is associated with specific problems in several psychosocial areas (Figure 27-6). Prolonged abuse or dependency on drugs or alcohol and the concomitant adverse behavioral changes that affect the person's life and well-being usually evolve into a self-destructive course unless the substance of abuse is discontinued or the lifestyle is altered.

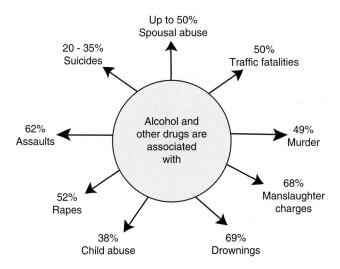

FIGURE 27-6 Association of alcohol and other drugs with specific problems. (From Office of Substance Abuse Prevention [1991].)

Ultimately, the individual who is substance dependent must learn to adapt to a life in which the substance is no longer the driving force, a challenging journey.

Although strides have been made in the diagnosis and treatment of substance use and abuse, more needs to be done. Substance abuse disorders often are difficult to treat, and most clients require several treatment episodes before they attain success. The prognosis for recovery from abuse and dependency on alcohol and other drugs is variable and depends on each individual's circumstances. Research is ongoing into the factors that affect relapse and recovery, such as personal resources, commitment, support for the rehabilitation process, stressors, and the individual's neuroregulatory makeup (Sinha, 2001; Weiss et al., 2001). A multidimensional approach is needed for individuals having these disorders. Healthcare professionals in all fields are uniting to combat abuse and dependency problems in psychological, physiologic, and social areas through treatment, research, and prevention.

Signs and Symptoms/ Diagnostic Criteria

Individuals who abuse or become dependent on substances are impaired physically, socially, and psychologically at some time during their disorder. The behaviors manifested by individuals who abuse drugs often are not tolerated or accepted in most cultures.

The *DSM-IV-TR* (APA, 2000) classifies the substance-related disorders into 12 categories (Box 27-4). All of these disorders share several common subdiagnostic categories (dependence, abuse, intoxication, and withdrawal) for which there are generic diagnostic criteria (Box 27-5).

BOX 27-4 ▼ *DSM-IV-TR Substance- Related Disorders*

1. Alcohol-Related Disorders
   a. Alcohol Use Disorders
      i. Alcohol Dependence
      ii. Alcohol Abuse
   b. Alcohol-Induced Disorders
2. Amphetamine (or Amphetamine-Like)-Related Disorders
3. Caffeine-Related Disorders
4. Cannabis-Related Disorders
5. Cocaine-Related Disorders
6. Hallucinogen-Related Disorders
7. Inhalant-Related Disorders
8. Nicotine-Related Disorders
9. Opioid-Related Disorders
10. Phencyclidine (or Phencyclidine-Like)-Related Disorders
11. Sedative–Hypnotic- or Anxiolytic-Related Disorders
12. Polysubstance-Related Disorder

Adapted with permission from American Psychological Association. (2000). *Diagnostic and statistical manual of mental disorders* (4th ed., text rev.). Washington, DC: Author.

ALCOHOL ABUSE AND DEPENDENCY

Alcohol abuse and dependency are among the most serious public health problems in the United States. The incidence of alcohol-related accidents resulting in fatalities or in permanent disabilities is enormous (see Figure 27-6). The social impact of the disorder on family members, especially children, is devastating. Many American adolescents are affected by destructive drinking patterns or experience alcoholism themselves; many children are born with abnormalities or have fetal alcohol syndrome (see Box 27-2).

Chemical Properties of Alcohol

The substance commonly referred to as alcohol is ethyl alcohol (C_2H_5OH). **Alcohol** also is known chemically as **ethanol** and sometimes is abbreviated as ETOH. It is a legal chemical substance or drug; that is, the commercial distribution of alcohol-containing beverages differs from the regulation and sale of other classes of drugs.

Ethyl alcohol has pharmacologic properties that produce mind- and mood-altering effects. It is a CNS depressant similar to barbiturates and ether.

Chloral hydrate and paraldehyde are sedative–hypnotic drugs derived from ethyl alcohol. Chloral hydrate has been used to induce sleep; paraldehyde was used in the medical management of alcohol withdrawal symptoms before the introduction of modern tranquilizers.

BOX 27-5 ▼ *DSM-IV-TR Substance-Related Disorders: Criteria for Dependence, Abuse, Intoxication, and Withdrawal*

Note: These criteria apply to all 12 categories of substances.

Dependence

A. The client's maladaptive pattern of substance use leads to clinically important distress or impairment as shown in a single 12-month period by one or more of the following:
  1. Tolerance, shown by either a markedly increased intake of the substance being needed to achieve the same effect, or
  2. With continued use, the same amount of the substance having a markedly lessened effect.
B. Withdrawal, shown by either manifestation of the substance's characteristic withdrawal syndrome, or the substance (or one closely related) being used to avoid or relieve withdrawal symptoms.
C. The amount or duration of use often is greater than intended.
D. The client repeatedly tries without success to control or reduce substance use.
E. The client spends much time using the substance, recovering from its effects, or trying to obtain it.
F. The client reduces or abandons important social, occupational, or recreational activities because of substance use.
G. The client continues to use the substance despite knowing that it probably has caused physical or psychological problems.

Abuse

A. The client's maladaptive substance use pattern causes clinically important distress or impairment as shown in a single 12-month period by three or more of the following:
  1. Because of repeated use, the client fails to carry out major obligations at work or at home.
  2. The client uses substances even when it is physically dangerous.
  3. The client repeatedly has legal problems from substance use.
  4. Despite knowing that it has caused or worsened social or interpersonal problems, the client continues to use the substance.
B. For this class of substance, the client has never fulfilled criteria for Substance Dependence.

Intoxication

A. The client develops a reversible syndrome because of recent use of or exposure to a substance.
B. During or shortly after using the substance, the client develops clinically important behavioral or psychological changes that are maladaptive.
C. This condition is neither the result of a general medical condition nor better explained by a different mental disorder.

Withdrawal

A. A syndrome specific to a substance develops when someone who has used it frequently and for a long time suddenly stops or markedly reduces its intake.
B. This syndrome causes clinically important distress or impairs work or social or personal functioning.
C. This syndrome is neither the result of a general medical condition nor better explained by a different mental disorder.

Adapted with permission from American Psychological Association. (2000). *Diagnostic and statistical manual of mental disorders* (4th ed., text rev.). Washington, DC: Author; and from Morrison, J. (1995). *The DSM-IV made easy.* New York: The Guilford Press.

Alcohol-containing beverages include beer, wine, and distilled spirits. The alcohol content of a beverage is expressed as **proof**, that is, the concentration of ethyl alcohol. In the United States, proof is twice the ethanol concentration (eg, 100 proof is 50% ethyl alcohol, and 80 proof is 40% ethyl alcohol). In contrast to other drugs that produce their effects from small quantities, alcohol usually requires large quantities used over a period of time to cause physical dependence.

Alcohol causes the following pattern of effects as the dose of the drug is increased: sedation, impaired mental and motor functioning, deepening stupor with a decrease in stimulation response (including painful stimulus response), coma, and eventually death from respiratory and circulatory collapse (Clark, Kanas, Smith, & Landry, 1995; Keltner & Folks, 1995).

Alcohol often is erroneously considered a stimulant. The reason for this misconception is that after drinking alcoholic beverages, some people may become more talkative or hyperactive, euphoric, self-confident, or aggressive. This behavior has been attributed to the disinhibiting effect produced by a low dose of alcohol.

Alcohol Concentration in the Body

The physical and behavioral manifestations of the effects of alcohol on the CNS are related directly to the level of alcohol in the blood and the concentration of alcohol in the brain. The **blood alcohol level** is expressed as milligrams of alcohol per milliliter of blood and is determined by a laboratory blood test to measure the degree of alcohol (ethanol) intoxication. It may be used in medicolegal procedures to rule out intoxication in a person who is comatose. A Breathalyzer also may measure the degree of intoxication. Hand-held breathalyzers that can be used at home or in other nonmedical settings have gained popularity.

Alcohol concentration in the blood depends on the rate of absorption, transportation to the CNS, redistribution to other parts of the body, metabolism, and elimination. Alcohol is absorbed through the mouth, stomach, and small intestine. It is absorbed unchanged into the blood and circulates throughout the body, including the brain. It also crosses the placenta into fetal circulation. Intoxication occurs when the circulating alcohol interferes with the normal functioning of brain nerve cells (Keltner & Folks, 1995).

The rate of absorption of alcohol into the blood varies with the following factors:

- Substances in the beverage, such as carbonation (CO_2) in champagne, increase absorption.
- The rate of alcohol ingestion can affect the rate of absorption. Drinking alcohol slowly over a long period may slow absorption and allow for metabolism by the liver. Because the body metabolizes alcohol at a steady rate, when a person drinks faster than the body can metabolize the alcohol, it accumulates in the blood.
- Food in the stomach (especially fatty foods) slows absorption, whereas an empty stomach increases absorption.
- The drinker's emotional state also may affect absorption of alcohol. For example, stress, fear, anger, and fatigue may increase or decrease absorption.

The drinker's body size affects the concentration of alcohol in the blood. The same amount of alcohol ingested by a 100-lb versus a 200-lb person results in greater blood alcohol concentration in the lighter person because the heavier person has more blood volume in which the alcohol is diluted. A person's body chemistry and cultural influences also may alter the behavioral effects of alcohol.

Oxidation, which occurs mainly in the liver, eliminates 90% of the alcohol absorbed by the body. The other 10% are eliminated unchanged through body fluids such as breath, sweat, and urine. The rate of drinking may vary, but the excretion of alcohol from the body remains at a fixed rate. The healthy liver metabolizes about 1 oz of alcohol per hour; the excess alcohol that the liver cannot metabolize continues to circulate in the blood.

Tolerance

Prolonged heavy drinking results in physical and behavioral **tolerance** to alcohol. Physical tolerance, or tissue adaptation, means that changes occur in the cells of the nervous system so that more of the drug is needed to achieve the desired effect. When physical tolerance develops, the person may experience withdrawal or abstinence syndrome after cessation or a decrease in alcohol consumption. Physical tolerance to alcohol never reaches the high-dose tolerance of the opiates. Cross-tolerance to sedative–hypnotics and other CNS depressants also occurs.

Behavioral tolerance to alcohol is manifested by the ability to mask the behavioral effects, for example, the acquired ability not to slur words, to walk straight, and to function in ways that would not be possible in a nondependent person who drinks. The drinking history of alcoholics often reveals the ability to increase tolerance and to maintain this increase for a long time, perhaps several years. Frequently, an irreversible drop in tolerance follows this increased tolerance; the person becomes intoxicated with smaller amounts of alcohol.

Blackout

Persistent, heavy drinking frequently results in the chemically induced alcoholic **blackout**. This is not the same as passing out, which is defined as a loss of consciousness. During a blackout, the person appears to function normally while drinking but later is unable to remember what occurred. The blackout may last a few hours or several hours. The person may come out of the blackout period and wonder, "Where did I leave my car last night?" He or she may wake up in a strange city unable to remember leaving home and wonder, "How did I get here?" or "Was I with someone?" These blackouts may be a symptom of alcohol abuse and dependency.

Alcohol-Induced Disorders

Intoxication. Intoxication occurs after drinking excessive amounts of alcohol and is evidenced in maladaptive behavior such as fighting, impaired judgment, or interference with social or occupational functioning. Physiologic signs, such as slurred speech, incoordination, unsteady gait, nystagmus, and flushed face, may accompany intoxication. Psychological signs also may be observed, such as mood changes, irritability, talkativeness, or impaired attention.

Alcohol Withdrawal. Alcohol withdrawal, also referred to as abstinence syndrome, occurs after a reduction in or a cessation of prolonged heavy drinking. A coarse tremor of hand, tongue, and eyelids may occur, as may nausea and vomiting, general malaise or weakness, autonomic nervous system hyperactivity (eg, increased blood pressure and pulse), anxiety, a depressed or irritable mood, and orthostatic hypotension. Sleep disturbances, insomnia, and nightmares also may occur during withdrawal. Alcohol withdrawal delirium, called **delirium tremens**, is the most serious form of withdrawal syndrome. It occurs after cessation of, or reduction in, prolonged heavy drinking and can occur as long as 1 week after cessation of drinking.

Alcoholic Hallucinosis. Alcoholic hallucinosis usually occurs within 48 hours after cessation of, or a reduction in, drinking. Vivid, perhaps threatening, auditory hallucinations may develop, but clouding of consciousness does not occur. The person's response to the hallucinations typically is anxiety or fear. Auditory hallucinations usually are experienced as voices but may be experienced as hissing or buzzing sounds.

Alcoholic Amnestic Disorder. The alcohol amnestic disorder results from heavy, prolonged drinking and is thought to be related to poor nutrition. If the disorder is related to thiamine deficiency, it is known as **Wernicke-Korsakoff syndrome**. Amnesia consists of impairment in the ability to learn new information (short-term memory) and to recall remote information (long-term memory). Other neurologic signs, such as neuropathy, unsteady gait, or myopathy, may be present.

Alcoholic Dementia. Alcoholic dementia is associated with prolonged, chronic alcohol dependence. Signs of dementia include loss of intellectual ability that is severe enough to interfere with social or occupational functioning and impairment in memory, abstract thinking, and judgment. The degree of impairment may range from mild to severe and may include permanent brain damage.

Medical Consequences of Alcohol Abuse and Dependency

Heavy consumption of alcohol adversely affects most body systems. Various medical conditions may alert the nurse to the early recognition of alcohol abuse problems. Gastrointestinal problems occur as a result of the irritating effects of alcohol on the gastrointestinal tract, resulting in gastritis or gastric ulcers. Acute or chronic pancreatitis may occur. Esophagitis may result from the direct toxic effects of alcohol on the esophageal mucosa, increased acid production in the stomach, or frequent vomiting. Alcohol cardiomyopathy results from the direct toxic effects of the substance and malnutrition.

The liver is highly susceptible to the damaging effects of alcohol because it is the primary organ that metabolizes alcohol. Alcohol is toxic to the liver, regardless of the person's nutritional status. Alcoholic hepatitis is a serious condition involving inflammation and necrosis of the liver cells and sometimes is reversible. Cirrhosis of the liver, the most serious condition, is irreversible. In cirrhosis, the liver cells are destroyed and replaced by scar tissue. About 90% of deaths from cirrhosis of the liver are related to chronic alcoholism (Antai-Otong, 1995). A high risk of cancer, especially of the mouth, pharynx, larynx, esophagus, pancreas, stomach, and colon, is associated with alcoholism.

CONTROLLED SUBSTANCES

Drugs other than alcohol are regulated by the Controlled Substance Act (Title II, Comprehensive Drug Abuse Prevention and Control Act of 1970; Public Law 91-513). This law was implemented to decrease the illegal use and abuse of drugs in the United States. Drugs that are controlled substances and are substances of abuse are categorized into classes, or categories, within which many of the symptoms, side effects, and withdrawal symptoms are similar (see Boxes 27-4 and 27-5). There often is confusion about which drugs belong in which classification because these drugs typically are sorted into different classifications throughout the literature. This chapter uses the *DSM-IV-TR* classifications throughout.

Table 27-1 includes eight major drug categories, examples of each, a description of the drug and its possible effects on the client, symptoms of overdose and withdrawal, and indicators of possible misuse (National Clearinghouse for Alcohol and Drug Information [NCADI], 2001). The table presents the specific drug names under *DSM-IV-TR* categories and also refers to categorizations that are published by the NCADI (2001).

The amphetamines/amphetamine-like drugs (eg, amphetamine, methamphetamine/ifosfamide, carboplatin, etoposide [ICE]), cocaine, and inhalants (eg, butyl nitrite, gasoline, toluene vapors such as in glue) have shared effects on the human body such as their effect on autonomic instability, irritability and anxiety, and loss of coordination and muscle control. Symptoms of overdose for the three categories also are similar, including agitation, hallucinations, and possible convulsions. These drugs often are not associated with a specific profile of "withdrawal symptoms," but their use, even on one occasion, can cause severe effects that can be life threatening. Cannabis (eg, marijuana and hashish) use results in euphoria, impaired cognitive function, disoriented behavior, and decreased appetite; this drug, similar to the hallucinogens, does not have a specific, well-defined withdrawal syndrome either. The hallucinogens (eg, lysergic acid diethylamide [LSD] and club drugs) and phencyclidines (eg, parachlorophenol [PCP] and angel dust) share common effects such as rapid emotional shifts, loss of coordination, irritation to lungs and respiratory system, fatigue, insomnia, and autonomic instability. These drugs can be dangerous because they often are obtained under questionable circumstances with unknown dose ranges and mixtures, such as in the case of "club drugs." The opioids (eg, morphine, codeine, and heroin) are used medicinally to relieve pain, and cause several life-threatening side effects. Withdrawal syndrome with these drugs includes severe cramping, tremors, panic, and chills and often requires medical management through the withdrawal phase. Sedative–hypnotics (eg, barbiturates, methaqualone, and tranquilizers) are used medicinally to relieve anxiety. They cause sensory alterations, relaxation, impaired judgment, and behaviors similar to alcohol intoxication. Withdrawal may be acute with this category of drug and can include autonomic instability, coma, and death; medical management is required. The medical management of withdrawal syndromes with each of these categories of drugs is based on the individual's response to the drug, the dose and type of drug being used, and the unique profile of withdrawal symptoms that occurs with each category of drug.

An enormous amount of information is available about drugs of abuse; therefore, Table 27-1 provides a

TABLE 27-1 ▼ Drug Categories, Names, Effects, and Withdrawal Syndromes for Substances of Abuse				
DRUG CATEGORY	**DRUG NAMES**	**WHAT ARE THEY?**	**POSSIBLE EFFECTS**	**SYMPTOMS OF OVERDOSE**
Amphetamines/ amphetamine-like (also called stimulants)	Amphetamine Benzedrine Benzphetamine Dextroamphetamine Methamphetamine/ ICE	Drugs used to in crease alertness, relieve fatigue, feel stronger and more decisive; used for euphoric effects or to counteract the "down" feeling of alcohol or tran-quilizers	Increases BP, HR, Resp; dilated pupils; decreased appetite; high doses may cause rapid/irregular heart beats, loss of coordination, collapse; may cause perspiration, blurred vision, dizziness, restless-ness, anxiety, delusions	Agitation, increased body tempera-ture, hallucina-tions, convul-sions, possible death
Cocaine (also may be classified as a stimulant or narcotic)	Cocaine	As with ampheta-mines, plus in crease carefree feeling, euphoria, relaxation, and a feeling of being in control	"High" lasts only 5– 20 minutes; may cause severe mood swings and irrita-bility; tolerance develops rapidly; increases BP, HR; one use can cause death	As with amphetamines
Inhalants (also called stimulants)	Butyl nitrite Amyl nitrite (gas in aerosol cans) Gasoline and toluene vapors (correction fluid, glue, marking pens)	Drugs that are used to get a "cheap high," a "quick buzz," and feelings of having fun	As with ampheta-mines, plus loss of muscle control, slurred speech, drowsiness or loss of consciousness, excessive secretions from nose and watery eyes, brain and lung damage	As with amphetamines
Cannabis	Marijuana Tetrahydro-cannabinol Hashish Hashish Oil	Hemp plant from which marijuana and hashish are produced; hashish consists of resinous secretions of the cannabis plant; marijuana is a tobacco-like sub-stance	Euphoria followed by relaxation, loss of appetite, impaired memory, concen-tration, knowledge retention; loss of coordination; more vivid sense of taste, sight, smell, hearing; strong doses cause fluctu-ating emotions, fragmentary thoughts, disori-ented behavior, psychosis; may cause irritation to lungs, respiratory system; may cause cancer	Fatigue, lack of coordination, paranoia, psychosis

(continued)

TABLE 27-1 ▼	**Drug Categories, Names, Effects, and Withdrawal Syndromes for Substances of Abuse** (Continued)			
DRUG CATEGORY	**DRUG NAMES**	**WHAT ARE THEY?**	**POSSIBLE EFFECTS**	**SYMPTOMS OF OVERDOSE**
Hallucinogens	LSD (acid, green/red dragon) Mescaline Peyote Psilocybin Designer drugs (ie, Ecstacy; these are phencyclidine analogs, amphetamine variants)	Drugs that produce behavioral changes that often are multiple and dramatic No known medicinal use; some block pain sensation and using may resut in self-inflicted injuries "Designer drugs" or "club drugs," made to imitate certain illegal drugs, often are significantly stronger than the drugs they imitate	Rapidly changing feelings, immediately and long after use; chronic use may cause persistent problems, depression, violent behavior, anxiety, distorted perception of time Large doses may cause convulsions, coma, heart/lung failure, ruptured blood vessels in brain May cause hallucinations, illusions, dizziness, confusion, suspicion, anxiety, loss of control Delayed effects: "flashbacks" may occur long after use Designer drugs: One use may cause irreversible brain damage	Longer, more intense "trip" episodes, psychosis, coma, death
Phencyclidine/phencyclidine-like (also classified as hallucinogens)	PCP Angel dust Love boat	As with hallucinogens	As with hallucinogens	As with hallucinogens
Opioids (also classified in narcotics)	Opium Morphine Codeine Heroin Hydromorphone Meperidine Methadone	Used medicinally to relieve pain; high potential for abuse; cause relaxation with an immediate "rush"; initial unpleasant effects of restlessness, nausea	Euphoria, drowsiness, respiratory depression, constricted (pinpoint) pupils	Slow, shallow breathing; clammy skin; convulsions; coma; possible death
Sedative-hypnotics (may be classified as depressants) or axiolytics	Barbiturates Methaqualone Tranquilizers Chloral hydrate Glutethimide	Drugs used medicinally to relieve anxiety, irritability, and tension; high potential for abuse, development of tolerance; produce state of intoxication similar to	Sensory alteration, anxiety reduction, intoxication Small amounts cause calmness, relaxation; larger amounts cause slurred speech, impaired judgment,	Shallow respirations, clammy skin, dilated pupils, weak and rapid pulse, coma, death

(continued)

				SYMPTOMS OF
DRUG CATEGORY	DRUG NAMES	WHAT ARE THEY?	POSSIBLE EFFECTS	OVERDOSE
		alcohol; when combined with alcohol, increases effects and multiplies risks	loss of motor coordination; very large doses may cause respiratory depression, coma, death
Newborn babies of abusers may show dependency and withdrawal symptoms, behavioral problems, birth defects	

TABLE 27-1 ▼ Drug Categories, Names, Effects, and Withdrawal Syndromes for Substances of Abuse (Continued)

BP, blood pressure; HR, heart rate; ICE, ifosfamide, carboplatin, etoposide; LSD, lysergic acid diethylamide; PCP, parachlorophenol; Resp, respiration.

focused, concise outline of the categories of drugs of abuse. However, students should make use of the web sites listed at the end of this chapter to gather more detailed information about specific drugs and their physiologic and behavioral affects. Interdisciplinary treatments, nursing assessment, and nursing interventions related to controlled substances are discussed later in this chapter.

Interdisciplinary Treatment

Various types of interdisciplinary treatment programs are available to clients who are addicted to substances. Professional treatment programs include detoxification programs and facilities, inpatient rehabilitation programs, outpatient rehabilitation programs, and private practice physician treatment. Paraprofessional or lay treatment includes programs such as AA, Cocaine Users Anonymous (CA), and NA. These programs are discussed later in Self-Help Groups.

Table 27-2, Phases of Treatment of Alcoholism and Drug Addiction, identifies four phases of treatment for drug and alcohol dependence. These phases need to be considered when treating clients' medical, social, and psychological needs. The client does not always need to enter treatment in this sequence (ie, phase 1 followed by 2, 3, and 4). Some clients may omit a phase; others may skip phases.

MEDICAL DETOXIFICATION FROM ALCOHOL

Most clients can be detoxified from alcohol in 3 to 5 days. The withdrawal time frame should be considered in the context of when the client will need the most support; for alcoholics, this is the second day after the last ingestion of alcohol. Other factors influencing the length of the detox-

ification period include the severity of the dependency and the client's overall heath status. Clients who are medically debilitated detoxify more slowly. Withdrawal needs to be carefully managed. Detoxification protocols have been developed through the Center for Substance Abuse Treatment (CSAT) as a Treatment Improvement Protocol (CSAT, 2001). Immediate goals and principles of detoxification are delineated in Box 27-6.

The American Society of Addiction Medicine has published evidenced-based practice guidelines for the medical treatment of alcohol withdrawal (Mayo-Smith et al., 1997). Benzodiazepines are recommended as first-line agents for alcohol withdrawal. All of the benzodiazepines are equally efficacious in reducing withdrawal signs and symptoms. Compared with nonbenzodiazepine sedative–hypnotics, they have better overall documented efficacy, a greater margin for safety, and lower abuse potential. The benzodiazepines reduce withdrawal severity, reduce the incidence of delirium, and reduce seizures. The choice of benzodiazepine is guided by the following:

- Long-acting agents may be more effective in preventing seizures during withdrawal.
- Long-acting agents may contribute to a smoother withdrawal with fewer rebound symptoms.
- Short-acting agents may have a lower risk of over sedation.
- Certain benzodiazepines carry a higher risk for abuse.
- The cost of benzodiazepines varies significantly.

β-Blockers, clonidine, and carbamazepine ameliorate withdrawal severity, but there is inadequate evidence to determine their effect on delirium and seizures. Phenothiazines ameliorate withdrawal symptoms but are less effective than benzodiazepines in reducing delirium. These

TABLE 27-2 ▼ Phases of Treatment for Alcoholism and Drug Addiction

PHASE OF TREATMENT	TYPICAL PROBLEMS	POSSIBLE SOLUTIONS
Phase 1 (acute crisis)	Biomedical: gastrointestinal bleeding (eg, alcohol); angina (eg, cocaine); coma (eg, opioids)	Appropriate medical intervention, which may include hospitalization
	Psychologic: hallucinosis (eg, alcohol, LSD, or stimulants); paranoia (eg, PCP, marijuana stimulants, alcohol); suicidal ideation (eg, stimulants, alcohol, LSD)	Appropriate psychiatric intervention, which may include hospitalization
	Social: family violence (eg, alcohol, stimulants, PCP)	Appropriate psychiatric intervention, which may include hospitalization, family therapy, home visit, domestic violence counseling
Phase 2 (withdrawal from substance abuse)	Biomedical: impending delirium tremens (eg, alcohol); impending seizures (eg, benzodiazepines); impending gastric distress (eg, opioids)	Medical or social model detoxification; outpatient detoxification; appropriate medical intervention
	Psychologic: denial, worry about health; stressful life events	Counseling; brief individual or group therapy; AA/NA/CA
	Social: inadequate food and shelter, financial problems	Counseling; social services referral
Phase 3 (sequelae of substance abuse)	Biomedical: chronic medical problems; malnutrition	Appropriate medical intervention; vitamin supplements, proper diet, and exercise; disulfiram (alcohol); methadone (opioid); naltrexone (opioid)
	Psychologic: denial, depression; guilt stressful life events; craving for alcohol or drugs	Counseling; brief individual or group therapy; antidepressants; behavior modification techniques
	Social: family, housing, vocational, and legal problems; loneliness; unfilled leisure time	Counseling; social services referral; family therapy; recreational therapy; AA/NA/CA, Al-Anon or Alateen; halfway house
Phase 4	Biomedical: genetic factors	Counseling
	Psychologic: neurotic and personality disorders; major affective disorders; schizophrenia	Long-term group therapy; antidepressants; major tranquilizers; therapeutic communities; individual therapy
	Social: sociocultural and familial influences	Counseling

From Clark, H. W., Kanas, N., Smith, D., & Landry, M. (1995). Substance-related disorders: Alcohol and drugs. In H. Goldman (Ed.), *Review of general psychiatry* (4th ed.). Norwalk, CT: Appleton & Lange.

medications may be used as adjunctive therapy but are not recommended as monotherapy for withdrawal.

Dose determinations for alcohol withdrawal must be made on an individualized basis so that clients can receive large amounts of medications rapidly if needed. Providing only a fixed standardized dose for all clients cannot adequately treat alcohol withdrawal. Specific clinical considerations that drive the choice of medication dosage in alcohol withdrawal may be found in the evidence-based practice guidelines (Mayo-Smith et al., 1997).

Individualizing therapy with withdrawal scales (eg, Clinical Institute Withdrawal Assessment—Alcohol, revised [CIWA-AR]) leads to significantly less medication use and shorter treatment. For treatment based on symptom monitoring, suggested regimens include administering one of the following medications every hour when the CIWA-AR is greater than, or equal to, 8 to 10:

Chlordiazepoxide, 50 to 100 mg
Diazepam, 10 to 20 mg
Lorazepam, 2 to 4 mg

For fixed-schedule regimens, one of the following medications may be given:

BOX 27-6 ▼ *Center for Substance Abuse Treatment Improvement Protocol for Detoxification*

Immediate Goals of Detoxification

- To provide a safe withdrawal from the drug(s) of dependence and enable the client to become drug free
- To provide withdrawal that is humane and protects the client's dignity
- To prepare the client for ongoing treatment for dependence on alcohol or other drugs of abuse

Principles of Detoxification

- Detoxification alone rarely is adequate treatment for substance dependencies.
- When using medication regimens or other detoxification procedures, clinicians should only use protocols of established safety and efficacy.
- Providers must advise clients when procedures are used that have not been established as safe and effective.

- During detoxification, providers should control clients' access to medication to the greatest extent possible.
- Initiation of withdrawal should be individualized.
- Whenever possible, clinicians should substitute a long-acting medication for short-acting drugs of addiction.
- The intensity of withdrawal cannot always be predicted accurately.
- Every means possible should be used to ameliorate the client's signs and symptoms of substance withdrawal.
- Clients should begin participating as soon as possible in follow-up support therapy such as peer group therapy, family therapy, individual counseling or therapy, 12-step recovery meetings, and drug recovery educational programs.

Chlordiazepoxide, 50 mg every 6 hours for four doses, then 25 mg every 6 hours for eight doses
Diazepam, 10 mg every 6 hours for four doses, then 5 mg every 6 hours for eight doses
Lorazepam, 2 mg every 6 hours for four doses, then 1 mg every 6 hours for eight doses

When symptoms are not controlled with these regimens, additional medication can be provided when needed (Mayo-Smith et al., 1997).

THE REHABILITATION PROCESS

The rehabilitation process usually focuses on the substance abuse or dependency disorder. Other problems encountered by the client, such as loss of job, marital conflicts, and legal problems, often result from the drug or alcohol abuse. Consequently, the client does not benefit from resolving these problems if the drug dependency continues. Conversely, many problems that stem directly from the drug use, such as physical illness or family or legal problems, diminish with rehabilitation and continued abstinence. Other significant problems, emotional and social, are treated concurrently with the substance abuse or dependency disorder.

The rehabilitation program usually involves detoxification, the restoring of physical and emotional stability, intervention methods to increase motivation to continue in treatment, confronting pathologic defenses, methods to increase self-esteem, facilitation of insight into problem areas, planning for discharge, and follow-up care. Table 27-3 lists commonly used interdisciplinary interventions and some important points regarding each.

An important aspect of any rehabilitation program is for the client to accept responsibility for their drug

abuse–dependency and to take needed actions toward their own recovery. Underlying the goal of discontinuing the substance abuse and maintaining abstinence is a change of the individual's behavior that will lead to a personal lifestyle of greater personal enrichment.

MEDICATIONS USED TO TREAT DRUG DEPENDENCY

Several medications currently are used to treat drug dependency. Table 27-4 lists medications, treatment mechanisms, and responses to the particular treatment. New medication treatments are being developed continuously, so it is important to seek updated information. The SAMSHA website (at end of this chapter) is an excellent resource for updated materials such as new psychotropic treatments for chemical and drug dependency.

One example of using medications to treat drug dependency is the methadone maintenance program. This program is useful for people who are dependent on opiates; it is used in conjunction with other treatment methods and is not a cure. Methadone is a long-acting narcotic that is substituted for the shorter acting opiates such as heroin. It has similar pharmacologic properties as heroin, including addiction, sedation, and respiratory depression. It blocks the euphoric effects of heroin and other opiates, thereby preventing the impulsive use of heroin (McGonagle, 1994). Methadone is administered in licensed clinics established to control its distribution and prevent its diversion for illegal use.

SELF-HELP GROUPS

The first, and perhaps most influential, of substance abuse self-help groups is AA. Two men—Dr. Bob, a surgeon, and Bill W., a New York stockbroker—founded this self-

TABLE 27-3 ▼ Selected Interdisciplinary Interventions in Treatment of Substance Abuse

INTERVENTION	DESCRIPTION AND TECHNIQUES
Breaking through defenses	The breakdown of the pathologic defense mechanisms manifested in the denial system is a gradual process. The care professional must recognize and understand the client's defensive maneuver; assist the client to come face to face with the objective reality that is being denied; maintain a consistent, persistent approach with the client, which conveys the message that there never is a valid reason for the client to use drugs or alcohol; refocus the client on the substance dependence problem and not become sidetracked around other problems.
Understanding and accepting the disorder	Assist the client who is dependent on substances to attain an intellectual comprehension of the disorder; disorders are illnesses, not mental problems; provide educational materials and clarification of misinformation; understanding the disease in an intellectual, factual manner helps client to accept the fact that the disorder is chronic and cannot be cured; disorder must be accepted on an emotional level and recover on a long-term, day-to-day basis; abstinence is a prerequisite to recovery.
Identification with peers	Peer group identification and confrontation are powerful in recovery. Assist clients to recognize and internalize that they are not alone in their suffering and that they can receive support and hope. Groups also allow for confrontation by peers who attack pathologic defense mechanisms and help each other in the process of obtaining insight into their behaviors.
Development of hope	Initial feelings of clients often include hopelessness, discouragement, and demoralization. The client needs to realize that it is possible to escape from what may be seen as a hopeless situation. Identifying with others who are going through recovery is significant in providing hope. Positive attitudes of caregivers also instill hope.
Resocialization	The pursuit of the addictive substance often causes the user's life to become drug-centered, and the client becomes self-centered. Social skills may be minimal to lacking. Assist the client to review and rebuild the capacity for establishing interpersonal relationship that the previously self-centered attitude has eroded.
Developing self-esteem and self-worth	Self-esteem and self-worth increase as the client is able to see the substance abuse problem as an illness. The client can be helped by taking responsibility for making changes in attitudes and actions and for getting satisfaction from achievements and relationships. Client also often needs help in developing self-discipline, such as organizing and adhering to a daily routine. Encourage positive efforts to change. Motivation is enhanced as involvement in the program increases.

help program in 1935. At the time, these men were unable to get help with their alcoholism. They found that by sharing their life experiences with each other and by identifying with each other in their common problems with alcohol, they were able to overcome their compulsion to drink. AA is a program that functions with a "12-step" model (Box 27-7).

Several programs now are based on the 12-step model, including Al-Anon (for families of substance abusers), Alateen (for teenagers who have a substance abuser in their life), NA (for narcotic abusers), CA (for cocaine abusers), and Adult Children of Alcoholics (ACOA). A first-hand account of a daughter with a father who is an alcoholic is presented in Box 27-8.

TABLE 27-4 ▼ Medications to Treat Substance Abuse Disorders

MEDICATION	PRIMARY THERAPEUTIC CATEGORY	DRUG ADDICTION TREATMENT MECHANISM	RESPONSE
For Cocaine			
desipramine (Norpramin, others)	Antidepressant	Counters decreased norepinephrine transmission by blocking its reuptake	Decrease craving during withdrawal
bromocriptine (Parlodel)	Dopamine receptor agonist for hyperprolactinemia	Counters decreased dopamine transmission by directly activating receptors	Decrease craving during withdrawal
amantadine (Symmetrel, others)	Antiparkinson	Counters dopamine depletion by releasing stored reserves	Decrease craving during withdrawal
phenylalanine and tyrosine	Amino acids; neurotransmitter precursors	Replete neurotransmitters, norepinephrine and dopamine	Decrease craving during withdrawal
For Narcotics			
methadone (Dolophine, others)	Narcotic analgesic	Substitutes for heroin at narcotic receptors	Less euphoria, less frequent dosing, and not injectable
clonidine (Catapres, others)	Antihypertensive	Inhibits central neural norepinephrine activity	Decrease discomfort during withdrawal
naltrexone (Trexan)	Narcotic antagonist	Blocks response to narcotics by binding to the receptors	No euphoria from consumed narcotics
For Alcohol			
disulfiram (Antabuse)	Interacts with alcohol	Interferes with alcohol metabolism	Distressing reaction to consumed alcohol
diazepam (Valium, others)	Antianxiety	Substitutes for alcohol depressant effects on central nervous system	Reduce symptoms of withdrawal

From Bender, K. (1990). *Psychiatric medications.* Newbury Park, CA: Sage Publications. Used with permission.

APPLICATION OF THE NURSING PROCESS TO THE CLIENT WITH A SUBSTANCE-RELATED DISORDER

The discussion of the use of the nursing process with clients who have substance abuse dependency and disorders focuses on psychological treatment that begins in the early stages of recovery and continues over time. Although the issue of rehabilitation is addressed in relation to psychiatric inpatient settings, nurses encounter problems of substance abuse and dependence in all areas of nursing.

Assessment

Nursing assessment of clients with substance abuse disorders focuses on assessment of physical status and psychosocial circumstances. Sometimes, there is a strong clinical suspicion of drug or alcohol use, but the client has not admitted to the problem. In that case, a screening tool is helpful in identifying clients with a probable abuse problem. The CAGE questionnaire is easy to administer and is included in general assessments in many areas of the inpatient hospital. The nurse asks four questions; a "yes" to any one of them indicates the need for further workup and referral (Box 27-9).

BOX 27-7 ▼ The 12 Steps of Alcoholics Anonymous

1. Admitted we were powerless over alcohol—that our lives had become unmanageable
2. Came to believe that a Power greater than ourselves could restore us to sanity
3. Made a decision to turn our will and our lives over to the care of God as we understood Him
4. Made a searching and fearless moral inventory of ourselves
5. Admitted to God, to ourselves, and to another human being the exact nature of our wrongs
6. Were entirely ready to have God remove all these defects of character
7. Humbly asked Him to remove our short-comings

8. Made a list of all persons we had harmed, and became willing to make amends to them all
9. Made direct amends to such people wherever possible except when to do so would injure them or others
10. Continued to take a personal inventory, and when we were wrong, promptly admitted it
11. Sought through prayer and meditation to improve our conscious contact with God as we understood Him, praying only for knowledge of His will for us and the power to carry that out
12. Having had a spiritual awakening as the result of these steps, we tried to carry this message to alcoholics and to practice these principles in all our affairs

BOX 27-8 ▼ The Al-Anon Family: A Daughter's Letter

The greatest fault of all is to be conscious of none.
—*Thomas Carlyle*

Dear Friends,

Your faces are not known to me, yet I know we share the same burden, because in our humanity, we share the same struggle to come to wholeness, to know, accept, and appreciate who we are, to take responsibility for our lives, and no matter what our calling is, to conduct our lives in such a way as to be a beacon of light.

Many years ago in search of a way to "save" my father from the scourge of alcoholism, I was introduced to the Twelve Steps of Alcoholics Anonymous through the Al-Anon program, a self-help support group for families and friends of alcoholics. In Al-Anon, I became conscious of my own weaknesses and shortcomings and experienced the humility to accept the fact that I was powerless over alcohol, that I could not make my father well or make well my husband who, I recognized from the knowledge and insight gained from the Al-Anon group, was in the early stages of alcoholism.

In Al-Anon I learned that the effects of alcoholism are pervasive; the entire family suffers; I learned that because of my Joan of Arc efforts to make things right, my continual failure to do so, my moldering sense of self-esteem in light of constant defeat, criticism, and confusion that I had become as sick as the alcoholic and that my life had become unmanageable. I came to believe that a Power greater than myself could restore me to sanity. I made a decision to turn my will and my life over to the care of God as I understood Him and in so doing embraced the Twelve-Step program.

Working the Twelve Steps, the constitution of all anonymous self-help groups, is not easy. It requires honesty and humility; it requires a commitment to grow in wholeness, to stay on the journey no matter what, and to trust that if we are faithful God will lead us to wellness, and to the peace and joy that comes when we accept the challenge "to grow," to take responsibility for our lives, and diligently work toward becoming the person we were created to be.

Growth requires change; it is often slow and sometimes painful; like the butterfly, we must gain strength from the struggle. The wisdom of the Al-Anon program, along with the dynamic interaction that happens in the honest and caring environment of a support group, has helped to give me the strength and the courage to undergo my own metamorphosis. Slowly I began to see that we change, our situation changes, as we become integrated, we become more secure and more loving and experience an inner harmony that affects all of our relationships. The family is the primary recipient of this blessed change in us.

Today there is more awareness than ever concerning alcoholism. What was once thought to be a disgrace is now known to be a disease, a disease of body, mind, and spirit. Tragically, my father died never knowing the serenity that can be found in Alcoholics Anonymous. Spiritually my husband was "reborn" and came to serenity through Alcoholics Anonymous. We have choices! Our choices make a difference!

Gratefully, JoAnn

BOX 27-9 ▼ *The CAGE Questionnaire for Substance Abuse Screening*

- Have you ever felt you should *C*ut down on your drinking?
- Have people *A*nnoyed you by criticizing your drinking?
- Have you ever felt bad or *G*uilty about your drinking?
- Have you ever had a drink (or *E*ye-opener) first thing in the morning to steady your nerves or to get rid of a hangover?

From Ewing, J. A. (1984). Detecting alcoholism: The CAGE questionnaire. *Journal of the American Medical Association, 252,* 1902–1907.

PHYSICAL EXAMINATION

For a client with a known substance abuse problem, the first hours and days of treatment involve assessing for withdrawal signs and symptoms. Abrupt cessation of a drug that has been used chronically and to which tolerance and dependence has been established may cause life-threatening withdrawal symptoms. Withdrawal is characterized initially by irritability, strong urges to use the drug of choice, and elevation in heart rate and blood pressure. For a guide to specific assessments and signs and symptoms of withdrawal based on drug category, refer to Table 27-1.

The client also should undergo an evaluation of baseline health status, including a physical examination, liver function studies, and possibly other diagnostic tests, depending on the preliminary findings. Because substance abuse is a risk factor for acquiring sexually transmitted diseases, including infection with HIV, the client also may undergo examination and testing for these disorders.

PSYCHOSOCIAL ASSESSMENT

The focus of the psychosocial assessment is to determine to what extent the addiction to alcohol, drugs, or both has disrupted family, social, and work relationships and to identify both resources for support and problem areas or relationships that may undermine treatment and recovery. For example, an alcoholic client whose job is tending bar will be confronted with powerful inducements to drink, and the treatment team will need to aggressively help the client manage this problem. Other potential problems might be the client whose spouse is abusing drugs or alcohol or for some reason does not support the treatment process. A thorough psychosocial assessment will identify these problems so that they may be confronted. See Box 27-10 for information about other assessment data concerning physiologic status, mental status, types and patterns of drug or alcohol use, and social information.

Nursing Diagnosis

Because of the wide range of physical and emotional needs of clients with substance abuse disorders, many nursing diagnoses apply. The following sections discuss several priority nursing diagnoses applicable to the initial and ongoing psychosocial recovery from substances:

- **Risk for Injury** related to substance withdrawal
- **Ineffective Denial** related to dysfunctional defense mechanisms associated with substance abuse
- **Anxiety** related to sudden loss of maladaptive coping strategy (drug or alcohol use)
- **Ineffective Coping** related to dysfunctional behavior patterns secondary to substance abuse
- **Dysfunctional Family Processes: Alcoholism** related to substance abuse
- **Chronic Low Self-Esteem** related to doubts and anxiety about self-worth and abilities
- **Risk for Spiritual Distress** related to history of substance abuse
- **Deficient Diversional Activity** related to loss of primary activity (substance abuse)

Planning

The goals for the client recovering from substance abuse touch every aspect of the client's life and vary according to the stage of recovery. Some goals for the early stages of recovery include the following:

- The client's withdrawal from substance of abuse will be managed successfully.
- The client will acknowledge alcohol or drug dependence and the need for treatment.
- The client will be able to identify and implement strategies for managing anxiety without using substances.
- The client will begin to develop adaptive coping strategies and will use them to manage stressors.
- The client will begin to rebuild damaged interpersonal and work relationships.
- The client will identify positive aspects of self.
- The client will develop alternative activities to replace time spent acquiring, using, or recovering from substance abuse.

See Nursing Care Plan 27-1.

Implementation

MAINTAINING SAFETY

The nursing role is a critical element of the inpatient treatment of detoxification from withdrawal and delirium; nurses often play a key role in assisting clients through this potentially life-threatening experience. Detoxification is

BOX 27-10 ▼ *Assessment Guidelines for the Client Who Is Abusing Substances*

Demographic data:
Name:
Age:
Sex:
Ethnic group:
Marital status:
Religious affiliation:
Significant other:

What is the reason for coming to the hospital (eg, symptoms of withdrawal, marital-family crisis, work problems, referred by legal source, wants to help to stop drinking or using drugs, medical problems)?

What is the motivation for treatment:
General observations:

Vital signs:	Blood pressure (hypotensive, hypertensive)
Pulse:	Rapid, regular, irregular
Temperature:	Elevated
Respirations:	Rapid, shallow, depressed
Appearance:	
Gait:	Unsteady, normal, weaving, shuffling
Eyes:	Conjunctival injection, bloodshot, dilated, pinpoint, normal pupils, lacrimation (tearing), vacant stare, poor eye contact, good eye contact
Skin:	Perspiration, cool, clammy, dry, bruises, needle tracks, scars, abrasions, gooseflesh, excoriations, reddened palms
Nose:	Running (rhinorrhea), congested, red
Presence of tremors:	Fine or coarse, slight-moderate or severe
Grooming:	Neat, unkempt, unshaven, odor (alcohol, foul)
Behavior:	
Speech:	Slurred, incoherent, loud, soft, normal, articulates clearly, monotone, hesitant, pressured, relevant, distractive
Attitude:	Quiet, calm, demanding, agitated, irritable, impatient, vague, withdrawn, suspicious, anxious, tearful, happy, silly
Dominant mood—Affect:	Euphoric, depressed, angry, sad, appropriate, inappropriate, normal
Sensorium:	Orientation to time, person, place; changes in memory
Perception:	The presence of illusions, hallucinations, delusions, hallucinosis
Potential for suicide:	Is the individual presently thinking about suicide? Is there a plan or a method to carry out that plan? Is there a history of previous suicide attempts or gestures? Were attempts in intoxicated state or sober state? Is there a family history of suicide? Is there a recent loss or anniversary of a loss? (Assess need for emergency consultation and intervention.)
Potential for violence:	Dose behavior indicate potential for violence (voice, manner, stance, verbal threats)? Assess need for consultation, emergency intervention if necessary. Ask if individual has a history of violence when taking substances or during withdrawal period.
Present drug history:	The areas that need specific assessment are the type of substance used, the amount taken, and the pattern of use.
Type:	Beer, wine, whiskey, cocaine, heroin, marijuana (cannabis), sedative-hypnotics, hallucinogens; one substance only, or a combination? This may mean combination within a class (ie, alcohol, beer, whiskey, and wine, or alcohol and sedative-hypnotics). It may be combinations in different classes (ie, heroin and alcohol and stimulants or narcotics and sedative-hypnotics). What is the predominant substance of choice? Does the individual use street drugs, prescription drugs?
Amount:	How much (approximate amount) does the individual drink? How many six packs, quarts, fifths? How much does he or she use, bags? What route (oral, intravenous, subcutaneous)? How many pills or hits daily?
Pattern of use:	Does drinking occur daily, several times a week? Is it increased on weekends or only occur weekends? Do binge or episodic drinking or runs occur? Is he or she intoxicated daily? Has individual ever tried to control or cut down drinking or substance use? How?

(continued)

BOX 27-10 ▼ *Assessment Guidelines for the Client Who Is Abusing Substances* (continued)

When was last drink?

When was last drug dose? How was it taken?

What drugs are currently being taken?

Has individual developed tolerance? (explain)

When did it begin?

Has there been a change in tolerance?

Are withdrawal symptoms present?

Is there a history of withdrawal?

Is there a history of seizures?

Is there a history of hallucinations? (explain)

Is there a history of hallucinosis?

Was individual ever hospitalized? If yes, for what?

Are there any present medical problems?

Are there any chronic medical problems?

Is there a history of the following: liver disease, hepatitis, diabetes, heart disease, anemia, drug overdose?

Have there been any recent falls, injuries, accidents?

Is the individual taking any prescribed medications?

Has the individual any known allergies?

Drug history:

Has the individual ever stopped drinking or using drugs?

How long was the period of abstinence?

Why did the individual abstain; what was the motivation?

At what age did the individual start abusing or using substances?

At what age did the individual first begin having difficulty in life circumstances due to drug intake?

Has the individual ever been in treatment for drug abuse or dependency?

What type of treatment: detoxification, rehabilitation?

How many times in treatment for the above?

Is there a family history of alcohol abuse or dependency?

Is there a family history of other substance abuse or dependency?

Psychosocial history:

Conjugal:	Married, separated, divorced, never married, widowed? What is spouse's reaction to client's abuse of substances? Does the spouse abuse substances? Is substance use causing marital conflicts?
Parenting:	Are there children? How many, ages, and sex? Have children had school problems, health problems, or physical, emotional, sleeping problems?
Intrapersonal:	What are the individual's leisure activities, hobbies? Has there been a change in participation in these activities? Has there been a change in friends or a loss of friendships? Do the social activities center on the substance use or abuse?
Occupation/employment:	What is individual's occupation and present employment? How long in present employment? Has the individual ever missed work from alcohol or drug use? Has the individual abused substances while working? Is substance use jeopardizing work or business? How long has individual been employed?
Finances and living conditions:	Approximate amount spent on substances. Source of income other than employment. Is the family suffering from less adequate housing or food due to substance abuse or purchases? What are present living conditions? Is individual living alone, in an apartment, own house, room; is there no address or no permanent living arrangement?
Legal problems:	Have there been any violations while intoxicated? Are any present legal offenses pending from substance abuse or dependency? Is present treatment court recommended?

Nursing Care Plan 27-1

THE CLIENT WITH ALCOHOLISM

During the admission interview, Eric verbalizes his need for treatment and has been able to discuss the increasingly negative impact that alcohol is having in his life. Eric reveals that he has been drinking a fifth of vodka per day in addition to several beers. The nurse checks the results of blood alcohol level that was drawn earlier in the day and finds it to be 0.05. Eric states that his last drink was 27 hours earlier at 7 PM. The nurse performs a physical examination, which reveals that Eric is underweight and deconditioned and has gum disease. The nurse also interviews Eric and his wife, Amanda, to obtain the psychosocial history. After the interview and examination, the nurse, Eric, and his wife identify problems and a plan of care.

Nursing Diagnosis: Risk for Injury related to impending alcohol withdrawal

Goals: The client's withdrawal from alcohol will be managed successfully.

Interventions	Rationales
Assess the client for signs and symptoms of impending withdrawal such as tachycardia, hypertension, tremors, anxiety, sweating, hallucinations, and psychomotor agitation.	Monitoring for the onset of symptoms allows for timely intervention.
Administer sedatives as ordered to control withdrawal symptoms.	Sedatives control the exaggerated sympathetic activity associated with withdrawal.
Continue frequent monitoring of vital signs, sensorium, and other variables. Report worsening of condition immediately.	Preventing alcohol withdrawal delirium is critical because of the associated mortality rate. Immediate intervention is required if Eric shows signs of delirium.

Evaluation: The plan of care can be evaluated using the following indicators:

- Alcohol withdrawal was recognized and treatment initiated promptly.
- The client experienced minimal discomfort related to alcohol withdrawal.
- Progression to alcohol withdrawal delirium was prevented or recognized and treated promptly.

Nursing Diagnosis: Ineffective Health Maintenance related to alcohol abuse as evidenced by poor state of health

Goals: The client will be well nourished and adopt health-seeking behaviors.

Interventions	Rationales
Provide vitamin and mineral supplements. Encourage consumption of well-balanced meals with minimal amounts of refined sugars and caffeine.	Alcohol depletes the body of essential nutrients, which must be replaced. Refraining from using caffeine or eating sugary foods can help manage anxiety and mood swings.
Arrange for dental care.	Gum disease places a burden on the immune system.
Encourage a physical exercise program.	Engaging in physical exercise increases stamina, helps balance mood, and aids in managing anxiety.

Nursing Diagnosis: Dysfunctional Family Processes: Alcoholism related to long-standing alcohol abuse

Goals: The family will demonstrate balanced and adaptive family functional and mature interpersonal relationships.

Interventions	Rationales
Teach family members effective communication skills and assertiveness.	Behavior that respects the rights and feelings of others leads to increased trust and intimacy.

(continued)

Nursing Care Plan 27-1 (Continued)

Interventions	Rationales
Help family members to clarify what they want, expect, and need from each other. Explore these topics to arrive at a means by which each member can support and meet the needs of the other. Help clients to recognize excessive dependency needs or unrealistic expectations.	Self-awareness and insight into others improves relationships.
Help clients explore appropriate expression of anger or other negative emotion. Teach problem-solving skills and conflict-management techniques.	Providing Eric and Amanda with new tools for interaction will help them abandon older, less functional behaviors.
Encourage client to assume functional parenting roles. Explore potential problems such as power struggles that may arise as client becomes more functional.	Amanda has been the responsible partner for many years. Although she may welcome Eric's sobriety and involvement, it represents a change in her role, which may be difficult for her.

Evaluation: The plan of care has been effective if Eric and Amanda demonstrate mature, respectful communication with each, collaboratively manage the functions of the family, handle conflict effectively, and support each other.

---

stressful and dangerous for the client. Alcohol withdrawal delirium can be a life-threatening emergency if not treated appropriately. Alcohol withdrawal occurs 24 to 48 hours after the last ingestion of alcohol, so clients should be placed on frequent observation for signs and symptoms of withdrawal on admission. Nursing care of the client experiencing withdrawal centers on safety first. The nurse must implement frequent vital sign assessment, seizure precautions, and fall precautions to ensure the client's safety. Close observation is critical. Monitoring symptoms and management over time provides data with which to implement and continue appropriate medication management.

Clients may experience hallucinations or illusions during withdrawal, which cause extreme anxiety. Phenothiazines may be helpful in ameliorating these symptoms. Speaking in a low, calm, reassuring voice assists the client to be relaxed. Reassurance of safety is important. Creating a comfortable, quiet, unthreatening environment assists the client by reducing anxiety-provoking stimuli.

BREAKING THROUGH DENIAL

Denial is a subconscious process that protects us from confronting painful or threatening realities. It can, in small doses, be helpful. For the substance abuser, however, denial of the problem is an impediment to recovery to the extent that there will be no recovery unless the client can first admit that he or she has a problem. Therefore, clients who are compelled to seek treatment by family, friends, employers, or the judicial system may be expected to be in denial about their problem. Even clients who seek treatment voluntarily have some degree of denial.

Denial may be obvious, for example, when the client denies having a problem outright. Denial may be subtler, and clients may make remarks such as, "Well, I drink a lot, but I've never been in trouble from it," or "I don't drink as much as my friends do"; or, they may minimize the amount of drugs or alcohol they typically use. People are not aware of being in denial; denial is not lying. Denial arises out of fear and a subconscious need to preserve the ego. When used to defend addictions, it is pathologic and perpetuates the addiction.

The nurse can begin to help the client relinquish denial first by establishing a relationship built on trust. Treating the client respectfully, maintaining a nonjudgmental attitude, and examining one's own attitudes toward substance abusers are critical components of care. To confront denial, the nurse can point to the evidence of severe dysfunction that inevitably appears in the substance abusers life. Job losses, financial problems, possible estrangement from family and friends, and legal problems are common, and the client can be respectfully but firmly reminded that many of these problems are a result of alcohol or drug abuse. For example, an alcoholic client may state that drinking excessively was related to job pressures. Instead of sympathizing with this rationalization, the nurse should point out that drinking excessively probably contributed to job performance difficulties.

Another approach to confronting denial includes educating clients about substance abuse as a disease. Accepting the disease concept rather than seeing substance abuse as a character flaw can alleviate the client's feelings of guilt and weakness and lessen the need for denial. Attending meetings for a 12-step program reinforces the disease concept of substance abuse and also helps the client relinquish denial as he or she hears the stories and comments of others who already have begun their recovery.

The nurse also can encourage clients to try consciously to have an open mind about the feedback provided by staff and others and to ask themselves the following questions when they find themselves challenging counselors or loved ones about their condition:

- Am I feeling defensive? What is it that is threatening to me?
- What will I lose if I accept their viewpoint?
- Why is this important to me?
- Have other people I trust said this to me?
- Is it possible that what they have said is true?

The nurse then can encourage the client to speak openly about the answers to these questions. An internal dialogue, that is, asking and answering the questions to oneself, may result in more rationalization and denial, but speaking openly with others will help expose the maladaptive thinking patterns and illogic that accompany addictive thinking. The nurse should bear in mind that breaking through these entrenched thinking patterns takes time. See Therapeutic Communication 27-1 for an example of effective communication about denial.

MANAGING ANXIETY

To the substance abuser, the drug of choice was the solution to all uncomfortable feelings. Anger, sadness, anxiety, frustration, and rejection were "managed" by substance abuse. When the client begins recovery, he or she may begin to experience these emotions unadulterated by mood altering substances. Not being able to "medicate" away these feelings and the meagerness of their coping skills secondary to the dysfunctional patterns that develop as a consequence of substance abuse leaves the newly sober client with anxiety and emotional discomfort. If these feelings become overwhelming, the client is at risk for drinking or using drugs. The nurse can encourage the client to learn stress management techniques such as aerobic activity, meditation, deep breathing or relaxation exercises, or talking with a staff member, friend or other recovering person.

TEACHING EFFECTIVE COPING STRATEGIES

We all use coping strategies to help manage stressful situations. Some of these are immature or maladaptive such as repressing uncomfortable feelings, blaming others, or avoiding stressful situations. The substance abuser typically has used similar maladaptive, immature coping strategies, particularly pathologic denial, projection, acting out, or complete avoidance. To experience recovery and personal growth, these coping strategies must be replaced by more mature ones.

The nurse can help in this process by teaching the client cognitive restructuring techniques. By reappraising a situation in a less ego-threatening way, the need to overly defend oneself is diminished. For example, a client may state that there always are problems during big family get-togethers because his father-in-law doesn't approve of him

and thinks his daughter married poorly. In the past, the client reacted by drinking heavily, treating his wife rudely, and leaving early. In cognitive restructuring, the client would be taught to become aware of the self-talk such as, "He thinks I'm a failure," or "I'll never be as good as his son," which is contributing to the situation. The client can be taught to stop these thoughts and replace them with more positive statements. The nurse can reinforce this concept by suggesting the client ask himself or herself the following questions when in a stressful situation:

- What assertive, positive action can I take to modify the situation so that it is less stressful to me?
- How can I look at this differently?
- What could I say to myself that would be more positive?
- Are others around me being negative? What can I do to avoid being affected by them?
- Are my expectations too high for this person or situation? What is more realistic?
- Am I blaming someone else for my problems?
- What can I do to take responsibility for my feelings and myself?

IMPROVING FAMILY PROCESSES

All members of the substance abuser's family are affected by the addiction. Often, one member, usually the spouse, may be referred to as an enabler or codependent. Generally, this refers to a pattern of behavior, sometimes described as "controlling" or over-responsible, which has arisen in response to the stress and self-perpetuating crises associated with the addict's or alcoholic's substance abuse. In addition to a host of personally self-defeating behaviors (feeling responsible for the client's substance abuse, living a life "walking on eggshells," and assuming many of the substance abusers responsibilities), the codependent functions as a rescuer, covering up for the substance abuser, making excuses, and taking the blame for missed appointments, absences, or failed responsibility. The net effect of this rescuing behavior is to enable the addiction to continue because it protects the substance abuser from feeling the full consequences of his or her behavior. The codependent family member also needs the attention of staff and counselors to learn to adjust to the sober spouse and to develop a less vigilant, more interdependent relationship. The nurse can recommend that family members begin their own recovery by attending support groups such as Al-Anon or Alateen.

ENHANCING SELF-ESTEEM

Whereas each client comes into recovery with a different personality and psychosocial history, the self-esteem of the newly recovering substance abuser may be low because he or she can no longer hide from the devastation caused by the substance abuse and related behaviors. Guilt, shame, embarrassment, and despair over current circumstances are common feelings experienced by substance abusers in the

THERAPEUTIC COMMUNICATION 27-1
A Cocaine Abuser in Denial

Tom, a 35-year-old black man, was admitted 2 weeks ago to the inpatient psychiatric hospital's substance abuse floor for assessment, stabilization, and referral for cocaine use after an automobile accident in which he ran off the road and hit a child, who later died. Tom has had no symptoms of withdrawal and stated that his most recent cocaine use occurred 2 days before his admission. The nurse has been working with Tom in several groups since his arrival to the unit and have observed that his level of denial is high regarding the circumstances under which he was admitted (eg, he has expressed no feelings about the child who was killed), about the extent of his cocaine use, or about the many problems that this drug dependency is creating in his everyday life.

Ineffective Dialogue

Tom: "Like I've said before, the cocaine was just a way to keep me occupied. It hasn't really caused any major problems for me."

Nurse: "Oh, I see. You use it just for, sort of, recreation? Just to keep your mind off other things? How does it help do that?" *(Nurse is reinforcing his denial through nonconfrontation and further exploration into the denial scenario Tom has created for himself.)*

Tom: "Well, when I'm high, I don't really have room in my head to think, so there you have it!"

Nurse: "OK. I understand. But the cocaine must cause some sort of problems for you in your daily life, doesn't it?" *(The nurse is nonconfrontive with Tom on the fact that he has reported numerous problems with the law, his family, the school, and his recent accident. Instead, he is approaching the topic with generalizations and abstract questions.)*

Tom: "Well, honestly, not really. I just take walks when I want some. My daughter doesn't really notice I'm gone because she's only 2. I leave her in the playpen, and she does just fine for 10 or 15 minutes. My wife doesn't even pay attention to me anymore, so that isn't affected either."

Nurse: "It sounds like your life is about the same as it was before your cocaine use, then?" *(The nurse ignores the serious content of Tom's message and rephrases or reframes the issue, almost minimizing circumstances that Tom mentioned.)*

Tom: "Yeah, I'd say so."

Effective Dialogue

Tom: "Like I've said before, the cocaine was just a way to keep me occupied. It hasn't really caused any major problems for me."

Nurse: "Tom, from what I understand, you were admitted because of a severe auto accident related to your cocaine use that killed a 3-year-old girl. I would say that was one example of a very serious consequence for you and for that child and her family as well." *(The nurse is using confrontation with a recent example to bring Tom to look at his cocaine use, as well as to link the drug to a serious consequence in his life. The nurse avoids being judgmental about the topic, but presents it in a neutral, yet firm manner.)*

Tom: "Well, that's true. But the car was actually out of balance, and it was raining. I don't see how that was really my fault."

Nurse: "This is one recent example of an accident that happened while you were using. The report states that you had white dust all over your shirt and that you were quickly moving straws and a bag around when they approached your car." *(The nurse does not accept Tom's excuse or his pattern of blaming someone or something else for his actions. Instead, the nurse ignores Tom's bringing up the car but continues to focus on Tom and the cocaine. He (nurse) gives more facts to Tom to drive home the point that it was Tom's actions that led to the accident, and no one else's.)*

Tom: "You know, cops have their own way of seeing things—and believe me, it's warped! I had a bag of candy in the car for my daughter, and I also had some of those sipper drinks that have the straws glued onto the box. The cops will find anything to haul me in. They just love doing that! And I'm getting really sick and tired of it."

(continued)

THERAPEUTIC COMMUNICATION 27-1 (CONTINUED)
A Cocaine Abuser in Denial

Effective Dialogue

Nurse: "Tom, you know that the drug test was done on that powder, and it was pure cocaine. I know you saw those results the other day when you and I were both in your room and the lawyer came to see you. Why are you continuing to deny it and to avoid taking responsibility for your own actions?" (*The nurse confronts Tom again on his denial and also provides more data, this time pointing out that Tom and he (the nurse) both were in the room and both witnessed these facts. The nurse follows up his observation with a direct question, pressing Tom to look at his behavior.*)

Tom: "Well, I . . . just don't know. I guess you have a point there." (*Period of silence follows.*)

Nurse: This is an old pattern that has created a very difficult situation for you, and this isn't the first time. As much as you try to deny, it can't be an easy thing for you to go through—especially with a child's death. Can we explore what you mean when you say I have a point?" (*The nurse continues pressing Tom and does not diverge from the topic at hand but also adds some empathy about the difficulty of this situation. He then continues on immediately by picking up on the small comment that Tom made, which could provide some way to open him up to discussing what he is thinking about his own responsibility.*)

Tom: "Well, I guess maybe there was something I did that might have contributed to the accident."

Reflection and Critical Thinking Questions

- If you were Tom's nurse, how would you feel about his accident and the child's death? Would you have personal reactions and ideas about Tom based on these events?
- If you had been trying to work on Tom's denial, think of the feelings you might have had and explore them.
- How might you have intervened therapeutically or nontherapeutically, and how would you analyze your interventions?

---

early stages of recovery. Repairing damaged relationships, making amends to those who have been harmed by the substance abuser, and maintaining sobriety are achievements that can help restore feelings of self-worth. The nurse assists in this process by counseling the client, listening and communicating therapeutically, teaching communication and relationship skills, and encouraging participation in the recovery program.

Other sources of poor self-esteem are negative self-talk and rumination. The nurse can help the client by break these self-defeating habits of thought by encouraging the client to use the following strategies:

- When negative self-talk begins, consciously say, "Stop!" This thought-stopping technique is surprisingly effective.
- Replace the negative self-talk with positive, kind, optimistic statements.
- Set realistic goals for yourself and take pride in your achievements.
- Examine your values and beliefs and make your actions congruent with those values.
- Find activities that are personally rewarding.
- Volunteer your time to help others.
- Spend time with positive, healthy people; avoid

people who can drag you down emotionally and spiritually.

- Participate in self-help groups.
- Don't compare yourself with others; you always will find someone who is better off or worse off. Compare yourself with yourself instead.

An addiction occupies a major role in the abuser's life and has been described as a relationship. As destructive as the abuse or relationship was, the abuser depends on it and returns to it for comfort. When this relationship is removed, and although the abuser may feel relief, the abuser often feels emotionally empty and spiritually bereft. These feelings of loss must be attended to in the early stages of recovery and new sources for emotional and spiritual connectedness established. AA addresses the spiritual aspect of recovery in a nonreligious way through its reliance on a higher power, which is defined differently and individually by each person. Recovery programs that use the 12 steps of AA incorporate this concept. The nurse should recognize that clients will be experiencing spiritual distress on some level and can assist by asking the client how he or she feels spiritually. Listening attentively and using therapeutic communication techniques are invaluable tools in helping clients work through such personal issues. The nurse also can help the client explore ways to feel connected that are culturally acceptable to the client.

PROMOTING HEALTHY ACTIVITIES

Alcoholics and substance abusers have typically devoted a great deal of their time to obtaining, using, and recovering from their drugs of choice. The substance becomes integral to their existence and occupies most of their leisure time and frequently their work time as well. When they begin recovery, clients can find themselves with time on their hands. They need to plan how they will use this time so that the temptation to revert to alcohol or drug use is minimized.

The nurse encourages clients to develop health-promoting habits that can occupy their time and also assist them in recovery. Exercise programs, yoga, or meditation are examples of useful activities. Clients also can resume pleasurable hobbies or pastimes that they once enjoyed before becoming addicted, or they may consciously develop new ones. Recommending attendance at AA or NA 12-step meetings, particularly during times of the day formerly devoted to drug or alcohol use, is an integral component in most recovery programs. The nurse encourages the client to be aware of how boredom, loneliness, or past habits can be overwhelming triggers to resuming drinking or drug abuse and to plan accordingly.

Evaluation

The effectiveness of the plan can be evaluated using the following criteria:

- Has the client remained safe through substance withdrawal?
- Has the client refrained from using drugs, alcohol, or both?
- Has the client acknowledged his addiction and dependence?
- Does the client use healthy stress management techniques?
- Has the client identified alternative activities to drinking or taking drugs?
- Is the client participating in the treatment plan?

▼ *Reflection and Critical Thinking Questions*

Now that you have completed this chapter, consider Clinical Example 27-1, which was presented at the beginning of the chapter, and the related nursing care presented in Nursing Care Plan 27-1. Answer the following questions.

1. List the symptoms that Eric has that lead you to think about alcohol dependence.

2. What other information would you need from Eric and his family?

3. List at least three NANDA nursing diagnoses that would be appropriate for Eric at this time.

4. What would be the immediate priorities in planning care for Eric if he were admitted to your inpatient treatment facility?

5. Discuss the longitudinal course of Eric's symptoms and talk about ways you might work with him to assist him in maintaining optimal functioning during times of relapse.

▼ CHAPTER SUMMARY

- Substance Use Disorders include both Substance Abuse and Substance Dependency. Substance Abuse occurs when an individual uses alcohol or other drugs repeatedly to the extent that functional problems occur; however, it does not include compulsive use or addiction. Conversely, Substance Dependency is diagnosed when the individual continues using alcohol or other drugs in spite of negative consequences such as significant functional problems in daily living. An individual with Substance Dependency is likely to experience tolerance as the use of the substance escalates and withdrawal when the drug of abuse is stopped.

- The Substance Abuse Disorders are classified by 12 categories of substances: alcohol, amphetamines, caffeine, cannabis, cocaine, hallucinogens, inhalants, nicotine, opioids, phencyclidines, sedative–hypnotics, and polysubstance abuse.

- All of the Substance Abuse Disorders may be associated with any of the four common subdiagnoses of Dependence, Abuse, Intoxication, and Withdrawal.

■ Substance Abuse Disorders are multidimensional and related strongly to neurophysiologic processes as well as to psychosocial and behavioral processes.

■ Alcohol abuse and dependency are among the most serious public health problems in the United States. The incidence and consequences of alcohol-related accidents resulting in fatalities or permanent injuries are enormous.

■ Individuals with drug or alcohol dependence or abuse are impaired in multiple areas, including physically, socially, and psychologically, at some time during their disorder. The behaviors manifested by these individuals often are not tolerated or accepted in most cultures. Signs and symptoms of abuse and dependence are specific to which drug is being used; however, functional impairment in several areas is a requisite for diagnosis.

■ Substance-related disorders are a major healthcare problem in America and globally. These disorders have a significant impact on the individual's physiology and behavior. The impact of drugs of abuse on society and family members, especially children, is devastating. Many American children and adolescents experience the effects of drug and alcohol abuse in multiple areas of functioning, and the incidence and prevalence of substance abuse disorders is high among adolescents themselves.

■ Many clients have **dual diagnosis**—coexistence of a substance abuse disorder and a major psychiatric disorder.

■ Interdisciplinary treatment of the client with a Substance Abuse Disorder is critical to a successful recovery process. There are various types of interdisciplinary treatment programs, including detoxification programs and facilities, inpatient rehabilitation, outpatient programs, and private practice physician treatment. In addition, there is a wide network of 12-step treatment programs throughout the world, which are led by lay or peers and paraprofessionals. These programs include AA, Al-Anon, ACOA, CA, and NA.

■ The nurse plays a critical role in the treatment and management of the client who is experiencing substance abuse or withdrawal from substances. The nursing process with clients with Substance Abuse Disorders provides a framework including assessment, planning, implementing care, and evaluation of the nursing care provided. The major issues in care of the client who is admitted for substance abuse include the following: (1) maintaining the client's safety; (2) breaking through denial; (3) managing anxiety; (4) teaching effective coping strategies; (5) improving family processes; (6) enhancing self-esteem; and (7) promoting healthy activities. Frequent reevaluation and assessment, with appropriate changes in care, are necessary to enhance treatment and ensure that clients successfully move toward healthier lifestyles that are free of substances of abuse.

▼ REVIEW QUESTIONS

1. A 48-year-old man is admitted to the emergency department with the following symptoms: fever, 101.5°F; pulse, 104; respirations, 28; blood pressure, 178/94; profuse perspiration and tremulousness. The mental status examination reveals confusion, disorientation, visual hallucinations, and agitation. His neighbor who accompanied him to the emergency department states that he stopped drinking 2 days ago after a long period of daily, heavy alcohol intake. What substance-induced disorder is this client experiencing?
   a. Wernicke-Korsakoff syndrome
   b. Alcohol amnestic disorder
   c. Alcohol withdrawal delirium
   d. Substance-induced psychotic disorder

2. When assessing the client for possible substance abuse, which of the following would alert the nurse to possible opiate abuse?
   a. Pupillary constriction
   b. Liver disease
   c. Reddened eyes
   d. Tactile hallucinations

3. The coexistence of substance abuse disorder and a major psychiatric disorder is called
   a. Primary disorder
   b. Addictive personality
   c. Dual diagnosis
   d. Substance psychosis

4. During the initial interview, the nurse asks the client if she has ever experienced blackouts. Blackouts are
   a. The denial of the unpleasant aspects of drinking and remembering only the pleasant experiences
   b. An inability to perform work requiring concentration
   c. Permanent amnesia for events that occurred while intoxicated
   d. A state of unconsciousness from an overdose of alcohol

5. Barbiturates and sedative–hypnotics taken in combination with alcohol will
   a. Decrease the effectiveness of alcohol
   b. Cause increased blood pressure
   c. Produce hyperactivity, restlessness, tactile hallucinations
   d. Potentiate the effects of the alcohol

6. Your client states that he snorts cocaine several times a day, spends all his money on ways to obtain the cocaine, and has been arrested once for threatening, abusive behavior. He could be said to have which disorder?
   a. Substance withdrawal
   b. Withdrawal delirium

and cannot focus or shift their attention readily. In addition, they experience difficulty attending to environmental stimuli. This diminished ability to control focus of attention and attention span fluctuates during the day and is more pronounced at night. Clients frequently are disoriented to time and sometimes to place and person. In more severe cases of delirium, clients mistake the unfamiliar for the familiar. For example, they may mistakenly identify and subsequently call healthcare personnel by the names of brothers, sisters, husbands, wives, or children.

Additional features of delirium may include (1) a reduced level of consciousness, (2) a disturbed sleep–wake cycle, and (3) an abnormality of psychomotor behavior. Change in level of consciousness may fluctuate between alertness and somnolence. The client often reverses the sleep–wake cycle and will nap and appear drowsy throughout the day. He or she may nap sporadically at night and awaken to become extremely agitated.

The client's psychomotor activity ranges from hypo-alert and hypoactive (which typically accompany metabolic dysfunction) to hyperalert and hyperactive (which typically occur during drug withdrawal) or any combination thereof. The hypoalert, hypoactive client exhibits minimal activity, appears stuporous, and is slow to respond to requests. This person often is mistakenly seen as depressed. The client in a hyperalert, hyperactive state is animated to the point of agitation and frequently has loud and pressured speech (Tueth & Cheong, 1993). The client in this agitated state often will try to remove intravenous (IV) lines and other tubes, "pick" at the air or the bed sheet, and try (often successfully) to climb over side rails or the end of the bed. In addition, the client often will exhibit the classic, autonomic response symptoms of dilated pupils, elevated pulse, and diaphoresis.

Implications and Prognosis

Delirium indicates the existence of a medical illness and should be considered a medically urgent condition. The prognosis for recovery from delirium is good if recognition and management of the underlying cause happen early. Depending on early recognition and management, the acute state of delirium can last for 3 to 5 days or, rarely, up to 3 weeks. Failure to deal with the underlying factors causing the delirium may result in irreversible brain damage or even death.

Interdisciplinary Goals and Treatment

The goals of the interdisciplinary team are to identify clients who are vulnerable to the development of delirium, recognize early signs of delirium, and institute measures quickly to correct underlying causes. In addition to early diagnosis and prompt medical treatment, therapeutic goals include managing the acute confusion to maximize cognitive functioning and prevent injury or further cognitive decline.

MEDICAL INTERVENTIONS

Medical interventions include treatment of the underlying cause. Therefore, treatment varies according to each client's physical condition. In cases of hypoperfusion or cerebral hypoxia, supplemental oxygen may significantly improve the acute symptoms of the disorder.

Physical restraints, chemical restraints, or both are used at times; however, such administration requires caution. The impetus for the use of chemical or physical restraints clearly must be to protect the client from harm rather than for staff convenience.

ENVIRONMENTAL INTERVENTIONS

The team must manipulate the client's environment to ensure safety as well as to maximize cognitive abilities and psychological comfort. A fine balance exists between environmental overstimulation and understimulation. Tailoring the environment to enhance the client's cognitive capability is essential. Having the client in a private room is beneficial so that staff can minimize the environmental stimuli to decrease the confusing environmental cues for the client. They cannot, however, completely extinguish environmental stimuli because doing so may cause the client to withdraw and attend more to internal stimuli. Television often inundates the client with confusing sensory input, whereas soft music provides appropriate environmental stimulation. Adequate lighting both during the day and evening is essential to promote the client's realistic perception of the environment. The client should use any other sensory aides (eg, eyeglasses, hearing aids) that he or she normally requires.

The client's safety during an acute episode of delirium must not be compromised. House staff must be alerted if the client is considered a candidate to leave the institution's premises. The client's propensity to pull tubes, climb over side rails, or fall may require the staff to institute a one-on-one observation or encourage the family to stay with the client. Consistency on the part of the staff in terms of an unhurried, daily routine, repeatedly assigned staff, and continuous visits by family members is helpful. Encouraging the family to bring in familiar objects from home (eg, personal effects, photographs) can increase the client's "comfort level" with the new environment.

COGNITIVE INTERVENTIONS

Staff members can try to direct the client's activity and cognitive focus by reorienting him or her to the environment with displays of calendars, clocks, and decorations commemorating upcoming holidays. Interactions between the staff and client are important. Therapeutic communications concerning the day's activities, repetition of facts concerning why the client is hospitalized, and even reassurance

Cognitive Disorders Information Map: Delirium

➡️ *Prevalence*

Adults age 18 years and older: 0.4%
Adults age 55 years and older: 1%
Prevalence rates are much higher in acute care settings and nursing homes

➡️ *Risk and Contributing Factors*

- Age: children and older adults are especially susceptible to delirium
- Gender: more cases occur in women; however, this is largely the result of women living longer than men
- Pre-existing illness or dementia
- Infection
- Fluid/electrolyte or metabolic imbalance
- Pain
- Use of medications

➡️ *Summary of DSM-IV-TR Diagnostic Criteria*

Delirium from a General Medical Condition

- Client has disturbed consciousness (reduced clarity of environmental awareness) and a reduced capacity to focus, sustain, or shift attention.
- Cognition changes (e.g., memory deficit, disorientation, language disturbance), or a perceptual disturbance develops that is not better explained by a preexisting, established, or evolving dementia.
- The change or disturbance develops quickly (usually hours to days) and tends to fluctuate.
- Evidence from the history, physical examination, or laboratory tests supports that the disturbance is caused by a general medical condition.

Substance Withdrawal Delirium

- Consciousness is disturbed, and ability to focus, sustain, or shift attention is reduced.
- Cognition changes, or a perceptual disturbance develops that is not better explained by a preexisting, established, or evolving dementia.
- The disturbance develops quickly (usually hours to days) and tends to fluctuate.
- Evidence from the history, physical examination, or laboratory tests supports that symptoms developed during or shortly after a withdrawal syndrome.

Substance Intoxication Delirium

- Consciousness is disturbed, and ability to focus, sustain, or shift attention is reduced.
- Cognition changes, or a perceptual disturbance develops that is not better explained by a preexisting, established, or evolving dementia.
- The disturbance develops quickly (usually hours to days) and tends to fluctuate.
- Evidence from the history, physical examination, or laboratory tests supports either:
  1. Symptoms developed during substance intoxication.
  2. Medication use is related to the disturbance.

Delirium Due to Multiple Etiologies

- Consciousness is disturbed, and ability to focus, sustain, or shift attention is reduced.
- Cognition changes, or a perceptual disturbance develops that is not better explained by a preexisting, established, or evolving dementia.
- The disturbance develops quickly (usually hours to days) and tends to fluctuate.
- Evidence from the history, physical examination, or laboratory tests supports more than one etiology (e.g., a medical condition and substance intoxication).

Delirium Not Otherwise Specified

The client's delirium does not meet criteria for any specific type of delirium. For example, a clinical presentation of delirium is suspected to result from a medical condition or substance, but evidence to establish a specific etiology is insufficient.

(continued)

Cognitive Disorders Information Map: Delirium *(Continued)*

➡️ *Prevention Strategies*

- Screen all clients, especially older adults, for signs and symptoms of delirium.
- Be sure to carefully review with all clients the medications they are using and any adverse effects they may be experiencing.
- If working in a nursing home or an acute care facility, monitor clients' neurologic status regularly.
- If working with a client who has delirium, avoid questions or tasks that require abstract thinking.
- For clients with delirium in long-term or acute settings, be sure that safety precautions are in place, the environment is free of clutter and dangerous objects, and that all measures possible are instituted to prevent falls.
- If a client is using medications, has an infection, or has a fluid and electrolyte imbalance or metabolic disturbance, be sure to teach the client and family signs and symptoms of delirium and measures to take if the client begins to exhibit them.

➡️ *Want to Know More?*

Children of Aging Parents (CAPs)
1609 Woodbourne Road
Suite 302A
Levitown, PA 19057
(800) 227-7294
http://www.aoa.dhhs.gov/coa/dir/77.html

National Alliance for the Mentally Ill
200 North Glebe Road
Suite 1015
Arlington, VA 22203-3754
(800) 950-6264
http://www.nami.org

National Institute on Aging
P. O. Box 8057
Gaithersburg, MD 20898-8057
(800) 222-2225
http://www/nih.gov/nia/

Diagnostic criteria adopted with permission from the American Psychiatric Association. (2000). *Diagnostic and statistical manual of mental disorders* (4th ed., text revision). Washington, DC: Author.

---

that the hallucinations and delusions experienced are part of the *transient* condition of delirium, are helpful.

PSYCHOLOGICAL INTERVENTIONS

The health team members' empathetic expression of concern for the client's fears and anxiety can address the memory impairment and emotional overtones that often are found in clients with delirium. It is better for healthcare team members to express empathy to the client rather than to be confrontational and, for instance, dispute any delusions that may be present.

Family members must be kept informed and included in the plans taken to resolve the delirium. They need to understand the biological basis for the behavior that they are witnessing in their loved one. This understanding will hopefully allay their fears that the delirium is a form of mental illness or dementia as well as motivate them to join the staff in efforts to reorient the client.

APPLICATION OF THE NURSING PROCESS TO THE CLIENT WITH DELIRIUM

Assessment

Early assessment of acute confusion is an essential part of nursing care for all hospitalized clients and, in particular, hospitalized older adults. Early recognition of delirium and subsequent identification and treatment of the underlying causes can prevent even more deleterious effects as well as the progression of acute confusion and all its ramifications.

All clients should have a baseline neurologic examination at the onset of care for any episode of illness. Clients at increased risk for delirium, for example, older adults or those with a head injury, should have mental status examinations routinely throughout the course of treatment. Clients who then have subtle or overt changes from their baselines in mental status, orientation, or level of consciousness should be evaluated for delirium. The Confusion Assessment Method (CAM) is a scale for assessing delirium and focuses on four domains:

1. Acute onset and fluctuating course of the condition
2. Inattention
3. Disorganized thinking
4. Altered level of consciousness

This tool is more specific to delirium. The Mini-Mental State Examination is an excellent tool for evaluating cognitive functioning; however, it cannot differentiate between delirium and dementia. It includes questions that test the client's orientation, attention span, recall, and ability to execute simple instructions that require cognitive integrity; it can be used in conjunction with the CAM and as a means of testing the delirious client's improvement or deterioration (Box 28-3). Once delirium is diagnosed and as treatment progresses, ongoing assessment of the client's mental status is necessary to monitor the client's recovery.

In addition to experiencing cognitive changes, the confused client often is anxious and emotionally distraught. The nurse assesses any changes in the client's anxiety level. If anxiety escalates to overt agitation, the client has the potential to become dangerous to self, other clients, and staff. Carefully assessing anxiety and

watching for signs of agitation (increased motor activity, labile mood, combativeness) can alert the staff to the need for interventions that will increase the client's psychological comfort and decrease the potential for dangerous behavior.

The nurse also monitors the client's ability to perform daily self-care needs. Confused clients may be too distracted to eat or drink adequately and may be inattentive to personal hygiene. Ongoing assessment of functional ability is necessary for the client's comfort and physical well-being.

Nursing Diagnosis

Nursing diagnoses that guide the planning of nursing interventions for the client experiencing delirium include the following:

- **Acute Confusion** related to delirium of known or unknown etiology
- **Risk for Injury** related to confusion and cognitive deficits
- **Bathing/Hygiene, Toileting, Feeding, and Dressing/Grooming Self-Care Deficit** related to cognitive impairment
- **Deficient Knowledge** of family related to client diagnosis, progression, and prognosis

Planning

Planning is a collaborative effort of the entire treatment team in conjunction with the family and the client as able. The plan of care must be deliberately designed to meet the client's unique needs. Major goals for the care of a client with delirium are as follows:

- The client will remain physically safe.
- The client's basic needs will be met until self-care ability resumes.
- The client will return to baseline cognitive functioning.
- The client will remain calm.

Implementation

Nursing Care Plan 28-1 illustrates the nursing process for Meredith, the client presented in Clinical Example 28–2.

MANAGING CONFUSION

Confusion and agitation can be easily worsened by too much unsettling stimuli, too little routine, abrupt changes in routine, poor sleep patterns, or insensitive approaches from others. The nurse can perform many activities to help promote a therapeutic climate for the client experi-

---

BOX 28-3 ▼ *Sample Mini-Mental Status Examination Questions*

- What is the year?
- What is today's date?
- In what city (town) are we?
- Spell "globe" backward.
- Repeat the following statement: "A rolling stone gathers no moss."
- Write a sentence of your own choice. (Nurse evaluates whether sentence has a subject, predicate [verb], and object.)

Questions adapted from Folstein, M. E., Folstein, S. E., & McHugh, P. R. (1975). Mini-Mental State: A practical method for grading the cognitive state of patients for the clinician. *Journal of Psychiatric Research, 12*(189). Used with permission.

Nursing Care Plan 28-1

THE CLIENT WITH DELIRIUM

As presented in Clinical Example 28-2, Meredith's mental status continues to fluctuate. She sometimes is quite confused and agitated. If left alone, she tries to get out of bed to go to the bathroom even though she is not steady enough to walk unassisted. She has lashed out at her husband, Frank, calling him names. Frank is very upset and asks if this is "permanent." He is afraid he will not be able to manage her at home. The nurse explains that recovery from delirium may occur quickly or make take a few weeks for full recovery.

In addition to implementing interventions designed to facilitate Meredith's recovery from hip surgery, the nurse develops a plan of care that addresses Meredith's neurologic condition and home care needs.

Nursing Diagnosis: Acute Confusion related to delirium and underlying infection

Goal: Meredith's mental status will return to baseline.

Interventions	Rationales
Monitor the client's neurologic status. Monitor level of consciousness, orientation, attention span, mood, affect, and behaviors. Report decline in neurologic functioning not attributable to expected fluctuation or "sundowning." Avoid confronting the client about the irrationality of her delusions. Offer an alternative explanation of events and acknowledge the emotional content reflected in the delusion (ie, fear).	Ongoing assessment is critical to determine Meredith's recovery from delirium or her deterioration, which would require an immediate change in the plan of care.
Reorient the client and provide environmental cues. Use calendars and clocks to help client remain oriented. Inform the client of time, place, and person often; try to do so in a conversational way. Keep familiar and needed objects visible. Remove confusing stimuli and make sure that the client wears her glasses or hearing aids. Supply a daily newspaper.	Reorienting Meredith and providing environmental clues will help her to feel more in control and will reduce her anxiety.
Provide information to the client and family. Tell the client often why she is in the hospital, what the medical problem is, and that the cognitive problems are temporary and a result of the medical condition. Remind the family that the behavior is transient. Provide reassurance as needed to both the family and the client.	Meredith, as with most clients with delirium, will respond better when factual information about the delirium is repeated as needed. It is a way of reorienting Meredith to her situation. Explaining the biologic basis of the delirium will help Frank understand that Meredith's words and actions are not intended to be hurtful.
Administer medication (haloperidol) when needed to control agitation and psychotic behavior. Monitor the client's affect, mood, and anxiety level. Observe for restlessness, signs of agitation, or hostile outbursts. Observe for unsafe behaviors that place the client at risk for self-injury or injury to others. If the client's agitation is increasing and reassurances and nonpharmacologic interventions are not effective, administer mediation as needed and observe for its effectiveness. Document the client's response to the medication.	Pharmacologic interventions are given to control agitation and psychosis in delirium and often are used concomitantly with other measures or while nonpharmacologic interventions are being implemented. Observing for and documenting the client's response to the medication informs the healthcare team of the usefulness of the medication. If the desired effect is not achieved, or if there are untoward side effects, the medication will be changed.

Evaluation: Meredith's confusion resolves and her cognitive abilities return to baseline. Her aggressiveness, hostility, delusions, and hallucinations subside, and she becomes oriented to person, place, and time.

Nursing Diagnosis: Risk for Injury to self or others related to impaired cognition, delusions, and hallucinations

Goal: Meredith will not sustain an injury attributable to her confused state, nor will she injure anyone else.

(continued)

Nursing Care Plan 28-1 (Continued)

Interventions	Rationales
Provide for around-the-clock observation by staff or arrange for a family member to stay with the client.	With a client who has severe delirium, one-on-one observation often is indicated. Observation of Meredith is essential and the only reliable way of preventing injury. Family members can provide psychological and practical support while observing.
Toilet the client frequently.	Clients with delirium often are incontinent or sustain falls attempting to get to the bathroom. Frequently toileting Meredith will help prevent a fall.
Avoid using restraints; administer antipsychotic or sedative medications judiciously as ordered.	Physical restraints increase the client's anxiety, sense of isolation, disorientation, and powerlessness. Many clients sustain injuries from restraint devices. Medication, which is considered "chemical restraint," should be used to control psychotic symptoms along with one-on-one observation. Using both should avert the need for physical restraints.
Make the environment safe and use a calm, empathetic approach. Approach the client with delirium using caution and never from behind. Move the client to a single room near the nurse's station. Explain all activities to the client. Discontinue any invasive lines that can be terminated.	Approaching Meredith calmly and reassuringly will lessen her anxiety and fearfulness, as will explaining what will happen during care activities and why they are being done. Moving her to a single room near the nurse's station will prevent isolation and keep other clients safe. Removing invasive lines, if possible, will prevent the client from forcefully removing them, which can cause internal injuries or bleeding.

Evaluation: Meredith and those around her are free from injury.

encing acute confusion. In fact, managing the environment is one of the most influential nursing interventions.

The confused client will be calmer when the nurse eliminates environmental stimuli that invite misinterpretation, such as abstract pictures on the wall or excessive background noise and television. Conversely, the nurse can provide environmental cues in the form of clocks, recognizable pictures, and calendars to help restore orientation to time and place. A caveat to reducing environmental stimuli is to not create an understimulating environment, which can be just as detrimental as an overstimulating one. The key is to remove abstract or difficult-to-interpret environmental cues and replace them with simple, easy-to-recognize ones.

The confused client also will benefit from a consistent daily routine created by familiar staff or family members. Staff and family should reinforce the predictability of the routine by telling the client what they are doing, what to expect, the time of day, and other relevant data as they proceed with these activities. Consistency is stabilizing for a client who has difficulty interpreting environmental cues.

The client will benefit from directed activity. Giving the agitated client psychomotor tasks may help him or her manage anxiety. Purses filled with familiar items for women to "pack" and "unpack," Velcro on which familiar objects can be stuck and unstuck, and zippers that can be opened and closed provide sensory stimulation and tasks to complete that are within the client's scope of cognitive function.

Nurses approach the client calmly and empathetically, calling him or her by name, and introducing themselves to help the client focus and correctly interpret events. They also are careful not to approach the client from behind, which gives the client minimal time to adjust to their presence. So that the client does not become frustrated, nurses avoid frequently quizzing him or her about orientation or posing questions that require decision making or abstract thinking. Instead, family and staff should communicate in simple, direct sentences and focus on what is meaningful to the client.

Because the clouded consciousness waxes and wanes, the nurse never should assume that the client does not need or will not understand explanations of what is happening. Recognizing the fears of the client is helpful. The nurse may reply to a client's fear with "It must be difficult to be so frightened, but I want you to know that I will not go far and I will do what needs to be done to keep you safe." The nurse must accept the client's sometimes bizarre behavior and not demean or correct him or her for behavior that he or she cannot control.

Occasionally, the client becomes so highly agitated that he or she needs medications. Staff members must seriously consider this option when the client's behavior is threatening to the safety of self, family, or staff. The neuroleptic medication haloperidol (Haldol), given either orally or by injection, is most commonly used to treat symptoms of delirium. It has minimal anticholinergic effects and does not cause the serious cardiovascular and respiratory side effects found with some other classes of antipsychotics, although extrapyramidal side effects are possible adverse reactions. Older adults should receive between 0.5 mg (for mild agitation) and 2 mg (for severe agitation). The younger client may be given 2 mg (for mild agitation) or up to 10 mg (for severe agitation). These doses can be repeated every 30 to 60 minutes until the agitated behavior has subsided and the client is calm or sedated. Other neuroleptics found useful in treating delirium are thiothixene (Navane) and droperidol (Wise, Gray, & Seltzer, 1999).

If the client has hepatic dysfunction, the treatment team may choose to use lorazepam (Ativan) orally, intramuscularly, or intravenously in doses ranging from 0.5 to 2 mg. This medication may be doubled every 30 to 60 minutes until the desired level of sedation is reached. Lorazepam can affect respiratory and cardiac function; therefore, the nurse must monitor the client while he or she is receiving lorazepam. In some instances, this medication may increase agitation in the delirious client and therefore must be discontinued.

PROVIDING A SAFE ENVIRONMENT

Because cognition is so clouded and the client is likely to misinterpret environmental clues, he or she is vulnerable to harm. The confused person also displays unsafe behavior such as pulling out tubes or wandering from a hospital unit because of his or her inability to think clearly. Making the environment safe helps to prevent harm that might result from the client's confusion. The nurse may provide this safety, in part, by placing personal and familiar items (eg, call light, water pitcher, eyeglasses) close at hand so that the client is not injured while attempting to get them.

Alerting staff and family to the possibility that the client may escape or wander away and arranging for continuous observation if necessary will help prevent a disastrous outcome. Clients with delirium have sustained significant injuries by wandering into traffic, falling down stairwells, or becoming lost.

Many clients with delirium, especially older adults, are injured climbing over raised bed rails. The bed should remain in its lowest position, and bed rails should remain down unless policy demands otherwise. Lighting in the environment needs to be bright enough so the client can see accurately. This is especially important at night and particularly significant for older adults who need brighter light to see.

The nurse must protect the client with clouded consciousness from as many environmental mishaps as possible. Restraints should be avoided if possible because the client may become agitated and fearful from the physical limitation, which increa... restraint-related injury.

Because foreseeing all the... environment of a client whose... impossible, the nurse must make re... on the client. At times, even this level o... cient. The nurse may ask family membe... their loved one, especially at night or during... tated periods of the delirium.

HELPING THE CLIENT WITH PERSONAL CARE

The distractibility and cognitive derangement of the client with delirium may seriously hamper his or her ability to maintain activities of daily living (ADLs). The nurse must support the client's efforts to carry out whatever ADLs he or she is capable of performing, as well as assume responsibility for those necessary activities that the client can no longer manage. Establishing a routine to carry out these activities also is helpful to the confused client.

PROVIDING CLIENT AND FAMILY EDUCATION

The client may be aware that his or her thinking is disordered; this realization will frighten him or her. The nurse must inform both the client and family about the nature of delirium. They need to realize that the confusion and abnormal behavior have a biological basis and are transient. Explaining the process, progress, and prognosis of the illness will alleviate some anxiety and apprehension. The healthcare team must continually update the family as to the state of the underlying illness and the progress being made to resolve it. The family needs to become partners with the healthcare team in planning the client's care and implementing some interventions, such as reorientation.

Evaluation

As stated previously, the signs and symptoms of delirium may fluctuate throughout the day. A perspective on how well the client is recovering may evolve over a period of days. Because clients have varying baseline cognitive function, the nurse evaluates each client's progress according to his or her previous level of functioning. Some indicators of resolving confusion include the following:

- Improved score on Mini-Mental State Examination
- Improved ability to communicate
- Increased ability to focus attention
- Increased ability to make decisions
- Reduced delusional behavior
- Improved ability to care for self
- Decreased anxiety and agitation

cognitive
ion, use of
Although
l forms of

ementia do
itions. The
ir differing
origins. Box 28-4 reveals the categories of dementia according to the *DSM-IV-TR,* which are differentiated from one another based on their etiology. Several of the dementia disorders are presented separately here.

LEARNING AND RETAINING NEW INFORMATION

The memory impairment of dementia is a deficit serious enough to significantly affect the social or occupational arena of the client's life (APA, 2000). Memory impairment in dementia encompasses the client's ability to learn and retain new material (short-term memory) as well as to recall previously learned material (long-term memory) (APA, 2000). The client becomes repetitive and has difficulty remembering recent conversations, events, and appointments. He or she repeatedly "loses" things. The client may attempt to compensate for these lapses (Costa et al., 1996).

HANDLING COMPLEX TASKS

The chronicity and degenerative nature of dementia result in significant deficiencies. These impairments are global, and the client's well-preserved social skills and mastery of confabulation (Morrison, 1995) often conceal the mental deterioration that is taking place. Family members first recognize cognitive problems in their loved ones when they have difficulties with such routine activities as meal planning, managing the checkbook, driving, and using familiar equipment such as the telephone.

REASONING ABILITY

Dementia affects the client's ability to reason. Clients no longer seem able to respond with a reasonable plan to problems that occur at work or in the home. Ultimately, their thought processes degenerate to the degree that they exhibit significant deficits in abstract thinking. Clients become so impaired that they cannot cognitively adapt to new situations. This impairment severely limits their competence to adjust to the dynamics of living (APA, 2000).

For example, if the bathroom at home floods, the client with dementia may be in a quandary as to how to respond to this household crisis. Clients also may begin to exhibit uncharacteristic disregard for rules of social conduct. For example, although they never may have used vile language publicly in the past, they may curse out their caregivers when frustrated. Families find this uncharacteristic behavior very distressing (Costa et al., 1996).

SPATIAL ABILITY AND ORIENTATION

Because their ability to process sensory information diminishes, clients gradually begin to experience confusion, which affects attentiveness to the environment and ultimately level of consciousness. As level of consciousness decreases, they cannot concentrate, their attention span progressively decreases, and they become distractible. They also may become disoriented. Eventually, they lose their ability to recognize or identify familiar objects (eg, the parts of a telephone), a condition called **agnosia**. When their sensory input falls below certain minimum need requirements and when the brain is affected structurally so that it can no longer perceive and interpret the stimuli adequately, decreased orientation results.

This disorientation and problems with spatial ability can make driving a car a point of contention with the family, as it becomes apparent that the affected individual is no longer a safe driver. Clients may drive around for hours, unable to find their way home, but they usually have little insight into this declining ability.

Affected individuals do not seem able to organize items around the house. They get lost and cannot find their way around familiar places such as their neighborhood or their own home (Costa et al., 1996). Disoriented clients do not know where they are, how they came to be there, why they are there, or how they fit into the environmental milieu.

LANGUAGE

Frequently, the client has difficulty with finding the words he or she wants to use (**aphasia**) in conversation (Costa et al., 1996). This difficulty can result in a frustrating process of charades, relying on others to guess the forgotten word (eg, referring to Thanksgiving Day as the time of the turkey or pumpkin). In addition, they may have difficulty *following* conversations (Costa et al., 1996).

BEHAVIOR

Behavior refers to an individual's responses to the continual changes in the internal and external environment and to the physiologic soundness of the brain. When something interferes with or interrupts the organic integrity of the brain, maladaptive behavior often follows. This behavior is not to be confused with that seen in delirium even though aberrant behavior is seen in both disorders. The client with dementia also may find that he or she cannot

Cognitive Disorders Information Map: Dementia

➡ *Prevalence*

Approximately 3%

➡ *Risk and Contributing Factors*

- Age: risk increases with aging; highest prevalence rates of Alzheimer's disease are found in people older than age 85 years
- Family history (with Huntington's disease, genetics are the dominant risk factor)
- Head trauma
- Low educational level
- High blood pressure (vascular dementia)

➡ *Summary of DSM-IV-TR Diagnostic Criteria*

Vascular Dementia

- Client develops multiple cognitive deficits manifested by both
  1. Impaired memory (for either new or previously learned information)
  2. One (or more) of the following:
     a. Aphasia
     b. Apraxia
     c. Agnosia
     d. Disturbed executive functioning
- Cognitive deficits significantly impair social or occupational functioning and represent a significant decline from previous functioning.
- Focal neurologic signs and symptoms (e.g., exaggerated deep tendon reflexes, extensor plantar response, pseudobulbar palsy, gait abnormalities, extremity weakness) or laboratory evidence indicate cerebrovascular disease (e.g., multiple infarctions involving cortex and underlying white matter) judged to be etiologically related to the disturbance.
- Deficits do not occur exclusively during delirium.

Substance-Induced Persisting Amnestic Disorder

- Memory is impaired as manifested by impaired ability to learn new information or recall previously learned information.
- The memory disturbance significantly impairs social or occupational functioning and represents a significant decline from previous functioning.
- The memory disturbance does not occur exclusively during delirium or dementia and persists beyond the usual duration of substance intoxication or withdrawal.
- Evidence from the history, physical examination, or laboratory tests supports that the memory disturbance is etiologically related to the persisting effects of substance use.

Dementia of the Alzheimer's Type

- Client has multiple cognitive deficits manifested by both:
  1. Impaired memory (either for new or previously learned information)
  2. One (or more) of the following:
     a. Aphasia (language disturbance)
     b. Apraxia (impaired ability to perform motor activities despite intact motor function)
     c. Agnosia (failure to recognize or identify objects despite intact sensory function)
     d. Disturbed executive functioning (i.e. planning, organizing, sequencing, abstracting)
- Cognitive deficits significantly impair social or occupational functioning and represent a significant decline from previous functioning.
- The course is characterized by gradual onset and continuing cognitive decline.
- The cognitive deficits are not from:
  1. Other central nervous system conditions that cause progressive deficits in memory and cognition (e.g., cerebrovascular disease, Parkinson's disease, Huntington's disease, brain tumor)
  2. Systemic conditions known to cause dementia (e.g. hypothyroidism, vitamin B_{12} or folic acid deficiency, HIV infection)
  3. Substance-induced conditions
- The deficits do not occur exclusively during delirium.
- The disturbance is not better explained by another Axis I disorder (e.g., schizophrenia).

Types are *with early onset* if onset is age 65 years or younger and *with late onset* if onset is after age 65.

(continued)

Cognitive Disorders Information Map: Dementia *(Continued)*

Dementia Due to Medical Conditions

- Client develops multiple cognitive deficits manifested by both:
  1. Impaired memory (for either new or previously learned information)
  2. One (or more) of the following:
     a. Aphasia
     b. Apraxia
     c. Agnosia
     d. Disturbed executive functioning
- The cognitive deficits significantly impair social or occupational functioning and represent a significant decline from previous functioning.
- Evidence from the history, physical examination, or laboratory tests indicates that the disturbance is caused by a medical condition other than Alzheimer's disease or vascular dementia (e.g., HIV infection, Parkinson's disease, Huntington's chorea, Pick's disease, Creutzfeldt-Jakob disease).
- The deficits do not occur exclusively during delirium.

Prevention Strategies

- For older adults, be sure to screen for signs and symptoms of Alzheimer's disease. When working with families, ask about the relationships between members. If stressors or problems have been developing, explore any changes that family members might have noticed in a loved one.
- If a client is diagnosed with early-stage Alzheimer's disease, be sure to encourage him or her to continue to engage in healthy behaviors (e.g., proper nutrition, exercise, adequate sleep). Optimal overall health may slow or delay the progression of symptoms.
- Discuss genetic screening for clients who have family members with Huntington's disease. Although this condition cannot be cured, knowledge of whether a client has the gene for this disorder may help him or her make informed decisions about having children, long-term care, and finances.

Want to Know More?

Alzheimer's Association
919 North Michigan Avenue
Suite 1000
Chicago, IL 60611–1676
(800) 272-3900
http://www.alz.org

Alzheimer's Disease Education and Referral (ADEAR)
   Center
P. O. Box 8252
Silver Spring, MD 20907–8252
(800) 438-4380
http://alzheimer's.org

Children of Aging Parents (CAPs)
1609 Woodbourne Road
Suite 302A
Levitown, PA 19057
(800) 227-7294
http://www.aoa.dhhs.gov/coa/dir/77.html

Eldercare Locator
1112 16th Street, NW
Washington, DC 20036
(800) 677-1116
http://www.aoa.dhhs.gov/elderpage/locator.html

Diagnostic criteria adapted with permission from the American Psychiatric Association. (2000). *Diagnostic and statistical manual of mental disorders* (4th ed., text revision). Washington, DC: Author.

BOX 28-4 ▼ *DSM-IV-TR Categories for Dementia*

Dementia of the Alzheimer's type
　With Early Onset
　Uncomplicated
　With Delirium
　With Delusions
　With Depressed Mood
Dementia of the Alzheimer's Type
　With Late Onset
　Uncomplicated
　With Delirium
　With Delusions
　With Depressed Mood
Vascular Dementia
　Uncomplicated
　With Delirium

　With Delusions
　With Depressed Mood
Dementia Due to HIV Disease
Dementia Due to Head Trauma
Dementia Due to Parkinson's Disease
Dementia Due to Huntington's Disease
Dementia Due to Pick's Disease
Dementia Due to Creutzfeldt-Jakob Disease
Dementia Due to General Medical Condition (specify if not listed above)
Substance-Induced Persisting Dementia
Dementia Due to Multiple Etiologies (code each of the specific etiologies)
Dementia Not Otherwise Specified

perform motor tasks (eg, brushing the teeth, combing the hair) despite intact motor function, a condition known as **apraxia** (APA, 2000; Morrison, 1995).

Clients with dementia display various behavioral changes. No key feature is characteristic of every client with dementia, but most behavior changes become more pronounced in the evenings after sunset (a phenomenon known as **sundowning**). They also may become more irritable and suspicious than usual and may misinterpret visual or auditory cues. Because of their diffuse cognitive impairment, clients can experience illusions and hallucinations (see Chap. 25). Family members report that their loved one is no longer responsive to discussion on topics in which they formerly were very interested. They also report noticeable changes in their loved one's behavior, dress, or both (Costa et al., 1996).

A comparison of some of the behaviors seen in delirium versus dementia is listed in Table 28-1.

Types of Dementia

ALZHEIMER'S DISEASE

Alzheimer's disease is the most prevalent of the dementias. An estimated 4 million Americans are victims of dementia, Alzheimer's type (DAT) (Ugarriza & Gray, 1993). The incidence and prevalence of DAT directly correlates with increased age. Alzheimer's disease is present in 1 of 10 people aged 65 years and older, with the incidence rising to 1 in 2 people aged 85 and older (Rocca, 1994). Incidence is higher in women than in men; however, this finding may be because women live longer than do men. Low educational levels may increase the risk for developing DAT and other dementias. Approximately 5% of cases of DAT clearly are familial. Familial DAT is more likely to have an early age

at onset (Lendon, Ashall, & Goate, 1997). See Historical Capsule 28-1.

The etiology of DAT is unknown, although studies have generated several theories. Some suggest that the etiology may be deficiencies in neurotransmitter acetylcholine (ACh). At the microscopic level, loss of neurons is seen and senile plaques occur in large numbers throughout the cortical regions of the brain. Neurofibrillary tangles are another neuropathologic feature of most clients with DAT, but both plaques and neurofibrillary tangles also are seen in the brains of older adult clients who did not have DAT.

Higher than normal amounts of aluminum deposits have been detected in the brains of clients with Alzheimer's disease. Some researchers believe that these deposits may be either a cause or at least a result of the disease. Some studies show abnormally high antibody titers, raising the possibility of an immunologic defect. A higher incidence of Alzheimer's disease has been associated with adult clients with Down syndrome and with close relatives of other clients with Alzheimer's disease, leading to the theory of a probable defect in at least chromosome 21 (if not another chromosome). Other genetic links also have been proposed. Some researchers believe that DAT, which has been seen as one disease entity, may be a group of disorders (Abraham & Neundorfer, 1990; Yi, Abraham, & Holroyd, 1994). See Research in Psychiatric-Mental Health Nursing 28-1.

DAT is considered to be clinically heterogeneous, that is, the symptomatology varies during the average 8- to 10-year course of the disease. There have been efforts to "stage" the progressive functional decline occurring with Alzheimer's disease (Table 28-2). Different staging formats are used to make some sense out of the disease progression. Doing so helps in planning for the future intensive care required by those who have Alzheimer's disease.

TABLE 28-1 ▼ **Delirium Versus Dementia**

CHARACTERISTIC	DELIRIUM	DEMENTIA
Onset	Rapid development	Gradual and insidious development
Duration	Brief duration of 1 month or less, depending on cause	Long, with progressive deterioration
Course	Diurnal alterations, more nocturnal exacerbations	Stable progression of symptomatology
Thinking and short-term memory	Disorganized and impaired	Short-term and long-term memory impairments, with eventual complete loss
Orientation	Markedly decreased, especially to environmental cues	Progressively decreases
Language	Rambling, pressured, irrelevant	Difficulty recalling the correct word; later may lose language
Perceptual disturbance	Environment unclear, progressing to illusions, hallucinations, and delusions	Often absent but can progress to paranoia, delusions, hallucinations, and illusions
Level of consciousness	Cloudiness that fluctuates; inattentiveness to hyperalert with distractibility	Not affected
Sleep	Day–night reversal, insomnia, vivid dreams and nightmares	Piecemeal
Psychomotor actions	Sluggish to hyperactive; change of range unpredictable	Not affected
Emotional status	Anxious with changes in sleep; fearful if experiencing hallucinations; weeping; yelling	Depression/anxiety when insight into condition is present; late in pathology, anger with outbursts, restless with pacing

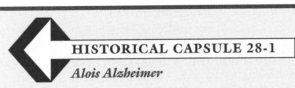

HISTORICAL CAPSULE 28-1

Alois Alzheimer

Alois Alzheimer was born in 1864 in Markbreit, Germany. An excellent student, he studied medicine in Berlin and graduated from the University of Wurzburg in 1887. Working at the Irrenanstalt Asylum in Frankfurt, Alzheimer began to focus his work and research on the cortex of the human brain in association with the renowned neurologist, Franz Nissl. Their collaborative efforts resulted in a six-volume reference work, *Histologic and Histopathologic Studies of the Cerebral Cortex.* Alzheimer pursued his love for scientific inquiry and clinical practice by becoming research assistant to the distinguished psychiatrist Emil Kraepelin at the Munich School of Medicine. In 1906, Alzheimer presented his famous case study of a 51-year-old woman with "an unusual disease of the cerebral cortex" whose symptoms included memory loss, disorientation, hallucinations, and depression. He also detailed his postmortem examination of the woman's brain that revealed a "paucity of cells in the cerebral cortex . . . and clumps of filaments between the nerve cells." He followed this presentation with a comprehensive paper in 1911 discussing the disease in detail. It was Kraepelin who proposed naming the disease after Alzheimer, who was the first person to present the syndrome to the scientific world.

Alzheimer was a punctilious researcher whose histologic studies extended into areas other than dementia. He made valuable scientific contributions to the area of histology with his work on the brains of persons who had the clinical symptomatology of epilepsy, tumors, Huntington's chorea, and alcoholic delirium. Known as a charitable teacher, his distinction in the scientific world was augmented by both his meticulous research as well as his inspiring influence on the researchers and physicians under his tutelage. He ended his career as professor of psychiatry and director of the Psychiatric and Neurologic Institute at the University of Breslau. He died in 1915 at 51 years of age. He is buried in Frankfurt am Main.

Research in Psychiatric-Mental Health Nursing 28-1
A FAMILY'S COMING TO TERMS WITH ALZHEIMER'S DISEASE

Purpose: To determine how family members are individually affected when one member has Alzheimer's disease.

Background: The researchers based their study on the ideas presented in Knafl and Deatricks's concept of family management style and Patterson's levels of family meaning.

Method and Sample: Using an exemplar family, the researchers conducted 10 in-depth interviews of five members of a family whose patriarch (husband, father, grandfather) had Alzheimer's disease in its middle stages.

Findings: Information gathered from the interviews supported the idea that each member interviewed experienced the same type of process as he or she came to terms with progressive changes in the Alzheimer's victim. Members (1) determined how their loved one was the same and how he was different since the onset of the disease, (2) redefined the identity of the person with Alzheimer's disease based on how they interpreted the changes, and (3) rewrote their relationship with the Alz[...] member based on the "newly defined ide[...]

Application to the Nursing Process: Nurses [...] realize that family members will experience the illne[...] of Alzheimer's differently and will uniquely redefine their roles in relation to the affected family member. These redefinitions then will have implications as to how the family members will interact with each other as well as to how they understand their new roles and the new roles of other family members. It is hard for the family to work cohesively and in a unified manner with all of the new role changes and individual interpretations of the situation. The nurse can assist the family immeasurably when he or she facilitates communication among family members so that they have insight into one another's definitions and beliefs of the situation. When family members share a common meaning of the situation, they can unite to construct a meaningful plan to deal with the illness.

From Perry, J., & Olshansky, E. (1996). *Western Journal of Nursing Research, 18*(1), 12–33.

TABLE 28-2 ▼ Stages of Alzheimer's Disease

STAGE	SYMPTOMATOLOGY
Mild	Frequently repeating oneself
	Regularly misplacing articles
	Inability to recall familiar words to use in conversation
	Withdrawal from formally enjoyed activities
	Awareness of and frustration with one's own "forgetfulness"
	Changes not readily apparent to many people and often are denied or excused by the family
Moderate	Decreased ability to carry out ADLs and IADLs
	Difficulty finding way around one's own neighborhood and home
	Disoriented to time and place
	Disruptive behaviors (wandering, pacing)
	Hallucinations and delusions
	Inability to perform complex motor activities
	Problems with visual perception (and thus susceptibility to accidents)
	Needs supervision frequently
	Temperament fluctuations from composed and tranquil to screaming and argumentative
	Deterioration apparent to friends and family
Severe	Lost capacity of self-care
	Lost use of language
	Only has minimal long-term memory
	Must have 24-hour, 7 days-a-week care

...s vascular to be con- ...llege that it ...ose older than ...dementia paral- ...(VA) and include ..., atrial fibrillation, ... scan and magnetic ...fy the brain disease in ...ve deficits arise from the multi... ...d the white matter of the brain after ... ...schemia inherent in a CVA. Historically, the c... ...nces a stepwise or fluctuating pattern of progression ...er than a steady and gradual deterioration. The client exhibits focal neurologic signs. The specific symptomatology seen with this dementia depends on the sectors of the brain infarcted and the extent to which they are damaged. Frequently, there is accompanying neurologic evidence of cerebrovascular disease, such as paresis or paralysis of a limb or headaches. Classically, the client with vascular dementia experiences impaired memory and manifests aphasia, apraxia, agnosia, and difficulties with executive functioning.

PARKINSON'S DISEASE

Parkinson's disease is a neurodegenerative illness that progresses slowly and has no known cure. This disease affects 1 million Americans and though its predominate clinical picture is that of immobility, the cognitive decline of dementia runs concurrently in more than 40% of affected clients. In Parkinson's disease, a decreasing number of brain cells in the substantia nigra results in a depletion of the neurotransmitter, dopamine. The client exhibits involuntary muscle movements at rest accompanied by overall slowness and rigidity. Most often seen in clients who display postural instability and gait disturbance, the intellectual deficits accompanying this disease vary, although their progression is predictably insidious and progressive. The dementia of Parkinson's disease does not impair the client's language capabilities as do many of the other dementias. It does not, however, spare the client's memory retrieval and executive functioning. The dementia seen in Parkinson's disease is unique and different from that seen in Alzheimer's disease, though sadly, some who have Parkinson's disease probably also have Alzheimer's disease (Scharre & Mahler, 1994).

HUNTINGTON'S CHOREA

Huntington's chorea is a familial disease passed on by an autosomal dominant trait. Children of affected parents have a 50% chance of inheriting the trait-carrying gene. Men and women are affected equally. The disease inevitably manifests itself in persons with the trait aged between 35

and 45 years. The course of the disease from onset to death is approximately 15 years (Kovach & Stearns, 1993). A genetic marker for Huntington's chorea makes presymptomatic and prenatal testing possible; however, the test is not always available. Moreover, when the test is available, it produces a high anxiety quotient for the at-risk person.

Autopsy typically reveals frontal cerebral atrophy. Research laboratory findings suggest that this disease may be the result of biochemical changes within the brain cells.

The person with Huntington's chorea experiences choreic movements that are intensified during stress, which can be as simple as having to wait for a need to be met. The jerking movements usually peak 10 years after onset and then stabilize or decrease. This particular dementia causes no aphasia, agnosia, and apraxia, but memory deficits, slowed thinking, problems with sustained attention span, and deficiency in judgment occur. An emotional component is apparent by the time clients reach their 20s or 30s. As the frontal lobe begins to deteriorate, the client becomes labile, impulsive, easily frustrated, irritable, hostile, and aggressive. The illness becomes more relentless with time, and the affected client often exhibits affective or intermittent explosive disorders (Kovach & Stearns, 1993).

HUMAN IMMUNODEFICIENCY VIRUS

AIDS dementia is seen more frequently in a younger population than the other dementias because HIV is more prevalent in the younger population. MRI of the brain often reveals some type of pathologic change, and the client usually manifests the other symptoms accompanying an incidence of full-blown AIDS. The client with HIV dementia has the typical dementia signs of memory loss, poor judgment, and decreased executive functions such as planning and reasoning. At times, clients have slowed motor movements. The progression of this dementia differs from other dementias that have a predictably steady mental deterioration. Some clients with HIV dementia have daily episodes of memory loss and confusion alternating with mental clarity. The dementia also can stabilize for months or even years on end before its downward progression resumes.

PICK'S DISEASE

Pick's disease accounts for about 5% of the progressive dementias. The onset of Pick's disease is between ages 40 and 60 years; studies show that it occurs slightly more often in men than women. Pick's disease is another degenerative cognitive disorder that so resembles Alzheimer's disease in its clinical picture that in several instances it is only at autopsy that differentiation can take place. The actual cause is unknown, but genetic factors are suspected. General microscopic findings include atrophy of the frontal and temporal lobes of the brain. Why this atrophy occurs is not clearly understood, but it is believed to be the reason for the aberrant behaviors seen in Pick's disease. In the beginning stages, the victims of this disorder have *less* disorientation and memory loss than those with Alzheimer's disease and *more* personality changes, including loss of social constraints (resulting in frequent behavioral problems).

CREUTZFELDT-JAKOB DISEASE

Creutzfeldt-Jakob disease is a rare disease that causes a cognitive disorder by targeting the central nervous system. With an incidence of about one new case per 1 million people per year, this rapidly progressive and ultimately fatal disease is caused by a protein-like agent called a prion (Anderson, 1998). One way that the disease is thought to be spread is through contact with contaminated human brain tissue or from improperly sterilized neurosurgical tools. The ingestion of certain neurologic parts of cows that have been infected with a prion similar to the one of Creutzfeldt-Jakob disease has been the source of contamination in recent outbreaks in Britain. The disease is termed "spongiform" because of the spongy appearance of the cerebral and cerebellar cortex. Creutzfeldt-Jakob disease is seen most frequently in middle-aged to older adults and often is initially misdiagnosed as Alzheimer's disease.

The client with Creutzfeldt-Jakob disease passes through three distinct stages. Initially, mental abnormalities progress into a rapidly deteriorating dementia. Later, a jerking, seizure-like activity appears. Many clients exhibit ataxia, dysarthria, and other cerebellar signs. Extrapyramidal signs, disruption in many of the senses, and seizures are other manifestations during the middle phase of this disease. The final phase usually is marked by coma, with the client dying from infections and respiratory problems (Chipps & Paulson, 1994).

Implications and Prognosis

The prognosis for those individuals with progressive dementia is very poor. Currently, no *cures* are available for the dementias; however, certain interventions appear to *delay* or *slow* the progression of some of the disorders.

Interdisciplinary Goals and Treatment

Clients with dementia and their caregivers truly need the participation of the whole healthcare team for a comprehensive treatment regimen. Overall goals of treatment for a client with dementia include the following:

- Physical care of the client
- Safe environment
- Behavior management
- Psychosocial support of client and family caregivers
- Education of client and family caregivers

The client with dementia benefits from as early a diagnosis as is possible to allow for interventions that slow the disorder's progression. An early diagnosis also gives family members time to adjust and rearrange their lives as they increasingly assume the caregiver role. The treatment team interacts most intensively with the client during the early stages of the dementia when he or she is still aware of and thus most frustrated and depressed about cognitive losses. As the disease becomes more incapacitating, the members of the healthcare contingent expand their involvement with family members to form a close-knit partnership. This partnership promotes the client's physical health and safety as well as supports the family itself.

As the client's cognitive abilities and behavior deteriorate, the needs of the client and family become more extensive. The family needs educative support from the physician and nurse on how to care for the loved one who can no longer meet his or her own physical needs or ADLs. Family members (most often a spouse or daughter) usually assume the role of primary caregiver. In taking on this role, they assume an exhaustive, 24-hour, 7 days-a-week job for someone who shows less and less appreciation for what they do, and with time, does not even recognize who they are. This is not only *physically* stressing to the caregiver but also *emotionally* distressing. The healthcare team must be a resource to the family for such things as innovative care tactics, community resources that offer respite care, home healthcare, information about support groups, and group or personal counseling. Such support helps the family to care for their loved one and delays or permanently postpones a client's institutionalization.

MEDICAL AND SUPPORTIVE INTERVENTIONS

Family caregivers need to know how to meet the physical needs of their loved one as his or her self-care capabilities diminish. Some caregivers can meet the client's physical needs with just a little information and guidance from the healthcare team; others require more tangible assistance (eg, home health aides).

Changing the environment often can assuage behavioral problems that occur during the progression of dementia. Sometimes, however, such behavioral problems are best dealt with pharmacologically. Those behaviors that warrant pharmacologic intervention include extreme agitation, depression, and disinhibition. Any medications given to a client with dementia need very careful monitoring because they can be causative agents of behavioral problems. Sometimes, merely lowering the dosage, discontinuing the medication, or substituting another medication can resolve behavioral issues.

Pharmacologic intervention also has proven moderately successful at slowing the cognitive decline of dementia. The treatment team needs to determine which medication is best suited to each client and to educate the family as to the dosage, schedule, and possible side effects.

The team also must take responsibility for assessing the response and any possible side effects of the prescriptive medications.

PSYCHOSOCIAL INTERVENTIONS

Because of the grim prognosis for clients with dementia, the client and the family members initially need the support of the interdisciplinary team to endure the shock of the diagnosis as well as to receive guidance for future planning. In the early stages, clients can be aware of the cognitive loses that are taking place and need emotional support. As the dementia progresses, the caregivers need increasing support from healthcare professionals to deal with their own exhaustion, depression, and frustration. The family needs to participate in the plan of the client's care and have educational input as to available resources to help them with the physical care that they render to their loved one as well as help to deal with their own emotional struggles.

APPLICATION OF THE NURSING PROCESS TO THE CLIENT WITH DEMENTIA

Assessment

The first step in determining treatment and nursing approaches for the client is assessment and screening for any underlying, treatable physical problems that accentuate or are comorbid with the cognitive disorder. Doing so involves taking an extensive history, physical examination (including an extensive neurologic and mental status examination), and diagnostic testing. Laboratory and diagnostic evaluation often includes the tests listed in Table 28-3. If the screening procedures reveal treatable illnesses, action needs to be initiated to resolve them. Treating underlying illnesses will

1. Expedite recovery from delirium, if present
2. Improve the symptomatology and delay further decline
3. Eliminate symptoms that can obscure the clinical picture of dementia and thus prevent a timely diagnosis

Once the client has been evaluated for underlying medical conditions, the nurse can proceed with an assessment of the client's cognitive functioning.

BEHAVIOR

The nurse assesses the client's behavior by separating it into components and assessing each (Box 28-5). The client's family is one of the most reliable sources of information because the client may have minimal or no insight into when the decline in cognitive abilities or change in behavior began. The nurse questions the client and fam-

ily in a nonjudgmental, nonthreatening way and recognizes that denial is common. The client may try to cover up for gaps in memory, and the family may have rationalized truly disruptive behavior as behavior that is just idiosyncratic of their loved one.

MENTAL STATUS

Using the various instruments and lab tests listed in Tables 28-4 and 28-5, the nurse can assess mental status. The classic assessment tool is the Short, Portable Mental Status Questionnaire (SPMSQ) developed by Pfeiffer. Lack of insight on the client's part is an early feature of dementia. The nurse can determine lack of insight by asking the client to explain what something like "a rolling stone gathers no moss" means. Failure to adequately explain such a proverb may indicate problems with abstract reasoning and concentration of executive functioning.

PERCEPTUAL PROBLEMS

The nurse may discover perceptual problems by observing the client's behavior and exploring strange or unusual comments that he or she has made. Family members may provide invaluable data associated with this area. They can contribute historical information about the client's unusual behavior and can relate any hallucinatory episodes (eg, a time where the client verbalized fears and concerns about seeing bugs that were not seen by anyone else).

ORIENTATION

Assessment should include evaluating the client's orientation to person, place, time, and date. The nurse must ask such questions skillfully so as not to insult the client. This can be accomplished by phrasing questions conversationally or informing the client that some basic questions will be asked as part of the examination. The nurse also should ask the family if the client "sundowns."

MEMORY

The client's memory is an important feature to evaluate during the nursing assessment. Incidents evoking remote memory usually are easy to elicit from the client. This is not always so with more current events. The nurse can assess recent memory by evaluating the client's response to questions that ask the client to recall events of the previous hour, day, or week.

FAMILY

The family, as indicated previously, is an invaluable resource for historical data. Family members often can provide much information concerning a client's ability to carry out ADLs and instrumental activities of daily living (IADLs). The interaction that takes place between the family and the client during the assessment interview also can reveal the

TABLE 28-3 ▼ Comparative Assessment for Cognitive Disorders

	COGNITION	LEVEL OF CON-SCIOUSNESS	MEMORY	APPEARANCE	EMOTIONS
Alzheimer's disease	Global intellectual impairment	Insidious onset characterized initially by "mistakes in judgment," progressing to inability to comprehend, agraphia, aphasia, and finally to unresponsiveness	Clouding late in disease; short-term memory loss initially progressing to both short-term and long-term loss	Progressive loss of grooming habits as a result of forgotten social behaviors and decreasing coordination required to dress	Initially depression and anxiety about recognized regression, progressing to loss or severe dampening of emotions Subtle loss of interest in work Inability to recognize family members
Pick's disease	Intellect intact	Lack of insight into disease process	Not affected	Slovenly	Dramatic personality changes Socially inappropriate behavior Flip beyond reasonable propriety
Huntington's chorea	Insight into the psychological degenerative changes	Increasingly a problem as pathology progresses but without aphasia, agnosia, or apraxia	Choreiform movements	Sloppy	Mood swings from apathy to aggressive behavior Inappropriate behavior Despair about changes taking place Suicidal tendencies Decreased interest in job
Wernicke-Korsakoff syndrome	Cannot learn new information because of an inability to retain facts	Alert	Suspended in time Recall limits to 2–3 min Extensive memory loss	Unsteady gait from peripheral neuropathies	Communication impaired related to memory gaps Confabulation
Vascular dementia	Not affected	Cannot learn new or recall previously learned material Proceeds in a stepwise progression as ministrokes occur	Does not handle new situations well	Deterioration of hygienic standards	Depression or pseudo-depression

BOX 28-5 ▼ *Assessment Guide*

I. Subjective data
   A. Behavioral changes (often asked of the family)
      1. Is there a change in behavior? If so,
         a. How does the present behavior differ from former behavior?
         b. When was this change in behavior first recognized?
   B. Emotional changes
      1. Are any of the following present?
         a. Depression
         b. Anxiety
         c. Paranoia
         d. Agitation
         e. Grandiosity
         f. Confabulation
      2. Does the client have insight into the fact that "things are not right"?
      3. Is the client complaining of many physical ailments for which there are no bases?
      4. Are certain previous personality traits becoming predominant or exaggerated?
   C. Social changes
      1. Is the client exhibiting embarrassingly loud and jocular behavior?
      2. Is there sexual acting-out beyond the bounds of propriety?
      3. Have the following developed?
         a. Short-temperedness
         b. Irritability
         c. Aggressiveness
      4. Is there an increasing inability to make social judgments?
   D. Intellectual behavior
      1. Has the ability to remember recent events decreased?
      2. Has the ability to problem solve decreased? (This might be especially apparent in the work or job area.)
      3. Do new environments or even old environments result in the client's disorientation?
      4. Is it difficult for the client to carry out complex motor skills? Do his or her efforts result in many errors?
      5. Are any of the following language problems present:
         a. Has the client's language changed?
         b. Does the client's language ramble and wander from the point of the conversation?

   c. Is the point of the conversation never clearly stated?
   d. Is there difficulty comprehending complex material?
   e. Does the client have trouble remembering names of people and objects?
   f. Does the client have difficulty writing?

II. Objective observations
   A. Level of consciousness
      1. Is the client confused, sleepy, withdrawn, adynamic, apathetic?
   B. Appearance
      1. Is there decreased personal hygiene?
   C. Attention
      1. Does the client have decreased ability to repeat digits after the interviewer?
      2. Do other stimuli in the environment easily distract the client from the interviewer?
      3. Does the client focus on only one of the stimuli in the environment and is he or she unable to turn attention from the one stimulus?
   D. Language
      1. Outflow of words decreases.
      2. Patterns of repetitive, tangential, or concrete speech appear.
      3. Writing skills decrease more rapidly than the spoken word.
   E. Memory—Tests client's ability to remember four unrelated words and recent events. (Confabulation and anger often will be used by the client to move the interviewer away from questions related to memory.)
   F. Constructional ability—The client is instructed to copy a series of line drawings; the client often is unable to do this or the ability to do so will decline dramatically over time.
   G. Cortical function
      1. The client's ability to perform arithmetic is faulty and reveals many errors.
      2. Proverb interpretation—Usually, the client will give only a concrete interpretation of the proverb.
      3. Similarities—The client often will deny similarities between two objects and instead will give a concrete answer. For example, when asked, "What is the similarity between a tiger and a cat?," the client may reply, "One is small and one is large. There is no similarity."

TABLE 28-4 ▼ Screening Tests

TEST	CLINICAL IMPORTANCE
1. WBC with differential	1. Infection
2. Sedimentation rate	2. Infection or vasculitis
3. Urine examination and toxicology test	
a. Sugar and acetone	a. Diabetes
b. Leukocytes	b. Infection
c. Barbiturates and other toxic substances	c. Toxicity
d. Albumin	d. Renal failure
e. Porphyria screen	e. Renal failure
4. Serum tests	
a. Blood urea nitrogen	a. Renal failure
b. Creatinine	b. Renal failure
c. Glucose	c. Diabetes, hypoglycemia
d. T_3, T_4	d. Thyroid disease
e. Electrolytes	e. Evaluation for imbalance including NA^+, K^+, Ca^{2+}, Cl^-, PO_4 = parathyroid-induced changes in calcium, phosphorus
f. Mg^+, Br^+	f. If available, bromides still are present in some common drugs and overuse may inadvertently lead to toxicity
g. Serum folate level	g. Nutritional problems, thiamin deficiency
h. AST, ALT	h. Liver failure
i. VDRL	i. Syphilis
j. Drug levels—specific search for evidence of drugs (eg, ETOH)	j. Barbiturate, other drug overdose
5. Routine radiographs	
a. Chest	a. Infection, heart failure
b. Skull	b. Evidence of increased intracranial pressure, fractures, and so forth
6. EEG	6. Ictal phenomenon
7. CT scan	7. Brain tumor, subdural hematoma, infection, hemorrhage
8. Spinal tap	8. Infection, hemorrhage
9. Invasive neuroradiologic procedures	9. Suspicion of tumors, vascular lesions, hydrocephalus

ALT, alanine aminotransferase; AST, aspartate aminotransferase; Br^+, bromide; Ca^{2+}, calcium; Cl^-, chloride; CT, computed tomography; EEG, electroencephalogram; ETOH, ethanol; K^+, potassium, Mg^+, magnesium; Na^+, sodium; PO_4, phosphorus; T_3, triiodothyronine; T_4, thyroxine; VDRL, Venereal Disease Research Laboratories; WBC, white blood cell count.
From Staub, R., & Black, F. (1981). Organic brain syndromes (pp. 109–110). Philadelphia: FA Davis.

condition of the client's social skills and the dynamics of the family group.

The nurse must assess family members, especially the caregivers, for the telltale signs of caregiver stress or burnout. Although this might not be an issue during the early stages of dementia, it becomes paramount as the client's state progressively degenerates, spiraling the demands for physical care onto the caregiver. It also becomes a factor as the "caregiver role" becomes an increasingly predominant part of the caregivers' lives while the roles of spouse, companion, confidante, and lover fade.

EDUCATION

The nurse must assess the family and client to d_____ their need for information and instruction abou_____ care of the client, and support for the care_____ giver can provide better care for the clie_____ knows what to expect as the disease pr_____ take care of the commonly seen b_____ Caregiver burnout, guilt, and f_____ rated when the family membe_____ ality of his or her feelings a_____

TABLE 28-5 ▼ **Testing for Cognitive Deficits**

FOCUS OF TEST	NAME OF TEST	WHAT IS MEASURED	ANALYSIS POTENTIAL
Intelligence, verbal performance	Wechsler Adult Intelligence Scale (WAIS)	Crystallized and fluid intelligence	Notes if client can pay attention and use memory
Memory	Wechsler Memory Scale–Revised California Verbal Learning Test		Alzheimer's Sensitive in early dementia If single finding, may indicate amnestic disorder
Language skills	Boston Diagnostic Aphasia Examination	Aphasia subtest—word finding ability (common in dementia)	Alzheimer's Single finding may indicate focal deficit
Conceptualization	WAIS-R Similarities Subtest	Abstract versus concrete thinking	
Visuospatial skills	Benton Visual Retention Test Block Design subtest of the WAIS-R		Alzheimer's
Attention	Digit Span Subtest of the WAIS-R		Single finding may indicate delirium disorder, focal frontal lesion

Compiled from Jutagir, K., Peterson, M. (1994). *Psychological aspects of aging: When does memory loss signal dementia? Geriatrics 49*(3), 45–51.

Nursing Diagnoses

There are as many nursing diagnoses for the client with cognitive disorders as there are possibilities of symptoms. Although nursing diagnoses must reflect the uniqueness of each client, a plan of care might include the following:

- **Chronic Confusion** related to cerebral degeneration
- **Self-Care Deficit** related to cognitive and motor impairments
- **Risk for Injury** related to cognitive and psychomotor impairments reducing ability to adapt to changing environment
- **Interrupted Family Processes** related to degen~~~~~ ~~~~~ nber

~~...~~tia is most
~~...~~idisciplinary
~~...~~alistic goals.
~~...~~uld include
~~...~~ness and sta-
~~...~~sponsibilities
~~...~~ite interven-

~~...~~dementia are

- The client's physical needs will be met.
- The client's environment will be safe and protected.
- The client will have infrequent episodes of agitation.
- The client's caregivers and family will have psychosocial support and resources for respite care.

Implementation

General interventions for clients with cognitive disorders are presented. Nursing Care Plan 28-2 illustrates the nursing process for Joe, the client presented in Clinical Example 28–1, who has Alzheimer's disease.

MANAGING THE CLIENT'S HEALTH

One of the most essential nursing actions for the client with a cognitive disorder is to facilitate optimal functioning by promoting physical health. Because exogenous substances can initiate or exacerbate aberrant behavior, the nurse must be sensitive to the client's response to prescribed medications. Besides knowing the side effects and toxic reactions of the specific drugs that the client is receiving, the nurse also must be alert to possible drug interactions.

The nurse also assesses the client for any symptoms of physical illness. Prompt recognition of symptoms and appropriate interventions may impede an episodic illness from becoming comorbid or a comorbid illness from accelerating the client's existing mental dysfunction. The

Nursing Care Plan 28-2

THE CLIENT WITH EARLY-STAGE ALZHEIMER'S DISEASE

Joe, from Clinical Example 28-1, is extremely upset by the diagnosis of Alzheimer's disease and at first denies that he has any problems. He initially becomes angry with the doctor and his daughter, Mandy, but then becomes tearful and admits that he has been concerned about his mental functioning. All agree that the biggest risks for Joe at this time are that he will accidentally injure himself, set a fire, or get lost as a result of his short-term memory loss and mild confusion.

After a long discussion, Mandy, Joe, and the doctor agree that Joe will need supervision. Joe's sister, Abby, who is 75 years old and also lives alone in the same town, agrees to move in with Joe to help monitor his behavior. Although Abby is in good physical health, the family realizes that she cannot provide physical care when it becomes necessary, nor can she manage Joe if he becomes hostile.

Nursing Diagnosis: Anticipatory Grieving related to expected loss of cognitive function and independence

Goal: Joe will work through his feelings of grief about his diagnosis.

Interventions	Rationales
Assist the client to identify his fears and express his feelings about the diagnosis. Listen carefully and empathetically. Remember that the loss of cognitive function is one of the most frightening changes a person can face and that the client will need much time to process his feelings.	Encouraging Joe to express his feelings and listening empathetically will help Joe release his feelings of sadness and fear and move through the grieving stages. It also will help him to feel that others understand as well.
Help the client identify existing coping strategies or learn new ones. Examples include living in the present, meditating, praying, and practicing deep breathing or relaxation techniques.	Establishing a plan for managing stress will help Joe during times of fearfulness and anxiety. Stress reduction techniques also may increase feelings of well-being.
Encourage the client to identify spiritual sources of support.	Many older adults experience a renewed connection with their spiritual selves as they age and confront death. Joe may find comfort by participating in spiritual practices.

Evaluation: Joe discusses his feelings of sadness and copes with them.

Nursing Diagnosis: Risk for Injury related to cognitive impairments

Goal: Joe will not incur any injury.

Interventions	Rationales
Identify danger areas in the home. Make the garage and basement unavailable to the client because dangerous items often are stored in these areas. Lock medications, poisons, cleaning agents, and other toxic fluids in secure containers or rooms. Lock doors leading to the outside or install alarms on them. Secure the windows and any balcony doors on the upper floors of the home.	Joe's decreasing cognitive skills make him prone to injury. Keeping certain areas off limits while keeping the rest of the house safe and secure will allow Joe freedom in his own home while protecting him.
Modify the environmental to make it safer. Plug electrical outlets and remove electrical items that pose hazards. Lower the thermostat on the hot water heater to its lowest setting. Remove all electrical appliances from counters and the control knobs from the stove and oven.	Although Joe is still at a high level of functioning, making the home environment safer will protect him and give Mandy and Abby some peace of mind. Monitoring the home environment is the best intervention for maintaining his safety. These interventions will help prevent accidental burns or fires.

Evaluation: Joe can live within the home environment with minimal threat to his safety.

(continued)

Nursing Care Plan 28-2 (Continued)

Nursing Diagnosis: **Chronic Confusion** related to Alzheimer's disease

Goal: Joe will remain calm and be able to function in his environment.

Interventions	Rationales
Establish a calm environment. Remove household clutter. Create predictability and simplify choices. Establish a daily routine for grooming, meals, and activities.	A routine and less clutter will help Joe feel safe and secure in his home. Simple choices and tasks that Joe can complete successfully will prevent frustration and loss of self-esteem.
Provide environmental memory cues. Cut out pictures from magazines and place them on cabinets and drawers to illustrate the contents. Place a large-print calendar in a conspicuous spot and record all appointments on the calendar. Encourage client to review the calendar daily.	Providing environmental cues will help jog Joe's memory and keep him as independent as possible for as long as possible.

Evaluation: Joe's demeanor remains calm throughout the day, and he can function within his environment.

Nursing Diagnosis: **Decisional Conflict** related to uncertainty about future health and available resources

Goal: Joe and his family will make plans for his future care.

Interventions	Rationales
Provide information. Describe the options available for care, including full-time nursing care in the home, adult day care centers, nursing homes, and other long-term care facilities. Help the family explore the advantages or disadvantages of each option. Supply all information as requested by the client and family but avoid portraying a hopeless prognosis.	Joe's family members need to have information so they can plan for the future. The current plan, caregiving by Joe's 75-year-old sister, will not be feasible if Joe's condition deteriorates. Joe still may be in denial about his condition; the healthcare team needs to respect his right to not receive information.
Help the client clarify his values and make important decisions while cognitive function remains high. Encourage the client and family to provide advanced directives and make any necessary legal decisions.	Encouraging Joe to make these decisions now will ensure that others can carry out his wishes if he becomes unable to make decisions in the future.

Evaluation: Joe and his family make plans for his future care.

Nursing Diagnosis: **Interrupted Family Processes** related to change in Joe's health status and alteration in family roles.

Goal: Joe, Mandy, and Abby will cope with the changes in family roles and Joe's health status.

Interventions	Rationales
Promote family cohesion. Help the family members, including the client, identify their feelings about role and health status changes. Help individuals resolve guilt feelings, if necessary. Identify effective coping mechanisms and encourage the family to use them as they adjust to the changes. Help the family resolve any conflicts and suggest attending an Alzheimer's support group.	Encouraging open communication about the effects of Alzheimer's disease will help Joe, Mandy, and Abby to adjust. Mandy and Abby may feel guilt about not being able to help more or resentment about increased responsibilities. Joe may feel guilty about becoming a "burden" on his family. Helping them resolve these feelings and identifying appropriate coping behaviors will decrease family stress. Support groups are a tremendous resource for sharing feelings and gaining insight and help.

Evaluation: Joe, Mandy, and Abby demonstrate ability to adjust to role changes and maintain family cohesiveness.

(continued)

Nursing Care Plan 28-2 (Continued)

Nursing Diagnosis: Risk for Caregiver Role Strain related to around the clock care responsibilities

Goal: Abby will express satisfaction with her life.

Interventions	Rationales
Provide practical support to caregiver. Explore caregiver's reaction to new role and help her identify the stressors, tasks, or behaviors that are most frustrating or anxiety producing. Help her develop a plan for managing these situations. Provide information about the disease process and local support groups.	Helping Abby become aware of her feelings, strengths, the progressive nature of the disease, and available social supports will empower her to manage the increasing demands of caregiving while protecting her emotional state. Thinking through and planning ahead will help Abby manage her caregiving responsibilities.
Provide emotional support to caregiver. Help the caregiver learn stress management techniques. Encourage her to get adequate rest and to maintain her own physical, emotional, and spiritual health. Help the caregiver recognize that caregiving is stressful. Encourage her to not feel ashamed or guilty if she experiences impatience, frustration, sadness, or anger.	Relaxation exercises such as deep breathing, meditation, and visualization, as well as physical exercise and adequate rest, can help Abby manage feelings of anxiety and stress. Finding sources for personal comfort and happiness will help Abby maintain her own identity separate from her caregiving role. Abby then can come to understand that these emotions are natural when caring for someone who may be unhappy, ungrateful, or difficult.
Establish a plan for respite care. Encourage caregiver to set realistic limits on what and how much she can do. Counsel the caregiver to avoid becoming isolated and to accept help from family or friends. Identify community resources for respite care or other family members or friends who are available to regularly relieve caregiver for a few hours at a time.	Abby will not be able to perform total full-time care and should not get pulled into doing more and more as Joe's condition declines. Respite care is essential to prevent "burnout," which is common among full-time caregivers, especially those who are socially isolated or have no relief from their duties.

Evaluation: Abby avails herself of respite care and Alzheimer's support groups and expresses satisfaction with plan of care and her role as caregiver.

nurse pays particular attention to the client's nutrition and hydration status, as well as to bowel and bladder elimination. Clients with dementia may resist eating or forget to eat, and poor hydration usually accompanies poor food intake. The nurse offers the client foods and fluids throughout the day. Presenting the food in small portions or offering finger foods may increase the likelihood that the client will eat.

Poor food and fluid intake can result in bowel and bladder problems. Constipation or impaction from insufficient bulk or water can have serious consequences if not treated promptly. The client may be unable to articulate feelings of fullness; caregivers should keep a record of the regularity of bowel movements. Insufficient intake of fluids can lead to urinary stasis and an environment conducive to urinary tract infection. Monitoring fluid intake so that the client receives at least 2000 mL/day (unless contraindicated by renal or cardiac disease) will help prevent infection and maintain health.

ENHANCING SENSORY CAPABILITIES

For the client who has trouble interpreting the environment, sensory aids, such as glasses and hearing aids, can be instrumental in helping the client feel more in control. The nurse can provide reading material in large type, if necessary, and speak to the client directly and carefully to further maximize the client's ability to process sensory input. The client's caregivers also need to be aware that sensory disturbances are not limited to sight and hearing. The client's perception of pain and temperature also may be altered. Thus, caregivers must take precautions with hot liquids and bath water to avoid burning the client. Diminished or altered pain perception further emphasizes the need for surveillance by the staff of the client's physical condition.

MEETING THE CLIENT'S PHYSICAL NEEDS

The ability of clients to care for themselves decreases as the severity of the cognitive order increases. The healthcare team and the family caregivers need to continually reevaluate the client's ability to meet self-care needs. Caregivers can help by enhancing the client's environment to facilitate his or her limited ability to perform ADLs and IADLs and by fulfilling unmet client needs themselves.

Sometimes, a client displays aberrant behavior because of unmet needs. An underlying medical problem may have gone undetected, or the client may be experiencing pain. As the ability to communicate decreases, the caregivers and the healthcare team may need to thoughtfully observe the client and play "detective" to try to discern the meaning behind the individual's actions. Problem behavior can be driven by something as basic as the discomfort of constipation. Problematic behavior may subside after a basic need has been met.

ENCOURAGING APPROPRIATE BEHAVIORS

A client with a cognitive disorder often cannot change his or her behavior. Therefore, the most successful intervention that nurses can implement is to change what the client experiences. Restructuring the environment to make it less formidable for the client whose cognitive function is impaired is especially helpful. Pharmacologic intervention may be necessary to manage behavior that is harmful to a client, family, or healthcare team.

Modifying the Environment

Environmental modification can be the key to managing behavior. The pathologic changes in the brain decrease the client's ability to interpret the environment accurately. Many clients overreact, especially when they are bombarded by multiple cues. Decreasing noise, choices, and overstimulating interactions can help the client maintain stable, appropriate behavior patterns. Instituting routines and keeping choices simple help the easily confused client.

Bath times or times when hands-on care is given seem to especially agitate a client. There often is a way to modify the environment to provide positive experiences for a client that does not inflame behavior. Sometimes, changing the site of the bath or giving a bed bath instead of a shower or tub bath in the bathroom of the home or the institution is helpful.

Enhancing environmental cues may be beneficial for the client. Clocks and calendars strategically placed in the environment may help to keep the client oriented. Reality orientation once was thought to be beneficial to orient the client, but recent thinking is that this type of orientation merely frustrates the client and causes more problems than it helps.

Simply controlling the light in the environment may decrease the perceptual difficulties of hallucinations or illusions. The nurse must eliminate any environmental hazards.

Those who are caring for clients with cognitive disorders can monitor their own interactions with them. Usually, a caregiver with a calm demeanor has more success handling or interacting with an individual who is manifesting problematic behavior. This is especially helpful when hands-on care is required. Bath times seem to be especially difficult.

At times, there may seem to be no way to resolve the emotional frustration, agitation, or outbursts of the client who is angry with the environment and those in it. The caregiver might find it beneficial to redirect or distract the client. This can be done by asking to see a client's personal items, such as photographs, and then talking about the family members and life events illustrated by the photographs in the book. See Therapeutic Communication 28-1.

Performing Pharmacologic Interventions

One of the findings in DAT is diminished activity in the cholinergic system. Some researchers believe that anything that activates or augments whatever activity remains in the cholinergic system will benefit cognitive function.

Tacrine (Cognex) is a centrally acting, noncompetitive inhibitor of acetylcholinesterase that helps to elevate the level of ACh in the system by decreasing the binding sites of acetylcholinesterase. This lengthens the potential for cholinergic activity. Tacrine is effective as long as at least some cells are producing ACh; consequently, tacrine is most efficacious in mild to moderate cases of DAT. Even then, the effects of this drug on cognition are modest, with only small improvements and possible slowing of deterioration of cognition.

The liver rapidly absorbs and metabolizes tacrine; therefore, the liver is most vulnerable to the drug's toxicity. Liver function tests, especially the level of alanine aminotransferase (ALT), must be monitored every week for the first 18 weeks. If it is necessary to increase the dosage, ALT must be monitored for 6 weeks. Once the dose is stable, monitoring can be done monthly.

The most common side effects involve the gastrointestinal system, with nausea and vomiting being the most prevalent complaints and elevated ALT level being the most common sign. Clients should be monitored for the development of peptic ulcer disease because the drug can increase gastric secretions. Antacids may be given to alleviate epigastric distress, especially if there is a history of ulcer disease or anti-inflammatory drug use.

Tacrine is contraindicated in any client sensitive to tacrine or acridine derivatives, with a history of liver disease or elevated ALT levels, or with a total bilirubin greater than 3.0 mg/dL. Clients with a history of stroke, subdural hematoma, or hydrocephalus are not candidates for this drug therapy.

Tacrine should not be given along with other drugs that have anticholinergic effects. Clients taking theophylline must be monitored carefully because theophylline levels can be elevated as a result of taking these two drugs concurrently (Davis & Powchik, 1990; Wood & Lantz, 1995).

Donepezil (Aricept) and rivastigmine (Exelon) are other cholinesterase inhibitors. These medications are prescribed for clients with Alzheimer's disease who have mild to moderate symptoms. In some individuals taking this medication, donepezil delays the progression of dementia for 6 to 12 months. It has a longer duration than tacrine, does not require monitoring liver function,

THERAPEUTIC COMMUNICATION 28-1
A Client With Dementia

Anne Tepsin, a 64-year-old woman with dementia, comes to the day care center three times a week. Today, Annie's husband tells Roy Smith, the nurse, that Annie was awake most of the previous night. After her husband leaves, Annie begins to follow Roy in and out of the day room, activity room, kitchen, and sunroom. Around 10:30 AM, she asks Roy, "Are we going to eat soon?"

Ineffective Communication

Roy: "It's too early to eat, Annie. You eat at 11:30, just after you paint ceramics."

Annie: *(Walks with Roy out of the day room)* "When will I eat? Do I eat soon?"

Roy: *(Looks at watch and shakes his head)* "You don't eat until later. I have to go into the sunroom to work on the plants."

Annie: *(Follows Roy to the sunroom)* "When will I eat?"

Roy: *(Sighs and continues to water the plants)* "Annie, are you hungry?"

Annie: "NO! I'm not hungry! Why do you ask that?"

Roy: *(Notices Annie's behavior is beginning to escalate and feels puzzled as to why she is getting upset)* "Annie, go back to the other room and look at your memory book." *(Points to Annie's pocketbook)* "It's in your purse. I'll walk you there." *(Walks Annie to the day room, sits her at a table near another client who is napping, and tells another nurse to keep an eye on Annie)*

Annie: *(Sits at the table, looking confused and sad)*

Effective Communication

Roy: "It's too early to eat, Annie. Lunch is at 11:30, just after ceramics."

Annie: *(Walks with Roy out of the day room)* "When will I eat? Do I eat soon?"

Roy: *(Stops, looks directly at Annie, and smiles)* "Annie, you eat at lunch time, 1 hour from now. Let's go into the sunroom. You can help me water the plants." *(Remains patient with Annie, sensing that she is trying to express something other than her words)*

Annie: *(Helps Roy bring plants to the sink in the sunroom)* "When did you say I will eat?"

Roy: *(Stops watering the plants, looks at Annie, and smiles)* "Annie, are you hungry?" *(Uses positive and "cueing" nonverbal behavior)*

Annie: "NO! I'm not hungry! Why do you ask that?" *(Gets louder)*

Roy: *(Realizes Annie's behavior is beginning to escalate)* "Annie, I remember seeing a picture of you working in your garden. Would you show me that picture again? I think it's in your memory book in your purse." *(Points to Annie's pocketbook)* "Would you show me the picture of you in your garden, Annie?"

Annie: *(Looks at her purse and then rummages through it and pulls out a little photo book)* "You want to see my pictures?"

Roy: "Yes, Let's go sit down on the sofa and look at them." *(Goes over to the sofa and sits down, patting the cushion for Annie to sit. Annie comes over and begins thumbing through the book, telling Roy about the pictures.)*

Reflection and Critical Thinking

- What types of communication did Annie exhibit in both scenarios? Assess the reason for Annie's repetitive speech. Why might she be more hungry, tired, or insecure this morning?
- What nonverbal cues did Roy give in the first scenario? How did these differ from his actions in the second scenario? What were the results of the differences?
- What methods of communication did Roy use in the second scenario that ultimately were more effective than those he used in the first?

and is administered only once a day, at bedtime. Clients usually start with 5 mg/day, increasing to 10 mg/day after 4 to 6 weeks. Higher doses may not help all individuals, and donepezil has an increased risk of cholinergic side affects (nausea, diarrhea, insomnia). Donepezil can cause irregular heartbeats in clients with heart conditions.

Other drugs that have some promise to modify the dementia by being neuroprotective in individuals with early signs of Alzheimer's or with a family history are estrogen therapy, vitamin E, and ginkgo biloba. Some research on the use of these drugs is promising; however, confirmatory studies have yet to follow up initial findings.

PREVENTING INJURY

Clients with dementia face multiple dangers resulting from their impaired cognitive abilities. Safety concerns include injury from falls, injury from ingesting dangerous substances, getting lost, and injury to self or others from dangerous objects. Starting fires or getting burned also are fairly common occurrences. All of these situations are made worse by the client's inability to respond quickly to emergencies. See Nursing Care Plan 28-2 for interventions for making the home a safer environment for the client with dementia.

PRESERVING THE FAMILY UNIT

Family members must be prepared for the personal toll that their new role as caregivers may take. The nurse can provide information concerning creative ways to care for the loved one, including providing counseling and information about respite care. Day care for the client is one possibility that gives family members a break from their extensive caregiving activities and allows them to continue with their own daily routines and responsibilities. Through day care, a spouse may be able to retain his or her job and income and have the energy to care for the client during evening and weekend hours. Some communities have overnight respite care to give the caregiver welcomed "down time."

Family support groups and individual family counseling may help some families experiencing stress or having difficulty coping. One of the most effective interventions ...bout the necessary skills ...rs families when he or ...e their problem-solving ...y have options and link- ...rvices are tremendous ...Given, 1994). The fam- ...ember with a cognitive ...Client and Family Edu-

...to keep their loved ones ...ust recognize that long- ...e family can make this decision, but the professional care providers should tactfully raise this issue occasionally.

Evaluation

Outcomes for this population of clients may focus less on improving cognition and more on maintaining the current level of functioning for as long as possible and on the client and family successfully adapting to the ongoing decline in levels of function. When evaluation of the plan of care reveals that interventions are no longer effective or feasible, the healthcare team and the family (and the client, if possible) will need to devise different interventions. Indicators that the care plan is effective include the following:

- The client's physical needs are met.
- The client is well nourished and well hydrated.
- The client does not sustain injuries.
- Episodes of wandering or agitation are infrequent and managed successfully.
- The caregiver reports satisfaction with his or her quality of life and has social supports and respite care options in place.

AMNESTIC DISORDERS

Amnestic disorders include conditions in which *short-term memory loss* is a hallmark. The deterioration of memory is so great that it prevents clients from functioning at previous levels of social and occupational performance and seriously deters them from learning new information. Clients typically cannot recollect any events as recent as 2 minutes before; they may have some difficulty recalling events or knowledge that they formerly knew to be fact. The acuity of remote memory recall varies, and clients become adept at confabulation to hide memory deficits.

The brain damage that causes the condition leaves the client disoriented to time and place to some degree, but not to personhood (APA, 2000; Morrison, 1995). Clients have a superficiality of emotions that precludes deep emotional ties with others. They frequently adopt an emotional blandness in their affect. The progression of the symptomatology depends on the underlying etiology and its severity.

The classifications of this disorder are listed in Box 28-6. Like the dementias, the symptomatology shares a commonality; the etiology is the differentiating factor.

Wernicke-Korsakoff syndrome, one of the substance-induced persisting amnestic disorders, has been known for years as Korsakoff syndrome. The two occur so frequently together that they present a classic picture and thus often are combined and referred to as Wernicke-Korsakoff syndrome. By itself, Wernicke syndrome produces physical symptoms of ataxia, confusion, and paralysis of some of the motor muscles of the eye. Both syndromes are caused

Client and Family Education 28-1

ALZHEIMER'S DISEASE: CARING FOR CLIENT AND FAMILY

The devastation of Alzheimer's disease is not limited to the client alone. Throughout the course of the disease, the client's family members suffer greatly, both from the anguish of seeing the decline of their loved one and from the stress of caring for him or her. Family members often feel inept and have feelings of guilt. They worry about the relationship that they have with their loved one as the dynamics of that relationship change; they are anxious about long-term care issues and how to deal with the extended family and their own coping skills.

The adversity encountered while caring for a person with Alzheimer's disease may produce health problems in caregivers. The nurse can help alleviate some of the family's difficulties by providing continuous education about the disease process and assisting with problem-solving of the situational difficulties and crises that arise.

Adult care centers in some communities offer families the opportunity for a few hours of respite care. Relatives responsible for or actually administering care should be aware of helpful books, such as *The 36-Hour Day: A Guide to Caring for Persons With Alzheimer's Disease and Related Dementing Illnesses and Understanding Alzheimer's Disease* (Aronson).

The Alzheimer's Disease Education and Referral Center (Box 8250, Silver Spring, MD 20907-8250, 1-800-438-4380, fax 301-495-3334, e-mail adear@alzheimers.org) is a service of the National Institute on Aging, which is a national resource for information on all aspects of Alzheimer's disease for both professionals and families.

This center also provides referrals to national and state resources.

Alzheimer's disease support groups are found throughout the country in large and small communities. Family members can find the support group closest to them (1) by calling the Alzheimer's Association chapters, which usually are listed in the phone book; (2) by calling the Alzheimer's Association for a chapter referral (1-800-272-3900, fax 312-335-1110); (3) by accessing their web site *http://www.alz.org*; or (4) by calling their Area Agency on Aging or the ElderCare Locator (1-800-667-1116). Families also may receive the Alzheimer's Association Newsletter to keep abreast of developments in research, legislation, and techniques of care.

The Corporation for National Service is another resource for families. It is a corporation that administers many federal service programs. Some of the programs provide supportive services to the adult experiencing difficulties, and some focus on preventing or delaying institutionalization. They can be reached at 1201 New York Ave. NW, Washington, DC 20525, 1-800-424-8867, or fax 202-565-2794.

The nurse must remember that the family needs as much nursing care as does the victim of dementia, especially because the disease progresses in such an agonizingly slow manner. By providing emotional support and counseling and serving as a coordinator of available community resources, the nurse can significantly help to relieve the stress on the family caregiver.

---

by the client's compulsion for ingestion of alcohol, which supersedes the need for nutritional intake. Indeed, this syndrome usually is found in the 40- to 70-year-old client with alcoholism and a history of steady and progressive alcohol intake. In time, this person develops a vitamin B_1 (thiamin) deficiency that directly interferes with the production of the brain's main nutrient, glucose, resulting in the symptomatology of this syndrome.

A client with this disorder has great difficulty with recent memory, specifically, the ability to learn *new* information. Because of the inability to recall recent events, the individual fills in memory gaps with fabricated or imagined data (**confabulation**). This is truly a case of anterograde amnesia, and the client has no idea that there is a memory defect, nor does he or she care.

The prognosis for an individual experiencing an amnestic disorder varies greatly. As with the other cognitive disorders, the *etiology* of an amnestic disorder determines the duration and the severity of the course of illness.

In the case of the amnestic disorder "type" presented here (Wernicke-Korsakoff syndrome), the administration of the B vitamin, thiamin, can help alleviate some of the ataxic symptomatology. For the most part, however, the memory impairment remains.

Reflection and Critical Thinking Questions

1. Reread Clinical Examples 28-1 and 28-2. Compare how the memory of each client is affected. What are the differences and similarities in behavior?

2. Compare and contrast the prognoses for both clients.

3. What nursing interventions would be appropriate for each client?

4. Would you work with the families differently? How and why?

Amnestic Disorders Information Map

Amnestic Disorder Due to a General Medical Condition (Specify)

- Memory is impaired as manifested by impaired ability to learn new information or inability to recall previously learned information.
- The memory disturbance significantly impairs social or occupational functioning and represents a significant decline from previous functioning.
- The memory disturbance does not occur exclusively during delirium or dementia.
- Evidence from the history, physical examination, or laboratory tests supports that the disturbance is directly caused by a medical condition (including physical trauma).

Specify if
Transient is if memory impairment lasts for 1 month or less.
Chronic is if it lasts for more than 1 month.

Substance-Induced Persisting Amnestic Disorder

- Memory is impaired as manifested by impaired ability to learn new information or recall previously learned information.
- The memory disturbance significantly impairs social or occupational functioning and represents a significant decline from previous functioning.
- The memory disturbance does not occur exclusively during delirium or dementia and persists beyond the usual duration of substance intoxication or withdrawal.
- Evidence from the history, physical examination, or laboratory tests supports that the memory disturbance is etiologically related to the persisting effects of substance use.

Diagnostic criteria adapted with permission from the American Psychiatric Association. (2000). *Diagnostic and statistical manual of mental disorders* (4th ed., text revision). Washington, DC: Author.

▼ CHAPTER SUMMARY

- Cognitive disorders appear not only in the aging population, but also in the general population.
- The possible etiologies of cognitive disorders include primary brain disease, systemic disturbances, influences of exogenous substances, and withdrawal and residual effects of exogenous substances.
- Aberrant behaviors associated with these disorders may include deficits in the sensorium, attention span, orientation, perception, and memory.
- Symptoms of cognitive disorders may be approached in terms of acute onset and chronic progression.
- Gathering and analyzing assessment data for a client with a cognitive disorder requires participation of family members or friends who have been in close contact with the client.

- Continuum of care involves the collaborative efforts of the entire interdisciplinary healthcare team.
- Goal-setting for the client with an organic disorder focuses on eliminating the organic etiology, preventing acceleration of symptoms, and preserving dignity.
- Specific nursing interventions strive to maintain the client's optimal physical health, structure the environment, promote socialization and independent functioning, and preserve the family unit.

▼ REVIEW QUESTIONS

1. A man brings his 75-year-old wife to the clinic. She has a history of Parkinson's disease and diabetes. Her husband states that she hasn't seemed herself for the last few days. He relates that she is very lethargic during the day and sometimes seems confused. He states her blood sugars have been elevated and that she frequently has been incontinent of small amounts of urine. The nurse evaluates the client's mental status and finds that the client is not sure of the day or year and has trouble with her short-term memory. Based on the data, which of the following is the most likely explanation for the client's cognitive condition?
   a. Chronic confusion secondary to Parkinson's disease
   b. Delirium related to underlying medical problem
   c. Depression related to declining health
   d. Dementia related to advancing age

BOX 28-6 ▼ DSM-IV-TR *Categories of Amnestic Disorders*

Amnestic Disorder Due to . . . (Indicate the General Medical Condition)
  (Specify if: Transient or Chronic)
Substance-Induced, Persisting
Amnestic Disorder Not Otherwise Specified

2. A 78-year-old man recovering from emergency hip surgery develops delirium. He seems to be hallucinating and is mildly confused. Which intervention should the nurse do first?
   a. Loosely apply a vest restraint
   b. Obtain an order for haloperidol
   c. Arrange for an unlicensed assistant to sit with the client
   d. Move the client to a room close to the nurse's station

3. A 74-year-old male client is delirious after a head injury. At 9 PM he tells the nurse to get his clothes because he has to leave for work. The nurse's most therapeutic response is
   a. "It isn't time for work yet. It's time to sleep."
   b. "Your clothes aren't here; they are at home. You'll be going back to work when you recover."
   c. "Do you work the night shift?"
   d. "You're in the hospital. You injured your head in a car accident."

4. An 82-year-old woman with no history of neurologic dysfunction is admitted to the hospital with a possible bowel obstruction. She has been vomiting for several days. In addition to managing her medical care, nurses are monitoring the client for signs of delirium. Which of the following suggests that the client may be becoming delirious?
   a. The client removes her IV line and tries to climb over the side rails to get out of bed.
   b. The client has trouble finding the right word when speaking.
   c. The client requests pain medication frequently.
   d. The client is not sleeping well at night.

5. A usually independent, ambulatory 85-year-old client has been hospitalized for 2 days with urosepsis. He is exhibiting signs of mild delirium such as occasional confusion about why he is in the hospital and what day of the week it is. When developing a care plan, the nurse identifies several strategies to improve the client's cognitive function. Which of the following interventions will be helpful to the client?
   a. Keeping the television on to provide stimulation
   b. Having someone play checkers with the client
   c. Making up a daily calendar for the client with the dates and times of scheduled activities
   d. Dimming the lights and pulling the curtains so the client can rest

6. A 75-year-old client is being evaluated for memory impairment. His wife asks the nurse to explain the term "dementia" to her. The nurse bases her response on the knowledge that
   a. Dementia is a primary brain disease.
   b. Dementia is secondary to a medical condition.
   c. Dementia often is reversible if diagnosed and treated quickly.
   d. Dementia does not always affect memory.

7. A 70-year-old woman with dementia, Alzheimer's type (DAT) lives at home with her husband who is her full-time caregiver. The nurse is teaching the husband about interventions to prevent injury. Which of the following suggestions should the nurse make?
   a. Put childproof looks on cabinets that contain cleaning fluids.
   b. Put cleaning fluids on a high shelf.
   c. Lock cleaning fluids in a cabinet in the kitchen.
   d. Store cleaning fluids in plain bottles in the garage.

8. The nurse questions the wife of a client with dementia to assess if she is at risk for depression or anxiety related to her caregiving activities. Which of the following statements or questions would be most useful in eliciting information?
   a. "You must feel overwhelmed by your caregiving responsibilities. Tell me about it."
   b. "Tell me about your usual day."
   c. "Do you feel stressed by your caregiving responsibilities?"
   d. "Do you wish you had more help with your husband?"

9. A client with cognitive dysfunction is exhibiting aggressive, hostile behavior. Staff members know that the behavior is worse at bath times and meet to develop a plan for ensuring that the client's hygiene is not neglected and that no one is injured. Which of the following strategies will most likely help?
   a. Put all supplies in the bathroom, lead the client to the bathroom, and allow him to wash independently.
   b. Establish an unrushed routine for bathing, based on the client's former habits.
   c. Remind the client frequently that bathing is important.
   d. Limit bathing to once a week, have several staff members available, and give the client a bed bath.

10. A client with early stage Alzheimer's disease is started on tacrine. The nurse is evaluating the caregiver's understanding of the medication and determines that the caregiver has understood the instructions when she makes which of the following statements?
    a. "My husband needs to have his blood checked every week for 18 weeks."
    b. "This medicine will not affect his stomach and can be taken between meals."
    c. "This medication will prevent my husband's memory problems from worsening."
    d. "This medication may cause urinary retention. I should monitor his intake and output."

▼ REFERENCES AND SUGGESTED READINGS

*Abraham, I., & Neundorfer, M. (1990). Alzheimer's: A decade of progress, a future of nursing challenges. *Geriatric Nurse, May–June*, 116–119.

Alzheimer's Disease and Related Disorders Association (2001). *General statistics and demographics*. Chicago: Author.

*American Psychiatric Association. (2000). *Diagnostic and statistical manual of mental disorders* (4th ed., text rev.). Washington, DC: Author.

*Andreson, G. (1998). Dx Dementia. But what kind? *RN, (June)*, 26–30.

Benson, S. (1999). Hormone replacement therapy and Alzheimer's disease: An update on the issues. *Health Care Women International, 20*(6), 619–638.

*Breitner, J., & Welsh, K. (1995). Diagnosis and management of memory loss and cognitive disorders among elderly persons. *Psychiatric Services, 46*(1), 29–35.

*Chipps, E., & Paulson, G. (1994). Creutzfeldt-Jakob disease: A review. *Journal of Neuroscience Nursing, 26*(4), 219–223.

*Collins, C., Given, B., & Given, C. (1994). Interventions with family caregivers of persons with Alzheimer's disease. *Nursing Clinics of North America, 29*(1), 195–207.

*Costa, P. T. Jr, Williams, T. F., Somerfield, M., et al. (1996). *Recognition and initial assessment of Alzheimer's disease and related dementias* (Clinical Practice Guideline No. 19). Rockville, MD: U.S. Department of Health and Human Services, Public Health Service.

*Davis, K., & Powchik, P. (1990). Tacrine. *Lancet, 345*(8950), 625–630.

Foreman, M. (1990). Complexities of acute confusion. *Geriatric Nurse, 11*(3), 139.

*Francis, J. (1992). Delirium in older clients. *Journal of the American Geriatric Society, 40*, 829–838.

Gearing, M., Mirra, S., Hedrien, J. C., et al. (1995). The consortium to establish a registry for Alzheimer's disease (DERAD): Part X. Neuropathology confirmation of the clinical diagnosis of Alzheimer's disease. *Neurology, 45*, 461–466.

Jutagir, R., & Peterson, M. (1994). Psychological aspects of aging: When does memory loss signal dementia? *Geriatrics, 49*(3), 45–51.

Kelley, L., et al. (2000). Family involvement in care for individuals with dementia protocol. *Journal of Gerontological Nursing, 2*, 13.

*Kovach, C., & Stearns, S. (1993). Understanding Huntington's disease: An overview of symptomatology and nursing care. *Geriatric Nurse, 14*(5), 268–271.

*Lendon, C. L., Ashall, F. D., & Goate, A. M. (1997). Exploring the etiology of Alzheimer's disease using molecular genetics. *Journal of the American Medical Association, 277*(10), 825–831.

Lipowski, Z. (1980). A new look at organic brain syndrome. *American Journal of Psychiatry, 137*, 674–677.

*Lipowski, Z. (1989). Delirium in the elderly patient. *New England Journal of Medicine, 320*(9), 578–582.

Ludwig, L. (1990). Acute brain failure in the critically ill patient. *Critical Care Nurse, 9*, 62.

Lyketsos, C. G., Steinberg, M., Tschanz, J. T., Norton, M. C., Steffan, D. C., & Breither, J. C. (2000). Mental and behavioral disturbances in dementia: Findings from the Cache County Study on memory in aging. *American Journal of Psychiatry, 157*, 707–714.

Mace, N., & Rabins, P. (1991). *The 36-hour day: A family guide to caring for persons with Alzheimer's disease and related dementing illnesses* (revised ed.). Baltimore: Johns Hopkins University Press.

Mantes, J. (1995). A nursing protocol to assess causes of delirium: Identifying delirium in nursing home residents. *Journal of Gerontological Nursing, 21*(2), 26–30.

Marcantonio, E. R., Flacker, J. M., Michaels, M., & Resnick, N. M. (2000). Delirium is independently associated with poor functional recovery after hip fracture. *Journal of the American Geriatrics Society, 48*(6), 618–624.

Mignor, D. (2000). Effectiveness of use of home health nurses to decrease burden and depression of elderly caregivers. *Journal of Psychosocial Nursing & Mental Health Services, 38*(7), 34–41.

*Morrison, J. (1995). *DSM IV made easy: The clinician's guide to diagnosis*. New York: Guilford Press.

Rabins, P. V., Black, B. S., Roca, R., et al. (2000). Effectiveness of a nurse-based outreach program for identifying and treating psychiatric illness in the elderly. *Journal of the American Medical Association, 283*, 2802–2809.

*Rocca, W. (1994). Frequency, distribution, and risk factors for Alzheimer's disease. *Nursing Clinics of North America, 29*(1), 101–111.

*Scharre, D., & Mahler, M. (1994). Parkinson's disease: Making the diagnosis, selecting drug therapies. *Geriatrics, 49*(10), 14–23.

Smith, G., Smith, M., & Toseland, R. (1991). Problems identified by family caregivers in counseling. *Gerontologist, 31*(1), 15–22.

Staub, R., & Black, F. (1981). *Organic brain syndromes*. Philadelphia: F. A. Davis.

*Tueth, M., & Cheong, J. (1993). Delirium: Diagnosis and treatment in the older patient. *48*(3), 75–80.

*Ugarriza, D., & Gray, T. (1993). Alzheimer's disease: Nursing interventions for clients and caretakers. *Journal of Psychosocial Nursing, 3*(10), 7–10.

*Wise, M. G., Gray, K. F., & Seltzer, B. (1999). Delirium, dementia, and amnestic disorders. In R. E. Hales, & S. C. Yudofsky (Eds.), *Essentials of clinical psychiatry* (3rd ed., pp. 149–184). Washington, DC: APA Press.

*Wood, J., & Lantz, M. (1995). Alzheimer's disease: How to give and monitor tacrine therapy. *Geriatrics, 50*(5), 50–53.

*Yi, E., Abraham, I., & Holroyd, S. (1994). Alzheimer's disease and nursing. *Nursing Clinics of North America, 29*(1), 85–99.

Starred references are cited in text.

For additional information on this chapter, go to *http://connection. lww.com*.

Need more help? See Chapter 28 of the *Study Guide to Accompany Mohr: Johnson's Psychiatric Mental-Health Nursing*, 5th ed.

Nursing Care for Special Populations

Working With Pediatric Clients

BARBARA SCHOEN JOHNSON,
WANDA K. MOHR, & SHERILL NONES CRONIN

▼ KEY TERMS

Adjustment disorder—A psychiatric disorder marked by clinically or behaviorally significant symptoms that develop within 3 months after the onset of an identifiable stressor.

Advocacy—Formal or informal promotion of children's rights.

Anhedonia—Loss of pleasure in hobbies or activities of interest; it is a characteristic of depression.

Attention-deficit disorder (ADD)—A psychiatric disorder characterized by inattention without hyperactivity or impulsivity.

Attention-deficit hyperactivity disorder (ADHD)—A psychiatric disorder characterized by inattention, impulsiveness, and hyperactivity.

Autism—A genetic disorder of neuronal organization that requires early detection and treatment.

Double depression—A diagnosis given when dysthymia and major depression occur together.

Dysthymia— A mild form of depression that lasts 1 year or more in a child or adolescent.

Obsessive-compulsive disorder (OCD)— A disorder characterized by recurrent intrusive thoughts (*obsessions*) and repetitive behaviors (*compulsions*) that the client realizes are senseless but feels he or she must perform.

Oppositional-defiant disorder (ODD)—A psychiatric disorder marked by negativistic, defiant behaviors such as stubbornness, resistance to directions, and unwillingness to negotiate with adults or peers.

Phobias—Morbid, irrational, and persistent fears.

Separation anxiety disorder—A child-

hood psychiatric disorder in which a child experiences severe anxiety to the point of panic when separated from a parent or attachment figure.

Systems of care—A comprehensive spectrum of mental health and other necessary services organized into a coordinated network.

Tic—A sudden repetitive movement, gesture, or utterance.

Tourette syndrome—The most severe tic disorder, characterized by multiple motor tics and one or more vocal tics occurring many times throughout the day for 1 year or more.

Trichotillomania—A chronic impulse-control condition in which clients have an irresistible urge to pull out their hair; they feel tension before pulling out the hair and relief or pleasure during and after pulling.

▼ LEARNING OBJECTIVES

On completion of this chapter, you should be able to accomplish the following:

- Discuss the effects of childhood mental illness.
- Identify factors that contribute to psychiatric disorders in children and adolescents.
- Describe general interventions available for children or adolescents with psychiatric disorders.
- Discuss the role of the psychiatric-mental health nurse in child and adolescent mental healthcare.
- Apply the nursing process to the care of children and adolescents with ADHD.
- Identify the most common childhood psychiatric illnesses.
- Discuss psychiatric nursing care for the child or adolescent facing a serious medical illness.

This chapter is divided into three sections: 1) an overview of mental health and psychiatric disorders in children and adolescents, 2) detailed discussions of common psychiatric disorders in children and adolescents, and 3) psychiatric nursing care for children facing serious medical illnesses. Because ADHD is commonly diagnosed in children and adolescents and is a disorder that nurses will commonly encounter in practice, it receives special focus within this chapter.

As you read the chapter, consider the case of Michael in Clinical Example 29-1. How do Michael's history and signs and symptoms relate to ADHD? You will learn more about the progression of Michael's care in Nursing Care Plan 29-1. You also will have the opportunity to apply your understanding of this client and others with

▼ *Clinical Example 29-1*

Michael, an 8-year-old boy, arrives at the pediatrician's office with his parents. During the interview, his mother (Melanie) explains to the nurse (Karen) that since Michael started the third grade 2 months ago, his teacher calls his parents several times each week to tell them that Michael is performing poorly at school, does not focus on or complete his work, gets out of his seat repeatedly, blurts out answers, fidgets, forgets to turn in his homework, and is disruptive in the classroom. Melanie goes on to explain that Michael has few friends because he changes the rules of games during play and does not share. If he does not get his way, he grabs the toys and interrupts the play. Lately, he told his parents that no one wants to play with him.

The parents report that Michael has always been hyperactive and has had problems paying attention. Rob, Michael's father, believes that Michael should "just mind" instead of taking medication. At home, his parents are constantly reminding him to finish an activity he's started. Every evening they struggle over homework. One day recently, after bringing home a daily behavior sheet to his parents, Michael told Rob, "Nobody likes me. I'm stupid and act bad at school."

Karen recognizes that Michael has symptoms consistent with ADHD; she tells Michael's parents that the physician will examine Michael and assures his parents that treatment is available.

ADHD in the Reflection and Critical Thinking Questions at the end of this chapter.

OVERVIEW OF MENTAL HEALTH AND PSYCHIATRIC DISORDERS IN CHILDREN AND ADOLESCENTS

Childhood traditionally has been perceived and portrayed as a time of innocence and uninterrupted happiness. The experience of many children, however, differs greatly—childhood is not a time of joy for all young people. Many children and adolescents live in less-than-nurturing homes, face traumatic events, suffer all types of abuse, become dependent on substances, fear that no one loves or will care for them, think of ways to hurt themselves, and develop illnesses such as mood and anxiety disorders.

Childhood mental illness has staggering effects. Untreated mental illness in childhood often results in long-term mental illness in adults. For example, children with untreated depression frequently develop dysthymia as adults, and almost 50% of children with conduct disorder become antisocial adults. The less-obvious results—conflict, shame, guilt, lowered self-esteem, blame, unmet needs of siblings, thwarted development, and diminished productivity—are just as debilitating. Families, communities, child welfare programs, special education services, juvenile justice, and healthcare systems bear the significant direct and indirect costs of mental illness in the young.

In December 1999, the first ever Surgeon General's report on the nation's mental health addressed mental health problems and treatment in children, adolescents, and their families (U.S. Department of Health and Human Services, 1999). This report emphasized that psychiatric disorders and problems occur in children from all socio-economic backgrounds. It also emphasized that children and adolescents have unique developmental needs, which providers must assess in terms of each child's familial, social, and cultural backgrounds. It further stated that some children are at an increased risk for developing a psychiatric disorder because of a family history of psychiatric and addictive disorders, physical health problems, intellectual deficits, low birth weight, multigenerational poverty, and separation from, or abuse or neglect by, caregivers.

Regarding treatment and interventions, the report stated the following:

- Those who work with children must be familiar with what is and is not developmentally "normal."
- Services must be culturally appropriate and accessible.
- Preventive programs, including parent education and early childhood intervention, can improve children's social and emotional development and reduce the risks of developing psychiatric disorders.
- Many interventions, both pharmacological and psychosocial, could significantly help children and adolescents with depression, ADHD, and disruptive disorders (U.S. Department of Health and Human Services, 1999).

On January 3, 2001, U.S. Surgeon General Dr. David Satcher released the *Report of the Surgeon General's Conference on Children's Mental Health: A National Action Agenda* (U.S. Department of Health and Human Services, 2001). The report called the state of U.S. children's mental health a "public health crisis" in which 10% of children and adolescents suffer from illnesses severe enough to cause some level of impairment. Sadly, only 20% of those needing treatment actually receive it. The human and economic costs of child and adolescent psychiatric disorders are enormous. This action agenda identified goals and strategies to improve services for children and adolescents with mental health problems and their families.

Theories of Child Development

Children and their behavior must be understood in a developmental context. When working with a child, providers must understand the point that child is at in his or her developmental trajectory and what influences are affecting that development.

There are many theories of child development, and new ones are emerging constantly, questioning and building on earlier discoveries. The National Academy of Sciences has recommended a developmental ecological theoretical framework for research and practice with children (Cicchetti, 1996; Sroufe, 1997). This perspective is useful for conceptualizing the influences of risk and protective factors on children's development. It simultaneously addresses child and environmental characteristics, emphasizing the interactive and reciprocal influences of the children themselves, family, culture, and community (Cicchetti, 1993). It is integrative, including the broader contexts of development and functioning. Additionally, it is informed by the genetic and neurophysiological ontogenic variables that each individual possesses. Underscoring the idea that the child's context affects his or her development, this perspective posits that contextual characteristics and events may enhance or impede a child's development and contribute to his or her adaptation or the emergence of psychopathology (Aber & Cicchetti, 1984; National Research Council, 1993). A detailed discussion of the developmental ecological perspective is provided in Chapter 3.

PSYCHOANALYTIC PERSPECTIVES

The *psychoanalytic perspective* of child development has made many important contributions to the field of child development and inspired a wealth of research on many topics in this area, including infant–caregiver attachment, aggression, sibling relationships, child-rearing practices, morality, gender roles, and adolescent identity. The psychoanalytic perspective, however, is no longer in the mainstream of child-development research, and several other perspectives have proven to have greater explanatory power. Two important psychoanalytic scholars bear mentioning: Sigmund Freud and Erik Erikson. Their theories are described in this chapter because of their historical importance.

Sigmund Freud's Psychosexual Theory

Sigmund Freud (see Chap. 3) constructed his psychosexual theory of development on the basis of adult remembrances. He emphasized that the way in which parents manage their child's sexual and aggressive drives in the first few years of life is crucial for healthy personality development. (See Table 3-3 for Freud's stages of development.)

Freud believed that over the course of childhood, children shift their sexual impulses from the oral to the anal to the genital regions of the body. In each stage, parents struggle between gratifying too many or too few of their children's basic needs. Either extreme can cause the child's psychic energies to become fixated or arrested at a particular stage. Too much satisfaction makes the child unwilling to progress to a more mature level of behavior.

Too little leads the child to continue seeking gratification of the frustrated drive. If parents find an appropriate balance, then children grow into well-adjusted adults with the capacity for mature sexual behavior, investment in family life, and rearing of the next generation.

Freud's psychosexual theory was important because it highlighted the role that family relations play in child development. But the theory is criticized for being too focused on sexual feelings and for being based on the problems of well-to-do, middle-class, Victorian women. Moreover, Freud never studied children directly.

Erik Erikson's Psychosocial Theory

Erik Erikson was an important disciple of Freud. He took what was useful from Freud's theory and rearranged it in ways that improved on the original vision.

Erikson accepted Freud's basic psychosexual framework; however, he emphasized the role of social processes and asserted that the ego was a positive force in development. According to Erikson, at each stage the ego acquires attitudes and skills that make the individual an active contributing member of society. How the person resolves basic psychosocial conflicts (such as strivings for autonomy versus feelings of dependence) along a positive–negative continuum determines his or her adjustment or maladjustment. Table 29-1 illustrates Erikson's psychosocial stages (Erikson, 1950).

PIAGET'S COGNITIVE-DEVELOPMENTAL THEORY

More than any other theorist, Jean Piaget has had the greatest historical influence on the field of child development, especially in the field of education. Piaget's main concern was intellectual competence and was influenced heavily by his background in biology. According to Piaget's *cognitive-developmental theory,* children are driven by heredity and environment. They construct knowledge actively as they manipulate and explore their worlds; their cognitive development occurs in stages. Children move through four broad stages, beginning with the infant's sensorimotor activity and ending with the adolescent's elaborate, abstract reasoning system. It is important to understand that Piaget's idea of "stage" is not descriptive but theoretical. It does not refer to some overt behavior but to a constellation of processes underlying a particular behavior. Piaget's stages of cognitive development are illustrated in Table 29-2.

In recent years researchers have challenged Piaget's theory, demonstrating that he underestimated the competencies of infants and preschoolers. Some adherents to Piaget's theory have modified their views of cognitive stages to suggest that changes in children's thinking are less sudden and more gradual than Piaget suggested. Others have abandoned the idea of cognitive stages in favor of a continuous "information-processing" approach (Case, 1992).

TABLE 29-1 ▼ Erikson's Psychosocial Stages

STAGE	PERIOD OF DEVELOPMENT	DESCRIPTION
Basic trust vs. mistrust	Birth–1 year	Infants gain a sense of trust or confidence that the world is a good place from warm and responsive care. Mistrust occurs when infants are handled harshly.
Autonomy vs. shame and doubt	1–3 years	Autonomy is fostered when children are permitted reasonable free choice and not forced or shamed into doing anything.
Initiative vs. guilt	3–6 years	Initiative develops when parents support their children's sense of purpose and direction. Guilt results from overcontrol.
Industry vs. inferiority	6–12 years	Capacity to work with others develops. Inferiority results from negative experiences at home or school.
Identity vs. identity diffusion	Adolescence	Adolescents try to answer questions about who they are and what their place is in society. Negative outcome is confusion about adult roles.

CONTEMPORARY APPROACHES TO CHILD DEVELOPMENT

Several contemporary theoretical perspectives bear mentioning. The *information-processing perspective* views children as active, sense-making beings who modify their own thinking in response to environmental demands. This perspective does not subscribe to the notion of stages; rather, it presumes that thought processes are similar for people of all ages. The same thought processes in adults are found in children, but to a lesser degree. Development is seen as continuous (Klahr, 1992).

Ethology theory stresses adaptation, survival, and the value of behavior in ensuring survival. This field has its origins in zoology and has become more influential in child development research in recent years (Dewsbury, 1992). Observations of ethology scholars have led to the important concept of the *critical period*, which refers to a limited time span during which a child is prepared biologically to acquire certain adaptive behaviors but needs the support of appropriate environmental stimuli to do so. See Chapter 2 for further discussion of critical periods.

Ecological systems theory, as developed by American psychologist Uri Bronfenbrenner (1995), views the child as developing within complex environmental systems. Bronfenbrenner expanded the idea of environment from a very narrow conceptualization to a series of nested structures that includes, but extends beyond, home, school, and neighborhood. Chapter 3 describes these levels in the discussion of the developmental ecological theoretical perspective.

TABLE 29-2 ▼ Piaget's Stages of Cognitive Development

STAGE	PERIOD OF DEVELOPMENT	DESCRIPTION
Sensorimotor	Birth to 2 years	Infants think by acting on the world through their senses and find ways of solving sensorimotor problems (eg, pulling a lever to hear music).
Preoperational	2–7 years	Children begin working with symbols to represent their earlier sensorimotor discoveries, but thinking lacks logical qualities of next two stages.
Concrete operational	7–11 years	Reasoning becomes logical. Children recognize hierarchies of class and subclass.
Formal operations	11 years and older	In this stage, there is reasoning with symbols that do not refer to objects in the real world; abstract thinking begins.

Finally, the contributions of the Russian psychologist Lev Semenovich Vygotsky have become increasingly important in child development theory. Vygotsky's perspective is sociocultural and focuses on how culture is transmitted intergenerationally. Vygotsky posited that children are active constructive beings. Unlike Piaget, he viewed cognitive development as being mediated socially and dependent upon support from adults. Rather than proceeding through stages, children acquire culturally relevant knowledge and skills gradually through cooperative dialogues with mature members of society. These dialogues become part of their thinking (Wertsch & Tulviste, 1992).

Risk Factors for Child and Adolescent Mental Disorders

No single cause can explain child and adolescent psychopathology. Risk factors that may cause a child to be more susceptible to psychopathology include family history of a mental illness; immature development of the brain; brain abnormality; family problems and dysfunction; poverty; mentally ill or substance-abusing parents; teen parents; abuse; discrimination based on race, creed, or color; chronic parental conflict or divorced parents; and chronic illness or disability.

BIOLOGICAL INFLUENCES

Biological factors, such as a family history of a certain disorder, will increase a child's likelihood to develop that disorder. For example, if one or both parents have depression, the child has an increased risk of developing a mood disorder.

Immature development of the brain also puts the child at risk. The prefrontal cortex of the brain, which is critical to good judgment and the suppression of impulses, is not fully developed until at least age 20 years. In recent shootings at schools, several of the shooters were age 15 years or younger; they are examples of individuals with immature prefrontal cortexes. Experts contend that they were not biologically ready to inhibit impulses, such as the impulse to harm others when angry (Weinberger, 2001).

Recent neuroimaging techniques have advanced the understanding of brain anatomy and physiology in mental illness. For example, in ADHD, there are brain abnormalities in the prefrontal cortex and striatum, as noted in decreased blood flow, less electrical activity in the frontal lobes, and a lack of normal asymmetry in the caudate nuclei and lateral ventricles (Wagner, 2000). Such studies are underway for most mental disorders (see Chap. 2).

Finally, the child's temperament, which is thought to be at least partly determined genetically, plays a role in whether he or she is at risk for maladjustment. An infant with a difficult temperament may be at risk for future maladjustment. It is important to remember, however, that responses from caregivers and others to the infant can modify the risk. Negative responses to an infant with a difficult temperament increase the risk for maladjustment.

PSYCHOSOCIAL INFLUENCES

Some people think that parents do things "to" a child that affects his or her development, as though parent–child transactions were one-way streets. In reality, they are two-way, reciprocal relationships. It is within the socialization context of the parent–child relationship that children largely acquire the coordination of affect, cognition, and behavior, which they need to successfully relate to others.

Families do not operate in a vacuum—the behavior of each family member affects the others, and each member is affected by other contexts to which he or she is exposed. Therefore, many situations affect family dynamics, and those dynamics may change from more to less adaptive depending on the nature of contextual factors. For example, a family may function adaptively given one set of circumstances (eg, death of a grandparent) but maladaptively given another (eg, sudden unemployment).

Because they function within a family that helps to buffer the effects of social change, children are less susceptible to sociocultural influences than are adults. As they grow and mature, however, children increasingly come into contact with the larger society. Stable, nurturing forces in the child's home protect him or her from outside harm. If the child does not have stable nurturing forces in the home, he or she is at risk for maladjustment (see Chap. 3).

Parents and families have powerful effects on children and adolescents. Parents' fears, anxiety, depression, and aggression, as well as their love, nurturance, and concern, shape the youth's developing sense of self and the world. Parenting is an extension of self. What parents believe about their world is often reflected in their child's skills or deficits.

Parents also help to maintain two important family boundaries: generational and gender. *Generational boundaries* divide the family into parents who nurture, lead, and direct and children who are nurtured, follow, and learn. *Gender boundaries* divide the family into females and males and promote gender awareness and identification.

STRESSORS

Exposure to stressors, especially multiple stressors over an extended period, can have damaging effects on development. Small amounts of manageable stress, however, can help "inoculate" the child to the effects of stress. Children with buffers and protective factors, such as a high IQ, stable family, and higher socioeconomic status, demonstrate greater adaptability under stress. Children with fewer protective factors and more risk factors, such as poverty and exposure to domestic violence, tend to be less adaptable under stress.

Divorce

Parental divorce affects children and adolescents in multiple ways, including increasing their vulnerability to physical and emotional disturbances. Divorce involves a series of changes, transitions, and adjustments. During their parents' divorce, children deal simultaneously with normal developmental stages and face the added stressors accompanying divorce. The father's or mother's absence, conflict between parents, financial difficulties, multiple changes (eg, geographical moves, poverty, remarriage), level of parent adjustment, and short-term crisis are all factors that contribute to the stress of divorce for children and teens.

Recent studies have shown that the effects of divorce are more detrimental than child development specialists once thought (Thompson, 1998). In the long term, there is the adverse effect of sustained stress. Children of divorce have decreased levels of well-being and poorer mental and social adjustment. Conflict between parents leads to anger and anxiety in children because they want to be loyal to and please both parents. This feeling of being "caught between parents" leads to depression, anxiety, and deviant behavior. Children often are exposed to a continuing demonstration of hostility, which results in aggressive behavior in the child. The less postdivorce conflict that occurs between parents, the greater is the children's well-being.

After divorce, many women and children move into poverty, with subsequent poor healthcare and nutrition, unsafe housing, and inferior schools. Problems such as inadequate social skills, a decline in academic performance, or drug and alcohol use may be identified. Children who are young at the time of divorce seem to suffer greater emotional and social effects. Gender-specific effects of divorce also have been identified; girls tend to engage in precocious sexual activity and have difficulty establishing lasting adult heterosexual relationships, while boys demonstrate an unstable sense of masculinity.

To reduce the negative effects of divorce, parents should reduce stressors in their children's and adolescents' lives, participate in divorce mediation to decrease conflict, and seek support for their children within schools and peer support groups. Referrals for therapy may be needed. Parents should be counseled to avoid hostile interactions with each other (Thompson, 1998).

Child Abuse

Each year about 1 million children are reported to Child Protective Services (CPS) as being abused or neglected (see Chap. 17). Many more cases go unreported. About 14 of every 1000 children are mistreated in some way. Estimates for sexual abuse number about one in four girls and one in eight to 10 boys. Exact figures are unknown.

Abuse has long been associated with psychopathology and maladjustment in children. Abused children learn that the world is unsafe and that people are not to be trusted. Sequelae of abuse include anxiety, depression, interpersonal difficulties such as mistrust, anger management problems, disruptive conduct, dissociative symptoms, somatization, sleep and eating disorders, chemical dependency, and sexual acting out and dysfunction. Sexually abused children are at risk for symptoms of post-traumatic stress disorder, dissociative disorders, and depression. Children who have been maltreated often are resistant to therapeutic interventions and are slow to trust; therapy may take many years.

Protective and Resilient Influences for Mental Health in Children and Adolescents

Several protective factors in children can increase their resistance to stress: personality factors, such as positive self-esteem and an easy temperament; family cohesion and absence of discord; and support from other significant persons in their lives to help the child learn to cope. In addition, a positive relationship with at least one parent has been shown to exert a protective effect on children. Children with positive parental relationships have greater resistance to the effects of stressors (Garmezy, 1985).

Developmental, ecological, and social systems theories emphasize the primary influence of the family on child functioning. The family and other systems can be seen as interdependent spheres of influence. Current research and theory indicate that children learn much of their social behavior from their families of origin, suggesting that early family experiences play a fundamental role in the development of children's social competence (Jacobson & Frye, 1991). Experiences in the primary social context of the parent–child relationship largely influence young children's abilities to prosper in any environment (Maccoby & Martin, 1983). Parenting styles are a specific aspect of the parent–child relationship and have been shown to relate to the quality of children's socioemotional functioning, such as in developing peer relations and transitioning into the school context (Hess, Holloway, Dickson, & Price, 1984).

In addition, family social support has been identified as an important factor in promoting positive outcomes for both parents and children and in mitigating the effects of environmental and situational stressors on families (Garbarino, 1977). For parents, a strong sense of external social support strengthens positive social networks and feelings of connectedness, fosters emotional well-being and ability to cope, provides healthy outlets for stress and frustration, and increases access to community resources (Thompson, 1995). These positive effects of social support for parents enable them to enhance their parenting skills, and, in turn, promote the socioemotional well-being of their children. Specific child outcomes that have been associated with strong family support include secure attachment with caregivers (Jacobson

& Frye, 1991), positive parent–child interactions (Jennings, Stagg, & Connors, 1991), healthy peer relationships (Melson, Ladd, & Hsu, 1993), and healthy behavior patterns (Dunst, Trivette, & Cross, 1986). Thus, research suggests that child well-being and success in developing competencies are nested in a strong support network of parents and families. Healthy, well-supported families give rise to healthy, well-supported children.

General Interventions for Child and Adolescent Mental Disorders

THE INTERDISCIPLINARY TEAM AND COORDINATION OF CARE

Many mental health professionals participate in the care of a mentally ill child or adolescent. They include child and adolescent psychiatrists, social workers, nurse psychotherapists, testing psychologists, direct care providers, recreational therapists, psychiatric nurses, and occupational therapists. Although some disciplines overlap in the care they provide, each discipline contributes a unique service. For example, reviewing psychological testing results helps the nurse develop a comprehensive picture of the client's diagnosis and condition.

Treatment Settings and Continuum of Care

Treatment for mentally ill children is provided in many different settings, from the most restrictive levels of care for seriously disturbed youth to the least restrictive level. Treatment services within these levels include preventive services, early intervention, crisis stabilization, inpatient hospitalization, crisis in-home services, residential treatment, partial hospitalization, day treatment, therapeutic foster care, case management, family support services, outpatient counseling, and medication management. Discharge planning, a collaborative process involving the youth, family, and mental health team, begins with admission to the inpatient unit or other treatment service.

Wrap-Around Services and Systems-of-Care Approaches

During the past 15 years, several initiatives to improve coordination among the agencies that provide services for children with emotional and behavioral disabilities and their families have been implemented. In the past these were called "wrap-around services," and the idea was that children and families were provided with the services needed to meet their needs.

Current structures of service provision are replacing the former wrap-around services concept and are referred to as systems of care. The term **systems of care** is defined as a comprehensive spectrum of mental health and other necessary services organized into a coordinated network. This network is dynamic and changes as the needs of the children and families change. Integral to the systems of care

concept is the belief that parents are full partners in the therapy and care of their children and are included in the decisions of what services are needed (Stroul & Friedman, 1986). Services may come from public or private mental healthcare, education, and juvenile justice (see Chap. 15).

PREVENTION AND EARLY IDENTIFICATION

Primary prevention refers to any activity undertaken before a child or adolescent is identified as a client. It would be wonderful if knowledge alone would lead to changes in behavior; however, increased knowledge does not necessarily indicate that a behavior change will occur (just as education about weight and diet does not prevent eating disorders). It is possible, however, that activities leading to feelings of self-efficacy and a positive outlook on life can help a child develop protective factors against eating and other disorders. For example, a web site developed by the U.S. Department of Health and Human Services called "Girl Power!" (*http://www.girlpower.gov/*) is intended to help girls form healthy attitudes about their bodies and themselves (White, 2000). This site includes assessment of risk factors, programs to educate parents about the effects of their attitudes and comments about appearance, body image classes, exercise programs for obese children and teens, and esteem-building programs.

Another example of primary prevention is preschool programs. Research has documented relationships between children's social and emotional competencies, early learning behaviors, language use, cognitive abilities, and behavioral difficulties, and their ability to successfully navigate present and future school environments. Success in school is a significant protective factor for children; poor outcomes at school are associated with maladjustment. Effective preschool programming is accordingly geared toward promoting developmental competencies. Head Start is the largest federally funded program committed to school readiness for children living in poverty. It has served more than 15 million children since its inception in 1965. A review of 36 studies of Head Start found that children who completed the program had lower rates of enrollment in special education and higher rates of high school graduation. Head Start and other early childhood programs produce other benefits that are less readily apparent, such as better peer relations, less truancy, and lower rates of antisocial behavior.

Early identification and treatment are the keys to reducing the harm caused by psychiatric disorders in children and adolescents. Nurses play integral roles in detecting early symptoms, such as depression, and referring children and families to appropriate psychiatric care providers. Screening for and prevention of psychiatric disorders needs to start during infancy. A study has shown that a fussy and demanding temperament in infancy predicts future maladjustment. When those demanding infants and their parents were provided in-home family counseling that focused on improving parent–child interaction, however, the children were less likely to exhibit maladjustment as adolescents (Teerikangas, Aronen, Martin, & Huttunen, 1998). In addition, early intervention with children and teens at risk can prevent more serious maladjustment and emotional turmoil later in life. For example, bereavement services through group sharing with peers can help ameliorate later adjustment difficulties for children whose parents have died.

TYPES OF THERAPIES

Several different forms of therapy may be used to treat the child or adolescent with a psychiatric disorder. Whichever type of therapy is used, it is important to consider the child's and family's culture (Implications for Nursing Practice 29-1) (see Chap. 5).

Individual therapy focuses on the needs and problems of the child or adolescent. The work accomplished depends on the therapist–client relationship, and the therapist must respect the child's unique nature. The therapist hopes to become an important person in the child's life, someone with whom the child can identify while growing and developing. It is a therapeutic challenge to gain adolescents' trust and motivate them to change. Improved self-understanding, symptom reduction, ability to use judgment and have fun, and enhancement of the ability to make healthy choices are desired outcomes.

Brief psychotherapy addresses a central issue in a specified time. The provider and child do not discuss extraneous issues. The provider openly explores the central problem with the child and family.

 Implications for Nursing Practice 29-1

Cultural Considerations for Mental Health Services

Lack of culturally competent services is a barrier to children and adolescents receiving needed mental health services. Minority children are less likely to seek and receive needed treatment than are nonminority children. Minority children usually drop out of treatment earlier, enter treatment at a later stage of the illness, and are misdiagnosed more often (Bush, 2000).

Different cultural groups have different mental health needs. Native Americans are at higher risk than most groups for the development of depression, substance abuse, anxiety, violence, and suicide. Services should be tailored to the needs of each distinct culture, which can be a formidable task. Asian Americans alone comprise at least 31 different ethnic groups. As minority populations increase, the demand for mental health services for children and adolescents will become critical. Nurses must refine their skills in providing culturally competent services to all clients (Bush, 2000).

Play therapy offers the child an opportunity to express his or her fears, anxieties, frustrations, and aggression. Play is the child's work and natural medium for expression. When a child expresses feelings through play, he or she allows them to surface and can face, manage, accept, or abandon them. Through this process, children learn that they are individuals who are capable of thinking and making decisions for themselves.

Family therapy is based on the premise that the behavior of one person in the family affects everyone else in the family. No behavior of an individual can be understood without understanding the behavior of other family members. Interventions are directed at the family as a whole and their behavior patterns, not at the identified client. Family therapy promotes family cohesion and addresses members' concerns and conflicts. Treating a child or adolescent successfully necessitates modifying how the home environment is reinforcing his or her behavior. Parents learn to become therapeutic agents of change.

Group therapy is especially helpful for adolescents for whom the influence of peers is strong; adolescents are more likely to accept feedback and suggestions from their peers than from adults. Group therapy is less threatening than individual therapy and allows the adolescent to identify with others who have similar problems. Groups provide opportunities to learn to identify and dismiss defeating cognitions and practice new behaviors.

Milieu therapy creates a therapeutic living environment through the setting, structure, and relationships with others. In a therapeutic milieu, every interaction becomes an opportunity for therapeutic intervention with the child or teen, and open, clear communication is modeled. Through the day-to-day living experiences of waking, dressing, eating, doing schoolwork, playing, interacting, and going to bed, the child or teen can learn how to manage activities, deal with feelings, and get along with others. Milieu staff members work to model supportive and respectful behavior, which illustrates cohesive adults dealing with youths and one another in healthy ways. Inpatient milieu settings must offer safety, security, clear and reasonable limits, behavioral consequences, age-appropriate activities, and 24-hour availability of mature, caring adults.

Behavioral and cognitive therapy is based on the concept that psychiatric disorders represent learned behavior. Thus, learning principles are applied to modifying these behaviors. Behavioral techniques include the use of token economies, time-out (from positive reinforcement), and rewards for and reinforcements of desired behaviors. Parents and teachers should learn and use these techniques. Participation in devising a written behavioral contract helps increase the adolescent's adherence to the treatment plan. Cognitive therapy, which assists with problem solving and stopping negative self-perceptions, is likely to work well with older adolescents who may view a behavioral management system as a type of adult control.

SPECIAL EDUCATION

Children or adolescents with mental illness have the same developmental strivings as all youth; they want to perform successfully in school and take pride in their accomplishments. The school's dilemma is how to manage the young person's disruptive behavior while teaching him or her academics.

The goals of special education for mentally ill youth are as follows:

- Decrease the child's disturbing behavior
- Increase the child's rate of learning to enable him or her to remediate and progress
- Reintegrate the child into regular classes as soon as possible

An essential classroom technique with disturbed youth is to provide a high degree of structure. Clear expectations and defined limits diminish the youth's anxiety. Another valuable approach is to maximize group cohesion and the influence of peer pressure in the classroom. Because youth with mental illness typically have experienced little success in school, it is difficult for them to approach their class work positively. The teacher's task is to help the child become motivated about learning. Coordination and collaboration between school and other care systems is critical.

COMMUNITY-BASED SERVICES

It is estimated that 8% to 10% of youth in juvenile justice facilities have serious mental illness and need immediate mental health treatment. School-based services, such as assessments of the child's emotional and academic status and educational modifications, are critical in treating children and teens with mental illness. In addition, career services are necessary for adolescents with mental illness, who typically drop out of school. These children and adolescents require coordination with mental health personnel and need intensive and comprehensive case management.

PHARMACOLOGIC THERAPY

Pharmacologic therapy is an important part of any treatment program for children and adolescents with mental illness. Medication does not solve all the child's or teen's problems. If it is combined with therapies, family education, parent guidance, and special education, however, medication improves the likelihood that the child's symptoms will decrease and his or her functioning will improve. Psychotropic medication must be given cautiously to children and adolescents because of the idiosyncratic reactions they can have (see Chap. 12).

NURSING CARE

Nursing care for children and adolescents with mental disorders will vary according to individual diagnoses, symptomatology, care settings, resources, and needs. All nursing care begins with assessment, and certain interventions are applicable in a wide variety of circumstances. Essentials of the psychiatric-mental health nursing assessment are presented in the following section, as is information about interventions that address common client and family needs or common clinical situations.

Assessment

Assessment sets the tone for the rest of the nursing interaction. The nurse welcomes the child or adolescent and family and clarifies that the whole family is involved in treatment, not just the identified child or teen client. The nurse allows time to answer family members' questions, support their desire to be good parents, alleviate their fears and guilt, and provide accurate information and teaching. Parents often worry that they "did something" to cause their child's problem. Explaining that multiple factors influence the development of mental disorders is helpful. Information from multiple informants, such as teachers and grandparents, gives a fuller picture of the issues.

Family Functioning. *Family assessment,* usually performed before assessment of the child, reinforces the concept that everyone in the family is involved in and expected to work on the identified problem. The nurse asks openended questions such as, "How are things for this family?" This form of questioning allows the family members to respond with whatever information they wish to share; it gives the nurse and other mental healthcare providers some insight into their perception of the problem.

The nurse also assesses family relationships, concern for one another, roles, empathy, decision making, and degree of autonomy or enmeshment. The nurse elicits how family members perceive the child and whether their perceptions are unrealistic or grounded in knowledge of growth and development. For example, some parents think that an infant cries on purpose to "get back at the parent" or that a 7-year-old boy should be "the little man of the family."

Current Problem. The nurse first gathers assessment information from the child or adolescent and family, including the nature, severity, and length of the *current problem* and any significant concomitant events. He or she always asks, "How upsetting is this problem to the child and family?" and "Does anything make this problem better or worse?" It is essential to obtain parents' descriptions of the child's behavior at home, to evaluate the child's response to discipline, and to learn whether the child is violent or defiant, cares about the rights of others, or has severe behavior problems (eg, cruelty to animals, fire-setting tendencies).

History. Next, the nurse inquires about the type, length, and outcomes of any *previous treatment,* testing results, and diagnoses. The *family history* reveals any medical and mental health problem or symptoms (psychiatric and substance abuse) of immediate and extended family members. *Developmental history* includes prenatal history (health or illness, substance use, physical abuse of the mother), neonatal history (birth complications, stability of newborn), and achievement of developmental milestones (sitting, walking, talking, self-care). The nurse questions the child's *social history* (names, ages, and relationships of people with whom the child lives; relationships with parents, siblings, other family members, and peers; activities or hobbies; legal charges against the child). The *abuse history* recounts the child's exposure to physical, sexual, or emotional abuse, whether CPS was notified, and what treatment was provided. Other important information to ask is whether the child is or has been exposed to family or community violence, as these are significant stressors for a developing youngster. The child's or adolescent's *chemical history,* as well as that of his parents and other caretakers, is significant.

The *medical history* includes a physical examination to rule out nonpsychiatric conditions, history of seizures, head injuries, acute illnesses, other injuries and accidents, surgeries, loss of consciousness, asthma and other chronic illnesses, and vision and hearing deficits. The nurse questions the child's current *medications,* their effects and side effects, and the names and effects of prior medications. It is essential to list all *allergies*—drug, food, and seasonal. The nurse elicits the child's or adolescent's *school history* by asking about the current grade, whether he or she attends regular or special education, if he or she has any learning difficulties, and if he or she exhibits behavior problems in school.

Mental Status Examination. The nurse conducts the mental status examination of a child or adolescent through observation, appropriate use of play, and questioning. He or she describes the client's behavior, orientation, memory, attention and concentration, speech, thought content and process, hallucinations, delusions, suicidal ideation, self-harm or homicidal thinking or actions, judgment, and insight (Falsafi, 2001).

The nurse asks children or teens what they do when they are angry, sad, or happy and tries to elicit their perception of their behavior. It is best to ask the child or teen privately about any drug or alcohol use and abuse experiences. Often a child will respond, "I hit," "I kick," "I cry," or "I go to my room and play video games," which are indications of their coping skills. The nurse notes any neurologic signs for further exploration.

Drawings are helpful as a tool to facilitate information gathering with children and adolescents. They are only a *tool* for communication, however, and nurses must take care not to overinterpret what a child has drawn. In addition, children tell their stories through games and toys, especially when they have limited vocabularies to communicate their feelings.

Interventions

Providing Medication Education. Few psychotropic medications have approval from the Food and Drug Administration (FDA) for use in children. Several of them, however, are prescribed "off label," because experience has proven them to effectively treat mental illness in children. The nurse explains the chemical basis for treating a disorder in simple terms. Parents, others caring for the child, and the child or teen himself or herself (if mature enough to understand) need information about the medication, its purpose and intended effects, how to administer it, side effects, and what to do if dangerous effects occur. The nurse also explains the importance of keeping the medication in a safe and secure place to which only adults have access. These medications should never be accessible to any child or teen, not just suicidal youths.

The nurse encourages honesty and openness about medication adherence. Adolescents and younger children may refuse to take or throw away their medicine for several reasons. In addition, some children may believe that medications are punishment for bad behavior. Sometimes the youth will agree to a time-limited trial of medication. At other times, the parent may decide not to adhere to the prescribing schedule out of fear, misinformation, or a belief system that is incompatible with pharmacotherapy for children. Therefore, teaching about psychotropic medications for children and adolescents and their parents is an important nursing action to promote accuracy and adherence with prescribed dosing schedules.

It also is important to teach about drug–drug and herb–drug interactions of the medication. Some people think that because they can buy St. John's wort and other products over the counter at health food stores, they must be "safe." These products can interact in dangerous ways, however, with prescribed medication (see Chap. 12).

Meeting Families' Needs. Families of children and adolescents with mental disorders need support, continuity of care, and information about their child's diagnosis and treatment as well as how to help their child. Parents also may have other concerns, such as future planning for the child's care, feeling helpless in helping their child, wanting to become an advocate for the child, respite, involvement in the school, financial support, and meeting the needs of siblings and themselves (Elder, 2001).

Evidence has shown that, in spite of efforts at education, nurses and other mental health care providers are not doing a stellar job at educating families. A recent study found that parents of children with pervasive developmental delay thought that their child's behavior was the result of his or her wanting "attention" or "to test people." They did not understand their child's frustration at being unable to communicate wants and needs (Elder, 2001).

Children or adolescents and their families need accurate information about their disorder and its treatment. Education should focus on correcting inaccurate beliefs

with limited distractions (closer to the teacher), providing a designated area where the child can move around freely when needed, and establishing a system of rules and rewards for desirable behaviors. Keeping a picture on the desk with specific rules for school behavior (such as raising a hand and being called on before speaking) will help the child remember the rules. The child also will need extra help with directions. Reviewing directions, listing the materials that will be needed, and breaking down tasks into smaller components helps the disorganized, inattentive child focus on and complete schoolwork.

TEACHING SOCIAL SKILLS

Various groups successfully advocated for the inclusion of mildly and moderately disabled children in the general education classroom. This inclusion has benefits as well as risks for children with ADHD. Positively, they may experience the same educational environment as other children their age. Negatively, they may be subjected to social pressures and possibly ridicule from those same peers.

Teaching the child with ADHD social skills and strategies is integral to his or her ability to maintain friendships. Childhood social skills include, among others, waiting for a turn, maintaining a conversation, sharing toys, asking for help, responding to teasing, playing cooperatively, handling frustration without aggressiveness, apologizing, and showing concern for others. Many children with ADHD are not attentive to verbal and nonverbal communications (ie, they do not "read" facial expressions or interpret tone of voice and language subtleties). While most children acquire these skills intuitively at an early age, albeit to varying degrees, the child with ADHD needs specific instruction and ample opportunities for practice to develop these skills. Nurses can coach parents in helping the child develop social skills or facilitate interactions with a group of children, which will help the children become more aware of their behaviors and the effects on others.

Social skills instruction should focus on one specific skill or behavior at a time. For example, the parents (or group facilitator) may choose hitting as the behavior or apologizing as the skill. The child can role-play or act out a scenario involving the target behavior. A discussion should follow in which the parents ask the child what happened, why they think it happened, how they felt, and what else might have been said or done. The role-playing can be videotaped and shown to the child to help him or her gain insight into the social situation. As the child makes progress in one area, the parents can then shift the focus to other areas.

Other strategies include developing a reward system, as described previously, or creating a script for potential social situations that the nurse anticipates the child will encounter, such as being wrongly accused of bad behavior, losing lunch money, or accidentally hurting someone. Practice and feedback from parents, teachers, siblings, and peers are fundamental to the success of teaching social skills.

IMPROVING SELF-ESTEEM

Children with ADHD are frequently the targets of negative assessments ("Can't you pay attention?", "He loses everything!", "She's disrupting the entire class."). Children internalize the opinions of others and form similar opinions of themselves, leading to negative self-assessments and low self-esteem. Additionally, all the problems discussed above—disruptive behavior, lack of social skills, poor academic performance—add to the child's feelings of inferiority.

Implementing a behavioral program that helps the child gain self-control and skills, uses his or her energy productively, and garners praise and rewards will help the child begin to mold a more positive self-image. Finding the child's strengths, perhaps in sports or creative arts, and focusing on skills and accomplishments in that arena is another source of self-pride.

Evaluation

The family needs to understand that the goals of treatment take time and that they will need to continue therapeutic approaches throughout childhood and adolescence. Indeed, the client with ADHD will continue to use strategies for overcoming ADHD or ADD into adulthood. Nevertheless, parents and teachers should see incremental improvement in the child as long as they implement behavioral strategies consistently. Indicators that the plan of care is effective include the following:

- The client can maintain friendships.
- Family functioning improves according to family report.
- The client's academic performance improves.
- The client can better manage responsibilities.
- The client experiences greater self-esteem.

OPPOSITIONAL-DEFIANT DISORDER

Oppositional-defiant disorder (ODD) is marked by negativistic, defiant behaviors such as stubbornness, resistance to directions, and unwillingness to negotiate with adults or peers. Children or adolescents with ODD persistently test limits, usually by ignoring directions, arguing, or failing to accept responsibility for behavior. They direct their hostility at adults or peers through verbal aggression or deliberately annoying actions. They do not see themselves as defiant but justify their behavior as a response to unreasonable demands. Symptoms may be present at home but not seen at school.

ODD is one of the more common disorders seen in adolescents, although children also have the disorder. Prevalence rates range from 2% to 16%. ODD is more common in boys before puberty but equally prevalent in both sexes after puberty. Symptoms are generally more confrontational and persistent in boys. There may be comorbid ADHD, depression, or learning problems.

School-age children with ODD are likely to exhibit low self-esteem; mood lability; low frustration tolerance; swearing; precocious use of alcohol, tobacco, and other drugs; and interpersonal conflicts. Parents and their children or adolescents often bring out the worst in one another. Youth with ODD are at risk for conduct disorder. Although adolescents are typically oppositional, those with ODD show more severe behaviors with more serious consequences and impairment in home, school, and social functioning.

Behavior modification techniques are effective in changing behaviors and violations of safety (eg, curfew violations and failure to report whereabouts). Family therapy can improve communication between parents and children or adolescents. Medication is used to treat comorbid conditions such as ADHD and depression. The nurse's role in caring for the child with ODD does not differ substantially from how the nurse will intervene in the child with ADHD; see the Application of the Nursing Process to a Client With ADHD for more nursing care strategies.

CONDUCT DISORDER

Adolescents with *conduct disorder* are often unmanageable at home and disruptive in the community. They have little empathy or concern for the feelings and well-being of others. They may be callous and lack appropriate feelings of guilt and remorse, although they may express remorse superficially to avoid punishment for their behavior. They often blame others for their actions. Risk-taking behaviors such as drinking, smoking, using illegal substances, experimenting with sex, and participating in criminal actions are common. Cruelty to animals or people, destruction of property, theft, and serious violation of rules are diagnostic criteria of conduct disorder.

The onset of conduct disorder is usually late childhood or early adolescence. Conduct disorder in adolescents is seen frequently in mental health treatment centers. Prevalence rates range from 6% to 16% in boys and 2% to 9% in girls younger than 18 years. A youth with conduct disorder may have comorbid ADHD, ODD, learning disorders, depression, anxiety disorders, and substance abuse. Risk factors for conduct disorder include physical and sexual abuse, inconsistent parenting with harsh discipline, lack of supervision, early institutional living, association with a delinquent peer group, and parental substance abuse.

Behavioral techniques may reduce some of the symptoms of conduct disorder; however, their application requires a great deal of consistency. Aggression and impulsivity can be treated with several medications, including the atypical antipsychotics, lithium, and other mood stabilizers such as valproic acid (see Chap. 12). Comorbid disorders must be treated with appropriate psychosocial and pharmacological means. The nurse's role in caring for the child with conduct disorder does not differ substantially from how the nurse will intervene in the child with ADHD; see Application of the Nursing Process to a Client With ADHD for more information.

ADJUSTMENT DISORDERS

An **adjustment disorder** is a psychiatric disorder marked by clinically or behaviorally significant symptoms that develop within 3 months after the onset of an identifiable stressor. Stress temporarily overwhelms the client's capacity to solve problems, resulting in impaired functioning. The course of adjustment disorders may be acute or chronic. An adjustment disorder may accompany depression, anxiety, or conduct disturbances.

The child or adolescent with adjustment disorder may have difficulty functioning at school or with peers or family members. Adjustment disorders are associated with an increased risk of suicidal actions. The response to the stressor is greater than normally expected. This maladaptive reaction may occur when a child becomes ill, is hospitalized, or faces surgery. Signs may include regressed, fearful, or acting-out behavior. After leaving the hospital, the child may cling to a parent, cry, have nightmares, eat poorly, and need a diaper even though he or she was formerly toilet trained.

Treating an adjustment disorder requires understanding, support, and encouragement to move beyond the event as the youth works out feelings associated with the stressor. The nurse teaches and reinforces adaptive coping skills. Specific symptoms of depression or anxiety are treated with appropriate medications.

ANXIETY DISORDERS

Children and adolescents experience several anxiety disorders, including obsessive-compulsive disorder, phobias, social anxiety disorder, generalized anxiety disorder, separation anxiety disorder, and post-traumatic stress disorder (see Chap. 18). Children with these types of disorders often have symptoms of fear, anxiety, physical complaints, and sleep disturbances, including nightmares and night terrors. In all age groups, sleep problems are associated with mental illness.

OBSESSIVE-COMPULSIVE DISORDER

Obsessive-compulsive disorder (OCD) is characterized by recurrent intrusive thoughts (*obsessions*) and repetitive behaviors that the person realizes are senseless but feels he or she must perform (*compulsions*). Obsessions and compulsions consume hours of the day and cause the child or teen great distress. OCD occurs in families; if a parent has OCD, the child has an increased likelihood to also have OCD.

Treatment of OCD in children and adolescents involves behavioral and psychopharmacological intervention. Behavioral techniques include *exposure* (deliberately confronting the client with stimuli that trigger obsessions and provoke the urge to perform rituals) and *response prevention* (either instructing the client to delay the ritual or blocking the child from performing the ritual). These two techniques allow the child to experience the rise and fall of anxiety. Effective medications for treating OCD symptoms are fluvoxamine, clomipramine, fluoxetine, and paroxetine (see Chaps. 12 and 18).

PHOBIAS

Phobias are morbid, irrational, and persistent fears. They are so common in childhood that mild, passing fears are considered part of normal development.

A child may express the anxiety of a specific phobia by crying, clinging, or having tantrums. Frequently, children fear animals, storms, or traveling in a certain vehicle. They may ask repeated questions about illness or death, kidnappers, or criminals. For example, the child with a phobia of dogs is preoccupied with the thought of possibly meeting a dog, feels constantly anxious about it, and may not want to leave the house for fear of encountering a dog. Phobias can be incapacitating.

Treatment of specific phobias includes pharmacotherapy with selective serotonin reuptake inhibitors (SSRIs)(see Chap. 12); preparation of children for traumatic experiences; behavioral training such as relaxation, desensitization, and modeling; and psychotherapy for youth who have experienced traumatic events (eg, an attack by a dog) (see Chap. 18).

SOCIAL ANXIETY DISORDER (SOCIAL PHOBIA)

Children and adolescents with *social anxiety disorder* avoid contact with unfamiliar people and performing or speaking in front of others. This behavior interferes with typical day-to-day functioning, such as with peers or at school. The youth appears socially withdrawn, embarrassed, shy, self-conscious, and anxious if asked to interact with strangers. The avoidance and anxious anticipation cause marked distress in new or forced social situations.

Treating social anxiety disorder requires both pharmacologic and psychosocial interventions. SSRIs, particularly paroxetine (Paxil), which has anxiety-reducing properties, is helpful in relieving the child's or adolescent's anxiety (see

Chap. 12). In addition, the youth needs support in learning and using social skills by means of role-playing and other forms of practice and reading and discussing books about children who have overcome their social reticence. Providers and family members should encourage the child to take calculated risks and reinforce his or her progress.

GENERALIZED ANXIETY DISORDER

Children with generalized anxiety disorder (GAD) have excessive or unrealistic anxiety; they worry about past and future events, the weather, their own school performance or health, the family's finances, and the welfare of others. For example, a child with GAD might say, "I'm worried about whether my father is going to get another kidney stone and whether we're going to have another tornado. I don't like it when there are clouds in the sky because there could be a storm." Physical symptoms of anxiety such as stomachache, headache, nausea, shortness of breath, and dizziness often accompany GAD.

The anxiolytic buspirone (BuSpar) or the SSRI paroxetine (Paxil) helps reduce anxiety and promotes a sense of well-being. In addition, reassuring the child or adolescent of his or her safety and that of his or her loved ones, teaching relaxation techniques, and helping the youth relax his or her standards to realistic levels of performance are appropriate nursing interventions.

SEPARATION ANXIETY DISORDER

A child or adolescent with **separation anxiety disorder** experiences severe anxiety to the point of panic when separated from a parent or attachment figure. When apart or threatened with separation from his or her parent, the child may be very fearful of accidents or injuries befalling the parent, may be extremely homesick, may cling to or shadow the parent, may have nightmares about separation, and may refuse to attend school or spend the night away from home. In addition, he or she may complain of headaches and stomachaches and may vomit when separated from the parent. Children with separation anxiety often have sleep disturbances such as being afraid to fall asleep apart from the parent. Adolescents usually complain of physical ailments and refuse to attend school. The prevalence of separation anxiety drops as the young person moves into adolescence.

Children and adolescents with separation anxiety usually respond well (ie, anxiety decreases) to SSRIs. Behavioral therapy includes imagery, self-talk, and cognitive techniques. Nursing interventions include reassuring the child and teaching the parents helpful responses to the child's fears and calming bedtime activities for the child.

POST-TRAUMATIC STRESS DISORDER

Post-traumatic stress disorder (PTSD) can result in children who are exposed to the pervasive trauma of inner-city life, suffer physical or sexual abuse, are exposed to community or family violence, or witness the wounding or death of a close family member. Whether a child or adolescent develops PTSD in response to a traumatic event depends on several factors, including the risk and protective factors in the child's environment, as well as individual vulnerabilities and strengths (Silva et al., 2000) (see Chap. 3).

Interventions for PTSD include psychotherapy with a skilled therapist and medications to treat symptoms. For example, a child or adolescent with PTSD may need an antipsychotic medication for auditory hallucinations, an antidepressant for depressive symptoms and thoughts of self-harm, or both types of medication.

MOOD DISORDERS

Mood disorders, including unipolar depression and bipolar disorder, occur in all age groups (see Chap. 24). The most prominent signs and symptoms are specific to the age and developmental level of the person with the mood disturbance. Some of the signs and symptoms of mood disorders in children and adolescents are similar to the normal mood swings that all people go through at different developmental stages. Therefore, mood disorders in children and adolescents are often unrecognized by families, physicians, and nurses. In fact, one research study found that adolescents were more likely to identify major depression in themselves than were their own parents (Fleming & Offord, 1990). Mood disorders in young people often co-occur with other mental disorders, such as anxiety, disruptive behavior, or substance abuse disorders and with physical illnesses, such as diabetes.

Several factors contribute to the failure to recognize depressive disorders in children and adolescents. The way that young people express symptoms is a function of their developmental stage. Adolescence is often a time of emotional turmoil, mood swings, and rebelliousness. Substance abuse also may contribute to a missed diagnosis of depression. Another problem is that children and adolescents sometimes have difficulty expressing their internal mood states and emotions. Sometimes, the only way they can express these emotions is through acting out and behaving inappropriately. Parents, teachers, and other adults, however, may misinterpret such clues as disobedience or insolent behavior.

Early diagnosis and treatment of mood disorders is essential for the continued healthy emotional, social, and behavioral development of children and adolescents.

Identifying and treating mood disorders early reduces their duration, severity, and resulting functional impairment.

DEPRESSION

Depression in children is often undiagnosed because many parents and other adults do not believe that childhood depression is real. Childhood depression, however, is real and takes a serious toll on the nation's youth. Mental health organizations and the U.S. Public Health Service estimate that at least 5% of children and adolescents are depressed at any point in time (Clinical Example 29-2). In fact, half of all adults with depression report that their depression started before age 20 years. Incidence of adolescent major depression is about 4.7%, although about one third to one half of adolescents report symptoms of depression. Adolescents disclose their depression more readily through self-reports than to their parents (Pullen, Modrcin-McCarthy, & Graf, 2000).

▼ *Clinical Example 29-2*

Eight-year-old Sarah and her parents came to the child outpatient clinic when she wrote a note to her father about how badly she feels when she bites herself; she asked him to forgive her. Sarah has bruised her arms and legs as a result of the biting that started about 3 months ago. She has a number of fears, including the dark, being alone, and getting sick and dying. Her parents say she is irritable, cries excessively, and "will cry over any little thing." Her parents have never seen her like this before this episode.

Her eating has lessened, and her sleeping is restless—she often awakens early in a "cranky mood." Her maternal grandmother died 1 year ago, and Sarah continues to talk about how much she misses her. She is demanding, has temper outbursts, and throws things in her room. She yells at her parents and 6-year-old sister. She "forgets things" and is inattentive and impulsive but not hyperactive.

The psychiatric nurse practitioner evaluated Sarah and gathered her history. Her diagnoses are Major Depressive Disorder, single episode, moderate; Attention-Deficit Disorder, inattentive type; Anxiety Disorder, NOS; and rule out Oppositional-Defiant Disorder.

Points for Reflection and Critical Thinking

- In order of priority, what are the mental health needs of Sarah and her family?
- Identify the appropriate level of treatment for Sarah. Justify your answer.
- Create a teaching plan for Sarah and her parents; include learning outcomes, teaching content, and strategies.

• How would you respond to Sarah's mother when she says, "Why is she depressed?" and "I don't want her to become addicted to any medicine."?

Dysthymia is a mild form of depression that lasts 1 year or more in a child or teen. Because the symptoms are less debilitating than with major depression, nurses in school and clinic settings may see youth with dysthymia. Youth with dysthymic disorder are at risk for developing major depression (Klein, Schwartz, & Rose et al., 2000). When dysthymia and major depression occur together, it is called **double depression**.

Etiology

Depression may result from underactivity of nerve cells whose neurotransmitters are the biogenic amines serotonin and norepinephrine. The cognitive-behavioral theory of depression holds that relying on approval from others for self-esteem puts a person at risk for depression. Often, a combination of biological and environmental factors contributes to the development of depression in children and adolescents. The risk of depression rises when close relatives have depressive disorders. For example, if one parent has depression, the child or adolescent has a 25% chance of developing the disorder. If both parents have depression, the risk rises to 75%. Stressful life events, such as conflict with parents, abuse, or academic problems, can precipitate a depressive episode in a child who is genetically vulnerable to the illness.

Signs and Symptoms

Depression affects children and teens in all areas of physical, emotional, and cognitive development. The duration and intensity of symptoms differentiate depression from sadness. Depressive behavior differs significantly from the child's usual behavior and interferes with his or her life in relation to family, schoolwork, and friends (Box 29-1).

Depression in children and adolescents is easily confused with other childhood disorders, such as ADHD. Because children often cannot tell adults what they are feeling, they communicate their feelings by acting out. A prepubertal child with depression often exhibits irritability and separation anxiety, whereas an adolescent may be negativistic, antisocial, defiant, socially withdrawn, and failing at school.

Signs of depression in children and adolescents are as follows:

• Depressed or irritable mood, low frustration level, overreaction to simple requests, loss of joy, and moodiness

---

BOX 29-1 ▼ *What Does a Child Have To Be Depressed About?*

Only decades ago, the general view held that children could not suffer depression. After all, what do they have to be depressed about? Children do not have to hold down a job to pay for food and shelter. All they must do is attend school and play. We idealize the period of childhood as a time of joy and learning.

Even today parents may ask, "What could he or she possibly have to be depressed about?" Depression does not only occur following a sad or traumatic event. Depression (like other mental disorders) "runs in families," just as heart disease and diabetes are familial disorders.

Children of any age can experience depression. However, the expression of mood disorders, depression, and bipolar disorder in children does not mirror the symptoms seen in adults. Whereas adults with depression are sad, children are usually irritable or angry. They may have rages. Adolescents may show disruptive behavior and end up in trouble at both home and school.

When parents have mood disorders such as depression, it is particularly crucial that their children be screened for a mood disorder. Early detection and treatment are essential to promote children's and adolescents' recovery from depression and return to wellness. Every October, National Depression Screening Day offers anyone the opportunity to take part in a screening.

• Psychomotor agitation or retardation; the child may talk slowly and pause before responding
• Changes in appetite and sleep; the child may eat everything or very little, not sleep restfully, have trouble falling or staying asleep, or awaken very early
• Physical complaints such as headache, stomachache, fatigue, and loss of energy
• Depressive themes expressed in play, dreams, or verbalizations; themes may include feeling worthless or guilty, minimizing one's own strengths and maximizing failures, and blaming self as the cause of problems in the family
• Social withdrawal
• Intense anger or rage
• **Anhedonia**—loss of pleasure in hobbies or activities of interest
• Acting-out behaviors, such as abusing drugs and alcohol, playing truant, dropping out of school, running away, exhibiting antisocial behavior, inflicting self-injury, or practicing sexual promiscuity
• Decreased ability to think, concentrate, or make

decisions; this often results in falling academic performance

- Thoughts of and verbalizations about death or wishing he or she had never been born; teens may express their thoughts through music, films, or writing with morbid themes
- Stressors, such as a breakup with a boyfriend or girlfriend, which may trigger suicidal thoughts (Kuchta, 2001)

Comorbidities

Half of children and adolescents with depression have another psychiatric illness, such as GAD, OCD, ADHD, or conduct disorder. In addition, adolescents with depression may abuse drugs or alcohol (see Chap. 27).

Prevention

Early identification and treatment are essential to prevent depression, especially long-term depression later in life. Facilitating a strong sense of self, trust, resiliency, and self-esteem; providing a stable home life; practicing open and honest communication; teaching how to deal with disappointment and frustration; and providing activities that build on the youth's abilities and talents may diminish the incidence of depression.

Interdisciplinary Goals and Treatment

The recovery rate from a single episode of major depression in children and adolescents is relatively high; 70% to 80% of youth with depression can be treated effectively. Episodes of depression, however, have a high rate of recurrence (Lewinsohn, Clarke, & Seeley et al., 1994); 40% of children with one depressive episode will experience another within 2 years. Therefore, the goal is no longer to help the child or teen respond to treatment; instead, it is for the child or teen to become well. In addition, youths with dysthymic disorder are at risk for developing major depression (Klein, Schwartz, & Rose et al., 2000). Anyone with depression needs to be monitored closely; ongoing treatment is needed to prevent recurrences of depression.

Cognitive-behavioral or play therapy for younger children, parent and family consultation, and medication constitute the necessary treatment for children and adolescents with depression. Neither therapy alone nor medication alone has been found to be as effective as the combination treatment.

COGNITIVE-BEHAVIORAL THERAPY AND FAMILY CONSULTATION

Cognitive-behavioral therapy can decrease errors in thinking and improve developmental skills. These include using self-talk to promote coping in certain situations, active participation in planning one's activities, and self-monitoring by writing about moods or feelings in a journal.

Family consultation helps family members understand mood disorders, support their child or adolescent with depression, and develop more effective parenting skills. Through consultation or parent education, parents learn strategies to develop and maintain effective communication within the family. Especially important is the need to listen to the adolescent and communicate openly and respectfully with him or her. Parents also learn to identify risk factors that will worsen depression, such as alcohol and nicotine use.

PHARMACOLOGIC THERAPY

The most commonly used antidepressant medications for children and adolescents are the SSRIs. Side effects, especially nausea, headache, and stomachache, are minimal, especially when the starting dose is low with a gradual increase to a therapeutic level. Although the youth and family may see improvement in 1 to 2 weeks, it may require 12 weeks to assess the full response to the medication. Antidepressants are given for 6 months to 2 years to treat the depression fully and decrease its likelihood of recurrence.

TCAs are older drugs with greater side effects, including potentially life-threatening dysrhythmias. Because of their potential lethality in an overdose, TCAs are rarely given to youth with depression. Imipramine (Tofranil) and amitriptyline (Elavil) are useful to treat both enuresis and ADHD symptoms (especially for a child in whom anxiety is also a problem) in children with depression.

For children with depression who also experience aggression, severe agitation, or the psychotic symptoms of delusions and hallucinations, antipsychotic medications, particularly the atypical antipsychotics, are used. The atypical antipsychotics most likely to be given to a child or teen are risperidone (Risperdal), quetiapine (Seroquel), and olanzapine (Zyprexa). They cause some sedation, especially initially. Of these three, quetiapine causes the least weight gain. Traditional antipsychotic medications are used less frequently in children because of the increased risk of tardive dyskinesia (see Chap. 12).

BIPOLAR DISORDER

When the book *The Bipolar Child* by Demitri and Janice Papolos was published in 1999, many parents of children with unusual patterns of disturbing behavior described a revelation in their lives. These authors have proposed a definition of juvenile-onset bipolar disorder that is marked by rapid, wide swings of emotion; arousal; excitability; and movement (see Chap. 24).

Etiology

Bipolar disorder has a strong familial component. When a parent has a history of bipolar disorder, the risk that his or her child will develop bipolar disorder is greatly increased. In addition, 20% to 40% of children with depression develop bipolar disorder. The prevalence of bipolar disorder in children is at least 1%, similar to the prevalence seen in adults.

Signs and Symptoms

Bipolar disorder is a mood disorder, and the primary symptoms are mood related. Severely irritable, dysphoric, and agitated children who have "affective (or emotional) storms" or rages (ie, prolonged, aggressive temper outbursts), are prone to violence, show poor school performance, have sleep disturbances, and experience rapid mood swings that may occur hourly or every 2 hours may have bipolar disorder. Children do not show the classic manic picture of elated mood seen in adults with bipolar disorder. Sometimes, it is difficult to identify episodes of cycling (ie, switching from one mood to another) because the symptoms seem to be chronic (Mohr, 2001). A child also may exhibit delusions, hypersexuality, pressured speech, or flight of ideas.

Adolescents may demonstrate hallucinations, delusions, labile mood, or idiosyncratic thinking (Mohr, 2001). Although adolescents may have symptoms that resemble those of adults, it is still difficult to determine cycling of moods. In addition, incidence of substance abuse is high in adolescents with bipolar disorder.

The symptoms of bipolar disorder overlap with those of ADHD, but children with bipolar disorder always have a mood disturbance. Childhood-onset bipolar disorder may have comorbidity with ADHD, ODD, and conduct disorder, or it may have features of ADHD, ODD, and conduct disorder.

Interdisciplinary Goals and Treatment

Children or adolescents with bipolar disorder and their families need several types of treatment including education, family therapy, special education or school modifications, support groups, individual or play therapy, and mood-stabilizing medication (Mohr, 2001). The goals of treatment for the child with bipolar disorder are to alleviate symptoms and improve day-to-day functioning.

IMPORTANCE OF EARLY IDENTIFICATION AND TREATMENT

Studies suggest that clients who have had prior episodes of bipolar disorder may have a poorer response to lithium and that a person's past history in terms of episodes and mood instability will affect treatment response (Swann, Bowden, Calabrese, Dilsaver, & Morris, 1999). Scientists believe that this results from neuronal sensitization that

can happen spontaneously as a progression of the illness and its cycles. If bipolar disorder remains unrecognized and unchecked in the child, future episodes of illness may occur independently of any stimulus, and they will occur with greater and greater frequency (Papolos & Papolos, 1999). Therefore, early identification of bipolar disorder in the child is urgent.

Strong evidence also suggests that medications such as TCAs and stimulants may induce sensitization (Post & Weiss, 1998). As stated previously, bipolar disorder appears to be comorbid with ADHD. Both stimulants and antidepressants are used in the treatment of ADHD; both may be implicated in the precipitation of mania in genetically vulnerable children (Geller, Fox, & Fletcher, 1993; Papolos & Papolos, 1999). In one study, Altshuler and colleagues (1995) found that 35% of clients with bipolar disorder had a manic episode rated as likely to have been induced by antidepressants. Moreover, an acceleration of cycling was associated with antidepressant treatment in 26% of subjects, and a younger age at first treatment was a predictor of vulnerability to antidepressant-induced cycle acceleration. Therefore, because of the confusion regarding diagnosis of bipolar disorder in children and adolescents, it is essential that the child undergo a detailed, thorough, longitudinal history before medications are prescribed. Rushing to judgment can have unintended consequences; medications that are completely appropriate for the treatment of ADHD may worsen the course and prognosis of bipolar disorder.

PHARMACOLOGIC THERAPY

Mood-stabilizing medications, including lithium, divalproex (Depakote), and carbamazepine (Tegretol), have calming and antiaggressive effects and help to prevent depressive and manic symptoms. Lithium, which affects serotonin, norepinephrine, and dopamine systems, is particularly effective in clients whose behavior is manic or elated rather than depressed. During mania, lithium diminishes the action of dopamine; during depression, it enhances the action of serotonin. The anticonvulsant mood stabilizers divalproex and carbamazepine are more effective in treating rapid cycling, angry, or depressed states. Children with bipolar disorder who also have psychosis may be given an antipsychotic medication, most likely an atypical antipsychotic (Mohr, 2001).

Although the medications discussed previously are used frequently in adults with bipolar disorder (see Chaps. 12 and 24), some concerns are specific to children and adolescents. For example, children and teens often spend more time outside playing and engaging in sports. Parents need to be careful that their children do not become dehydrated while taking lithium because it could elevate their lithium levels. Many schools allow children and teens taking lithium to keep a water bottle with them in class to maintain hydration. Other side effects of lithium are nausea, polyuria with resulting enuresis, and polydipsia.

AUTISM SPECTRUM DISORDERS

Autism spectrum disorders, also called *pervasive developmental disorders,* have the following core features:

- Impairments in socialization
- Impairments in communication
- Restricted repertoire of behaviors

Autism spectrum disorders are found in about one out of 300 to 500 children between the ages of birth to 3 years. The intelligence of these children is usually in the average to above-average range.

AUTISM

Autism is a genetic disorder of neuronal organization that requires early detection and treatment. Chromosomal abnormalities are present in 5% to 6% of children with autism. A child with autism develops language slowly or not at all. He or she may use words without attaching meaning to them or communicate with gestures or noises instead of words. He or she spends time alone and shows little interest in making friends. Children with autism are less responsive to social cues such as smiles or eye contact. There is often some degree of sensory impairment, including sensitivity in the areas of sight, taste, hearing, touch, or smell.

Children with autism do not play spontaneously or imaginatively. They act socially aloof and indifferent. They do not imitate others' actions or participate in pretend games. They may act aggressively and throw tantrums for no obvious reason. In addition, they may *perseverate;* that is, show an obsessive interest in some item or activity and engage in ritualistic behavior. They often adhere to routines and do not tolerate changes in routine well. These characteristics are evident in children with autism before the age of 3 years.

ASPERGER SYNDROME

Asperger syndrome is a severe developmental disorder characterized by major difficulties in social interaction and restricted and unusual interests and behavior. Although there is not a significant general delay in language, people with Asperger syndrome use monotone speech and rigid language. They cannot understand jokes and are taken advantage of easily. In spite of not grasping nonverbal communication cues and an inability to show empathy to others, they want to meet people and make friends.

Persons with Asperger syndrome have an obsession with facts about circumscribed and odd topics. For example, they may have a tremendous interest in, and talk incessantly about, a topic that would not appeal to another child (eg, deep-fat fryers, the counties of their state, or lists of every character in every video game played). They are often perfectionists and hate to fail.

Interdisciplinary Goals and Treatment

Improved outcomes are achieved with early detection. An easy screening tool for 18-month-olds is the Checklist for Autism in Toddlers (CHAT), which is used to evaluate the child's ability to pretend, enjoyment in peekaboo games, attempts to engage the parent, and eye contact.

Treatment for clients with autism, Asperger syndrome, and related disorders centers on behavioral interventions, particularly cognitive and behavior therapy, special education, social skills training in groups, language therapies, occupational therapy, and sometimes pharmacotherapy. Behavior modification techniques include those used to enhance and reduce certain behaviors. For example, social skills training:

- Uses role-playing, coaching, and social stories to help the child play like other children of his or her age
- Teaches flexibility in how to engage in an activity and how to recognize cues and actions for specific social situations
- Teaches ways to reduce stress, anxiety, and inattention

Medication may be needed to manage the symptoms of hyperactivity, irritability, aggression, self-injury, ritualistic behavior, and obsessive-compulsive behavior. These can span a wide range of psychoactive medications, including the neuroleptics, anticonvulsants, and mood stabilizers.

Treatment needs change according to the age of the developing child. Speech and language therapy and assistance to parents are critical when the child is very young. An older child or adolescent may need cognitive-behavioral therapy and medication to deal with obsessive-compulsive symptoms. The child's prognosis is more positive when language development and social interaction are less impaired. Researchers hope that, at some point in the future, it may be possible to treat autism with neuronal growth factors.

Children with autism spectrum disorders need a structured environment and social-emotional training. The goal may be to learn to imitate social behavior that other children learn intuitively. In addition, special education placement in public school settings with measurable goals and objectives for the child is necessary. Public Law 94–142, the Education for All Handicapped Children Act of 1975, requires that all children between 3 and 21 years with diagnosed autism or a pervasive developmental disorder receive free, appropriate education. A newer law ensures that services be provided from birth, although they may be provided by an agency outside the school system.

Parents need accurate information, training in becoming advocates for their child, respite programs, and inclusion in individualized, collaborative treatment planning to understand and help their child. Future needs of the child with autism spectrum disorder might include vocational training and placement, use of sheltered workshops, supported employment, and community-based programs such as group home or supervised apartment living.

EATING DISORDERS

Adolescents and sometimes children develop eating disorders of anorexia and bulimia. The prevalence among adolescents is estimated to be 0.5% for anorexia and between 0.5% and 5.8% for bulimia. Many girls have some eating disordered symptoms but do not meet all criteria for the illness (White, 2000). These disorders are long-term, complex problems, affecting both physical and psychological well-being. Eating disorders are discussed in depth in Chapter 23.

SUBSTANCE ABUSE

Adolescents are polysubstance abusers, primarily. They most widely use tobacco, alcohol, and marijuana. Nicotine and alcohol are termed "gateway" drugs because they often "open the gates" to further and heavier drug use for teens. The young person's choice of a drug often is related to "drug fashions" such as "club drugs." Club drugs refer to dangerous, even lethal, substances that young people use at all-night parties, called "raves" or "trances," dance clubs, or bars. Examples of club drugs are 3,4-methylene-dioxymethamphetamine (MDMA), or Ecstasy, gamma hydroxybutyric acid (GHB), Rohypnol, ketamine, methamphetamine, and lysergic acid diethylamide (LSD).

Substance abuse is associated with other problem behaviors such as criminality and sexual promiscuity. It provides the teen with a maladaptive way to escape frustration, disappointment, boredom, and emptiness. Teens who abuse drugs and alcohol are at higher risk for physical health problems, depression, suicidal ideation, and conduct disorder (Box 29-2). In addition, teen substance abusers are more likely to drive while intoxicated, putting them at great risk for fatal motor vehicle accidents. Adolescent substance abuse is related to premature involvement in sex, higher incidence of sexually transmitted diseases, and teen pregnancy. Prevalence of alcohol and drug-use disorders among adolescents is 32% and higher among teens with mental illness. Mood disorders, anxiety disorders, and disruptive behavior disorders are comorbid conditions.

BOX 29-2 ▼ *Signs and Symptoms of Substance Abuse in Adolescents*

All of the following can be signs that an adolescent is using substances:

- Poor academic performance, failure, or truancy
- Withdrawal from family and friends
- Change in or loss of friends
- Physical complaints
- Aggression or risk-taking behavior
- Depression and suicidal thoughts or actions
- Continuous use of the substance, even though it interferes with the adolescent's ability to perform at school, home, or work and causes interpersonal or social problems
- Use of the substance in situations in which it is dangerous, for example, when driving a car, which may lead to legal problems (eg, driving while intoxicated [DWI])

Etiology

Children growing up in families with alcohol abuse often have guilt and anxiety, may be confused about parental inconsistency, may have difficulty establishing close relationships, and may exhibit anger, depression, or both. The likelihood is high that a person will abuse substances if one or both parents are or were substance abusers. In fact, children of alcoholics have a four times higher risk of alcohol abuse than do children of nonalcoholic parents. Whether peers are involved in substance abuse is a critical factor in the adolescent's decision regarding drug use. Societal values, media, and the adolescent's role models also affect his or her decision about use of drugs and alcohol.

Prevention of Drug and Alcohol Abuse

According to the Partnership for a Drug-Free America, "Communication is the anti-drug." Children and teens are somewhat "protected" from drug and alcohol use when they have positive relationships with their parents, attend religious services, are involved in activities that instill values, and perceive that their basic needs are met (Mainous, Mainous, Martin, Oler, & Haney, 2001). High-risk youth whose parents are substance abusers must be identified and given prevention education and support. The goals should be to improve self-esteem, impulse control, and coping through behavioral and cognitive measures.

Interdisciplinary Goals and Treatment

The first step in treating adolescent substance abuse is awareness and recognition of the problem, especially considering that parents, teachers, and communities frequently deny or underestimate the problem. It is critical that nurses ask direct questions of the child or adolescent and his or her family about the child's substance use; embarrassment or fear should not be used as excuses for not asking these questions (Therapeutic Communication 29-1). Nurses and other mental health professionals must aim to change the substance-abusing family's direction back to health and strength.

Interventions should address the reasons teens give for using substances, including avoiding peer pressure, getting "high," cheering up, getting rid of boredom, having more energy (cocaine or stimulant users), and escaping from problems. Adolescents also may express feelings of unmet needs as important factors in their substance abuse (Mainous et al., 2001). Substance abuse and its treatment are presented fully in Chapter 27.

TIC DISORDERS

A **tic** is a sudden repetitive movement, gesture, or utterance. Tics are brief and may occur in bouts. They tend to

---

THERAPEUTIC COMMUNICATION 29-1
Discussing Peer Pressure and Substance Use With Adolescents

Luis is a 14-year-old boy who has come for a regular physical examination. The nurse is interviewing him before the physical assessment.

Ineffective Dialogue

Nurse: "How are things going for you at school?"

Client: (Shrugs) "Okay."

Nurse: "Have you been facing any peer pressure lately?"

Client: (Looks confused) "No."

Nurse: "A lot of kids your age start using drugs. I'm giving you a bunch of pamphlets about the dangers of drinking and doing drugs. Please read them. If you have questions, let me know."

Client: (Seems to stifle a laugh) "Okay."

Effective Dialogue

Nurse: "How are things going for you at school?"

Client: (Shrugs) "Okay."

Nurse: "Many teenagers face issues involving peer pressure, especially related to drugs and alcohol. *(Pauses)* Have you used any of these substances recently?"

Client: (Looks down at the floor) "Well, a few weeks ago, my friend tried to get me to drink beer with him. I took a sip, but I didn't like it. I don't want to do it again."

Nurse: "Were there reasons why you didn't say no?"

Client: (Smiles weakly) "I didn't want to seem like a nerd or have him laugh at me."

Nurse: "It's very difficult to say no to friends. We all want to fit in and be part of the crowd. Let's talk more about how to handle these situations and why drugs and alcohol can be dangerous. I also have pamphlets that you can read on your own. What questions do you have?"

Client: (Begins to ask the nurse questions about the effects of drugs)

Reflection and Critical Thinking

- Why do you think the first nurse failed to learn the information that the client divulged to the second nurse?
- How did the second nurse achieve rapport with the client? Cite specific ways in which the nurse made the client feel comfortable and encouraged him to share information.
- What assumptions about teenagers do nurses need to try to avoid? How can such assumptions block communication?

increase during periods of stress and lessen during absorbing activities. Tics can be motor or vocal, simple or complex.

Tourette syndrome is the most severe tic disorder. It is characterized by multiple motor tics and one or more vocal tics many times throughout the day for 1 year or more. The disorder impairs functioning at home, in school, and with peers. Obsessions, compulsions, hyperactivity, disinhibited speech or behavior, and impulsivity may be associated features. The child may also have depression and school and behavioral problems.

Tic disorders are treated with supportive counseling, school modifications, parent guidance, and individual therapy, as needed. Pharmacotherapy with haloperidol, pimozide, clonidine, clomipramine, desipramine, fluoxetine, and sertraline is useful to diminish tics. Anticipatory guidance will help the child or teen and family learn that tics get better and worse in response to many variables and stressors in the young person's life.

TRICHOTILLOMANIA

Clients with **trichotillomania** have an irresistible urge to pull out their hair; they feel tension before pulling out the hair and relief or pleasure during and after pulling. They may then examine, chew on, or eat the hair. The hair loss is noticeable. Trichotillomania is a chronic impulse control condition, and it impairs the child's or adolescent's social or school life. Typically, people with trichotillomania try to deny or hide their behavior; hair pulling is done privately. This results in social withdrawal because the person fears that he or she may have a strong urge to pull hair while with others. Feelings of shame and humiliation, poor self-image, and problems with mood, anxiety, or addictions are common (Enos & Plante, 2001).

At least 2.5 million people in the United States have trichotillomania. Boys and girls develop it with equal frequency. The average age of onset is 12 to 13 years, although many younger children have trichotillomania. Children and adults most commonly pull out their scalp hair, then eyelashes, eyebrows, and pubic hair. The person may pull hair in certain circumstances, such as while watching television, reading or studying, or lying in bed waiting to fall asleep. Causes for the disorder seem to be biological (links have been seen between trichotillomania and Tourette syndrome) and behavioral (eg, the client relies on hair pulling as a tension-reducing action, and it becomes a habit).

Treatment for trichotillomania includes both behavior therapy and pharmacotherapy with clomipramine, fluvoxamine, fluoxetine, or another SSRI. *Habit reversal therapy* (HRT) is the method used to increase awareness of the hair pulling. In addition, teaching alternative coping activities (eg, relaxing, pulling weeds) and maintaining motivation through social support are methods useful for treating children and adults with trichotillomania (Enos & Plante, 2001).

SUICIDE

Another major concern among adolescent youth is suicide. Although children and adolescents with depression are at risk for suicide, they are not alone. Young people with bipolar disorders, those who abuse substances, and gay and lesbian youths also are at risk for self-harm. Those younger than age 25 years (35% of the population) account for approximately 15% of all suicide deaths in the United States. Suicide is the second leading cause of death among college students, third among youths from 15 to 24 years, and sixth among children younger than 15 years. The Surgeon General has noted that the suicide rate in children aged 10 to 14 years has increased by 100% since 1980 (U.S. Department of Health and Human Services, 1999). Some estimate that as many as 10% of children make one suicide attempt by the end of high school. Children often fantasize about suicide by violent means—stabbing or hanging themselves, jumping from heights, or drowning.

Risk factors for suicide among children and adolescents include the following:

- Family history of depression, suicide, or physical or sexual abuse
- Exposure to violence
- Impulsivity
- Loss of a loved one before age 12 years
- Violent behavior
- Diminished sense of connection to family
- Increased family pressures

Signs

It is often hard for parents, teachers, and other adults to see the warning signs of suicidal thoughts or behavior. They include the following:

- Statements such as, "I won't be around for you to yell at," or "You won't have to worry about me much longer"
- Lack of emotional responsiveness
- Social withdrawal
- Inability to enjoy previously enjoyed activities
- Drug or alcohol abuse
- Threat making and giving away of possessions
- Sudden cheerfulness after being depressed

Prevention

There is a nationwide call for increased awareness, focus, and interventions targeted at decreasing the rates of suicide in the general population, particularly within the adolescent population (Center for Mental Health Services, 2001).

The rising incidence of suicide in youth must be lowered through early screening and prompt intervention. The American Foundation for Suicide Prevention aims to teach the nation that suicide is the result of undiagnosed or untreated mental illness.

Interdisciplinary Goals and Treatment

Safety concerns are the priority when a child or teen is suicidal. Nurses must take all threats of self-harm seriously. They must help parents to establish a safety plan that encompasses provision of a safe and unrestrictive environment, action alternatives to self-harm, and directions to take the child in crisis to a hospital emergency room. If the child cannot contract to refrain from self-harm, then parents will need to take the child for an appropriate level of care assessment (Kuchta, 2001).

To assess suicide risk, the nurse talks openly with the child or adolescent and family to determine certain risk factors. These include the presence of a suicide plan, the plan's lethality, the availability of lethal methods such as a gun, a history of substance abuse, prior suicide attempts, exposure to suicidal people that could result in imitative behavior, and level of depression and hopelessness. Children and adolescents, like adults, require close observation and monitoring when recovering from a depressive episode, because they may have regained enough energy to carry out a suicidal thought or plan.

A safety contract is the youth's written promise not to hurt self or another intentionally or accidentally for a specific time period and a list of actions or coping skills to prevent suicidal behavior. The young person may need to be taught how to differentiate his or her feelings and to rank their intensity.

CHILDREN WITH MEDICAL ILLNESS OR DISABILITY

Medical illness is a stressor in the life of a child and family system. Whether the illness is congenital, acute, or chronic, it interrupts the developmental process and disrupts the lives of both child and family. The child may regress to earlier forms of behavior (eg, throwing tantrums, refusing to use the toilet, demanding a bottle). Visits to healthcare settings alter the family's daily routines. Hospital stays can affect the parents' sleeping arrangements and family responsibilities. Siblings experience disruptions as they become secondary to the ill child and are cared for by neighbors or relatives. Hospital bills, medication costs, and time away from work result in financial strains. As one

child assumes the client role, other family members shift in their roles and functions within the family. These disruptions in the family's daily living, routines, and roles require adaptation by all family members (Baker, 1996).

How the child and family perceive these stresses influences how they cope. Benefits can occur when the child and family view the illness as a stressful event that can result in positive adaptation and that can lead to more self-confidence, self-esteem, and mastery. By providing support and assistance in mastering stress, the nurse mediates the family's adaptive responses.

APPLICATION OF THE NURSING PROCESS TO THE CHILD OR ADOLESCENT WITH MEDICAL ILLNESS OR A DISABILITY

Assessment

Assessment begins with determining the child's developmental level. An understanding of age-related capabilities helps the nurse determine the child's perceptions of the illness and associated stressors, formulate appropriate explanations, design strategies to lessen anxiety, and evaluate responses. Table 29-3 outlines common healthcare-related fears and anxieties of children at various stages.

Nurses must remember that a child may regress to a previous developmental level in response to illness. Regression is particularly common in toddlers, since almost any additional stressor threatens their autonomy and developmental mastery. The nurse explains to the family that regression is a feature of illness so that they do not view it as abnormal.

The nurse also assesses for previous experiences with stress and determines how the child has dealt with them. For some children, hospitalization is the first stressful experience they encounter. In such cases, the child's repertoire of coping responses and skills may be limited because of little experience in responding to stress. A child who has faced many recent changes in his or her life may have intensified feelings of vulnerability and insecurity.

Information about the child's personality and temperament also helps the nurse understand the child's response to stress. For example, some children are adventurous and actively seek out new experiences; others are shy and more withdrawn. Knowing what the child was like before the illness helps distinguish between responses that are usual and those that may indicate ineffective coping.

CHARACTERISTICS OF THE DISEASE

Research has not substantiated a causal relationship between a specific illness or disability and a psychological disorder in a child. Nevertheless, knowledge about spe-

TABLE 29-3 ▼ Common Fears and Anxieties of Children in Healthcare

DEVELOPMENTAL PHASE	FEARS AND ANXIETIES
Infancy	Separation anxiety
Toddlerhood	Separation anxiety Fear of the unknown Fear of strangers
Preschool age	Separation anxiety Anxiety about body intrusions, intense need for body intactness Anxieties aroused by egocentric thought, fantasies, magical thinking Fear of punishment aroused by guilt, as child feels he or she is the cause of the illness or disability Fear of body mutilation
School age	Fear of body injury Fear of pain Fear of loss of respect, love, and emerging self-esteem Anxiety related to guilt Fear of anesthesia
Adolescence	Fear of loss of identity and control Anxiety about body image and changes in physical appearance Fear of loss of status in peer group Anxiety related to long-term implications of illness or disability

cific diagnoses provides the nurse with information about the kind of hospitalization required, treatments prescribed, and medical events that the child will encounter; anticipated pain and physical discomfort he or she will experience; type and number of intrusive procedures expected; outward physical signs that will result from the disease or disability; and required treatments to which the child and family must adjust.

Illnesses that require admission to a hospital carry the potential for psychological upset, which may disrupt the child's development. Children with multiple admissions during the first 4 years of life are most vulnerable to the effects of psychological upset.

If the illness is a chronic condition or disability, the risk for psychological disturbance is increased, and coping becomes more complex. The family unit must make ongoing adjustments with each phase of the illness and with each developmental phase through which the child passes. Stress, disequilibrium, adjustment, and adaptation may recur several times as the disease process and treatments progress. For example, the child with congenital abnormalities may have to cope with frequent disruptions in daily living resulting from staged surgical corrections. As the child gets older, the evolving processes of body image, sexual identification, self-esteem, and mastery take on different emphases with each stage of psychosexual development.

The parents' feelings of grief and guilt for what the child is or could have been may further complicate the family's adaptation. The family may mourn the loss of a fantasized child. Their feelings about the child's disability and their perceptions of the stresses caused by the disability may influence their adjustment.

FAMILY ASSESSMENT

The greatest environmental influence on a child is the family. The family's ability to organize daily activities, socioeconomic level, culture, religious beliefs, life experiences, and hardiness influence responses to stress and may affect the child's vulnerability to psychological disturbance resulting from medical illness. For example, the family who has recently undergone significant changes to which members are still adjusting may have depleted their resources for dealing with the stress of the child's illness (Heath, 1996). Members may be less emotionally available than the child needs while he or she is experiencing the stresses of illness, disability, and hospitalization.

The family serves a particularly important role in preventing psychosocial maladjustment in children with chronic illnesses. Protective factors found in a wide range of studies include family functioning with harmony, self-esteem, mastery behaviors, and available social support systems. Families with higher adaptation have been identified as having more family cohesion and greater moral or religious emphasis. The latter characteristic gives positive attribution (meaning) to the chronic illness and provides a belief system that gives support and makes sense of what has happened.

The nurse also determines the family's expectations and desires regarding participation in their child's care. While healthcare providers often assume that parents want to be involved in caregiving activities, research evidence suggests wide variations in the amount of care that parents may be willing or able to undertake (Coyne, 1995;

Marchant, 1996). Determining the family's wishes in advance helps to avoid confusion and conflict.

Nursing Diagnosis

Appropriate nursing diagnoses may include the following:

- **Delayed Growth and Development** related to prolonged or repeated hospitalizations, chronic illness, or physical disability
- **Fear** related to inadequate comprehension of invasive or painful procedures, lack of opportunity to use medical play to work through the procedure or event, or parental anxiety
- **Ineffective Coping** related to overwhelming stimuli of the medical environment
- **Compromised Family Coping** related to serious illness of child, separation of siblings, or absence of parent from home during hospitalization
- **Deficient Diversional Activity** related to separation from siblings and peer group, separation from home and usual activities, or restrictions of illness and treatment

Planning

The primary goal is to minimize the potential for psychosocial disturbance in the child as the state of physical health is restored or supported. A secondary goal is to maximize opportunities for psychosocial benefit: to help the child develop trust, understanding, and mastery of the stressful experiences of healthcare.

Nurses must also direct planning toward family support (Box 29-3). Evidence clearly indicates the importance of the child's primary emotional support figure being present during hospitalization (Endacott, 1998). Anxiety aroused by unfamiliar surroundings and painful events will be compounded by the anxiety aroused by separation from the child's primary source of support. This is true not only for young children, but also for older children for whom regression is a normal response to the physical and emotional demands of illness and hospitalization. Usually this primary attachment is to the parents, particularly the mother. On the child's entry into healthcare, the nurse explains to the parents the value of *rooming-in;* that is, unlimited stay in the child's room. A referral to the social work department to acquire financial assistance or other services, such as child care, may be needed to make the parents' rooming-in possible.

Implementation

The nurse helps the child and family achieve positive psychosocial outcomes through efforts to reduce anxiety,

---

BOX 29-3 ▼ *Family-Centered Care*

The Association for the Care of Children's Health has identified key elements of family-centered care. By incorporating these elements into the delivery of care, the nurse provides psychosocial support to families and decreases risk to children receiving healthcare.

- Recognize that the family is the constant in the child's life.
- Facilitate parent–professional collaboration in healthcare decisions.
- Share unbiased and complete information with parents about their child's care in appropriate, supportive ways on an ongoing basis.
- Recognize family strengths and respect different methods of coping.
- Understand and incorporate developmental needs of children and their families into nursing care delivery.
- Encourage and facilitate parent-to-parent support.

---

develop understanding, and promote positive coping. Therapeutic use of self when working with the child at risk is a primary organizing factor in the nursing process. Conveying an openness, acceptance, and warmth actualizes the development of trust. Ego strength in the nurse is necessary to allow and accept the child's negative feelings.

▼ *Clinical Example 29-3*

Brian, 16 years old, was critically injured in an automobile accident. The accident occurred 60 miles from the nearest trauma center, so Brian was flown to the center by helicopter. On arrival, he had multiple fractures, including both legs, ribs, and right arm, and a closed head injury with loss of consciousness. Brian was quickly moved to the intensive care unit (ICU) for treatment. He was intubated, placed on a ventilator, and given vasopressors to maintain his blood pressure.

His mother is notified of the accident by the county sheriff. She cannot reach her husband and drives to the hospital alone. On arrival, she is directed to the ICU where she sees her son intubated, unconscious, and attached to multiple monitors and intravenous lines.

Points for Reflection and Critical Thinking

- Discuss the possible stressors that Brian's mother might be experiencing.
- What immediate needs of his mother should the nurse assess?

- What actions could friends and family members take to help Brian's family during the initial crisis?
- Discuss interventions the nurse could initiate to facilitate the family's adaptation.

Anxiety may be reduced through *stress immunization;* that is, preparation and play activities that give the child an opportunity to anticipate a stressful event. Stress immunization allows the child to mentally rehearse the event, become desensitized, and practice effective coping strategies. For example, to decrease anxiety and fear and increase cooperation during injections, the nurse may combine reading a story about the event, drawing pictures, discussing fears and fantasies, reading a poem, and playing with examining medical instruments.

Thought stopping involves substituting reassuring information each time the child begins to think about an upcoming stress event. The child, with help from parents and the nurse, generates the reassuring information and memorizes short phrases that convey the meaning. For example, a child with daily venipunctures may use positive statements such as: "It doesn't take too long; I get a prize when it is over; it will help the doctors help me; my mother can stay with me; I can go to the playroom when it's over." Using thought stopping gradually weakens fear responses. In addition, the child develops a resource that decreases feelings of helplessness and increases mastery.

Relaxation training teaches the child to focus attention on his or her body, tighten and relax different muscles, and breathe deeply. The nurse should use the same progression each time so that the process becomes familiar. The training should take place in a nonstressful setting. When the child has learned the process of relaxation, the parent can coach the child in the process during a stressful event.

Sensory preparation has also been found to decrease children's anxiety during healthcare procedures. Children's fantasies of what will happen can often be more frightening than the real events. Through sensory preparation, the child learns about the reality—what he or she will see, hear, feel, and be expected to do. For example, while preparing a child for surgery, the nurse could explain that a mist that feels cool and soft will be blowing in his or her face when awakening after surgery. Experiencing the feeling of the mist during presurgery preparation enhances sensory preparation for the child.

Answering the question of "why" is important to developing the child's understanding. Giving suitable explanations for healthcare events lets the child know that there is a plan for care, that he or she is not being subjected to disturbing events at the whim of more powerful individuals, and that boundaries and limits are known and shared. Children's concepts of illness and causality follow developmental trends aligned with cog-

nitive development. Young children functioning at the concrete operational level need brief, specific, unambiguous, object-related explanations of why things are being done to them. A common misconception among young children is that they have somehow caused their illness. Telling the child many times in different ways that he or she did not cause the illness develops appropriate intellectualization, which reduces guilt and anxiety.

Older children who can grasp cause-and-effect relationships benefit from simple analogies. Adolescents who have begun abstract thinking may require more detailed information with explanations of the implications for treatment. Nevertheless, the nurse also must consider the effects of regression, as the child may regress to a lower level of cognition during stress.

Numerous movies, filmstrips, coloring books, and children's books have been developed for pediatric preparation and parent education. Materials that most closely approximate reality and provide behavioral modeling for the child most effectively decrease children's anxiety.

Understanding is also promoted through the structuring of events. As much as possible, the nurse structures routines of care to follow a course that is known to the child. It is desirable, wherever possible, to follow routines the child experiences at home living (eg, meals, naps, bathing, bedtime). This is especially true for toddlers, who rely on the consistency and familiarity of daily rituals to provide stability and control. Disruption of these routines may result in regressive behavior. For school-age children, simple charts of daily activities and calendars to mark the days and special events will help them understand the process and reinforce the ending of the hospitalization.

Interventions to guide positive coping efforts may include the promotion of cognitive avoidance or distraction. The use of humor, daydreaming, watching television, listening to music, or visualizing helps to divert attention from painful sensations. These strategies are particularly helpful in situations that are beyond the child's control (eg, undergoing a painful procedure).

Idiosyncratic rituals are patterns of behavior developed to cope with, or get through, particular aspects of illness or treatments. Unless the ritual interferes with the child's care, the nurse should not disrupt it, because it offers a playful yet formalized sequence that provides boundaries for the child's anxiety and enhances the child's feeling of belonging and personal distinctiveness. For example, a 6-year-old boy having difficulty with intravenous injections may begin chanting, "I think I can, I think I can, I think I can," throughout the procedure. At the conclusion of the procedure, the child and nurse exclaim together, "I knew I could!"

The use of play supports positive coping by affording the child the opportunity to be actively involved in structuring, controlling, and recreating the stresses of hospital and illness events. This is particularly true of *medical play,* dramatic play using props of real medical equipment in which the child plays being a client and a caregiver. This play facilitates the child's mastery of aggressive, angry feelings. The presence of the nurse during medical play provides support and boundaries for the child's expression of feelings.

Another intervention that supports positive coping is encouraging the child to express feelings through symbolic or creative means. Traditional methods include art, music, storytelling, books, and peer-group discussions. Newer methods include the use of videotherapy (video essays, performance videos, video letters) (Rode, Capitulo, Fishman, & Holden, 1998). Efforts that facilitate the expression of feelings between parents and the child help overcome the "conspiracy of silence" that may develop during a child's illness and lead to shared mastery. In most facilities, child life specialists are available to facilitate expressive efforts (Box 29-4).

Providing school activities for the child who is hospitalized or homebound builds the child's self-esteem as he or she learns new academic skills and information. This intervention enhances the child's internal perceptions.

One of the newest interventions to promote positive coping is the use of computer technology and the Internet. An example is "Starbright World" (*http://www.starbright.org/*), a private computer network where seriously ill children interact in a virtual community, articulating their experiences and escaping the day-to-day trials of hospitalization (Rode et al., 1998). This project, which began in 1995, has more than 25 hospitals online. Through the network, children can get answers to their medical questions, find explanations of upcoming procedures, and communicate through videoconferencing and audio conferencing, chat rooms, bulletin boards, and e-mail. Positive outcomes of the program include reduced feelings of anxiety and isolation, increased levels of activity and interaction, and diversion of attention from pain and discomfort (Stephenson, 1995).

Evaluation

The nurse determines the effectiveness of the treatment plan by observing the child's and family's behaviors and analyzing their meaning and probable causes. Successful outcomes for the child include minimal fear and anxiety, developmentally appropriate behavior, cooperation with ongoing treatment, maintenance of relationships with family and friends, and for school-age children, return to school activities after the acute phase of illness. Successful family coping is characterized by participation in the child's treatment planning and care, management of the usual problems of daily family life, and appropriate use of available resources.

Before discharge, the nurse instructs the family about possible changes in the child's behavior, either specific to the diagnosis or as common reactions to hospitalization. These may include sleep disturbances, developmental task regression, and behavior problems. With chronic illness or disability, anticipatory guidance regarding what to expect at various stages of the illness is also important. The family may need follow-up contact to assess the child's adjustment and any parental concerns.

At discharge, the nurse addresses the concept of *closure*, the ending of an experience marked by a sense of

---

BOX 29-4 ▼ *Child Life Programs*

Hospitalization and illness can be traumatic for anyone—especially children. When they are routinely subjected to complex and invasive procedures, children sometimes feel isolated, scared, and may undergo depersonalization. The meaning an illness holds for someone in the context of his or her life can be easily overlooked in healthcare settings. Child life specialists help children adjust.

Child life specialists—child development experts who are trained and certified in special education and in early childhood, creative arts, or recreation therapies—provide psychosocial assessment as well as therapeutic activities in group contexts, such as pediatric unit playrooms, and individually. These specialists collaborate with a patient's interdisciplinary health team.

During the past 25 years, the child life profession has developed in response to children and families who seek psychosocial guidance in handling illness and hospitalization. Today, child life programs exist in 98% of pediatric medical-surgical settings throughout the U.S. The child life specialist joins the pediatrician, the child psychiatrist, the pediatric nurse, and the medical social worker in an interdisciplinary approach to offering comprehensive services within pediatrics. Using creative arts, child life specialists provide developmentally appropriate therapy and education to children in an effort to minimize psychological trauma. The program encourages children to master creative skills, learn about their illnesses, interact with peers, and express themselves through play.

Visit the web site of the Child Life Program at Mount Sinai Medical Center, at *http://www.mssm.edu/peds/spec-clife.shtml* or the Child Life Council web site, at *http://www.childlife.org*.

From Rode, D., Capitulo, K. L., Fishman, M., & Holden, G. (1998). The therapeutic use of technology. *American Journal of Nursing, 98*(12), 33–35.

resolution, which can include feelings that the individuals involved express toward one another. Closure is particularly important for a child who has experienced a lengthy hospitalization. Closure of the hospital experience gives the child permission to move on in the process of adaptation—to return to usual family and other relationships while retaining the esteem of the people left behind in the healthcare setting. A simple closure device is saying to the child, "You have done it! You have been here with people you didn't know, and you had things done to you that hurt, but you did it! Now you get to go home. You helped us help you. Thank you!"

NURSES' SELF-CARE

Working with children and adolescents with mental disorders and their families is emotionally draining. The very idea of children having such severe mental problems is appalling to some and frightening to others. Nurses are no different than other people. They come from backgrounds and upbringings that range from optimal to destructive. They carry with them many messages that were handed to them when they were young. They may see themselves in the youths with whom they work.

Nurses may find the care of ill or disabled children in a hospital or healthcare setting particularly difficult and emotionally draining. There are times of helplessness: The child's physical pain continues, the disability cannot be reversed, the disease progress cannot be arrested, or death is an approaching reality. Anger is a natural expression of helplessness. How and where the nurse directs anger is important.

To care for themselves, nurses need to recognize and discuss the stressors they face as part of their job. They need to acknowledge and deal with the issues that remind them of their own childhood and adolescence. And, just as important, they need to take excellent care of their physical and mental health. Proper nutrition, rest and sleep, exercise, healthcare, maturity, and balance in personal and professional lives will maximize the energy available to work therapeutically with youth and their families. Furthermore, in the clinical setting, nurses must consider whether their expectations are realistic for the child or adolescent and his or her family and what the nurse can accomplish realistically.

The concept of hardiness may play an important role in preventing caregiver burnout. Nurses can assess their own hardiness and determine ways to increase it. To establish a sense of control and minimize the effects of uncertainty, the nurse needs adequate educational preparation and continued mentoring in any nursing situation. Orientation programs that facilitate the development of mentoring relationships are the most advantageous. The importance of a relationship between the novice nurse and a more experienced nurse cannot be overemphasized.

This relationship builds personal hardiness by nurturing competent clinical practice. The verbal and nonverbal support of a mentor can reduce the uncertainty of a situation and increase the novice nurse's sense of mastery.

▼ *Reflection and Critical Thinking Questions*

1. Reread Clinical Example 29–1 and Nursing Care Plan 29-1. Develop a rewards-based program for school performance for Michael.

2. Based on all the information in this chapter, identify what you think is the most pressing mental health issue confronting children and adolescents. Identify ways in which the social environment contributes both positively and negatively to this issue.

3. Discuss how families from various cultural backgrounds approach mental health issues in children and adolescents. Compare and contrast the suicide and depression rates in the United States with those of other countries. Suggest reasons why rates may differ.

▼ CHAPTER SUMMARY

- The effects of child and adolescent mental illness include the increased likelihood of the disorder continuing into later life, feelings of guilt and blame, unmet needs of siblings and other family members, marital stress and conflict, diminished productivity of lives, and direct and indirect costs.

- Factors placing the child or adolescent at risk for development of mental health disorders include biological ones, such as a family history of a mental illness, immature development of the brain, or a brain abnormality; psychological ones, including family problems and dysfunction; and stressors, including poverty, mentally ill or substance-abusing parents, teen parents, abuse, discrimination because of race, creed, or color, chronic parental conflict or divorced parents, and chronic illness or disability.

- Early intervention with children and adolescents at risk can prevent more serious mental disturbance later in life. Child and adolescent mental illness is treated by biological interventions such as psychotropic medication, psychosocial interventions such as therapies, therapeutic approaches designed for each client, school modifications, and community-based services.

- The role of the nurse in child and adolescent mental healthcare is essential. The nurse performs a thorough assessment, including an assessment of family functioning and current problems; a history; and a mental status examination. The nurse also provides medication education, meets the needs of the families, and promotes the rights of children in treatment settings, which includes avoiding seclusion and restraints and providing advocacy.

■ Children and adolescents are affected by many psychiatric illnesses, including ones that are usually first diagnosed during infancy, childhood, or adolescence and ones that, although common in adults, have different manifestations and require different treatment in children and adolescents. The most common from each category include ADHD, conduct disorder, ODD, adjustment disorder, OCD, phobias, social anxiety disorder, GAD, separation anxiety disorder, PTSD, depression, bipolar disorder, autism spectrum disorders, eating disorders, substance abuse, trichotillomania, and tic disorders.

■ Nursing care of the child with ADHD focuses on the family as a whole and involves educating them about treatment and behavioral strategies, helping the family cope, managing developmental and academic issues, teaching social skills, and improving self-esteem.

▼ R E V I E W   Q U E S T I O N S

1. Which of the following statements accurately reflects Erikson's theory of child development?
    a. Children move through four broad steps of cognitive development.
    b. A balance between too little or too much gratification of the child's sexual and aggressive drives results in a well-adjusted child.
    c. Successful development consists of mastering the skills and attitudes of successive developmental stages.
    d. Children acquire culturally relevant skills through cooperative dialogue with mature members of society.

2. Divorce affects children and adolescents in many ways. Which of the following factors affecting the child describes why divorce has such a powerful effect?
    a. Witnessing parental conflict and wanting to be loyal to both parents
    b. Experiencing a disruption of social activities
    c. Adjusting to new routines imposed by the divorce
    d. Having to cope with normal developmental issues as well as the divorce

3. Which of the following factors has been shown to have the strongest buffering effect on childhood stress?
    a. Strong social and family support
    b. High economic status
    c. Good educational systems
    d. Good physical health

4. A 6-year-old girl was hospitalized for a bowel obstruction. After discharge to home, the child exhibited a flat affect, had nightmares, and began wetting the bed. These symptoms suggest which of the following psychiatric problems?

    a. Conduct disorder
    b. Adjustment disorder
    c. Dysthymia
    d. Generalized anxiety disorder

5. The parents of a child newly diagnosed with ADHD relate that their son cannot focus on school activities for more than a minute or two at a time. Which of the following responses by the nurse reflects an accurate comment about treatment?
    a. "We can develop a system of negative consequences for inattentive behavior that will help your son focus on schoolwork."
    b. "A system of rewards will be the most helpful intervention for improving his ability to focus."
    c. "Medication can help improve your son's ability to focus."
    d. "Social skills training can help improve his behavior at school."

6. The nurse is interviewing a family whose youngest child, a 4-year-old boy, has ADHD. The nurse obtains information about the child's behaviors and what strategies the parents are using to manage unwanted behavior. Which of the following other variables should the nurse assess?
    a. Onset of symptoms
    b. Siblings' feelings about their brother
    c. Problems during childbirth
    d. Food and food additives allergies

7. Children with ADHD or other disorders that affect development often require social skills training. Which of the following represents social skills training?
    a. Offering the child a favorite food for "being nice" to other children
    b. Teaching the child how to interpret facial expressions
    c. Putting the child on time-out for "bad behavior"
    d. Withholding television time when the child pushes or hits another child

8. Depression among children and adolescents is often undiagnosed. Which of the following reasons best explains why this may be true?
    a. Teenagers and children often deliberately cover up their true feelings.
    b. Transient depression is a normal part of growing up.
    c. Teenagers and children may be unable to verbally express their feelings and act out instead.
    d. Healthcare providers do not believe childhood depression is real.

9. Substance abuse is a significant problem among adolescents, one that puts them at risk for other mental health disorders, negative life events, and injury. When assessing the adolescent client for signs and

symptoms of substance abuse, the nurse should consider which of the following as a possible indicator of a substance problem?

a. Change in or loss of friends

b. Family history of substance abuse

c. Sleep disturbances and rapid mood swings

d. Avoidance of contact with unfamiliar people

10. What is the *most* important intervention to decrease emotional upset in a child who is in a hospital or healthcare setting?

a. Presence of his or her primary emotional support person

b. Preparation for medical events

c. Age-appropriate and clear communication

d. Availability of play materials

▼REFERENCES AND SELECTED READINGS

*Aber, J. L., & Cicchetti, D. (1984). The social-emotional development of maltreated children: An empirical and theoretical analysis. In H. Fitzgerald, B. Lester, & M. Yogman (Eds.), *Theory and research in behavioral pediatrics* (pp. 123–145). New York: Plenum.

*Altshuler, L. L., Post, R. M., Leverich, G. S., Mikalauskas, K., Rosoff, A., & Ackerman, L. (1995). Antidepressant-induced mania and cycle acceleration: A controversy revisited. *American Journal of Psychiatry, 152*(8), 1130–1138.

American Psychiatric Association. (2000). *Diagnostic and statistical manual of mental disorders* (4th ed., text rev.). Washington, DC: Author.

Anderson, C. A., & Dill, K. E. (2000). Video games and aggressive thoughts, feelings, and behavior in the laboratory and in life. *Journal of Personality and Social Psychology, 78*(4), 772–790.

Arnold, L. E., Aman, M. G., Martin, A., et al. (2000). Assessment in multisite randomized clinical trials (RCTs) of patients with autistic disorder. *Journal of Autism Development, 30,* 99–111.

*Association of Child and Adolescent Psychiatric Nurses. (1999). *On the rights of children in treatment settings: Position paper.* Philadelphia: Author.

*Baker, N. (1996). Psychosocial adaptation of the child, adolescent, and family with physical Ilness. In P. D. Barry (Ed.), *Psychosocial nursing: Care of physically ill patients and their families* (pp. 505–524). Philadelphia: Lippincott Williams & Wilkins.

*Barkley, R. A. (1996). Attention deficit hyperactivity disorder. In E. J. Mash & R. A. Barkley (Eds.), *Childhood psychopathology* (pp. 63–112). New York: Guilford Press.

Barkley, R. A. (1998). *Attention deficit hyperactivity disorder: A handbook for diagnosis and treatment.* New York: Guilford Press.

*Berrios, C. D., & Jacobowitz, W. H. (1998). Therapeutic holding: Outcomes of a pilot study. *Journal of Psychosocial Nursing, 36*(8), 14–18.

*Bronfenbrenner, U. (1995). The bioecological model from a life course perspective: Reflections of a participant observer.

In P. Moen, G. H. Elder, Jr., & K. Luscher (Eds.), *Examining lives in context* (pp. 599–618). Washington, DC: American Psychological Association.

*Bush, C. T. (2000). Cultural competence: Implications of the Surgeon General's Report on Mental Health. *Journal of Child and Adolescent Psychiatric Nursing, 13*(4), 177–178.

*Case, R. (1992). *The mind's staircase.* Hillsdale, NJ: Erlbaum.

*Center for Mental Health Services. (2001). National strategy for suicide prevention (NSSP). [On-line.] Available: www.mentalhealth.org.

Chakrabarti, S., & Fombonne, E. (2001). Pervasive developmental disorders in preschool children. *Journal of the American Medical Association, 285*(24), 3093–3142.

*Cicchetti, D. (1993). Developmental psychopathology: Reactions, reflections, projections. *Developmental Review, 13,* 471–502.

*Cicchetti, D. (1996). Development theory: Lessons from the study of risk and psychopathology. In S. Matthysse & D. Levy (Eds.), *Psychopathology: The evolving science of mental disorder* (pp. 253–284). New York: Cambridge University Press.

*Coyne, I. T. (1995). Parental participation in care: A critical review of the literature. *Journal of Advanced Nursing, 21,* 716–722.

*Dewsbury, D. A. (1992). Comparative psychology and ethology: A reassessment. *American Psychologist, 47,* 209–215.

*Dunst, C. J., Trivette, C. M., & Cross, A. H. (1986). Mediating influences of social support: Personal family and child outcomes. *American Journal of Mental Deficiency, 90,* 403–417.

*Edwards, A. (1999). Attention-deficit hyperactivity disorder. *Advance for Nurse Practitioners, 7*(5), 47–50.

*Elder, J. H. (2001). A follow-up study of beliefs held by parents of children with pervasive developmental delay. *Journal of Child and Adolescent Psychiatric Nursing, 14*(2), 55–60.

*Endacott, R. (1998). Needs of the critically ill child: A review of the literature and report of a modified Delphi study. *Intensive and Critical Care Nursing, 14,* 66–73.

*Enos, S., & Plante, T. (2001). Trichotillomania: An overview and guide to understanding. *Journal of Psychosocial Nursing, 39*(5), 10–18.

*Erikson, E. (1950). *Childhood and society.* New York: Norton.

*Falsafi, N. (2001). Pediatric psychiatric emergencies. *Journal of Child and Adolescent Psychiatric Nursing, 14*(2), 81–88.

*Feinberg, A. G. (2000). Diagnosis and treatment of AD/HD in adults. *Attention,* March/April, 20–22.

*Fleming, J. E., & Offord, D. R. (1990). Epidemiology of childhood depressive disorders: A critical review. *J Am Acad Child Adolesc Psychiatry 29*(4), 571–580.

*Garbarino, J. (1977). The human ecology of child maltreatment: A conceptual model of research. *Journal of Marriage and the Family, 39,* 721–735.

*Garmezy, N. (1985). Stress resistant children: The search for protective factors. In J. Stevenson (Ed.), *Recent research in developmental psychology.* Oxford: Pergamon Press.

*Geller, B., Fox, L. W., Fletcher, M. (1993). Effects of tricyclic antidepressants on switching to mania and on the onset of bipolarity in depressed 6- to 12-year olds. *Journal of the American Academy of Child and Adolescent Psychiatry, 32,* 43–50.

*Harmon, P. L. (2000). One-on-one with Russell Barkley. *Attention,* March/April, 12–14.

*Heath, S. (1996). Childhood cancer—a family crisis: Coping with diagnosis. *British Journal of Nursing, 5,* 790–793.

*Hess, R. D., Holloway, S. D., Dickson, W. P., & Price, G. G. (1984). Maternal variables as predictors of children's school readiness and later achievement in vocabulary and mathematics in 6th grade. *Child Development, 55,* 1902–1912.

*Jacobson, S. W., & Frye, K. F. (1991). Effect of maternal social support on attachment: Experimental evidence. *Child Development, 62,* 572–582.

*Jennings, K. D., Stagg, V., & Connors, R. E. (1991). Social networks and mothers' interactions with their preschool children. *Child Development, 62,* 572–582.

*Kendall, J. (1999, Spring). Sibling accounts of ADHD. *Family Process, 38,* 117–136.

*Klahr, D. (1992). Information processing approaches to cognitive development. In M. H. Bornstein & M. E. Lamb (Eds.), *Developmental psychology: An advanced textbook* (pp. 273–335). Hillsdale, NJ: Erlbaum.

*Klein, D. N., Schwartz, J. E., Rose, S., et al. (2000). Five-year course and outcome of dysthymic disorder: A prospective, naturalistic follow-up study. *American Journal of Psychiatry, 157*(6), 931–939.

*Krueger, M., & Kendall, J. (2001). Descriptions of self: An exploratory study of adolescents with ADHD. In *Journal of Child and Adolescent Psychiatric Nursing, 14*(2), 61–72.

*Kuchta, M. (2001). Depression in pre-teen and adolescent children. *Nursing in Pediatrics,* Spring/Summer, 4–7.

Leckman, J. F., & Cohen, D. J. (1999). *Tourette's syndrome. Tics, obsessions, compulsions:* Developmental psychopathology and clinical care. New York: John Wiley & Sons.

*Mainous, R. O., Mainous, A. G., Martin, C. A., Oler, M. J., & Haney, A. S. (2001). The importance of fulfilling unmet needs of rural and urban adolescents with substance abuse. *Journal of Child and Adolescent Psychiatric Nursing, 14*(1), 32–40.

*Marchant, J. (1996). Review of the literature relating to parent participation in the care of the hospitalised child. *Paediatric Nursing Review, 9*(1), 3–7.

*Martinez, R. J., Grimm, M., & Adamson, M. (1999). From the other side of the door: Patient views of seclusion. *Journal of Psychosocial Nursing, 37*(3), 13–22.

*Melson, G. F., Ladd, G. W., & Hsu, H. (1993). Maternal social support networks, maternal cognitions, and young children's social and cognitive development. *Child Development, 64,* 1401–1417.

*Mohr, W. K. (2001). Bipolar disorder in children. *Journal of Psychosocial Nursing, 39*(3), 12–23.

*Mohr, W. K., & Anderson, J. A. (2001). Faulty assumptions associated with the use of restraints with children. *Journal of Child and Adolescent Psychiatric Nursing, 14*(3), 141–151.

*Mohr, W. K., Mahon, M. M., & Noone, M. J. (1998). A restraint on restraints: The need to reconsider the use of restrictive interventions. *Archives of Psychiatric Nursing, 12*(2), 95–106.

*Mohr, W. K., & Mohr, B. D. (2000). Mechanisms of injury and death proximal to restraint use. *Archives of Psychiatric Nursing, 14*(6), 285–295.

*National Research Council. (1993). *Understanding child abuse and neglect.* Washington, DC: National Academy of Sciences.

*Papolos, D., & Papolos, J. (1999). *The bipolar child.* New York: Broadway Books.

Piacentini, J. (1999). Cognitive behavioral therapy of childhood OCD. *Child and Adolescent Psychiatric Clinics of North America, 8*(3), 599–616.

*Pliszka, S. R., Browne, R. G., Olvera, R. L., & Wynne, S. K. (2000). A double-blind, placebo-controlled study of Adderall and methylphenidate in the treatment of attention-deficit/hyperactivity disorder. *Journal of the American Academy of Child & Adolescent Psychiatry, 39*(5), 619–626.

*Pliszka, S. R., Greenhill, L. L., Crismon, M. L., Sedillo, A., Carlson, C., Conners, K., et al. (2000). The Texas Children's Medication Algorithm Project: Report of the Texas Consensus Conference Panel on medication treatment of childhood attention-deficit hyperactivity disorder. Part I. *Journal of the American Academy of Child and Adolescent Psychiatry, 39*(7), 908–919.

*Post, R. M., & Weiss, S. R. (1998). Sensitization and kindling phenomena in mood, anxiety, and obsessive compulsive disorders. The role of serotonergic mechanisms in illness progression. *Biological Psychiatry, 44,* 193–206.

*Pullen, L. M., Modrcin-McCarthy, M. A., & Graf, E. V. (2000). Adolescent depression: Important facts that matter. *Journal of Child and Adolescent Psychiatric Nursing, 13*(2), 69–75.

*Rode, D., Capitulo, K. L., Fishman, M., & Holden, G. (1998). The therapeutic use of technology. *American Journal of Nursing, 98*(12), 32–35.

Scahill, L., Chappell, P. B., King, R. A., & Leckman, J. F. (2000). Pharmacologic treatment of tic disorders. *Child and Adolescent Psychiatric Nursing Clinics of North America, 9*(1), 99–117.

Scharer, K. (1999). Nurse-parent relationship building in child psychiatric units. *Journal of Child and Adolescent Psychiatric Nursing, 12*(4), 153–167.

*Silva, R. R., Alpert, M., Munoz, D. M., Singh, S., Matzner, F., & Dummit, S. (2000). Stress and vulnerability to posttraumatic stress disorder in children and adolescents. *American Journal of Psychiatry, 157*(8), 1229–1236.

*Sroufe, L. A. (1997). Psychopathology as an outcome of development. *Development and Psychopathology, 9,* 251–268.

St. John Seed, M. (1999). Identification and measurement of maladaptive behaviors in preschool children: Movement toward a preventive model of care. *Journal of Child and Adolescent Psychiatric Nursing, 12*(2), 62–69.

*Stephenson, J. (1995). Sick kids find help in a cyberspace world. *Journal of the American Medical Association, 274*(24), 1899–1901.

*Stroul, B., & Friedman, R. M. (1986). *A system of care for children and youth with severe emotional disturbances* (revised edition). Washington, DC: Georgetown University Child Development Center, CASSP Technical Assistance Center.

*Swann, A. C., Bowden, C. L., Calabrese, J. R., Dilsaver, S. C., & Morris, D. D. (1999). Differential effect of number of previous episodes of affective disorder on response to lithium or divalproex in acute mania. *American Journal of Psychiatry, 156*(8), 1264–1266.

*Teerikangas, O. M., Aronen, E. T., Martin, R., & Huttunen, M. O. (1998). Effects of infant temperament and early intervention on the psychiatric symptoms of adolescents. *Journal of the American Academy of Child and Adolescent Psychiatry, 37*(10), 1070–1076.

*Thompson, P. (1998). Adolescents from families of divorce:

Vulnerability to physiological and psychological disturbances. *Journal of Psychosocial Nursing, 36*(3), 34–39.

*Thompson, R. A. (1995). *Preventing child maltreatment through social support: A critical analysis.* Thousand Oaks, CA: Sage.

*U.S. Department of Health and Human Services. (1999). *Mental health: A report of the surgeon general.* Rockville, MD: U.S. Department of Health and Human Services, Substance Abuse and Mental Health Services Administration, Center for Mental Health Services, National Institutes of Health, National Institute of Mental Health.

*U.S. Department of Health and Human Services. (2001). *Report of the Surgeon General's Conference on Children's Mental Health: A national action agenda.* Rockville, MD: U.S. Department of Health and Human Services, Substance Abuse and Mental Health Services Administration, Center for Mental Health Services, National Institutes of Health, National Institute of Mental Health.

Velosa, J. F., & Riddle, M. A. (2000). Psychopharmacologic treatment of anxiety disorders in children and adolescents. *Child and Adolescent Psychiatric Clinics of North America, 9*(1), 119–133.

*Wagner, B. J. (2000). Attention deficit hyperactivity disorder: Current concepts and underlying mechanisms. *Journal of Child and Adolescent Psychiatric Nursing, 13*(3), 113–124.

*Weinberger, D. R. (2001, March 10). A brain too young for good judgment. *New York Times* [op-ed].

*Wertsch, J. V., & Tulviste, P. (1992). L. S. Vygotsky and contemporary developmental psychology. *Developmental Psychology, 28,* 548–557.

*White, J. H. (2000). The prevention of eating disorders: A review of the research on risk factors with implications for practice. *Journal of Child and Adolescent Psychiatric Nursing, 13*(2), 76–88.

*Zametkin A. J., & Liotta, W. (1998). The neurobiology of attention-deficit/hyperactivity disorder. *Journal of Clinical Psychology, 59*(Suppl. 7), 17–23.

* *Starred references are cited in text.*

For additional information on this chapter, go to *http://connection.lwm.com.*

Need more help? See Chapter 29 of the *Study Guide to Accompany Mohr: Johnson's Psychiatric-Mental Health Nursing,* 5th edition.

TABLE 30-1 ▼ Aging Terminology

DO NOT USE	SUBSTITUTE
Adult day care (similar to child care)	Adult day services (may include needed health care)
Adult diaper (implies being a baby)	Pants, pads, briefs, trade name (product)
Afflicted	Affected by
Aged	Older people
Bed bound (not tied to the bed)	In bed much of the time
Bed sore	Pressure ulcer (area)
Bib	Clothes protector
Cerebral palsied	People with cerebral palsy
Childish, childlike	None (never use)
Convalescent home	Nursing facility (home)
Crazy	Mentally ill (often with a physical cause)
Crippled	Disabled
Deaf and dumb	Hearing and speech impaired
Elderly (implies people age 50–110 all alike)	Older people
First name or familial title (granny)	Only if the family, friend, or by request
Formula (relates to babies)	Nutritional supplement
Frail, fragile (What does this mean?)	Disabled, or description of specific problem
Golden agers	None (never use)
Greedy geezers (odd character)	None (never use)
Handicapped	Disabled
Homebound, shut-in (not tied to the house)	Rarely leaves home
Honey, deary, sweetie, grandpa, grandma	Mr., Ms.
Incompetent	Incapacitated (legal term)
Little old lady (man)	Older woman (man)
Older generation	Older people
Oldsters	Older people
Old-timer's disease (implying Alzheimer's)	None (never use)
Poor	Low income
Rest home	Nursing facility (home)
Role reversal	Role reversal (dependent parent becomes child) does not occur; a mature adult-to-adult relationship.
Senile	None (never use)
Senior	Older adult
Senior moment (implies forgetfulness)	Never use (all ages forget at times)
Sitter (used for babies)	Companion
Suffers (from a disease)	Has a disease
Symptoms or problems due to age	Diagnose symptoms and treat
Victim (of a disease)	None (never use)
Wheelchair bound (not tied to the wheelchair)	Wheelchair user
Young man (lady)—when obviously older	None (never use)

Nurses should be aware of several words and terms not to use when talking with or about or writing about disabled or older people. Many of the *terms are disrespectful and demeaning.* Others have unclear meanings open to various interpretations.

Note: Some words have been contributed by REACH Resource Center on Independent Living, in Fort Worth, Texas.

Adapted from Hogstel, M. O. (1998). *Community resources for older adults: A guide for case managers.* St. Louis: Mosby. Used with permission.

los, 2001). Epidemiological studies since the 1950s have documented a 15% to 25% prevalence rate of serious mental disorders in clients 65 years of age or older. Estimates are that approximately 25% of older adults in the community and more than 50% of those in nursing homes have symptoms of mental illness.

Identifying and treating mental disorders in the older population are especially challenging for nurses. Failure to distinguish disease-related psychiatric symptoms from manifestations of normal aging may blur the understanding of mental functioning in healthy older adults (Abrams et al., 1995). Health professionals cannot treat the mental health problems of older adults when they view the behavior a client exhibits as normal aging. For example, a healthcare professional may find it difficult to determine if a client is experiencing dementia or depression. The distinction is important, however—unlike dementia—depression can be successfully treated. On the other hand, dementia and depression may be misdiagnosed as physical problems because mental and physical illnesses in older people often occur simultaneously. Furthermore, each tends to mimic or exacerbate the symptoms of the other.

Often healthcare professionals tend to focus on physical problems when treating older adults rather than considering mental health issues. Many older people are reluctant to seek assistance, particularly for mental or emotional disorders, because they grew up at a time when people talked about mental problems only in a derogatory manner. The need for self-determination and independence often impedes their willingness to seek care. They may endure problems in an attempt to ensure that they preserve their independence. Those with cognitive disturbances may not be motivated or aware of the need for care.

Approximately 40% to 70% of all nursing home residents have a chronic mental condition. Nursing home staff members frequently are unprepared to deal with the challenging needs of clients with mental illness. Some facilities have used a combined consultation and training program to meet these clients' needs. Although such programs cannot completely replace direct professional intervention, they may help nursing home staff effectively manage behavioral problems (Smith, Mitchell, Buckwalter, & Garand, 1994).

Ageism, Myths, and Prejudices

Sometimes healthcare providers, family members, and older people themselves incorrectly believe that depression, confusion, memory loss, and other mental or emotional problems are simply a normal part of aging. These attitudes prevent older people and their family members from seeking treatment and, unfortunately, some healthcare providers from aggressively diagnosing and treating emotional and behavioral problems. For example, depression is the most common disorder in older adults, but depression is not part of normal aging and can be diagnosed and treated.

Settings for Care

Because of evolving changes in the healthcare delivery system in the United States, essential mental health services are sometimes difficult for clients to locate and finance. Few mental illnesses are being treated in a hospital inpatient setting for several reasons. Some people prefer and can stay at home and receive treatment on an outpatient basis in a physician's office or clinic, especially if they have available supportive family members, friends, or both. Some home health agencies also have psychiatric-mental health nurses on their staffs to provide mental healthcare for clients in their homes on a limited schedule of visits.

Some hospitals and community clinics provide partial hospitalization on a day basis, which Medicare covers. Geriatric psychiatrists, geriatric nurses, and social workers provide diagnosis, medication management, various forms of counseling and therapy, nutrition, and activities. Decreasing coverage for such services by Medicare and Medicare health maintenance organizations, however, has led to decreased availability. Nursing facilities (homes) in some areas have become more aware of the mental health needs of their residents and are employing, either as part-time staff persons or consultants, geriatric psychiatrists, gerontological clinical psychologists, and geropsychiatric or mental health nurses.

Specific Mental Health Disorders

Many mental health disorders are seen across the life span. As clients age, some disorders become more prevalent, and the resulting prognoses are more serious. Distinguishing those disorders that are reversible or at least controllable so that immediate action can be taken is essential to ensure a positive outcome. Table 30-2 shows those conditions that are most prevalent in older adults. It includes the usual onset, identifying symptoms, assessment techniques, treatment options, and prognosis. Although many of these disorders are discussed in other areas of this book (especially Chapters 24 and 28), nurses must understand that the presentation in older adults often differs from that found in the general population. The seriousness of the illness and treatment modalities may differ as well.

Treatment

In the last 5 years, researchers have conducted many studies regarding psychotropic medications for older adults. Findings from such research have resulted in new medications for cognitive disorders, which are used more com-

TABLE 30-2 ▼ Common Psychiatric Disorders in Older Adults

DISORDER	ONSET	SYMPTOMS	ASSESSMENT AND TREATMENT	PROGNOSIS
Delirium	Rapid (from hours to days)	Fluctuating loss of concentration, confusion, disorientation, disturbed sleep, impaired memory and cognition, incoherent speech, good insight when lucid	Score on Mini-Mental Status Examination improves as condition improves. Treatment should address underlying medical condition as indicated.	Reversible
Dementia, Alzheimer's type	Gradual (from months to years)	Confusion, disorientation, labile affect, impaired memory and cognition, disorganized speech and behavior, delusions, poor insight and judgment	Score on Mini-Mental Status Examination decreases over time. Treatment aims at controlling psychosis.	Irreversible: mental condition deteriorates, as does physical condition eventually.
Vascular dementia	Rapid—immediately following vascular incident (eg, cerebrovascular accident and transient ischemic attack)	Confusion, disorientation, labile affect, impaired memory and cognition, delusions, poor insight and judgment	Score on Mini-Mental Status Examination decreases over time. Treatment aims at controlling psychosis. Condition remains the same over time, unless there is an additional vascular incident.	Irreversible: initial improvement is possible with therapeutic intervention, but condition tends to stabilize and becomes irreversible after 3 to 6 months.
Delusions	Fluctuates: can be gradual or rapid	Possible visual or auditory hallucinations, often paranoia, difficulty distinguishing between reality and delusions	Good physical examination is necessary to rule out medical conditions (usually infections). Treatment aims at eliminating the delusions through medication and reality orientation.	Reversible
Depression	Usually gradual, unless there is a sudden personal loss	Sleep disturbance, appetite changes, decreased pleasure in usual activities, feelings of sadness, worthlessness, and guilt	Use of a depression scale is essential, as is assessment of suicidal ideation and lethality. Treatment may include antidepressants, psychotherapy, and various somatic therapies.	Improvement occurs with medication and psychotherapy; somatic therapies also may be needed. Without treatment, deterioration to the point of suicide is a risk.

(continued)

TABLE 30-2 ▼ **Common Psychiatric Disorders in Older Adults (Continued)**

DISORDER	ONSET	SYMPTOMS	ASSESSMENT AND TREATMENT	PROGNOSIS
Anxiety	Usually rapid	Feelings ranging from apprehension, to dread, to panic	Treatments include psychotherapy, antianxiety agents, and biofeedback.	Improvement occurs with treatment but can recur with increased stressors.
Schizophrenia	Usually develops over 6 months; usually first noted in client's early 20s	Delusions, hallucinations, flat affect, disorganized speech and behaviors	Mini-Mental Status Examination is necessary. Treatment includes antipsychotic medication and psychotherapy aimed at adherence to medication regimen.	Remission is possible with adherence to treatment plan.
Mental retardation	Usually present at birth; may be secondary to injury (trauma) or disease (tumor)	Developmental delay, inability to meet learning expectations of age group	Intelligence scale testing and developmental and social history will reveal the diagnosis. Treatment consists of an individualized learning plan focused on meeting capabilities.	Irreversible
Substance abuse (drugs, alcohol, caffeine, tobacco)	May be rapid or gradual	Inability to hold a job or meet obligations, substance use in dangerous situations (driving, caring for children, operating machinery), legal problems related to substance use	Thorough psychosocial assessment, history, and physical examination are needed to rule out emergency and other secondary medical conditions. Treatment includes detoxification, psychotherapy, and medication management.	Remissions are possible with treatment; however, relapses are common. There can be long-term medical consequences of any substance abuse. Suicidal and homicidal ideation is not uncommon during initial treatment.
Elder abuse	May be rapid or gradual	Unexplained bruising, malnutrition, social isolation, and withdrawal	A detailed history and physical examination are necessary, as is a psychosocial assessment. Treatment can include removal of client from residence and appropriate medical and legal interventions.	With quick, appropriate interventions, prognosis is positive. There may be long-term consequences of injuries and malnutrition.

Adapted from Margolis, S. E. (1999). *Mental health disorders and their effect on the older adult.* Unpublished manuscript, Texas Woman's University at Denton.

monly in this population, as well as many dosage alterations of long-established medications. Length and quality of life have improved dramatically as healthcare professionals have integrated research findings into the care that they provide. Nurses need to learn about changing treatments and to advocate the highest level of care for their older clients.

Recognizing the physical changes of aging is important, because these factors play an important role in assessment and treatment. Many factors can cause such changes, including heredity, environment, and chronic medical conditions. There are often overlaps between these changes and concurrent medical processes. A gradual hearing deficit combined with tinnitus can result in not only additional hearing problems but also problems with equilibrium, increasing the potential risk of falling. Visual problems such as cataracts can impair sight to the degree that self-medicating becomes dangerous with potentially fatal consequences. On the cellular level, the regeneration of some cells is decreased, as well as the efficiency of the cells produced. There is a deterioration of highly specialized cells that do not divide, such as skeletal muscle cells and neurons. This process alone can lead to a functional deficit. Entire organ systems experience changes caused by connective tissue alterations that lead to decreased elasticity and thus increased rigidity (Leventhal, 1991).

When combining the previously mentioned concerns with medical issues (eg, diabetes, arthritis, malnutrition), psychosocial concerns (eg, moving, loss of spouse, increased dependence on others), and cognitive changes (eg, Alzheimer's disease and vascular disorders), it is clear that a comprehensive assessment and care plan is imperative for this population. Creative treatment options are essential. This section will discuss assessment, methods of drug administration, polypharmaceutical risks, pharmacokinetics, pharmacodynamics, and medication side effects and adverse reactions.

ASSESSMENT

Obviously a comprehensive assessment is the first thing that the nurse must perform (see Chap. 6). The assessment should include not only a detailed history and physical examination, but also a mental state examination and a review of psychosocial factors, including guardianship and power-of-attorney issues (see Chap. 28). The documentation should include certified copies of all legal papers as well as advance directives and living wills. If the nurse finds a client to be cognitively impaired to the point of being unable to make competent healthcare decisions, the family (or the treating institution if no family is available) must take legal action immediately to ensure appropriate and timely treatment (see Chap. 7).

PSYCHOTROPIC MEDICATIONS

When discussing mental health disorders, treatment options almost always come under the heading of pharmacotherapy and psychotherapy. Some adjunct somatic therapies also are mentioned. Problems arise when prescribed treatments cannot be administered because of physical and cognitive barriers. These barriers can range from inability to swallow secondary to a stroke to the client's refusal to swallow a pill because of a delusional belief that the pill is poison. To stay within the legal and ethical parameters of good care, it is important to anticipate and resolve possible barriers before they inhibit needed care.

Methods of Administration

Routes of medication administration have expanded dramatically over the past several years. Oral medications are available in tablet, capsule, chewable, and liquid forms. Many of these drugs are also available as injections, intravenous solutions, suppositories, drops (eye, ear, nose), sprays, aerosols, ointments, creams, and patches. Which method is best? The answer depends on many factors, including the specific medication ordered and routes of administration available, the client's physical and cognitive abilities, caregiver abilities, and cost of medications.

Many institutionalized older adults have some type of feeding tube. Nurses must use careful consideration if feeding tubes are to be the chosen delivery route. Not all oral medications (such as time-release capsules) may be put in a feeding tube. Also, the distal end of the tube may be in the stomach, duodenum, or jejunum, which would affect the absorption amount and rate. Because of physical impairments (such as hepatic or renal insufficiency) alternate dosing schedules might be required to avoid toxicity (Chernoff, 1999).

The number of physical problems a person has tends to increase with age. The number of physician specialists seeing the client increases. Clinical Example 30-2 illustrates this problem.

▼ Clinical Example 30-2

Graham, 77 years old, experiences an episode of decreased level of consciousness and syncope. After calling emergency services, his frantic wife gathers all his medications, which she takes with her in the ambulance as she accompanies her husband to the emergency department. Upon arrival, the triage nurse empties the sack of medications and discovers the following:

- Lasix, Trental, Clinoril (prescribed by Dr. Abruzzi)
- NPH insulin (prescribed by Dr. Elihu)
- Prozac, Desyrel, Aricept (prescribed by Dr. Perkins)
- Depakote, Dilantin (prescribed by Dr. Neville)
- Zantac, Reglan (prescribed by Dr. Goldberg)
- Aspirin, one-a-day vitamins, Benadryl, and Milk of Magnesia

The nurse approaches the wife and asks what medications Graham had taken prior to fainting. The wife looks bewildered and states that she is unsure because her husband took his own medications. The wife reports that the client has taken vitamins daily for more than 40 years. She also states that for the past several days, he had been complaining of allergies and had been taking aspirin and over-the-counter allergy medications several times a day. He also had complained of stomach problems and had taken at least one full bottle of Milk of Magnesia over the past day.

Situations like the one presented in Clinical Example 30-2 are, unfortunately, becoming daily occurrences at hospitals across the country. There are many frightening facts to consider. One of the first concerns is that this client, who obviously has some type of cognitive impairment (as evidenced by taking Aricept), is taking his own medications. One would guess from the information provided that the client probably also has congestive heart failure (Lasix), hypertension (Trental), some type of arthritic condition (Clinoril), diabetes (NPH insulin), seizure disorder (Depakote, Dilantin), and some type of gastrointestinal disorder (Zantac, Reglan).

What is wrong with the client? Aside from the current medical emergency, which could be several conditions simultaneously, there are many overt concerns. First, five different physicians have written prescription medications. They are all probably specialists in their fields, but do they each know what other medications have been prescribed? Has anyone checked for drug compatibility? Is the client capable of measuring and giving his own insulin? Is the client adhering to his medication regimen? How would the nurse know? Does the client have a history of a bleeding ulcer, stroke, heart attack, or diabetic coma? Are any of the client's physicians aware of his over-the-counter (OTC) medication use?

Polypharmacy

The term for many drugs being used simultaneously in the same client is **polypharmacy** (see Chap. 12). Because many clients have several different medical conditions that require treatment, this seems like a sensible approach. The problems start when there is not one particular physician overseeing all the medications for compatibility and client adherence. When the client adds the use of OTC medications, severe medical repercussions can occur.

Can the nurse do anything about polypharmacy? The nurse is in a position to help resolve the polypharmacy issue and help prevent future problems. The first step is the *all* system. The nurse should request that *all* clients bring in *all* the medications they are taking (including OTC medications) at *all* visits. Health conditions can change often (such as seasonal allergies, trauma from a fall, a spicy meal), and clients buy many OTC medications to relieve temporary conditions. These conditions could influence

other medical conditions. An example would be a client with diabetes taking an OTC medication for nausea and vomiting following a day of spicy foods. The nurse should be concerned about the client's blood sugar and suggest that during this period, the client use a sliding scale to determine an appropriate insulin dosage.

Once the nurse has noted all of the medications, the next step would be to list the medications, the times for administration, the route of administration, and the name and phone number of each physician who ordered medications. He or she also should list OTC medications. Obviously, it is important to have this information documented in the client's chart. It is possibly more important for the client (and family) to have a copy of this list. If Graham in Clinical Example 30-2 had had such a list, it would have been faster for the triage nurse to notify the client's physicians about the medication information. Another important thing to add to this medication card would be a list of medical conditions. In an emergency this could be vital.

Pharmacokinetics and Pharmacodynamics

Pharmacokinetics refers to the metabolism and actions of medications on a person, related to absorption, duration of action, distribution, and excretion. Even if the same medication is given for the same condition to two people of the same age and gender, the absorption, actions, and possible side effects could be very different (Lee, 1996). Even if they were the same age and gender, their weight and relative height could influence metabolism and thus absorption.

Assessment of activity level is also important. Other medical conditions, allergies, and food or alcohol intake could also influence medication effects. An important consideration is client adherence. This alone can make the difference in drug efficacy.

Pharmacodynamics refers to actions of medications on the body. It is important to know what organs and body systems are involved for a particular medication and the implications. For instance, acetaminophen is metabolized (broken down) in the liver. If a person has a hepatic (liver) disorder this might not be the drug of choice. When medications are not metabolized as they are intended to be, the drug could accumulate and cause a toxic or overdosed situation in the body. So, if there is a liver disorder it is important to consider possible alternatives.

For any medication to be effective, it has to bind to appropriate receptor sites. Chapter 12 addresses psychopharmacology in great detail; however, it is important to understand this action in specific reference to the older adult. Because of the prevalence of Alzheimer's disease that results in the dysfunction and loss of cholinergic neurons, this phenomenon is important because of current medication treatments.

Messages travel from the end of one neuron (brain cell) to the start of another neuron. Acetylcholine is released from the presynaptic (first cell) neuron. It travels to specific receptors on the postsynaptic (receiver cell) neuron. In the space between the neurons, called the synapse, the enzyme acetylcholinesterase (AchE) is released and rapidly breaks down the acetylcholine before it can all bind to the receptor sites on the postsynaptic neuron. Acetylcholine is a necessary component of clear thoughts. Without it, confusion and eventually delusions take over thought processes. In Alzheimer's disease, the number of functioning neurons is significantly decreased, and this situation gets worse over the progression of the disease. It is important to keep as much acetylcholine between the neurons as possible. Blocking the production of AchE is not feasible at this time; however, there are drugs that inhibit the AchE and allow the acetylcholine to bind with their receptor sites on the postsynaptic neuron. These medications are called AchE inhibitors and are the cornerstone of current Alzheimer's treatments (Thelan, Urden, Lough, & Stacy, 1998).

Because the need to preserve acetylcholine in the synaptic junction is so important, nurses should be aware of drugs that interfere with this process. One of the most common anticholinergic medications is Benadryl. This medication is now available OTC and is used for allergy reactions and is in many sleep aids. Many people begin to feel dizzy and light-headed, get a dry mouth, and sometimes get confused and disoriented. Imagine an older adult who already has confusion and disorientation secondary to Alzheimer's disease who takes an anticholinergic medication. Physiologically the uptake of acetylcholine has been blocked. Some of the side effects of this process are already evident in the client but are not intensified. What if this client tries to get out of bed alone to get a drink of water because of his dry mouth? Because of the side effect of dizziness, there is an increased risk of falling. Confusion is also worse, so even if the client does not fall, he may be inclined to wander off.

Why are anticholinergic effects so dangerous? Many nursing home clients are given Benadryl to aid in sleep. It is also a common treatment for seasonal allergies. Anticholinergics are often given preoperatively to decrease oral secretions and thus decrease the chance of aspiration. Even if a client does not have Alzheimer's disease, it is a dangerous practice to give anticholinergics routinely to any older adult. The nurse should be aware of the effects of anticholinergics to prevent dangerous situations from occurring.

Like acetylcholine, dopamine is another messenger that travels between neurons. Lack of dopamine results in parkinsonian symptoms such as rigidity and gait disturbance. Medications that inhibit dopamine to reach their receptor sites can increase the risk of falls. In clients with Parkinson's disease, dopamine inhibitors can send the client into a parkinsonian crisis (Thelan, Urden, Lough, & Stacy, 1998). In clinical practice it has been observed that some selective serotonin reuptake inhibitors (SSRIs) inhibit dopamine uptake.

Adverse and Side Effects

All medications have side effects and adverse reactions. Because of polypharmacy in the older adult, it is vital to check on drug compatibility. Even when a medication is not contraindicated secondary to drug interactions or known allergies, it is important to be aware of potential problems. Teaching clients about their medications is a serious responsibility. Besides a medication list, as suggested earlier in this chapter, it might be helpful to devise a medication administration sheet. This plan not only serves as a client reminder about when and what to take, but also because of the check-off format, it allows for supervision of medication adherence. This form, along with the client's current medications, should be brought to all healthcare and hospital visits.

Neuroleptic malignant syndrome (NMS) is a potentially fatal condition that is a reaction to antipsychotic medication use. Although this symptom is rare, it is usually not immediately recognized in the older adult. The antipsychotic could be a new prescription, something that has been taken for days or weeks, or even a medication taken for months or years. NMS is characterized by intense body rigidity and a sudden high temperature not explained by any other disorder (such as an urinary tract infection). It is crucial to stop the antipsychotic medication and transport the client to the hospital immediately for supportive therapy. A delay in hospitalization usually results in death.

ROLE OF THE NURSE

Care of older adults has become a highly sophisticated area of practice. The number of nurses who have focused their practice on the care of older adults has grown enormously. Several hundred nurses every year achieve certification in gerontological nursing from the American Nurses Credentialing Center. There is national certification in psychiatric and mental health nursing and three types of gerontological nursing but none in geropsychiatric nursing. The specialty has advanced rapidly and will continue to grow as the challenges of and demand for specialized nursing of older adults become more apparent.

Nurses need to consider the importance of maintaining their own personal mental and emotional health, especially when caring for clients who have multiple health problems including physical and mental health symptoms. Caring for severely depressed or aggressive clients on a daily basis can be challenging. For protection of self and others when clients are physically aggressive, a decrease in sensory stimulation (eg, noise and light), seclusion to an area of decreased stimulation, and appropriate referral to a geropsychiatric specialist (eg, geriatric psychiatrist, gerontological clinical nurse specialist, or gerontological nurse practitioner) should be considered. For self-protection, the nurse should keep a clean exit path, request assistance from other staff, and maintain a quiet, calm demeanor.

...owledge about mental health ...opulation, experience in caring ...support group for staff in the ...e helpful. If there is no such a sup-...nurses could initiate and plan such ...chnical and support staff members ...uraged to participate in these support g... ...ey have less education and experience in caring ...ts who exhibit difficult behaviors, they often become withdrawn, terminate their employment, or even physically or psychologically abuse their clients. Also, selecting and using personal strategies, such as family visits, activities with friends, and exercise that can reduce stress, help individuals to cope when working conditions become difficult.

PROMOTING MENTAL HEALTH AND WELLNESS IN OLDER ADULTS

In addition to caring for clients with diagnosed mental health problems, nurses in all settings where they have contact with older people must teach and promote activities that will help these clients maintain mental health and wellness. For clients of all ages, mental health and wellness depend greatly on and are interrelated with physical health and wellness. Physical concerns for older adults especially involve the areas of nutrition, activity, and relationships. Older people who eat poorly, are inactive, and have no close family members or friends are more likely to become lonely and depressed, experience more physical and mental health problems, and possibly become suicidal. These areas are discussed in more detail in the following sections. In addition, overall strategies to promote healthy aging are presented in Boxes 30-2 and 30-3.

Nutrition and Fluids

Good nutrition and fluids are essential to physical health. Decreasing calories, fats, salt, and sugar and increasing complex carbohydrates, fresh vegetables, fruits, and calcium-rich foods are basic suggestions. Eating four to five small meals a day is better than eating two or three large meals. Moderation is essential to healthy eating habits. Clients must obtain essential vitamins and minerals from foods. Because of various factors related to aging, including decreased absorption of some substances, most older people probably should take at least one basic multivitamin and mineral supplement.

Some older people are increasing their use of alternative medicines, including large doses of some vitamins. Nurses should caution all clients that excessive doses could be dangerous, and some herbs and other health-

---

BOX 30-2 ▼ Ten Tips for Healthy Aging

1. Eat a balanced diet.
2. Exercise regularly.
3. Get regular checkups.
4. Do not smoke. It is never too late to quit.
5. Practice safety habits at home to prevent falls and fractures. Add grab bars, bath mats, and rails in the bathroom as needed. Always wear your seat belt when traveling by car.
6. Maintain contacts with family and friends, and stay active through work, recreation, and community.
7. Avoid overexposure to the sun and the cold.
8. If you drink, do so in moderation. When you drink, let someone else drive.
9. Keep personal and financial records in order to simplify budgeting and investing. Plan long-term housing and financial needs.
10. Keep a positive attitude toward life. Do things that make you happy.

Adapted from the National Institute on Aging, National Institutes of Health. (n.d.). Rockville, MD: Author.

---

food products could react with prescription medications and cause dangerous adverse effects.

Mental and Physical Activities

Physical activity remains an important aspect of healthy aging throughout the life span. Simple walking is probably best. The nurse may wish to suggest to most clients (unless contraindicated because of other physical factors) that they exercise at least 30 minutes a day, three times a week.

Keeping active mentally is also important. More and more older people are working after retirement, participating in volunteer organizations and activities in the community and being actively involved in church and political groups. A basic recommendation related to muscles and bones as well as mental functioning is "use it or lose it." Multiple sensory stimulations may help clients to maintain and enhance brain function.

Support Systems

The third major criteria for healthy aging is a good support system, which means that the older person needs family members, friends, neighbors, and church or other organizations to provide support and assistance. The person may benefit from a daily telephone call from people who care about them or assistance with transportation for

BOX 30-3 ▼ *Suggestions About Mental Wellness*

Nurses should teach clients as follows:

- Keep active, both mentally and physically. Reduce stress.
- Take as few medicines as possible, but do not stop taking any medication without discussing it with the physician. Discuss the possible need for a vitamin, mineral, and calcium supplement with the physician.
- Ask the physician for a written explanation of the benefits and risks of specific medicines, treatments, and surgery.
- Prepare for all physician's office visits by writing down questions and concerns a few days before

the visit and do not leave until questions have been answered.
- Keep a written record of the dates of physician visits.
- Select physicians and hospitals that have the special services, staff, and equipment to provide quality care to older people, noting that a quality to look for in a physician and nurse is the ability to listen well.
- Be *assertive* in seeking quality healthcare.
- Report poor care to the appropriate person or agency.
- Take responsibility for your own health.
- Do not sign anything that you do not completely understand.

shopping. Family caregivers may also need education about aging and mental health issues as well as participation in a support group.

▼ *Reflection and Critical Thinking Questions*

1. What factors may cause a society to neglect mental health problems in older adults?

2. What factors interfere with accurate mental status assessments of older adult clients?

3. How can nurses become more interested in and committed to the field of geropsychiatric nursing?

▼ CHAPTER SUMMARY

- The age 65 years has arbitrarily become the point at which a person is considered old.

- To be more precise about the relationship between age and needs, the National Institute on Aging has defined chronological categories of the young old (ages 65 to 74 years), the middle old (ages 75 to 84 years), the old old (ages 85 to 94 years), and the elite old (ages 95 and older).

- As more people live longer, there will be a greater diversity of physical and mental health needs for society to recognize.

- Tasks of aging include conserving strength and resources as necessary and adapting to changes and losses that accompany the normal aging process.

- Changes and issues that most older adults confront include retirement, relocation, and bereavement.

- Effective communication with older adults is one of the most important nursing interventions. Nurses will need to use specific techniques for those who have a hearing, visual, or cognitive deficit or display aggres-

sive tendencies as a result of their condition. They also must avoid using any forms of degrading terminology.

- Approximately 25% of older adults in the community and more than 50% of those in nursing homes have symptoms of mental illness. Identifying and treating mental disorders in the older population is challenging, because healthcare providers may confuse signs of normal aging with problems in mental functioning or may misdiagnose physical problems as mental illness.

- Geriatric psychiatrists, geriatric nurses, and social workers can provide diagnoses, medication management, various forms of counseling and therapy, nutrition, and activities for older adults. Medicare and Medicare health maintenance organizations, however, have decreased coverage for such services in recent years.

- Nurses must understand that the presentation of several psychiatric disorders can differ in older adults from findings in the general population. A comprehensive assessment is vital.

- When administering and monitoring psychopharmacotherapy to older adults, nurses must handle issues involving adjustments in the method of administration, polypharmacy, age-related differences in pharmacokinetics and pharmacodynamics, and increased possibility of adverse and side effects.

- Areas of mental health promotion for nurses to address when working with older adults include maintaining adequate nutrition and fluids, engaging in mental and physical activities, and ensuring adequate support systems.

▼ REVIEW QUESTIONS

1. When preparing a class discussion for a group of nursing students on the demographics of the older adult population, which of the following would the nursing instructor include?

a. The fastest growing group of older adults is those 75 to 84 years of age.

b. The majority of older adults live in some type of institutionalized facility.

c. Although aging varies with an individual, it usually occurs at a similar rate for most persons.

d. Availability of Medicare and Social Security are the major determinants for the onset of older age.

2. Which of the following, if stated by an older adult couple in which the husband is to retire in 2 weeks, would alert the nurse to the possibility of future problems?

a. "She's going to do some volunteer work while I help out with some household chores."

b. "We're going to travel and travel all year long to all sorts of foreign and exotic places."

c. "I'm finally going to be able to learn how to play golf like I've wanted all these years."

d. "Even though I get a good pension, we're planning a budget so that we don't overspend."

3. Which of the following would be most appropriate to write in an older client's chart?

a. Client incontinent for four episodes. Adult diaper applied.

b. Formula infusing via NG tube at 80 cc per hour.

c. Client's daughter reports history of hearing impairment.

d. Client demonstrating childish behavior.

4. An 80-year-old woman who wears a hearing aid in her left ear is being admitted to an extended care facility. When obtaining the client's history, which of the following would be most appropriate for the nurse to do?

a. Keep the television on to provide stimulation during the interview.

b. Hug the client as part of the introduction and greeting.

c. Speak calmly but loudly, directing the voice to the client's left ear.

d. Ask one question at a time, allowing the client ample time to answer.

5. Which of the following assessment findings would lead the nurse to suspect that a client is experiencing delirium?

a. Gradual onset of progressive confusion and disorientation

b. Recent history of a cerebrovascular accident

c. Difficulty distinguishing between reality and delusions

d. Incoherent thoughts but good insight when lucid

6. Which of the following older adults would the nurse assess as being at greatest risk for mental health problems?

a. A 72-year-old man with severe degenerative joint disease, who is recently widowed and lives alone

b. A 67-year-old man, who lives with his daughter and volunteers twice a week at a community center

c. A 70-year-old woman, who lives with her 72-year-old husband in an assisted living community

d. A 68-year-old woman with a history of osteoporosis, who lives with her 74-year-old spouse and works part time

7. The nurse is completing the assessment of an 84-year-old client with Alzheimer's type dementia. Which of the following statements by the client's son would alert the nurse to a potential problem?

a. "He has a night-light in his bedroom, and there's one in the hallway on the way to the bathroom."

b. "We make sure that somebody is in the house with him at all times, day or night."

c. "He's been having trouble sleeping over the past week or so, so we're giving him Benadryl."

d. "I've been giving him a liquid nutritional supplement because he's such a poor eater."

8. When evaluating the effectiveness of drug therapy for an older client, which of the following would be most important to address?

a. Activity

b. Adherence

c. Weight

d. Alcohol use

9. A recently widowed 73-year-old woman with a history of hypertension and diabetes has just moved to an assisted living facility. While assessing the client on a home visit, the client states, "I can't eat. I can't sleep. I get up so early in the morning. I don't know how much longer I can live like this." Further assessment reveals that the client has not been taking her antihypertensive medications. Which of the following would the nurse identify as a priority need for this client?

a. Lack of medication compliance

b. Difficulty sleeping

c. Inadequate nutrition

d. Feelings of loss

10. After teaching a class on mental health promotion to a group of older adults, which of the following, if stated by a member of the group, indicates the need for additional teaching?

a. "We should eat a big breakfast and light lunch and dinner."

b. "Taking a multivitamin and mineral supplement is a good thing."

c. "We need to stay active because if we don't use it, we'll lose it."

d. "My wife and I plan to walk for about 1/2 hour, three times a week."

performance fell below the standard of care, the substandard care resulted in injury, the injury was foreseeable, and permanent injury was established. *Rationales for Incorrect Answers:* a. The nurse followed hospital policy for assessments but did not exercise clinical judgment by removing the restraint when evidence of impaired circulation (dusky color) was clear. b. The reasonable person test would not be met. Prudent nurse behavior would dictate removal of the restraint to prevent impaired blood flow to the extremity. c. All five elements must exist for malpractice.

3. **The correct answer is a. As the client's advocate, the nurse is obligated to assess the client's legal capacity when that client is asked to give consent.** *Rationales for Incorrect Answers:* b. The nurse makes sure that the client has the opportunity and power to revoke consent at any time during treatment. c. It is always the primary provider's obligation to obtain consent, not the nurse's. d. Clients should not be persuaded or influenced in any way when seeking consent.

4. **The correct answer is b. The nurse should have told the client that their conversations were not protected as privileged and that the nurse might be required to repeat them in court.** *Rationales for Incorrect Answers:* a. The nurse should not have encouraged the client to reveal incriminating information. Instead, the nurse should have focused on the specific issues that brought the client into psychiatric care. c. All people whose conversations are not privileged by state law are ethically obligated to tell the truth and legally obligated in a court of law. d. The nurse has a duty to report to the authorities certain dangerous or illegal circumstances (e.g., child abuse, threats on the life of another) but is not required to draw out incriminating evidence about other criminal behavior. The nurse's duty is to provide psychiatric mental healthcare.

5. **The correct answer is c. Clients are considered to have emergency admission status when they behave in ways that indicate that they are mentally ill and may be a danger to themselves or others.** *Rationales for Incorrect Answers:* a. A person who refuses psychiatric hospitalization, poses a danger to self or others, is mentally ill, and for whom less drastic measures are unsuitable may be legally remanded to the hospital as an involuntary admission. b. Clients who present themselves at psychiatric facilities and request hospitalization are considered voluntary admissions. The fact that the client did not resist is not the same as presenting herself voluntarily for treatment. d. Urgent admission has clinical (not legal) relevance in medical-surgical healthcare, and is not a term relevant to psychiatric admissions.

6. **The correct answer is c. The concept of autonomy,** or the right to self-determination, conflicts with the concept of paternalism, or the belief that the medical professional knows what is best for the client (overriding or ignoring the client's autonomous wishes). *Rationales for Incorrect Answers:* a, b, and d. The concept of autonomy, or the right to self-determination, conflicts with the concept of paternalism, or the belief that the medical professional knows what is best for the client (i.e., overriding or ignoring the client's autonomous wishes).

7. **The correct answer is d. Fidelity is faithfulness to duties, obligations, and promises. The nurse has a duty to the client to maintain the boundaries of the nurse-client relationship.** *Rationales for Incorrect Answers:* a. Veracity is consistent truthfulness and honesty. While the nurse was truthful in her response, her honesty served the higher concept of fidelity. b. Beneficence is the principle of doing good, not harm. The opinions of the nurse and client may differ about what is good in this situation; in fact, the nurse, who likes the client very much, may regret that she cannot continue the relationship as friends. The nurse's behavior is most explicitly governed by the concept of fidelity, or her faithfulness to her duty to the client to maintain the boundaries of the nurse-client relationship. c. Autonomy is the right to self-determination and is not really an issue in this scenario.

8. **The correct answer is a. Justice refers to equitable healthcare. Although it is often referred to in economic discussions and healthcare, it also applies to the care individual practitioners supply to their clients. The nurse is limiting her involvement with the client, depriving him of his right to her time. This violates the principle of justice.** *Rationales for Incorrect Answers:* b. Veracity refers to truthfulness and is not an issue in this scenario. c. Beneficence is the principle of doing good, not harm. The nurse is not directly harming the client; rather, she is knowingly limiting her time with him. d. Paternalism is the belief by a medical professional that he or she knows what is best for the client (i.e., overriding or ignoring the client's autonomous wishes). This is not an issue in this scenario.

9. **The correct answer is b. The dilemma is whether to tell the truth (veracity) or to make a decision for the client (paternalism).** *Rationales for Incorrect Answers:* a. Justice refers to the equitableness of healthcare and is not an issue in this scenario. c. Beneficence is the principle of doing good not harm. It is certainly a consideration; however, the specific dilemma is whether to tell the client the truth or to decide for the client (paternalism). d. Fidelity is faithfulness to one's duties and obligations. Staff members are behaving with fidelity as they try to meet their obligation to the client in the most ethical way possible.

10. The correct answer is a. Everyday ethics is best described as focusing on interpersonal relationships, respect, and caring; involving unconditional positive regard; and requiring a search for human dignity. *Rationales for Incorrect Answers:* b. Everyday ethics certainly involves maintaining the client's autonomy; however, it also focuses on interpersonal relationships, respect, and caring; involves unconditional positive regard; and requires a search for human dignity. c. Nurses strive for beneficence in their actions; however, paternalism deprives the client of autonomy. Nurse should very carefully and cautiously consider its use. d. To the extent that they are able, nurses advocate for and ensure the just provision of healthcare; however, everyday ethics focuses on interpersonal relationships, respect, and caring; involves unconditional positive regard; and requires a search for human dignity.

CHAPTER 8—WORKING WITH INDIVIDUALS

1. The correct answer is c. When entering into the nurse-client relationship, the nurse believes that the client is capable and competent. *Rationales for Incorrect Answers:* a, b, and d. When entering into the nurse-client relationship, the nurse believes that the client is competent and capable and that, together, they will identify solutions.

2. The correct answer is a. Free association is a technique in which the client unrestrictedly says the first thing that comes to his or her mind in response to something the therapist says. *Rationales for Incorrect Answers:* b. Countertransference refers to a therapist's response to a client because of feelings that the client triggers from the therapist's past. c. Cognitive triad refers to the three areas of negative view: self, world, and future. All issues and problems can be subsumed under one or a combination of these three areas. d. Schema refers to the client's core beliefs or basic rules of life.

3. The correct answer is d. Overgeneralization is a cognitive distortion in which the client feels that his or her choices or activities are always wrong. *Rationales for Incorrect Answers:* a. Catastrophizing is a cognitive distortion in which the client believes that if he or she does something, it will fail or the results will be horrific or terrible. b. All-or-nothing thinking is a cognitive distortion in which the client views things in extremes (e.g., either a complete success or an absolute failure). c. Perfectionism is a cognitive distortion in which the client believes that he or she must do everything perfectly or else will be criticized and viewed as a failure.

4. The correct answer is b. A token economy system is a component of behavioral therapy in which a client receives tokens for performing specific behaviors. The client can exchange these tokens for reinforcers of the client's choice. *Rationales for Incorrect Answers:* a. Choice therapy focuses on the present as the only reality to consider. Looking at the past is fruitless. c. The major concept of rational emotive behavioral therapy (REBT) is that people are disturbed not by things and events, but by their view of those things and events. d. Brief, solution-focused therapy emphasizes identifying past successes and behaviors that are maintaining the problem, which arises from mishandling life's difficulties.

5. The correct answer is d. Milton Erickson's theory is the basis for the goals of the Alliance of the Mentally Ill (AMI). *Rationales for Incorrect Answers:* a. Sigmund Freud is responsible for developing psychoanalysis. b. Abraham Maslow's theory emphasizes the strengths and capabilities of individuals. c. Thomas Szasz believed that when others treat a person as normal, then that person will act in socially acceptable ways.

6. The correct answer is d. Irrational beliefs are dogmatic; expressed as rigid "musts, shoulds, oughts, or have tos"; and lead to negative emotions that interfere with the pursuit and attainment of goals. *Rationales for Incorrect Answers:* a. Rational beliefs are evaluative cognitions that are preferential and expressed as wishes, dislikes, and likes, which may or may not be attained. b. Rational beliefs, not irrational beliefs, can lead to the achievement of goals. c. Rational beliefs, or healthy beliefs, form the foundation of functional behavior.

7. The correct answer is b. The focus of choice therapy is building a more effective present by doing rather than feeling and taking self-responsibility. *Rationales for Incorrect Answers:* a. Psychoanalysis explores the client's conscious and unconscious conflicts and past coping patterns. c. Behavioral therapy uses positive and negative reinforcers to modify behavior. d. Cognitive-behavioral therapy focuses on changing current ways of thinking and behavior and learning new skills.

8. The correct answer is c. Setting the agenda is the first step in the process of solution-focused therapy. Asking the client what would be helpful to know is a general question that sets the agenda and tone for the interaction. *Rationales for Incorrect Answers:* a. Asking about ways the problem is still interfering with the client's life is appropriate once the problem has been identified and the agenda has been set. This question is appropriate when attempting to understand the effects of the problem. b. Asking about when the problem doesn't happen is important once the agenda has been set and the effects of the problem have been identified. This question helps to identify exceptions to the problem. d. Asking about the spouse's interpretation of the effect is appropriate once the problem has been identified and the agenda has been set. This question is appropriate when attempting to understand the effects of the problem.

9. **The correct answer is d. A psychiatric nurse practicing at the basic level is a licensed RN with a baccalaureate degree in nursing and demonstrates clinical skill within the specialty.** *Rationales for Incorrect Answers:* a. The advanced practice nurse functions as a primary mental healthcare provider, practicing autonomously within applicable state laws. b. The advanced practice nurse has the basic knowledge as well as expertise in psychotherapy and psychobiologic interventions. c. The advanced practice nurse can function as an individual therapist.

CHAPTER 9—WORKING WITH GROUPS

1. **The correct answer is b. Members of primary groups have fact-to-face contact, boundaries, norms, and explicit and implicit interdependent roles. The family is an example of a primary group.** *Rationales for Incorrect Answers:* a. Formal, not primary, groups are characterized primarily by their fixed structure and authority. c. Secondary, not primary, groups are large and impersonal. d. Informal groups provide much of a person's education and contribute greatly to his or her cultural values, such as friendship and hobby groups.

2. **The correct answer is b. Group norms influence a group's patterns of interaction and behavioral expectations.** *Rationales for Incorrect Answers:* a. Group norms influence role expectations in the group. c. Group norms develop over time. d. Group norms are connected to sanctions, taboos, or reference power.

3. **The correct answer is c. The autocratic leader exerts significant authority and control over group members and rarely seeks or uses input from the group. Developing and assigning tasks rather than seeking input from the group reflects an autocratic style.** *Rationales for Incorrect Answers:* a. In a laissez-faire style, group members are free to operate as they choose. b. The democratic leader encourages group interaction and participation in group problem solving and decision making. This leader, by developing and assigning tasks for the group, demonstrates an autocratic style. d. The terms "egalitarian" and "democratic" are synonyms. This leadership style is autocratic.

4. **The correct answer is a. Major group roles are categorized as (1) group task roles, (2) group building and maintenance roles, and (3) individual roles. Each category contains various types that operate at one time or another in all groups.** *Rationales for Incorrect Answers:* b. Harmonizer, gatekeeper, and follower are examples of group building and maintenance roles, but are not the major group role categories. c. Aggressor, recognition seeker, and blocker are examples of individual roles, but are not the major group role categories. d. Information-giver, coordinator, and information seeker are examples of group task roles, but are not the major group role categories.

5. **The correct answer is c. Supportive, empathetic relationships and the ability to problem solve in the face of group crisis are characteristics of mature groups.** *Rationales for Incorrect Answers:* a. Uncertainty and dependence on the leader are characteristics of groups in the initial stage. b. Conflict tempered by cooperativeness and willingness to problem solve are characteristics of the working stage. d. This group has regressed in the face of group crisis and is no longer functioning at the mature stage.

6. **The correct answer is c. Providing feedback and offering a safe place to model new behaviors are advantages of a therapeutic group.** *Rationales for Incorrect Answers:* a. Sharing their experiences with their in-laws may help; however, the most therapeutic intervention is to provide feedback and an opportunity to try new behaviors. b. Support from group members at difficult times may help; however, this approach is not likely to have a lasting effect on the client's relationship with her in-laws. d. Confrontation is an important component of group therapy, but it is not indicated at this time. Helping the client work through feelings of shame and develop a more assertive, self-affirming communication style is most therapeutic.

7. **The correct answer is a. Clients in psychotherapeutic groups may have limiting or maladaptive-to-severe emotional disorders. Thus, their ability to benefit from a growth group is limited.** *Rationales for Incorrect Answers:* b. While educational preparation may vary, this is not a factor in differentiating between a psychotherapeutic group and a growth group. c. Members must be able to tolerate a group setting for both psychotherapeutic and growth groups. d. Group members do not become co-therapists in psychotherapeutic groups; however, this is because of the impaired member's capacity to do so, not to the leader's willingness or lack of willingness.

8. **The correct answer is d. Alcoholics Anonymous is an example of a community support group.** *Rationales for Incorrect Answers:* a. Alcoholics Anonymous is not a psychotherapeutic group. b. Alcoholics Anonymous is not a T group. c. Alcoholics Anonymous is not an encounter group.

9. **The correct answer is b. Group therapy should not function as individual therapy. A therapist who allows this to happen does not understand group dynamics and processes as integral to the therapeutic process. The effective group leader must be skilled in techniques and interventions that foster group interaction and that shape group behavior and growth.** *Rationales for Incorrect Answers:* a. Confrontation is an important component of group communication. c. One advantage of groups is that members learn about the functional roles of people in the group and sometimes share the responsibility as the co-therapist. d. Exposure to the problems of others helps each member feel less isolated and alone.

10. The correct answer is a. Topics such as responsibility, mortality, and freedom of choice are examples of existential (involving "existence") factors that operate during group interactions. *Rationales for Incorrect Answers:* b. Expression of deep emotions refers to the therapeutic factor of catharsis. c. Lessening of feelings of isolation refers to the therapeutic factor of universality. d. Bonding and solidarity refers to the therapeutic factor of group cohesion.

CHAPTER 10—WORKING WITH FAMILIES

1. The correct answer is c. The mother's most predominant concern will be what will become of her son after she dies. *Rationales for Incorrect Answers:* a. Although important, her most predominant concern will be what will become of her son after she dies. b. This is not likely to be the primary concern; the welfare of her son with schizophrenia is more important. d. Mrs. Owens has likely confronted and handled the concern about getting the doctor to talk to her after 38 years of managing her son's care. Her predominant concern will be what will become of her son after she dies.

2. The correct answer is a. Family consultation does not involve vocational rehabilitation. It involves helping families deal with their feelings, find focus, and find solutions. *Rationales for Incorrect Answers:* b. Providing information about the illness is a component of family consultation. c. Teaching effective communication is a component of family consultation. d. Helping families problem solve is a component of family consultation.

3. The correct answer is b. Grief is a subjective burden. Subjective burdens are the emotions that families experience in response to a loved one's mental illness. *Rationales for Incorrect Answers:* a. Financial drain is an objective burden. c. Daily hassles are the minor stressors that all people and families encounter in the course of daily living. d. Conflict with the police is an objective burden.

4. The correct answer is d. A nurse calling a client's spouse an enabler and a flawed mental health system are both iatrogenic burdens. Iatrogenic burdens refer to the problems that families encounter when dealing with the mental health system and its practitioners. *Rationales for Incorrect Answers:* a. This is one example of an iatrogenic burden. b. This is one example of an iatrogenic burden. c. Guilt is an example of a subjective burden.

5. The correct answer is d. The average time lapse before members received the correct diagnosis was 10 years. *Rationales for Incorrect Answers:* a, b, and c. The average time lapse before members received the correct diagnosis was 10 years.

6. The correct answer is b. Improved quality of life is the primary goal of family education. *Rationales for Incorrect Answers:* a. Symptom reduction was one goal of family psychoeducation, not family education. c. Increased knowledge about mental illness may accompany family education, but is not a goal of it; improved quality of life and reduced family burden are the goals. d. Improved caregiving skills may accompany family education, but is not a goal of it; improved quality of life and reduced family burden are the goals.

7. The correct answer is d. Family consultation is based on the assumptions that the family dealing with the mental illness of a loved one is healthy and competent, lacks knowledge and skills about how to manage the ill member, and has the client's best interests at heart. *Rationales for Incorrect Answers:* a, b, and c. This is only one component of family consultation.

8. The correct answer is b. In Marsh's study of siblings and offspring, 77% said they had participated in therapy. *Rationales for Incorrect Answers:* a, c, and d. In Marsh's study of siblings and offspring, 77% said they had participated in therapy.

9. The correct answer is d. Historically, the target of violence is a family caregiver. *Rationales for Incorrect Answers:* a. Historically, the target of violence is a family caregiver, not a mental health professional. b. Historically, the target of violence is a family caregiver, not a police officer. c. Historically, the target of violence is a family caregiver, not a stranger.

10. The correct answer is b. The need for clarity is important because family members are under stress, preoccupied, and anxious. Therefore, they may not fully remember everything that is said. *Rationales for Incorrect Answers:* a. The need for clarity is not about language barriers; it is about a family's stress level when a member is in crisis. c. Communication deviance is an outdated concept. Family members of a client in crisis are anxious, preoccupied, and stressed; they may struggle with their own cognitive issues. d. The object of clarity in communication is the client's family, not the consultant.

CHAPTER 11—WORKING WITH SPECIAL ENVIRONMENTS: FORENSIC CLIENTS, CRISIS INTERVENTION, AND THE HOMELESS

1. The correct answer is c. Governmental institutions in a democratic society typically reflect its social and political convictions. *Rationales for Incorrect Answers:* a. The latest developments in healthcare technology are typically not found in forensic institutions.

b. Meeting the treatment needs of the population being served is an unmet challenge in most forensic institutions. d. Forensic institutions do not have a holistic approach to those in their care for multiple economic, social, and political reasons.

2. **The correct answer is a. The increased graying population has resulted in the need for special adaptations to address the health and psychosocial needs of older adults.** *Rationales for Incorrect Answers:* b. The number of minority ethnic offenders is disproportionately high in forensic facilities. c. The number of female offenders has increased, not decreased. d. Although drug abusers represent the majority of clients in forensic facilities, this phenomenon is not new.

3. **The correct answer is d. The nurse's action reflects appropriate self-awareness. She seeks to avoid bringing her own emotional past into the therapeutic relationship.** *Rationales for Incorrect Answers:* a. All psychiatric mental health professionals must demonstrate self-awareness in all settings. Working with clients can be emotionally taxing. The fact that the client reminds this nurse of someone from the past does not mean the nurse cannot work in the forensic milieu. b. The fact that the client reminds the nurse of someone from the past does not mean the nurse needs psychotherapy. c. This issue is not related to boundaries. The nurse has behaved appropriately.

4. **The correct answer is d. Primary prevention is reducing the incidence of a mental health problem. Therefore, participating in a multidisciplinary committee focusing on domestic violence is an example of primary prevention.** *Rationales for Incorrect Answers:* a. Tertiary prevention is reducing the residual effects of a mental health problem by preventing complications or by promoting rehabilitation. Therefore, conducting a relapse prevention program for sexual offenders is an example of tertiary prevention. b. Secondary prevention is reducing the prevalence of a mental health problem by shortening its duration. Therefore, applying principles of crisis management following a suicide attempt is an example of secondary prevention. c. Developing a medication management program for an offender with schizophrenia is an example of secondary prevention.

5. **The correct answer is a. Factors contributing to the significantly higher rate of suicide in the forensic population include history of a psychiatric illness, difficulties facing the crime, and actual or perceived victimization by other offenders.** *Rationales for Incorrect Answers:* b. An associated risk factor is the inability to cope within a confined environment, not the ability to do so. c. An associated risk factor is the lack of communication with family members, not open communication with them. d. Factors contributing to the significantly higher rate of suicide include history of a psychiatric illness, difficulties facing the crime and actual or perceived victimization by other offenders. Other factors include substance abuse, inability to cope within a confined environment, and lack of communication with family.

6. **The correct answer is a. Increased anxiety level (from baseline) characterizes the first phase of the crisis.** *Rationales for Incorrect Answers:* b. A person in crisis tries to use problem-solving and coping techniques in the first phase of a crisis; however, if they are effective, then there is no crisis. c. Reaching out for help characterizes the third phase of a crisis. d. Short attention span and rumination characterize the fourth phase of a crisis.

7. **The correct answer is c. Resolution of the immediate problem and reestablishment of pre-crisis level of functioning are the goals of crisis intervention.** *Rationales for Incorrect Answers:* a. Resolution of long-term problems may be a benefit of the crisis intervention; however, it is not the goal. b. Gaining insight into past problems may be a benefit of the crisis intervention; however, it is not the goal. d. Resolving the crisis is a goal; however, resolving a crisis within 24 hours may be unrealistic.

8. **The correct answer is b. Maturational crises are part of normal development.** *Rationales for Incorrect Answers:* a. Situational crises are precipitated by sudden traumatic events. c. A crisis of values is not a crisis defined in crisis theory. d. A crisis of spirit is not a crisis defined in crisis theory.

9. **The correct answer is a. Amelioration of factors related to the nursing diagnosis will increase the likelihood of positive outcomes. Therefore a decrease in feelings of anxiety will increase the client's ability to think logically and make decisions, thereby resolving the problem of Disturbed Thought Processes.** *Rationales for Incorrect Answers:* b. The client's use of the agreed upon coping (problem solving) strategies is not a goal relative to Disturbed Thought Processes. This would be a goal for Ineffective Coping. c. The client's ability to give a realistic interpretation of the crisis is not as helpful a criterion for evaluation of Disturbed Thought Process related to impaired ability to make decisions as is a reduction in the client's level of anxiety. High levels of anxiety impair thinking ability. d. The client's recognition of personal capabilities is an important goal; however, a decrease in anxiety level must precede this higher level of functioning.

10. **The correct answer is c. An increase in U.S. immigration is not a factor in the number of mentally ill living outside the hospital. The introduction of major tranquilizers, the civil rights movement,**

and the reduction in low-income housing are factors that have influenced the deinstitutionalization of the mentally ill. *Rationales for Incorrect Answers:* a. The introduction of major tranquilizers is a factor in the number of mentally ill living outside the hospital. b. Reduced low-income housing has increased the numbers of mentally ill people living outside the hospital. d. The civil rights movement is a factor in the number of mentally ill living outside the hospital.

11. **The correct answer is b. Families are the fastest growing subpopulation of the homeless.** *Rationales for Incorrect Answers:* a. Veterans are a subpopulation of the homeless, but do not represent the fastest growing group. c. Street youth are a subpopulation of the homeless, but do not represent the fastest growing group. d. The mentally ill are a subpopulation of the homeless, but do not represent the fastest growing group.

12. **The correct answer is d. A higher incidence of schizophrenia, a greater likelihood to have a diagnosis of an addictive disorder, and a higher incidence of major affective disorders are all characteristics of the homeless population.** *Rationales for Incorrect Answers:* a. The homeless population has a greater likelihood to have a diagnosis of an addictive disorder and a higher incidence of major affective disorders, not just a higher incidence of schizophrenia. b. The homeless population has a higher incidence of major affective disorders and schizophrenia, not just a greater likelihood of having an addictive disorder. c. The homeless population has a greater likelihood to have a diagnosis of an addictive disorder and a higher incidence of schizophrenia, not just a higher incidence of major affective disorders.

13. **The correct answer is c. Eligibility criteria, specifically the requirement of a permanent address, are barriers to homeless people seeking services.** *Rationales for Incorrect Answers:* a. Symptoms experienced are not barriers to care. b. Family history of disease is not a barrier to care. d. Length of time being homeless is not a barrier to care.

14. **The correct answer is a. Health problems specific to urban homeless people are related to exposure, high population density, poor ventilation, and dependent positioning.** *Rationales for Incorrect Answers:* b. Inadequate hygiene is not a significant factor contributing to the health issues of the homeless. c. Drug abuse and irregular eating habits contribute to health issues for subpopulations (i.e., drug abusers and clients with diabetes). They are not general factors for the entire population. d. Shelter rules and anonymity do not create health issues.

15. **The correct answer is b. The nurse avoids metaphors and uses short concrete sentences until he** or she understands the client's level of cognitive function. *Rationales for Incorrect Answers:* a. The nurse is sensitive to the client's possible desire of not wanting to be identified with a mental health program. c. Beginning with a discussion of basic needs rather than a discussion of symptoms is best. d. The nurse confronts suicidal ideation directly.

CHAPTER 12— PSYCHOPHARMACOLOGY

1. **The correct answer is b. Drug therapy may affect a client's symptoms in one area as well as the same target receptors in other parts of the body, resulting in dysfunction and discomfort (side effects) in an entirely new area.** *Rationales for Incorrect Answers:* a. Psychoactive medications have a wide strike zone, hitting the specific target area but also affecting everything else around that area to some degree. c. Psychoactive medications have a wide strike zone, hitting the specific target area but also affecting everything else around that area to some degree. d. Drug therapy is inexact. Although beneficial effects are possible, so too are side effects. In addition, factors such as age and use of alternative therapies can influence the drug's action and effect.

2. **The correct answer is b. Refractoriness, also called down regulation, generally occurs when drugs (agonists) continually stimulate cells, which ultimately results in desensitization or diminished effectiveness of the drug with repeated exposure at the same concentrations. Over time, the effectiveness may diminish, resulting in the appearance of symptoms that first necessitated treatment.** *Rationales for Incorrect Answers:* a. Affinity refers to the chemical properties of a drug that make the drug associate with or bind to the receptors. c. Potency is related to the concentration of the drug in plasma. d. Polypharmacy refers to the use of two or more psychotropic drugs, the use of two or more drugs of the same chemical class, or the use of two or more drugs with the same or similar pharmacologic action to treat different conditions.

3. **The correct answer is a. Changing positions slowly is most important when beginning TCA therapy because orthostatic hypotension is possible. In addition, the client may experience anticholinergic side effects such as blurred vision, dizziness, and fainting, which increase the risk of falling.** *Rationales for Incorrect Answers:* b. The clinical effectiveness of TCAs (i.e., mood elevation) usually takes 2 to 6 weeks and thus would not be seen when therapy begins. c. Orthostatic hypotension, not hypertensive crisis, is possible when beginning TCA therapy. Hypertensive crisis is associated with the use of MAOIs and ingestion of foods containing tyramine or the concomitant use of TCAs and MAOIs. d. Constipation,

not diarrhea, is a possible side effect of TCAs. Thus, the client may need a laxative, not an antidiarrheal agent.

4. **The correct answer is c. Because phenelzine (Nardil) is an MAOI, the client must avoid foods with tyramine to prevent hypertensive crisis. Sour cream and guacamole (made from avocados) both contain tyramine. Therefore, the client needs more teaching.** *Rationales for Incorrect Answers:* a. The client is correct. Aged cheeses, such as blue cheese, contain tyramine. b. Salami, like any processed meat, contains tyramine. d. Drinks such as coffee, tea, and caffeinated colas contain tyramine. Orange juice would be an appropriate substitute.

5. **The correct answer is d. Sexual dysfunction, including delayed or impaired orgasm or interference with sexual performance, response, and arousal, is a common complaint of clients, cited as having the greatest effects on adherence to therapy.** *Rationales for Incorrect Answers:* a. Although nausea is a possible bothersome side effect, it is less commonly cited than is sexual dysfunction. b. Although agitation is a possible bothersome side effect, it is less commonly cited than is sexual dysfunction. c. Although drowsiness is a possible bothersome side effect, it is less commonly cited than sexual dysfunction.

6. **The correct answer is a. Because lithium alters sodium transport in nerve and muscle cells, maintaining adequate hydration (such as by not becoming overheated outside) is important to minimize the risk for toxicity.** *Rationales for Incorrect Answers:* b. Frequent evaluations of serum drug levels are necessary to decrease the risk of toxicity. Early on, levels are obtained two times per week prior to the morning dose of medication. Maintenance therapy requires levels to be checked at least every 2 months. c. Limiting water intake to 2 to 3 glasses per day predisposes the client to possible toxicity. Adequate hydration with approximately 2 to 3 L per day is required. d. Weight gain, not weight loss, is a possible side effect of lithium therapy.

7. **The correct answer is c. A lithium blood level of 1.6 mEq/L is considered mild to moderate toxicity. The nurse would expect assessment findings such as coarse hand tremors, mental confusion, drowsiness, lack of coordination, gastrointestinal upset, and ECG changes.** *Rationales for Incorrect Answers:* a. Ataxia is seen with a lithium blood level ranging from 2.0 to 2.5 mEq/L. b. Stupor is seen with a lithium blood level ranging from 2.0 to 2.5 mEq/L. d. Slurred speech, along with lethargy, muscle weakness, nausea, vomiting, or diarrhea are seen with lithium blood levels above the therapeutic level but less than 1.5 mEq/L.

8. **The correct answer is d. Diazepam (Valium), a benzodiazepine, acts directly on GABA receptors and is thought to increase GABA available, thereby dampening neural overstimulation.** *Rationales for Incorrect Answers:* a. Benzodiazepines, such as diazepam, have no effect on serotonin. b. Benzodiazepines, such as diazepam, have no effect on norepinephrine. c. Benzodiazepines, such as diazepam, have no effect on dopamine.

9. **The correct answer is a. Fine wormlike movements of the tongue may be the first sign of tardive dyskinesia (TD).** *Rationales for Incorrect Answers:* b. In akathisia, a movement disorder associated with neuroleptic therapy, the client cannot sit still and is often seen pacing, rocking, marching in place, or crossing and uncrossing the legs. c. Extrapyramidal syndrome refers to a group of acute movement disorders associated with long-term neuroleptic administration. d. Pseudoparkinsonism, a movement disorder associated with neuroleptic therapy, is characterized by rigidity, slowed movements, and tremors.

10. **The correct answer is b. Neuroleptic malignant syndrome is characterized by hyperpyrexia, severe muscle rigidity, altered consciousness, stupor, catatonia, and labile pulse and blood pressure.** *Rationales for Incorrect Answers:* a. Severe muscle rigidity, not flaccidity, is seen with neuroleptic malignant syndrome. c. Labile pulse, not bradycardia, is seen with neuroleptic malignant syndrome. d. Altered level of consciousness, stupor, and catatonia, not hyperalertness, are seen with neuroleptic malignant syndrome.

11. **The correct answer is c. Use of clozapine (Clozaril) requires weekly monitoring of the client's WBC count to assess for agranulocytosis. If the WBC levels decrease significantly from the baseline, the drug should be discontinued.** *Rationales for Incorrect Answers:* a. Clozapine (Clozaril) produces little to no TD, so assessing for this would not be most important. b. Refractory dysrhythmias are associated with the use of haloperidol (Haldol), a high potency typical antipsychotic agent, not clozapine (Clozaril). d. Orthostatic hypotension is associated with the use of numerous agents, including low potency typical antipsychotics such as chlorpromazine (Thorazine) and atypical antipsychotics such as olanzapine (Zyprexa) and quetiapine (Seroquel).

12. **The correct answer is b. If insomnia occurs, the mother should give the last dose of the medication before 6 p.m. to minimize the risk for insomnia. In this way, the medication's peak time has passed, and the time of duration is almost complete by the time the child is ready to go to bed.** *Rationales for Incorrect Answers:* a. The drug should be given 30 minutes before meals, not after meals. Timing with meals, however, would have no effect on the development of insomnia. c. Switching to a sustained release form may or may not improve the child's insomnia. Moreover, the physician would

need to be contacted to order this formulation. d. Insomnia is not a temporary side effect. The best action is to readjust the dosing schedule so that the last dose is given before 6 p.m.

13. **The correct answer is d. When planning medication administration, nurses are responsible for knowing essential information about the prescribed drug prior to administering it. This information includes knowledge about the prescribed dose and maximum dose of the drug that is ordered.** *Rationales for Incorrect Answers:* a. Community and family supports are important information to be collected during assessment. b. The client's perception of the problem is important information to obtain during assessment. c. The client's previous history of psychiatric problems is important information to obtain during assessment.

14. **The correct answer is c. The most frequent reason clients discontinue medication is the adverse side effects, many of which can be debilitating or difficult to manage.** *Rationales for Incorrect Answers:* a. Although the social stigma of long-term illness may contribute to nonadherence, the most frequent reason clients discontinue medication is the adverse side effects, many of which can be debilitating or difficult to manage. b. Although loss of control over life may contribute to nonadherence, the most frequent reason clients discontinue medication is the adverse side effects, many of which can be debilitating or difficult to manage. d. Although fear of addiction may contribute to nonadherence, the most frequent reason clients discontinue medication is the adverse side effects, many of which can be debilitating or difficult to manage.

15. **The correct answer is b. In older adults, kidney function declines, which affects drug absorption and subsequently the pharmacologic action of psychotropic medications.** *Rationales for Incorrect Answers:* a. In older adults, decreased gastrointestinal motility affects drug absorption and subsequently the pharmacologic action of psychotropic medications. c. In older adults, fatty tissue increases, affecting drug absorption and subsequently the pharmacologic action of psychotropic medications. d. In the elderly, decreased plasma protein levels impact drug absorption and subsequently the pharmacologic action of psychotropic medications.

CHAPTER 13—SPIRITUALITY

1. **The correct answer is b. Spirituality is described as a person's experience of or belief in a power apart from his or her own existence (greater than himself or herself).** *Rationales for Incorrect Answers:* a. Religion refers to the outward practice of a spiritual system of beliefs, values, codes of conduct, and rituals. c. Values refer to the ideals or beliefs that a person considers important and that often determine how he or she will act or behave. d. Worship refers to the devotion a person accords to a higher power or deity.

2. **The correct answer is c. According to Richards and Bergin, scholars who are committed to using spiritual strategies in psychotherapy, spiritual interventions are contraindicated specifically for clients who are psychotic or delusional.** *Rationales for Incorrect Answers:* a. Spiritual interventions are appropriate for clients with depression. b. Spiritual interventions are appropriate for clients with self-esteem disturbance. d. Spiritual interventions are appropriate for clients with moderate anxiety.

3. **The correct answer is d. Empirical literature suggests a positive benefit between spirituality and religious beliefs and health. The findings are inconsistent, however, making it difficult to support recommendations for clinical interventions.** *Rationales for Incorrect Answers:* a. A problem associated with research involving spirituality and health is the lack of specific definitions of religious and spiritual activities. b. Lack of consistency in research involving spirituality and health is characteristic, possibly the result of differences in study design, definitions of religious and spiritual variables, and outcome variables. c. Published works on religion and health have been criticized on methodological grounds, with researchers failing to control confounding variables.

4. **The correct answer is b. Spiritual care and health have been linked throughout history. Over the past 2 decades, interest in this area has resurged. Although factors involved are numerous, a heightened awareness of complimentary and alternative healthcare practices is cited as one important reason.** *Rationales for Incorrect Answers:* a. Acknowledgement that medical care is limited, not unlimited, has led to renewed interest in spiritual aspects of healthcare. c. Research suggests that the health benefits of a spiritual life have been cited as a reason for the change in attitudes and philosophies associated with spiritual care. d. Historically, increased scientific and technological advances making medical care more effective have resulted in a drifting apart of religion or spirituality and medicine.

5. **The correct answer is a. The nurse's question is attempting to clarify the client's values. Clarifying values helps uncover what a person believes and what is important to him or her. Doing so helps nurses become more conscious of what clients value and how such values influence attitudes and behaviors in the clinical setting.** *Rationales for Incorrect Answers:* b. Determining the client's rituals would involve questions pertaining to any ceremonies, rites, or acts that the client uses to express his or her devotion to a deity. The nurse would typically focus on

areas such as prayer, worship, or sacramental emblems. c. Assisting the client with meditation would involve the nurse helping the client with a mental exercise that limits thought and attention. All forms of meditation involve isolation from distraction, active focusing, muscle relaxation, release, and surrender of control. d. Bibliotherapy involves the use of literature to help clients gain insight into feelings and behavior (e.g., providing the client with sacred writings to use as a source of comfort, insight, or wisdom).

6. **The correct answer is c. Asking the client about what being ill means is an open-ended question that allows him or her to discuss the illness and provide the nurse with information about personal views and beliefs. In addition, the client can choose the information he or she shares with the nurse.** *Rationales for Incorrect Answers:* a. Asking the client about going to church is a closed-ended question, easily answered with a yes or no and providing little information about spirituality. b. Although asking a client about practicing religion may provide some information about one aspect of the client's spirituality, this type of question is closed ended and offers little information about overall beliefs and views. d. Although asking about participating in rituals may provide some information about one aspect of the client's spirituality, this type of question is closed ended and offers little information about the client's overall beliefs and views.

7. **The correct answer is d. Although a person involved in a 12-step program may use meditation, it is not a significant spiritual intervention associated with such programs.** *Rationales for Incorrect Answers:* a. Bibliotherapy with sacred writings is a significant aspect of 12-step programs. b and c. Repentance and forgiveness are integral parts of 12-step programs, demonstrated in public confessions and recounting of wrongs done.

8. **The correct answer is b. Altruistic service helps reduce client isolation and self-preoccupation.** *Rationales for Incorrect Answers:* a. Bibliotherapy helps clients gain insight into their feelings. c. Bibliotherapy helps clients learn new ways to cope with difficult situations. d. Meditation involves a surrender of control.

9. **The correct answer is a. Fasting on the eve of a holiday is an example of a ritual, or a ceremony, rite, or action that serves to express a person's devotion to a deity.** *Rationales for Incorrect Answers:* b. Providing food for the needy in a soup kitchen is an example of altruistic service. c. Practicing guided imagery is an example of meditation. d. Reading bible stories for insight is an example of bibliotherapy.

10. **The correct answer is c. When a nurse plans to use a spiritual or religious intervention, he or she should always obtain informed consent from the** client and the client's parents when appropriate. **The nurse implements such interventions only when clients have explicitly stated their desire for them.** *Rationales for Incorrect Answers:* a. Suggesting that religious practice is highly and positively linked with better health outcomes represents a departure from the nurse's specialized knowledge or area of expertise. This would be considered an abuse of the nurse's status as a professional. b. The client could view receiving literature about the nurse's own religion as a violation of boundaries. d. Nurses must use spiritual interventions with children and adolescents with caution because of the potential for perceived governmental influence and violation of work setting (church-state) boundaries.

CHAPTER 14—COMPLEMENTARY AND ALTERNATIVE MEDICINE

1. **The correct answer is b. Increasing reimbursement for services is one of the three goals of the National Center for Complementary and Alternative Medicine (NCAAM).** *Rationales for Incorrect Answers:* a. The NCCAM does not promote a single type of alternative medicine. c. The concept that people can be responsible for their own healing is an underlying principle of CAM, but is not a goal of the NCCAM. d. The NCCAM does not advocate decreasing reliance on allopathic medicine.

2. **The correct answer is a. Low personal interactions between physician and client is one reason cited for the growing interest in CAM.** *Rationales for Incorrect Answers:* b. While many herbs are thought to be safe, little research has been done on them. Also, reports that some herbs contain only minute concentrations of the active ingredient or are tainted with chemicals or contaminants call into question the reliability of herbal remedies. c. While poor coordination of traditional healthcare services can be a major problem for healthcare consumers, it has not been singled out as contributing to the interest in CAM. d. While evidence supports the efficacy of some alternative treatments, by no means have most botanicals, natural remedies, and alternative treatments been evaluated.

3. **The correct answer is d. Back and neck problems are cited 42% of the time as reasons for seeking alternative or complementary healthcare.** *Rationales for Incorrect Answers:* a. Depression is not the most cited problem. b. Hypertension is not the most cited problem. c. Irritable bowel syndrome is not the most cited problem.

4. **The correct answer is c. Since herbals cannot be patented, no drug company can exclusively market that product and therefore cannot charge exorbitant prices that partly help them recoup research**

expenses. **Pricing would be determined by competitive forces in the market and would therefore likely be low.** *Rationales for Incorrect Answers:* a. Drug companies may have similar products, or rather, products that treat the same problem, but that is not the reason for their disinterest in conducting expensive research. b. Drug companies spend a great deal of money on research but are more likely to put their money into a product that they can patent. d. On the contrary, there is a very large market for herbal remedies.

5. **The correct answer is a. Homeopathy is based on the concept that illness can be treated with minute quantities of substances that cause the same symptoms.** *Rationales for Incorrect Answers:* b. Chiropractors and osteopaths support the concept that spinal misalignment causes medical illness. c. Many advocates of CAM embrace the concept that pessimistic thought patterns can be reversed to cure illness; however, this concept is not the basis of homeopathy. d. The concept of energy imbalances causing illness is the foundation of both Chinese and Ayurvedic medicine.

6. **The correct answer is c. Concomitant intake of St. John's wort is a concern because of the potential for serotonin syndrome.** *Rationales for Incorrect Answers:* a. Ginseng is not implicated in serotonin syndrome. b. Gingko biloba is not implicated in serotonin syndrome. d. Rosemary is not implicated in serotonin syndrome.

7. **The correct answer is c. Kava-kava has been linked with liver disorders and failure.** *Rationales for Incorrect Answers:* a. Kava-kava has not been linked with pulmonary hypertension. b. Kava-kava has not been linked with bowel obstruction. d. Kava-kava has not been linked with renal failure.

8. **The correct answer is a. SAMe is thought to regulate the actions of serotonin and dopamine and is therefore potentially useful in the treatment of depression.** *Rationales for Incorrect Answers:* b. SAMe has been used to treat depression. c. SAMe is not used to treat phobias. d. SAMe is not used for short-term memory loss.

9. **The correct answer is c. 5-hydroxytryptophan is a precursor to serotonin and may contribute to dangerously high levels of serotonin when combined with an SSRI.** *Rationales for Incorrect Answers:* a. Valerian is a mild sedative and is not implicated in the development of serotonin syndrome. b. Guarana is a stimulant and is not implicated in the development of serotonin syndrome. d. Passion flower is a mild sedative and is not implicated in the development of serotonin syndrome.

10. **The correct answer is b. Herbal remedies and other complementary and alternative medicines have been used for centuries.** *Rationales for Incorrect Answers:* a. The use of CAM therapies is fairly common, not uncommon. c. CAM may be as effective as pharmaceutical drugs; however, sufficient research has not been performed to make such a general statement. d. CAM has governmental backing and funding through the NCCAM.

CHAPTER 15—COMMUNITY MENTAL HEALTH, SUPPORT, AND REHABILITATION

1. **The correct answer is a. Planning activities that will enhance health in the absence of disease is an example of primary prevention.** *Rationales for Incorrect Answers:* b. Secondary prevention focuses on early detection of mental illness; the nurse is helping him plan for how he will use his time after retirement. This will help prevent depression. c. Tertiary prevention focuses on rehabilitation and reduction of residual effects of mental illness. d. Evaluation is a step of the nursing process that occurs after implementation of a plan of care. This action is an intervention.

2. **The correct answer is a. The concept of community mental health represents the change in focus from the individual to the interaction of the individual with his or her community.** *Rationales for Incorrect Answers:* b. Community mental health is not a place where care is delivered; it is a conceptual shift from the individual as a client to the community as a client. c. Community mental health is not just about services available in the community; it is a conceptual shift from the individual as a client to the community as a client. d. Self-help groups are an example of services available to individuals. They are not a definition of the term community mental health.

3. **The correct answer is d. An effective community support system includes both the needs and functioning level of people with serious mental illness and a philosophy of care based on values and guiding principles.** *Rationales for Incorrect Answers:* a and b. An effective community support system includes both the needs and functioning level of people with serious mental illness and a philosophy of care based on values and guiding principles. c. An effective community support system does not use one specific program model; rather, it uses several to best meet the needs of the community.

4. **The correct answer is d. A community support system delivers community-based care through linkages to a network of agencies that provide mental health services, rehabilitation services, and social support services.** *Rationales for Incorrect Answers:* a, b, and c. A community support system delivers community-based care through linkages to a network of agencies that provide mental health services, rehabilitation services, and social support services.

5. **The correct answer is b. The primary focus of a**

community support system is to improve functioning. *Rationales for Incorrect Answers:* a. Elimination of symptoms is a secondary goal. c. Rehabilitation is an example of tertiary prevention; community support systems are involved in all levels of prevention. d. The primary focus of a community support system is to improve functioning.

6. **The correct answer is b. The nurse does not provide individual therapy.** *Rationales for Incorrect Answers:* a. Medication monitoring is an appropriate community-based intervention. c. System advocacy is an appropriate community-based intervention. d. Mental health teaching is an appropriate community-based intervention.

7. **The correct answer is b. Full participation of parents and caregivers in all aspects of their children's services is an important component of children's mental healthcare.** *Rationales for Incorrect Answers:* a. Children's mental healthcare services focus on the least restrictive setting for care. c. The case manager is responsible for ensuring the cost effectiveness of a plan of care. d. A single approach that serves all families equally well is unrealistic.

8. **The correct answer is c. Unfortunately, many psychiatric mental health clients are reinstitutionalized through the legal system into jails.** *Rationales for Incorrect Answers:* a. Reinstitutionalization refers to placement in a confined environment; mental health clinics, by definition, are part of the network of ambulatory community services. b. Fairweather lodges are group homes within the general community. d. Community support programs are networks of services that support the needs of the community; they are not places in which clients are housed.

9. **The correct answer is b. The case manager coordinates the various services that address the needs of a mentally ill client.** *Rationales for Incorrect Answers:* a. Home care nurses provide care in the home and may arrange for some other services; however, the case manager is responsible for the coordination of these services. c. Although client participation in care is crucial, the coordination of a complex system of services is the responsibility of the case manager. d. The social worker may address many diverse needs; however, the case manager is responsible for coordinating all the services the client needs.

10. **The correct answer is d. A group that has at least one commonality among its members is called an aggregate group. It is not an organized group.** *Rationales for Incorrect Answers:* a. A support group is an organized group that meets to provide its members with a place for sharing feelings. b. A self-help group is similar to a support group; it is an organized and self-directed group. c. An advocacy group is a highly organized that works on behalf on vulnerable individuals.

CHAPTER 16—BEHAVIORAL HEALTH HOME CARE

1. **The correct answer is c. Behavioral health home care is more cost effective than inpatient hospitalization, not more expensive.** *Rationales for Incorrect Answers:* a. It is true that behavioral health home care is less threatening and restrictive than hospitalization. b. It is true that behavioral health home care is more comfortable than hospitalization. d. It is true that behavioral health home care can be part of a discharge plan.

2. **The correct answer is b. Homebound means unable to travel outside the home for physical or psychiatric reasons. Therefore, clients with severe depression or paranoia who are psychologically incapable of leaving their homes meet the criterion for homebound status.** *Rationales for Incorrect Answers:* a. Frequent absences from the home for shopping would indicate that the client is not homebound. c. Attending a day treatment program for socialization purposes would indicate that the client is not homebound. d. Driving a car would indicate that the client is not homebound.

3. **The correct answer is d. Former behavioral health home care clients, members of the clergy, and hospital-based psychiatric nurses are all potential referral sources for behavioral health home care.** *Rationales for Incorrect Answers:* a, b, and c. Former behavioral health home care clients, members of the clergy, and hospital-based psychiatric nurses are all potential referral sources for behavioral health home healthcare.

4. **The correct answer is a. Psychiatric and chemical dependency treatments are not accomplished through home visits.** *Rationales for Incorrect Answers:* b. Behavioral aspects of primary care can be accomplished through home visits. c. Cognitive-behavioral programs can be accomplished through home visits. d. Health teaching and wellness can be accomplished through home visits.

5. **The correct answer is d. Home care is one of the most rapidly growing and changing fields in healthcare today.** *Rationales for Incorrect Answers:* a. Home care services are not limited or few in number. On the contrary, many services formerly provided only in inpatient settings are now are offered through home care. b. Clients who live in residential care facilities or group homes are eligible for home care. c. Home care is not an alternative to institutional care.

6. **The correct answer is b. Home care has been delivered in the United States since the 1950s.** *Rationales for Incorrect Answers:* a, c, and d. Home care has been delivered in the United States since the 1950s.

7. **The correct answer is b. Sigmund Freud did not develop models for behavioral health home care programs.** *Rationales for Incorrect Answers:* a. Behavioral health home care programs do supply 24-hour telephone triage and on-site or contracted emergency response teams. c. Behavioral health home care programs do provide scheduled and immediate follow-up in the client's home after discharge from more restrictive levels of care. d. Behavioral health home care programs use quality improvement programs and outcome measurement systems to evaluate clinical effectiveness, clinical and financial outcomes, client/family/caregiver levels of functioning and satisfaction, and resource use.

8. **The correct answer is a. The correct term for a master's-prepared nurse with psychiatric and mental health assessment and intervention skills who is eligible for, or has already received, certification from the American Nurses Association (ANA) as a specialist in adult psychiatric and mental health nursing is a behavioral health clinical nurse specialist.** *Rationales for Incorrect Answers:* b, c, and d. The correct term for a master's-prepared nurse with psychiatric and mental health assessment and intervention skills who is eligible for, or has already received, certification from the American Nurses Association (ANA) as a specialist in adult psychiatric and mental health nursing is a behavioral health clinical nurse specialist.

9. **The correct answer is d. Sexual dysfunction is not an indication for behavioral health home nursing care. It is possible for a certified sex therapist to see a client in the home environment for therapy; however, that is unusual, and such therapy would not typically come under the purview of behavioral home healthcare.** *Rationales for Incorrect Answers:* a. A change in mental health status is an indication for behavioral health home nursing care. b. An emotional crisis is an indication for behavioral health home nursing care. c. A change in the home environment is an indication for behavioral health home nursing care.

10. **The correct answer is c. For home care services to remain focused and cost effective, the nurse begins discharge planning early in the course of home care, ideally during the initial visit.** *Rationales for Incorrect Answers:* a. Ideally, discharge planning begins early in the course of home care. b and d. The provider should initiate discharge planning early in the course of home care.

CHAPTER 17—VIOLENCE WITHIN THE COMMUNITY

1. **The correct answer is d. Attachment behaviors result from the infant's innate behaviors to elicit maternal responses and the ways that parents meet** such attachment-seeking behavior. This level is called *ontogenic*, indicating a view of development as an ongoing interaction between a person's emerging capabilities and the environment's response to them. *Rationales for Incorrect Answers:* a. The macrosystem level includes societal beliefs and cultural norms that foster violence within families and communities. b. The microsystem level includes the formal and informal social structures that make up children's and their family's world: neighborhood, schools, workplaces, churches, and social service agencies. c. The exosystem represents the community level of influences. It includes those institutions and neighborhood contexts to which all people are exposed.

2. **The correct answer is c. One example of an individual risk factor is an aggressive youth's tendency to misread a situation and attribute hostile intent to benign situations.** *Rationales for Incorrect Answers:* a. Using aggression to gain status or acceptance is a manifestation of peer associations and peer status risk factors. In this situation, the child has misread and interpreted the situation as a deliberately hostile act. This is an example of an individual cognitive bias. b. Family risk factors include attachment problems, family stress, and parenting styles. d. Neighborhood risk factors include high levels of transience, family disruption, firearm ownership, drug distribution networks, high rates of school dropout, substance use, and unemployment.

3. **The correct answer is a. A problem-solving program for all students is the intervention most likely to help reduce the use of violence as a strategy for managing conflict.** *Rationales for Incorrect Answers:* b. Hoping to involve in therapy all families of students who have engaged in fighting is unrealistic and would be prohibitively costly. c. Referral of students involved in fighting to the school counselor will help on an individual basis, but a school-wide program dealing with problem-solving skills may be most beneficial in changing the climate of violence and fostering more mature coping strategies. d. Distribution of handouts about youth violence may be a starting point or a component of a larger program, but by itself is unlikely to have great influence.

4. **The correct answer is b. Knowledge deficits and biases of healthcare professionals are factors contributing to the underreporting of intimate partner violence (IPV). Healthcare workers may believe that IPV is a personal matter or that IPV is restricted to particular socioeconomic groups. Also, healthcare providers receive little education or instruction in how to identify and manage clients they suspect of being abused.** *Rationales for Incorrect Answers:* a. Providers can accomplish screening using the two-questions method; therefore, lack of screening tools is not a factor contribut-

ing to the underdetection of IPV. c. When people do not seek treatment after an incident of IPV, providers may fail to detect that incident; however, failure to screen for IPV during routine healthcare assessments or when physically injured men and women present to emergency services with improbable excuses for their injuries contribute more to the problem of underdetection of IPV. d. Although clients may try to conceal the true causes of their injuries, the most significant barrier to detection is healthcare providers' lack of knowledge about IPV and personal biases that make them unwilling to confront the issue.

5. **The correct answer is d. The mother's explanations for the injuries are plausible; however, the nurse should inform the physician that she suspects possible child abuse. The nurse and the physician can assess the situation to obtain more data.** *Rationales for Incorrect Answers:* a. Falling down the steps and off a swing in a 5 year old are not uncommon and do not suggest a neurological problem. b. Reporting the mother for suspected child abuse would be premature. The child's injuries are not that suspicious. The nurse should inform the physician, and they should conduct an assessment sensitive to possible child abuse. c. The mother's explanations for the injuries are plausible; however, the nurse should inform the physician that she suspects possible child abuse. The nurse and the physician can assess the situation to obtain more data.

6. **The correct answer is c. These are signs of physical neglect.** *Rationales for Incorrect Answers:* a. The client's age and weakness may make it difficult for him to care for himself; however, the client's condition suggests neglect of many of his physical needs. b. The client's condition suggests neglect, not abuse. Physical abuse would result in injuries. d. Although the client's physical condition may predispose him to pressure ulcers, the fact that he is unkempt and dehydrated suggests neglect of his physical needs.

7. **The correct answer is a. Once a healthcare professional has detected elder abuse, he or she has a responsibility to report the mistreatment. Each state has its own guidelines for reporting.** *Rationales for Incorrect Answers:* b. Family counseling may be a helpful intervention; however, the law requires healthcare professionals to report the abuse. c. A state protective services worker will meet with the victim and will begin to develop plans for the older adult's care and safety after the abuse has been reported. d. Education may be helpful; however, the healthcare professional must report the abuse to the state so that a protective services worker can meet with the victim and develop plans for the older adult's care and safety.

8. **The correct answer is a. Contrary to widespread** misconceptions, rape by a stranger accounts for only 15% of total rapes. *Rationales for Incorrect Answers:* b, c, and d. Rape by a stranger accounts for only 15% of total rapes.

9. **The correct answer is a. Rape trauma syndrome refers to a two-phase process including an acute disorganization phase and a long-term reorganization phase.** *Rationales for Incorrect Answers:* b. Rape trauma syndrome is not an abnormally severe reaction to sexual assault; it is a process that affects most victims of sexual assault. c. This four-phase process is typically associated with the emotional responses a person with a terminal illness experiences. d. Rape trauma syndrome refers to a two-phase process including an acute disorganization phase and a long-term reorganization phase, not physical injuries.

10. **The correct answer is d. Some clients may appear unaffected emotionally by the trauma; however, this does not mean that they are handling the situation well, that they have an emotional problem, or that they are more concerned about their physical status. This reaction may represent an effort to regain emotional control in the face of a devastating emotional and physical assault.** *Rationales for Incorrect Answers:* a. This does not mean that the client is handling the situation well. This reaction may represent an effort to regain emotional control in the face of a devastating emotional and physical assault. b. This response does not suggest that the client has an emotional problem. It may represent an effort to regain emotional control in the face of a devastating emotional and physical assault. c. This reaction does not mean that the client is more concerned about her physical status. It may represent an effort to regain emotional control in the face of a devastating emotional and physical assault.

CHAPTER 18—THE CLIENT WITH AN ANXIETY DISORDER

1. **The correct answer is b. Anxiety is a sense of psychological distress. It is neither normal nor abnormal in and of itself; its amount and duration in relation to the stressor determine whether the anxiety is normal or abnormal.** *Rationales for Incorrect Answers:* a. The amount and duration of anxiety in relation to the stressor determine whether the anxiety is normal or abnormal. c. Anxiety may cause the fight-or-flight physiological response; however, anxiety is a feeling of psychological distress. d. The amount and duration of anxiety in relation to the stressor determine whether the anxiety is normal or abnormal.

2. **The correct answer is a. Mild anxiety results in a heightened sense of awareness.** *Rationales for Incorrect Answers:* b. Distorted sensory awareness is a fea-

ture of severe anxiety. c. Forgetfulness occurs with moderate or severe anxiety. Mild anxiety tends to improve cognitive function. d. Impaired ability to concentrate is seen as anxiety levels increase. Mild anxiety tends to improve cognitive function.

3. **The correct answer is a. Excessive worry or anxiety lasting more than 6 months is the hallmark feature of GAD.** *Rationales for Incorrect Answers:* b. Flashbacks and feelings of unreality are associated with post-traumatic stress disorder (PTSD). c. Fear of going outdoors is called agoraphobia. d. Repetitive, ritualized behavior is the hallmark feature of obsessive- compulsive disorder (OCD).

4. **The correct answer is b. Clients with social phobia intensely fear being scrutinized by others.** *Rationales for Incorrect Answers:* a. Clients with agoraphobia fear being in public. c. Clients with claustrophobia fear closed spaces. d. Clients with acrophobia fear heights.

5. **The correct answer is d. Benzodiazepines potentiate the effects of alcohol.** *Rationales for Incorrect Answers:* a. Serotonin syndrome is a potential problem for clients taking selective serotonin reuptake inhibitors (SSRIs). b. SSRIs, not benzodiazepines, interact with monoamine oxidase inhibitors (MAOIs). c. Tardive dyskinesia is a potential side effect of neuroleptic drugs.

6. **The correct answer is c. Memory, ability to concentrate, and thinking patterns are cognitive functions.** *Rationales for Incorrect Answers:* a. Affective symptoms relate to mood and are assessed through facial expression, tone of voice, and demeanor. b. Physiologic symptoms are bodily sensations or physical changes in response to an emotional state. d. Behavioral symptoms are actions that indicate anxiety (e.g., pacing, wringing hands).

7. **The correct answer is c. Asking the client nonjudgmental, open-ended questions will promote the client's reflection, which may lead to insight about the worrying.** *Rationales for Incorrect Answers:* a. This comment, although intended to be supportive, may block further discussion because it does not acknowledge the primary problem–the client's worrying. b. Pat reassurances dismiss the client's problem and are a barrier to communication. d. This question challenges the client to defend her thinking, which will indulge her tendency to catastrophize without helping her gain insight into her worrying.

8. **The correct answer is d. Controlled breathing techniques may be very beneficial to this client because they can dampen the sympathetic arousal and correct the hyperventilation that occur during a panic attack. In addition, regular practice may help prevent panic attacks.** *Rationales for Incorrect Answers:* a. Desensitization is used for clients with phobias. b. Nothing in the data provided suggests lifestyle changes. c. Panic attacks usually have no identifiable

trigger. Problem-solving techniques are more beneficial for clients with GAD, who tend to catastrophize about decision-making.

9. **The correct answer is c. Systematic desensitization is an integral part of treatment for clients with specific phobias.** *Rationales for Incorrect Answers:* a. Psychoanalysis is not particularly helpful in overcoming a specific phobia. b. SSRIs may be prescribed, but medication is not the primary form of treatment for clients with specific phobias. d. Problem-solving techniques are more useful for clients with GAD, not specific phobias.

10. **The correct answer is c. Acute stress disorder is characterized by hyperarousal, sensory distortions, nightmares, and flashbacks within 3 months of the event.** *Rationales for Incorrect Answers:* a. PTSD shares the same symptomatlogy as acute stress disorder but occurs about 6 months after the event. b. Anxiety after such a traumatic event is certainly normal; however, without treatment acute stress can worsen into PTSD, depression, or another disorder. Therefore, characterizing these findings as "normal" is unwise, because clients may not seek treatment for "normal" conditions. d. GAD is characterized by extreme worrying without cause that lasts at least 6 months.

CHAPTER 19—THE CLIENT WITH A SOMATOFORM DISORDER

1. **The correct answer is b. Clients with somatization disorder have difficulty expressing their feelings and needs openly; instead, they express these emotions physically in the form of various bodily symptoms.** *Rationales for Incorrect Answers:* a. Clients with somatization disorder often relate an exaggerated and detailed medical history as their bodily sensations and complaints become the major focus of their lives. c. Because symptoms persist though there is usually nothing physically wrong with clients with somatization disorder, they often have a history of going to many different providers without satisfaction. d. Clients with somatization disorder do unconsciously express emotions through physical symptoms.

2. **The correct answer is c. Clients with a factitious disorder consciously and purposefully manipulate symptoms to gain attention. Clients with a somatoform disorder are not consciously aware of what they are doing.** *Rationales for Incorrect Answers:* a. The conscious desire to obtain attention is the basis of factitious, not somatoform, disorder. b. In somatoform disorder, clients are unaware that their symptoms have no physical cause. d. Neither factitious disorder nor somatization disorder responds readily to psychopharmacologic treatment.

3. **The correct answer is b. The calm, unconcerned demeanor of clients with conversion disorder has**

been termed *la belle indifference.* *Rationales for Incorrect Answers:* a, c, and d. The calm, unconcerned demeanor of clients with conversion disorder has been termed *la belle indifference.*

4. **The correct answer is d. Priority interventions when managing the care of the client with a somatoform disorder are developing trust and establishing a therapeutic relationship.** *Rationales for Incorrect Answers:* a. Interventions are not aimed at reducing symptoms per se; they are aimed at helping the client express emotional content verbally rather than physically, which can be accomplished only within the context of a trusting therapeutic relationship. b. Enhancing the client's ability to make connections between emotions and body is an important, even critical goal of treatment; however, the first focus is on establishing a trusting therapeutic relationship. c. While assessing for thoughts of suicide is always important and should be a part of all initial psychiatric evaluations, clients with somatoform disorder do not typically present with suicidal ideation. The first focus is on establishing a trusting therapeutic relationship.

5. **The correct answer is a. Assessing mood in clients with a somatoform disorder is important because clients with somatoform disorders often experience co-morbid depressive illnesses that frequently are undiagnosed and untreated.** *Rationales for Incorrect Answers:* b. It is not known that somatoform disorders result from depression; however, depression often does coexist with somatoform disorder. c. Being depressed does not automatically correlate with suicidal ideation. The reason for assessing mood in clients with a somatoform disorder is that somatoform disorder has been clinically shown to coexist with major depression and other psychiatric disorders. d. It is inaccurate to state that clients with somatoform disorders often have underlying bipolar disorders.

6. **The correct answer is b. Although all the diagnoses may apply in certain circumstances, Ineffective Coping related to unresolved psychological issues as evidenced by inability to express feelings verbally and difficulty establishing trust with others best addresses the underlying causes associated with somatoform disorders.** *Rationales for Incorrect Answers:* a, c, and d. Ineffective Coping related to unresolved psychological issues as evidenced by inability to express feelings verbally and difficulty establishing trust with others best addresses the underlying causes associated with somatoform disorders.

7. **The correct answer is a. Women experience somatoform disorders about 10 times more often than do men.** *Rationales for Incorrect Answers:* b. This statement is inaccurate; women experience somatoform disorders about 10 times more often than men. c. This

statement is inaccurate; somatoform disorders have been shown to have familial links. d. This statement is inaccurate; age of onset for somatoform disorders is adolescence or early to middle adulthood.

8. **The correct answer is a. The plan has been ineffective if the client experiences increased self-esteem from the increased attention received during physician visits. Self-esteem is not built on nor should it depend on external sources of attention. Self-esteem reflects positive self-assessments related to personal accomplishments or other internal variables the person deems important.** *Rationales for Incorrect Answers:* b. Establishing a trusting relationship with the psychotherapist and physician indicates that the plan of care has been effective. c. The client's ability to focus on symptoms less indicates that the plan of care has been effective. d. Increased participation in ADLs indicates that the plan of care has been effective.

9. **The correct answer is c. Ignoring the remark and trying to refocus on a neutral topic are important. It would then be appropriate to begin discussing how the client has been feeling from an emotional, not a physical, standpoint.** *Rationales for Incorrect Answers:* a. This response focuses on Bob's somatizing. The nurse should ignore the remark and try to refocus on a neutral topic. b. This comment is too abrupt and judgmental. It makes the client "wrong" and is a barrier to communication and trust. d. This comment indirectly contradicts the client and invites further discussion about bodily symptoms.

10. **The correct answer is c. Somatoform disorders generally are very difficult to treat, often are intransigent, and always require long-term interventions and management.** *Rationales for Incorrect Answers:* a. Somatoform disorders generally are very difficult to treat, often are intransigent, and always require long-term interventions and management. b. Frequent changes of therapists will completely undermine the plan of care, which is based upon a trusting, long-term, therapeutic relationship. d. Somatoform disorders generally are very difficult to treat, often are intransigent, and always require long-term interventions and management.

CHAPTER 20—THE CLIENT WITH A SEXUAL OR GENDER DISORDER

1. **The correct answer is a. Sexuality is defined as the experience of the sexual self. It is inextricably connected with awareness of the total self. It is not limited to only overtly sexual behaviors and feelings—it is part of every experience.** *Rationales for Incorrect Answers:* b. Desire for sexual activity is a component of, but does not alone define, sexuality. c. How a person defines masculine and feminine sex-

ual roles is a component of, but does not alone define, sexuality. d. How attractive a person feels is a component of, but does not alone define, sexuality.

2. **The correct answer is b. Sexual expression between two consenting adults that is not harmful (physically or psychologically) to either party, does not involve any form of force or coercion, and occurs in private is thought to be within the range of acceptable sexual expression. It is appropriate to ask if both partners consent to the activity and find it pleasurable.** *Rationales for Incorrect Answers:* a. Nurses should be aware of their own values and not impose them on clients seeking help. Calling an activity demeaning is judgmental and may, in fact, be demeaning to the clients. c. It has not been established that this activity harms either party. The nurse should first explore if both partners consent to and find the activity pleasurable. d. Bringing one's own sexual preferences into the conversation is completely inappropriate.

3. **The correct answer is d. Sexual orientation encompasses sexual preference, gender role, and sexual identity.** *Rationales for Incorrect Answers:* a. Heterosexuality, bisexuality, and homosexuality are terms used to describe sexual preferences. b. Sexual expression is not a component of sexual orientation; rather, sexual orientation is a component of sexual expression. c. Cultural mores influence sexual expression; however, sexual orientation refers to sexual preference, gender role, and sexual identity.

4. **The correct answer is c. The most appropriate response is to apologize, leave, and provide privacy.** *Rationales for Incorrect Answers:* a. The need for sexual release is normal and does not cease because a person is ill or incapacitated in some way. Pretending not to notice and continuing with nursing activities is unfair to the client. He is entitled to privacy, and the nurse should provide it. b. The client's behavior is not inappropriate. The nurse should recognize the client's need for privacy, apologize for the invasion, and provide the necessary privacy. The nurse also should convey respect and appreciation for the client's needs and values. d. It is not appropriate for the nurse to suggest other times for this activity unless the client is disoriented and masturbates when others are present.

5. **The correct answer is b. Telling the client his symptoms sound like normal age-related changes and exploring his concerns about his performance both provide facts that may alleviate his concerns and allow the client an opportunity to further discuss any concerns.** *Rationales for Incorrect Answers:* a. The client's symptoms do not suggest erectile dysfunction but are normal age-related changes. c. The nurse should first address the client's symptoms before exploring other issues. d. This response dismisses the client's concerns, even though the statement is technically accurate.

6. **The correct answer is a. Sexual dysfunction disorders include pain during intercourse and disturbances in the sexual response cycle.** *Rationales for Incorrect Answers:* b. Decreased desire and aversion to sexual activity are subtypes of sexual dysfunction, but there are many others as well. Sexual dysfunction disorders include pain during intercourse and disturbances in the sexual response cycle. c. Inability to achieve an orgasm is a subtype of sexual dysfunction, but there are many others as well. Sexual dysfunction disorders include pain during intercourse and disturbances in the sexual response cycle. d. Confusion over gender identification is a gender identity disorder, which is characterized by strong and persistent cross-gender identification accompanied by persistent discomfort with assigned sex. In addition, there must be evidence of clinically significant distress or impaired social, occupational, or other important areas of functioning.

7. **The correct answer is c. The client needs an opportunity to verbalize her feelings surrounding the sexual dysfunction. Beginning with a discussion of her beliefs about her sexuality is appropriate.** *Rationales for Incorrect Answers:* a. This approach minimizes and dismisses the client's concerns. b. It is too soon in the therapeutic discussion to raise this topic. The nurse should begin with general questions and discussion about sexuality. d. This approach cuts off all discussion and makes the client "wrong" for feeling how she does.

8. **The correct answer is c. Self-reports about frequency of orgasm are good indicators of the effectiveness of the treatment plan. Follow-up long after therapy terminates is critical to determining the true effectiveness of the interventions.** *Rationales for Incorrect Answers:* a. This indicator suggests only that the couple has made a cognitive gain. The evaluation should be based on whether the female partner is sufficiently aroused to achieve orgasm. b. This indicator suggests the plan has been effective; however, frequency of orgasm is more conclusive for the purposes of evaluation. d. This indicator suggests the plan has been effective, but a report of increased frequency 6 months after discharge is a more reliable indicator.

9. **The correct answer is d. Paraphilias refer to sexual expressions for at least 6 months that are characterized by intense sexually arousing fantasies, urges, or behaviors generally involving 1) nonhuman objects, 2) suffering or humiliation of oneself or one's partner, or 3) children or other nonconsenting persons.** *Rationales for Incorrect Answers:* a. Sexual behavior with members of one's own sex is homosexual behavior, not a paraphilia. b. Sexual behavior with members of the opposite sex is

AMPHETAMINE-INDUCED DISORDERS

292.89 Amphetamine Intoxication
   Specify if: With Perceptual Disturbances
292.0 Amphetamine Withdrawal
292.81 Amphetamine Intoxication Delirium
292.xx Amphetamine-Induced Psychotic Disorder
   .11 With Delusions[I]
   .12 With Hallucinations[I]
292.84 Amphetamine-Induced Mood Disorder[I, W]
292.89 Amphetamine-Induced Anxiety Disorder[I]
292.89 Amphetamine-Induced Sexual Dysfunction[I]
292.89 Amphetamine-Induced Sleep Disorder[I, W]
292.9 Amphetamine-Related Disorder NOS

Caffeine-Related Disorders

CAFFEINE-INDUCED DISORDERS

305.90 Caffeine Intoxication
292.89 Caffeine-Induced Anxiety Disorder[I]
292.89 Caffeine-Induced Sleep Disorder[I]
292.9 Caffeine-Related Disorder NOS

Cannabis-Related Disorders

CANNABIS USE DISORDERS

304.40 Cannabis Dependence*
305.20 Cannabis Abuse

CANNABIS-INDUCED DISORDERS

292.89 Cannabis Intoxication
   Specify if: With Perceptual Disturbances
292.81 Cannabis Intoxication Delirium
292.xx Cannabis-Induced Psychotic Disorder
   .11 With Delusions[I]
   .12 With Hallucinations[I]
292.89 Cannabis-Induced Anxiety Disorder
292.9 Cannabis-Related Disorder NOS

Cocaine-Related Disorders

COCAINE USE DISORDERS

304.20 Cocaine Dependence*
305.60 Cocaine Abuse

COCAINE-INDUCED DISORDERS

292.89 Cocaine Intoxication
   Specify if: With Perceptual Disturbances
292.0 Cocaine Withdrawal
292.81 Cocaine Intoxication Delirum
292.xx Cocaine-Induced Psychotic Disorder
   .11 With Delusions[I]
   .12 With Hallucinations[I]
292.84 Cocaine-Induced Mood Disorder[I, W]
292.89 Cocaine-Induced Anxiety Disorder[I, W]
292.89 Cocaine-Induced Sexual Dysfunction[I]
292.89 Cocaine-Induced Sleep Disorder[I, W]
292.9 Cocaine-Related Disorder NOS

Hallucinogen-Related Disorders

HALLUCINOGEN-USE DISORDERS

304.50 Hallucinogen Dependence*
305.30 Hallucinogen Abuse

HALLUCINOGEN-INDUCED DISORDERS

292.89 Hallucinogen Intoxication
292.89 Hallucinogen Persisting Perception Disorder (Flashbacks)
292.81 Hallucinogen Intoxication Delirium
292.xx Hallucinogen-Induced Psychotic Disorder
   .11 With Delusions[I]
   .12 With Hallucinations[I]
292.84 Hallucinogen-Induced Mood Disorder[I]
292.89 Hallucinogen-Induced Anxiety Disorder[I]
292.9 Hallucinogen-Related Disorder NOS

Inhalant-Related Disorders

INHALANT USE DISORDERS

304.60 Inhalant Dependence*
305.90 Inhalant Abuse

INHALANT-INDUCED DISORDERS

292.89 Inhalant Intoxication
292.81 Inhalant Intoxication Delirium
292.82 Inhalant-Induced Persisting Dementia
292.xx Inhalant-Induced Psychotic Disorder
   .11 With Delusions[I]
   .12 With Hallucinations[I]
292.84 Inhalant-Induced Mood Disorder[I]
292.89 Inhalant-Induced Anxiety Disorder[I]
292.9 Inhalant-Related Disorder NOS

Nicotine-Related Disorders

NICOTINE USE DISORDER

305.10 Nicotine Dependence*

NICOTINE-INDUCED DISORDER

292.0 Nicotine Withdrawal
292.9 Nicotine-Related Disorder NOS

Opioid-Related Disorders

OPIOID USE DISORDERS

304.00 Opioid Dependence*
305.50 Opioid Abuse

OPIOID-INDUCED DISORDERS

292.89 Opioid Intoxication
   Specify if: With Perceptual Disturbances
292.0 Opioid Withdrawal
292.81 Opioid Intoxication Delirium
292.xx Opioid-Induced Psychotic Disorders
   .11 With Delusions[I]
   .12 With Hallucinations[I]
292.84 Opioid-Induced Mood Disorder[I]
292.89 Opioid-Induced Sexual Dysfunction[I]

292.89 Opioid-Induced Sleep Disorder[I, W]
292.9 Opioid-Related Disorder NOS

Phencyclidine (or Phencyclidine-Like)-Related Disorders

PHENCYCLIDINE USE DISORDERS
304.90 Phencyclidine Dependence*
305.90 Phencyclidine Abuse

PHENCYCLIDINE-INDUCED DISORDERS
292.89 Phencyclidine Intoxication
        Specify if: With Perceptual Disturbances
292.81 Phencyclidine Intoxication Delirium
292.xx Phencyclidine-Induced Psychotic Disorders
    .11 With Delusions[I]
    .12 With Hallucinations[I]
292.84 Phencyclidine-Induced Mood Disorder[I]
292.89 Phencyclidine-Induced Anxiety Disorder[I]
292.9 Phencyclidine-Related Disorder NOS

Sedative-Hypnotic- or Anxiolytic-Related Disorders

SEDATIVE-HYPNOTIC- OR ANXIOLYTIC USE DISORDERS
304.10 Sedative, Hypnotic, or Anxiolytic Dependence*
305.40 Sedative, Hypnotic, or Anxiolytic Abuse

SEDATIVE, HYPNOTIC, OR ANXIOLYTIC-INDUCED DISORDERS
292.89 Sedative, Hypnotic, or Anxiolytic Intoxication
292.0 Sedative, Hypnotic, or Anxiolytic Withdrawal
        Specify if: With Perceptual Disturbances
292.81 Sedative, Hypnotic, or Anxiolytic Intoxication Delirium
292.81 Sedative, Hypnotic, or Anxiolytic Withdrawal Delirium
292.82 Sedative-, Hypnotic-, or Anxiolytic-Induced Persisting Delirium
292.83 Sedative-, Hypnotic-, or Anxiolytic-Induced Persisting Amnestic disorder
292.xx Sedative-, Hypnotic-, or Anxiolytic-Induced Psychotic Disorder
    .11 With Delusions[I, W]
    .12 With Hallucinations[I, W]
292.84 Sedative-, Hypnotic-, or Anxiolytic-Induced Mood Disorder[I, W]
292.89 Sedative-, Hypnotic-, or Anxiolytic-Induced Anxiety Disorder[W]
292.89 Sedative-, Hypnotic-, or Anxiolytic-Induced Sexual Dysfunction[I]
292.89 Sedative-, Hypnotic-, or Anxiolytic-Induced Sleep Disorder[I, W]
292.9 Sedative-, Hypnotic-, or Anxiolytic-Induced Disorder NOS

Polysubstance-Related Disorder

304.80 Polysubstance Dependence*

OTHER (OR UNKNOWN) SUBSTANCE-RELATED DISORDERS

OTHER (OR UNKNOWN) SUBSTANCE USE DISORDERS
304.90 Other (or Unknown) Substance Dependence*
305.90 Other (or Unknown) Substance Abuse

OTHER (OR UNKNOWN) SUBSTANCE-INDUCED DISORDERS
292.89 Other (or Unknown) Substance Intoxication
        Specify if: With Perceptual Disturbances
292.0 Other (or Unknown) Substance Withdrawal
        Specify if: With Perceptual Disturbances
292.81 Other (or Unknown) Substance-Induced Delirium
292.82 Other (or Unknown) Substance-Induced Persisting Dementia
292.83 Other (or Unknown) Substance-Induced Persisting Amnestic Disorder
292.xx Other (or Unknown) Substance-Induced Psychotic Disorder
    .11 With Delusions[I, W]
    .12 With Hallucinations[I, W]
292.84 Other (or Unknown) Substance-Induced Mood Disorder[I, W]
292.89 Other (or Unknown) Substance-Induced Anxiety Disorder[I, W]
292.89 Other (or Unknown) Substance-Induced Sexual Dysfunction[I]
292.89 Other (or Unknown) Substance-Induced Sleep Disorder[I, W]
292.9 Other (or Unknown) Substance-Induced Disorder NOS

SCHIZOPHRENIA AND OTHER PSYCHOTIC DISORDERS

295.xx Schizophrenia
The following Classification of Longitudinal Course applies to all subtypes of Schizophrenia:
    Episodic With Interepisode Residual Symptoms
        (*Specify if:* With Prominent Negative Symptoms)/
    Episodic With No Interepisode Residual Symptoms/
    Continuous
        (*Specify if:* With Prominent Negative Symptoms)
    Single Episode in Partial Remission
        (*Specify if:* With Prominent Negative Symptoms)
    Single Episode in Full Remission
    Other or Unspecified Pattern
    .30 Paranoid Type
    .10 Disorganized Type
    .20 Catatonic Type
    .90 Undifferentiated Type
    .60 Residual Type
295.40 Schizophreniform Disorder
        Specify if: Without Good Prognostic Features/ With Good Prognostic Features

NANDA-Approved Nursing Diagnoses

This list represents the NANDA-approved nursing diagnoses for clinical use and testing.

Activity Intolerance
Activity Intolerance, Risk for
Adjustment, Impaired
Airway Clearance, Ineffective
Allergy Response, Latex
Allergy Response, Risk for Latex
Anxiety
Anxiety, Death
Aspiration, Risk for
Attachment, Risk for Impaired Parent/Infant/Child
Autonomic Dysreflexia
Autonomic Dysreflexia, Risk for
Body Image, Disturbed
Body Temperature, Risk for Imbalanced
Bowel Incontinence
Breastfeeding, Effective
Breastfeeding, Ineffective
Breastfeeding, Interrupted
Breathing Pattern, Ineffective
Cardiac Output, Decreased
Caregiver Role Strain
Caregiver Role Strain, Risk for
Comfort, Impaired
Communication, Impaired Verbal
Conflict, Decisional
Conflict, Parental Role
Confusion, Acute
Confusion, Chronic
Constipation
Constipation, Perceived
Constipation, Risk for
Coping, Ineffective
Coping, Ineffective Community
Coping, Readiness for Enhanced Community
Coping, Defensive
Coping, Compromised Family
Coping, Disabled Family
Coping, Readiness for Enhanced Family
Denial, Ineffective
Dentition, Impaired

Italicized diagnoses are the most recent additions. Copyright © 2001 by the North American Nursing Diagnosis Association.

Development, Risk for Delayed
Diarrhea
Disuse Syndrome, Risk for
Diversional Activity, Deficient
Energy Field, Disturbed
Environmental Interpretation Syndrome, Impaired
Failure to Thrive, Adult
Falls, Risk for
Family Processes: Alcoholism, Dysfunctional
Family Processes: Interrupted
Fatigue
Fear
Fluid Volume, Deficient
Fluid Volume, Excess
Fluid Volume, Risk for Deficient
Fluid Volume, Risk for Imbalanced
Gas Exchange, Impaired
Grieving
Grieving, Anticipatory
Grieving, Dysfunctional
Growth and Development, Delayed
Growth, Risk for Disproportionate
Health Maintenance, Risk for Ineffective
Health-Seeking Behaviors
Home Maintenance, Impaired
Hopelessness
Hyperthermia
Hypothermia
Identity, Disturbed Personal
Incontinence, Functional Urinary
Incontinence, Reflex Urinary
Incontinence, Risk for Urge Urinary
Incontinence, Stress Urinary
Incontinence, Total Urinary
Incontinence, Urge Urinary
Infant Behavior, Disorganized
Infant Behavior, Readiness for Enhanced Organized
Infant Behavior, Risk for Disorganized
Infant Feeding Pattern, Ineffective
Infection, Risk for
Injury, Risk for
Injury, Risk for Perioperative-Positioning
Intracranial, Adaptive Capacity, Decreased
Knowledge, Deficient
Loneliness, Risk for
Memory, Impaired

Mobility, Impaired Bed
Mobility, Impaired Physical
Mobility, Impaired Wheelchair
Nausea
Neglect, Unilateral
Noncompliance
Nutrition: Less Than Body Requirements, Imbalanced
Nutrition: More Than Body Requirements, Imbalanced
Oral Mucous Membrane, Impaired
Pain, Acute
Pain, Chronic
Parenting, Impaired
Parenting, Risk for Imparied
Peripheral Neurovascular Dysfunction, Risk for
Poisoning, Risk for
Post-Trauma Syndrome
Post-Trauma Syndrome, Risk for
Powerlessness
Powerlessness, Risk for
Protection, Ineffective
Rape-Trauma Syndrome
Rape-Trauma Syndrome; Compound Reaction
Rape-Trauma Syndrome; Silent Reaction
Relocation Stress Syndrome
Relocation Stress Syndrome, Risk for
Role Performance, Ineffective
Self-Care Deficit
Self-Care Deficit, Bathing/Hygiene
Self-Care Deficit, Feeding
Self-Care Deficit, Toileting
Self-Esteem, Chronic Low
Self-Esteem, Situational Low
Self-Esteem, Risk for Situational Low
Self-Mutilation
Self-Mutilation, Risk for

Sensory Perception, Disturbed
Sexual Dysfunction
Sexuality Patterns, Ineffective
Skin Integrity, Impaired
Skin Integrity, Risk for Impaired
Sleep Deprivation
Sleep Pattern, Disturbed
Social Interaction, Impaired
Social Isolation
Sorrow, Chronic
Spiritual Distress
Spiritual Distress, Risk for
Spiritual Well-Being, Readiness for Enhanced
Suffocation, Risk for
Suicide, Risk for
Surgical Recovery, Delayed
Swallowing, Impaired
Therapeutic Regimen Management, Effective
Therapeutic Regimen Management, Ineffective
Therapeutic Regimen Management, Ineffective
    Community
Therapeutic Regimen Management, Ineffective Family
Thermoregulation, Ineffective
Thought Processes, Disturbed
Tissue Perfusion, Ineffective
Transfer Ability, Impaired
Trauma, Risk for
Urinary Elimination, Impaired
Urinary Retention
Ventilation, Impaired Spontaneous
Ventilatory Weaning Response, Dysfunctional (DVWR)
Violence, Risk for Other-Directed
Violence, Risk for Self-Directed
Walking, Impaired
Wandering

Canadian Standards of Psychiatric and Mental Health Nursing Practice (2nd ed.)[1]

BELIEFS ABOUT PSYCHIATRIC AND MENTAL HEALTH NURSING

Psychiatric and mental health nursing is a specialized area of nursing that has as its focus the promotion of mental health, the prevention of mental illness, and the care of clients experiencing mental health problems and mental disorders.

The psychiatric and mental health nurse works with clients in a variety of settings, including institutional facility and community settings. Clients may be unique in their vulnerability as, in this area of nursing practice, they can be involved involuntarily and can be committed to an institution under the law. Further, clients may receive treatment against their will. This fact affects the nature of the nurse-client relationship and often raises complex ethical dilemmas.

The centrality of PMHN practice is the therapeutic use of self; nurse-client interactions are purposeful and goal directed. The psychiatric and mental health nurse understands how the psychiatric disease process, the illness experience, the recuperative powers and the perceived degree of mental health are affected by contextual factors. Advances in knowledge (for instance, the current increase in understanding the biological basis of mental disorders, and the sociological determinants of behaviour) require that psychiatric and mental health nurses continually incorporate new research-based findings into their practice. PMH nurses acknowledge a responsibility to promote evidence-based, outcomes-oriented practice to enhance knowledge and skill development within the specialty. PMH nurses also acknowledge a responsibility to personal mental health promotion and maintenance.

PMHN knowledge is based on nursing theory, which is integrated with physical science theory, social science theory and human science theory. PMHN shares with other mental health disciplines a body of knowledge based on theories of human behaviour. As well, "reflection on practice" continues to develop the nurses habitual practices and skills of being truly present to the client situation at hand (Benner et al., 1996, p. 325). In some settings there may be an overlapping of professional roles and/or a sharing of competencies. PMH nurses recognize their accountability to society for both the discrete and shared functions of practice.

STANDARD I: PROVIDES COMPETENT PROFESSIONAL CARE THROUGH THE HELPING ROLE

The helping role is fundamental to all nursing practice. PMH nurses "enter into partnerships with clients, and through the use of the human sciences, and the art of caring, develop helping relationships" (CNA, 1997b, p. 43) and therapeutic alliances with clients. A primary goal of psychiatric and mental health nursing is the promotion of mental health and the prevention or diminution of mental disorder.

The Nurse:

1. Assesses and clarifies the influences of personal beliefs, values and life experiences on the therapeutic relationship.
2. Establishes and maintains a caring goal directed environment.
3. Uses a range of therapeutic communication skills, both verbal and nonverbal, including core communication skills (eg, empathy, listening, observing).
4. Makes distinctions between social and professional relationships.
5. Recognizes the influence of culture and ethnicity on the therapeutic process and negotiates care that is culturally sensitive.
6. Mobilizes resources that increase clients' access to mental health services.
7. Understands and responds to human responses to distress such as: anger, anxiety, fear, grief, helplessness, hopelessness and humour.
8. Guides the client through behavioral, developmental, emotional, or spiritual change while acknowledging and supporting the client's participation, responsibility and choice in own care.
9. Supports the client's sense of resiliency, for example self-esteem, power and hope.
10. Offers supportive and therapeutic care to the client's significant others.

---

[1]Standards Committee of the Canadian Federation of Mental Health Nurses. (1998). *Canadian Standards of Psychiatric Mental Health Nursing Practice* (2nd ed.). Ottawa, Ontario: Canadian Nurses Association.

11. Reflectively critiques therapeutic effectiveness of nurse-client relationships by evaluating client responses to therapeutic processes, and by evaluating personal responses to client. Seeks clinical supervision with ongoing therapeutic skill development.

STANDARD II: PERFORMS/REFINES CLIENT ASSESSMENTS THROUGH THE DIAGNOSTIC AND MONITORING FUNCTION

Effective diagnosis and monitoring is central to the nurse's role and is dependent upon theory, as well as upon understanding the meaning of the health or illness experience from the perspective of the client. This knowledge, integrated with the nurse's conceptual model of nursing practice, provides a framework for processing client data and for developing client-focused plans of care. The nurse makes professional judgements regarding the relevance and importance of this data, and acknowledges the client as a valued and respected partner throughout the decision-making process.

The Nurse:

1. Collaborates with clients to gather holistic assessments through observation, examination, interview, and consultation, while being attentive to issues of confidentiality and pertinent legal statutes.
2. Documents and analyzes baseline data to identify health status, potential for wellness, health care deficits, potential for danger to self and others; alterations in thinking, perceiving, communicating and decision-making abilities; substance abuse and dependency; and history of abuse (emotional, physical, sexual or verbal).
3. Formulates and documents a plan of care in collaboration with the client and with the mental health team, recognizing variability in the client's ability to participate in the process.
4. Refines and extends client assessment information by assessing and documenting significant change in the client's status, and by comparing new data with the baseline assessment and intermediate client goals.
5. Anticipates problems in the futures course of the client's functional status: eg, shifts in mood indicative of change in potential for self-harm; effects of "flashbacks."
6. Determines most appropriate and available therapeutic modality that will potentially best meet client's needs, and assists the client to access these resources.

STANDARD III: ADMINISTERS AND MONITORS THERAPEUTIC INTERVENTIONS

Due to the nature of mental health problems and mental disorders, there are unique practice issues confronting the psychiatric and mental health nurse in administering and monitoring therapeutic interventions. Safety in psychiatric and mental health nursing has unique meaning since many clients are at risk for self-harm and/or self-neglect. Clients may not be mentally competent to participate in decision-making. The PMH nurse needs to be alert to adverse reactions as client's ability to self-report may be impaired. The PMH nurse uses evidence-based and experiential knowledge from nursing, health sciences and related mental health disciplines to both select and tailor nursing interventions. This is accomplished in collaboration with the client to the greatest possible extent.

The Nurse:

1. Assists and educates clients to select choices which will support positive changes in their affect, cognition, behavior and/or relationships (CNA, 1997b, p. 68).
2. Supports clients to draw on own assets and resources for self care and mental health promotion (CNA, 1997b, p. 68).
3. Makes discretionary clinical decisions, using knowledge of client's unique responses and paradigm cases as the basis for the decision, eg, frequency of client contact in the community.
4. Uses appropriate technology to perform safe, effective and efficient nursing intervention (CNA, 1997b, p. 68).
5. Administers medications accurately and safely, monitoring therapeutic responses, reactions, untoward effects, toxicity and potential incompatibilities with other medications or substances.
6. Assesses client responses to deficits in activities of daily living and mobilizes resources in response to client's capabilities.
7. Provides support and assists with protection for clients experiencing difficulty with self protection.
8. Utilizes therapeutic elements of group process.
9. Incorporates knowledge of family dynamics and cultural values and beliefs about families in the provision of care.
10. Collaborates with the client, health care providers and community to access and coordinate resources.

STANDARD IV: EFFECTIVELY MANAGES RAPIDLY CHANGING SITUATIONS

The effective management of rapidly changing situations is essential in critical circumstances which may be termed psychiatric emergencies. These situations include self harm and other assaultive behaviours and rapidly changing mental health states. This domain also includes screening for risk factors and referral related to psychiatric illnesses and social problems, ie, substance abuse, violence/abuse and suicide/homicide (SERPN, 1996, p. 41).

The Nurse:

1. Assesses clients for risk of substance use/abuse, victim violence/abuse, suicide or homicide.
2. Knows resources required to manage potential emergency situations and plans access to these resources.
3. Monitors client safety and utilizes continual assessment to detect early changes in client status, and intervenes in situations of acute agitation.
4. Implements crisis intervention as necessary.
5. Commences critical procedures: in an institutional setting, eg, suicide precautions, emergency restraint, elopement precautions, when necessary; in a community setting, uses appropriate community support systems, eg, police, ambulance services, crisis response resources.
6. Coordinates care to prevent errors and duplication of efforts where rapid response is imperative.
7. Considers the legal and ethical implications of responses to rapidly changing situations; invokes relevant provisions in mental health acts as necessary.
8. Evaluates the effectiveness of the rapid responses and modifies critical plans as necessary.
9. Explores with the client and/or family the precipitates of the emergency event and plans to minimize risk of recurrence.
10. Participates in "debriefing" process with team (including client and family) and other service providers, eg, reviews of critical event and/or emergency situation.
11. Incorporates knowledge of community needs or responses in the provision of care.
12. Encourages and assists clients to seek out support groups for mutual aid and support.
13. Assesses the client's response to, and perception of, nursing and other therapeutic interventions.

STANDARD V: INTERVENES THROUGH THE TEACHING-COACHING FUNCTION

All nurse-client interactions are potentially teaching/learning situations. The PMH nurse attempts to understand the life experience of the client and uses this understanding to support and promote learning related to health and personal development. The nurse provides mental health promotion information to individuals, families, groups, populations, and communities.

The Nurse:

1. In collaboration with the client, determines client's learning needs.
2. Plans and implements, with the client, health education while considering the context of the client's life experiences on readiness to learn. Plans teaching times and strategies accordingly.
3. Provides anticipatory guidance regarding the client's situational needs, eg, assists the client in identifying living, learning or working needs and ways in which to access available community or other resources.
4. Facilitates the client's search for ways to integrate mental illness, chronic illness or improved functioning into lifestyle.
5. Considers a variety of learning models and utilizes clinical judgement when creating opportunities with clients regarding their learning needs.
6. Provides relevant information, guidance and support to the client's significant others within the bounds of any freedom of information legislation.
7. Documents the teaching/learning process (assessment, plan, implementation, client involvement and evaluation).
8. Evaluates and validates with the client the effectiveness of the educational process, and seeks client's input into developing other means of providing teaching opportunities.
9. Engages in learning/teaching opportunities as partners with consumer groups.

STANDARD VI: MONITORS AND ENSURES THE QUALITY OF HEALTH CARE PRACTICES

Clients may be particularly vulnerable as recipients of health care, because of the nature of mental health problems and mental disorders. Mental health care is conducted under the provisions of provincial/territorial Mental Health Acts and related legislation. It is essential for the PMH nurse to be informed regarding the interpretation of relevant legislation and its implications for nursing practice. The nurse has a responsibility to advocate for the client's right to receive the least restrictive form of care and to respect and affirm the client's right to pursue individual goals of equality and justice.

The Nurse:

1. Identifies limitations in the workplace or care setting that interfere with the nurse's ability to perform with skill, safety and compassion and takes appropriate action.
2. Identifies limitations at a community level that interfere with the entire health of the community, eg, poverty, malnutrition, unsafe housing.
3. Expands knowledge of innovations and changes in mental health and psychiatric nursing practice to ensure safe and effective care.
4. Critically evaluates current mental health and psychiatric research findings and uses research findings in practice.
5. Ensures and documents ongoing review and evaluation of psychiatric and mental health nursing care activities.
6. Understands and questions the interdependent functions of the team within the overall plan of care.

7. Advocates for the client within the context of institutional, professional, family and community interests.

8. Follows agency/institutional procedures when dissatisfied with the safety of a treatment plan and/or management interventions of other mental health care providers.

9. Uses sound judgement in advocating for safe, competent and ethical care for clients and colleagues even when there are system barriers to enacting an advocacy function.

10. Maintains and monitors confidentiality of client information.

11. Attends to changes in the mental health services system by recognizing changes that affect practice and client care, and by developing strategies to manage these changes (CNA, 1997b, p. 79).

STANDARD VII: PRACTICES WITHIN ORGANIZATIONAL AND WORK-ROLE STRUCTURES

The PMHN role is assumed within organizational structures, both community and institutional, particular to the provision of health care. In PMHN, the ethic of care is based on thoughtful and wise practice judgements within multiple, complex situations. As mental health care in Canada evolves into community based care, the psychiatric and mental health nurse needs to be skilled in collaborative partnering and decision-making, mental health promotion and community development.

The Nurse:

1. Collaborates in the formulation of mental health promotion, and in activities and overall treatment plans and decisions with the client and treatment team and, throughout the continuum of care (primary, secondary and tertiary).

2. Recognizes and addresses the impact of the dynamic of the treatment team on the therapeutic process.

3. Uses conflict resolution skills to facilitate interdisciplinary health team interactions and functioning.

4. Uses computerized and other mental health and nursing information systems in planning, documenting and evaluating client care.

5. Demonstrates knowledge of collaborative strategies in working with consumer/advocacy groups (SERPN, 1996, p. 50).

6. Actively participates in developing, implementing and critiquing mental health policy in the workplace.

7. Acts as a role model for nursing students and the beginning practitioner in the provision of psychiatric and mental health nursing care.

8. Practices independently within legislated scope of practice.

9. Supports professional efforts in psychiatric and mental health practice to achieve a more mentally healthy society.

The Academy for Guided Imagery
P.O. Box 2070
Mill Valley, CA 94942
(800) 726-2070
FAX: (415) 389-9342
http://www.healthy.net/agi

Academy of Psychosomatic Medicine
5824 North Magnolia
Chicago, IL 60660
(773) 784-2025
FAX: (773) 784-1304
http://www.apm.org/

Action on Smoking and Health (ASH)
2013 H Street, NW
Washington, DC 20006
(202) 659-4310
http://www.ash.org

Administration on Aging
U.S. Department of Health and Human Services
330 Independence Avenue, SW
Washington, DC 20201
(202) 619-0724 or (800) 677-1116
FAX: (202) 260-1012
http://www.aoa.dhhs.gov

Adopt a Special Kid
7700 Edgewater Drive, Suite 320
Oakland, CA 94621
(888) 680-7349
FAX: (510) 553-1747
http://www.adoptaspecialkid.org

Adoption Service Information Agency, Inc.
8555 16th Street, Suite 600
Silver Spring, MD
(301) 587-7068
FAX: (301) 587-3869
http://www.asia-adopt.org/

Adoption World, Inc.
820 South 4th St., 2nd Floor
Philadelphia, PA 19147
(215) 336-5135
http://adoptionworld.org

Adult Children of Alcoholics
P. O. Box 3216
Torrance, CA 90510
(310) 534-1815
http://www.adultchildren.org/

Agency for Healthcare Research and Policy
Executive Office Center
2101 East Jefferson Street, Suite 501
Rockville, MD 20852
(301) 594-7195
http://www.ahcpr.gov/

AIDS Drug Assistance Programs (ADAP)
Critical Path AIDS Project
2062 Lombard Street
Philadelphia, PA 19146
(215) 545-2212
FAX: (215) 735-2762
http://www.critpath.org/docs/adap.htm

Al-Anon Family Group Headquarters, Inc.
1600 Corporate Landing Parkway
Virginia Beach, VA 23454-5617
(757) 563-1600
FAX: (757) 563-1655
http://www.al-anon.alateen.org/

Alcoholics Anonymous
Box 449, Grand Central Station
New York, NY 10163
(212) 870-3400
FAX: (212) 870-3003
http://www.alcoholics-anonymous.org

Alliance for Aging Research
2021 K Street, NW, Suite 305
Washington, DC 20006
(202) 293-2856
FAX: (202) 785-8574
http://www.agingresearch.org/

Alzheimer's Association
919 North Michigan Avenue, Suite 1100
Chicago, IL 60611-1676
(800) 272-3900
FAX: (312) 335-1110
http://www.alz.org

Alzheimer's Disease Education and Referral (ADEAR)
Center
P. O. Box 8250
Silver Spring, MD 20907-8250
(800) 438-4380
http://www.alzheimers.org

American Association of Managed Care Nurses, Inc.
(AAMCN)
4435 Waterfront Drive, Suite 101
Glen Allen, VA 23060
(804) 747-9698
FAX: (804) 747-5316
www.aamcn.org

American Association of Retired Persons
601 E. Street, NW, Washington, DC 20049
(800) 424-3410
http://www.aarp.org/

American Board of Electroencephalography and
Neurophysiology
1701 West Charleston Avenue, Suite 105
Las Vegas, NV 89102
(702) 388-4244
FAX: (702) 388-0333
http://www.ecnsociety.com/aben.htm

American Dietetic Association
216 West Jackson Blvd.
Chicago, IL 60606
(312) 899-0040
http://www.eatright.org/

American Holistic Nurses' Association
P. O. Box 2130
Flagstaff, AZ 86003-2130
(800) 278-2462
http://ahna.org

The American Nurses Association
600 Maryland Avenue, SW, Suite 100 West
Washington, DC 20024
(800) 274-4262
FAX: (202) 651-7001
www.nursingworld.org/

American Psychiatric Association
1400 K Street, NW
Washington, DC 20005
(888) 357-7924
FAX: (202) 682-6850
http://www.psych.org/

American Psychological Association
750 First Street, NE
Washington, DC 20002-4242
(202) 336-5510
http://www.apa.com

American Psychosomatic Society
6728 Old McLean Village Drive
McLean, VA 22101-3906
(703) 556-9222
FAX: (703) 556-8729
http://www.psychosomatic.org/

The American Self-Help Clearinghouse
http://mentalhelp.net/selfhelp/

American Social Health Association
P.O. Box 13827
Research Triangle Park, NC 27709
(919) 361-8400
FAX: (919) 361-8425
http://www.ashastd.org/

Anxiety Disorders Association of America
8730 Georgia Avenue, Suite 600
Silver Spring, MD 20910
(240) 487-0120
http://www.adaa.org/

Association for the Advancement of Behavior Therapy
305 7th Avenue, 16th Floor
New York, NY 10001-6008
(212) 647-1890
FAX: (212) 647-1865
http://www.aabt.org

Association for Applied Psychophysiology and
Biofeedback
10200 W. 44th Avenue, Suite 304
Wheat Ridge, CO 80033-2840
(303) 422-8436
FAX: (303) 422-8894
http://aapb.org/

The Association for Integrative Medicine
Box 1
Mont Clare, PA 19453
(610) 933-8145
http://www.integrativemedicine.org/

Association for Rehabilitation Nurses
4700 West Lake Avenue
Glenview, IL 60025
(800) 229-7530 or (847) 375-4710
FAX: (877) 734-9384
http://www.rehabnurse.org/

Bioethics Network
www.bioethics.net

Center for the Study of Anorexia and Bulimia
1 West 91st Street
New York, NY 10024
(212) 595-3449
http://www.4woman.gov/nwhic/references/mdreferrals
/csab.htm

Centers for Disease Control and Prevention
1600 Clifton Road, NE
Atlanta, GA 30333
(800) 311-3435
http://www.cdc.gov

Children of Aging Parents (CAPs)
1609 Woodbourne Road, Suite 302A
Levitown, PA 19057
(800) 227-7294
http://www.caps4caregivers.org/

Cultural Diversity in Health Care
http://www.ggalanti.com/index.html

Eldercare Locator
927 15th Street, NW, 6th Floor
Washington, DC 20005
(800) 677-1116
http://www.eldercare.gov/

Families USA
1334 G Street, NW
Washington, DC 20005
(202) 628-3030
FAX: (202) 347-2417
http://familiesusa.org

The Gerontological Society of America
1030 15th Street, NW, Suite 250
Washington, DC 20005
(202) 842-1275
FAX: (202) 842-1150
http://www.geron.org

Health Resources and Services Administration
Division of Transplantation
5600 Fishers Lane, Room 7C22
Rockville, MD 20857
(301) 443-7577
http://www.hrsa.gov/OSP/dot/dotmain.htm

Healthy People 2010
http://www.health.gov/healthypeople

International Food Information Council Foundation
1100 Connecticut Avenue, NW, Suite 430
Washington, DC 20036
(202) 296-6540
FAX: (202) 296-6547
http://www.ific.org/

The International Society of Psychoneuroendocrinology
c/o Dirk Hellhammer, Ph.D.
Center for Psychobiological & Psychosomatic Research
Trier University
Universitaetsring 15
Trier 54286
Germany
49-651-201-2929
FAX: 49-651-201-2934
http://www.ispne.org/

The Joint Council on International Children's Services
1320 Nineteenth St., NW, Suite 200
Washington, DC 20036
(202) 429-0400
FAX: (202) 429-0410
http://www.jcics.org

Mental Health Infosearch
http://www.mhsource.com

The Mind/Body Medical Institute
110 Francis Street
Boston, MA 02215
(617) 632-9530
FAX: (617) 632-9545
http://www.mbmi.org/

Mind-Brain Society
http://www.brown.edu/Students/Mind-Brain/

Mothers Against Drunk Driving (MADD)
P.O. Box 541688
Dallas, TX 75354
(800) 438-6233
http://www.madd.org

Narcotics Anonymous
P. O. Box 9999
Van Nuys, CA 91409
(800) 773-9999
FAX: (818) 700-0700
http://www.na.org

National Aging Information Center
330 Independence Avenue, SW
Room 4656
Washington, DC 20201
(202) 619-7501
FAX: (202) 401-7620
http://aoa.dhhs.gov/naic/

National Alliance for the Mentally Ill
Colonial Place Three
2107 Wilson Blvd., Suite 300
Arlington, VA 22201
(703) 524-7600
http://www.nami.org

National Anxiety Foundation
3135 Custer Drive
Lexington, KY 40517-4001
(859) 272-7166
http://lexington-on-line.com/naf.html

National Aphasia Association
29 John St., Suite 1103
New York, NY 10038
(800) 922-4622
FAX: (212) 267-2812
http://www.aphasia.org/

National Association for Anorexia and Associated
  Disorders
P. O. Box 7
Highland Park, IL 60035
(847) 831-3438
FAX: (847) 433-4632
http://www.anad.org/

National Association of Area Agencies on Aging
927 15th Street, NW, 6th Floor
Washington, DC 20005
(202) 296-8130
FAX: (202) 296-8134
http://www.n4a.org/

National Association of Clinical Nurse Specialists
3969 Green Street
Harrisburg, PA 17110
(717) 234-6799
http://www.nacns.org/

National Association of Hispanic Nurses
1501 16th Street, NW
Washington, DC 20036
(202) 387-2477
FAX: (202) 483-7183
http://www.thehispanicnurses.org/

National Association of Rehabilitation Agencies
11250 Roger Bacon Drive, Suite 8
Reston, VA 20190
(703) 437-4377
FAX: (703) 435-4390
http://www.naranet.org/

National Black Nurses Association
8630 Fenton Street, Suite 330
Silver Spring, MD 20910-3803
(301) 589-3200
FAX: (301) 589-3223
http://www.nbna.org/

National Center for Cultural Competence
Georgetown University
Child Development Center
3307 M Street, NW, Suite 401
Washington, DC 20007-3935
(800) 788-2066
FAX: (202) 687-8899
http://www.georgetown.edu/research/gucdc/nccc/index.
  html

National Center for Environmental Health
Mail Stop F-29
4770 Buford Highway, NE
Atlanta, GA 30341-3724
(888) 232-6789
http://www.cdc.gov/nceh/default.htm

National Clearing House for Alcohol and Drug
  Information (NCADI)
P.O. Box 2345
Rockville, MD 20847-2345
(800) 729-6686
http://www.samhsa.gov/centers/clearinghouse/clearing
  houses.html

National Coalition Against Domestic Violence
P.O. Box 18749
Denver, CO 80218
(303) 839-1852
FAX: (303) 831-9251
http://www.ncadv.org/

National Commission for Acupuncture and Oriental
  Medicine
11 Canal Center Plaza, Suite 300
Alexandria, VA 22314
(703) 548-9004
FAX: (703) 548-9079
http://www.nccaom.org

National Council for Adoption
1930 17th St., NW
Washington, DC 2009-6207
(202) 328-1200
FAX: (202) 332-0935
http://www.ncfa-usa.org/

National Council on Alcoholism and Drug Dependence
20 Exchange Place, Suite 2902
New York, NY 10005
(212) 269-7797
FAX: (212) 269-7510
http://www.ncadd.org

National Depressive and Manic Depressive Association
730 North Franklin, Suite 501
Chicago, IL 60610
(800) 826-3632
FAX: (312) 642-7243
http://ndmda.org/

National Domestic Violence Hotline
PO Box 161810
Austin, Texas 78716
(800) 799-7233
http://www.ndvh.org/

National Eating Disorders Association
603 Stewart Street, Suite 803
Seattle, WA 98101
(206) 382-3587
http://www.nationaleatingdisorders.org

National Foundation for Depressive Illness
P.O. Box 2257
New York, NY 10116
(800) 239-1265
http://www.depression.org

National Institute of Mental Health (NIMH)
NIMH Public Inquiries
6001 Executive Boulevard, Rm. 8184, MSC 9663
Bethesda, MD 20892-9663
(301) 443-4513
FAX: (301) 443-4279
http://www.nimh.nih.gov/

National Institute of Neurological Disorders and Stroke
    (NINDS)
National Institute of Health
P.O. Box 5801
Bethesda, MD 20824
(800) 352-9424
http://www.ninds.nih.gov/

National Institute on Aging
Building 31, Room 5C27
31 Center Drive, MSC 2292
Bethesda, MD 20892
(301) 496-1752
http://www.nia.nih.gov/

National Institute on Alcohol Abuse and
    Alcoholism
6000 Executive Boulevard, Willco Building
Bethesda, MD 20892-7003
http://www.niaaa.nih.gov

National Institute on Drug Abuse
National Institutes of Health
6001 Executive Boulevard, Room 5213
Bethesda, MD 20892-9561
(301) 443-1124
http://www.nida.nih.gov

National Mental Health Association
1021 Prince Street
Alexandria, VA 22314-2971
(703) 684-7722
FAX: (703) 684-5968
http://www.nmha.org/

National Mental Health Consumers' Self-Help
    Clearinghouse
1211 Chestnut Street, Suite 1207
Philadelphia, PA 19107
(215) 751-1810 or (800) 553-4539
FAX: (215) 636-6312
http://www.mhselfhelp.org/

National Rehabilitation Association
633 South Washington Street
Alexandria, VA 22314
(703) 836-0850
FAX: (703) 836-0848
http://www.nationalrehab.org/

NCCAM Clearinghouse
P.O. Box 7923
Gaithersburg, Maryland 20898
(301) 519-3153 or (888) 644-6226
FAX: (866) 464-3616
http://nccam.nih.gov/

North American Nursing Diagnosis Association
1211 Locust Street
Philadelphia, PA 19107
(215) 545-8105
FAX: (215) 545-8107
www.nanda.org

Nursing Ethics Network
http://www.nursingethicsnetwork.org/

Office of Minority Health
P.O. Box 37337
Washington, D.C. 20013-7337
(800) 444-6472
FAX: (301) 230-7198
http://www.omhrc.gov/

Organization for Human Brain Mapping
5841 Cedar Lake Road, Suite 204
Minneapolis, MN 55416
(952) 646-2029
FAX: (952) 545-6073
http://www.humanbrainmapping.org/

Overeaters Anonymous
6075 Zenith Court, NE
Rio Rancho, NM 87124
(505) 891-2664
FAX: (505) 891-4320
http://www.overeatersanonymous.org/

Pan American Health Organization
Regional Office of the World Health Organization
525 23rd Street, NW
Washington, DC 20037
(202) 974-3000
FAX: (202) 974-3663
http://www.paho.org

Philippine Nurses Association of America
151 Linda Vista Drive
Daly City, CA 94014
(415) 468-7995
FAX: (415) 468-7995
http://www.pna-america.org/

P.R.I.D.E. Foundation (Promote Real Independence for
    the Disabled and Elderly)
391 Long Hill Road
Groton, CT 06340
(860) 445-1448
http://members.aol.com/sewtique/pride.htm

Recovery, Inc.
802 Dearborn Street
Chicago, IL 60610
(312) 337-5661
FAX: (312) 337-5756
http://www.recovery-inc.com

Schizophrenia.com
http://www.schizophrenia.com

Sex Information and Education Council of the United
    States (SIECUS)
130 West 42nd Street, Suite 350
New York, NY 10036
(212) 819-9770
FAX: (212) 819-9776
http://www.siecus.org

Society for Light Treatment and Biological Rhythms
P. O. Box 591687
174 Cook Street
San Francisco, CA 941159-1687
FAX: (415) 751-2758
http://www.sltbr.org

Society for Neuroscience
11 Dupont Circle, NW, Suite 500
Washington, DC 20036
(202) 462-6688
http://www.sfn.org/

Transcultural Nursing Society
c/o Madonna University College of Nursing and Health
36600 Schoolcraft Road
Livonia, MI 48150-1173
(734) 432-5470 or (888) 432-5470
FAX: (734) 432-5463
http://www.tcns.org

Translation Services
AT&T Language Line Services
(800) 752-6096
Provides written and oral translation in 140 languages
U. S. Census Bureau
Washington, DC 20233
Street address: 4700 Silver Hill Road
Suitland, MD 20746
(301) 763-4636
http://www.census.gov/

Volunteers of America
1660 Duke Street
Alexandria, VA 22314-3421
(703) 341-5000 or (800) 899-0089
FAX: (703) 341-7000
http://www.voa.org/

World Health Organization
Avenue Appia 20
1211 Geneva 27
Switzerland
(00 41 22) 791 21 11
FAX: (00 41 22) 791 3111
http://www.who.int/home-page/

Chapter 18—The Client With an Anxiety Disorder

NIC
Anticipatory Guidance
Anxiety Reduction
Behavior Modification: Social Skills
Calming Technique
Cognitive Restructuring
Complex Relationship Building
Coping Enhancement
Decision-Making Support
Emotional Support
Impulse Control Training
Security Enhancement
Self-Awareness Enhancement
Simple Guided Imagery
Simple Relaxation Therapy
NOC
Aggression Control
Anxiety Control
Coping
Decision Making
Impulse Control
Information Processing
Role Performance
Sleep
Social Interaction Skills

Chapter 19—The Client With a Somatoform Disorder

NIC
Anxiety Reduction
Body Image Enhancement
Calming Technique
Cognitive Restructuring
Coping Enhancement
Emotional Support
Security Enhancement
Self-Awareness Enhancement
Self-Esteem Enhancement
NOC
Body Image
Coping
Decision Making
Self-Esteem

Chapter 20—The Client With a Sexual or Gender Disorder

NIC
Anxiety Reduction
Calming Technique
Cognitive Restructuring
Coping Enhancement
Emotional Support
Security Enhancement
Self-Awareness Enhancement
NOC
Anxiety Control
Coping
Rest
Self-Esteem
Sleep
Social Interaction Skills
Social Support

Chapter 21—The Client With a Dissociative Disorder

NIC
Behavior Management: Self-Harm
Body Image Enhancement
Delusion Management
Environmental Management: Violence Prevention
Hallucination Management
Reality Orientation
Self-Esteem Enhancement
NOC
Aggression Control
Distorted Thought Control
Identity
Impulse Control
Self-Mutilation Restraint

Chapter 22—The Client With a Personality Disorder

NIC
Anxiety Reduction
Behavior Modification
Impulse Control Training
Limit Setting
Mutual Goal Setting
Self-Responsibility Facilitation

NOC

Adherence Behavior
Compliance Behavior
Symptom Control

Chapter 23—The Client With an Eating Disorder

NIC

Body Image Enhancement
Cognitive Restructuring
Eating Disorders Management
Fluid Monitoring
Life Span Care
Nutrition Management
Nutrition Monitoring
Self-Esteem Enhancement
Weight Gain Assistance

NOC

Body Image
Nutritional Status: Food & Fluid Intake
Nutritional Status: Nutrient Intake
Self-Esteem
Weight Control

Chapter 24—The Client With a Mood Disorder

NIC

Active Listening
Behavior Management: Overactivity
Behavior Management: Sexual
Cognitive Restructuring
Coping Enhancement
Guilt Work Facilitation
Hallucination Management
Limit Setting
Mood Management
Self-Esteem Enhancement
Simple Guided Imagery
Simple Relaxation Therapy
Socialization Enhancement
Spiritual Support
Suicide Prevention
Teaching: Disease Process

NOC

Anxiety Control
Coping
Rest
Self-Esteem
Sleep
Social Interaction Skills
Social Support

Chapter 25—The Client With a Thought Disorder

NIC

Active Listening
Anxiety Reduction

Complex Relationship Building
Delusion Management
Energy Management
Environmental Management: Violence Prevention
Family Integrity Promotion
Family Involvement
Hallucination Management
Self-Care Assistance
Socialization Enhancement
Suicide Prevention

NOC

Aggression Control
Cognitive Ability
Cognitive Orientation
Concentration
Decision Making
Distorted Thought Control
Family Coping
Family Normalization
Identity
Impulse Control
Information Processing
Self-Mutilation Restraint

Chapter 26—The Client Who Displays Angry, Aggressive, or Violent Behavior

NIC

Abuse Protection
Abuse Protection: Child
Abuse Protection: Elder
Anger Control Assistance
Environmental Management: Violence Prevention
Impulse Control Training
Rape-Trauma Treatment
Support Groups

NOC

Abuse Cessation
Abusive Behavior Self-Control
Aggression Control
Impulse Control

Chapter 27—The Client Who Abuses Drugs or Alcohol

NIC

Hope Instillation
Impulse Control Training
Nutrition Management
Spiritual Support
Substance Use Treatment: Alcohol Withdrawal
Substance Use Treatment: Drug Withdrawal

NOC

Acceptance: Health Status
Anxiety Control
Family Coping
Risk Control
Substance Addiction Consequences

Chapter 28—The Client With a Cognitive Disorder

NIC
Delirium Management
Dementia Management
Environmental Management
Reality Orientation

NOC
Cognitive Ability
Cognitive Orientation
Communication Ability
Distorted Thought Control
Information Processing
Memory

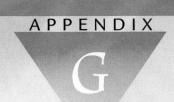

Commonly Used Assessment Tools

HAMILTON RATING SCALE FOR DEPRESSION

Clinic No._____ Date_____ Rating No._____ Code Number_____

Sex_____ Age_____ Patient's Name_____

Patient's Address_____ Tel_____

Item	Range	Score
1. Depressed mood	0–4	
2. Guilt	0–4	
3. Suicide	0–4	
4. Insomnia initial	0–2	
5. Insomnia middle	0–2	
6. Insomnia delayed	0–2	
7. Work and interest	0–4	
8. Retardation	0–4	
9. Agitation	0–4	
10. Anxiety (psychic)	0–4	
11. Anxiety (somatic)	0–4	
12. Somatic gastrointestinal	0–2	
13. Somatic general	0–2	
14. Genital	0–2	
15. Hypochondriasis	0–2	
16. Insight	0–4	
17. Loss of weight	0–2	
	Total score	
Diurnal variation (M.A.E)	0–2	
Depersonalization	0–4	
Paranoid symptoms	0–4	
Obsessional symptoms	0–4	

The scale is designed to measure the severity of illness of patients already diagnosed as suffering from depressive illness. It is obviously not a diagnostic instrument because that requires much more information (eg, previous history, family history, precipitating factors).

As far as possible, the scale should be used in the manner of a clinical interview. The first time the interview should be conducted in a relaxed, free, and easy manner, giving the patients time to unburden themselves and giving them the opportunity to speak of their problems and ask whatever questions they wish. It may then be necessary to obtain further information by asking them questions. At subsequent assessments, the interview can be briefer and more to the point.

An observer rating scale is not a checklist in which each item is strictly defined. The raters must have sufficient clinical experience and judgment to be able to interpret the patients' statements and reticences about some symptoms, and to compare them with other patients. They should use all sources of information (eg, from relatives and nurses).

The scale consists of 17 items, the scores on which are summed to give a total score. These are four other items, one of which (diurnal variation) is excluded on the grounds that it is not an additional burden on the patient. The last three are excluded from the total score because they occur infrequently, although information on them may be useful for other purposes.

The method of assessment is simple. For some symptoms it is difficult to elicit such information as will permit full quantification. If present, score 2; if absent, score 0; and if doubtful or trivial, score 1. For those symptoms where more detailed information can be obtained, the score of 2 is expanded into 2 for mild, 3 for moderate, and 4 for severe. In case of difficulty, the raters should use their judgment as clinicians.

Hamilton, M. (1960). A rating scale for depression. *Journal of Neurology, Neurosurgery and Psychiatry, 23,* 56.

I. **Symptom Rating Scale (0=Not Present, 4=Disabling)**
  A. Anxious Mood
     1. Worries
     2. Anticipates worst
  B. Tension
     1. Startles
     2. Cries easily
     3. Restless
     4. Trembling
  C. Fears
     1. Fear of the dark
     2. Fear of strangers
     3. Fear of being alone
     4. Fear of animal
  D. Insomnia
     1. Difficulty falling asleep or staying asleep
     2. Difficulty with Nightmares
  E. Intellectual
     1. Poor concentration
     2. Memory Impairment
  F. Depressed Mood
     1. Decreased interest in activities
     2. Anhedonia
     3. Insomnia
  G. Somatic Complaints: Muscular
     1. Muscle aches or pains
     2. Bruxism
  H. Somatic Complaints: Sensory
     1. Tinnitus
     2. Blurred vision
  I. Cardiovascular Symptoms
     1. Tachycardia
     2. Palpitations
     3. Chest Pain
     4. Sensation of feeling faint
  J. Respiratory Symptoms
     1. Chest pressure
     2. Choking sensation
     3. Shortness of Breath
  K. Gastrointestinal symptoms
     1. Dysphagia
     2. Nausea or Vomiting
     3. Constipation
     4. Weight loss
     5. Abdominal fullness
  L. Genitourinary symptoms
     1. Urinary frequency or urgency
     2. Dysmenorrhea
     3. Impotence
  M. Autonomic Symptoms
     1. Dry Mouth
     2. Flushing
     3. Pallor
     4. Sweating
  N. Behavior at Interview
     1. Fidgets
     2. Tremor
     3. Paces

II. **Interpretation**
  A. Above 14 symptoms are graded on scale
     1. Not present: 0
     2. Very severe symptoms: 4
  B. Criteria
     1. Mild Anxiety (minimum for Anxiolytic): 18
     2. Moderate Anxiety: 25
     3. Severe Anxiety: 30

BRIEF PSYCHIATRIC RATING SCALE

DIRECTIONS: Place an X in the appropriate box to represent level of severity of each symptom.

	Not Present	Very Mild	Mild	Moderate	Mod. Severe	Severe	Extremely Severe
SOMATIC CONCERN—preoccupation with physical health, fear of physical illness, hypochondriasis.	☐	☐	☐	☐	☐	☐	☐
ANXIETY—worry, fear, overconcern for present or future, uneasiness.	☐	☐	☐	☐	☐	☐	☐
EMOTIONAL WITHDRAWAL—lack of spontaneous interaction, isolation deficiency in relating to others.	☐	☐	☐	☐	☐	☐	☐
CONCEPTUAL DISORGANIZATION—thought processes confused, disconnected, disorganized, disrupted.	☐	☐	☐	☐	☐	☐	☐
GUILT FEELINGS—self-blame, shame, remorse for past behavior.	☐	☐	☐	☐	☐	☐	☐
TENSION—physical and motor manifestations of nervousness, over-activation.	☐	☐	☐	☐	☐	☐	☐
MANNERISMS AND POSTURING—peculiar, bizarre unnatural motor behavior (not including tic).	☐	☐	☐	☐	☐	☐	☐
GRANDIOSITY—exaggerated self-opinion, arrogance, conviction of unusual power or abilities.	☐	☐	☐	☐	☐	☐	☐
DEPRESSIVE MOOD—sorrow, sadness, despondency, pessimism.	☐	☐	☐	☐	☐	☐	☐
HOSTILITY—animosity, contempt, belligerence, disdain for others.	☐	☐	☐	☐	☐	☐	☐
SUSPICIOUSNESS—mistrust, belief others harbour malicious or discriminatory intent.	☐	☐	☐	☐	☐	☐	☐
HALLUCINATORY BEHAVIOR—perceptions without normal external stimulus correspondence.	☐	☐	☐	☐	☐	☐	☐
MOTOR RETARDATION—slowed weakened movements or speech, reduced body tone.	☐	☐	☐	☐	☐	☐	☐
UNCOOPERATIVENESS—resistance, guardedness, rejection of authority.	☐	☐	☐	☐	☐	☐	☐
UNUSUAL THOUGHT CONTENT—unusual, odd, strange, bizarre thought content.	☐	☐	☐	☐	☐	☐	☐
BLUNTED AFFECT—reduced emotional tone, reduction in formal intensity of feelings, flatness.	☐	☐	☐	☐	☐	☐	☐
EXCITEMENT—heightened emotional tone, agitation, increased reactivity.	☐	☐	☐	☐	☐	☐	☐
DISORIENTATION—confusion or lack of proper association for person, place, or time.	☐	☐	☐	☐	☐	☐	☐

Global Assessment Scale (Range 1–100)

Reprinted with permission from Overall J. E. (1988). The Brief Psychiatric Rating Scale (BPRS): Recent developments in ascertainment and scaling. *Psychopharmacology Bulletin, 24,* 97–99.

CHILD BEHAVIOR CHECKLIST FOR AGES 4–18

Please print. Make dark marks.

Fill bubbles completely ●

Child's Full Name: First   Middle   Last

Child's Age [ ][ ]

Today's Date

month
○ Jan
○ Feb
○ Mar
○ Apr
○ May
○ Jun
○ Jul
○ Aug
○ Sep
○ Oct
○ Nov
○ Dec

day year [ ][ ] [ ][ ]

office use only
○○ 0 ○○
○○ 1 ○○
○○ 2 ○○
○○ 3 ○○
○ 4 ○○
○ 5 ○○
○ 6 ○○
○ 7 ○○
○ 8 ○○
○ 9 ○○

Child's Birthdate

month
○ Jan
○ Feb
○ Mar
○ Apr
○ May
○ Jun
○ Jul
○ Aug
○ Sep
○ Oct
○ Nov
○ Dec

day year [ ][ ] [ ][ ]

office use only
○○ 0 ○○
○○ 1 ○○
○○ 2 ○○
○○ 3 ○○
○ 4 ○○
○ 5 ○○
○ 6 ○○
○ 7 ○○
○ 8 ○○
○ 9 ○○

Child's Sex
○ Boy
○ Girl

office use only—center label within box

Age	Identification Number	Eval ID	SES	Agency	User Defined
[ ]	[ ][ ][ ][ ][ ][ ][ ][ ][ ][ ]	[ ][ ][ ]	[ ]	[ ][ ]	[ ][ ][ ][ ]
○○ 0	○○○○○○○○○○○○	0 ○○○	○○	○○○	○○○○○
○○ 1	○○○○○○○○○○○○	1 ○○○	○○	○○○	○○○○○
○ 2	○○○○○○○○○○○○	2 ○○○	○○	○○○	○○○○○
○ 3	○○○○○○○○○○○○	3 ○○○	○○	○○○	○○○○○
○ 4	○○○○○○○○○○○○	4 ○○○	○○	○○○	○○○○○
○ 5	○○○○○○○○○○○○	5 ○○○	○○	○○○	○○○○○
○ 6	○○○○○○○○○○○○	6 ○○○	○○	○○○	○○○○○
○ 7	○○○○○○○○○○○○	7 ○○○	○○	○○○	○○○○○
○ 8	○○○○○○○○○○○○	8 ○○○	○○	○○○	○○○○○
○ 9	○○○○○○○○○○○○	9 ○○○	○○	○○○	○○○○○

Grade in School
○ Preschool
○ Kindergarten
○ 1   ○ 5   ○ 9
○ 2   ○ 6   ○ 10
○ 3   ○ 7   ○ 11
○ 4   ○ 8   ○ 12
○ Post High School
○ Not Attending School

Ethnic Group
○ African American
○ Asian
○ Latino, Latina
○ Native American
   (American Indian)
○ Pacific Islander
○ White Non-Latino
○ Other (specify):

Parents' Usual Type of Work:

Enter parents' usual type of work, even if they are not working now. Please be specific—for example, auto mechanic, homemaker, laborer, high school teacher, lathe operator, shoe salesperson, army sergeant.

Father's type of work:

Mother's type of work:

This form filled out by:

Your Full Name

Your gender: ○ Male   ○ Female

Your relation to the child:
○ Biological Parent   ○ Foster parent
○ Adoptive Parent   ○ Grandparent
○ Other (specify):   ○ Stepparent

Please fill out this form to reflect your view of the child's behavior even if other people might not agree.

○ None

	Don't Know	Less Than Average	Average	Above Average	Don't Know	Less Than Average	Average	Above Average
a.	○	○	○	○	○	○	○	○
b.	○	○	○	○	○	○	○	○
c.	○	○	○	○	○	○	○	○

○ None

	Don't Know	Less Than Average	Average	Above Average	Don't Know	Less Than Average	Average	Above Average
a.	○	○	○	○	○	○	○	○
b.	○	○	○	○	○	○	○	○
c.	○	○	○	○	○	○	○	○

○ None

	Don't Know	Less Active	Average	More Active	
a.	○	○	○	○	
b.	○	○	○	○	
c.	○	○	○	○	

Glossary

Action potential The change in electrical potential on the surface of a nerve or muscle cell, often initiated by a change in cellular ionic balance.

Acute stress disorder An anxiety disorder in which symptoms of post-traumatic stress disorder appear within 4 weeks of exposure to the trauma and usually last less than 3 months.

Adaptive plasticity An irreversible change in nervous tissue that usually affects the expression of a genotype into a phenotype.

Adherence A client's willingness to receive recommended drug treatment as prescribed by a caregiver.

Adjustment disorder A psychiatric disorder marked by clinically or behaviorally significant symptoms that develop within 3 months after the onset of an identifiable stressor.

Adventitious crisis A crisis precipitated by an unexpected event (eg, natural disasters,. bombings, mass shootings).

Advocacy Formal or informal promotion of children's rights.

Affect An observable behavior that expresses feeling or emotional tone; it refers to more fluctuating changes in emotional "weather." It is of shorter duration, more variable, and more reactive than underlying mood, which is more pervasive and stable.

Affective flattening A reduced intensity of emotional expression and response.

Affinity A drug's tendency to be found at a given receptor site.

Aggregate group A group identified as having at least one commonality among its members.

Aggregate mental health The degree to which families and groups within a given environment contribute to, enhance, or intensify interaction among individuals along the mental health-illness continuum.

Aggression Harsh physical or verbal responses that indicate rage and a potential for destructiveness.

Agnosia An inability to recognize or identify familiar objects (eg, the parts of a telephone).

Agonist A drug that initiates a therapeutic effect by binding to a receptor.

Agoraphobia A marked fear of being alone or in a public place from which escape would be difficult or help would be unavailable in the event of becoming disabled.

Alcohol (ethanol) A legal chemical substance (drug) that commonly leads to abuse and dependency.

Alogia A poverty of thinking that is inferred from observing the client's language and speech.

Alter Two or more identities or personality states.

Altruism The desire to contribute something valuable to society.

Amenorrhea Absence of or abnormal cessation of menstruation.

Anger An emotional response to perceived frustration of desires or needs.

Anhedonia Loss of pleasure in hobbies or activities of interest; a characteristic of depression.

Anorexia nervosa A life-threatening eating disorder characterized by disturbed body image, emaciation, and intense fear of becoming obese.

Antagonist A drug that binds to receptors without causing any regulatory effect; its action is to block the binding of an endogenous agonist.

Anxiety A sense of psychological distress that may or may not have a focus; it is a state of apprehension that may represent a response to environmental stress or a physical disease state.

Anxiety disorder A group of conditions in which the affected person experiences persistent anxiety that he or she cannot dismiss and that interferes with his or her daily activities.

Apathy A sense of detachment and the belief that nothing a person does makes any difference, leading to a lack of concern about the problem or outcome.

Aphasia Difficulty with finding the appropriate words in conversation.

Applied behavior analysis A systematic way of examining and analyzing behaviors as they relate to the environment and basing appropriate interventions on this analysis.

Apraxia An inability to perform motor tasks despite intact motor function.

Aromatherapy The use of essential oils to treat symptoms for physiological and psychological benefits.

Arousal Physiological stimulation, such as touching, kissing, fondling, licking, or biting erogenous body parts, that causes changes in the genitals.

Assertiveness A technique by which a person communicates what he or she thinks, feels, or wants directly and respectfully.

Assessment Gathering, classifying, categorizing, analyzing, and documenting information about a client's health status.

Assimilation The prevailing expectation during most of the 20th century for immigrants and minority groups in the United States to become like the majority (white) culture.

Attention-deficit disorder (ADD) A psychiatric disorder characterized by inattention without hyperactivity or impulsivity.

Attention-deficit hyperactivity disorder (ADHD) A psychiatric disorder characterized by inattention, impulsiveness, and hyperactivity.

Autism A genetic disorder of neuronal organization that requires early detection and treatment.

Autocratic leader A leader who exercises significant authority and control over group members; rarely, if ever, seeks or uses input from the group; and does not encourage participation or interaction from the group.

Autonomy The right to make decisions for oneself.

Avolition The inability to start, persist in, and carry through to its logical conclusion any goal-directed activity.

Axon A cylindrical neuron structure that relays information away from the cell body.

Battery Touching another person without his or her permission.

Behavioral health clinical nurse specialist A master's-prepared nurse with skills in psychiatric and mental health assessment and intervention who is eligible for, or has already received, ANA certification as a specialist in adult psychiatric and mental health nursing.

Behavioral statement A statement in a nursing plan of care in which the verb represents an observable behavior.

Beneficence The principle of doing good, not harm.

Bibliotherapy The use of literature to help clients gain insight into feelings and behavior and learn new ways to cope with difficult situations.

Binge eating Uncontrollable consumption of large amounts of food.

Binge eating disorder An eating disorder characterized by recurrent episodes of binge eating, with accompanying marked distress and impaired control over such behavior.

Bisexuality An equal or almost equal attraction to or preference for either sex as a sexual partner.

Blackout A phenomenon in which a person functions normally while drinking but later has no memory of what occurred during that period, with no accompanying loss of consciousness.

Blood alcohol level (BAL) Milligrams of alcohol per milliliter of blood.

Blood-brain barrier A protective system in the lining of blood vessels composed of endothelial cells with tight junctions, thus limiting access of blood constituents to the central nervous system.

Blunting A reduced intensity of emotional expression and response.

Body dysmorphic disorder A somatoform disorder in which the client is preoccupied with an imagined defect in his or her appearance (eg, a facial flaw or spot) when no abnormality or disturbance actually exists.

Bulimia nervosa An eating disorder characterized by binge eating, followed by purging.

Caring A core value of nursing that consists of three primary behaviors: (1) giving of self, (2) meeting the client's needs in a timely manner, and (3) providing comfort measures for clients and family members.

Case manager A person who coordinates the various services that address the individual needs (eg, housing, healthcare, mental health treatment, social contacts, work-ups) of a mentally ill client.

Channel The route or method a communicator chooses to convey his or her message.

Circadian rhythm A rhythmic activity cycle lasting approximately 24 hours.

Club drugs A group of synthetic drugs used commonly in nightclubs and as recreational drugs.

Cognitions Beliefs and thoughts that color a person's construction of his or her world.

Cognitive mental disorders A group of disorders characterized by a disruption of or deficit in cognitive functioning.

Communication The process of conveying information through a complex variety of verbal and nonverbal behaviors.

Communicator A person who simultaneously sends and receives messages through words and nonverbal behaviors.

Community support system A network of caring and responsible people committed to assisting a vulnerable population to meet its needs and develop its potential without becoming unnecessarily isolated or excluded from the community.

Compulsions Ritualistic behaviors that a person feels compelled to perform either in accord with a specific set of rules or in a routine manner.

Concepts The building blocks of theories.

Concordance rate The rate at which a trait expressed in one twin is expressed in another.

Conditioning A basic form of learning by which a subject begins to associate a behavior with a previously unrelated stimulus. There are two kinds of conditioning: operant and respondent.

Confabulation A characteristic of cognitive disorders in which an affected individual fills in gaps in memory with fabricated or imagined data.

Confrontation The skill of pointing out, in a caring way, concern about another person's behavior or discrepancies between what the other person says and what he or she does.

Contemplation and meditation Types of mental exercises that involve calmly limiting thought and attention.

Conversion disorder A somatoform disorder in which the client has at least one symptom or deficit of sensory or voluntary motor function (eg, paralysis) that cannot be explained by a neurologic or general medical condition.

Countertransference The feelings and thoughts that a mental-health service provider has toward a client that may be related to the provider's own unconscious or repressed emotions, feelings, and experiences.

Crisis intervention Methods and techniques used to assist a person in distress to resolve the immediate problem and regain emotional equilibrium.

Critical periods Periods during which children should be most exposed to certain stimuli for optimum development to take place. These periods vary according to different domains of functioning.

Cultural competence The skills, both academic and interpersonal, that allow persons to understand and appreciate cultural differences and similarities within, between, and among groups.

Culturally competent care Care provided in a manner acceptable to a client's cultural background, regardless of whether the healthcare professional who delivers the care is from the same ethnic or minority group as the client.

Culture The integration of human behavior (including thoughts, communications, actions, customs, beliefs, values, and institutions) of a racial, ethnic, religious, or social group.

Culture bound A term used to describe a person whose understanding of other cultures is limited because he or she refuses to go beyond the parameters of his or her personal culture.

Culture-bound syndromes Forms of mental illness found only in one particular culture, symbolizing that culture's unique expression of physical or mental distress.

Culture care theory A theory developed by Dr. Madeleine Leininger that emphasizes learning principles related to culture care, culturalogical assessments, the universality of culture care diversity, and the importance of fit between the client's healthcare values and services provided.

Cyclothymia A disorder resembling bipolar disorder, with less severe symptoms, characterized by repeated periods of nonpsychotic depression and hypomania for at least 2 years (1 year for children and adolescents).

Decoding The process by which one communicator discerns or interprets what another communicator is saying.

Defense mechanisms Unconscious measures that people use to defend their personal stability and protect against anxiety and threat resulting from conflicts between the id, ego, and superego.

Deinstitutionalization The massive discharge of clients from state hospitals that began in the 1950s, accelerated in the 1960s and 1970s, and continues today as psychiatric treatment continues to move from inpatient to outpatient settings.

Delirium A cognitive disorder caused by an acute disruption of brain homeostasis that is characterized by a rapid onset of cognitive dysfunction and disruption in consciousness; when the cause of that disruption is eliminated or subsides, the cognitive deficits usually resolve within a few days or sometimes weeks.

Delirium tremens (DTs) Most serious form of withdrawal from alcohol; occurs after cessation or reduction in prolonged heavy drinking; can be a medical emergency and needs immediate treatment.

Delusions Fixed, false beliefs about external reality that reasoning cannot correct; these include, but are not limited to the following types: grandiose (beliefs involving inflated self-worth, power, or knowledge); persecutory (belief that one is being attacked, harassed, cheated, or conspired against); and somatic (beliefs that give false attributions to the appearance or functioning of one's body).

Dementia A cognitive disorder resulting from primary brain pathology that is usually not amenable to treatment; prognosis depends on whether the cause can be identified and the condition reversed.

Democratic leader A leader who encourages group interaction and participation in group problem-solving and decision-making, values the input and feedback of each group member, seeks spontaneous and honest interaction among group members, creates an atmosphere that rewards members for their contributions, solicits the group's opinions, and tailors the group's work to their common goals.

Dendrites Branched processes that extend from and relay information to the cell body and receive signals from numerous neurons.

Depersonalization disorder A dissociative disorder characterized by a recurring or persistent feeling that one is detached from one's own thinking. Affected clients feel that they are outside their mind or body, much like an observer.

Depressive/Manic Depressive Association (DMDA) A national support and advocacy association with regional chapters for people with depressive and bipolar disorders and their families.

Desire Activation of areas in the brain that produce sexual appetite or drive.

Diagnostic and Statistical Manual of Mental Disorders (DSM) A criteria-based psychiatric diagnostic system that specifies the type, intensity, duration, and effect of the various behaviors and symptoms required for the diagnosis.

Discrimination (1) Differential treatment based on race, class, gender, or other variables rather than on individual merit. (2) The process by which a person learns to distinguish between and respond differently to similar stimuli.

Dissociation Altering one's usual level of self-awareness in an effort to escape an upsetting event or feeling.

Dissociative amnesia A dissociative disorder characterized by loss of memory that is not organic and involves an inability to recall events or facts too extensive to be labeled as mere forgetfulness.

Dissociative disorders A disruption in the usually integrated functions of consciousness, memory, identity, or perception, causing disturbance that may be sudden or gradual, transient or chronic.

Dissociative fugue A dissociative disorder that involves sudden travel away from home coupled with an inability to remember the past and confusion about identity or the adoption of a new identity.

Dissociative identity disorder A dissociative disorder in which the person acquires two or more identities or personality states (alters), who take control over the client's behavior.

Dissociative trance A dissociative state in which a person's awareness of his or her immediate surroundings narrows, and he or she exhibits stereotyped behaviors, such as immobilization, collapse, or loud, uncontrollable shrieking.

Double depression A diagnosis given when dysthymia and major depression occur together.

Dual diagnosis A diagnosis of a coexisting substance abuse or dependency disorder and a major psychiatric disorder; the disorders are unrelated and meet the *DSM-IV-TR* diagnostic criteria for each specific disorder.

Dyspareunia Genital pain associated with sexual intercourse in either a man or woman.

Dysthymia A mild form of depression that lasts 1 year or more in a child or adolescent.

Ecological model A perspective that holds that certain behaviors result from the interaction of individuals' traits with contextual factors arising from the family, community, and culture in which they reside.

Efficacy The information encoded in a drug's chemical structure that causes the receptor to change accordingly when the drug is bound.

Elder abuse Mistreatment of older adults, which includes physical abuse, physical neglect, sexual abuse, psychological abuse or neglect, financial abuse, and violation of personal rights

Electroconvulsive therapy (ECT) A therapy that involves the application of a small dose of electricity to one or both sides of the brain to induce a seizure.

Elite old A chronological category used to designate those 95 years of age or older.

Emergency admission Admission to a psychiatric hospital that occurs when a client acts in a way that indicates that he or she is mentally ill and, as a consequence of the particular illness, is likely to harm self or others. State statutes define the exact procedure for the initial evaluation and the possible length of detainment.

Emotional reasoning A cognitive distortion by which a person relies on his or her subjective emotions to determine reality.

Empathy Emotional knowing of another person.

Encoding The process by which a communicator puts into words or behaviors the ideas or feelings that he or she is trying to convey.

Environment In communication, the personal experiences and cultural background that a communicator brings to an interaction.

Ethical dilemma A situation in which there are conflicting moral claims or in which two ethical principles conflict.

Ethics Principles that serve as a code of conduct about right and wrong behavior to guide the actions of individuals.

Ethnocentrism The belief that one's own cultural practices and values are inherently correct or superior to those of others.

Excitement Psychological stimulation during the desire phase such as sexual fantasies or romantic communication.

Expressive violence Interpersonal violence, usually between people known to one another and of similar age, ethnicity, and cultural background.

External noise Factors outside a communicator that create distractions.

Extrapyramidal side effects (EPS) The most common and distressing side effects associated with traditional antipsychotic medications; they include akathisia (severe restlessness), dystonia (muscle spasm or contraction), chronic motor problems such as tardive dyskinesia, and the pseudoparkinsonian symptoms of rigidity, mask-like facies, and stiff gait.

Family burden The effects of serious mental illness on the family (see iatrogenic burden, objective burden, and subjective burden).

Family consultation A professional service offered to families to reduce family burden; a type of secondary prevention, originally called supportive counseling.

Family education Educational programs of varying duration to increase family members' knowledge about mental illness, caregiving, and self-care, with the objective of improving the entire family's quality of life.

Family psychoeducation A lengthy educational program for families (including the client) that is team-taught by professionals and includes, in addition to didactic content about mental illness, extensive training in behavioral skills intended to create a home environment conducive to reducing relapse and recidivism.

Family support services Opportunities for mutual support available without cost to families through groups organized by family organizations (eg, NAMI, DMDA).

Feedback The discernible response that a receiver makes to a sender's message when communicating.

Fetal alcohol syndrome A syndrome characterized by a group of congenital birth defects caused by the mother's drinking while pregnant.

Fidelity Faithfulness to duties, obligations, and promises.

First messengers Neurotransmitters that are responsible for transmitting impulses between nerve cells.

Flexibility The ability to embrace change by modifying expectations, readjusting old operating norms and stereotypes, and trying new behavior

Foreplay Petting and fondling behaviors that cause arousal during the excitement phase.

Formal group A group with structure and authority, which usually emanates from above; interaction in the group is usually limited.

Free association A technique in which a client says the first thing that comes to his or her mind, without restrictions, in response to something the therapist says.

Gang violence Violence associated with group membership and committed for retaliation or revenge (Labecki, 1994; Sigler, 1995).

Generalization The process by which a person learns to associate a conditioned response with similar stimuli.

Generalized anxiety disorder An anxiety disorder characterized by chronic and excessive worry and anxiety more days than not for at least 6 months and involving many aspects of the person's life; the worry and anxiety cause such discomfort as to interfere with daily life and relationships.

Genuineness A nursing value that involves being a real person and truly engaged in knowing the client in open, human exchanges.

Glial cells In the nervous system, non-neural cells that serve supporting and nutritive roles for neurons.

Group Three or more people with related goals.

Group norm The development, over time, of a pattern of interaction within a group to which certain behavioral expectations are attached.

Hallucinations Sensory perception with a compelling sense of reality; types include auditory (involving the perception of sound); gustatory (involving the perception of taste); olfactory (involving the perception of odor); tactile (involving the perception of being touched or of something under the skin; visual (involving sight—such as seeing images, people, flashes of light); and somatic (involving perception of a physical experience localized within the body).

Healing touch Two methods of energetic healing that incorporate the therapist's intention to heal, through either actual touch or non-touch re-patterning, energy fields around the person.

Heterosexuality An attraction to and preference for members of the opposite sex as sexual partners.

Home care Part of a comprehensive healthcare and mental healthcare system that aims to provide an array of health-related services to clients and families in their places of residence.

Homosexuality An attraction to and preference for members of the same sex as sexual partners.

Horizontal violence Anger or negativity a nurse directs toward another nurse.

Hostility-related variables Emotions, attitudes, and behaviors that occur regularly and predictably in people prone to aggression and violence.

Hypervigilance A common symptom of somatoform disorders in which the client's heightened focus on the body and its sensations leads to chronic, prolonged misinterpretation and overreaction to physical signs.

Hypochondriasis A somatoform disorder characterized by a client's unwarranted fear or belief that he or she has a serious disease, without significant pathology.

Hypomania A subcategory of mania, slightly less severe and without the psychotic features or severely impaired functioning that would require hospitalization.

Hypothesis An assumptive statement about the relationship between two or more concepts (or variables).

Hysteria An historical term (preceding somatoform disorder) coined in the early 1900s by Sigmund Freud to describe a condition in which people could not use certain body parts despite having no physiological damage or dysfunction.

Iatrogenic burden Iatro, from Greek *iatros* (physician) and *iasthai* (to heal). Used here to mean family burden exacerbated by the mental health system or mental health professionals.

Impulsivity A symptom of an underlying disorder or a pervasive personality trait that causes a person to perform actions with little or no regard for the consequences.

Informal group A group that provides much of a person's education and contributes greatly to his or her cultural values; members do not depend on one another.

Informed consent Consent that a recipient of healthcare gives to treating providers that enables the recipient to understand a proposed treatment, including its administration, prognosis after treatment, side effects, risks, possible consequences of refusal, and other alternatives.

Instrumental violence Violent acts that are usually premeditated and motive driven (frequently economic gain), usually involving people unknown to one another.

Intimate partner violence Violence occurring between persons (same or opposite sex) who have a current or former relationship (ie, dating, marital, or cohabiting). Violent acts include both physical and sexual violence as well as threats and psychological/emotional abuse.

Involuntary admission Admission to a psychiatric hospital that occurs when a person with mental illness who refuses psychiatric hospitalization or treatment poses a danger to self or others and cannot safely be cared for in a less restrictive setting.

La belle indifference In conversion disorder, a remarkable lack of affect or concern shown by a client despite a symptom that imposes significant physical disability (eg, paralysis).

Laissez-faire leader A leader who allows group members to operate as they choose.

Learning A process that occurs when organisms take in and store information as a function of experience.

Licensure A nonvoluntary process through which a government agency regulates a profession.

Listening Focusing on all behaviors exhibited by a person who is communicating.

Loss of efficacy The loss of ability to achieve a drug's maximum benefit.

Malpractice A tort action that a consumer plaintiff brings against a defendant professional from whom the plaintiff believes that he or she has received injury during the course of the professional–consumer relationship; professional negligence.

Maltreatment Behavior toward another person that is outside the norms of conduct and involves a significant risk of causing physical or emotional harm; four categories are recognized: physical abuse, sexual abuse, neglect, and emotional maltreatment.

Manic episodes Periods of abnormally and persistently elevated, expansive, or irritable mood.

Mantras Sounds, short words, or phrases repeated in the mind.

Masturbation Self-stimulation of erogenous areas to the point of orgasm.

Maturational or **developmental crisis** A crisis precipitated by the normal stress of development.

Maturity The ability to integrate aspects of life into a whole and find balance in one's outlook and attitudes toward others.

Maximal efficacy The maximal effect a drug can produce.

Medication adherence The actual taking of medications as prescribed; also called medication compliance.

Meditation A state of consciousness and an experience of the mind in which one tries to achieve awareness without thought.

Memory Information that is stored as a result of learning.

Mental disorders Health conditions marked by alterations in thinking, mood, or behavior that cause distress, impair ability to function, or both.

Mental health The successful performance of mental function, resulting in productive activities, fulfilling relationships, and the ability to adapt to change and cope with adversity.

Mental health nursing The care of well and at-risk populations to prevent mental illness or provide immediate treatment for those with early signs of a psychiatric disorder.

Mental illness A clinically significant behavioral or psychological syndrome experienced by a person and marked by distress, disability, or the risk of suffering, disability, or loss of freedom.

Mental status examination A tool for assessing objective and observational data that yields information about the client's appearance, level of consciousness, motor status and behavior, affect and mood, attitude, intellectual functioning, speech, cognitive status (including attention and concentration), judgment, abstraction, content of thought, and insight.

Middle old A chronological category used to designate those 75 to 84 years of age.

Modeling The demonstration of desired behavior patterns to a learner.

Mood A pervasive, sustained emotional coloring of one's experience; a sustained emotional "climate."

NAMI, The Nation's Voice on Mental Illness Formerly known as the National Alliance for the Mentally Ill, a national advocacy organization with state and local affiliates dedicated to improving the lives of persons with serious mental illness and their families.

Naturopathy An umbrella term used in most Western countries to cover a range of therapies referred to as natural medicine; a way of life wherein the body innately knows how to maintain health and heal itself.

Negative reinforcement Removal of an aversive stimulus that results in an increase in behavior or response.

Neuroleptic malignant syndrome A serious and potentially fatal side effect that accompanies use of certain antipsychotic agents. Characteristics include severe muscular rigidity, altered consciousness, stupor, catatonia, hyperpyrexia, and labile pulse and blood pressure.

Neurons Nerve cells; the fundamental units of the nervous system.

Neuropeptides The newest class of neurotransmitters, which includes endorphins and enkaphalins, vasoactive intestinal peptide, cholecystokinin, and substance P.

Neuroplasticity The ability of nervous tissue to change in its structure and functioning.

Neurotransmitters Chemical substances that relay messages between presynaptic and postsynaptic cells and are synthesized, stored, and released by neurons.

Noise Any forces within communicators or in the environment that interfere with effective communication.

Nontherapeutic communication Interactions in which the nurse uses ineffective responses that result in clients feeling defensive, misunderstood, controlled, minimized, alienated, or discouraged from expressing their thoughts and feelings.

Nursing diagnosis A clinical judgment about individual, family, or community responses to actual or potential health problems or life processes—it is the product of the analysis of data collected during the assessment step of the nursing process.

Nursing process A problem-solving method of five steps (assessment, nursing diagnosis, planning, intervention, and evaluation) that nurses systematically apply to the care of clients.

Objective burden The practical problems associated with caregiving (eg, employment issues, financial drain).

Objective data Phenomena that a person other than the client observes to be present.

Obsessions Recurrent, intrusive, and persistent ideas, thoughts, images, or impulses.

Obsessive-compulsive disorder An anxiety disorder marked by recurrent obsessions or compulsions that are time-consuming (taking more than 1 hour per day) or cause significant impairment or distress.

Old old A chronological category used to designate those 85 to 94 years of age.

Operant conditioning A type of conditioning by which a subject responds to a stimulus to achieve something rewarding or to avoid something aversive.

Oppositional-defiant disorder (ODD) A psychiatric disorder marked by negativistic, defiant behaviors such as stubbornness, resistance to directions, and unwillingness to negotiate with adults or peers.

Orgasm The peak of sexual pleasure. In the female, it consists of 3 to 15 strong rhythmic contractions of the orgasmic platform of the vagina. In the male, it consists of emission and ejaculation.

Panic attack A discrete period of intense apprehension or terror without any real accompanying danger, accompanied by at least 4 of 13 somatic or cognitive symptoms.

Panic disorder An anxiety disorder marked by recurrent, unexpected panic attacks that cause the affected person to persistently worry about recurrences or complications from the attacks or to undergo behavioral changes in response to the attacks for at least 1 month.

Paraphilias Sexual expressions for at least 6 months that are characterized by recurrent, intense sexual urges, fantasies, or behaviors that generally involve nonhuman objects or animals, suffering or humiliation of self or partner, or children or other nonconsenting persons.

Passive-aggressive communication Communication that uses indirect aggression through backstabbing, sabotaging, ignoring, or "forgetting" to do something.

Paternalism An ethical principle by which the intent is to do good; however, the professional determines what is considered "good" and may override a client's wishes and self-determination.

Perception check A confrontational communication technique that uses a three-step formula to clarify another person's behavior. The three steps are to (1) describe the inconsistent or confusing behavior, (2) offer at least two possible interpretations of that behavior, and (3) ask for feedback.

Personality The totality of a person's unique biopsychosocial characteristics that consistently influences his or her inner experience and behavior across the lifespan.

Personality disorder A collection of personality traits that have become fixed and rigid to the point that they impair the affected client's functioning and cause distress; also can be considered a lifelong pattern of behavior that affects many areas of the client's life, causes problems, and is not produced by another disorder or illness.

Phobia A persistent, irrational fear attached to an object or situation that objectively does not pose a significant danger.

Phototherapy Use of artificial light therapy to prevent and treat depression with a seasonal pattern.

Physiologic noise Physical factors within a communicator that detract from effective communication.

Polypharmacy Use of two or more psychotropic drugs, two or more drugs of the same chemical class, or two or more drugs with the same or similar pharmacologic actions to treat different conditions.

Positive reframing A communication technique in which the mental healthcare provider specifically states the behavior changes a client should make rather than criticizing the client's negative behavior.

Positive reinforcement The addition of something that increases the probability of a behavior or response.

Possession trance A dissociative state that involves acquiring a new identity attributed to the influence of a spirit, power, deity, or other person.

Post-traumatic stress disorder An anxiety disorder marked by the development of characteristic symptoms after exposure to a severe or extraordinary stressor (eg, natural disasters, accidental or intentional human-made disasters), in which there is actual or threatened death, serious injury, or maiming to the self or others; occurs only in response to a traumatic life experience.

Potency The concentration of a drug in plasma.

Power The perceived ability to control appropriate reward, therefore lending influence.

Prayer A kind of communication or conversation with a power that a person recognizes as divine.

Prejudice Negative preconceived opinions about other people or groups based on hearsay, perception, or emotion.

Premature ejaculation A persistent or recurrent onset of orgasm and ejaculation with minimal sexual stimulation before, on, or shortly after penetration and before the person wishes it.

Primary gain The main benefit a person derives from the "sick role," which, in the case of somatoform disorders, is the blocking of psychological conflict from conscious awareness.

Primary group A group that has face-to-face contact, boundaries, norms, and explicit and implicit interdependent roles.

Primary prevention Healthcare interventions designed to prevent mental disorders or to reduce identified mental disorders and disabilities within a population.

Professional A person who applies a specific background of knowledge and skills.

Professional certification A voluntary process that grants recognition to people for having met certain qualifications.

Proof Concentration of ethyl alcohol in a beverage.

Psychiatric nursing The care and rehabilitation of people with identifiable mental illnesses or disorders.

Psychiatric-mental health nursing The diagnosis and treatment of human responses to actual or potential mental health problems.

Psychological noise Emotional and cognitive forces within a communicator that interfere with accurately expressing or understanding a message.

Psychoneuroimmunology An emerging field that focuses on the links between a person's emotions, the functioning of his or her immune system, and how both factors alter central nervous system functioning.

Psychopharmacology The study of the chemistry, disposition, actions, and clinical pharmacology of drugs used to treat psychiatric disorders.

Psychosocial assessment The assessment of psychological, sociological, developmental, spiritual, and cultural data commonly derived from interviews with a client.

Psychosomatic medicine The clinical and scientific study of the connections between the mind and body.

Public health approach A method of addressing social problems that holds that multiple causes of the phenomena must be met with solutions that address each level of the problem.

Punishment Presentation of a negative or aversive stimulus or event that results in a decrease in a response or behavior.

Purging Attempting to eliminate the body of excess calories; examples of purging methods include self-induced vomiting, use of laxatives, and excessive exercise.

Rape A crime of forced or coerced sexual penetration (oral, anal, or vaginal) of a nonconsenting person.

Reactive plasticity A rapid, usually reversible, functional change in nervous tissue.

Reasonable person test A legal concept that refers to how a reasonable and prudent healthcare professional is expected to perform with regard to his or her professional role in a practice situation.

Respondeat superior A Latin term meaning that acts of employees are attributable to their employer, whom the court also will find responsible for damages to injured third parties.

Receptor A component of the cell membrane with the capacity to bind to a specific neurotransmitter.

Refractoriness A state of desensitization in which a drug's effect diminishes with repeated or subsequent use of the same concentration.

Refractory mania Bipolar disorder with mania that is completely unresponsive or marginally responsive to drug therapy with conventional mood-stabilizing agents.

Reinforcement The process by which a stimulus, whether pleasant (positive) or aversive (negative), strengthens a new response by its repeated association with that response.

Reinforcer A stimulus that strengthens a new response (behavior) by its repeated association with that response.

Religion The outward practice of a spiritual system of beliefs, values, codes of conduct, and rituals.

Repressed Pushed out of consciousness.

Resilient families Families who are able to rebound from the effects of mental illness.

Respondent conditioning The process by which a response and a stimulus become connected.

Restraint The use of a physical or mechanical device to involuntarily restrict the free movement of all or a portion of a person's body to control his or her physical activity.

Reuptake The process of the terminal of a presynaptic nerve cell taking back released neurotransmitter molecules for storage and subsequent release.

Ritual abuse A severe form of abuse in which a child is repeatedly physically and sexually abused in ceremonies by an organized group of perpetrators.

Rituals Ceremonies, rites, or acts such as prayer, singing hymns, fasting, or abstaining from food, water, or sexual relations, and partaking of sacramental emblems.

Schema or core beliefs An accumulation of the person's learning and experience within the family, religion, ethnicity, gender, regional subgroups, and broader society.

Schizophrenia A heterogeneous disorder of the brain with features including thought disturbances and preoccupation with frightening inner experiences (eg, delusions and hallucinations), affect disturbances (eg, flat or inappropriate affect), and behavioral/social disturbances (eg, unpredictable, bizarre behavior or social isolation).

Seclusion The placement of a client alone in a hazard-free room that is often locked and in which others can maintain direct observation of him or her.

Second hit Environmental factors hypothesized to contribute to the expression and characteristics of a person's illness.

Second messengers Secondary chemicals produced by the binding of a neurotransmitter to a receptor coupled with a G protein.

Secondary gain Additional benefits that a person derives from the "sick role"; examples include being released from expected responsibilities and receiving attention from others.

Secondary group A group that usually is larger and more impersonal than a primary group; members do not have the relationship bonds or emotional ties of members of a primary group.

Secondary prevention (1) An intervention to prevent further damage after a traumatic event; in this context, interventions to prevent families subjected to the trauma of mental illness from experiencing further adverse consequences (eg, caregiver burnout, disrupted interpersonal relationships, psychiatric and medical health problems). (2) Healthcare interventions designed to identify mental health problems early and reduce their duration and prevalence.

Separation anxiety disorder A childhood psychiatric disorder in which a child experiences severe anxiety to the point of panic when separated from a parent or attachment figure.

Serious mental illness A term given to a psychiatric disorder that meets the criteria for duration (at least 1 year), disability (relatively severe functional impairment), and diagnosis (including schizophrenia, bipolar disorder, and major depression) (National Advisory Mental Health Council, 1993).

Sexual assault Forced or coerced sexual acts performed on a nonconsenting person.

Sexual dysfunction Sexual expressions characterized by a disturbance in the processes that characterize the sexual response cycle or by pain associated with sexual intercourse.

Sexual intercourse (coitus) Penetration of the vagina by the penis.

Sexuality The experience of the sexual self.

Shaping A procedure employed in behavioral therapy when a person lacks a certain behavior in his or her inventory, so that reinforcement of that behavior might take place.

Sick role The role that all chronically ill clients assume that releases them from usual responsibilities; in somatoform disorders, clients unconsciously assume the sick role to meet their dependency needs.

Side effects Dysfunctions and discomforts that a client experiences directly as a result of taking a medication.

Situational crisis A crisis precipitated by a sudden traumatic event (eg, job loss).

Social phobia An anxiety disorder characterized by a persistent, irrational fear of and compelling desire to avoid situations in which the person may be exposed to unfamiliar people or to the scrutiny of others; fear of behaving in a way that may prove humiliating or embarrassing.

Somatization disorder A somatoform disorder characterized by many physical complaints over several years that cannot be explained by pathology or a general medical condition.

Somatoform disorders A group of psychiatric disorders in which clients complain of extreme physiologic discomfort or disability without any identifiable pathology on testing or examination.

Spirituality A person's experience of, or a belief in, a power apart from his or her own existence; an individual search for meaning.

Splitting Perceiving people and life experience in terms of "all good" or "all bad" categories.

Statutory rape Rape of a minor.

Stereotyping Believing that one member of a cultural group will display certain behaviors or hold certain attitudes (usually negative) simply because he or she is a member of that cultural group.

Stigmatization The attribution of negative characteristics or identity to one person or group, causing the person or group to feel rejected, alienated, and ostracized from society.

Structural and functional analysis An assessment of the functional relationships between various purported motivational variables and the rate of occurrence of certain behaviors.

Subjective burden The emotional response the client and family have to mental illness and caregiving (eg, grief, fear, guilt, anger). (Note: Some researchers define subjective burden differently, as perceived objective burden.)

Subjective data Data that the nurse gathers by interviewing the client.

Substance abuse Use of alcohol or other drugs repeatedly to the extent that functional problems occur; it does not include compulsive use or addiction.

Substance dependency Continued used of alcohol or other drugs despite negative consequences, such as significant functional problems in daily living.

Substituted consent Authorization that another person gives on behalf of a client who needs a procedure or treatment but cannot provide consent for it independently.

Sundowning A characteristic feature of dementia by which most behavior changes are more pronounced in the evenings after sunset.

Synapse The area involving the membrane of a presynaptic neuron (sender), the synaptic cleft, and the membrane of the postsynaptic neuron (receiver), across which a nerve impulse passes.

Synaptic cleft A gap between the cellular membranes of the terminal of the presynaptic neuron and dendritic processes of the postsynaptic neuron.

Systems of care Comprehensive spectrums of mental health and other necessary services organized into coordinated networks so that providers can more appropriately address the various and changing needs of children and adolescents with serious emotional disturbances and their families.

Tai' Chi A Chinese blend of exercise and energy work with a series of choreographed, continuous slow movements performed with mental concentration and coordinated breathing.

Tardive dyskinesia The most serious side effect of long-term use of neuroleptics (extrapyramidal symptom), with often irreversible and severely disabling effects that include involuntary choreoathetotic movements affecting the face, tongue, perioral, buccal, and masticatory muscles.

Target symptoms The specific symptoms that a medication aims to change.

Tautology A logical error in reasoning.

Taxonomy A classification system that uses a hierarchical structure.

Temperament Constitutional or biologically based personality dispositions that are partly inherited, evident early in life, and somewhat stable across situations and over time.

Tertiary prevention Healthcare interventions designed to provide rehabilitation for clients with diagnosed disorders and to minimize the residual effects for people within a community who have encountered mental health problems.

Theory One person's or group's beliefs about how something happens or works.

Therapeutic communication A planned process of interaction in which the nurse demonstrates empathy, uses effective communication skills, and responds to the client's thoughts, needs, and concerns.

Therapeutic touch Two methods of energetic healing that incorporate the therapist's intention to heal, through either actual touch or non-touch re-patterning, energy fields around the person.

Thought disorders Serious and often persistent mental illnesses characterized by disturbances in reality orientation, thinking, and social involvement.

Tic A sudden repetitive movement, gesture, or utterance.

Tolerance A phenomenon that occurs after heavy drug or alcohol use in which the user needs more of the drug to achieve the same effect.

Tourette syndrome The most severe tic disorder, characterized by multiple motor tics and one or more vocal tics many times throughout the day for 1 year or more.

Transactional analysis An assertive communication technique by which a persons speaks from the adult ego state to others in the adult ego state.

Transcription Process whereby a DNA sequence is copied onto RNA.

Transference Feelings and thoughts that a client has toward the nurse, psychiatrist, or other service provider that are rooted in the client's unconscious or repressed emotions and feelings toward people in his or her past (eg, parents, teachers).

Translation Process by which information in RNA produces amino acids (which make up proteins).

Transsexual A person who identifies with and lives as if he or she is of the opposite gender.

Transvestite A person who cross-dresses for the purpose of sexual arousal.

serotonin syndrome and, 234, 365,
    496, 496t
side effects of, 227–232, 228t–232t,
    233–234, 252
  sexual, 409
for somatoform disorders, 383, 384t
suicide risk and, 504–509
tetracyclic, 229t, 232
tricyclic, 227–232, 228t–229t, 233b,
    497, 497f
Antihistamines, for antipsychotic side
    effects, 539b
Antipsychotics, 239–245, 537–540. *See
    also* Drug therapy
  for aggression, 562t
  atypical, 538t, 539–540
    for bipolar disorder, 499–500
  cardiotoxicity of, 251–252
  client teaching for, 249b
  decanoate injections of, 252b
  deinstitutionalization and, 171b
  for delirium, 616–617
  for mania, 237
  neuroleptic malignant syndrome and,
    240, 539, 695
  nonadherence to, 253
  for schizophrenia, 537–540
    adherence to, 547–549
    client teaching about, 548–549
  side effects of, 538–539, 539t
    extrapyramidal, 240, 243t, 249,
      250f–251f, 538
    motor, 240, 244t, 249, 250f–251f,
      538–539, 538t
    treatment of, 539t
  sudden death and, 251–252
  tardive dyskinesia and, 240, 243t,
    538t, 539
  typical, 240–244, 241t–242t,
    537–539, 538t
Antisocial personality disorder, 440b,
    442, 445t, 450b–451b. *See also*
    Personality disorder(s)
Anxiety, 350–351
  cognitive effects of, 350–351
  continuum of, 350–351
  coping with, 351, 351b
  definition of, 350
  drug therapy for, 237–239,
    238t–239t
  fight-or-flight reaction and, 350
  in hospitalized children, 675t
  medical disorders causing, 353b
  in mood disorders, 512
  normal vs. abnormal, 351
  in older adults, 692t
  physiologic responses to, 350
  sensory effects of, 350
  separation, 656, 665
  in somatoform disorders, 384, 391
  vs. stress, 350

in substance abuse, 600
substances causing, 353b
therapeutic communication in, 72
verbal ability and, 351
Anxiety disorders, 351–369
  acute stress disorder, 354
  agoraphobia, 355
  breathing retraining for, 363–364
  in children, 656, 664–666
  clinical example of, 349b–350b
  cognitive-behavioral therapy for,
    362–363, 363b
  cognitive reframing in, 368
  comorbidities and, 361
  complications of, 361
  coping strategies for, 368–369
  diagnostic criteria for, 353–361,
    354–356
  drug therapy for, 364–365
  dual diagnoses and, 361
  etiology of, 352
  exposure treatment for, 363
  generalized anxiety disorder,
    353–357, 354
    in children, 665
  hyperventilation in, 368
  information map for, 354b–357b
  learning theory and, 352
  medical disorders and, 352, 353b
  neurobiological theories of, 352,
    353b
  nursing process in, 366–369
  obsessive-compulsive disorder,
    355–356. *See also* Obsessive-
    compulsive disorder
  overview of, 351–352
  panic attack, 356
  panic disorder, 354
  post-traumatic stress disorder, 355. *See
    also* Post-traumatic stress disorder
  prevalence of, 351–352
  prevention of, 356–357
  prognosis of, 361
  psychodynamic therapy for, 362–363
  psychological theories of, 352
  relaxation techniques for, 363–364,
    364b, 368–369
  risk/contributing factors for, 354
  signs and symptoms of, 353–361, 366
  social phobia, 356
    in children, 665
  specific phobia, 356
    in children, 665
  substance abuse and, 352, 353b
  systematic desensitization for, 363
  therapeutic communication in, 367,
    367b
  treatment of, 362–365
    barriers to, 352
Anxiolytics. *See* Antianxiety agents
Apathy, 57

Aphasia, in dementia, 618
Apomorphine (Uprima), 409
Appearance
  in mental status examination, 100b,
    503
  in mood disorders, 512
  in schizophrenia, 532
Applied behavior analysis, 44
Apraxia, 621
Arachnoid mater, 25
Aricept (donepezil), 634–635
Aromatherapy, 280–283
Arousal, sexual, 402
  disorders of, 403–405, 406b, 409
Arrhythmias, antipsychotics and,
    251–252
Art therapy, for dissociative disorders,
    427–428
Asendin (amoxapine), 227, 228t, 497
Asian and Pacific Islanders. *See also*
    Culture; Racial/ethnic groups
  culturally congruent care for, 89b
  health beliefs and practices of, 81t,
    86–87, 88
Asperger syndrome, 655, 670–671
  schizophrenia and, 524, 526b
Assault, sexual, 335–339
Assertive community treatment, 299,
    542
Assertiveness, in therapeutic
    communication, 70
Assertiveness training, 569
Assessment, 97–102
  contextual factors in, 49–50
  definition of, 97, 97b
  exosystem factors in, 49
  health history in, 97–99, 98t–99t
  importance of, 49b
  interview in, 97, 97b
  mental status examination in, 99–102,
    100b–101b
  microsystem factors in, 49
  multidimensional, 49–50
  nursing diagnosis in, 102–106. *See
    also* Nursing diagnosis(es)
  nutritional, 464
  spiritual, 267
  transcultural, 90
Assimilation, 80
Ataque de nervios, 375, 423
Ativan. *See* Lorazepam (Ativan)
Attention-deficit disorder, 658
Attention-deficit/hyperactivity disorder,
    658–663
  academic issues in, 662–663
  behavior therapy for, 660
  client/family teaching for, 660–663,
    662b
  clinical example of, 644b
  comorbidities in, 658–659, 668, 669
  definition of, 658

Attention-deficit/hyperactivity disorder (*continued*)
developmental factors in, 662–663
diagnostic criteria for, 654, 658
drug therapy for, 245–246, 246t, 659, 662b
etiology of, 658
family concerns in, 662
nursing care plan for, 661
nursing process in, 659–663
self-esteem in, 663
signs and symptoms of, 654, 658
social skills training in, 663
treatment of, 659
Attention deficits
in delirium, 610–611
in dementia, 618
Attributions, anger and, 558–559
Atypical antidepressants, 229t, 232. *See also* Antidepressants
Autism, 655, 670–671
schizophrenia and, 524, 526b
Autocratic leader, 153
Automatic thought, anger and, 558–559, 569
Autonomy, 126
Aventyl (nortriptyline), 227, 228t
Aversion therapy, for paraphilias, 417
Avoidant personality disorder, 440b–441b, 443, 445t. *See also* Personality disorder(s)
Avolition, in schizophrenia, 531b, 534
Axon, 22, 24f
Ayurvedic medicine, 278

B

Barbiturates, abuse of, 588t. *See also* Substance abuse
Basal ganglia, 28, 28t
Battery, 120
Beck, Aaron, 138, 139, 493
Behavioral assessment
in dementia, 626, 628b
in mental status examination, 100b, 503
Behavioral care plan, for violent/aggressive client, 509
Behavioral change, in twelve-step programs, 582
Behavioral change theories, of substance abuse, 582
Behavioral health clinical nurse specialist, 314–315
Behavioral health home care, 311–321
advantages and disadvantages of, 315
assessment in, 315–317, 317b
client populations for, 313–314
clinical example of, 311

cultural factors in, 316b
documentation in, 316–317
evaluation in, 319–320
goals of, 313
historical perspective on, 312
implementation in, 319
indications for, 315–316
nurse's skills and attitudes in, 315
nursing diagnoses for, 317, 318b
nursing process in, 315–320
outcomes in, 318–319
overview of, 311–312
planning in, 317–319
political influences on, 320
principles of, 312
professional support in, 315
providers of, 313
referral sources for, 314b
reimbursement for, 314b, 320
safety concerns in, 317b, 319
services offered in, 312–313
societal influences on, 320
trends in, 320
Behavioral inhibition, 658
Behavioral statement, client outcomes and, 106
Behavior family systems therapy, for eating disorders, 463
Behaviorism, 41–44, 42t
cognitions and, 44–45, 45b
Behavior modification, 44–45, 45t, 46t
Behavior therapy, 137t, 139–143
for attention-deficit/hyperactivity disorder, 660
for children and adolescents, 650
for eating disorders, 462
rational emotive, 45, 137t, 143–144
token economy in, 142–143, 560–561
Beliefs
distorted, 44–45, 45b
religious. *See* Religious beliefs
Benadryl (diphenhydramine), for aggression, 562t
Beneficence, 126
Benson, Herbert, 364
Benzedrine, abuse of, 587t
Benzodiazepines, 237–239, 238t–239t
for alcohol withdrawal, 589, 590t
for antipsychotic side effects, 539b
for anxiety disorders, 365
guidelines for, 365b
Benzphetamine, abuse of, 587t
Bereavement, in older adults, 687
Beta blockers
for aggression, 564t
for antipsychotic side effects, 539b
for anxiety disorders, 365
Bibliotherapy, with sacred writings, 268
Binge-eating disorder, 456, 457b. *See also* Eating disorders

Bioelectromagnetic therapy, 285
Biofield therapies, 284–285
Biogenic amine hypothesis, 482–483
Biophysiological perspective, 46–47
Bipolar disorder, 489
antidepressants in, 494–495, 495f
anxiety and agitation in, 512
assessment in, 501–504
attention-deficit/hyperactivity disorder and, 669
in children, 480–481, 668–669
client/family teaching in, 505b
cognitive problems in, 512
diagnostic criteria for, 488b, 489b, 490–492
dissociative disorders and, 424
drug therapy for, 234–237, 235t–236t, 494–495, 495f, 497–500
adherence to, 513
epidemiology of, 480–481
etiology of, 481–486
evaluation in, 513
family issues in, 504
genetic factors in, 482
hypomania in, 491
implementation in, 504–513
mania in, 490–491
drug therapy for, 234–237, 235t–236t
nursing care plan for, 507b–509b
refractory, 237–238, 499–500
signs and symptoms of, 490–491
mental status examination in, 502–503
nursing care plan for, 105b–106b, 507b–509b
nursing diagnoses for, 504
nursing process in, 501–513
personal hygiene in, 512
physical health concerns in, 509–512
physiological stability in, 503–504
planning in, 504
prognosis of, 492
risk factors for, 488b
self-care in, 491b
self-esteem in, 512
sleep deprivation in, 509–511
suicide in, 501–502, 502b, 504–509, 510b–511b. *See also* Suicide
treatment of, 492, 493b
type I, 490–491
type II, 491–492
vegetative signs in, 503–504
violence assessment in, 502
Bisexuality, 399–400
sexual assessment and, 414b
Blackouts, alcoholic, 585
Bleuler, Eugen, 527b
Blocking, 351
Blood alcohol level, 584–585

Blood-brain barrier, 25
Blood phobia, 358
Body-based therapies, 283–284
Body dysmorphic disorder, 376t, 377t, 378t, 381, 384t. *See also* Somatoform disorders
Body image, in eating disorders, 469f, 472
Borderline personality disorder, 440b, 442, 445t. *See also* Personality disorder(s)
Botanicals, 280–283, 281t–283t. *See also* Complementary/alternative medicine
Boundary issues, 55, 56t, 127–129
  family, 647
  in forensic nursing, 199, 200b
  sexual acting out and, 400, 401b
  in spiritual care, 269
Brain
  development of, 28–29
  plasticity of, 29–30
  structure and function of, 25–30, 27f, 27t–29t
Brain fag, 375
Brain lesions, aggression and, 558
Brainstem, 26, 27f, 28t
Breast-feeding, drug therapy and, 255
Breathing retraining, 363, 368–369
Brief Psychiatric Rating Scale (BPRS), 225, 226f
Brief psychotic disorder, 523b, 525
Brief solution-focused therapy, 138t, 144, 145b
  for children and adolescents, 650
  for eating disorders, 463
Briquet's syndrome, 376t, 377–380, 378t
Bromocriptine (Parlodel), for cocaine addiction, 593t
Bronfenbrenner, Uri, 48
Brujas/brujos, 86b
Bulimia nervosa, 455–474, 671. *See also* Eating disorders
  clinical example of, 461b–462b
  definition of, 456
  diagnostic criteria for, 459b
  nonpurging type, 460
  purging type, 460
Bupropion (Wellbutrin), 231t, 233–234, 497
  for attention-deficit/hyperactivity disorder, 659
Burland, Joyce, 184
Burnout, 17–18
  caregiver, 679
  prevention of, 17, 18b
Buspirone (BuSpar), 237, 238t
  for aggression, 563t
  for anxiety disorders, 365
Butyl nitrate, abuse of, 587t

C

CAGE questionnaire, 595b
California poppy, 281t
Canterbury vs. Spence, 120
Carbamazepine (Tegretol), 234, 235t
  for aggression, 563t
Cardiotoxicity, of psychotropic drugs, 251–252
Caregiver burnout, 679
Caregiving, family, 170–178. *See also* Family burden
Care maps, 108, 108b
Care plan. *See* Nursing care plan; Planning
Caring, in therapeutic relationship, 56–57
Cartesian dualism, 23b
Case management, 147
  in community mental health, 295
  for homeless, 217
  in schizophrenia, 535, 536t–537t, 542
Catapres. *See* Clonidine (Catapres)
Catastrophizing, in eating disorders, 468t
Catatonic schizophrenia, 524, 532. *See also* Schizophrenia
Catharsis, in group therapy, 161
Caudate, 28
Celexa (citalopram), 231t, 233–234
Center for Mental Health Services, 297, 325
Central nervous system
  development of, 28–29
  endocrine system and, 33
  immune system and, 33
  structure and function of, 24, 26f, 27f, 27t–29t, 30
Cerebellum, 26, 27f, 28t
Cerebral cortex, 26, 27f
Cerebrum, 26, 27f
Chakras, 284
Change, resistance to, 62b
Channels, communication, 63
Checklist for Autism in Toddlers (CHAT), 670
Child abuse and neglect, 331–333, 648
  repressed memory syndrome and, 426–427, 426b
Child Abuse and Trauma Questionnaire, 429
Child Abuse Prevention and Treatment Act of 1984, 331
Child and Adolescent Service System Program (CASSP), 292, 297, 300
Child Behavior Checklist, 429
Child development, 644–647. *See also* Development
Child life programs, 678b

Children. *See also* Adolescents
  adjustment disorders in, 656, 664
  advocates for, 653
  antidepressants for, 668, 669
  anxiety disorders in, 656, 664–666
  Asperger syndrome in, 655, 670–671
    schizophrenia and, 524, 526b
  attention-deficit/hyperactivity disorder in, 658–663
  autism in, 655, 670–671
    schizophrenia and, 524, 526b
  bipolar disorder in, 480–481, 668–669
  chronic illness/disability in, 674–679
  community support systems for, 300–301
  conduct disorder in, 654, 664
  depression in, 480–481, 666–668
    in bipolar disorder, 668–669
    suicide and, 673–674
  disruptive behavior disorders in, 658–664
  dissociative disorders in, 429
  divorce and, 648
  domestic violence and, 328–329
  drug therapy for, 256
  educational needs of, 302, 303
  hospitalization of, 674–679
  incarcerated, 194
  maltreatment of, 331–333, 648
    ritualized abuse and, 423b, 426b
  mania in, drug related, 669
  medical illness/disability in, 674–679
  mental illness in
    assessment in, 651–652
    biological factors in, 647
    classification of, 6
    common types of, 653–674
    community-based services for, 651
    cultural considerations in, 650b
    developmental ecological model of, 47–50, 48t, 49f
    diagnosis of, 6
    drug therapy for, 651, 652
    early identification of, 649–650
    family concerns in, 652–653
    family dynamics and, 647, 648–649
    history taking in, 651–652
    information map for, 654–657
    interventions for, 649–653, 652–653
    nurse's self-care and, 679
    nursing care in, 651–653
    patient rights in, 653
    prevalence of, 6
    prevention of, 649–650
    protective factors for, 648–649
    psychosocial factors in, 647
    risk factors for, 647–648
    special education for, 651
    stressors in, 647–648

Children, mental illness in (*continued*)
  therapeutic approaches in, 650
  mood disorders in, 480–481,
    666–669
  obsessive-compulsive disorder in,
    664–665
  oppositional-defiant disorder in, 656,
    663–664, 669
  parental mental illness and, 172
  peer pressure and, 672b
  pervasive developmental disorders in,
    655, 670
    schizophrenia and, 524, 526b
  phobias in, 665
  post-traumatic stress disorder in, 666
  psychiatric–mental health disorders in,
    643–679
  restraint/seclusion of, 564, 653
  schizophrenia in, 523, 526
  separation anxiety disorder in, 665
  social anxiety disorder in, 665
  substance abuse in, 671–672
  suicide in, 673–674
  tic disorders in, 672–673
  Tourette syndrome in, 673
  trichotillomania in, 673
Chinese medicine, traditional, 277
Chloral hydrate
  abuse of, 588t. *See also* Substance
    abuse
  for aggression, 562t
Chlordiazepoxide (Librium), 237–239,
    238t–239t
  for alcohol withdrawal, 590
Chlorpromazine (Thorazine), 240–244,
    241t
  for aggression, 562t
  for schizophrenia, 538t
Choice therapy, 137t, 144
Chromosomes, 30–31
Chronic illness, in children and
    adolescents, 674–679
Cicchetti's developmental ecological
    model, 47–50, 48t, 49f
Cigarette smoking, in pregnancy,
    578–579
Circadian rhythms, 32–33
Cirrhosis, alcoholic, 586
Citalopram (Celexa), 231t, 233–234
Clanging, 531, 532b
Classical conditioning, 43, 141–142
Class issues, 47
Claustrophobia, 358
Clergy, in mental healthcare, 266–267
Client adaptation model, 11, 12t
Client advocacy, 11, 118, 119t
  for children and adolescents, 653
  in forensic nursing, 201
  for homeless, 217
Client autonomy, 126
Client/family teaching, 147

  for antipsychotics, 10b, 249b
  for attention-deficit/hyperactivity
    disorder, 660–663, 662b
  for bipolar disorder, 492, 505b
  for delirium, 617
  for dementia, 629
  for drug therapy, 10b, 252b
    in children and adolescents, 652
  for eating disorders, 472b
  for homeless, 217
  for mood disorders, 492, 505b
  for personality disorders, 445
  for problem-solving skills, 369
  for relaxation techniques, 364b,
    368–369
  for schizophrenia, 543, 548–549, 550
  simultaneous, 184
Client records. *See also* Documentation
  client's rights to, 121
  legal issues involving, 121
Clinical maps, 108, 108b
Clinical nurse specialist, behavioral
    health, 314–315
Clinical nursing practice, levels of,
    145–146
Clinical pathway, 108, 108b
  for schizophrenia, 535, 536t–537t
Clinical trajectories, 108, 108b
Clomipramine (Anafranil), 227, 229t
Clonazepam (Klonopin), for aggression,
    562t
Clonidine (Catapres)
  for attention-deficit/hyperactivity
    disorder, 659
  for narcotic addiction, 593t
Clozapine (Clozaril), 236, 242t,
    244–245, 496–497, 499
  for aggression, 562t
  agranulocytosis and, 244–245
  for schizophrenia, 538t, 539
Club drugs, 577, 577f, 586, 588t, 671.
    See also Substance abuse
Clubhouse model, 299
Coaching, 146
Cocaine abuse, 587t. *See also* Substance
    abuse
  drug therapy for, 593t
  fetal effects of, 579, 580b
Codeine, abuse of, 588t. *See also*
    Substance abuse
Code of Ethics for Nurses (ANA), 125b
Cognex (tacrine), 634
Cognitions, 44–45, 138
  anxiety and, 350–351
Cognitive-behavioral theory, 42t,
    44–45, 46t
Cognitive-behavioral therapy, 137t, 143
  for anxiety disorders, 362–363, 363b,
    368
  for children and adolescents, 650, 668
  for eating disorders, 462

  for mood disorders, 492–494
  for schizophrenia, 540
  for somatoform disorders, 383
Cognitive deficits
  in delirium, 610–611
  in dementia, 618
  in schizophrenia, 530–534, 531b,
    532b
    assessment for, 542
    interventions for, 546–547
  tests for, 630t
Cognitive development, 645, 646t
Cognitive distortions, 139, 140t
  in depression, 493–494, 494f, 512
  in eating disorders, 468t
  in mood disorders, 485, 493–494,
    494f, 512
Cognitive mental disorders, 607–638
  amnestic disorders, 636–637, 638b
  assessment for, 627t, 628b, 629t,
    630t
  definition of, 608
  delirium, 609–617. *See also* Delirium
  dementia, 618–636. *See also*
    Dementia
  epidemiology of, 608
  etiology of, 608–609
  evaluation in, 636
  implementation in, 630–636
  medical problems in, 629b, 630–634
  nursing diagnoses for, 630
  overview of, 608–609
  planning in, 630, 631–632
Cognitive reframing, 363
  in anxiety disorders, 363
Cognitive relabeling, 46t
Cognitive restructuring, 42t, 44–45
  in anger management, 569
Cognitive theories, 42t
  of aggression, 558–559
  of anxiety, 352
  of substance abuse, 582
Cognitive therapy, 137t, 138–139,
    140t, 141b
  for anxiety disorders, 362–363
  for depression, 493–494, 494f
  for eating disorders, 462
Cognitive triad, 139
  of depression, 493, 494f
Commission for the Prevention of
    Youth Violence, 326
Commitment. *See also* Hospitalization
  conditional release from, 559
  decline in. *See* Deinstitutionalization
  involuntary, 117–118, 122, 123–124,
    303
    least restrictive environment and,
      559
  legal aspects of, 115–116, 117–118,
    122–124
  outpatient, 559

preventive, 559
racial bias and, 85
voluntary, 122–123
Communication
with aggressive clients, 569
assertive, 70
content, 154–155
decoding in, 63
definition of, 63
encoding in, 63
environment for, 63
family, schizophrenia and, 529–530
feedback in, 63
in groups, 154–157, 155t–156t, 157b
intercultural, 89–90
latent, 154
listening in, 64, 67b, 68b
manifest, 154
in mental status examination, 100b
noise in, 63–64
nontherapeutic, 64, 66t
with older adults, 687–688, 688b, 689t
passive-aggressive, 70
privileged, 121
process, 154–155
about religion/spirituality, 265–266
in schizophrenia, 530–531, 546, 548–549
about sexual expression, 409–410, 411t, 412b, 413b, 414–416
therapeutic, 63–72. See also Therapeutic communication
Communication channels, 63
Communicator, definition of, 63
Community mental health care, 294–297
assessment in, 304–305, 305b
case manager in, 295
for children and adolescents, 651
definition of, 294
deinstitutionalization and, 171b. See also Deinstitutionalization
ethical issues in, 127
evaluation in, 306
funding for, 302
goals of, 305–306
government involvement in, 295, 303–304
health promotion in, 296–297, 296b, 296t
historical perspective on, 294–295, 294b
homelessness and, 210–218
implementation in, 306
legislation affecting, 303
levels of prevention in, 295–297, 296t, 306
nurse's role in, 304–306
nursing diagnoses for, 305
nursing process in, 304–306

planning in, 305–306
populations served by, 294
poverty and, 302
public policy and, 303–304
reforms needed in, 303–304
reinstitutionalization and, 302
safety net services in, 303
for schizophrenia, 541–542
Community Mental Health Center Act of 1963, 171b, 211, 295, 541–542
Community mental health centers, 115, 295
Community support groups, 162, 163t
Community support program (CSP), 300
Community support systems, 297–304
child and adolescent, 300–301
community support program model for, 300
community worker models for, 299–300
components of, 297–298. See also Community mental health care
consumer-run alternative models for, 299
definition of, 297
Fairweather lodge model for, 299
funding for, 302
principles of, 298
program models for, 298–301
psychosocial rehabilitation model for, 299
training in community living model for, 299
Community worker models, 299–300
Comorbidity, 6, 535, 582. See also Substance abuse
in children and adolescents, 671
definition of, 582
Compeer program, 301
Complementary/alternative medicine, 257
acupuncture in, 277–278
aromatherapy in, 280–283
ayurvedic medicine in, 278
bioelectromagnetic therapy in, 285
biofield therapies in, 284–285
biologically based, 280–283, 281t–283t
classification of, 277
vs. conventional medicine, 278t
energy therapies in, 284
ethical aspects of, 276–277
federal funding for, 276
healing touch in, 284–285
herbal therapies in, 280, 281t–283t
homeopathy in, 278–279
imagery in, 279
legal aspects of, 277
licensure in, 277

manipulative/body-based methods in, 283–284
meditation in, 279
mind-body interventions in, 279–280
music therapy in, 279
naturopathy in, 278
nurse's role in, 285
overview of, 275–276
prayer in, 279–280
prevalence of, 276
professional certification in, 277
Reiki in, 285
research studies of, 276
spiritual healing in, 279–280. See also Spirituality
therapeutic touch in, 284–285
traditional Chinese medicine in, 277
types of, 277–279
Compliance, with drug therapy, 10, 253–254, 254b, 547–549
Compulsions, 358. See also Obsessive-compulsive disorder
Computed tomography (CT), 34t
Concepts, 38
Concerta (methylphenidate), 245–246, 246t, 659, 662b
Concordance rate, 31–32
Conditional release, 559
Conditioning, 43. See also Behavior therapy
classical, 141–142
in substance abuse, 582
Conduct disorder, 654, 664
Confabulation, 637
Confidentiality, 119t
trust and, 55
Conflict avoidance, eating disorders and, 473
Confrontation, in therapeutic communication, 70–71
Confusion Assessment Method (CAM), 614
Consensus, 153
Consent, 118–121, 119t, 303
fiscal, 121
substituted, 120–121
Consumer-run alternative models, 299
Contemplation, spiritual, 268
Contemporary nursing groups, 164
Content communication, 154–155
Contracts, in eating disorders, 469
Controlled substances, 586–589, 587t–589t. See also Substance abuse
Conversion disorder, 376t, 378t, 379b, 380–381. See also Somatoform disorders
Coping skills
assessment of, 207
in eating disorders, 473
for hospitalized children, 677–678

Coping skills (*continued*)
for nurse, 17–18, 18f
in personality disorders, 447
in schizophrenia, 549
spiritual, 268
in substance abuse, 600
Core beliefs, 139
Corporation for National Service, 637b
Corpus callosum, 28t
Correctional facilities. *See* Forensic
psychiatric nursing
Cortisol, 369
Counseling, by nurse, 147
Countertransference, 40, 60, 138
in groups, 156–157, 157b
Covert rehearsal, 363
Covington v. Harris, 122
Creutzfeldt-Jakob disease, 625
Crime, homelessness and, 215
Criminality
clinical example of, 193b–194b
forensic nursing and, 191–201. *See
also* Forensic psychiatric nursing
incarceration and, 192–193
population characteristics and,
193–196
substance abuse and, 193
Crisis
adventitious, 203–204
definition of, 201, 202
maturational, 203
phases of, 202–203
situational, 203
stress and, 201–202
types of, 203
Crisis group, 205–206
Crisis intervention, 204–210
assessment in, 206–207
clinical example of, 201b
crisis groups in, 205–206
definition of, 204
evaluation in, 210
family involvement in, 206
goals of, 208–209
implementation in, 209–210
nurse's role in, 147
nursing diagnoses in, 207
nursing process in, 206–210
planning in, 208–209
skills for, 205
team approach in, 205
telephone counseling in, 206
vs. traditional therapies, 205
Crisis prevention, 204, 204b
Crisis theory, 202–204, 202b
Critical pathways, 108, 108b
Critical periods, of brain development,
29
Cross-cultural understanding, 89
Cultural awareness, 79–80
development of, 90–91

Cultural barriers, to mental health care,
85
Cultural-bound concepts, 88
Cultural congruence, 83–84
Cultural factors
affecting older adults, 687
in behavioral home health care, 316b
in dissociative disorders, 423
in eating disorders, 458
in health beliefs and practices, 81t,
86–87, 86b
in health promotion/health
maintenance, 81t
in mental health promotion, 81t
in pediatric mental illness, 650b
in psychiatric–mental health care,
77–92
in somatoform disorders, 375
in substance abuse, 87, 581
Culturally competent care, 10, 81–84,
88–91
assessment in, 90
challenges in, 80
clinical example of, 77–79
communication in, 89–90
cultural awareness and, 79–80, 90–91
cultural self-awareness and, 90–91
culture care theory and, 84
definition of, 81
elements of, 82–83, 83f, 88–91
essential skills in, 88–90
example of, 83b
flexibility in, 90
folk healing in, 86b. *See also*
Complementary/alternative
medicine
health promotion in, 81t
knowledge base for, 90
model of, 83f
need for, 84–87
recommendations for, 82
religious/spiritual beliefs and, 86–87
research in, 90b
transcultural focus in, 88
treatment disparities/barriers and,
84–87
Cultural self-awareness, 91, 91b
Culture, 47, 77–92
assimilation and, 80
definition of, 79
demographic trends and, 79–80, 80t
health beliefs and practices of, 81t
health concepts and, 81t
medical anthropology and, 47
Culture-bound syndromes, 47, 375,
423
Culture care theory, 84
Curanderismo, 86b
Cyclothymic disorder, diagnostic criteria
for, 489b, 492
Cyproheptadine (Periactin), 409

D

Dalmane (flurazepam), 239t
Data, objective, for nursing diagnosis,
103
Date rape, 335
Dawn Project, 301
Decanoate injections, 249b
Decision making, group, 153
Declarative memory, 32
Decoding, 63
Defense mechanisms, 40, 41t
Deinstitutionalization, 115
aggressive/violent behavior and, 557
community mental health centers and,
115, 295. *See also* Community
mental health care
drug therapy and, 253, 254, 254b
failure of, 171b
family burden and, 170, 175. *See also*
Family burden
historical perspective on, 170, 171b
homelessness and, 211, 213–214
incarceration and, 192–193
reinstitutionalization and, 302
Delirium, 609–617
agitation in, 611, 614–617
clinical example of, 609
confusion in, 610–611, 614–617
definition of, 609
vs. dementia, 622t
diagnostic criteria for, 610–611,
610b, 612
environmental interventions for, 611
etiology of, 609, 610b
illness-related, 612
information map for, 612–613
nurse's response to, 609
nursing care plan for, 615–616
nursing process in, 613–617
in older adults, 691t
prevalence of, 612
prevention of, 612
prognosis of, 611
safety concerns in, 611, 617
signs and symptoms of, 610–611,
610b, 622t
in substance intoxication, 612
in substance withdrawal, 612
treatment of, 611–613
Delirium tremens, 585
Delusional disorder, 523b, 525
Delusions
in older adults, 691t
vs. religious beliefs, 266
in schizophrenia, 531b, 533
Dementia
AIDS-related, 624
alcoholic, 586
Alzheimer's, 619b, 621. *See also*
Alzheimer's disease

assessment in, 626–629, 627t, 628b, 629t, 630t
behavior problems in, 618–621
classification of, 621, 621b
client/family teaching in, 629
clinical example of, 607–608
in Creutzfeldt-Jakob disease, 625
vs. delirium, 622t
diagnostic criteria for, 618, 619–620
drug therapy for, 634–636
environmental modifications for, 634
evaluation in, 636
family concerns in, 623b, 625, 626–629, 636
in Huntington's chorea, 624, 627t
implementation in, 630–636
language deficits in, 618
learning deficits in, 618
medical interventions in, 625–626
medically caused, 620b
medical problems in, 629b, 630–634
memory deficits in, 618–621
nurse's response to, 609
nursing diagnoses for, 630
nursing process in, 626–636
in older adults, 691t
in Parkinson's disease, 624
in Pick's disease, 624–625, 627t
planning in, 630, 631–633
prevention of, 620
prognosis of, 625
psychosocial interventions in, 626
safety concerns in, 636
screening for, 629t
signs and symptoms of, 618–621, 622t
therapeutic communication in, 635b
treatment of, 625–626
types of, 621–625, 621b
vascular, 619b, 624, 627t, 691t
in Wernicke-Korsakoff syndrome, 586, 627t, 636–637
Democratic leader, 153
Demographic trends, 79–80, 80t
aging and, 686
Dendrites, 22, 24f
Denial, 41t
by family, 170
in substance abuse, 599–600, 601b–602b
Depakene (valproic acid), for aggression, 563t
Depakote (divalproex), 235t, 236, 498
Dependence
in alcohol abuse, 577, 584b
in substance abuse, 584b
Dependency, in somatoform disorders, 384–385, 391
Dependent personality disorder, 441b, 443, 445t. See also Personality disorder(s)

Depersonalization disorder, 424, 425b. See also Dissociative disorders
Depression, 479–514
anxiety and agitation in, 512
assessment in, 501–504
attention-deficit/hyperactivity disorder and, 668
biogenic amine hypothesis for, 482–483
in bipolar disorder, 491–492. See also Bipolar disorder
brain areas involved in, 482f
bulimia nervosa and, 459–462
in children and adolescents, 480–481, 666–668
in bipolar disorder, 668–669
suicide and, 673–674
classification of, 7
clinical example of, 479b–480b
cognitive distortions in, 493, 494f, 512
cognitive factors in, 485
cognitive therapy for, 138–139, 140t, 141b
cognitive triad of, 493, 494f
in cyclothymia, 489b, 492
diagnostic criteria for, 486–487
dissociative disorders and, 424
double, 667
drug therapy for, 227–234, 228t–232t, 494–497. See also Antidepressants
adherence to, 513
dysthymia and, 667
electroconvulsive therapy for, 500
endogenous, 486
epidemiology of, 480–481
etiology of, 481–486
evaluation in, 513
exogenous, 486
family issues in, 504
financial impact of, 492
genetic factors in, 481–482
hypochondriasis and, 381
implementation in, 504–513
learned helplessness and, 485
mental status examination in, 502–503
nursing care plans for, 506b–507b
nursing diagnoses for, 504
nursing process in, 501–513
nursing research in, 491b
in older adults, 481, 691t
personal hygiene in, 512
physical health concerns in, 509–512
physiological stability in, 503–504
physiologic factors in, 482–484
planning in, 504
postpartum, 490b
prognosis of, 492
psychodynamic factors in, 485
psychological factors in, 484–485, 484–486

reactive, 486
St. John's wort for, 257
in schizophrenia, 534
seasonal, 33, 500
self-care in, 491b
self-esteem in, 512
signs and symptoms of, 486–487
somatoform disorders and, 381
suicide in, 501–502, 502b, 504–509, 510b–511b. See also Suicide
treatment of, 492–501
vegetative signs in, 503–504
violence assessment in, 502
in women, 486, 486b
Depressive/Manic Depressive Association (DMDA), 171, 188
Descartes, René, 23b
Desensitization, systematic, 363
Designer drugs, 577, 577f, 586, 588t, 671. See also Substance abuse
Desipramine (Norpramin, Pertofrane), 227, 228t
for cocaine addiction, 593t
Desire phase, of sexual response cycle, 402
disorders of, 403, 406b, 409
Desyrel (trazodone), 231t, 233–234, 496, 563t
Detoxification
in alcohol abuse, 589–591, 590t, 591b, 595–599
in drug abuse, 591b, 595–599
Development
brain, 28–29
child, 644–647
cognitive, 28–29, 645, 646t
contemporary theories of, 646–647
ecological systems theory of, 646
ethology theory of, 646
information-processing theory of, 646
psychosexual, 645
Freud's model of, 40–41, 41t
psychosocial, 91, 203, 645, 646t, 662
in attention-deficit/hyperactivity disorder, 662–663
Vygotsky's theory of, 647
Developmental crisis, 203
Developmental ecological model, of mental illness, 47–50, 48t, 49f
Dextroamphetamine (Dexedrine), 245–246, 246t
Dextroamphetamine abuse, 587t. See also Substance abuse
Diagnosis
DSM-IV-TR categories and, 6–7
nursing, 102–106. See also Nursing diagnosis(es)
psychiatric, 103–106
Diagnostic and Statistical Manual of Mental Disorders (DSM-IV-TR), 6–7, 103–106

Diazepam (Valium), 237–239, 238t, 593t
for alcohol withdrawal, 590, 591
Dibenzothiazine (quetiapine), 243t, 245
Dichotomous thinking, in eating disorders, 468t
Diencephalon, 26, 27f, 28t
Diet, monoamine oxidase inhibitors and, 232–233
Diphenhydramine (Benadryl), for aggression, 562t
Disability, in children and adolescents, 674–679
Discharge planning, 106
for aggressive/violent clients, 564–565
Discrimination, racial, 44, 80, 85, 85b
Disease
chronic, in children and adolescents, 674–679
factitious, 377. *See also* Somatoform disorders
in homeless, 214–215
sexual expression and, 400–401, 404b
Disease prevention, 295
Disorientation
in delirium, 611–612, 614–616
in dementia, 618, 626
Disruptive behavior disorders, 658–664
Dissociation
continuum of, 422f
definition of, 422
vs. repression, 422
Dissociative amnesia, 424, 425b
Dissociative disorders, 421–433
clinical example of, 421
comorbidities and, 424
cultural aspects of, 423
definition of, 422
diagnostic criteria for, 424, 425
dual diagnoses and, 424
epidemiology of, 422–423
etiology of, 423–424
family dynamics and, 424
information map for, 425
nurse's attitude toward, 433b
nursing care plan for, 430b–431b
nursing process in, 428–431
risk/contributing factors for, 425
ritual abuse and, 423b, 426b
signs and symptoms of, 424
therapeutic communication in, 432b
treatment of, 424–428
Dissociative fugue, 424, 425b
Dissociative identity disorder, 422–423, 425b, 426b
Dissociative trance, 423
Disulfiram (Antabuse), 593t
Divalproex (Depakote), 235t, 236, 498
Divorce, 648
Dix, Dorothea, 115, 170, 171b
Documentation. *See also* Records

in behavioral home health care, 316–317
legal aspects of, 121
Domestic violence, 328–331
screening for, 329–330
Donepezil (Aricept), 634–635
Dopamine
in anorexia nervosa, 457
in depression, 483
in schizophrenia, 528–529
Dopamine agonists, for antipsychotic side effects, 539b
Double depression, 667
Down-regulation, 225
Doxepin (Sinequan), 227, 228t
Drug abuse. *See* Substance abuse
Drug therapy, 223–258. *See also specific drugs*
adherence to, 10, 253–254, 254b, 547–549
adverse effects of, 224, 240, 243t, 249–251, 250f–251f
affinity in, 224–225
for aggression, 561, 562t–564t
for agitation, 616–617
agonists in, 224
alternative agents and, 257
antagonists in, 224
for anxiety, 237–239, 238t–239t
assessment in, 247
for attention-deficit/hyperactivity disorder, 245–246, 246t, 659, 662b
for bipolar disorder, 234–237, 235t–236t, 494–495, 497–500
cardiotoxicity of, 251–252
for children and adolescents, 256, 651, 652
mania and, 669
client teaching for, 10b, 252b
costs of, 8
decanoate injections in, 249b
for delirium, 616–617
for dementia, 634–636
for depression, 227–234, 228t–232t, 494–497. *See also* Antidepressants
in children, 668
development of, 247b
for dissociative disorders, 427
down-regulation in, 225
drug interactions in, 225
for eating disorders, 463
efficacy of, 225
evaluation in, 255
expected drug reaction in, 249
family involvement in, 254, 255b–256b
for family members, 185
homelessness and, 214b, 217
implementation of, 252–255
loss of efficacy of, 225

maximal efficacy of, 225
method of administration in, 248
for mood disorders, 227–237, 492–494
nursing diagnoses for, 248, 248b
nursing process in, 246–255
nursing research in, 257
for older adults, 256, 693–695
for personality disorders, 444, 446b
planning in, 248–252
polypharmacy in, 225
potency in, 225
in pregnancy and lactation, 255, 255b
prescribed maximum dose in, 248
principles of, 224–225
receptor binding in, 224
refractoriness in, 225
right to refuse, 115, 122
for schizophrenia, 239–245, 537–540, 538t, 539b. *See also* Antipsychotics
adherence to, 547–549
client teaching about, 548–549
self-clarification and, 254–255
side effects of, 10b, 224, 240, 243t, 249, 250f–251f
in older adults, 695
sexual, 405t
stimulants in, 245–246, 246t
for substance abuse, 591, 592t
target symptoms for, 225
DSM-IV-TR (Diagnostic and Statistical Manual of Mental Disorders), 6–7, 103–106
Dual diagnosis, 6, 535, 582. *See also* Substance abuse
in children and adolescents, 671
Dualism, Cartesian, 23
Due process, 303
Duman, Rhetaugh, 82b
Dura mater, 25
Duty to warn, 121, 559
Dyslexia, genetic factors in, 32
Dyspareunia, 405, 407b
Dysrhythmias, antipsychotics and, 251–252
Dysthymia
in children, 667
depression and, 667
diagnostic criteria for, 487–488
Dystonia, antipsychotics and, 240, 243t, 538

E

Eating disorders, 455–474, 671
anorexia nervosa, 456
assessment in, 464–467, 465b, 466t–467t
binge-eating disorder, 456, 457b

bulimia nervosa, 456
client/family teaching in, 472b
clinical example of, 461b–462b
cognitive distortions in, 468t
comorbidities and dual diagnoses for, 459–462
diagnostic criteria for, 459
dissociative disorders and, 424
etiology of, 456–459, 458f
evaluation in, 473–474
implementation in, 469–473
information map for, 460b–461b
nursing care plan for, 470b–471b
nursing diagnoses for, 467–468
nursing process in, 464–474
nutritional assessment in, 464
planning in, 468, 470b–471b
prevention of, 460b–461b, 472
prognosis of, 462
risk/contributing factors in, 460b
signs and symptoms of, 459
therapeutic communication in, 465b
treatment of, 462–463
Ecological factors, in mental illness, 48–50, 48t, 49f
Ecological model
definition of, 324
of violence, 324–325
Ecological systems theory, 646
Ecstasy, 577, 577f, 586, 588t, 671. See also Substance abuse
Education
family, 183–185. See also Client/family teaching
nursing
group process in, 162–164
needed improvements in, 177–178
Educational needs
in attention-deficit/hyperactivity disorder, 662–663
of hospitalized children, 678
of mentally ill children, 302
Efficacy, drug, 225
Ego, 40, 40t
Ejaculation, premature, 405, 406b
Elavil. See Amitriptyline (Elavil)
Elder abuse, 333–334, 692t
Elderly. See Older adults
Electroconvulsive therapy, 500
Electroencephalography, 34t
Elite old, 686
Ellis, Albert, 143–144
Emergency admission, 123
Emergency department
screening for domestic violence in, 329–330
treatment of rape victims in, 338–339
Emotional maltreatment
of children, 331–333
of older adults, 333–334

Emotional reasoning, in eating disorders, 464, 468t
Empathy, 57, 108
Employment problems, 302
Encoding, 63
Encounter groups, 162
Endocrine system, nervous system and, 33
Endocrine treatment, for gender identity disorders, 417
Energy therapies, 284–285
Enmeshed families, eating disorders and, 473
Environment
communication, 63
heredity and, 32
Environmental modifications
for delirium, 611, 616, 617
for dementia, 634
Epilepsy, aggression and, 558
Erectile dysfunction, 403–405, 406b, 409, 410t
nursing care plan for, 415b
Erikson, Milton, 136b, 144
Erikson's developmental theory, 91, 203, 645, 646t, 662
Ethanol. See Alcohol
Ethical dilemmas, 126, 127
Ethical issues, 125–129
autonomy, 126
beneficence, 126
boundary-related, 55, 56t, 127–129
in community mental health, 127127
in complementary/alternative medicine, 276–277
fidelity, 126
justice, 127
paternalism, 126
in spiritual care, 269–270
veracity, 126
Ethics
definition of, 125
everyday, 125
Ethnic groups. See Racial/ethnic groups
Ethnocentrism, 80
Ethology theory, 646
Evaluation, 109–110
Everyday ethics, 125
Evil eye, 86b
Excitement phase, of sexual response cycle, 402
Exelon (rivastigmine), 634–636
Exercise, compulsive, in anorexia nervosa, 464, 469
Exhibitionism, 407b, 416
Existential factors, in group therapy, 161
Explicit memory, 32
Expressed emotion, 183
Expressive violence, 194
External noise, 63–64

Extrapyramidal symptoms, antipsychotic, 240, 244t, 249, 250f–251f, 538, 538t
Eye movement desensitization and reprocessing, 337

F

Factitious disorder, 377
Fairweather lodge model, 299
False memory syndrome, 426–427, 426b
False pregnancy, 381
Family
in attention-deficit/hyperactivity disorder, 662
as cause of mental illness, 175–178, 180
in crisis intervention, 206
in dementia, 623b, 625, 626–629, 636, 637b
drug therapy for, 185
in eating disorders, 458–459, 473
empowerment of, 183
enmeshed, 473
in forensic nursing, 200
of hospitalized child, 674–679
involvement of in treatment, 176b–177b
in medication management, 254, 255b–256b
mentor, 179
in mood disorders, 504
pediatric mental illness and, 647, 648–649
psychotherapy for, 185
resilient, 178, 179b
response of to mental illness, 11, 11t, 172b. See also Family burden
risk factors for, 178–179
secondary prevention for, 178–185
support services for, 183. See also Support groups
teaching of. See Client/family teaching
therapeutic communication with, 72, 176b–177b
Family adaptation model, 11, 11t
Family advocacy movement, 11, 11t
Family assessment, in pediatric mental illness, 675–676
Family burden, 170–178
health consequences of, 178–179
iatrogenic, 175
objective, 171–173
as risk factor, 178–179
subjective, 173–175
Family caregiving, 170–178. See also Family burden
historical perspective on, 170
Family-centered care, 676b

Family communication patterns, schizophrenia and, 529–530
Family consultation, 179–180
  clinical example of, 180b
  components of, 180
  vs. family therapy, 180
  nurse's role in, 180–183
  research in, 181b
Family education, 183–185
  nurse's role in, 184
  peer-taught, 184–185
Family psychoeducation, 183
Family support services, 183
Family systems model, 458–459
Family teaching. *See* Client/family teaching
Family therapy, 180
  for aggression, 561
  for children and adolescents, 650
  for eating disorders, 463
  for mood disorders, 492
  for pediatric depression, 678
  for personality disorders, 445
Family to Family Education Program (NAMI), 184–185, 184b
Family violence, 328–334
  child maltreatment, 331–333, 648
  elder abuse, 333–334, 692t
  intimate partner, 328–331, 335–336
FAST TRACK, 325
Father. *See* Family
FDA, in complementary/alternative medicine, 276–277
Fears. *See also* Anxiety
  of family members, 173
  of hospitalized children, 675t
Feedback, 63
Fellowship, 269
Female offenders, 194, 195b
Female orgasmic disorder, 405, 406b
Female sexual arousal disorder, 403, 406b, 409
Fetal alcohol syndrome, 579, 580b
Fetishism, 407b, 416
  transvestic, 407b–408b, 416
Fidelity, 126
Fight-or-flight reaction, 350, 369
First messengers, 23–24
Fiscal informed consent, 121
Flattened affect, in schizophrenia, 531b, 533–534
Flexibility, 90
Flooding, 363
Fluoxetine (Prozac), 231t–232t, 233–234
  for aggression, 563t
  for obsessive-compulsive disorder, 359
Fluphenazine (Prolixin), 241t, 244
  for schizophrenia, 538t
Flurazepam (Dalmane), 239t
Folie à deux, 523b, 525

Folk healers, 86b
Food and Drug Administration, in complementary/alternative medicine, 276–277
Forbidden love, 199
Forensic psychiatric nurses
  attitudes of, 196–197
  dual responsibilities of, 196
  skills of, 197
Forensic psychiatric nursing, 191–201
  assessment in, 198
  boundary issues in, 199, 200b
  causes of incarceration and, 192–193
  client advocacy in, 201
  client characteristics in, 193–196
  clinical example of, 193b–194b
  continuity of care in, 200–201
  evaluation in, 201
  family concerns in, 199, 200
  female offenders and, 194, 195b
  health promotion in, 199–200
  HIV/hepatitis-infected offenders in, 195–196
  homelessness and, 215
  implementation in, 199–201
  juvenile offenders and, 194
  levels of prevention in, 197b
  mentally ill offenders and, 193–194
  nursing diagnoses in, 198
  nursing process in, 198–201
  nursing research in, 195b
  older adult offenders and, 194–195
  planning in, 198–199
  safety issues in, 194
  settings for, 192
  stressors in, 196b
  subspecialties of, 192b
  suicide in, 198
  team approach in, 199, 200
  therapeutic relationship in, 199
  violent offenders and, 194
Foreplay, 402
Forgiveness, 268–269
Formal groups, 152
Fornix, 28
Fountain House, 299
Free association, 138
Freud, Sigmund, 39, 39f, 136, 136b, 137t, 138, 374b, 527b
Freudian theory, 39–41, 645
Frontal lobe, 26, 27f, 27t
Frotteurism, 407b, 416
Fugue, dissociative, 424, 425b
Functional health patterns assessment guide, 466t–467t

G

Gabapentin (Neurontin), 234, 235t, 237, 500

Gang violence, 194. *See also* Violence
  risk factors for, 326–327
Gay/lesbian sexual preference, 399–400
Gender boundaries, 647
Gender identity disorders, 407b, 408b, 417
Gender roles, 400
Generalization, behaviorist view of, 43–44
Generalized anxiety disorder, 353–357, 363t
  in children, 665
General personality disorder, 439b
Generational boundaries, 647
Genetics, 30–32
Genital stage, 41t
Genuineness, 57
Geodon (ziprasidone), 538t, 540
Ginkgo biloba, 281t
Ginseng, 281t
Glasser, W., 144
Glial cells, 22
Globus pallidus, 28
Glutethimide, abuse of, 588t. *See also* Substance abuse
Goals, long- vs. short-term, 107t
Graduated exposure, 363
Grief
  in family members, 173
  in older adults, 687
Grooming
  in mental status examination, 100b, 503
  in mood disorders, 512
  in schizophrenia, 532
Group(s), 151–164
  characteristics of, 152
  cohesiveness of, 161
  communication in, 154–157, 155t–156t, 157b
  community support, 162, 163t. *See also* Support groups
  crisis, 205–206
  decision-making in, 153
  definition of, 152
  development of, 157, 158t
  encounter, 162
  formal, 152
  informal, 152
  mature, 157, 158t
  nursing, historical perspective on, 164
  in nursing education, 162–164
  in nursing practice, 164
  power in, 152
  primary, 152
  roles in, 154
  secondary, 152
  structure of, 153–154
  study, 163–164
  T, 152–153, 162

transference/countertransference in, 156–157, 157b
types of, 152
Group leadership, 152–153, 152–154
Group norms, 152
Group therapy, 158–164
  advantages and disadvantages of, 158–160
  for aggression, 561
  for children and adolescents, 650
  common problems in, 159t–160t
  for dissociative disorders, 427
  for eating disorders, 463
  growth-oriented, 162
  nurse's role in, 164
  for personality disorders, 445
  psychotherapeutic, 161–162
  purposes of, 158
  for schizophrenia, 540
  therapeutic factors in, 160–161
  types of, 161–162
Growth groups, 162
Guarana, 281t
Guided discovery, 560
Guided imagery, 268
Guilt, in family members, 173
Gypsies, health beliefs and practices of, 81t

H

Habit reversal therapy, 673
Haley, Jay, 136b
Hallucinations
  alcohol-induced, 585–586
  in delirium, 610
  in schizophrenia, 531b, 533, 546–547
Hallucinogens, 588t. *See also* Substance abuse
Haloperidol (Haldol), 242t, 244
  adverse effects of, 10b
  for aggression, 562t
  for delirium, 616–617
  for schizophrenia, 538t
Hardiness, 679
  in older adults, 686
Harper, Mary, 82b
Hatfield, Agnes, 183–184
Head Start, 649
Healing touch, 284–285
Health. *See also* Mental health
  definition of, 3
Health beliefs and practices
  assessment of, 90
  cultural factors in, 81t, 86–87, 86b
  knowledge of, 90
  religious beliefs and, 86–87, 86b
Health history, 97–99, 98t–99t

Health promotion/health maintenance
  in community mental health, 295, 296t
  cultural factors in, 81t
  in forensic nursing, 199
  nurse's role in, 146
Health teaching, 147
Hepatitis
  alcoholic, 586
  in incarcerated population, 195–196
Herbal remedies, 257. *See also* Complementary/alternative medicine
Heroin, 588t. *See also* Substance abuse
Heterosexuality, 399
Heterozygosity, 31
Hippocampus, 26
  anxiety and, 352
Hispanic Americans. *See also* Culture; Racial/ethnic groups
  folk healers of, 86, 86b
  health beliefs and practices of, 81t, 88
  increasing population of, 79–80, 80t
History
  abuse, 652
  developmental, 652
  family, 651–652
  health, 97–99, 98t–99t
  pediatric, 651–652
  school, 652
  sexual, 410–411, 412b, 413b
  social, 652
  spiritual, 267
Histrionic personality disorder, 440b, 442–443, 445t. *See also* Personality disorder(s)
HIV infection. *See* Human immunodeficiency virus infection
Hoff's crisis paradigm, 209
Holistic health, 294
Holistic medicine. *See* Complementary/alternative medicine
Home care
  behavioral, 311–321. *See also* Behavioral health home care
  definition of, 311–321, 312
Homelessness, 210–218
  advocacy for, 217
  assessment in, 215, 216b
  case management in, 217
  clinical example of, 210b
  contributing factors in, 211b, 212–213
  crime and, 215
  deinstitutionalization and, 211, 213–214
  demographics of, 210
  evaluation in, 217–218
  historical perspective on, 211b
  implementation in, 217

medication management and, 214b, 217
  mental health care and, 213–215
  mental illness and, 210–215
  nursing diagnoses for, 215–216
  nursing process and, 215–218
  physical disorders and, 214–215
  planning in, 216–217
  shelter system and, 214
  substance abuse and, 211, 213
  therapeutic communication and, 216b
  therapeutic relationship and, 217
Homeopathy, 278–279
Homosexuality, 399–400
  sexual assessment and, 414b
Homozygosity, 31
Hope, 161
Hops, 281t
Horizontal violence, 17
Hormone treatment, for gender identity disorders, 417
Hospitalization. *See also* Commitment
  of children, for medical illness/disability, 674–679
  deinstitutionalization and. *See* Deinstitutionalization
  delirium and, 609–617
  emergency, 123
  historical perspective on, 115
  intake screening/evaluation in, 147
  involuntary, 117–118, 122, 123–124, 303
    least restrictive environment and, 559
  legal aspects of, 117–118, 122, 123
  racial bias and, 85
  revolving door, 9, 171
    incarceration and, 192
  sexual expression and, 400–401
  voluntary, 122–123
Hostility, aggression and, 556. *See also* Aggression
Hotlines, crisis, 206
5-HT. *See* Serotonin
Huffing, 587t. *See also* Substance abuse
Human immunodeficiency virus infection
  dementia in, 624
  in incarcerated population, 195–196
  prevention of, safer sex practices for, 399b
Humanism, 45–46
Human sexual response cycle, 401–402
Huntington's chorea, 624, 627t
Hya-byung, 375
Hydromorphone, abuse of, 588t. *See also* Substance abuse
5-Hydroxytryptophan. *See* Serotonin
Hyperactivity. *See* Attention-deficit/hyperactivity disorder

Hypertensive crisis, monoamine oxidase inhibitors and, 498

Hyperventilation, in anxiety disorders, 368

Hypervigilance, hypochondriasis and, 381

Hypnotics. *See* Sedative-hypnotics

Hypoactive sexual desire disorder, 403, 406b, 409

Hypochondriasis, 376t, 378t, 380b, 381, 384t. *See also* Somatoform disorders

Hypomania, 491
    in cyclothymia, 489b, 492

Hypothalamic-pituitary-adrenal axis, 483–484, 483f, 484f

Hypothalamus, 28t

Hypothesis, 38

Hysteria, 374b

I

Ice, 587t

Id, 40, 40t

Identification, 41t

Illness
    chronic, in children and adolescents, 674–679
    factitious, 377. *See also* Somatoform disorders
    in homeless, 214–215
    sexual expression and, 400–401, 404b

Illusions, in delirium, 610

Imagery, 279, 369

Imipramine (Tofranil), 227, 228t

Immune system, nervous system and, 33

Implementation. *See also* Interventions
    in nursing process, 108–109

Implicit memory, 32

Impotence, 403–405, 406b, 409, 410t
    nursing care plan for, 415b

Imprisonment, 192–193. *See also* Forensic psychiatric nursing

Impulse-control disorders, 556

Impulsivity
    aggression and, 556
    in attention-deficit/hyperactivity disorder, 654, 658

Incarceration, 192–193. *See also* Forensic psychiatric nursing
    mental health effects of, 196, 196b

Inderal (propranolol), for aggression, 564t

Individual roles, 154

Individual therapy, 135–148. *See also* Psychotherapy

Informal groups, 152

Information-processing perspective, developmental, 646

Information technology, in crisis intervention, 209–210

Informed consent, 118–121, 119t, 303
    fiscal, 121
    substituted, 120–121

Inhalant abuse, 587t. *See also* Substance abuse

Injections, decanoate, 249b

Insight
    in mental status examination, 101b, 503
    in schizophrenia, 534

Instrumental violence, 194

Intake screening/evaluation, 147

Intellectualization, 41t

Intensive case management, for schizophrenia, 542

Intercultural communication, 89–90

International Association of Forensic Nurses (IAFN), 192

International Society of Psychiatric Nurses (ISPN), 653

Internet resources
    in crisis intervention, 209–210
    for hospitalized children, 678

Interpersonal perspective, 46

Interpersonal therapy, 46
    for eating disorders, 462–463

Interventions, 107–109. *See also* Treatment
    advanced, 108b
    basic, 108b
    for beginning practitioner, 109
    levels of prevention and, 295–296, 296t
    selection of, 106–108
    supervision in, 109

Interview, 97, 97b
    of homeless, 216b

Intimate partner violence, 328–331
    screening for, 329–330

Intoxication
    in alcohol abuse, 585
    in substance abuse, 584b
    delirium in, 612

Involuntary admissions, 117–118, 122, 123–124, 303
    decline in. *See* Deinstitutionalization
    least restrictive environment and, 559

Irrational beliefs, 44–45, 45b

Irtazapine (clozapine). *See* Clozapine (Clozaril)

Islam, 77–79

Isocarboxazid (Marplan), 230t, 232–233

J

Jo, Jeanni, 82b

Job-related problems, 302

Joint Commission on Accreditation of Healthcare Organizations (JCAHO), 118, 121

Journal writing, 269

Judgment, in mental status examination, 101b, 503

Judgmental attitudes, 57–58

Jung, Carl, 527b

Justice, 127

Juvenile offenders, 194

K

Kava kava, 281t–282t

Kent, Elizabeth Lipford, 82b

Kindling, 558

Klonopin (clonazepam), for aggression, 562t

Knuz, Dora, 284–285

Koro, 47

Korsakoff syndrome, 586, 636–637

Kraepelin, Emil, 527b

Krieger, Dolores, 284–285

L

La belle indifference, 381, 385

Lactation, drug therapy in, 255

Laissez-faire leader, 153

Lamotrigine (Lamictal), 236t, 237, 499

Language problems
    in autism, 670
    in dementia, 618
    in schizophrenia, 530–531, 546, 548–549

Latency stage, 41t

Latent communication, 154

Latinos. *See* Hispanic Americans

Lawyers, utilization of, 117

Leadership
    autocratic, 153
    democratic, 153
    group, 152–153
    laissez-faire, 153
    power and, 152–153

Learning
    in children, 30b
    neuroplasticity and, 30, 32

Learning disabilities
    in attention-deficit/hyperactivity disorder, 662–663
    genetic factors in, 32

Learning theory, 44–45
    anxiety disorders and, 352
    substance abuse and, 582

Least restrictive environment, 122, 559

Legal counsel, utilization of, 117

Legal issues, 114–125
    battery, 120

client rights, 117–118, 118b
clinical example of, 114
in community mental health, 303
in complementary/alternative
medicine, 277
confidentiality, 119t, 121
expanded role of nursing, 116
forensic clients, 124
historical perspective on, 115–116
informed consent, 118–121, 119t,
303
involuntary admissions, 117, 122,
123–124, 303, 559–560
least restrictive environment, 122,
559
malpractice, 116–117, 117b
medical records, 121
need for legal counsel, 117
nurse practice acts, 116
preventive admissions, 559
restraint, 117–118, 118b, 561–564,
653
right to aftercare, 122
right to treatment, 122
treatment of minors, 124–125
treatment refusal, 115, 122
voluntary admissions, 122–123, 559
Leininger, Madeleine, 82, 84, 90
Lesbians, 399–400
Liability, malpractice and, 116–117
Librium. *See* Chlordiazepoxide
(Librium)
Licensure, in
complementary/alternative
medicine, 277
Light therapy, for depression, 500
Limbic system, 26–28, 27f, 28t
Limit setting, for aggression, 560, 568
Listening skills, 64, 67b, 68b
in psychotherapy, 136
Lithium, 234–237, 235t, 498, 499t
for aggression, 563t
arrhythmias and, 252
for children, 669
toxicity of, 498, 499t
Liver disease, alcoholic, 586
Living wills, 303
Locus ceruleus, 352
Loose associations, 530, 532b
Lopressor (metoprolol), 564t
Lorazepam (Ativan), 237–239, 238t
for aggression, 562t
for alcohol withdrawal, 590, 591
for delirium, 617
for obsessive-compulsive disorder,
359
Loss of drug efficacy, 225
Louisville Behavior Checklist, 429
Low serotonin syndrome, 558
Loxapine (Loxitane), for schizophrenia,
538t

LSD, 588t. *See also* Substance abuse
Ludiomil (maprotiline), 229t, 232, 497

M

Magnetic resonance imaging (MRI), 34t
Magnification, in eating disorders, 468t
Major depressive disorder. *See also*
Depression; Mood disorders
diagnostic criteria for, 486–487
Majority vote, 153
Mal aire, 86b
Male erectile dysfunction, 403–405,
406b, 409, 410t
nursing care plan for, 415b
Male orgasmic disorder, 405, 406b, 409
Malingering, 377
Mal ojo, 86b
Malpractice, 116–117, 117b
Maltreatment. *See* Abuse
Managed care, 8, 115–116
Mania, 490–491. *See also* Bipolar
disorder
drug-related, in children, 669
drug therapy for, 234–237, 235t–236t
nursing care plan for, 105b–106b,
507b–509b
refractory, 237–238
treatment of, 499–500
signs and symptoms of, 490–491
Manifest communication, 154
Manipulative therapies, 283–284
Mantras, 279
Maprotiline (Ludiomil), 229t, 232, 497
Marijuana, 587t. *See also* Substance
abuse
Marital rape, 335
Marplan (isocarboxazid), 230t,
232–233
Marriage
divorce and, 648
mental health and, 47
mental illness and, 185
in children, 648–649
violence in, 328–331
Maslow, Abraham, 136b
Maslow's hierarchy of needs, 58–59, 60f
Masochism, 407b, 416
Massage, 284
Masturbation, by client, 400–401
Maturational crisis, 203
Mature group, 157, 158t
Maturity, self-awareness and, 60
Maximal drug efficacy, 225
Medical anthropology, 47
Medical conditions
chronic, in children and adolescents,
674–679
factitious, 377. *See also* Somatoform
disorders

in homeless, 214–215
sexual expression and, 400–401, 404b
Medical model, 47
Medical play, 674–675
Medical records. *See also*
Documentation
client's rights to, 121
legal issues involving, 121
Medicare/Medicaid, 302
for behavioral health home care, 320
for community mental health care, 320
Medications. *See* Drug therapy
Meditation, 268, 279
Medulla oblongata, 26
Mellaril (thioridazine). *See* Thioridazine
(Mellaril)
Memory, 32
assessment of, 101b
repressed, 422, 426–427, 426b
Memory deficits
alcohol-related, 586
in amnestic disorders, 636–637, 638b
in delirium, 610–611
in dementia, 618, 626
Mendel, Gregor, 31
Meninges, 25
Mental disorders, definition of, 4
Mental health, 4
elements of, 5, 5f
influences on, 5, 5f
Surgeon General's report on, 4, 6
*Mental Health: A Report of the Surgeon
General,* 4, 6
Mental health care. *See*
Psychiatric–mental health care;
Treatment
Mental health-illness continuum, 4
Mental health nursing, 12. *See also*
Psychiatric–mental health nursing
Mental health promotion
in community mental health,
295–196
cultural factors in, 81t
in forensic nursing, 199
nurse's role in, 146
Mental Health Study Act, 295
Mental Health Systems Act, 295
Mental illness
in children, 643–679. *See also*
Children
classification of, 6–7
definition of, 4
developmental ecological model of,
47–50, 48t, 49f
diagnosis of, 6–7
distal factors for, 48
etiology of, 6
family as cause of, 177–178
genetic factors in, 31–32
homelessness and, 210–218. *See also*
Homelessness

Mental illness (*continued*)
  incidence and prevalence of, 5–6
  mind-body connection and, 23b
  occupational problems and, 302
  in older adults, 680–687. *See also*
    Older adults; Older adults,
    mental illness in
  poverty and, 302
  protective factors for, 48, 48t
  proximal factors for, 48
  in racial/ethnic minorities, 84–85
  risk factors for, 48, 48t
  serious, 170
  severe, chronicity of, 301–302
  social disability due to, 301–302
  stigma of, 8–9, 302–303
  substance abuse and, 6, 535, 582
  treatment of, 8–11. *See also*
    Intervention; Psychiatric–mental
    health care *and under*
    Therapeutic
Mental retardation, in older adults, 692t
Mental status examination, 99–102,
    100b–101b
  in delirium, 614, 614b
  in dementia, 626, 629t, 630t
  in mood disorders, 502–503
  pediatric, 652
Mental stimulation, in older adults, 696,
    697b
Mentgen, Janet, 285
Mentor families, 179
Meperidine, abuse of, 588t. *See also*
    Substance abuse
Mescaline, 588t. *See also* Substance abuse
Methadone, 593t
  abuse of, 588t. *See also* Substance
    abuse
Methamphetamine, 587t. *See also*
    Substance abuse
Methaqualone, 588t. *See also* Substance
    abuse
Methylphenidate (Ritalin), 245–246,
    246t, 659, 662b
Metoprolol (Lopressor), 564t
Mexican Americans. *See* Hispanic
    Americans
Meyer, Adolf, 527b
Midbrain, 26
Middle old, 686
Milieu management, 428
  for schizophrenia, 540
Milieu therapy, for children and
    adolescents, 650
Mind-body connection, 23b
Mind-body interventions, 279–280
Mini-Mental Status Examination. *See*
    also Mental status examination
  in delirium, 614, 614b
Minority groups. *See* Racial/ethnic
    groups

Minority vote, 153
Mint, 282t
Mirtazapine (Remeron), 227, 229t,
    232, 496–497
Modeling, 44
Molindone (Moban), for schizophrenia,
    538t
Moller, Mary, 184
Monoamine oxidase, aggression and, 558
Monoamine oxidase inhibitors
    (MAOIs), 229t–230t, 232–233,
    233b, 497, 498f. *See also*
    Antidepressants
Mood
  vs. affect, 532
  assessment of
    in mental status examination, 100b,
      503
    in schizophrenia, 542
  definition of, 480
  depression of, 489
Mood disorders. *See also* Bipolar
    disorder; Depression; Dysthymia
  anxiety and agitation in, 512
  assessment in, 501–504
  in children and adolescents, 480–481,
    666–669
  cognitive problems in, 485, 493,
    494f, 512
  definition of, 480
  diagnostic criteria for, 486–492
  drug therapy for, 227–237, 494–500
    adherence to, 513
  epidemiology of, 480–481
  etiology of, 481–486
  evaluation in, 513
  family issues in, 504
  implementation in, 504–513
  information map for, 488b–489b
  learned helplessness and, 485
  mental status examination in,
    502–503
  mood stabilizers for, 234–237,
    235t–236t
  nursing care plans for, 506b–509b
  nursing diagnoses for, 504
  nursing process in, 501–513
  nursing research in, 491b
  in older adults, 481
  personal hygiene in, 512
  physical health concerns in, 509–512
  physiological stability in, 503–504
  planning in, 504
  prevalence of, 488b
  prognosis of, 492
  psychodynamic factors in, 485
  psychological factors in, 484–485
  risk factors for, 488b
  self-care in, 491b
  self-esteem in, 512
  signs and symptoms of, 486–492

somatic nonpharmacologic treatment
    for, 500–501
  suicide in, 501–502, 502b, 504–509,
    510b–511b. *See also* Suicide
  treatment of, 492–501
  violence in, 502, 509, 511b. *See also*
    Violence
  in women, 486, 486b
Mood stabilizers, 234–237, 235t–236t,
    497–500
  for aggression, 563t
  for children, 669
Morphine, abuse of, 588t. *See also*
    Substance abuse
Mother. *See* Family
Motor side effects, of antipsychotics,
    240, 244t, 249, 250f–251f,
    538–539, 538t
Multidisciplinary approach, 47–48
Multiple personality disorder, 422
Murillo-Rohde, Ildaura, 82b
Music therapy, 279
Muslims, 77–79
Mysoline (primidone), 236t, 237

N

Naltrexone (Trexan), 593t
NAMI, 177–178, 183, 188–189, 295
  Caring/Sharing groups of, 206
  Family to Family Education Program
    of, 184–185, 184b
Narcissistic personality disorder, 440b,
    443, 445t. *See also* Personality
    disorder(s)
Narcotic abuse/addiction, 588t. *See also*
    Substance abuse
  drug therapy for, 593t
Narcotics Anonymous (NA), 582
Nardil (phenelzine sulfate), 229t–230t,
    232–233
National Alliance for Mental Patients
    (NAMP), 295
National Alliance for the Mentally Ill
    (NAMI). *See* NAMI
National Center for Complementary
    and Alternative Medicine
    (NCCAM), 257, 276
National Formulary, 280
National Institute of Mental Health
    (NIMH), 295, 297
National Institutes of Health (NIH), 276
Nation's Voice on Mental Illness
    (NAMI). *See* NAMI
Native Americans. *See also* Racial/ethnic
    groups
  discrimination against, 84
  health beliefs and practices of, 81t,
    87–88
  mental illness in, 84

Naturopathy, 278. *See also*
    Complementary/alternative
    medicine
Navane (thiothixene), 242t, 244
    for schizophrenia, 538t
Nefazodone (Serzone), 230t–231t, 233,
    495
Negative emotionality, aggression and,
    558
Negative reinforcement, 43, 142
Negative symptoms, in schizophrenia,
    530, 531t, 533–534
Neglect
    child, 331–333
    elder, 333–334
Negligence, 116–117
Neologisms, 531, 532b
Nervous system
    development of, 28–29
    endocrine system and, 33
    immune system and, 33
    structure and function of, 24, 26f,
        27f, 27t–29t, 30
Neuroanatomy, 22–32
Neuroendocrine system, 33
Neuroglia, 25
Neuroimaging techniques, 33, 34t
Neuroleptic malignant syndrome, 240,
    539
    in older adults, 695
Neuroleptics. *See* Antipsychotics
Neurologic examination
    in delirium, 614, 614b, 626, 630t
    in dementia, 626, 629t, 630t
Neurons, 22, 24f
Neurontin (gabapentin), 234, 235t,
    237, 500
Neuropeptides, 33
Neurophysiology, 22–32
Neuroplasticity, 24, 29–30
    learning and, 30, 32
    memory and, 32
Neurotransmitters, 22–24, 24f, 25t
    aggression and, 558
    in depression, 483, 483f
    in eating disorders, 457
    reuptake of, 23
    in schizophrenia, 528–529
Nimodipine (Nimotop), 236t
Noise, in communication, 63–64
Nonadherence, to drug therapy, 10,
    253–254, 254b, 547–549
Nontherapeutic communication, 64,
    66t
Norepinephrine
    aggression and, 558
    in depression, 483, 483f
    in schizophrenia, 529
Norms, group, 152
Norpramin. *See* Desipramine
    (Norpramin, Pertofrane)

North American Nursing Diagnosis
    Association (NANDA),
    102–103, 102f, 110f
Nortriptyline (Aventyl, Pamelor), 227,
    228t
Nurse. *See also* Psychiatric–mental health
    nurse
    advanced practice, 146
Nurse'self-care, in pediatric mental
    health care, 679
Nursing
    mental health, 12
    psychiatric, 12. *See also*
        Psychiatric–mental health nursing
Nursing care plan. *See also* Planning
    for aggression, 567–568
    for alcohol abuse, 598–599
    for Alzheimer's disease, 631–633
    for anorexia nervosa, 470–471
    for attention-deficit/hyperactivity
        disorder, 661
    for bipolar disorder, 105–106,
        507–509
    in community mental health care,
        305–306
    in crisis intervention, 208
    for delirium, 615–616
    for depression, 507–509
    example of, 105–106
    for personality disorders, 448
    for post-traumatic stress disorder,
        360–361
    for rape/sexual assault, 340
    sample, 104–105
    for schizophrenia, 544–546
    for sexual dysfunction disorders,
        415
    for somatoform disorders, 387–388
    standardized, 107–108
Nursing diagnosis(es), 102–107
    axes of, 102–103
    correct vs. incorrect, 104t
    definition of, 102
    examples of, 104t
    flowchart for, 110f
    objective data for, 103
    selection and formulation of, 103
    taxonomy of, 102–103, 103f
Nursing education
    group process in, 162–164
    needed improvements in, 177–178
Nursing groups
    contemporary, 164
    historical perspective on, 164
Nursing history, 97–99
Nursing knowledge, transcultural, 90
Nursing process, 12, 95–110
    assessment in, 97–102. *See also*
        Assessment
    clinical example of, 95b–96b
    evaluation in, 109

implementation in, 106–109. *See also*
    Interventions
nursing diagnosis in, 102–106. *See
    also* Nursing diagnosis(es)
planning in, 106–108. *See also*
    Planning
steps in, 96
Nutrition, in mood disorders, 509
Nutritional history, in eating disorders,
    464

O

Obesity
    binge eating and, 456
    eating disorders and, 456, 467
Objective burden, on family, 171–173
Objective data, for nursing diagnosis,
    103
Obsessions, 358
Obsessive-compulsive disorder,
    355–356, 358–359, 363t. *See
    also* Anxiety disorders
    bulimia nervosa and, 457
    in children, 664–665
    vs. obsessive-compulsive personality
        disorder, 358
Obsessive-compulsive personality
    disorder, 441b, 443–444, 445t.
    See also Personality disorder(s)
    vs. obsessive-compulsive disorder, 358
Occipital lobe, 26, 27f, 28t
Occupational problems, 302
O'Connor v. Donaldson, 122
Office of Alternative Medicine (OAM),
    276
Olanzapine (Zyprexa), 237, 242t–243t,
    245, 499–500
    for schizophrenia, 538t, 540
Older adults, 685–697
    abuse of, 333–334, 692t
    anxiety in, 692t
    bereavement of, 687
    care of, 695–697
    classification of, 686
    communication with, 687–688, 688b,
        689t
    cultural factors affecting, 687
    delirium in, 609–617, 691t
    delusions in, 691t
    dementia in, 618–636. *See also*
        Dementia
    demographic trends affecting, 686
    depression in, 691t
    drug therapy for, 256, 693–695
    exercise by, 696
    fluid balance in, 696
    incarcerated, 194–195
    mental illness in, 6, 688–697
        ageism and, 690

Older adults, mental illness in (*continued*)
  myths and prejudices about, 690
  prevalence of, 6
  settings for care in, 690
  treatment of, 690–696
  types of, 691t–692t
    mental retardation in, 692t
    mental stimulation in, 696, 697b
    mood disorders in, 481
    nutrition in, 696
    psychosocial concerns of, 686–687
    relocation and, 686–687
    retirement and, 686, 687b
    schizophrenia in, 692t
    sexuality of, 402
    spirituality of, 687
    substance abuse in, 692t
    support systems for, 696–697
    terminology for, 689t
    wellness for, 696–697, 696b
Old old, 686
Omega-3 fatty acids, 257
Operant conditioning, 43
Opioid abuse, 588t. *See also* Substance abuse
  drug therapy for, 593t
Opium, 588t. *See also* Substance abuse
Oppositional-defiant disorder, 656, 663–664
  attention-deficit/hyperactivity disorder and, 669
Oral stage, 41t
Orbitofrontal syndrome, aggression and, 558
Orgasmic phase, 402
  disorders of, 405, 406b, 409
Orientation
  in delirium, 611–612, 614–616
  in dementia, 618, 626
  environmental modifications for
    in delirium, 611, 616, 617
    in dementia, 634
  in mental status examination, 100b
Osiris complex, 426b
Outcome identification, 104
Overgeneralization, in eating disorders, 468t
Overprotectiveness, eating disorders and, 473

P

Pain, during intercourse, 405
Pain disorder, 376t, 378t, 381. *See also* Somatoform disorders
Pamelor (nortriptyline), 227, 228t
Panic attacks, 358, 363t. *See also* Anxiety disorders

Panic disorder, 354, 357, 358. *See also* Anxiety disorders
Paranoid personality disorder, 439b, 442, 445t. *See also* Personality disorder(s)
Paranoid schizophrenia, 524, 534. *See also* Schizophrenia
Paraphilias, 407b, 416–417
Parens patriae, 115
Parents. *See* Family
Parietal lobe, 26, 27f, 27t
Parkinsonian reactions, antipsychotics and, 240, 243t
Parkinson's disease, 624
Parlodel (bromocriptine), for cocaine addiction, 593t
Parnate (tranylcypromine), 230t, 232–233
Paroxetine (Paxil), 232t, 233–234
Parson's sick role theory, 377
Partnership, in therapeutic relationship, 57
Passion flower, 282t
Passive-aggressive behavior, by nurse, 17
Passive-aggressive communication, 70
Paternalism, 126
PATHS, 327
A Patient's Bill of Rights, 121
Patient Self-Determination Act (PSDA), 120
Pavlov, Ivan, 141
Paxil (paroxetine), 232t, 233–234
PCP (phencyclidine), 588t. *See also* Substance abuse
Pediatric disorders. *See* Children
Pedophilia, 407b, 416
Peer pressure
  response to, 672b
  violence and, 327
Peer-taught family education, 184–185
Peplau, Hildegarde, 54, 164
Perception, in mental status examination, 101b
Perception check, 70–71
Perceptual problems
  alcohol-incuded, 585–586
  in dementia, 626
  in mental status examination, 503
  in schizophrenia, 531b, 533, 546–547
Periactin (cyproheptadine), 409
Perphenazine (Trilafon), for schizophrenia, 538t
Perseveration, 531, 670
Personal hygiene
  in mood disorders, 512
  in schizophrenia, 532
Personality
  definition of, 437
  development of, 437–438

psychoanalytic view of, 40, 41t
  theories of, 437–438
Personality disorder(s), 437–452, 444–445, 446b, 449
  antisocial, 440b, 442, 445t
  assessment in, 446–447
  avoidant, 440b–441b, 443, 445t
  borderline, 440b, 442, 445t
  clinical examples of, 437, 446b
  cluster A, 438–442
  cluster B, 442–443
  cluster C, 443–444
  comorbidities and dual diagnoses in, 444
  definition of, 438
  dependent, 441b, 444, 445t
  diagnostic criteria for, 438–444, 439–441
  dissociative disorders and, 424
  etiology of, 438
  evaluation in, 450
  family issues in, 448, 449b
  general, 439b
  histrionic, 440b, 442–443, 445t
  implementation in, 447–449
  narcissistic, 440b, 443, 445t
  nurse's self-care for, 451
  nursing care plan for, 448b
  nursing diagnoses for, 447
  nursing process in, 446–451
  obsessive-compulsive, 440b–441b, 443–444, 445t
    vs. obsessive-compulsive disorder, 358
  paranoid, 439b, 442, 445t
  planning in, 447, 448b
  prognosis of, 444
  schizoid, 439b–440b, 442, 445t, 448b
  schizotypal, 439b, 442, 445t
  signs and symptoms of, 438–444
  therapeutic communication in, 450b–451b
  treatment of, 444–446, 445t
Personalization, in eating disorders, 468t
Pertofrane. *See* Desipramine (Norpramin, Pertofrane)
Pervasive developmental disorders, 655, 670
  schizophrenia and, 524, 526b
PET scans, 34t
  in schizophrenia, 528, 528f
Peyote, 588t. *See also* Substance abuse
Phallic stage, 41t
Pharmacodynamics, in older adults, 694–695
Pharmacokinetics, in older adults, 694–695
Phencyclidine (PCP), 588t. *See also* Substance abuse

Phenelzine sulfate (Nardil), 229t–230t, 232–233
Phenotype, 31
Phenylalanine, for cocaine addiction, 593t
Phobias, 357–358. *See also* Anxiety disorders
   agoraphobia, 355, 357
   in children, 665
   definition of, 357
   social, 356, 357–358, 363t
      in children, 665
   specific, 356, 357, 358, 363t
Phototherapy, for depression, 500
Physiologic noise, 64
Phytomedicine, 280
Piaget's cognitive-developmental theory, 645, 646t
Pia mater, 25
Pick's disease, 624–625, 627t
Pindolol (Visken), for aggression, 564t
Pituitary, 483–484, 483f, 484f
Planning, 104–108. *See also* Nursing care plan
   critical pathways in, 108, 108b
   discharge, 106
   in forensic psychiatric nursing, 198–199
   intervention selection in, 106–108, 108b
   long- vs. short-term goals in, 106, 107t
   outcome identification in, 106
Plasticity, neuronal, 24
Play, medical, 674–675
Play therapy, 650
Polypharmacy, 225, 694
Polysomnography, 34t
Positive reframing, 71, 71t
Positive reinforcement, 43, 142
Positron emission tomography (PET), 34t
   in schizophrenia, 528, 528f
Possession trance, 423
Postpartum depression, 490b
Post-traumatic stress disorder, 355. *See also* Anxiety disorders
   causes of, 359b
   child abuse and, 332, 332b
   in children, 666
   cognitive-behavioral therapy for, 363t
   diagnostic criteria for, 355
   eye movement desensitization and reprocessing for, 337
   general counseling for, 362b
   nursing care plan for, 360b–361b
   after sexual assault/abuse, 332, 332b, 336–337
   symptoms of, 355, 359
   trauma therapy for, 337, 362b
Potency, drug, 225

Poverty
   homelessness and, 212
   mental illness and, 47, 302
   youth violence and, 327
Power, 152
Powerlessness
   in eating disorders, 473
   in somatoform disorders, 391
Practice standards, 116
Pramipexole (Mirapex), 236t, 237
Prana, 278, 284
Prayer, 268, 279–280
Predicted deterioration standard, 559
Pregnancy
   drug therapy in, 255
   false, 381
   postpartum depression and, 490b
   substance abuse in, 578–579, 580b
Prejudice, 80
Premature ejaculation, 405, 406b
Preschool programs, 649
Prevention
   in community mental health, 295–296, 296b, 296t
   in forensic nursing, 197b
   primary, 197b, 296t
   secondary, 197b, 296t
   tertiary, 197b, 296t
Preventive commitment, 559
Primary gain, in somatoform disorders, 377
Primary groups, 152
Primary prevention, 197b, 296t
   in community mental health, 295–297, 296t, 306
   in forensic nursing, 197b
Primidone (Mysoline), 236t, 237
Prisons. *See* Forensic psychiatric nursing
Privacy, 119t
   masturbation and, 400–401
   trust and, 55
Private speech, anger and, 558–559, 569
Privileged communication, 121
Probing, excessive, 58–59
Problem-solving skills, teaching of, 369
Procedural memory, 32
Process communication, 154–155
Professional, definition of, 55
Professional certification, in complementary/alternative medicine, 277
Professionalism, 55
Progressive relaxation, 363–364, 364b
Projection, 41t
Prolixin (fluphenazine), 241t, 244
   for schizophrenia, 538t
Proof, alcoholic, 584
Propranolol (Inderal), for aggression, 564t
Proselytizing, 269

Protriptyline (Vivactil), 227, 228t
Prozac. *See* Fluoxetine (Prozac)
Pseudocyesis, 381
Psilocybin, 588t. *See also* Substance abuse
Psychiatric advance directives, 11, 559–560
Psychiatric diagnoses, 103–106
   vs. nursing diagnoses, 102–106
Psychiatric disorders. *See* Mental illness
Psychiatric–mental health care. *See also* Intervention; Psychotherapy; Treatment
   access to, 8, 9, 85
   advances in, 8, 9b
   barriers to, 8–9
   for children and adolescents, 649–653
   client's view of, 17
   community-based. *See* Community mental health care
   costs of, 8
   cultural factors in, 10, 77–92. *See also* Culturally competent care
   drug therapy in, 8. *See also* Drug therapy
   family-centered, 676b
   goals of, 9–10
   historical perspective on, 115
   home-based, 311–321. *See also* Behavioral health home care
   least restrictive environment for, 122
   legal aspects of, 114–125
   managed care and, 115–116
   parity for, 9, 10
   racial bias in, 85, 85b
   response to, cultural factors in, 87–88
   revolving door treatment in, 9, 171, 192
   right to, 122
   right to aftercare in, 122
   right to refuse, 115, 122
   role of clergy in, 266–267
Psychiatric–mental health nurse
   burnout in, 17–18, 679
   as client advocate, 11, 118, 119t, 201. *See also* Client advocacy
   inexperienced, problems and concerns of, 16–17, 16f
   passive-aggressive behavior of, 17
   response of to disturbed behavior, 16, 17
   stress management for, 17–18, 18f
   supervision of, 109
Psychiatric–mental health nursing, 12–18
   assisting with self-care in, 147
   case management in, 147
   counseling in, 147
   crisis intervention in, 147
   forensic, 191–201. *See also* Forensic psychiatric nursing

Psychiatric–mental health nursing
(*continued*)
general, 145
group processes in, 164
health promotion/health
maintenance in, 146
health teaching in, 147. *See also*
Client/family teaching
history of, 14b
intake screening and evaluation in,
147
levels of practice in, 12–13, 145–146
minorities in, 82b
nursing process in, 12, 95–110. *See
also* Nursing process
phenomena of concern in, 13b
principles of, 13
psychiatric rehabilitation in, 148
psychobiological interventions in, 147
specialized, 146
standards of care in, 12, 14b–16b
team approach in, 13–16, 16f
therapeutic interventions in, 146–148
understanding client's life experience
in, 146
Psychiatric rehabilitation, 148
psychosocial model of, 299
Psychoanalysis, 40, 136, 136b, 137t, 138
Psychoanalytic theory, 39–41, 40t
Psychobiological interventions, 147
Psychoeducation, family, 183
Psychological abuse
of children, 331–333
of older adults, 333–334
Psychological noise, 64
Psychomotor activity, in delirium, 611
Psychoneuroendocrine systems, in
depression, 483–484
Psychoneuroimmunology, 33
Psychopathic personality disorder, 442
Psychopharmacology. *See* Drug therapy
Psychosexual development, 645
Freud's model of, 40–41, 41t
Psychosis. *See also* Schizophrenia
postpartum, 490b
therapeutic communication in, 72
Psychosocial assessment, 97–102. *See
also* Assessment
Psychosocial development
in attention-deficit/hyperactivity
disorder, 662–663
Erikson's theory of, 91, 203, 645,
646t, 662
Psychosocial rehabilitation model, 299
Psychotherapy. *See also under*
Interventions; Psychiatric–mental
health care; Therapeutic
behavioral, 137t, 139–143. *See also*
Behavior therapy
brief solution-focused, 138t, 144,
145b, 650

changing focus of, 136b
for children and adolescents, 650
choice, 137t, 144
cognitive, 137t, 138–139, 140t,
141b. *See also* Cognitive therapy
cognitive-behavioral, 137t, 143. *See
also* Cognitive-behavioral therapy
collaborative goals of, 136
for dissociative disorders, 427–428
educational aspects of, 30
for family members, 185
for gender identity disorders, 417
group, 161–162. *See also* Group
therapy
historical perspective on, 136b
individual, 135–148
listening in, 136
for mood disorders, 492
overview of, 135–136
for personality disorders, 444–445,
446b
physiologic effects of, 30
for post-traumatic stress disorder, 337
psychoanalytic, 136, 136b, 137t, 138
rational emotive behavior, 45, 137t,
143–144
reality, 137t, 144
for schizophrenia, 540
for somatoform disorders, 383
types of, 136–145, 137t–138t
Psychotic disorder not otherwise
specified, 523b
Psychotropic drugs. *See* Drug therapy
and specific drugs
Public health approach
definition of, 325
to violence, 325
Punishment
behaviorist view of, 43
in classical conditioning, 142
Purging, in bulimia nervosa, 456
Putamen, 28

Q

Qi, 277
QT prolongation, antipsychotics and,
251–252
Quetiapine (Seroquel), 243t, 245
for schizophrenia, 538t

R

Racial bias, in psychiatric–mental health
care, 44, 85, 85b
Racial/ethnic groups. *See also* Culture
and specific groups
assimilation of, 80
attitudes toward, 80

criminality in, 195
demographic trends among, 79–80
health beliefs and practices of, 81t
mental health care for, 84–87. *See also*
Culturally competent care
mental illness in, 47, 84–85
older adults in, 687
prejudice against, 80
in psychiatric nursing, 82b
religious/spiritual beliefs of, 86–87
stereotyping of, 80
stigmatization of, 80
substance abuse in, 577, 581
Ramadan, 78–79
Rape, 335–339
acquaintance, 335
date, 335
definition of, 335
marital, 335–336
post-traumatic stress disorder and,
336–339
prevention of, 337–338
in sexual history, 412b
statutory, 335
stranger, 335
substance abuse and, 336
victim of
client teaching for, 341b
nursing care plan for, 340b
psychological problems in,
336–337
treatment of, 337–339, 338b,
340b, 341b
Rape trauma syndrome, 336–339
client teaching for, 341b
nursing care plan for, 340b
Rating disorders, epidemiology of,
456
Rational emotive behavior therapy, 45,
137t, 143–144
Rational problem solving, 46t
Reaction formation, 41t
Reactive depression, 486
Reactive plasticity, 30
Reality therapy, 137t, 144
Reasonable person test, 117
Receptor binding, in drug therapy, 224
Receptors, neurotransmitter, 23
Records. *See also* Documentation
client's rights to, 121
legal issues involving, 121
Recovered memory syndrome,
426–427, 426b
Refeeding, in eating disorders, 469
Refractoriness, to drug effects, 225
Refractory period, in sexual response
cycle, 402
Reframing, 363
in anxiety disorders, 363
positive, 71, 71t
Regression, 41t

Rehabilitation
  psychiatric, 148
  psychosocial, 299
  vocational, in schizophrenia, 540–541
Reiki, 285
Reinforcement, 42t, 43, 142
Reinstitutionalization, 302
Relaxation response, 364
Relaxation techniques, 363, 364b,
    368–369
  for aggressive clients, 569
  for children, 674
Religious beliefs, 264. *See also*
    Spirituality
  definition of, 264
  vs. delusions, 266
  ethical issues and, 269–270
  health beliefs and practices and,
    86–87
  prayer and, 268
  repentance and forgiveness and,
    269–270
  sacred writings and, 268
  worship and rituals and, 269
Religious proselytizing, 269
Remeron (mirtazapine), 227, 229t,
    232, 496–497
Repentance, 268–269
Repressed memory syndrome, 426, 426b
Repression, 41t
  vs. dissociation, 422
Resilience, family, 178, 179b
Respect, in therapeutic relationship,
    55–56
Respite care, for Alzheimer's disease,
    637
Respondeat superior, 117
Respondent conditioning, 43
Restraint, 561–564
  for children, 564, 653
  legal aspects of, 117–118
Restriction fragment length
    polymorphisms, 31
Reticular formation, 26
Retirement, 686, 687b
Reuptake, 23
Revolving door hospitalization, 9, 171
  incarceration and, 192
Rhinelander model, 301
Richards, Hilda, 82b
Rigidity, eating disorders and, 473
Risk factors, for mental illness, 48, 48t,
    49–50
Risperidone (Risperidal), 242t, 245,
    499
  for aggression, 562t
  for schizophrenia, 538t, 540
Ritalin (methylphenidate), 245–246,
    246t, 659, 662b
Ritual abuse, dissociative disorders and,
    423b, 426b

Rituals
  for hospitalized children, 674
  spiritual/religious, 269
Rivastigmine (Exelon), 634–636
Roles
  group, 154
  individual, 154
Rosemary, 282t

S

Sacred writings, in bibliotherapy, 268
Sadism, 407b, 416
Safer sex practices, 399b
Safety
  in behavioral home health care, 317b,
    319
  in delirium, 611, 617
  in dementia, 636
  of family members, 577
  in forensic nursing, 194
  in mood disorders, 501–502, 502b.
    See also Suicide
  of other clients, 566
  personality disorders and, 449
  of staff, 559, 566
  in substance abuse, 595–599
Safety contract, for suicide, 674
Safety net services, 303
St. Augustine, 136b
St. John's wort, 257, 282t–283t
SAMe, 283t
Satanic cults, child abuse and, 423b,
    426b
Satiation therapy, 417
Schema, 139
Schizoaffective disorder, 523b, 525
Schizoid personality disorder,
    439b–440b, 442, 445t. *See also*
    Personality disorder(s)
  nursing care plan for, 448b
Schizophrenia, 521–551
  assertive community treatment for,
    542
  assessment in, 542–543
  case management for, 542
  catatonic, 524, 532, 534
  childhood, 523, 526
  client/family teaching in, 543,
    548–549, 550
  clinical example of, 522
  cognitive-behavioral therapy for, 540
  cognitive problems in, 530–534,
    531b, 532b
    assessment of, 542
    interventions for, 546–547
  community mental health care for,
    541–542
  comorbidities/dual diagnosis in, 535
  continuum of care in, 541–542

  coping skills in, 549
  definition of, 522
  delusions in, 531b, 533
  depression in, 534
  diagnostic criteria for, 524–525, 530
  discharge planning for, 541
  disorganized, 524, 534
  disorganized behavior in, 532
  disorganized speech in, 530–531,
    546, 548–549
  dopamine hypothesis for, 528–529
  drug therapy for, 240–245,
    242t–243t, 537–540, 538t,
    539b. *See also* Antipsychotics
    adherence to, 547–549
  etiology of, 523–530
  evaluation in, 550
  family communication patterns and,
    529–530
  family needs in, 549–550
  financial impact of, 523
  genetic factors in, 31–32, 526–528
  hallucinations in, 531b, 533,
    546–547
  historical perspective on, 527b
  homelessness and, 210–211. *See also*
    Homelessness
  imaging studies in, 528–529, 528f
  implementation in, 543–550
  incongruous affect in, 532–533
  information map for, 524–525
  language problems in, 530–531, 546,
    548–549
  late-onset, 526
  milieu management for, 540
  negative symptoms in, 530, 531b,
    533–534
  neurochemical/neuroanatomic
    changes in, 528–529, 528f
  nursing care plan for, 544–546
  nursing diagnoses for, 543
  nursing process in, 542–550
  in older adults, 692t
  onset of, 523, 526
  overview of, 522–523
  paranoid, 524, 534
  pervasive developmental disorder and,
    524
  physical health problems in, 541b
  planning in, 543, 544–546
  prognosis of, 535
  psychosocial theories of, 529–530
  psychotherapy for, 540
  psychotic dimension of, 533
  reality reinforcement in, 546
  residual, 524, 534
  signs and symptoms of, 524–525,
    530, 531t
  social support in, 543, 547
  stigma of, 523
  substance abuse in, 535

Schizophrenia (*continued*)
  subtypes of, 524, 534
  suicide in, 535
  treatment of, 535–542
  undifferentiated, 524, 534
  violence in, 542–543, 547
  vocational rehabilitation in, 540–541
  vulnerability model of, 529
  water intoxication in, 534
Schizophreniform disorder, 524
Schizotypal personality disorder, 439b, 442, 445t. *See also* Personality disorder(s)
School history, 652
School needs
  in attention-deficit/hyperactivity disorder, 662–663
  of hospitalized children, 678
  of mentally ill children, 302
Scientific method, 96
Scope and Standards of Psychiatric–Mental Health Nursing Practice (ANA), 125
Screening
  community, 297
  for dementia, 629t
  intake, 147
Seasonal affective disorder, 33, 500
Seclusion, 561–564
  for children, 564, 653
  legal aspects of, 117–118
Secondary gain, in somatization disorders, 377
Secondary groups, 152
Secondary prevention, 197b, 296t
  in community mental health, 296t, 297, 306
  for families, 178–185
  in forensic nursing, 197b
Second hits, 32
Second messengers, 24
Sedative-hypnotics
  abuse of, 588t–589t. *See also* Substance abuse
  for aggression, 562t–563t
Seizures
  aggression and, 558
  induced, for depression, 500
Selective abstraction, in eating disorders, 468t
Selective reuptake inhibitors, 230t–231t, 233. *See also* Antidepressants
Selective serotonin reuptake inhibitors, 231t–232t, 233–234, 233b, 495–496, 495f. *See also* Antidepressants
  for aggression, 563t
  for anxiety disorders, 364–365
  for somatoform disorders, 383, 384t

Self-awareness
  cultural, 91, 91b
  development of, 59–60
Self-care
  assistance with, 147
  in mood disorders, 491b
Self-disclosure, in therapeutic communication, 71–72
Self-esteem
  in attention-deficit/hyperactivity disorder, 663
  in eating disorders, 472–473
  in mood disorders, 512
  sexual dysfunction and, 415–416
  in substance abuse, 600–603
Self-harm. *See also* Suicide
  risk assessment for, 207
Self-help programs, 11, 299
  for alcohol/drug abuse, 582, 591–592, 594b, 603
Self-medication, substance abuse in, 535
Self-talk, anger and, 558–559, 569
Sensation, anxiety and, 350
Sensory aids, in dementia, 633
Sensory function, in mental status examination, 100b
Sensory preparation, for children, 674
Separation anxiety disorder, 656
  in children, 665
Serious mental illness, 170
Seroquel. *See* Quetiapine (Seroquel)
Serotonin
  aggression and, 558
  in depression, 483, 484f
Serotonin syndrome, 234, 365, 496, 496t
  St. John's wort and, 257
Sertraline (Zoloft), 232t, 233–234
  for aggression, 563t
Serzone (nefazodone), 230t–231t, 233, 495
Sex reassignment surgery, 417
Sex therapy, 409
Sexual abuse
  of children, 331–333
  of older adults, 333
Sexual assault, 335–339. *See also* Rape
  in sexual history, 412b
Sexual assessment, 409–410, 411t, 412b, 414b
Sexual aversion disorder, 403, 406b, 409
Sexual dysfunction disorders, 403–416
  arousal, 403–405
  assessment in, 409–410, 411t, 412b, 414b
  client counseling/teaching in, 414
  definition of, 403
  desire, 403
  diagnostic criteria for, 403, 406–408, 406b–407b

  etiology of, 403, 404b–405b
  evaluation in, 416
  implementation in, 414–416
  information map for, 406–408
  nursing diagnoses for, 412–413
  nursing process in, 409–416
  orgasmic, 405
  pain, 405
  planning in, 413–414, 415b
  prevalence of, 406
  signs and symptoms of, 403, 406b–407b
  treatment of, 405–409
  types of, 403–405, 404b–405b
Sexual expression, 398–401
  age-related changes in, 402
  communication about, 409–410, 411t, 412b, 413b
  cultural aspects of, 400
  harmful forms of, 398
  physical illness and, 400–401, 404b
  sexual orientation and, 399–400
Sexual identity, 400
Sexual intercourse, painful, 405
Sexuality
  definition of, 398
  normal, 398–402
  of older adults, 402
Sexually inappropriate behavior, by client, 400, 401b
Sexually transmitted diseases, in incarcerated population, 195–196
Sexual masochism, 407b, 416
Sexual preference, 399–400
Sexual response, phases of, 401–402
Sexual sadism, 407b, 416
Shaping, 44
Shared psychotic disorder, 523b, 525
Shelters, homeless, 214
Shenjing shuairuo, 375
Short Portable Mental Status Questionnaire, 626
Siblings. *See also* Family
  responses of to mental illness, 172, 173
Sick role, 377
Side effects, in drug therapy, 10b, 224, 240, 243t, 249–252, 250f–251f
Signaled punishment, 417
Sildenafil (Viagra), 409, 410t
Simultaneous family/patient education, 184. *See also* Client/family teaching
Sinequan (doxepin), 227, 228t
Single photon emission computed tomography, 34t
Situational crisis, 203
Skinner, B.F., 141–142
Sleep, circadian rhythms and, 33
Sleep deprivation

in bipolar disorder, 509–511
in depression treatment, 501
Sleep disturbances
    in delirium, 611
    in mood disorders, 504, 509–512
Smoking, in pregnancy, 578–579
Sobardoras, 86b
Social assessment, in somatoform
        disorders, 385–386
Social class, mental health and, 47
Social disability, due to mental illness,
        301–302
Social phobia, 356, 363t
    in children, 665
Social relationship, vs. therapeutic
        relationship, 55, 56t, 127–129
Social skills training, in attention-
        deficit/hyperactivity disorder,
        663
Social support, assessment for, in
        schizophrenia, 543
Sociocultural perspective, 47
Socioeconomic status
    aggression/violence and, 556
    homelessness and, 212
    mental illness and, 47, 302
    youth violence and, 327
Sociopathic personality disorder, 442
Solution-focused brief therapy, 138t,
        144, 145b
    for eating disorders, 463
Solvent abuse, 587t. *See also* Substance
        abuse
Somalia, 77–79
Somatic therapies, for somatoform
        disorders, 383
Somatization disorder, 376t, 377–380,
        378t, 384t
Somatoform disorders, 373–393
    assessment in, 383–386
        physical, 385–386
        psychological, 383–385
        social, 385–386
    body dysmorphic disorder, 376t,
        378t, 381
    classification of, 375
    clinical example of, 374b
    comorbid conditions in, 375, 381
    conversion disorder, 376t, 378t,
        379b, 380–381
    cultural aspects of, 375
    definition of, 374
    diagnostic criteria for, 377, 379–380,
        379b–380b
    dual diagnoses in, 375, 381
    epidemiology of, 375, 376t–377t
    etiology of, 375–377
    evaluation in, 392
    vs. factitious disorder, 377
    family issues in, 391–392
    historical perspective on, 374b

hypochondriasis, 376t, 378t, 380b,
        381
    information map for, 379–380
    interaction with medical system in,
        388–391
    vs. malingering, 377
    nursing care plan for, 386,
        387b–388b
    nursing diagnoses for, 386
    nursing process in, 383–392
    pain disorder, 376t, 378t, 381
    planning in, 386, 387b–388b
    primary/secondary gain in, 377
    prognosis of, 381–382
    psychosocial factors in, 375
    risk/contributing factors for, 379
    sick role and, 377
    signs and symptoms of, 377,
        379b–380b
    somatization disorder, 376t,
        377–380, 378t
    therapeutic relationship in, 386–388,
        389b–390b
    treatment of, 382–383, 382b, 384t,
        386–392
    undifferentiated somatoform disorder,
        379b, 380
Spatial ability, in dementia, 618
Special education, 651
Specific phobias, 356, 357, 358, 363t
    in children, 665
SPECT (single photon emission
        computed tomography), 34t
Speech
    disorganized, in schizophrenia,
        530–531, 546, 548–549
    in mental status examination, 100b
    private, 558–559
Speed, 587t
Spinal cord, structure and function of,
        25, 26f
Spiritual assessment, 267
Spiritual care, 279–280
    clergy's role in, 266–267
    ethical concerns in, 269–270
    nurse's role in, 267–269
Spiritual coping
        strategies/interventions,
        268–269
Spiritual Distress, 102
Spiritual history, 267
Spirituality, 263–286
    communication about, 265–266, 267
    definition of, 264
    health beliefs and practices and,
        86–87
    illness prevention and, 264–265
    mental health and, 265
    mental illness and, 265–266
    nursing process and, 267–269
    nursing research on, 265, 269

of older adults, 687
    overview of, 263–264
    physical health and, 264
    religion and, 264. *See also* Religious
        beliefs
    substance abuse and, 265
    in twelve-step programs, 269
    values and, 266
Splitting, 442
Spousal abuse, 328–331
    screening for, 329–330
Spouse. *See also* Family
    responses of to mental illness, 172,
        174b
Staff, safety concerns of, 559, 566
Standardized care plans, 107–108
Standard of care, negligence and,
        116–117
*Standard of Nursing Practice in
        Correctional Facilities* (ANA),
        196
Standards of nursing practice, 116
Standards of Practice for Home Health
        Care (ANA), 315, 316b
Starbright World, 678
Statutory rape, 335
Stelazine (trifluoperazine), 241t, 244
    for schizophrenia, 538t
Stereotyping, 80
Stigmatization
    of mentally ill, 121, 302–303
    of minorities, 80
Stimulants, 245–246, 246t. *See also*
        Drug therapy
    abuse of, 587t. *See also* Substance
        abuse
    for attention-deficit/hyperactivity
        disorder, 245–246, 246t, 659,
        662b
    for children, mania and, 669
Stimulus-response theories, 42t, 44–45
Stress
    vs. anxiety, 350
    balancing factors in, 208–209, 208f
    caregiver, 679
    crisis and, 201–202
    fight-or-flight reaction and, 350, 369
    in forensic settings, 196b
    of hospitalization, in children,
        674–679
Stress immunization, for children, 674
Stress management. *See also* Coping
        skills
    for nurse, 17–18, 18f
    in schizophrenia, 549
Stress-vulnerability model, for
        schizophrenia, 529
Striatum, 352
Study groups, 163–164
Subjective burden, on family, 173–175
Sublimation, 41t

Substance abuse, 575–603
  anxiety disorders and, 352, 353b
  anxiety in, 600
  assessment in, 593–595, 595b–597b
  behavioral factors in, 581
  biologic factors in, 581
  case management in, 535, 536t–537t
  in children and adolescents, 671–672
  classification of, 583b
  coexistent mental illness and, 6, 535, 582
  cognitive theory of, 582
  comorbidities and dual diagnoses in, 6, 582, 583f
  coping skills in, 600
  criminality and, 193
  cultural aspects of, 87, 581
  delirium in, 612
  denial in, 599–600, 601b–602b
  dependence in, 576, 584b
  detoxification in, 591b, 595–599
  diagnostic criteria for, 583, 583b, 584b
  dissociative disorders and, 424
  drugs of abuse in, 583t, 586–589, 587t–589t
  dual diagnosis and, 6, 535, 582
  epidemiology of, 576–578, 577b, 579f
  etiology of, 581–582
  family concerns in, 600
  genetic factors in, 581
  historical perspective on, 576
  homelessness and, 211, 213. See also Homelessness
  implementation in, 595–603
  intoxication in, 584b
  nursing diagnoses for, 595
  nursing process in, 593–603
  in older adults, 692t
  overdose in, 588t–589t
  personality disorders and, 444
  physical examination in, 595
  planning in, 595
  prevalence of, 576–578, 577b, 577f–579f
  prognosis of, 582–583
  psychosocial factors in, 581
  by rape victims, 336
  rehabilitation in, 591
  religion and, 265
  risk factors for, 581
  in schizophrenia, 535
  in self-medication, 535
  theoretical concepts of, 582
  therapeutic communication in, 602b–603b
  tolerance in, 585
  treatment of, 589–592
    phases of, 590t
    team approach in, 589
  types of, 583b
  withdrawal in, 584b, 595–599

Substance dependency, 576, 584b
Substance-induced persisting amnestic disorder, 619b, 636–637, 638b
Substituted consent, 120–121
Suicide, 172–173
  in children and adolescents, 673–674
  prevention of, 504–509, 510b. See also Crisis intervention
    telephone counseling in, 206
  risk assessment for, 207, 501–502, 502b
    in forensic nursing, 198
  in schizophrenia, 535
  therapeutic communication and, 504–509, 510b
Suicide contract, 674
Suicide survivors, 481b
Sullivan, Harry Stack, 527b
Sundowning, 621
Superego, 40, 40t
Supervision, 109
Support groups, 11, 162, 163t
  for alcohol/drug abuse, 582, 591–592, 594b, 603
  for Alzheimer's disease, 637b
  in crisis intervention, 205–206
Support services, family, 183
Support systems, assessment of, 207
Surmontil (trimipramine), 227, 229t
Susto, 86b, 375
Symmetrel (amantadine), for cocaine abuse, 593t
Synapses, 22, 24f
Synaptic cleft, 22, 24f
Systematic desensitization, 363
Systematic rational restructuring, 46t
Systems of care, 300–301
  in pediatric mental health care, 649
Szasz, Thomas, 136b

T

Tacrine (Cognex), 634
T'ai chi, 283–284
Tarasoff v. Board of Regents of University of California, 121, 559
Tardive dyskinesia, 240, 243t, 249–250, 250f–251f, 538t, 539
Target symptoms, 225, 226f
Task roles, group, 154
Tautology, 6
Taxonomy
  definition of, 102
  of nursing diagnoses, 102–103, 103f, 110f
  of psychiatric diagnoses, 103–106
Teaching. See Client/family teaching
Tegretol. See Carbamazepine (Tegretol)
Telephone counseling, in crisis intervention, 206

Temperament
  aggression and, 558
  pediatric mental illness and, 647
Temporal lobe, 26, 27f, 28t
Temporal lobe epilepsy, aggression and, 558
Tertiary prevention, 197b, 296t, 306
  in community mental health, 296t, 297
  in forensic nursing, 197b
Tetracyclic antidepressants, 229t, 232. See also Antidepressants
T groups, 152–153, 162
Thalamus, 28t
Theories
  concepts and, 38
  definition of, 38
  of human behavior, 39–47
  importance of, 38–39
  utility of, 39
Therapeutic communication, 63–72. See also Communication
  in antisocial personality disorder, 450b–451b
  in anxiety disorders, 367, 367b
  with anxious clients, 72
  assertiveness in, 70
  confrontation in, 70–71
  definition of, 64
  in dementia, 635b
  in dissociative disorders, 432b
  in eating disorders, 465b
  examples of, 67b–70b
  excessive probing in, 58–59
  with families, 72, 176b–177b
  in family consultation, 182b
  with homeless, 216b
  judgmental attitudes in, 57–58
  listening in, 64, 67b, 68b
  noise in, 63–64
  vs. nontherapeutic communication, 64, 66t
  with older adults, 687–688, 687b, 689t
  about peer pressure, 672
  positive reframing in, 71, 71t
  with psychotic clients, 72
  in schizophrenia, 548–549
  self-disclosure in, 71–72
  about sexual expression, 409–410, 411t, 412b, 413b, 414–416
  in somatoform disorders, 386–388, 389b–390b
  in substance abuse, 602b–603b
  with suicidal client, 504–509, 510b
  techniques of, 65t
Therapeutic holding, 653
Therapeutic relationship, 53–72. See also Psychotherapy
  acting-out behavior in, 60–61
  caring in, 56–57

clinical examples of, 54, 59b
coaching in, 146
communication in. *See* Therapeutic
communication
confidentiality and, 55
definition of, 54
essential elements of, 54–57
in forensic nursing, 199
with homeless, 217
introductory phase of, 60–62
middle (working) phase of, 62–63
mutual respect in, 55–56
obstacles to, 57–60
partnership in, 57
phases of, 60–63
positive connectedness in, 58b
professionalism and, 55
resistance to change and, 62b
vs. social relationship, 55, 56t
termination phase of, 63
trust in, 55
understanding client's life experience
in, 146
Therapeutic touch, 284–285
Thinking, in mental status examination,
100b–101b
Thioridazine (Mellaril), 240, 241t
for schizophrenia, 538t
Thiothixene (Navane), 242t, 244
for schizophrenia, 538t
Thorazine. *See* Chlorpromazine
(Thorazine)
Thorndike, E.L., 141
Thought broadcasting, 533
Thought content, in mental status
examination, 503
Thought disorders, 521–551. *See also*
Schizophrenia
definition of, 522
information map for, 524–525
types of, 523b
Thought processes
anxiety and, 350–351
in mental status examination, 503
Thought stopping, for children, 674
Thought withdrawal, 533
Tic disorders, 672–673
Tofranil (imipramine), 227, 228t
Token economy, 142–143, 560–561
Tolerance, in alcohol abuse, 585
Torrey, Fuller, 527b
Torsades de pointes, antipsychotics and,
251
Tourette syndrome, 656, 673
Traditional Chinese medicine, 277
Traditional healers, 86b. *See also*
Complementary/alternative
medicine
Training (T) groups, 152–153, 162
Training in community living model,
299

Trance
dissociative, 423
possession, 423
Tranquilizers, abuse of, 588t. *See also*
Substance abuse
Transactional analysis, passive-
aggressive, 70
Transcendental Meditation, 279
Transcranial magnetic stimulation, 501
Transcription, 30–31, 31f
Transcultural assessment, 90
Transcultural nursing knowledge, 90
Transference, 40, 138
in groups, 156–157, 167b
Translation, 31, 31f
Transsexuals, 417
Transvestites, 417
Transvestic fetishism, 407b–408b, 416
Tranylcypromine (Parnate), 230t,
232–233
Trauma. *See also* Post-traumatic stress
disorder
general counseling for, 362b
Trauma therapy, for sexual assault
victims, 337
Traumatic Events Drawing Series, 429
Trazodone (Desyrel), 231t, 233–234,
496, 563t
for aggression, 563t
Treatment. *See also under* Interventions;
Psychiatric–mental health care;
Psychotherapy; Therapeutic
community-based. *See* Community
mental health care
family involvement in, 176b–177b
refusal of, 115
Trexan (naltrexone), 593t
Trichotillomania, 673
Tricyclic antidepressants, 227–232,
228t–229t, 233b, 497, 497f. *See
also* Antidepressants
for aggression, 563t
for anxiety disorders, 365
for attention-deficit/hyperactivity
disorder, 659
Trifluoperazine (Stelazine), 241t, 244
for schizophrenia, 538t
Triggers, behavioral, 142, 143
Trilafon (perphenazine), for
schizophrenia, 538t
Trimipramine (Surmontil), 227, 229t
Trust
confidentiality and, 55
in therapeutic relationship, 55
Truth, Sojourner, 82b
Truth serum, 427
Twelve-step programs, 582, 591–592,
594b, 603. *See also* Support
groups
for alcoholism, 591–592, 594b, 603
repentance and forgiveness in, 269

Twin studies, of schizophrenia, 31–32
Tyrosine, for cocaine addiction, 593t

U

Unconditional positive regard, 57
Unconscious, 40
Undifferentiated somatoform disorder,
379b, 380
Universal Bill of Rights for Mental
Health Patients, 118b
Universality, 161
Uprima (apomorphine), 409
Utility, 39

V

Vaginismus, 405
Vagus nerve stimulation, 501
Valerian, 283t
Valium. *See* Diazepam (Valium)
Valproic acid (Depakene), for
aggression, 563t
Values, spirituality and, 266
Variance, in critical pathway, 108
Vascular dementia, 619b, 624, 627t,
691t. *See also* Dementia
Vegetative signs, in depression, 503–504
Veracity, 126
Verbal ability. *See also* Language problems
anxiety and, 351
Viagra (sildenafil), 409, 410t
Violence, 323–339. *See also* Aggression;
Forensic psychiatric nursing
behavioral care plan for, 509
definition of, 324, 556
discharge planning for, 564–565
ecological model of, 324–325
expressive, 194
family, 328–334. *See also* Family
violence
family factors in, 557
gang, 194, 327
horizontal, 17
inpatient factors in, 557
instrumental, 194
intimate partner, 328–331
legal aspects of, 559–560
marital, 328–331
outpatient factors in, 557
prevention of, 325, 509
public health approach to, 325
risk assessment for, 502
in mood disorders, 502
in schizophrenia, 542–543
risk factors for, 566t
in schizophrenia, 542–543, 547
sexual, 331–333, 335–338
sociodemographic factors in, 556–557

Violence (*continued*)
  threats of, duty to warn of, 121, 559
  youth, 325–328
Visken (pindolol), for aggression, 564t
Visualization techniques, 279, 369
Vivactil (protriptyline), 227, 228t
Vocational rehabilitation, for
    schizophrenia, 540–541
Voyeurism, 408b, 416
Vulnerability model, for schizophrenia,
    529
Vygotsky, L.S., 647

W

Water intoxication, in schizophrenia, 534
Watson, John B., 141
Waxy flexibility, 532
Wellbutrin. *See* Bupropion (Wellbutrin)
Wer, Jo Ann, 184

Wernicke-Korsakoff syndrome, 586,
    627t, 636–637
WIAG, 173
Widows/widowers, 687
Wilson, Junius, 85b
Wintersteen, Richard T., 184
Withdrawal
  in alcohol abuse, 585, 589–591,
    590t, 595–599
  in substance abuse, 584b, 595–599
    delirium in, 612
Women, mood disorders in, 486, 486b
Word salad, 531, 532b
Worship, 269
Wrap-around services, 649
Wyatt v. Stickney, 122

X

Xanax (alprazolam), 237–239, 238t

Y

Yoga, 284
Young old, 686
Youth violence, 325–328. *See also*
    Violence
  prevention of
    nurse's role in, 328
    public health approach to,
      327
  protective factors for, 327
  risk factors for, 326–327

Z

Ziprasidone (Geodon), 538t, 540
Zoloft. *See* Sertraline (Zoloft)
Zyban (bupropion), 231t, 233–234,
    497
Zyprexa. *See* Olanzapine (Zyprexa)